WALTERS AND KARRAM

UROGYNECOLOGY AND RECONSTRUCTIVE PELVIC SURGERY

WALTERS AND KARRAM

UROGYNECOLOGY AND RECONSTRUCTIVE PELVIC SURGERY

FIFTH EDITION

Matthew D. Barber, MD, MHS
E.C. Hamblen Professor and Chair
Department of Obstetrics and Gynecology
Duke University Medical Center
Durham, North Carolina

Catherine S. Bradley, MD, MSCE
Professor
Department of Obstetrics and Gynecology
University of Iowa Carver College of Medicine
Iowa City, Iowa

Mickey M. Karram, MD
Director of Urogynecology and Clinical Professor of Obstetrics and Gynecology
Department of Obstetrics and Gynecology
The Christ Hospital and University of Cincinnati
Cincinnati, Ohio

Mark D. Walters, MD
Professor of Obstetrics, Gynecology and Reproductive Biology
Ob/Gyn and Women's Health Institute
Cleveland Clinic
Cleveland, Ohio

ELSEVIER

Elsevier
1600 John F. Kennedy Blvd.
Ste 1800
Philadelphia, PA 19103-2899

WALTERS AND KARRAM UROGYNECOLOGY AND RECONSTRUCTIVE PELVIC SURGERY, FIFTH EDITION

ISBN: 978-0-323 697835

Notice

Practitioners and researchers must always rely on their own experience and knowledge in evaluating and using any information, methods, compounds or experiments described herein. Because of rapid advances in the medical sciences, in particular, independent verification of diagnoses and drug dosages should be made. To the fullest extent of the law, no responsibility is assumed by Elsevier, authors, editors or contributors for any injury and/or damage to persons or property as a matter of products liability, negligence or otherwise, or from any use or operation of any methods, products, instructions, or ideas contained in the material herein.

Library of Congress Control Number: 2021935504

Content Strategist: Nancy Duffy
Content Development Specialist: Casey Potter
Publishing Services Manager: Deepthi Unni
Project Manager: Beula Christopher
Design Direction: Ryan Cook

Printed in Canada

Last digit is the print number: 9 8 7 6 5 4 3 2 1

To my current and former fellows,
I have learned far more from you than you have from me.
And to my wife Heather, for all her love and support.
Matthew D. Barber

To my husband Phil, with love and gratitude
for his unwavering support of me and my work.
Catherine S. Bradley

In memory of my parents Mike and Mary Karram,
for their love, kindness, and unselfish support, as well as
for instilling in me the values of education,
discipline, and hard work.
Mickey M. Karram

To ginny, my best friend, with love and respect.
Mark D. Walters

CONTRIBUTORS

Cindy L. Amundsen, MD
Roy T. Parker Professor
Division of Urogynecology and Reconstructive Pelvic Surgery
Department of Obstetrics and Gynecology
Duke University
Durham, North Carolina

Yehudith Assouline Dayan, MD
Staff Gastroenterologist
Pentucket Medical Associates
Mass General Brigham Community Physicians
Haverhill, Massachusetts

Marjan Attaran, MD
Assistant Professor
Ob/Gyn and Women's Health Institute
Cleveland Clinic
Cleveland, Ohio

Matthew D. Barber, MD, MHS
E.C. Hamblen Professor and Chair
Department of Obstetrics and Gynecology
Duke University Medical Center
Durham, North Carolina

Liliana Bordeianou, MD, MPH
Professor of Surgery
Harvard Medical School;
Director
Massachusetts General Hospital (MGH) Center for Pelvic Floor Disorders,
Chair
MGH Colorectal Surgery Program
Boston, Massachusetts

Catherine S. Bradley, MD, MSCE
Professor
Department of Obstetrics and Gynecology
University of Iowa Carver College of Medicine
Iowa City, Iowa

Megan S. Bradley, MD
Assistant Professor
Obstetrics, Gynecology, and Reproductive Sciences
Division of Urogynecology
University of Pittsburgh - Magee Women's Hospital
Pittsburgh, Pennsylvania

Geoffrey W. Cundiff, MD, FACOG, FRCSC
Professor
Department of Obstetrics and Gynecology
University of British Columbia
Vancouver, British Columbia, Canada

Roger R. Dmochowski, MD, MMHC, FACS
Professor of Urology
Department of Urology,
Professor of Surgery
Section of Surgical Sciences
Vanderbilt Medical Center
Nashville, Tennessee

Denicia S. Dwarica, MD MS
Assistant Professor
Obstetrics and Gynecology, Female Pelvic Medicine and Reconstructive Surgery
University of Missouri School of Medicine
Columbia, Missouri

Brittany R. Egnot, MS
Student
School of Medicine
University of Pittsburgh
Pittsburgh, Pennsylvania

Cecile A. Ferrando, MD, MPH
Associate Professor of Surgery
Ob/Gyn and Women's Health Institute
Cleveland Clinic
Cleveland, Ohio

Ian C. Fields, MD, MCR
Assistant Professor
Division of Urogynecology
Department of Obstetrics and Gynecology
Oregon Health and Science University
Portland, Oregon

John B. Gebhart, MD, MS
Professor of Obstetrics and Gynecology and Surgery
Department of Obstetrics and Gynecology
Mayo Clinic
Rochester, Minnesota

W. Thomas Gregory, MD
Professor
Division of Urogynecology
Department of Obstetrics and Gynecology
Oregon Health and Science University
Portland, Oregon

Tamara Grisales, MD
Assistant Clinical Professor
Department of Obstetrics and Gynecology
University of California Los Angeles
Los Angeles, California

Victoria L. Handa, MD, MHS
Professor
Department of Gynecology and Obstetrics
Johns Hopkins School of Medicine
Baltimore, Maryland

Siobhan M. Hartigan, MD
Director of Reconstructive Urology and Pelvic Health
Hunterdon Urological Associates
Flemington, New Jersey

Lisa C. Hickman, MD
Assistant Professor
Division of Female Pelvic Medicine and Reconstructive Surgery
Department of Obstetrics and Gynecology
Ohio State University Wexner Medical Center
Columbus, Ohio

Mallorie L. Hoover, DO
Fellow
Female Pelvic Medicine and Reconstructive Surgery
The Christ Hospital
Cincinnati, Ohio

John Eric Jelovsek, MD, MMEd, MSDS
Associate Professor
Department of Obstetrics and Gynecology
Duke University
Durham, North Carolina

Mickey M. Karram, MD
Director of Urogynecology and Clinical Professor of Obstetrics and Gynecology
Department of Obstetrics and Gynecology
The Christ Hospital and University of Cincinnati
Cincinnati, Ohio

Erika L. Kelley, PhD
Psychologist
Obstetrics and Gynecology, Division of Behavioral Medicine
University Hospitals MacDonald Women's Hospital;
Assistant Professor
Reproductive Biology
Case Western Reserve University
Cleveland, Ohio

Kimberly A. Kenne, MD, MCR
Clinical Assistant Professor
Department of Obstetrics and Gynecology
University of Iowa Hospital and Clinics
Iowa City, Iowa

Sheryl A. Kingsberg, PhD
Chief, Division of Behavioral Medicine
Department of Obstetrics and Gynecology
University Hospitals Cleveland Medical Center;
Professor
Reproductive Biology and Psychiatry
Case Western Reserve University School of Medicine
Cleveland, Ohio

Katrina M. Knight, PhD
Assistant Professor
Department of Bioengineering
University of Pittsburgh
Pittsburgh, Pennsylvania

Joseph T. Kowalski, MD
Clinical Assistant Professor
Department of Obstetrics and Gynecology
University of Iowa Hospitals and Clinics
Iowa City, Iowa

Stephen R. Kraus, MD, MBA
Professor and Vice Chairman
Department of Urology
University of Texas Health Science Center at San Antonio
San Antonio, Texas

Frank C. Lin, MD, MS
Assistant Professor
Department of Urology
University of Wisconsin School of Medicine and Public Health
Madison, Wisconsin

Ayman Mahdy, MD, PhD
Associate Professor of Urology
Department of Urology,
Interim Chief of Urology
Department of Surgery,
Director of Voiding Dysfunction and Female Urology
University of Cincinnati College of Medicine
Cincinnati, Ohio

Deepali Maheshwari, DO, MPH
Fellow
Department of Urogynecology and Reconstructive Pelvic Surgery
University of Massachusetts Medical School
Worcester, Massachusetts

Catherine A. Matthews, MD, FACOG, FACS
Professor, Division Head and Fellowship Director
Department of Urology and Obstetrics and Gynecology
Wake Forest Baptist Health
Winston-Salem, North Carolina

Neil Mendhiratta, MD, MS
Resident Physician
Department of Urology
University of California Los Angeles
Los Angeles, California

Kate V. Meriwether, MD
Assistant Professor
Department of Obstetrics and Gynecology
University of New Mexico
Albuquerque, New Mexico

Pamela A. Moalli, MD, PhD
Professor
Department of Obstetrics, Gynecology and Reproductive Sciences
University of Pittsburgh
Pittsburgh, Pennsylvania

Elizabeth R. Mueller, MD, MSME
Professor
Department of Urology and Obstetrics and Gynecology
Loyola University Chicago
Maywood, Illinois

Tristi W. Muir, MD
Alan L. Kaplan, M.D. Chair in Obstetrics and Gynecology
Chairwoman
Department of Obstetrics and Gynecology,
Professor of Clinical Obstetrics and Gynecology
Institute for Academic Medicine, Houston Methodist, Weill Cornell Medical College
Houston, Texas;
Adjunct Professor
Department of Obstetrics and Gynecology
Texas A&M University, College of Medicine
Bryan, Texas

Diane K. Newman, DNP, ANP-BC, FAAN
Adjunct Professor of Urology in Surgery
Division of Urology,
Research Investigator Senior
Perelman School of Medicine
University of Pennsylvania;
Co-Director
Penn Center for Continence and Pelvic Health
Division of Urology
Penn Medicine
Philadelphia, Pennsylvania

Victor W. Nitti, MD
Professor
Division of Female Pelvic Medicine and Reconstructive Surgery
Department of Urology
University of California Los Angeles
Los Angeles, California

Ian M. Paquette, MD
Associate Professor of Surgery
Division of Colorectal Surgery, Department of Surgery
University of Cincinnati College of Medicine
Cincinnati, Ohio

Danielle Patterson, MD, SM
Assistant Professor
Department of Gynecology and Obstetrics
Johns Hopkins School of Medicine
Baltimore, Maryland

Karina Pedersen, BS
College of Medicine
Northeast Ohio Medical University
Rootstown, Ohio

Thythy T. Pham, MD, MA
Assistant Professor
Departments of Obstetrics and Gynecology and Urology
Loyola University Medical Center
Maywood, Illinois

Lieschen H. Quiroz, MD
Professor
Department of Obstetrics and Gynecology,
Section Chief of Female Pelvic Medicine and Reconstructive Surgery
University of Oklahoma Health Sciences
Oklahoma City, Oklahoma

Roya L. Rezaee, MD, FACOG
Female Genital Disorder and Sexual Health Consultant
Cleveland, Ohio

Holly E. Richter, PhD, MD
Professor
Department of Obstetrics and Gynecology, Urology and Geriatrics
University of Alabama at Birmingham
Birmingham, Alabama

Beri M. Ridgeway, MD
Academic Chair
Ob/Gyn and Women's Health Institute
Cleveland Clinic
Cleveland, Ohio

Amy Rosenman, MD
Health Sciences Clinical Professor
Department of Obstetrics and Gynecology
David Geffen School of Medicine at University of California Los Angeles
Los Angeles, California

Elizabeth Rourke, DO MPH
Assistant Professor of Urology
Louisiana State University
New Orleans, Louisiana

Megan R. Routzong, BS
PhD Candidate
Bioengineering
University of Pittsburgh
Pittsburgh, Pennsylvania

Rebecca Shaffer, MD
Assistant Professor
Urogynecology
University of Vermont
Colchester, Vermont

Nazema Y. Siddiqui, MD, MHSc
Associate Professor
Division of Urogynecology and Reconstructive Pelvic Surgery
Department of Obstetrics and Gynecology
Duke University
Durham, North Carolina

Gennady Slobodov, MD
Professor
Department of Urology
University of Oklahoma Health Sciences Center
Oklahoma City, Oklahoma

Ellen R. Solomon, MD
Assistant Professor
Female Pelvic Medicine and Reconstructive Surgery
University of Massachusetts Medical School – Baystate
Springfield, Massachusetts

Vivian W. Sung, MD, MPH
Professor
Department of Obstetrics and Gynecology
Alpert Medical School of Brown University
Women and Infants Hospital
Providence, Rhode Island

Elizabeth B. Takacs, MD
Clinical Associate Professor
Department of Urology
University of Iowa Hospitals and Clinics
Iowa City, Iowa

Christopher Tarnay, MD
Division Chief, Female Pelvic Medicine and Reconstructive Surgery
Department of Obstetrics and Gynecology
David Geffen School of Medicine at University of California Los Angeles
Los Angeles, California

Sandip P. Vasavada, MD
Professor of Surgery (Urology)
Glickman Urological Institute
Cleveland Clinic
Cleveland, Ohio

Anthony G. Visco, MD
Professor of Obstetrics and Gynecology
Duke University Medical Center
Durham, North Carolina

Mark D. Walters, MD
Professor of Obstetrics, Gynecology and Reproductive Biology
Ob/Gyn and Women's Health Institute
Cleveland Clinic
Cleveland, Ohio

Hoi Tik Hyde Yuen, MD
Fellow
Female Pelvic Medicine and Reconstructive Surgery
The Christ Hospital
Cincinnati, Ohio

ACKNOWLEDGMENTS

We would like to acknowledge the exemplary work of Laverne Alston, who provided outstanding administrative support in the creation of this new edition, and Dr. Elizabeth Howell, who expertly curated more than a hundred videos, allowing us to select only the best for this edition.

CONTENTS

PART 6 Lower Urinary Tract Disorders, 494

PART 7 Specific Conditions, 587

PART 8 Research Methods, 650

PART 1

Basic Science

1

Anatomy of the Lower Urinary Tract, Pelvic Floor, and Rectum

Matthew D. Barber and Mark D. Walters

CHAPTER OUTLINE

PELVIC ANATOMY

Bones of the Pelvis

The bones of the pelvis are the rigid foundation to which all the pelvic structures are ultimately anchored. In the standing position, forces are dispersed to minimize pressures on the pelvic viscera and musculature and to transmit forces to bones that are better suited to the long-term, cumulative stress of daily life. In the upright position, the pubic rami are oriented in an almost vertical plane. Similar to the supports of an archway or bridge, the body weight is transmitted along these bony supports to the femurs. Where the pubic rami articulate in the midline, they are nearly horizontal. Much of the weight of the abdominal and pelvic viscera is inferiorly supported by the bony articulation.

The pelvic bones are the ilium, ischium, pubic rami, sacrum, and coccyx (Fig. 1.1A and B). The sacrum is composed of five sacral vertebrae that are fused together. The nerve foramina are positioned anterior and laterally. Overlying the middle of the sacrum is a rich neurovascular bed. The coccyx is inferiorly attached and is the posterior border of the pelvic outlet.

Several landmarks are important to the pelvic surgeon. The anterior superior iliac spine (ASIS) is easily identifiable and is anterior and laterally located on the superior ileum. The ischium is fused to the ilium. The medial surface of the ilium forms the lateral borders of the pelvic outlet. The superior greater sciatic notch and inferior lesser sciatic notch are medially separated by a projection, the ischial spine. The sacrospinous ligament, which is triangular in form, is laterally attached by its apex to the ischial spine; its broader base arises from the side of the lower sacral and coccygeal segments. This ligament converts the greater sciatic notch into the greater sciatic foramen (see Fig. 1.1B). Through this foramen pass the piriformis muscle and all of the vessels and nerves that leave the pelvis for the gluteal region and back of the thigh. The sacrospinous ligament and the dorsal sacrotuberous ligament also convert the lesser sciatic notch to the lesser sciatic foramen. Through this foramen pass the tendon and nerve of the internal obturator muscle, the pudendal nerve, and the internal pudendal vessels.

The ischial spine can be palpated easily through a vaginal, rectal, or retropubic approach, and many supportive structures attach to it. The ischial spine is useful as a fixed point to describe the relative position of other anatomic structures and as a landmark in various reconstructive surgeries for pelvic organ prolapse. The superior and inferior pubic rami are anteriorly located and articulate in the midline at the pubic symphysis. The ridge along the superior, medial surface of the superior pubic rami is called the iliopectineal line, or Cooper's ligament.

In the standing position, the ASIS and pubic symphysis are in the same vertical plane (see Fig. 1.1B). This directs the pressure of the intraabdominal and pelvic contents toward the bones of the pelvis instead of the muscles and endopelvic fascia attachments of the pelvic floor. The posterior surface of the pubic symphysis is located in a plane approximately 2 to 3 cm inferior to the ischial spine. Therefore, a line drawn connecting the two structures would be almost horizontal in the standing

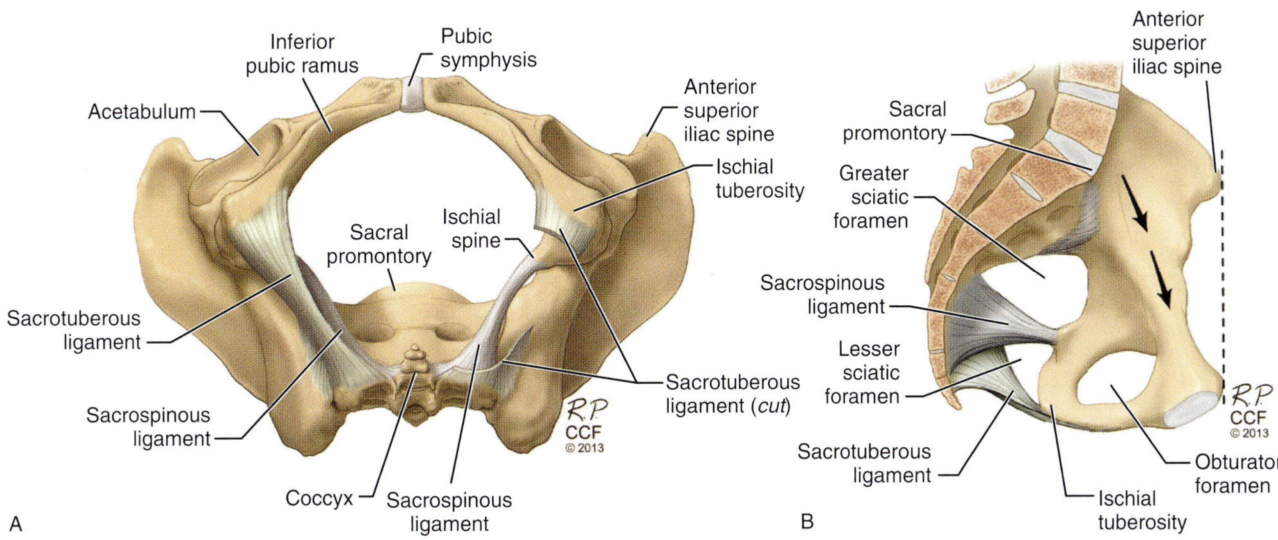

Fig. 1.1 **A**, Bones and ligaments of the pelvis. Lithotomy view shows the relationships of the ligaments to the pelvic outlet and bony structures. **B**, Bones and ligaments of the pelvis. Sagittal view shows the nearly vertical distribution of weight (*arrows*) toward the pubic symphysis. The ischial spine is at approximately the level of the pubic symphysis. The dashed line indicates the vertical axis in a standing woman.

position. This has important implications for the support of pelvic organs, and will be discussed later in the chapter.

Pelvic Floor and Sidewalls

The obturator internus and piriformis make up the pelvic sidewalls (Fig. 1.2). The obturator membrane is a fibrous membrane that covers the obturator foramen. The obturator internus muscle lies on the superior (intrapelvic) side of the obturator membrane. The obturator internus origin is on the inferior margin of the superior pubic ramus and the pelvic surface of the obturator membrane. Its tendon passes through the lesser sciatic foramen to insert onto the greater trochanter of the femur to laterally rotate the thigh. The obturator internus receives its innervation from the obturator nerve originating from L5 to S2. The obturator vessels and nerve pass through the anterior and lateral border of the obturator membrane, in the obturator canal, to their destination in the adductor compartment of the leg.

The piriformis is part of the pelvic sidewall and is located dorsal and lateral to the coccygeus. It extends from the anterolateral sacrum to pass through the greater sciatic foramen and insert onto the greater trochanter. Lying on top of the piriformis is a particularly large neurovascular plexus, the lumbosacral plexus.

There is a linear thickening of the fascial covering of the obturator internus muscle called the arcus tendineus levator ani. This thickened fascia forms an identifiable line from the ischial spine to the posterior surface of the ipsilateral superior pubic ramus. The muscles of the levator ani originate from this musculofascial attachment.

The pelvic diaphragm is defined as the levator ani muscles and the coccygeus muscle. It is stretched hammock-like between the pubis in front and the coccyx behind, and is attached along the lateral pelvic walls to the arcus tendineus levator ani. The puborectalis, pubococcygeus, and iliococcygeus are the three components of the levator ani muscle recognized by *Terminologia Anatomica* (see Fig. 1.2). The more medial puborectalis arises from the posterior inferior pubic rami and passes posteriorly, forming a sling around the vagina, rectum, and perineal body to form the anorectal angle and contribute to fecal continence. The pubococcygeus has a similar origin, but it inserts in the midline onto the anococcygeal raphe and the anterolateral borders of the coccyx. The pubococcygeous muscle further subdivides into fibers that blend with the muscularis of the vagina (*pubovaginalis m.*), perineal body (*puboperineal m.*), and anal sphincter muscle (*puboanalis m.*). Because of the significant attachments of the pubococcygeus to the walls of the pelvic viscera, the term "pubovisceral muscle" is frequently used to describe it, although this term is not officially recognized by *Terminologia Anatomica*. The iliococcygeus extends along the arcus tendineus levator ani from the pubis to the ischial spine to insert in the midline onto the anococcygeal raphe and coccyx.

The coccygeus, although not part of the levator ani, does make up the posterior part of the pelvic floor, and it plays a role in support. Its origin is on the ischial spine and sacrospinous ligament. It inserts on the lateral lower sacrum and coccyx, and it overlies the sacrospinous ligament. The muscle becomes thin and fibrous with age. The coccygeus often blends with the sacrospinous ligament, and it can be difficult to distinguish the two because they have the same origin and insertion.

The space between the levator ani musculature through which the urethra, vagina, and rectum pass is called the levator hiatus. The fusion of the levator ani where they meet in the midline creates the levator plate. The levator plate forms the basis for pelvic support. The levator ani may be very thin and attenuated, especially in elderly patients and those with pelvic organ prolapse.

With the change from plantigrade to erect posture, the human pelvis and vertebral column underwent various evolutionary changes that restored the balance between intraabdominal pressure and visceral support. The lumbosacral curve, a specific human characteristic, directs abdominal pressure forward onto

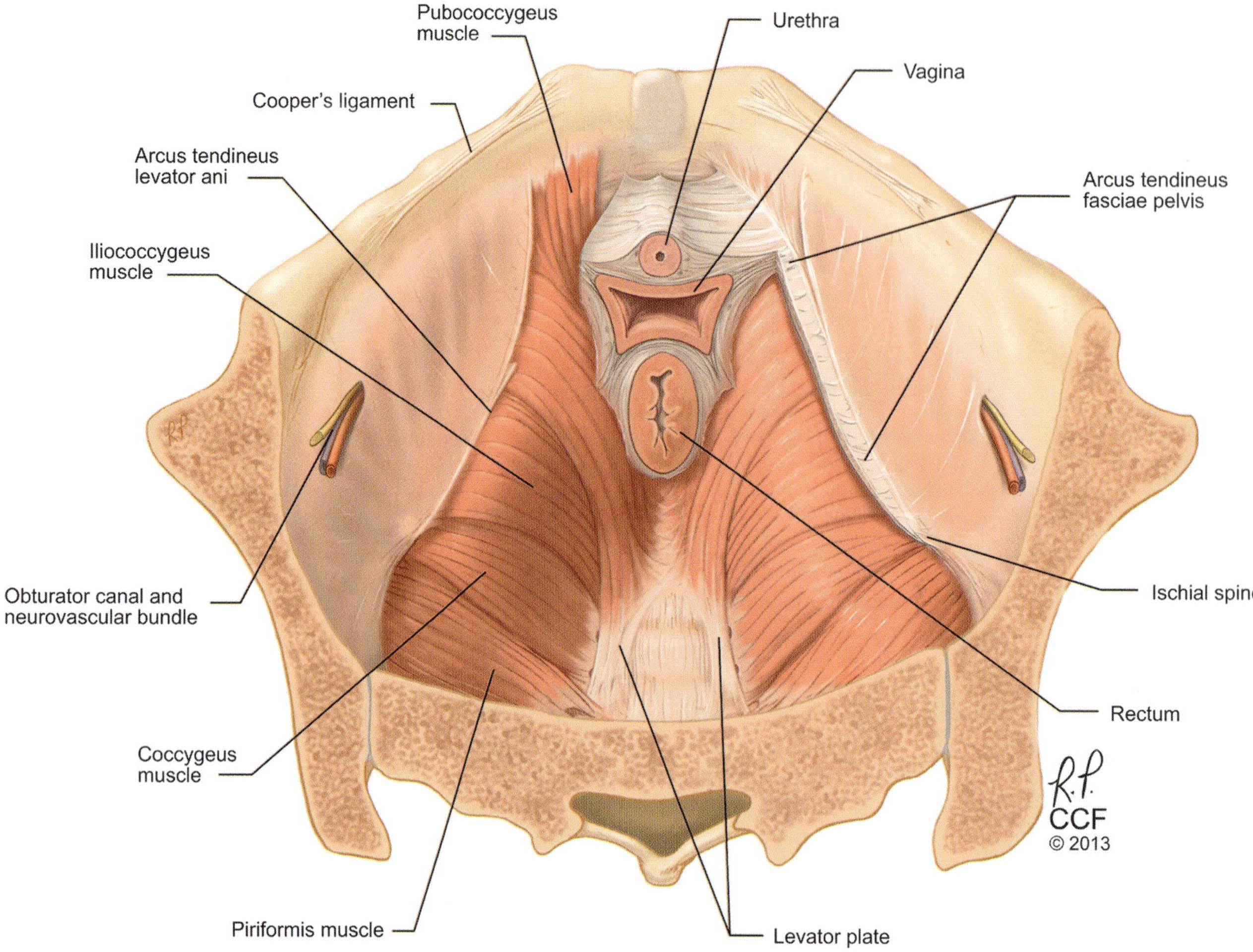

Fig. 1.2 The relationships of the muscles of the pelvic floor and sidewalls and their attachments from an abdominal view. The arcus tendineus fasciae pelvis has been removed on the left, showing the origins of the levator ani muscles. On the right, the arcus tendineus fasciae pelvis remains intact, showing the attachment of the lateral vagina via the endopelvic fascia (cut away).

the abdominal wall and the nearly horizontal, flattened pubic bones. Downward pressure is directed backward onto the sacrum and the rearranged pelvic muscles, which now fill in the pelvic cavity to form the pelvic floor and sidewalls.

The pelvic floor and sidewalls are made up of muscular and fascial structures that enclose the abdominopelvic cavity, the external vaginal opening (for intercourse and parturition), and the urethra and rectum (for elimination). The fascial components consist of two types of fascia: parietal and visceral (endopelvic). Parietal fascia covers the pelvic skeletal muscles and provides attachment of muscles to the bony pelvis; it is characterized histologically by regular arrangements of collagen. Visceral endopelvic fascia is less discrete and exists throughout the pelvis as a meshwork of loosely arranged collagen, elastin, and adipose tissue through which the blood vessels, lymphatics, and nerves travel to reach the pelvic organs, similar to the mesentery of the intestines. By surgical convention, condensations of the visceral endopelvic fascia of the pelvis have been described as discrete "ligaments," such as the cardinal or uterosacral ligaments. The role of the endopelvic fascia in pelvic organ support will be discussed in detail later in this chapter.

The pelvic floor muscles have constant tone except during voiding and defecation, and they can be voluntarily contracted. This activity serves to close the urethral and anal sphincters, narrow the urogenital hiatus, and provide a constant support for the pelvic viscera. The levator muscles and the skeletal components of the urethral and anal sphincters all have the ability to contract quickly at the time of an acute stress, such as a cough or sneeze, to maintain continence. The muscles contain type I (slow-twitch) fibers to maintain constant tone and type II (fast-twitch) fibers to provide reflex and voluntary contractions.

Although most anatomy and surgical texts depict the levator ani muscles as a bowl or as "funnel-shaped," this reflects the uncontracted state of the muscles, as might be seen in a cadaver dissection, and not that of a normally functioning levator. In a woman with normal pelvic floor function, the levator ani muscle complex in its tonically contracted state has an intricate three-dimensional structure in which the anterior portion of the muscle complex (pubococcygeus and puborectalis muscles) is oriented vertically as a sling around the midurethra, vagina, and anorectum, and the posterior portion (iliococcygeus muscle) has a horizontal, upwardly biconvex shape with a "butterfly wing" appearance (Fig. 1.3). Thus, the anterior portion of the levator ani complex serves to close the urogenital hiatus and pull the urethra, vagina, perineum, and anorectum toward the pubic bone, while the horizontally oriented posterior portion (levator plate) serves as a supportive diaphragm or "backstop" behind the pelvic viscera. Loss of normal levator ani tone, through denervation or direct muscle trauma, results in a more open urogenital hiatus, loss of the horizontal orientation of the levator plate, and a more bowl-like configuration. These changes can be bilateral or asymmetric. Such configurations are seen more often in women with pelvic organ prolapse than in women with normal pelvic organ support.

Nerves of the Pelvis

The sacral plexus is formed by the nerve roots of L4, L5, and S1 to S4 and is located on the anterior surface of the piriformis muscle on the lateral pelvic floor and sidewalls. The sacral plexus gives rise to multiple nerve branches, including the sciatic nerve, the superior gluteal nerve, the pudendal nerve, and the nerve to the levator ani. The pudendal nerve innervates the striated urethral and anal sphincters as well as the deep and superficial perineal muscles and provides sensory innervation to the external genitalia. Although there is variability in the branching patterns of the pudendal nerve, it consistently originates from the S2 to S4 (with S3 providing the largest contribution) sacral nerve trunks. Together, the pudendal vessels and nerve follow a complex course as they leave the pelvis. With the nerve oriented medially and the vessels laterally, the pudendal neurovascular bundle travels behind the sacrospinous ligament at the ischial spine, exiting the pelvis through the greater sciatic foramen (Fig. 1.4). It then enters the ischioanal fossa through the lesser sciatic foramen and travels through the pudendal canal (Alcock's canal) on the medial aspect of the obturator internus muscles before emerging in the perineum, where the bundle separates into several branches that terminate within the muscles and skin of the perineum and the clitoris. The neuroanatomy of the perineum, including the pudendal nerve branches, are described later in the chapter.

Although the muscles of the pelvic floor were initially thought to have innervation from direct branches of the sacral nerves on the pelvic surface and via the pudendal nerve on the perineal surface, evidence indicates that these standard descriptions are inaccurate, and that the levator ani muscles are innervated primarily, if not solely, by a nerve traveling on the superior (intrapelvic) surface of the muscles, without contribution of the pudendal nerve (Fig. 1.5). Other lumbosacral branches include the nerves to the piriformis and obturator internus, the pelvic splanchnic nerves, and the cutaneous nerves.

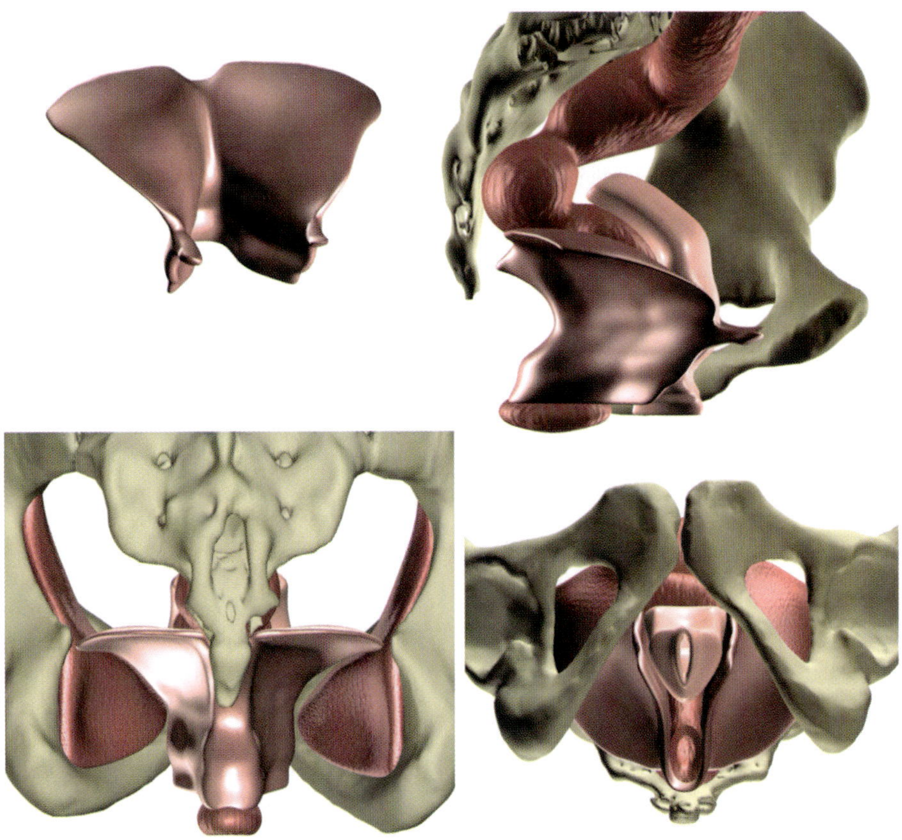

Fig. 1.3 Digitally enhanced three-dimensional reconstructions of the female pelvic floor from a magnetic resonance image of the pelvis in a healthy, nulliparous 23-year-old woman. *Upper left:* anterior view of the levator ani muscle with normal resting tone. *Upper right:* sagittal view of the levator ani muscle, bony pelvis, vagina, and rectum. *Lower left:* posterior view of the levator ani muscle, obturator internus muscles, and bony pelvis. *Lower right:* lithotomy view. (From Barber MD. Contemporary views on female pelvic anatomy. *Cleve Clin J Med.* 2005;72:S3.)

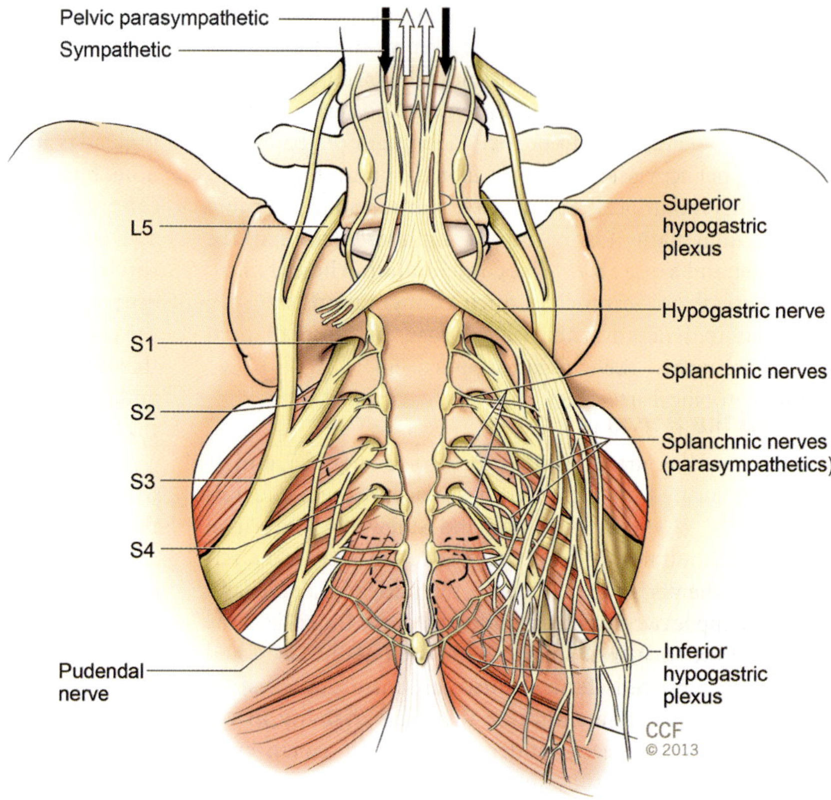

Fig. 1.4 The sympathetic and parasympathetic nerves entering the pelvis. The superior hypogastric plexus can be seen lying directly over the sacral promontory until it divides to the right and left sides of pelvis. The pudendal nerve originates from S2–S4 sacral nerve trunks, travels behind the sacrospinous ligament at the ischial spine, and exits the pelvis through the greater sciatic foramen.

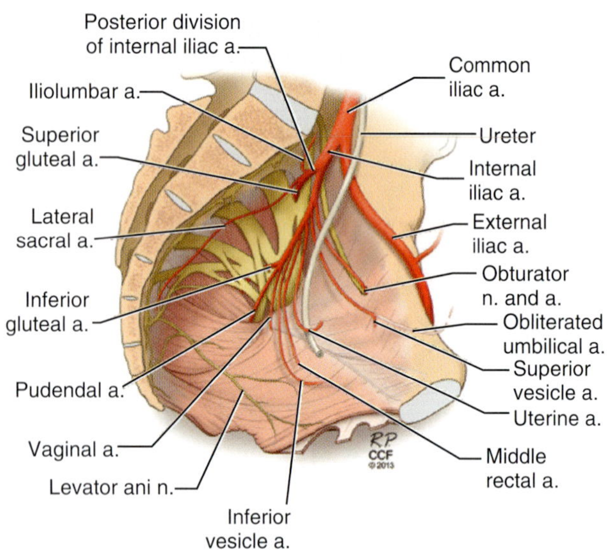

Fig. 1.5 View of the nerves and blood vessels of the lateral wall of the pelvis. The sacral plexus is shown in *yellow*. The smaller branches innervating the muscles of the pelvic floor can be seen supplying the levator ani muscles (S3, S4). The uterine artery originates from the anterior division of the internal iliac artery. *a.*, artery; *n.*, nerve.

The autonomic nervous system innervates the pelvis through the superior and inferior hypogastric (or pelvic) plexuses (see Fig. 1.4). The superior hypogastric plexus receives sympathetic input from the thoracic and lumbar splanchnic nerves (T5–L2) and afferent pain input from the pelvic viscera. It lies over the bifurcation of the aorta in the presacral space and splits into two hypogastric nerves that run along the internal iliac vessels. This sympathetic innervation promotes organ storage by causing relaxation of the bladder and rectum and contraction of the smooth-muscle components of the urethral and anal sphincters. Parasympathetic input derives from S2 to S4 via the pelvic splanchnic nerves that travel to join the hypogastric plexus through the lateral pelvic wall and promote evacuation of the bladder and rectum. When the hypogastric nerves are joined by the pelvic splanchnic nerves, the pelvic plexuses (inferior hypogastric plexus) are formed. The pelvic plexuses consist of three areas: the vesical plexus, the uterovaginal plexus, and the middle rectal plexus extending bilaterally to provide autonomic innervation of their corresponding viscera.

Uterus and Ovaries

The uterus is a muscular organ consisting of the uterine fundus, isthmus, and cervix. The uterus and cervix are continuous with the anterior apical portion of the vagina and are connected superiorly to the ovaries via the uteroovarian ligaments. The ovaries receive their blood supply from the ovarian (gonadal) vessels that originate from the aorta. The uterus receives most of its blood supply bilaterally from the uterine arteries (see Fig. 1.5). The uterine arteries originate at the anterior division of the internal iliac arteries and reach the lower uterine segment within the cardinal ligament. The arteries caudally give off the vaginal branches and continue along the lateral surface of the uterus to anastomose with the ovarian blood supply.

The uterus is a midline organ positioned posterior to the bladder and anterior to the rectum. Condensations of peritoneum form the cardinal and broad ligaments, the round ligaments, and the suspensory ligaments of the ovary (infundibulopelvic ligament). The cardinal ligaments are a condensation of the endopelvic fascia, which is part of the supportive structure of the uterus. They extend outward and laterally from the uterine isthmus and cervix in a three-dimensional fan-like manner and are continuous with the endopelvic fascia of the pelvic sidewall. In addition to playing a role in upper vaginal support, they divide the deeper pelvis into avascular planes anteriorly called the paravesical space and posteriorly called the pararectal space. The retropubic space (space of Retzius) is continuous with the paravesical space. The borders of the paravesical space are the obturator internus and neurovascular bundle laterally, the cardinal ligament posteriorly, the pubic symphysis anteriorly, and the obliterated umbilical artery medially. The borders of the pararectal space are the cardinal ligament anteriorly, the rectum medially, the internal iliac artery laterally, and the sacrum posteriorly.

Vagina

The vagina is a hollow, fibromuscular tube with rugal folds that extends from the vestibule to the uterine cervix. In the standing woman, the upper two-thirds of the vagina is almost horizontal, whereas the lower one-third is nearly vertical. The vaginal wall is histologically composed of three layers. It is lined by a nonkeratinized stratified squamous epithelium that lies over a thin, loose layer of connective tissue, the lamina propria. The lamina propria contains no glands. Coursing through the lamina propria are small blood vessels. Vaginal lubrication is via a transudate from the vessels, the cervix, and the Bartholin's and Skene's glands. Beneath the lamina proppria is the vaginal muscularis, a well-developed fibromuscular layer consisting primarily of smooth muscle with smaller amounts of collagen and elastin. The muscularis is surrounded by an adventitial layer, which is a variably discrete layer of collagen, elastin, and adipose tissue containing blood vessels, lymphatics, and nerves. The adventitia represents an extension of the visceral endopelvic fascia that surrounds the vagina and adjacent pelvic organs and allows for their independent expansion and contraction.

The walls of the vagina are in contact except where its lumen is held open by the cervix. The vaginal lumen is H-shaped, with the principal dimension being transverse. In addition, the upper vagina is supported by connective tissue attachments to the sacrum, coccyx, and lateral pelvic sidewalls; these are identified at surgery as the cardinal and uterosacral ligament complex.

There is considerable variability in vaginal length, size, and width among women. Based upon magnetic resonance imaging studies of women with normal support, the average length of the anterior vaginal wall is 6.3 cm, with a wide range of 4.4 to 8.4 cm. Similarly, the average length of the posterior vaginal wall is 9.8 cm, with a range of 5.1 to 14.4 cm (Luo et al., 2016). The vaginal width is greatest at its cranial portion and decreases as it passes through the pelvic diaphragm, to its smallest width at the introitus. There are large variations in transverse dimensions; in one study, as much as a five-fold variation was seen in total vaginal surface area (34–164 cm^2) (Luo et al., 2016). In women with normal vaginal support, there are three major vaginal axes, with an average angle of 90 degrees relative to the horizontal for the lower vagina, 72 degrees for the middle vagina, and 41 degrees for the upper vagina; however, these angles vary significantly among women (Luo et al., 2016; Fig. 1.6).

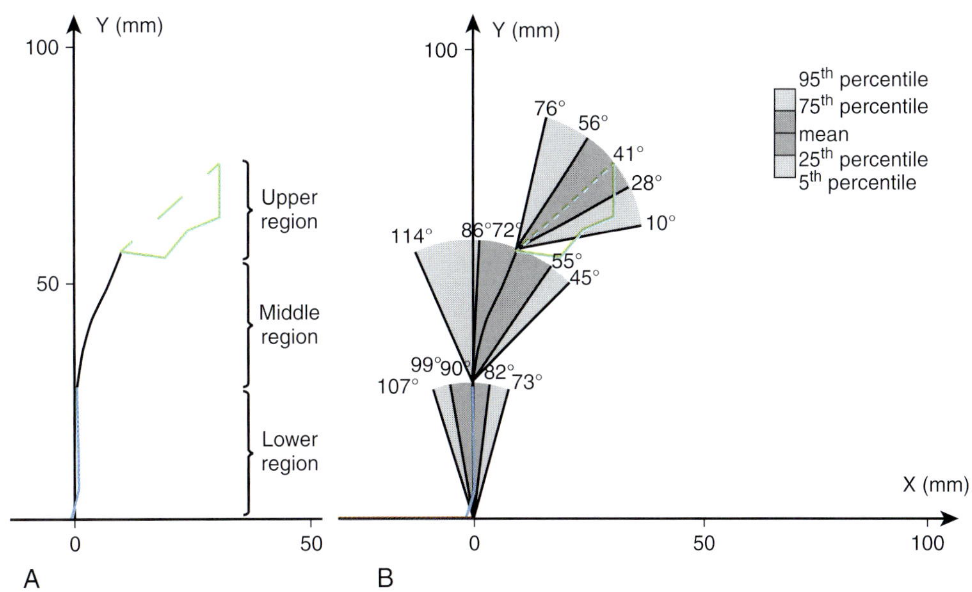

Fig. 1.6 Vaginal axis in a standing woman. **A**, Mean midsagittal shapes of the anterior vaginal wall and cervix are shown relative to fixed bony landmarks. The y-axis corresponds to how "high" or "low" the organ is along the line of the body axis, and the x-axis describes the anterior and posterior axis (see Luo et al., 2016 for details). Three contiguous vaginal axes were defined as follows: the lower region (*blue*), the middle region (*black*), and the upper region with a line showing the cervical axis (*green dashed line*) connecting the anterior and posterior margins. **B**, Variation in vaginal axis orientation is shown by the 5th, 25th, mean, 75th, and 95th percentile axis angles. (From Luo J, Betschart C, Ashton-Miller JA, DeLancey JO. Quantitative analyses of variability in normal vaginal shape and dimension on MR images. *Int Urogynecol J.* 2016;27:1087.)

The presence of a true fascia between the vagina and adjacent organs has been debated. Surgical terms such as pubocervical fascia and rectovaginal fascia refer to layers that are developed as a result of separating the vaginal epithelium from the muscularis or by splitting the vaginal muscularis layer. Anteriorly, the vagina lies adjacent to and supports the bladder base, from which it is separated by the vesicovaginal adventitia (endopelvic fascia). The urethra is fused with the anterior vagina, with no distinct adventitial layer separating them. The terminal portions of the ureters cross the lateral fornices of the vagina on their way to the bladder base. Posteriorly, the vagina is related to the cul-de-sac, to the rectal ampulla, and inferiorly to the perineal body. Embryologically, an extension and fusion of the peritoneum from the cul-de-sac attached to the posterior surface of the vaginal muscularis forms the rectovaginal septum. A layer of adventitia separates the muscular layer of the rectum from the posterior vaginal wall, except at the level of the perineal body, where there is fusion of the vaginal muscularis and connective tissue of the perineal body. The dense connective tissue of the perineal body extends 2 to 3 cm cephalad from the hymenal ring along the posterior vaginal wall and forms what some have called the rectovaginal fascia. Although at the time of surgery there appears to be an identifiable fascial plane, Weber and Walters (1997), DeLancey (1999), and Maldonado et al. (2020) have each concluded that between the adjacent organs is primarily vaginal muscularis or loose fibroadipose tissue, and that no fascia is histologically present.

Perineum

The perineum is divided into two compartments: superficial and deep. These are separated by a fibrous connective tissue layer called the perineal membrane. The perineal membrane is a triangular sheet of dense fibromuscular tissue that spans the anterior half of the pelvic outlet. It was previously called the urogenital diaphragm; this change in name reflects the appreciation that it is not a two-layered structure with muscle in between, as was previously thought. The perineal membrane provides support to the vagina and urethra as they pass through it. Cephalad to the perineal membrane lies the striated urogenital sphincter muscle, which compresses the mid- and distal urethra (Fig. 1.7). The borders of the perineum are the ischiopubic rami, the ischial tuberosities, the sacrotuberous ligaments, and the coccyx (Fig. 1.8A). A line connecting the ischial tuberosities divides the perineum into the urogenital triangle anteriorly and the anal triangle posteriorly. The perineal body marks the point of convergence of the bulbospongiosus muscles, the superficial and deep transverse perinei, the perineal membrane, the external anal sphincter, the posterior vaginal muscularis, and the insertion of the puborectalis and pubococcygeus (puboperinealis) muscles. The bulbospongiosus originates on the inferior surface of the superior pubic rami and the crura of the clitoris. It inserts on the perineal body, where its fibers blend with the superficial transverse perinei and the external anal sphincter. The superficial transverse perinei are bilateral muscles that extend from the medial ischial tuberosities to insert on the perineal body. The ischiocavernosus muscles originate from the medial ischial tuberosities and ischiopubic rami. They insert on the inferior aspect of the pubic angle.

The deep perineal compartment is composed of the deep transverse perineus muscle, portions of the external urethral sphincter muscles (compressor urethrae and urethrovaginal sphincter), portions of the anal sphincter, and the vaginal musculofascial attachments.

The neurovascular anatomy of the perineum is illustrated in Fig. 1.8A and B. The motor and sensory innervation of the

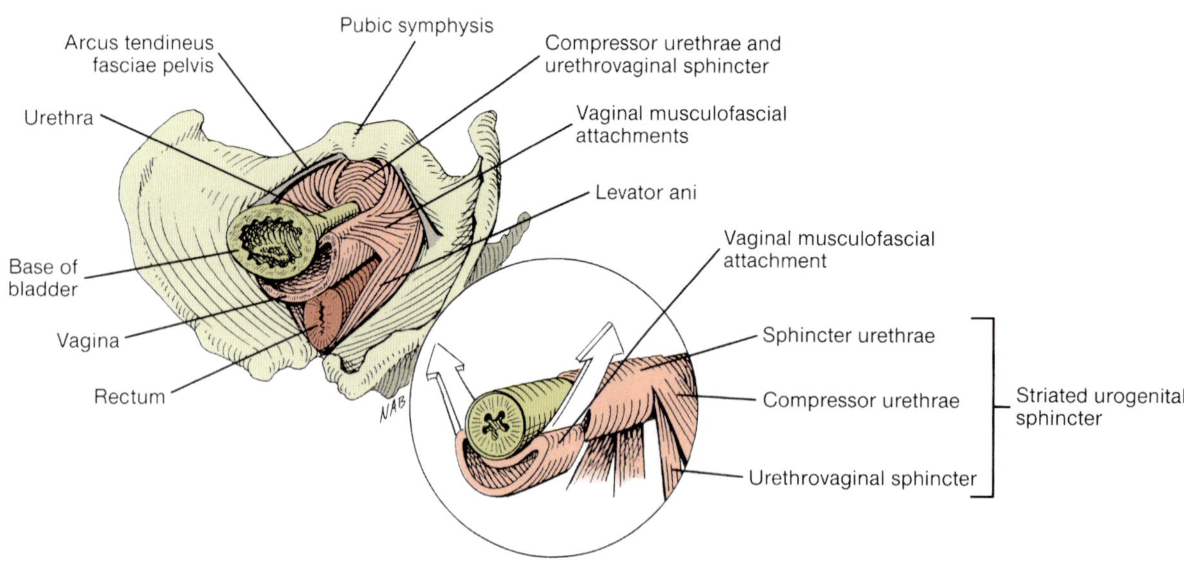

Fig. 1.7 Diagrammatic representation showing the component parts of the urethral support and sphincteric mechanisms. Note that the proximal urethra and bladder neck are supported by the anterior vaginal wall and its musculofascial attachments to the pelvic diaphragm. *Inset,* Contraction of the levator ani muscles elevates the anterior vagina and overlying bladder neck and proximal urethra, contributing to bladder neck closure. The sphincter urethrae, urethrovaginal sphincter, and compressor urethrae are all parts of the striated urogenital sphincter.

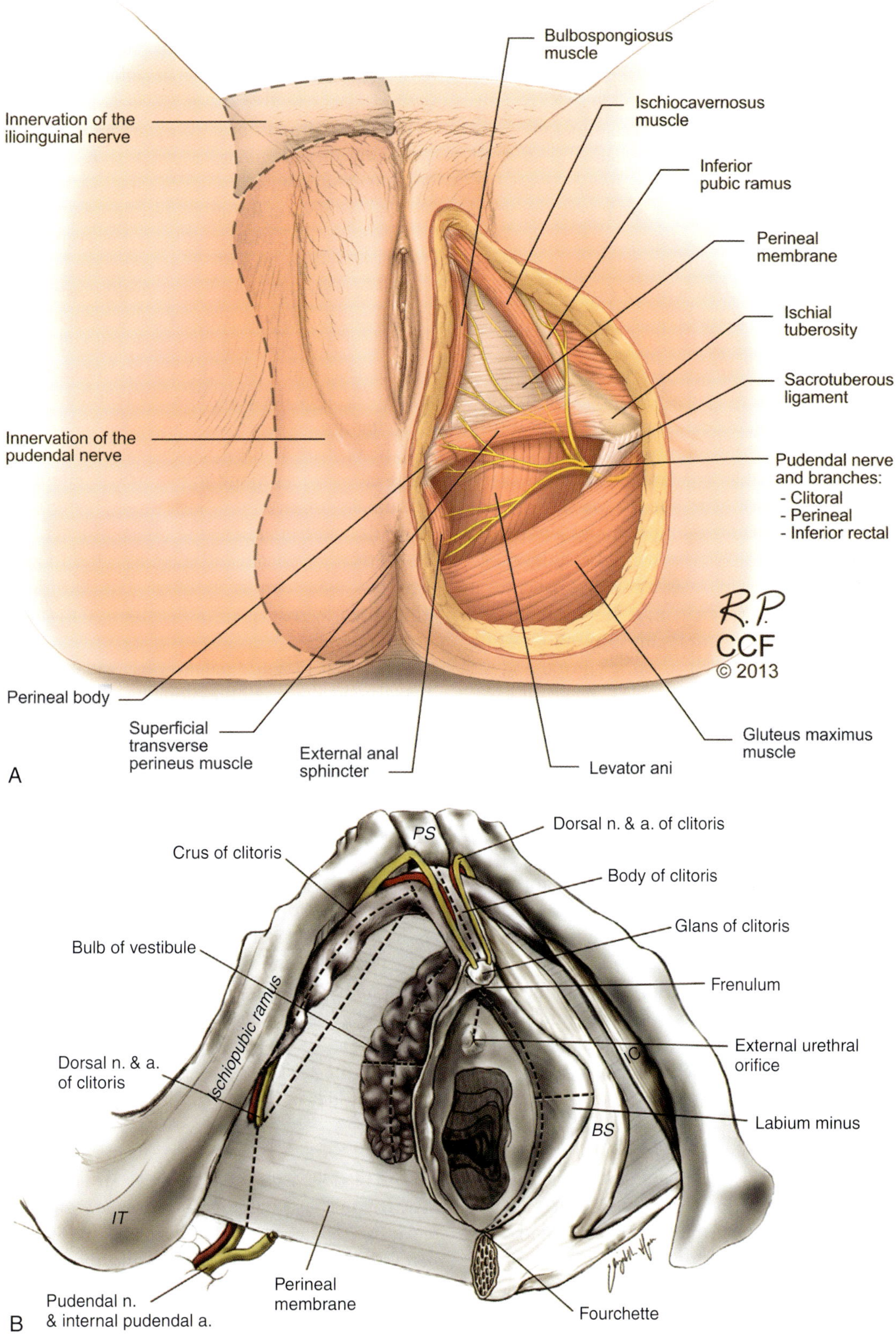

Fig. 1.8 **A**, Neurovascular anatomy of perineum, illustrating the muscles and nerves of the perineum, including the distribution of the pudendal and ilioinguinal innervation (shaded on left). **B**, Schematic view of exposed superficial space of anterior perineal triangle showing vulvar structures including the clitoris and the path of the dorsal nerve and artery of the clitoris. *a.*, Artery; *BS*, bulbospongiosus muscle; *IC*, ischiocavernosus muscle; *IT*, ischial tuberosity; *n.*, nerve; *PS*, pubic symphysis. (From Jackson LA, Hare AM, Carrick KS, et al. Anatomy, histology, and nerve density of the clitoris and associated structures: clinical applications to vulvar surgery. *Am J Obstet Gynecol*. 2019;221:519.e1.)

perineum is via the pudendal nerve. The pudendal nerve originates from S2 to S4, exits the pelvis through the greater sciatic foramen, hooks around the ischial spine, and then travels along the medial surface of the obturator internus through the ischiorectal fossa in a thickening of fascia called Alcock's canal. It emerges posterior and medial to the ischial tuberosity and divides into three branches to supply the perineum: the clitoral, perineal, and inferior rectal (inferior hemorrhoidal) branches. The inferior rectal nerve provides innervation to the external anal sphincter. The blood supply to the perineum is from the pudendal artery, which travels with the pudendal nerve to exit the pelvis. Similar to the nerve, there are three main branches, with rich collateral anastomoses.

Vulva

The female external genitalia or vulva include: labia majora, labia minora, clitoris, vulvar vestibule, external urethral meatus, and vaginal orifice. The labia minora bifurcate anteriorly to form medial and lateral folds. The lateral folds unite ventrally over the clitoris to form the prepuce of the clitoris. The components of the clitoris include the glans, body, and paired crura. The clitoral body is comprised of paired erectile tissue structures that originate from each crus. The proximal clitoral body is cephalad to the midpubic arch, on the anterior surface of the pubic symphysis. The crura run bilaterally along the ischiopubic rami. The mean length of the clitoral body is 2.9 cm (range 1.3–5.9 cm), and the length of the crura is on average 5.0 cm (range 2.5–6.8 cm) (Jackson et al., 2019b). The dorsal nerve of the clitoris and the associated artery can consistently be found posterior to the midsegment of the crus. They emerge into the anterior perineal triangle by piercing the perineal membrane adjacent to the medial surface of the ischiopubic rami (Fig. 1.8B).

The labia minora fuse posterior to the vestibule to form the posterior fourchette or frenulum of the labia minora. Erectile tissue is present in the clitoral body, crura, and vestibular bulbs but is absent in the glans and labia minora. The labia majora are lateral to the labia minora and unite anteriorly to form the mons pubis. The mons pubis is a fat pad that overlies the inferior aspect of the pubic symphysis. The vulvar vestibule is the area enclosed by the labia minora into which the urethra and vagina open. Within the vestibule, the ducts of the Skene's (paraurethral) glands open on each side of the lateral margin of the urethra. The ducts of the Bartholin's glands (greater vestibular glands) open on the posterior lateral margin of the vaginal opening at the four and eight o'clock positions. The hymen is a ring-like membrane that surrounds the vaginal orifice and typically has one or more central perforations. After rupture of the hymen, from sexual intercourse or trauma, fringe-like hymenal remnants persist surrounding the vaginal opening. Congenital anomalies of the hymen, such as imperforate hymen, can occur that may require surgical correction (see Chapter 2).

Bladder

The bladder is a hollow, muscular organ that is the reservoir for the urinary system. The bladder is flat when empty and globular when distended. The superior surface and upper 1 to 2 cm of the posterior aspect of the bladder are covered by peritoneum, which sweeps off of the bladder into the vesicouterine pouch. The anterior bladder is extraperitoneal and adjacent to the retropubic space (space of Retzius). Between the bladder and pubic bones, within the retropubic space, lie adipose tissue, pubovesical ligaments, muscle, and a prominent venous plexus. The bladder rests inferiorly on the anterior vagina and lower uterine segment, separated by an envelope of adventitia (endopelvic fascia).

The epithelium lining the bladder lumen is loosely attached to the underlying musculature, except at the trigone, where it is firmly adherent. The bladder lining consists of a transitional epithelium (urothelium) supported by a layer of loose connective tissue, the lamina propria. The internal surface of the bladder has a rugose appearance formed by mucosal folds in the contracted state. In the distended state, a variably prominent mesh-like appearance is formed by mucosa-covered detrusor musculature.

The bladder wall musculature is often described as having three layers: inner longitudinal, middle circular, and outer longitudinal. However, this layering occurs only at the bladder neck; the remainder of the bladder musculature is composed of fibers that run in many directions within and between layers. This plexiform arrangement of detrusor muscle bundles is ideally suited to reduce all dimensions of the bladder lumen on contraction.

The inner longitudinal layer has widely separated muscle fibers that course multidirectionally. Near the bladder neck, these muscle fibers assume a longitudinal pattern that is contiguous through the trigone and, according to Tanagho (1986), into the inner longitudinal muscular layer of the urethra. The middle circular layer is prominent at the bladder neck, where it fuses with the deep trigonal muscle, forming a muscular ring. This layer does not continue into the urethra. The outer longitudinal layer forms a sheet of muscle bundles around the bladder wall above the level of the bladder neck. Anteriorly, these fibers continue past the vesical neck as the pubovesical muscles and insert into tissues on the posterior surface of the pubic symphysis. The pubovesical muscles may facilitate bladder neck opening during voiding. Posteriorly, the longitudinal fibers fuse with the deep surface of the trigonal apex and communicate with several detrusor muscle loops at the bladder base; these loops probably aid in bladder neck closure.

Trigone

In the bladder base is a triangular area known as the trigone. The trigone has a flattened appearance with a smooth epithelial covering. The corners of the trigone are formed by three orifices: the paired ureteral orifices and the internal urethral orifice. The superior boundary of the trigone is a slightly raised area between the two ureteric orifices called the interureteric ridge. The two ureteral openings are slit-like and, in an undistended organ, lie approximately 3 cm apart.

The trigone has two muscular layers: superficial and deep. The superficial layer is directly continuous with longitudinal fibers of the distal ureter and is continuous posteriorly with the smooth muscle of the proximal urethra. The deep muscular layer of the trigone forms a dense, compact layer that fuses somewhat with the detrusor muscle fibers. The deep layer is in direct communication with a fibromuscular sheath, Waldeyer's sheath, in the intravesical portion of the ureter. The deep trigonal muscle has autonomic innervation identical to that of the detrusor, being rich in cholinergic (parasympathetic) nerves and sparse in noradrenergic (sympathetic) nerves. In contrast, the superficial trigonal muscle has few cholinergic nerves but more noradrenergic nerves.

Urethra

The female urethra is approximately 3.5 to 4 cm long and averages 6 mm in diameter. Its lumen is slightly curved as it passes from the retropubic space, perforates the perineal membrane, and ends with its external orifice in the vestibule directly above the vaginal opening. Throughout its length, the urethra is embedded in the adventitia of the anterior vagina. Its blood supply consists of extensions of the pudendal vessels and the vesical vessels.

Histologically, the urethra has four distinct layers: mucosa, submucosa, internal urethral sphincter (smooth muscle), and striated external urethral sphincter. The urethral epithelium has longitudinal folds and many small glands that open into the urethra throughout its entire length. It is primarily stratified squamous epithelium that becomes transitional near the bladder. The submucosal layer is highly vascular. These vascular cushions, along with the urethral mucosa, account for approximately one-third of the urethral resting tone; the internal and external urethral sphincters account for the remainder.

The internal urethral sphincter is composed primarily of oblique and longitudinal smooth muscle fibers, with a smaller amount of circularly oriented outer fibers. This smooth muscle is usually noted to be under alpha adrenergic and cholinergic control. The longitudinally directed muscles probably shorten and widen the urethral lumen during micturition, whereas the circular smooth muscle (along with the striated urogenital sphincter muscle) contributes to urethral resistance to outflow at rest.

The striated urethral and periurethral muscles form the extrinsic urethral sphincter mechanism. It has two components: an inner portion, which lies within and adjacent to the urethral wall, and an outer portion composed of skeletal muscle fibers of the pelvic diaphragm. The inner portion is made up of the sphincter urethrae, a striated band of muscle that surrounds the proximal two-thirds of the urethra, and the compressor urethrae and urethrovaginal sphincter, which consist of two strap-like bands of striated muscle that arch over the ventral surface of the distal one-third of the urethra (see Fig. 1.7). These three muscles, which function as a single unit, have been called by Oelrich (1983) the striated urogenital sphincter. The striated urogenital sphincter is primarily composed of small-diameter, slow-twitch muscle, making it ideally suited to exert tone on the urethral lumen over prolonged time periods. These muscles may also contribute (along with the levator ani) to voluntary interruption of the urine stream and to urethral closure with stress via reflex muscle contraction.

Pelvic Ureter

As it courses retroperitoneally from the renal pelvis to the bladder, the ureter is divided anatomically into abdominal and pelvic segments, which are approximately equal in length, at 12 to 15 cm each. The ureter enters the pelvis by crossing over the iliac vessels where the common iliac artery divides into the external iliac and internal iliac (hypogastric) artery. It travels lateral to the hypogastric artery, but eventually crosses to lie medial to the branches of the anterior division of the hypogastric artery and lateral to the peritoneum of the cul-de-sac. It is attached to the peritoneum of the lateral pelvic wall. As it proceeds more distally, the ureter courses along the lateral side of the uterosacral ligament and enters the endopelvic fascia of the parametrium (cardinal ligament). The ureter courses medially as the uterosacral ligament is traced from the sacrum toward the vagina. At the level of the ischial spine, the ureter is approximately 1.5 to 2 cm lateral to the uterosacral ligament (Siff et al., 2018). The ureter is closest to the uterosacral ligament at its distal end, at approximately 1 cm. It then dives medially in a deep trajectory to enter the parametria and courses inferior to the uterine artery ("water under the bridge"), approximately 1.5 to 2 cm lateral to the uterine isthmus or, in women with prior hysterectomy, approximately 1.3 cm from the vaginal cuff. The ureter passes through the tunnel of Wertheim (i.e., the cardinal ligament/anterior bladder pillar) then travels medially and anteriorly over the vaginal fornix to enter the trigone of the bladder. The ureters perforate the bladder 5 to 6 cm apart and run obliquely through the bladder wall for 1.5 cm before terminating at the trigone (Fig. 1.9).

The ureter has only one muscular coat that forms an irregular, helical pattern of muscle bundles with fibers oriented in almost every direction. As the ureter approaches and enters the bladder wall, its helical fibers elongate and become parallel to its lumen. The intravesical ureter is approximately 1.5 cm long and is divided into an intramural segment that is totally surrounded by the bladder wall and a submucosal segment directly under the urothelium. The longitudinal muscle fibers of the distal ureter proceed uninterrupted into the superficial trigonal muscle.

Rectum and Anal Sphincters

The rectum extends from its junction with the sigmoid colon to the anal orifice. The distribution of smooth muscle is typical for the intestinal tract, with inner circular and outer longitudinal layers of muscle. At the perineal flexure of the rectum, the inner circular layer increases in thickness to form the internal anal sphincter. The internal anal sphincter is under autonomic control (sympathetic and parasympathetic) and is responsible for 80% of the resting anal pressure. The outer longitudinal layer of smooth muscle becomes concentrated on the anterior and posterior walls of the rectum, with connections to the perineal body and coccyx, and then passes inferiorly on both sides of the external anal sphincter.

The external anal sphincter is composed of striated muscle that is tonically contracted most of the time and can also be voluntarily contracted. Various divisions of the external anal sphincter have been described, and although there is no consensus, recent descriptions favor superficial (combining the previous superficial and subcutaneous components) and deep compartments. The external anal sphincter functions as a unit with the puborectalis portion of the levator ani muscle group.

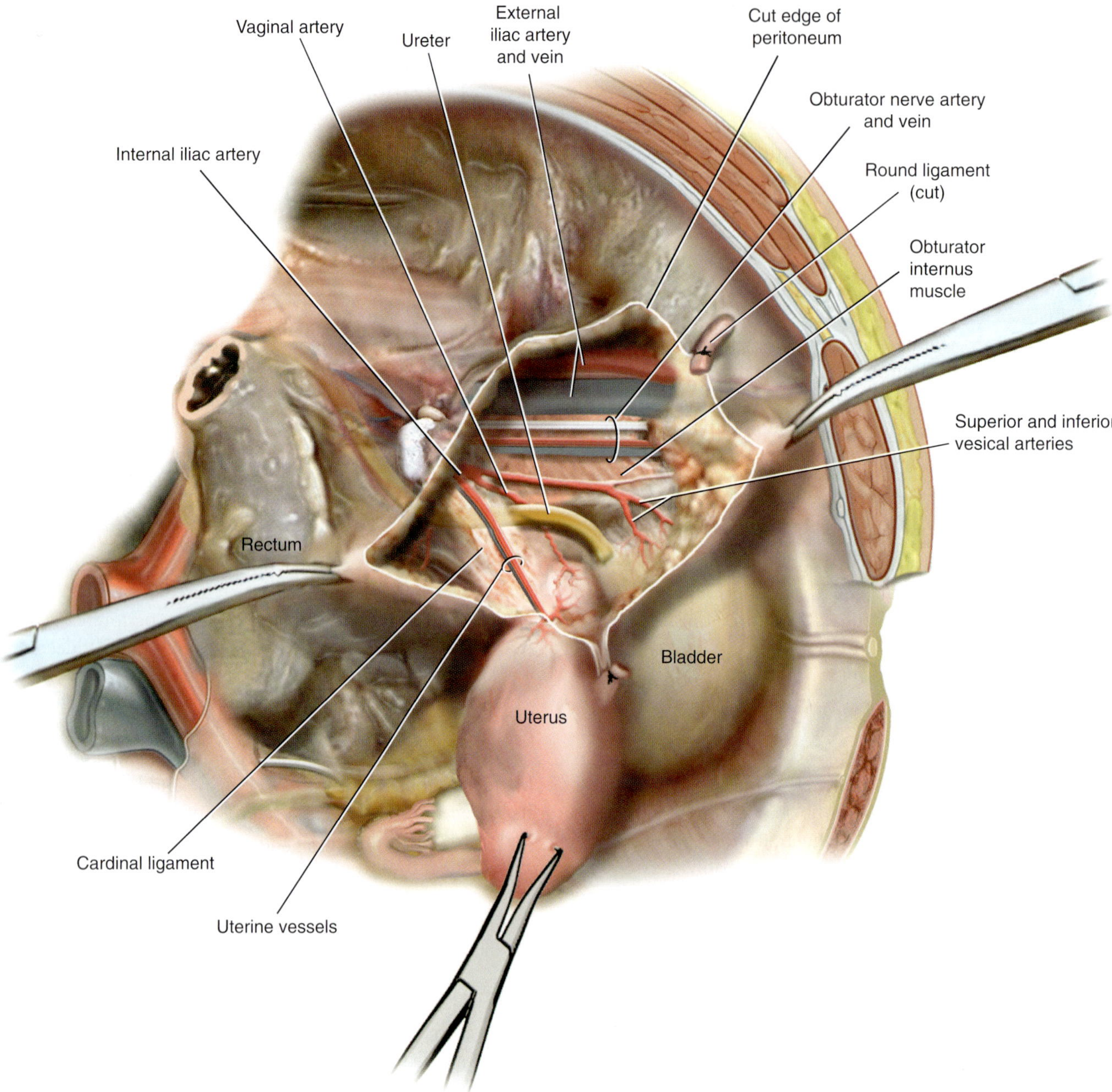

Fig. 1.9 Pelvic retroperitoneal anatomy *(left)* demonstrating course of the pelvic ureter from the pelvic brim to insertion into the bladder relative to vascular and neurologic structures. The uterus is retracted medially.

The anal sphincter mechanism comprises the internal anal sphincter, the external anal sphincter, and the puborectalis muscle (Fig. 1.10). As with the bladder neck and urethra, a spinal reflex causes the striated sphincter to contract during sudden increases in intraabdominal pressure, such as coughing. The anorectal angle is produced by the anterior pull of the puborectalis muscles. These muscles posteriorly form a sling around the anorectal junction. The anorectal angle was previously thought to be important in maintaining fecal continence, but its importance has been questioned. More recent studies suggest that fecal incontinence in women is often related to denervation of the muscles of the pelvic diaphragm and to disruption and denervation of the external anal sphincter.

SURGICAL SPACES

Retropubic Space

The retropubic space, also known as the prevesical space or space of Retzius, is a potential space between the bladder and the pubic bone (Fig. 1.11). It is bounded by the pubic bone, the peritoneum, and muscles of the anterior abdominal wall. Its lateral borders are the pelvic sidewall muscles (obturator internus, levator ani m.), arcus tendineus fasciae pelvis, and the ischial spines. Surgically, this space can be entered by perforating the transversalis fascial layer of the anterior abdominal wall. Within this space lie the dorsal clitoral neurovascular bundle, located in the midline, and the obturator neurovascular bundle,

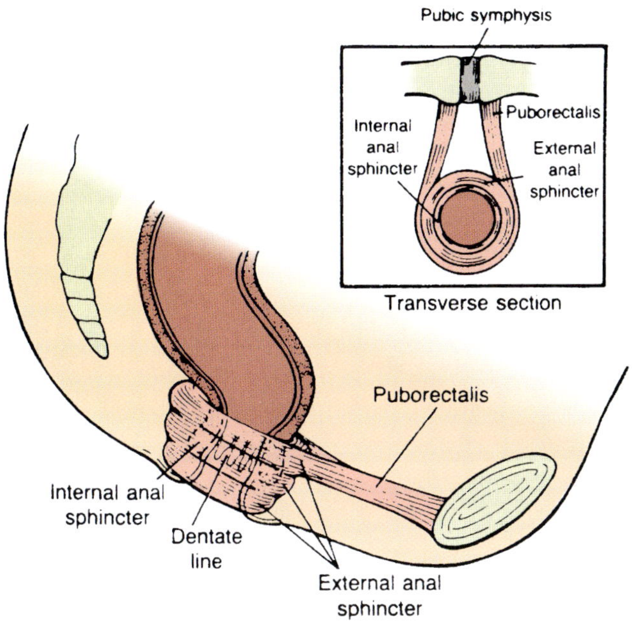

Fig. 1.10 Diagram of the rectum, anal canal, and surrounding muscles. The puborectalis muscle posteriorly forms a sling around the anorectal junction. The external anal sphincter (skeletal muscle) surrounds the anal canal and is closely associated with the puborectalis muscle. The internal anal sphincter muscle (smooth muscle) lies within the ring of the external sphincter muscle and is a continuation of the inner circular layer of the smooth muscle of the rectal wall. (From Madoff RD, Williams JG, Caushaj PF. Fecal incontinence. *N Engl J Med.* 1992;326:1003).

located laterally as it enters the obturator canal. The retropubic space is a highly vascular space with considerable variation in vascular structures, particularly venous plexuses. An accessory obturator artery can usually be found arising from the external iliac or inferior epigastric artery to cross the superior pubic rami and connect with the obturator vessels near the obturator canal. The space lateral to the bladder neck and urethra contain nerves innervating the bladder and urethra, as well as a venous plexus (venous plexus of Santorini). The iliopectineal line, or Cooper's ligament, runs along the superior border of the ischiopubic rami bilaterally and is used for suture placement during Burch retropubic colposuspension. The obturator canal is located approximately 5 to 6 cm from the midline of the pubic symphysis and 1 to 2 cm below the upper margin of the iliopectineal ligament. Although some have described condensations of periurethral tissue extending from the lateral walls of the retropubic urethra to the pubic bones that have been labeled "periurethral ligaments," histologic studies have failed to identify these ligaments as unique structures or to differentiate them from the arcus tendineus fasciae pelvis, and as such they are not recognized as a unique structure by *Terminologia Anatomica.*

Presacral Space

The presacral space is a retroperitoneal space anterior to the sacrum and posterior to the rectosigmoid. It is bounded by the aortic bifurcation superiorly, the internal iliac vessels and ureters laterally, and the pelvic floor inferiorly. The superior hypogastric

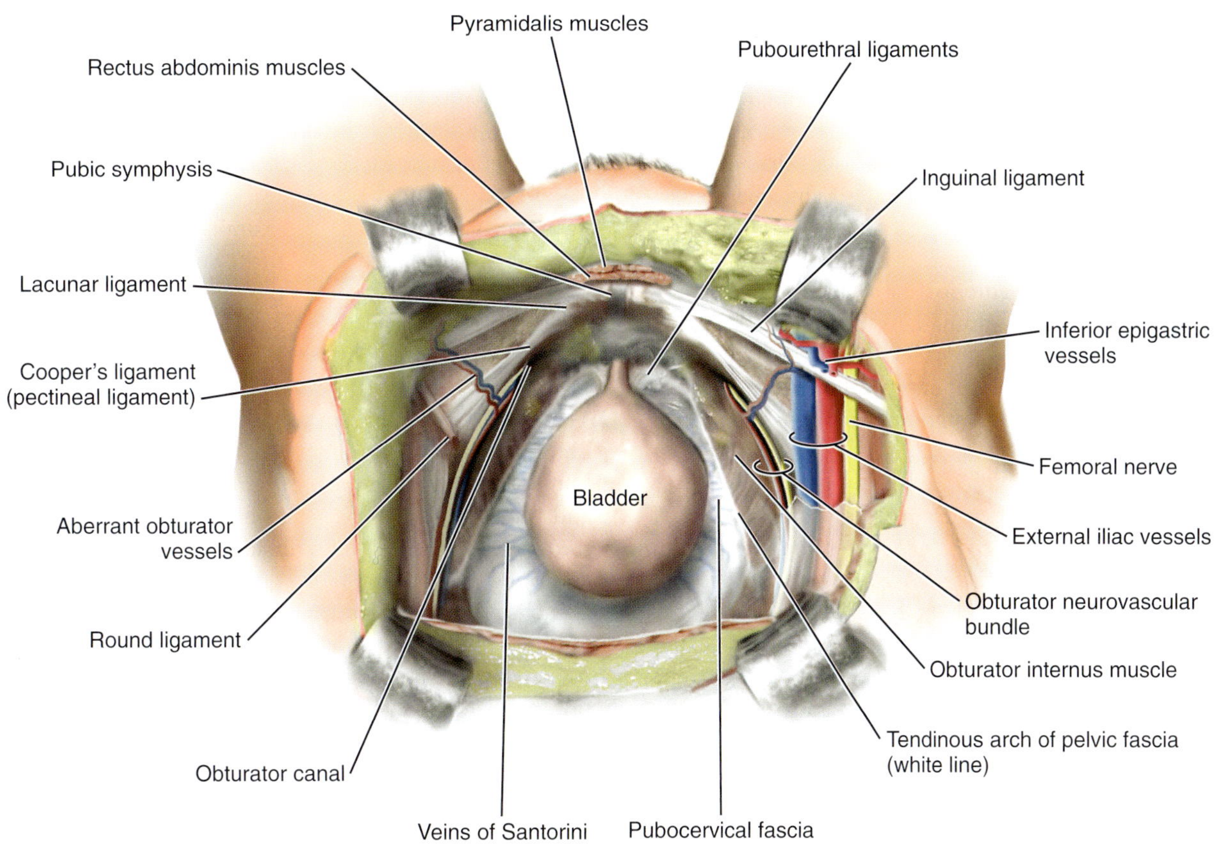

Fig. 1.11 Retropubic space anatomy.

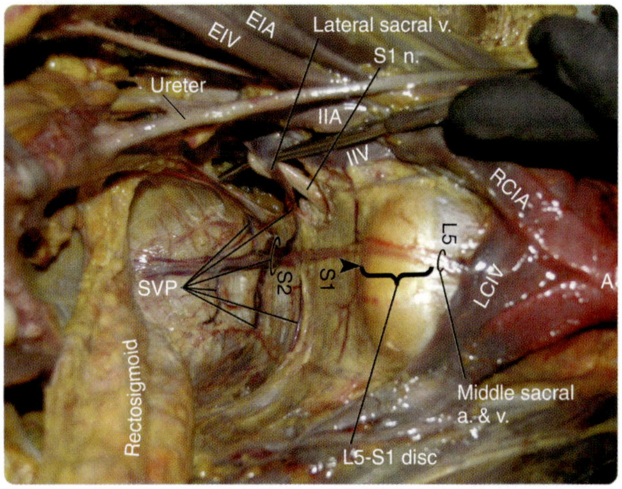

Fig. 1.12 Presacral anatomy in an embalmed cadaver. The rectosigmoid is reflected caudad, demonstrating the retroperitoneal structures. The midpoint of the sacral promontory is indicated by the *black arrowhead*. Note that, in the shown supine position, the most prominent vertebral structure in the presacral space is the L5–S1 disc. *A*, Distal aorta; *a.*, artery; *EIA*, external iliac artery; *EIV*, external iliac vein; *IIA*, internal iliac artery; *IIV*, internal iliac vein; *L5*, fifth lumbar vertebra; *n.*, nerve; *RCIA*, right common iliac artery; *SVP*, sacral venous plexus; *v.*, vein. (From Good MM, Abele TA, Balgobin S, et al. Vascular and reteral anatomy relative to the midsacral promontory. *Am J Obstet Gynecol.* 2013;486.e1.)

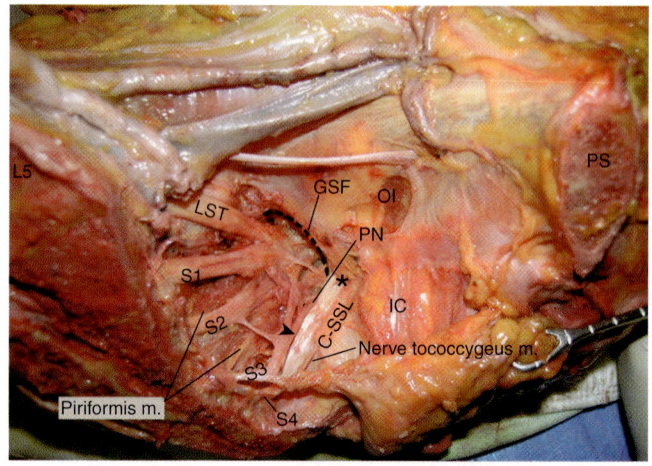

Fig. 1.13 Coccygeus and sacrospinous ligament anatomy. Medial view of dissected left hemi pelvis demonstrating coccygeus sacrospinous ligament complex and surrounding structures. The *black arrow* indicates the superior border of the sacrospinous ligament at its midpoint; the *asterisk* indicates the ischial spine. *C-SSL*, Coccygeus-sacrospinous ligament complex; *GSF*, greater sciatic foramen; *IC*, iliococcygeous muscle; *LST*, lumbosacral trunk; *m*, muscle; *OI*, obturator internus muscle; *PN*, pudendal nerve; *PS*, pubic symphysis; *S1–S4*, first through fourth sacral nerves. (From Florian-Rodriguez ME, Hare A, Chin K, et al. Inferior gluteal and other nerves associated with sacrospinous ligament: a cadaver study. *Am J Obstet Gynecol.* 2016;646.e1.)

plexus, hypogastric nerves, and portions of the inferior hypogastric plexus can be found within this space, as can the sacral promontory and anterior longitudinal ligament of the sacrum (presacral fascia), which are commonly used sites of fixation for sacrocolpopexy (Fig. 1.12). Entry into the presacral space is achieved by pulling the rectosigmoid to the left and incising the peritoneum vertically just to the right of the sigmoid peritoneal attachment over the sacrum. The most vulnerable structure during this initial dissection is the left common iliac vein as it crosses the sacral promontory from left to right. The presacral space has a complex vasculature that includes an extensive sacral venous plexus formed by anastomoses of the middle and lateral sacral veins on the anterior surface of the sacrum. The middle sacral artery arises from the posterior distal portion of the abdominal aorta and courses down the middle of the sacrum. The middle sacral vein courses next to the middle sacral artery and drains into the left common iliac vein.

Sacrospinous Ligament

The sacrospinous ligament is a strong, triangularly-shaped ligament whose apex attaches to the ischial spine laterally and whose base attaches to the distal sacrum and coccyx medially. Its average length is 5.3 cm (range 4.4–6.6 cm). This ligament divides the lateral pelvic outlet into two foramina: the greater sciatic foramen superiorly and the lesser sciatic foramen inferiorly. The coccygeus muscle lies on the superior surface of the sacrospinous ligament. This ligament is a common attachment point for the vaginal apex for the treatment of vaginal vault prolapse (i.e., sacrospinous ligament fixation). A number of important structures lie in close proximity to the sacrospinous ligament that must be avoided when placing sutures in this ligament (Fig. 1.13). The pudendal neurovascular bundle passes behind the ischial spine and lateral aspect of the sacrospinous ligament as it exits the pelvis and enters the ischioanal fossa (see above for further details of the course of the pudendal neurovascular bundle). The S3 sacral nerve root and/or the pudendal nerve course parallel over the superior border of the sacrospinous ligament. The inferior gluteal artery, a branch of the posterior trunk of the internal iliac, is located, on average, 2.4 cm from the ischial spine and a mean vertical distance of 3.4 mm (range 1–5 cm) above the superior border of the sacrospinous ligament. Given the close proximity of these structures, the recommended location for suture or trocar placement is at least two fingerbreadths medial to the ischial spine and ideally in the middle third of the ligament, safely below its superior border.

Obturator Space

The obturator membrane is a fibrous sheath that spans the obturator foramen through which the obturator neurovascular bundle penetrates via the obturator canal. The obturator artery and vein originate as branches of the internal iliac vessels. As they emerge from the inferior side of the obturator membrane and enter the obturator space, they divide into many small branches supplying the muscles of the adductor compartment of the thigh. Cadaver work by Whiteside et al. (2004) has contradicted previous reports of the obturator vessels bifurcating into medial and lateral branches. Rather, the vessels are predominantly small (<5 mm in diameter) and splinter into variable courses. The muscles of the medial thigh and adductor compartment are, from superficial to deep: the gracilis, the adductor longus, the adductor brevis, the adductor magnus, and the obturator externus muscles (Fig. 1.14).

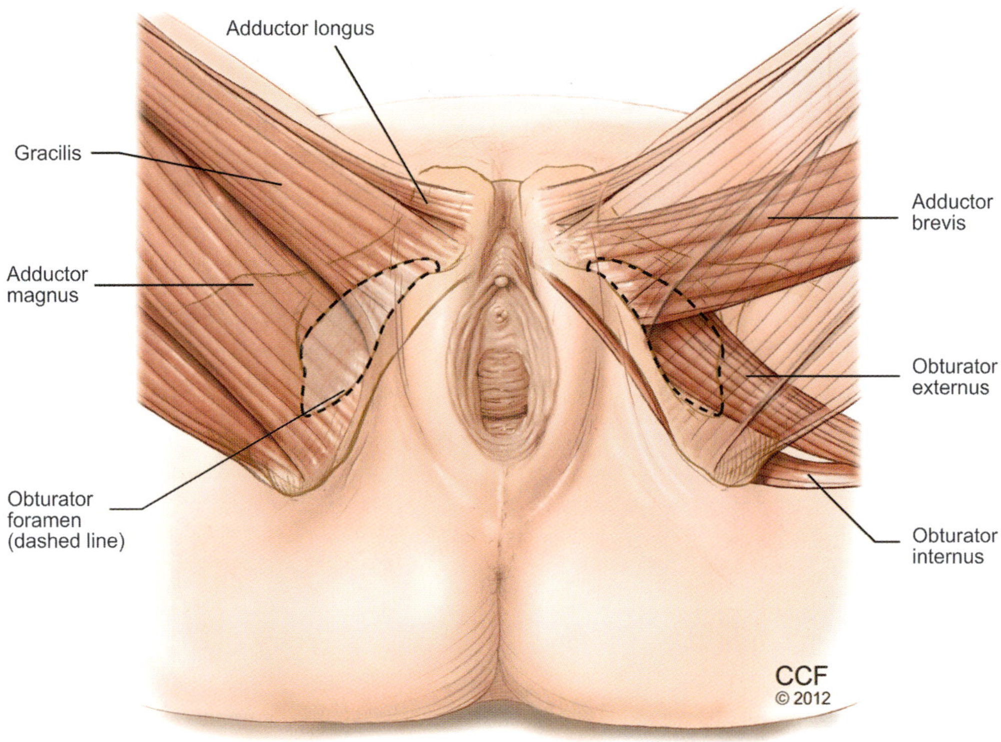

Fig. 1.14 Transobturator anatomy. Diagrammatic representation showing the muscles of the obturator compartment. The superficial muscles are illustrated on the left. On the right, the superficial muscles have been made transparent to illustrate the deeper muscles.

In contrast to the vessels, the obturator nerve emerges from the obturator membrane and bifurcates into anterior and posterior divisions traveling distally down the thigh to supply the muscles of the adductor compartment. With the patient in dorsal lithotomy position, the nerves and vessels follow the thigh and course laterally away from the ischiopubic ramus.

PELVIC ORGAN SUPPORT

Support of the Uterus and Vagina

Normal pelvic support is provided by interaction between the pelvic floor muscles and connective tissue attachments. Under most conditions, the pelvic muscles are the primary support for the pelvic organs, providing a firm yet elastic base on which they rest. The connective tissue (endopelvic fascia) attachments keep the pelvic organs in the proper orientation so that they may be supported by the pelvic floor musculature. When the pelvic muscles are relaxed, as during micturition or defecation, the connective tissue attachments temporarily hold up the pelvic organs.

The endopelvic fascia is a connective tissue network of the retroperitoneum that envelopes the pelvic organs and connects them loosely to the supportive musculature and bones of the pelvis. The term "endopelvic fascia" is used here to describe the tissues located between the surfaces of the peritoneum, muscles, and pelvic organs. Histologically, it is composed of collagen, elastin, adipose tissue, nerves, vessels, lymph channels, and smooth muscle. It provides stabilization and support but allows for mobility, expansion, and contraction of the viscera to permit urine and stool storage, coitus, parturition, voiding, and defecation.

Other than the cervix, the uterus does not have fixed supports, as indicated by its ability to enlarge without restriction during pregnancy. Several areas of the endopelvic fascia (and its associated peritoneum) have been named by anatomists. These are really condensations of the endopelvic fascia and not true ligaments, and include the uterosacral ligament, cardinal ligament, broad ligament, mesoovarium, mesosalpinx, and round ligament. The broad ligament, mesoovarium, mesosalpinx, and round ligament do not play a role in support of the pelvic organs.

Connective tissue attachments stabilize the vagina at different levels, as described by DeLancey (1992) and others (Fig. 1.15). Level I refers to the uterosacral ligament/cardinal ligament complex and represents the most cephalad supporting structures. Level II support is provided by the anterior and posterior paravaginal attachments along the length of the vagina. Level III support describes the most inferior or distal portions of the vagina, including the perineum. Each of these areas plays a significant role in maintaining pelvic organ support and will be discussed individually. However, it is important to remember that levels I, II, and III are all connected through a continuation of the endopelvic fascia.

Comprising level I support, the cardinal and uterosacral ligaments attach to the cervix from the lateral and posterior sides, respectively, with fibers intermingling. The cardinal ligaments blend with the uterosacral ligaments, and they are difficult, if not impossible, to precisely delineate from one another. Fibers traveling predominately laterally make up the cardinal ligaments, whereas fibers going to the sacrum make up the

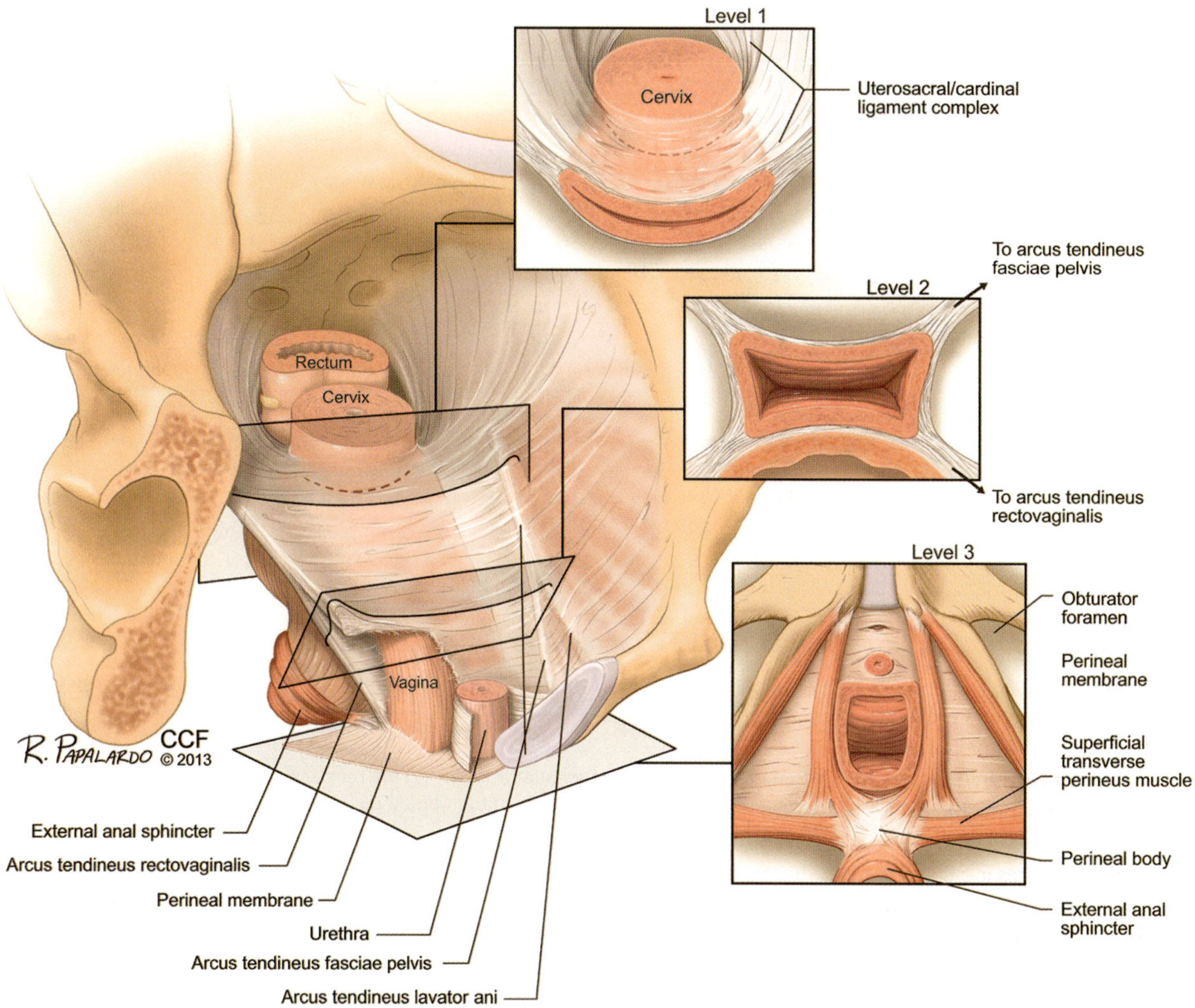

Fig. 1.15 Integrated levels of pelvic organ support. Illustrates the three levels of support of the vagina and uterus as described by DeLancey (1992) and shows the continuity of supportive structures throughout the entire length of the genital tract. In level I, the endopelvic fascia suspends the upper vagina and cervix from the lateral pelvic walls. The fibers of level I extend vertically and posteriorly toward the sacrum. In level II, the vagina is attached to the arcus tendineus fasciae pelvis and to the superior fascia of the levator ani muscles. In level III, the distal vagina is supported by the perineal membrane and muscles.

uterosacral ligaments. These fibers form a three-dimensional complex attaching the upper vagina, cervix, and lower uterine segment to the sacrum and lateral pelvic sidewalls at the piriformis, coccygeus, levator ani, and perhaps the obturator internus fascia overlying the ischial spine. Together, the uterosacral/cardinal ligament complex supports the cervix and upper vagina to maintain vaginal length and to keep the vaginal axis nearly horizontal so that it rests on the rectum and can be supported by the levator plate. This keeps the cervix just superior to the level of the ischial spine.

Contiguous with the cardinal/uterosacral ligament complex at the location of the ischial spine is level II support—the paravaginal attachments. These are the connections of the lateral vagina and endopelvic fascia anteriorly to the arcus tendineus fasciae pelvis and posteriorly to the arcus tendineus rectovaginalis. Level II support functions to keep the vagina midline, directly over the rectum.

The arcus tendineus fasciae pelvis, or "white line," is a thickened condensation of parietal fascia into which the paravaginal endopelvic fascia connects, supporting and creating the anterior lateral vaginal sulci. Similar to the arcus tendineus levator ani, it originates on the ischial spine. However, as it approaches the pubic symphysis, the arcus tendineus fasciae pelvis travels medially and inferiorly to the arcus tendineus levator ani, inserting on the inferior aspect of the superior pubic rami over the origin of the puborectalis muscle. The axes of the arcus tendineus levator ani and the arcus tendineus fasciae pelvis are nearly horizontal in the standing woman, establishing the normal axis of the upper vagina.

Similar to the anterior paravaginal supports, there are also posterior lateral supports. The endopelvic fascia extends posteriorly from the posterior lateral vagina sulci around the rectum to attach the vagina to the pelvic floor. These fibers blend with the vaginal muscularis anteriorly, the rectal muscularis posteriorly, and the perineal body inferiorly. The lateral endopelvic fascia attachments of the posterior vaginal wall do not have significant connections across the midline. Rather, they anchor the posterior lateral vaginal sulci to the ipsilateral levator ani. The posterior vaginal muscularis is attached through this endopelvic fascia to the fascia of the levator ani laterally at the arcus tendineus rectovaginalis. The arcus tendineus rectovaginalis represents a condensation of the parietal fascia of the levator ani coursing from the perineal body inferiorly, along the levator ani laterally, where it intersects the midpoint of the arcus tendineus fasciae pelvis (see Fig. 1.15). The arcus tendineus rectovaginalis is approximately 4 cm in length. The connection to the arcus tendineus rectovaginalis creates the change in axis toward vertical of the distal vagina.

Level III support is provided by the perineal body, the perineal membrane, the superficial and deep perineal muscles, and the endopelvic fascia. These structures support and maintain the normal position of the distal one-third of the vagina and introitus. The endopelvic fascia anteriorly blends with the vaginal muscularis and is continuous with the supportive structures of the urethra. The perineal body is critical for support of the lower part of the vagina and proper function of the anal canal. The perineal membrane anchors the perineal body and distal vagina laterally and anteriorly to the ischiopubic rami. Separation of the perineal body from the perineal membrane results in perineal decent and can contribute to defecatory dysfunction.

The three levels of support are connected and interdependent. Level III structures are connected to the endopelvic fascia that surrounds the vagina and rectum; therefore, they are continuous with level II support. Level II support is connected to level I support through the confluence of the lateral endopelvic fascia attachments and the uterosacral ligament/cardinal ligament complex. Adequate support at all levels maintains the pelvic organs in their normal anatomic positions.

When the vagina, bladder, and rectum are kept in the horizontal plane over the levator plate and pelvic floor muscles, intraabdominal and gravitational forces are applied perpendicular to the vagina and pelvic floor, while the pelvic floor musculature counters those forces with its constant tone. It is this horizontal position and support by the levator ani that maintain pelvic organ support. With proper tone of the pelvic floor muscles (levator ani), stress on the lateral paravaginal attachments is minimized. Furthermore, in times of acute stress such as a cough or sneeze, there is a reflex contraction of the pelvic floor musculature, countering and further stabilizing the viscera. The genital hiatus also responds by narrowing to maintain level III support. With pelvic floor weakness, such as with neuropathic injury or mechanical muscular damage, the endopelvic fascia becomes the primary mechanism of support. Over time, this stress can overcome the endopelvic fascial attachments and result in loss of the normal anatomic position through breaks, stretching, or attenuation of endopelvic fascia supports. This can result in changes in the vector forces applied to the viscera and may lead to pelvic organ prolapse and/or visceral dysfunction. Recreation of these supportive connections and proper position of the organs while maintaining adequate vaginal length to keep the vaginal apex in a natural position should be the goal of reconstructive pelvic surgery.

Urethral Support

When the vagina is normally supported, it provides support to the bladder and urethra. Support of the urethra and bladder neck was traditionally thought to be provided by the interaction of the pubourethral ligaments, the perineal membrane, and the muscles of the pelvic floor. Numerous investigators have described the so-called pubourethral ligaments as extending from the inferior surface of the pubic bones to the urethra. Milley and Nichols (1971) found bilaterally symmetric anterior, posterior, and intermediate pubourethral ligaments and stated that the anterior and posterior ligaments were formed, respectively, by the inferior and superior fascial layers of the perineal membrane. An anatomic defect of the pubourethral ligaments has been cited as a contributing factor to stress urinary incontinence in women.

Studies by DeLancey (1986, 1988, 1989, 1992) provide a more complete view of urethral support. Rather than being suspended ventrally by ligamentous structures, the proximal urethra and bladder base are supported in a sling-like fashion by the anterior vaginal wall, which is attached bilaterally to the muscles of the pelvic diaphragm (levator ani muscles) at the arcus tendineus fasciae pelvis. Similar anatomic connections between the pelvic diaphragm and vagina were described by Olesen and Grau (1976) and others. These attachments extend caudally and blend with the superior fibers of the perineal membrane. The tissues, described as pubourethral ligaments, are made up of the perineal membrane and the most caudal portion of the arcus tendineus fasciae pelvis, which fix the distal urethra beneath the pubic bone. Fig. 1.7 illustrates the anatomic structures that contribute to urethral support and closure.

Anterior vaginal attachment at the arcus tendineus fasciae pelvis may contribute to urethral closure by providing a stable base onto which the bladder neck and proximal urethra are compressed with increases in intraabdominal pressure. These attachments also are responsible for the posterior movement of the vesical neck seen at the onset of micturition (when the pelvic floor relaxes) and for the elevation noted when a patient is instructed to arrest her urinary stream (see Fig. 1.7, *inset*). Defects in these attachments probably result in proximal urethral support defects (urethral hypermobility) and anterior vaginal prolapse (cystocele), conditions associated with stress urinary incontinence. These defects also correspond to the paravaginal fascial defects, with detachment of the vagina from its lateral connective tissue supports, described by Richardson et al. (1976).

BIBLIOGRAPHY

Aronson MP, Lee RA, Berquist TH. Anatomy of anal sphincters and related structures in continent women studied with magnetic resonance imaging. *Obstet Gynecol.* 1990;76:846.

Baggish MS, Karram MM. *Atlas of Pelvic Anatomy and Gynecologic Surgery*. 4th ed. Philadelphia: Elsevier; 2015.

Barber MD, Bremer RE, Thor KB, et al. Innervation of the female levator ani muscles. *Am J Obstet Gynecol.* 2002;187:64.

Barber MD. Contemporary views on female pelvic anatomy. *Cleve Clin J Med.* 2005;72:S3.

Barber MD. Surgical Urogenital Anatomy. In: Barbieri R, ed. *UpToDate*. Waltham, MA: UpToDate, 2021. Accessed May 8, 2021.
Berger MB, Doumouchtsis SK, DeLancey JO. Are bony pelvic dimensions associated with levator ani defects? A case-control study. *Int Urogynecol J*. 2013;24:1377.
Betschart C, Chen L, Ashton-Miller JA, Delancey JO. On pelvic reference lines and the MR evaluation of genital prolapse: a proposal for standardization using the Pelvic Inclination Correction System. *Int Urogynecol J*. 2013;24:1421.
Brown KM, Handa VL, Maruca KJ, DeLeon VB. Three-dimensional shape differences in the bony pelvis of women with pelvic floor disorders. *Int Uroygnecol*. 2013;J 24:431.
Buller JL, Thompson JR, Cundiff GW, et al. Uterosacral ligament: description of anatomic relationships to optimize surgical safety. *Obstet Gynecol*. 2001;97:873.
Corton MM. Anatomy of Pelvic Floor Dysfunction. *Obstet Gynecol Clin N Am*. 2009;36:401.
Curtis AH, Anson BJ, Ashley FL. Further studies in gynecological anatomy and related clinical problems. *Surg Gynecol Obstet*. 1942;74:709.
Curtis AH, Anson BJ, McVay CB. The anatomy of the pelvic and urogenital diaphragms, in relation to urethrocele and cystocele. *Surg Gynecol Obstet*. 1939;68:161.
Dalley AF. The riddle of the sphincters: the morphophysiology of the anorectal mechanism reviewed. *Am Surgeon*. 1987;53:298.
DeLancey JOL. Correlative study of paraurethral anatomy. *Obstet Gynecol*. 1986;68:91.
DeLancey JOL. Structural aspects of the extrinsic continence mechanism. *Obstet Gynecol*. 1988;72:296.
DeLancey JOL. Pubovesical ligament: a separate structure from the urethral supports ("pubo-urethral ligaments"). *Neurourol Urodyn*. 1989;8:53.
DeLancey JOL. Anatomic aspects of vaginal eversion after hysterectomy. *Am J Obstet Gynecol*. 1992;166:1717.
DeLancey JOL. Anatomy of the pelvis. In: Thompson JD, Rock JA, eds. *Telinde's Operative Gynecology*. 7th ed. Philadelphia: JB Lippincott; 1992.
DeLancey JOL, Starr RA. Histology of the connection between the vagina and levator ani muscles. *J Reprod Med*. 1990;35:765.
DeLancey JOL. Structural anatomy of the posterior pelvic compartment as it relates to rectocele. *Am J Obstet Gynecol*. 1999;180:815.
DeLancey JOL. Anatomy. In: Cardozo L, Staskin D, eds: *Textbook of Female Urology and Urogynecology*. 3rd ed. London, UK: Informa Healthcare; 2010.
Dickinson RL. Studies of the levator ani muscle. *Am J Obstet Dis Women Child*. 1889;22:897.
Elbadawi A. Neuromorphologic basis of vesicourethral function: I. Histochemistry, ultrastructure and function of the intrinsic nerves of the bladder and urethra. *Neurourol Urodyn*. 1982;1:3.
Florian-Rodriguez ME, Hare A, Chin K, et al. Inferior gluteal and other nerves associated with sacrospinous ligament: a cadaver study. *Am J Obstet Gynecol*. 2016;646.e1.
Funt MI, Thompson JD, Birch H. Normal vaginal axis. *South Med J*. 1978d;71:1534.
Good MM, Abele TA, Balgobin S, et al. Vascular and reteral anatomy relative to the midsacral promontory. *Am J Obstet Gynecol*. 2013;486.e1.
Gosling JA, Dixon JS, Critchley HO, et al. A comparative study of the human external sphincter and periurethral levator ani muscles. *Br J Urol*. 1981;53:35.
Gosling JA, Dixon JS, Humpherson JR. *Functional anatomy of the urinary tract: an integrated text and color atlas*. Baltimore: University Park Press; 1982.
Halban J, Tandler J. Anatomie und Atiologie der Genital-prolapse (Translated by Porges RF, Porges JC. The anatomy and etiology of genital prolapse in women). *Obstet Gynecol*. 1960;15:790.
Hamner JJ, Carrick KS, Ramirez DM, Corton MM. Gross and histologic relationships of the retropubic urethra to lateral pelvic sidewall and anterior vaginal wall in female cadavers: clinical applications to retropubic surgery. *Am J Obstet Gynecol*. 2018;219:597.e1.
Handa VL, Pannu HK, Siddique S, et al. Architectural differences in the bony pelvis of women with and without pelvic floor disorders. *Obstet Gynecol*. 2003;102:1283.
Jackson LA, Ramirez DMO, Carrick KS, et al. Gross and histologic anatomy of the pelvic ureter. *Obstet Gynecol*. 2019;133:896.
Jackson LA, Hare AM, Carrick KS, et al. Anatomy, histology, and nerve density of the clitoris and associated structures: clinical applications to vulvar surgery. *Am J Obstet Gynecol*. 2019;221:519.e1.
Jeppson PC, Balgobin S, Washington BB, et al. Recommended standardized terminology of the anterior female pelvis based on a structured medical literature review. *Am J Obstet Gynecol*. 2018;219:26.
Kearney R, Sawhney R, DeLancey JOL. Levator ani muscle anatomy by origin-insertion pairs. *Obstet Gynecol*. 2004;104:168.
Krantz KE. The anatomy of the urethra and anterior vaginal wall. *Am J Obstet Gynecol*. 1951;62:374.
Lawson JO. Pelvic anatomy. I. Pelvic floor muscles. *Ann R Coll Surg Engl*. 1974;52:244.
Leffler KS, Thompson JR, Cundiff GW, et al. Attachment of the rectovaginal septum to the pelvic sidewall. *Am J Obstet Gynecol*. 2001;185:41.
Luo J, Betschart C, Ashton-Miller JA, DeLancey JO. Quantitative analyses of variability in normal vaginal shape and dimension on MR images. *Int Urogynecol J*. 2016;27:1087.
Lund CJ, Fullerton RE, Tristan TA. Cinefluorographic studies of the bladder and urethra in women. *Am J Obstet Gynecol*. 1959;78:706.
Madoff RD, Williams JG, Caushaj PF. Fecal incontinence. *N Engl J Med*. 1992;326:1003.
Maldonado PA, Carrick KS, Montoya TI, Corton MM. Posterior vaginal compartment anatomy: Implications for surgical repair. *Female Pelvic Med Reconstr Surg*. 2020;26:751.
Margulies RU, Hsu Y, Kearney R, et al. Appearance of the levator ani muscle subdivisions in magnetic resonance images. *Obstet Gynecol*. 2006;107:1064.
Mattox TF, Lucente V, McIntyre P, et al. Abnormal spinal curvature and its relationship to pelvic organ prolapse. *Am J Obstet Gynecol*. 2000;183:1381.
McGuire EJ. The innervation and function of the lower urinary tract. *J Neurosurg*. 1986;65:278.
Mengert WF. Mechanics of uterine support and position. *Am J Obstet Gynecol*. 1936;31:775.
Milley PS, Nichols DH. The relationship between the pubo-urethral ligaments and the urogenital diaphragm in the human female. *Anat Rec*. 1971;170:281.
Nguyen JK, Lind LR, Choe JY, et al. Lumbosacral spine and pelvic inlet changes associated with pelvic organ prolapse. *Obstet Gynecol*. 2000;95:332.
Oelrich TM. The striated urogenital sphincter muscle in the female. *Anat Rec*. 1983;205:223.
Olesen KP, Grau V. The suspensory apparatus of the female bladder neck. *Urol Int*. 1976;31:33.
Pierce LM, Reyes M, Thor KB, et al. Innervation of the levator ani muscles in the female squirrel monkey. *Am J Obstet Gynecol*. 2003;188:1141.

Redman JF. Anatomy of the genitourinary system. In: Gillenwater JY, Grayhack JT, Howards SS, Duckett JW, eds. *Adult and Pediatric Urology*. Vol. 1. Chicago: Mosby; 1987.

Richardson AC, Lyon JB, Williams NL. A new look at pelvic relaxation. *Am J Obstet Gynecol.* 1976;126:568.

Ridgeway BM, Arias BE, Barber MD. Variation of the obturator foramen and pubic arch of the female bony pelvis. *Am J Obstet Gynecol.* 2008;198:546.e1.

Siff LN, Jallad K, Hickman LC, Walters MD. Surgical anatomy of the uterosacral ligament colpopexy. *Female Pelvic Med Reconstr Surg.* 2018;24:380.

Singh K, Jakab M, Reid WM, et al. Three-dimenstional assessment of levator ani morphologic features in different grades of prolapse. *Am J Obstet Gynecol.* 2003;188:910.

Sze EH, Kohli N, Miklos JR, et al. Computed tomography comparison of bony pelvic dimensions between women with and without genital prolapse. *Obstet Gynecol.* 1999;93:229-232.

Tanagho EA. Anatomy of the lower urinary tract. In: Walsh PC, Gittes RF, Perlmutter AD, Stamey TA, eds. *Campbell's Urology*. 5th ed. Philadelphia: WB Saunders; 1986.

Weber AM, Walters MD. Anterior vaginal prolapse: review of anatomy and techniques of surgical repair. *Obstet Gynecol.* 1997;89:331.

Whiteside JL, Barber MD, Walters MD, Falcone T. Anatomy of ilioinguinal and iliohypogastric nerves in relation to trocar placement and low transverse incisions. *Am J Obstet Gynecol.* 2003;189:1574.

Whiteside JL, Walters MD. Anatomy of the obturator region: relations to a transobturator sling. *Int Urogynecol J.* 2004;15:223.

Wood BA, Kelly AJ. Anatomy of the anal sphincters and pelvic floor. In: Henry MM, Swash M, eds. *Coloproctology and The Pelvic Floor*. 5th ed. Oxford: Butterworth-Heinemann; 1992.

Woodburne RT. Anatomy of the bladder and bladder outlet. *J Urol.* 1968;100:474.

Woodburne RT. *Essentials of Human Anatomy.* 5th ed. New York: Oxford University Press; 1976.

Zacharin RF. The suspensory mechanism of the female urethra. *J Anat.* 1963;97:423.

2

Embryology and Congenital Anomalies of the Urinary Tract, Rectum, and Female Genital System

Beri M. Ridgeway and Marjan Attaran

CHAPTER OUTLINE

EMBRYOLOGY

Formation of the Mesoderm

The period of organogenesis, also called the embryonic period, spans the third to the eighth week of development. At approximately 15 days after fertilization, invagination and lateral migration of mesodermal cells occur between the ectodermal and endodermal layers of the embryo. At about the sixteenth day of development, the posterior wall of the yolk sac forms a small diverticulum, the allantois, which extends into the connecting stalk. The hindgut undergoes slight dilation to form the cloaca; it receives the allantois ventrally and the two mesonephric ducts laterally. By the seventeenth day of development, the endoderm and ectoderm layers are separated entirely by the mesoderm layer, with the exception of the prochordal plate cephalad and the cloacal plate caudal. The cloacal plate consists of tightly adherent endodermal and ectodermal layers. With ventral bending of the embryo, the connecting stalk and contained allantois, as well as the cloacal membrane, are displaced onto the ventral aspect of the embryo.

A spur of mesodermal tissue migrates from the base of the allantois toward the cloacal membrane around 28 days after fertilization, forming the urorectal septum (Fig. 2.1). This structure partitions the cloaca into a ventral urogenital sinus and a dorsal rectum. Following this, each of the three germ layers, the endoderm, mesoderm, and ectoderm, give rise to specific tissues and organs. The intermediate mesoderm differentiates into the urogenital structures. Other portions of the mesoderm form multiple structures, including the vascular system, the spleen, the connective tissue, and the wall of the gut tube.

At birth, the urogenital system can be divided functionally into two different systems: the urinary system and the genital system. However, embryologically and anatomically they are intimately connected because both develop from a common mesodermal ridge known as the intermediate mesoderm. Both systems share a common origin, with significant interaction between the components of each system during the later stages of development. Epithelial-mesenchymal interactions are primarily responsible for the maintenance and differentiation of many of the structures of the urogenital system. Furthermore, male and female sexual differentiation is dependent on the presence of specific promoting or inhibiting factors.

This chapter will explore the embryology and basic congenital anomalies of the urinary tract, rectum, and anal sphincters. It will detail the embryology of female genital organs and discuss congenital anomalies and their treatments.

Urinary System

Kidney and Ureter. The urinary system begins to take shape before any gonadal development is evident. The kidney exists in three distinct but slightly overlapping forms during development. The first is the pronephros, which is present at approximately 22 days of gestation and is rudimentary and nonfunctioning. The second form, the mesonephros, likely functions for a short time during the early fetal period. The excretory tubules of the mesonephros enter the longitudinal

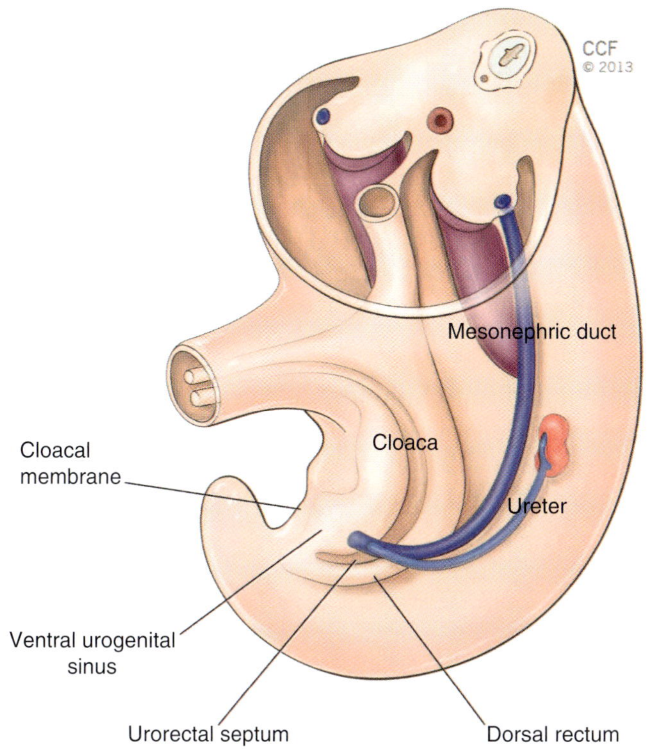

Fig. 2.1 Embryo approximately 32 days (8-mm crown–rump length) after fertilization. The urorectal septum is shown dividing the cloaca into a ventral urogenital sinus and dorsal rectum. Definitive ureter and mesonephric ducts share a common opening into partially divided cloaca. Note the ureter has induced formation of a kidney from metanephrogenic blastema.

collecting duct (primary nephric duct). These formations go on to form the mesonephric duct, which is crucial in the formation of the male genital system but disappears in the female. By the end of the fourth week, the mesonephric ducts attach to the cloaca, and a continuous lumen is present. The ureteric bud is an epithelial outgrowth of the mesonephric duct near the attachment to the cloaca that penetrates the mesodermal tissue and ultimately forms the renal calyces, ureter, renal pelvis, and collecting tubules. Interactions between the mesoderm and ureteric bud form the third and permanent form of kidney, the metanephros (Fig. 2.2). The excretory units of the kidney develop from the metanephric mesoderm.

The definitive kidney, formed from the metanephros, begins to function around the twelfth week of development. Urine is passed and mixes with amniotic fluid. The fetus swallows this and recycles it through the kidney. During fetal life, the placenta is responsible for waste excretion, not the kidney.

Initially the kidney is positioned in the pelvic region, but it begins a caudal ascent secondary to lumbar and sacral body growth in the late embryonic and early fetal periods. If a kidney fails to ascend, it remains close to the iliac vessels and is known as a pelvic kidney. Occasionally, the kidneys are so close in proximity that the lower poles fuse, leading to development of a horseshoe kidney. This structure often cannot ascend completely, as it cannot pass the inferior mesenteric artery root.

Bladder, Trigone, and Urethra. During the fourth to seventh week of development, the cloaca divides into two separate structures: the urogenital sinus (anteriorly) and the anal canal

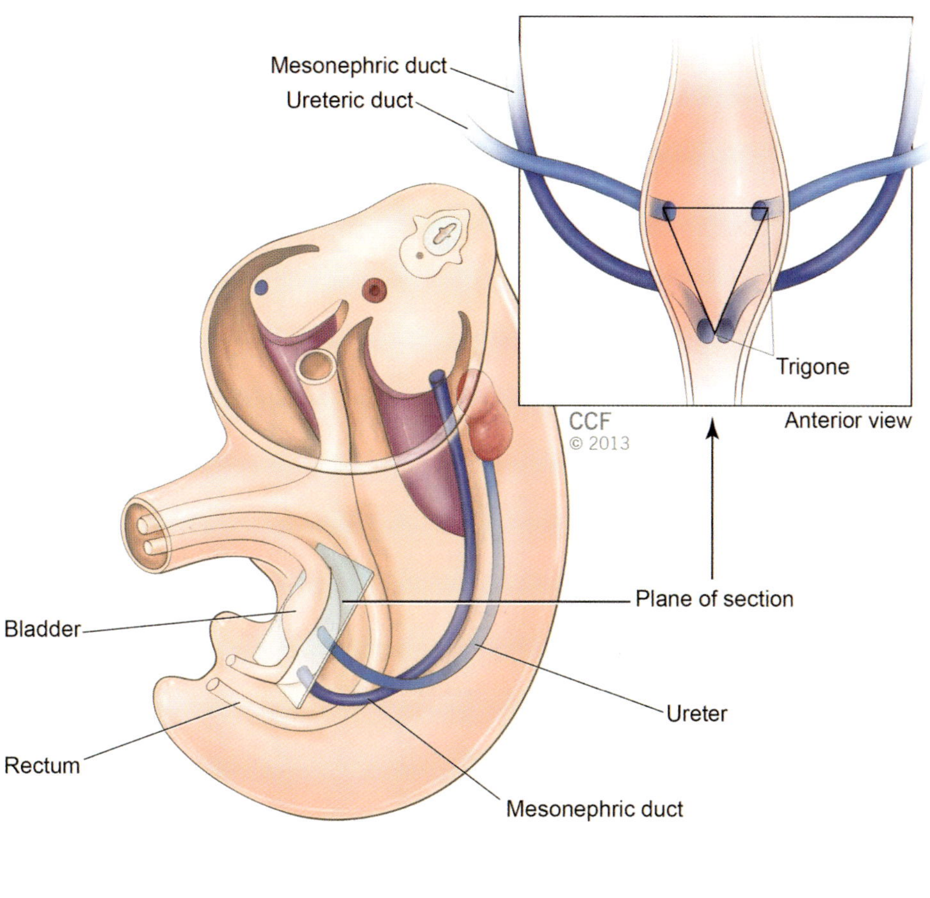

Fig. 2.2 By day 37 to 40, the kidney has continued to ascend and undergo medial rotation, and the mesonephric ducts and future ureter have separated. Also, the cloaca has been divided into ventral urogenital and dorsal alimentary parts. The *inset* demonstrates the urogenital sinus and associated ducts at approximately 40 days (17-mm crown–rump length) after fertilization. The trigone lies between the separate ureteric and mesonephric ducts.

(posteriorly). These structures are separated by a mesodermal structure, the urorectal septum. The tip of this septum eventually forms the perineal body. The upper and largest portion of the urogenital sinus forms the urinary bladder, which is of endodermal origin. Initially, the bladder is continuous with the allantois (rudimentary structure primarily involved in nutrition and waste excretion in the embryo), but the lumen of the allantois becomes obliterated and forms a fibrous cord called the urachus, which runs from the bladder dome to the umbilicus and is called the median umbilical ligament in the adult. The middle portion of the urogenital sinus forms the prostatic and membranous parts of the urethra, and the distal portion forms the phallic portion.

The expanding wall of the bladder grows and incorporates the mesonephric ducts and ureteric buds, forming the bladder trigone. This structure provides a mesodermal contribution to the endodermal wall of the vesicourethral canal. At about 42 days after fertilization, the trigone may be defined as the region of the vesicourethral canal lying between the ureteric orifices and the termination of the mesonephric ducts (see Fig. 2.2). The caudal portion of the vesicourethral canal remains narrow and forms the entire urethra. The urethra consists of epithelium that is derived from endoderm, whereas the surrounding connective tissue and smooth muscle are mesodermal in origin. In females, the cranial portion of the urethra gives rise to the urethral and paraurethral glands. A timetable and schematic representation of the embryologic contributions of the various structures of the urogenital system are shown in Table 2.1 and Fig. 2.3, respectively.

The separate development of the trigone and bladder may explain why the muscle laminae of the trigone are contiguous with the muscle of the ureter, but not with the detrusor muscle of the bladder. This separate development also may account for pharmacologic responses of the musculature of the bladder neck and trigone, which differ partially from those of the detrusor. Because of its embryonic origins (mesonephric ducts and ureters), initially the bladder mucosa is mesodermal, but with time this lining is replaced by endodermal epithelium from the hindgut.

TABLE 2.1 Timetable of Events in the Development of the Lower Urinary Tract

Time After Fertilization	Event
15 days	Ingrowth of intraembryonic mesoderm
16–17 days	Allantois appears
17 days	Cloacal plate forms
22 days	Pronephros present
28 days	Mesonephric duct reaches cloaca; ureteric bud appears
28–49 days	Partitioning of cloaca by urorectal septum
30–37 days	Ureteric bud initiates formation of metanephros (permanent kidney)
41 days	Lumen of urethra is discrete; genital tubercles prominent
42–44 days	Urogenital sinus separates from rectum; mesonephric ducts and ureters drain separately into urogenital sinus, defining boundaries of trigone
51–52 days	Kidneys in lumbar region; glomeruli appear in kidney
12 weeks	Renal function initiates
13 weeks	Bladder becomes muscularized
20–40 weeks	Further growth and development complete the urogenital organs

Congenital Anomalies of the Urinary Tract. Anomalies of the urinary system are common (3%–4% of live births). Knowledge of the embryology of the genitourinary system is necessary for understanding the causes of the multiple congenital anomalies of the upper and lower urinary tracts. Selected congenital anomalies of the urinary tract and their embryologic causes are shown in Table 2.2.

Rectum and Anal Sphincters

Normal Development of the Hindgut. In the early embryo, the caudal portion of the primitive gut forms the hindgut. The hindgut extends from the posterior intestinal portal to the cloacal membrane and gives rise to the distal third of the transverse colon, the descending colon, the sigmoid, the rectum, and the upper part of the anal canal. The terminal portion of the hindgut enters into the cloaca, an endoderm-lined cavity that is in direct contact with the surface ectoderm. This boundary between the endoderm and ectoderm forms the cloacal membrane.

During further development, a transverse ridge called the urorectal septum arises from mesoderm between the allantois and the hindgut. This septum gradually grows caudad, thereby dividing the cloaca into an anterior portion, the primitive urogenital sinus, and a posterior portion, the anorectal canal. The primitive perineum is formed when the urorectal septum reaches the cloacal membrane when the embryo is 7 weeks old. At this time, the cloacal membrane ruptures, creating an anal opening for the hindgut and a ventral opening for the urogenital sinus.

Ectoderm on the surface portion of the cloaca proliferates and invaginates to create the anal pit. Degeneration of the anal membrane (formerly cloacal membrane) establishes continuity between the upper and lower anal canal. The upper part of the anal canal is thus endodermal in origin; the lower third of the anal canal is ectodermal. The junction between these regions is delineated by the pectinate line. The embryologic origin of the anus explains the differing blood and nerve supplies and epithelial cell types of the upper and lower anal canal.

The external anal sphincter appears in human embryos at approximately 7 to 8 weeks. This sphincter, together with the levator ani, is believed to originate from hypaxial myotomes. Although the anal sphincter and levator ani may arise from distinct primordia, their relationship is very close.

Congenital Anomalies of the Rectum and Anal Sphincters. Imperforate anus is one of the more common abnormalities of the hindgut. In simple cases, the anal canal ends blindly at the anal membrane, which then forms a diaphragm between the endodermal and ectodermal portions of the anal canal. This occurs when the anal membrane fails to break down. In more severe cases, a thick layer of connective tissue may be found between the terminal end of the rectum and the surface because of either a failure of the anal pit to develop or atresia of the rectal ampulla. Vascular accidents in this region are the likely

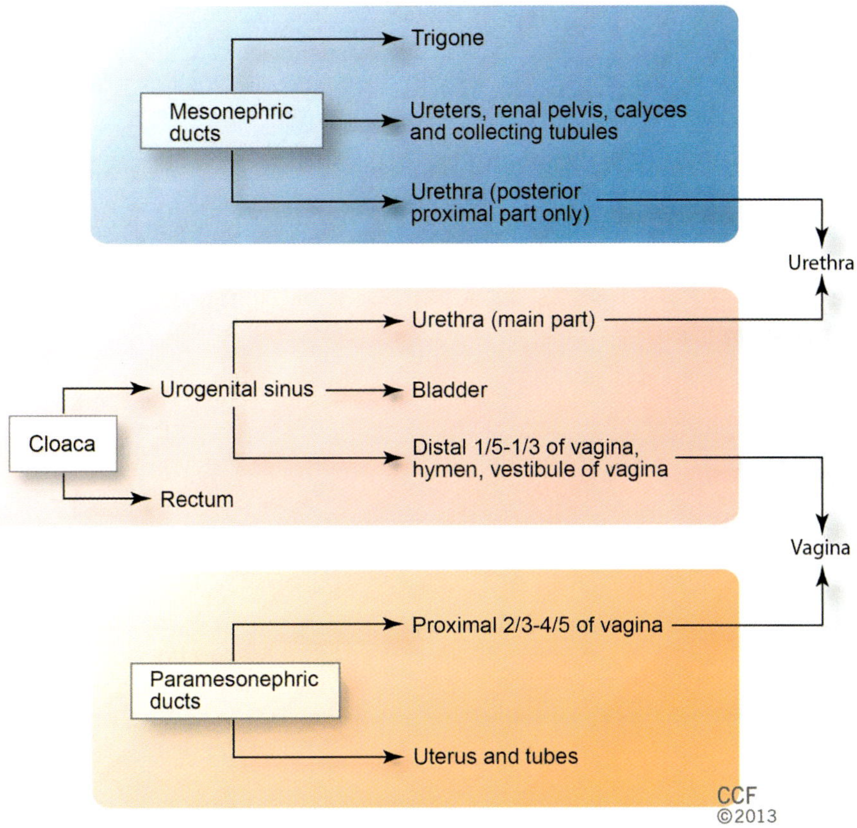

Fig. 2.3 Schematic representation of the embryologic contributions of various structures of the female urogenital system.

TABLE 2.2 Selected Congenital Anomalies of the Urinary Tract and Their Embryologic Causes

Condition	Embryologic Cause
Renal agenesis	Faulty interaction between the ureteric bud and metanephrogenic mesenchyme
Pelvic kidney	Failure of kidney to ascend to the lumbar region
Horseshoe kidney	Fusion of lower poles of both kidneys; ascent to lumbar region prevented by root of inferior mesenteric artery
Urachal fistula, cyst, sinus	Variable persistence of the intraembryonic portion of allantois, from bladder to umbilicus
Double ureter	Early splitting of the ureteric bud
Ectopic ureter	Two ureteric buds develop from one mesonephric duct. One bud is in normal position; the abnormal bud moves downward with the mesonephric duct to enter into the urethra, vagina, vestibule, or uterus
Bladder exstrophy	Insufficiency of mesoderm of the ventral abdominal wall leading to abdominal ectodermal breakdown and degeneration of the anterior bladder wall; the bladder opens broadly onto the abdominal wall

cause of rectoanal atresias. These vary greatly and present as a fibrous remnant or loss of a segment of the rectum or anus.

Rectourethral and rectovaginal fistulas are likely caused by abnormalities in the formation of the cloaca or urorectal septum. If the urorectal septum does not extend far enough caudally or shifts anteriorly, then the hindgut opens into the urethra or vagina, creating a fistula.

Female Genital System

Gonads. Gonads appear in early development as a pair of longitudinal ridges of steroidogenic mesoderm called the genital or gonadal ridges, which are formed by proliferation of the epithelium and condensation of the underlying mesenchyme. These initially do not contain germ cells. Primordial germ cells originate in the epiblast, migrate through the primitive streak, and by the third week reside in the posterior wall of the yolk sac (Fig. 2.4). They then migrate along the dorsal mesentery of the hindgut and arrive at the primitive gonads at the beginning of the fifth week and invade the genital ridges in the sixth week. Approximately 1000 to 2000 primordial germ cells enter the genital ridges. If the primordial germ cells fail to reach the genital ridge, the gonads do not develop. In the female, once the primordial germ cells reach the genital ridge, they are called oogonia. Oogonia begin to proliferate at this stage and continue into the fourth month. Once these cells proliferate via mitosis, they are called oocytes.

In the absence of the Y chromosome (XX or XO) and in the presence of the appropriate somatic cell environment, primitive sex cords (medullary cords) regress (Fig. 2.5A). However, the surface epithelium continues to proliferate and develops a second generation of cords called cortical cords. Cells in these cords surround each oocyte with a layer of epithelial cells called follicular cells. Together, the oocyte and follicular cells constitute a primary follicle (Fig. 2.5B). These enter meiosis until prophase I, when meiosis is arrested. The oocytes remain in this phase until ovulation, which may occur up to 50 years later.

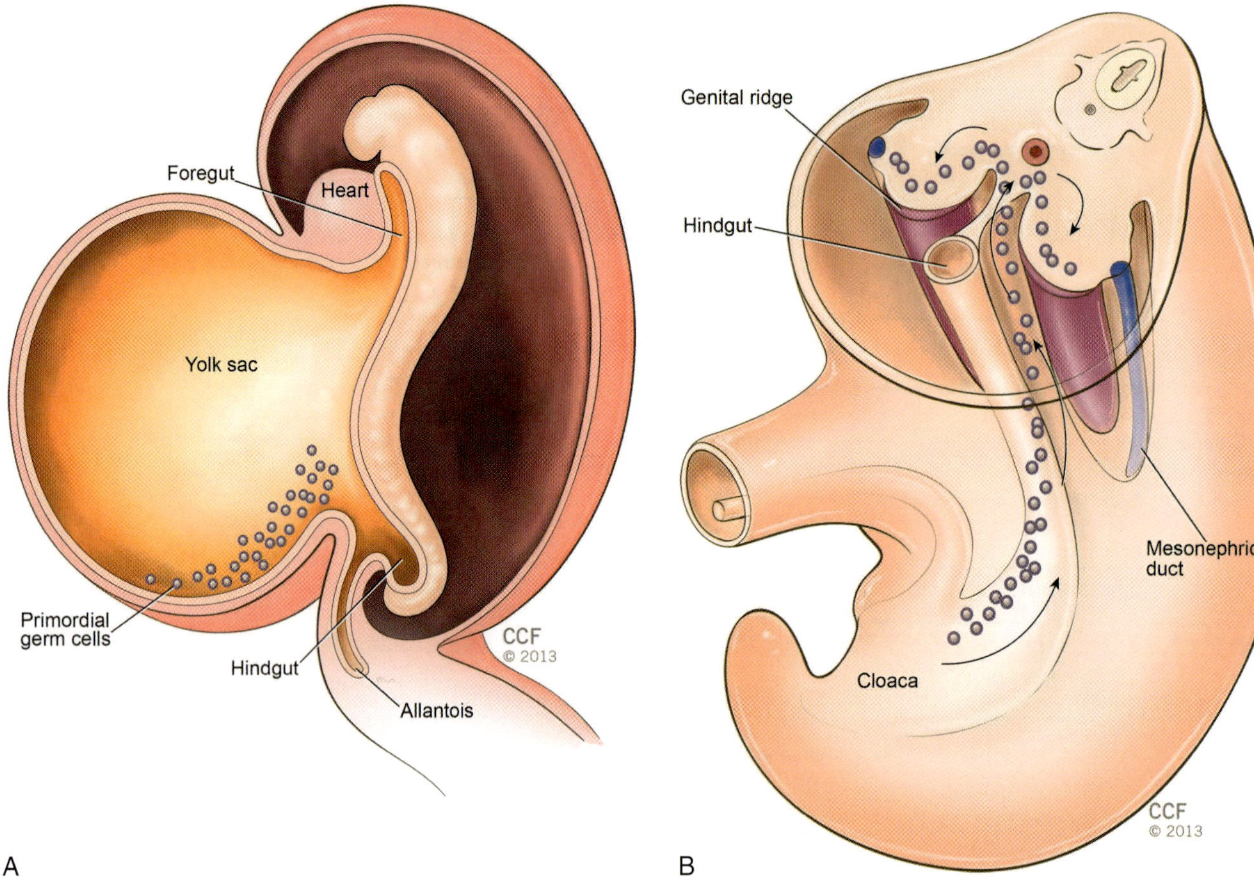

Fig. 2.4 A, A 3-week-old embryo showing the primordial germ cells in the wall of the yolk sac close to the attachment of the allantois. **B**, Migrational path of the primordial germ cells along the wall of the hindgut and the dorsal mesentery into the genital ridge. This takes place approximately 4 to 6 weeks after fertilization.

Genital Ducts, Sexually Indifferent Stage. As in gonadal development, the embryo genital ducts go through a sexually indifferent stage. Until approximately 8 weeks, both male and female embryos contain two pairs of genital ducts: paramesonephric (Müllerian) ducts and mesonephric (Wolffian) ducts. The paramesonephric ducts are a longitudinal invagination of the epithelium of the urogenital ridge. The ducts open cranially into the intraabdominal cavity and extend caudally. The paramesonephric ducts travel lateral to the mesonephric ducts and move medially, crossing the mesonephric ducts ventrally and coming into close contact in the midline. The paired paramesonephric ducts initially are separated by a septum but later fuse to form the uterine canal. Once these ducts are combined, the fused tip projects into the posterior wall of the urogenital sinus, where it causes a small swelling called the paramesonephric tubule. The mesonephric ducts open into the urogenital sinus on either side of this tubercle.

Sexual Differentiation. Sexual differentiation is determined genetically at the time of fertilization, but the gonads do not acquire sex-specific morphologic characteristics until the seventh week of development. Sexual differentiation is a complex process that depends on the presence or absence of the Y chromosome, which contains the testis-determining gene, *SRY* (sex determining region on Y). Under its influence male development occurs, and in its absence female development occurs.

The way in which the genital ducts undergo sexual differentiation is an intricate process that involves multiple levels of molecular regulation, of which is only partially understood. *SRY*, autosomal gene *SOX9*, and Müllerian inhibiting substance (MIS) all play important roles. SRY is a transcription factor that acts in conjunction with SOX9. When the Y chromosome is present, SRY and SOX9 influence multiple pathways that lead to testes development and testosterone production in the male. SOX9 is also known to bind to the promoter region of the gene encoding MIS. MIS is critical in sexual differentiation, as its presence leads to regression of the paramesonephric ducts (Fig. 2.6). When the Y chromosome is not present, WNT4, which is encoded by a gene called the ovary-determining gene, inhibits the function of SOX9 and regulates the expression of other genes responsible for ovarian differentiation. Estrogens are also important in sexual differentiation, as they stimulate the paramesonephric ducts to form the uterus, fallopian tubes, cervix, and upper vagina. They also act on external genitalia.

Once sexual differentiation begins, at approximately 7 to 8 weeks, the paramesonephric ducts develops into three main sections: the cranial portion that opens into the abdominal cavity, the horizontal portion that crosses the mesonephric duct,

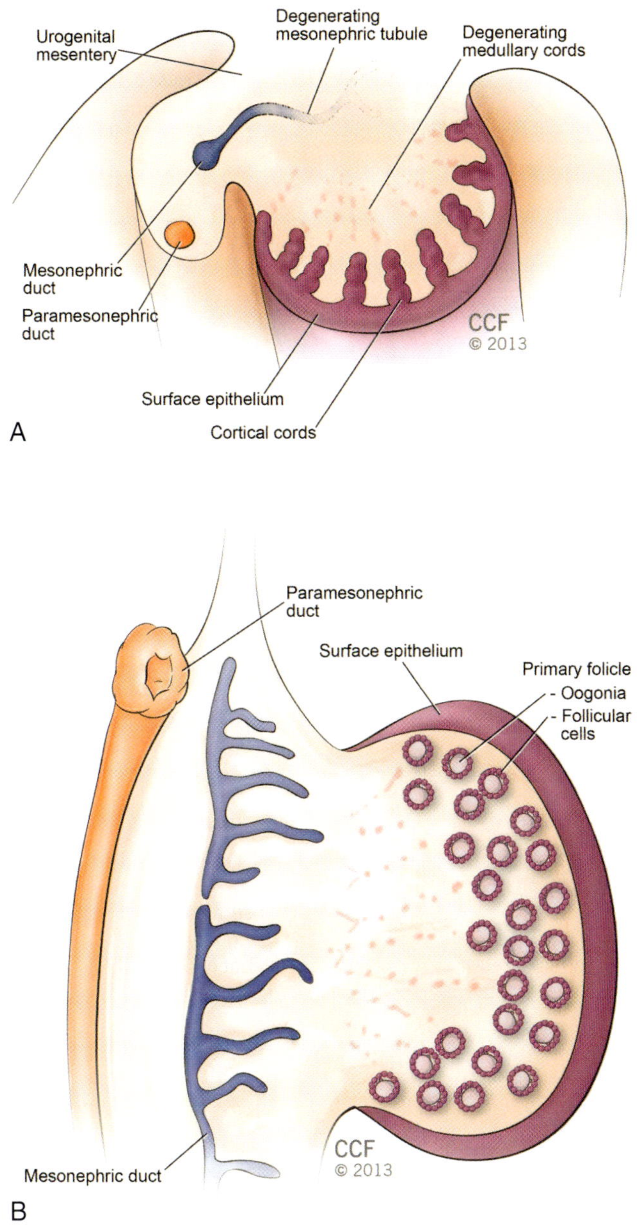

Fig. 2.5 **A**, Transverse section of the ovary at the seventh week showing degeneration of the primitive (medullary) sex cords and formation of the cortical cords. **B**, Ovary and genital ducts in the fifth month. Note degeneration of the medullary cords. The cortical zone of the ovary contains a group of oogonia surrounded by follicular cells.

and the fused caudal portion located medial to the mesonephric duct (Fig. 2.7A). As the paramesonephric ducts move medially, a pelvic fold is formed from the pelvis to the fused paramesonephric ducts, forming the broad ligament. The two most cranial portions develop into the fallopian tubes and the fused distal portion forms the uterus and cervix (Fig. 2.7B).

Vagina. After the solid tip of the paramesonephric ducts reaches the urogenital sinus, two solid evaginations known as the sinovaginal bulbs grow out from the pelvic part of the sinus (Fig. 2.8A). These bulbs proliferate and form the solid vaginal plate. Proliferation continues at the cranial plate, which increases the distance between the uterus and urogenital sinus (Fig. 2.8B). The solid plate becomes canalized by the fifth month of development (Fig. 2.8C). This demonstrates that the vagina has two origins: the upper vagina originates from the paramesonephric ducts, and the lower vagina from the urogenital sinus. The lumen of the vagina remains separated from the urogenital sinus by the hymen, which consists of the epithelial lining of the sinus and a thin layer of vaginal cells.

Though the mesonephric ducts regress in a developing female embryo, in some females a remnant of these ducts persists. If a small cranial portion persists, it forms the epoohoron, whereas the caudal portion forms the paroophoron. Most of these regress during further embryonic development, but the most cranial portion (found in the epoophoron) and most caudal portion (found in wall of uterus or vagina and called Gartner's cyst) may be found in adult women (see Fig. 2.7B).

External Genitalia. Cloacal folds form around the cloacal membrane in the third week of development. Cranial to the cloacal membrane, these folds fuse to form the genital tubercle (Fig. 2.9A). Caudally, the folds are subdivided into urogenital folds anteriorly and anal folds posteriorly. A second set of tissue elevations, the genital swellings, becomes visible on each side of the urogenital folds (Fig. 2.9B). When the original cloacal membrane breaks down during the eighth week, the urogenital sinus opens between the genital folds directly to the outside. Estrogens further stimulate development of the external genitalia. The genital tubercle elongates and forms the clitoris. The urogenital folds form the labia minora, and the genital swellings form the labia majora. The urogenital sinus remains open and forms the vestibule, into which the urethra and vagina open (Fig. 2.9C). Table 2.3 delineates the embryologic origin of the major female genital structures. Video 2.1 provides an overview of the embryology and congenital anomalies of the lower urogenital tract.

CONGENITAL ANOMALIES OF THE FEMALE GENITAL SYSTEM

Congenital Anomalies of the Female Genital System Presenting as Congenital Absence of the Vagina and Uterus

Malformations of the Müllerian ducts and the external genitalia can have significant impact on both reproductive potential and sexual function. When a patient presents with such an abnormality, it is important to put significant thought and time into determining the correct diagnosis and subsequent treatment.

The literature reports the rate of female congenital anomalies at between 0.2% to 0.4% of the general population. However, the prevalence of female congenital anomalies may be as high as 7% when using some of the newer diagnostic methods. These rates are much higher when looking at subgroups of patients with recurrent pregnancy loss and infertility. However, in many instances women with these anomalies are asymptomatic.

Though sex steroid receptor abnormalities and enzyme deficiencies are not considered malformations of the Müllerian ducts, they often have similar clinical presentations and should be considered in the differential. The workup and diagnosis of

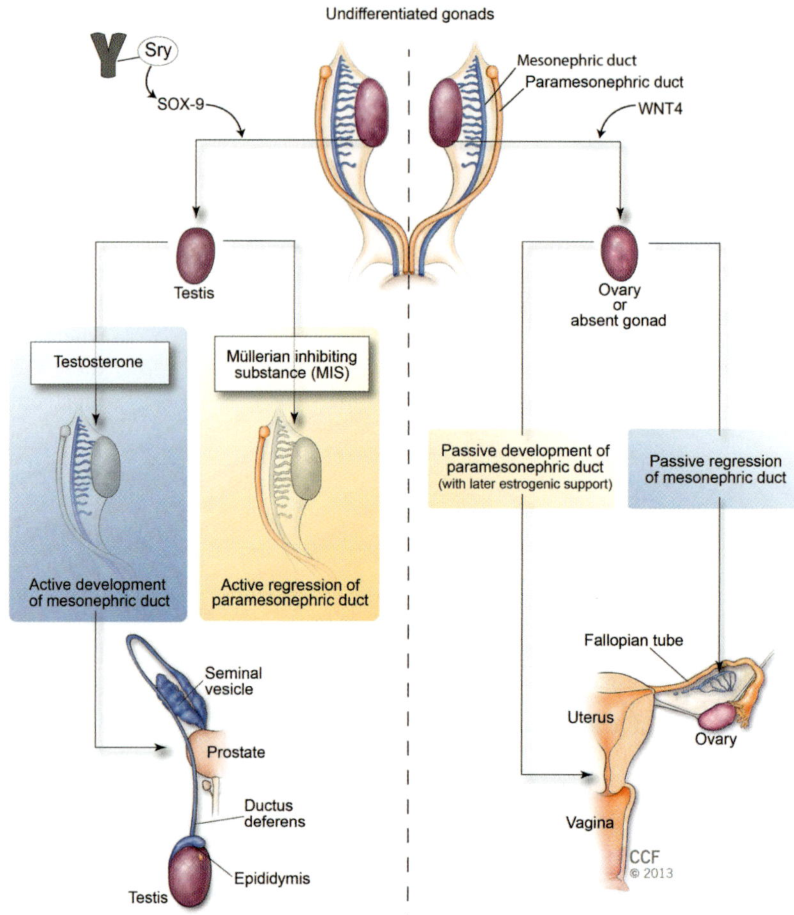

Fig. 2.6 Factors involved in sexual differentiation of the genital tract.

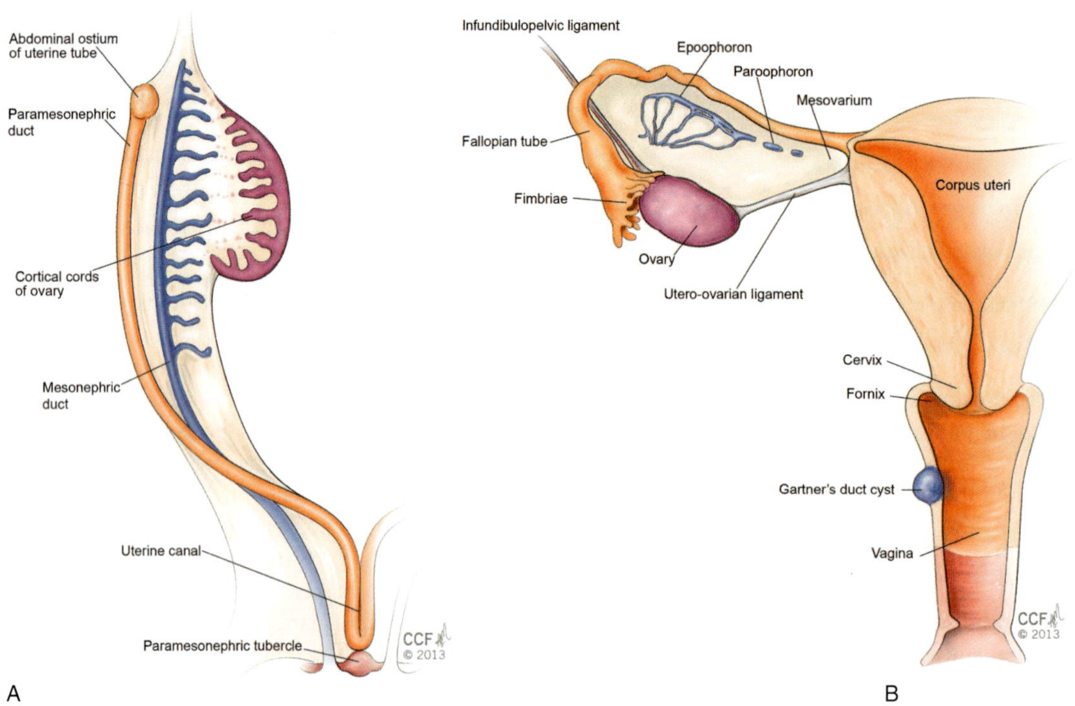

Fig. 2.7 **A**, Genital ducts in the female at the end of 8 weeks. The paramesonephric ducts cross the mesonephric ducts to fuse in the midline and form the uterine canal. **B**, Genital ducts after descent of the ovary. The only parts remaining from the mesonephric duct system are the epoohoron, paroophoron, and Gartner's cyst.

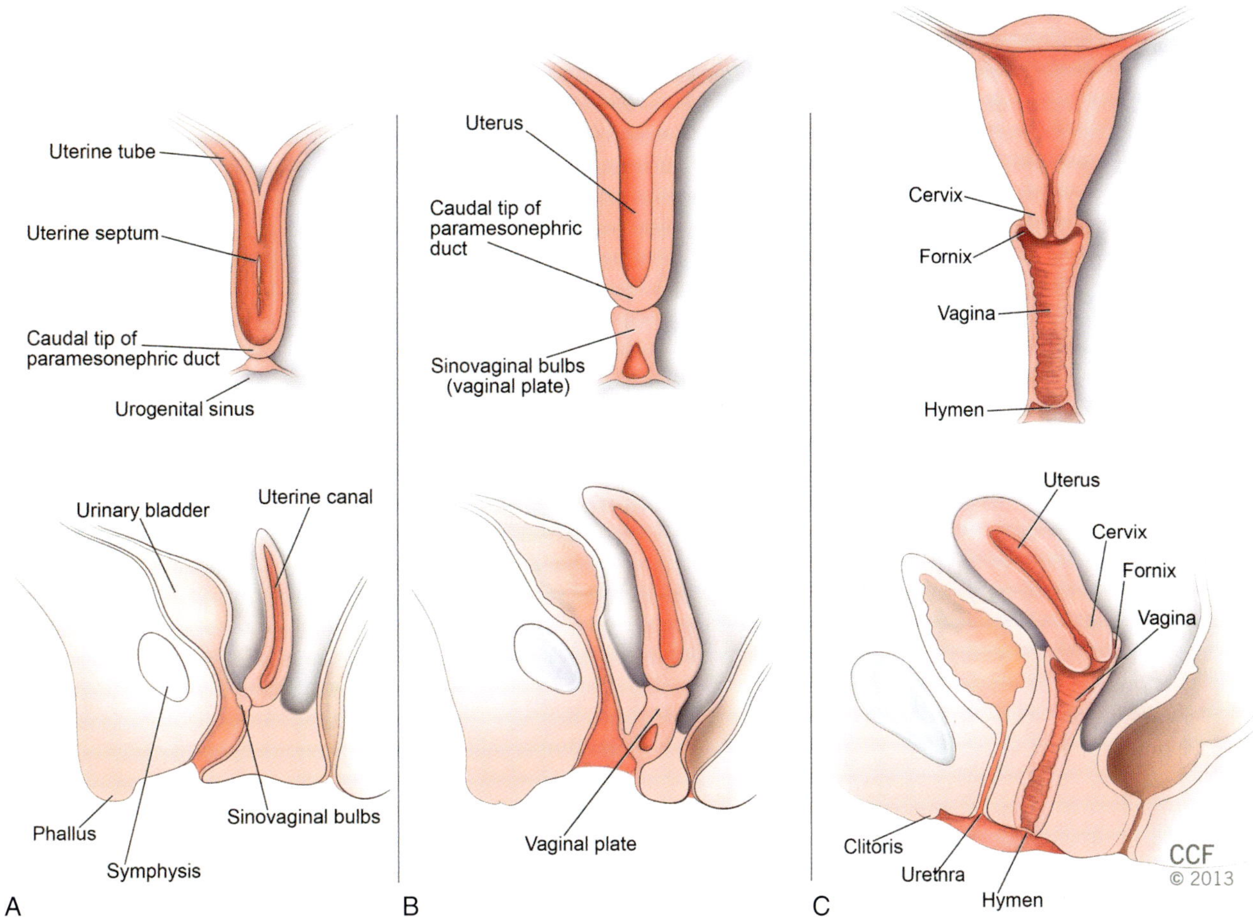

Fig. 2.8 Coronal and sagittal sections demonstrating the formation of the uterus and vagina **A**, At approximately 9 weeks the paramesonephric ducts meet the urogenital sinus. Also, the uterine septum begins to degenerate. **B**, At 12 weeks the sinovaginal bulbs proliferate, creating a solid vaginal plate, which increases the distance between the uterus and urogenital sinus. **C**, The fornices and upper portion of the vagina are formed by vacuolization of the paramesonephric tissue, while the lower portion of the vagina is formed by vacuolization of the sinovaginal bulbs.

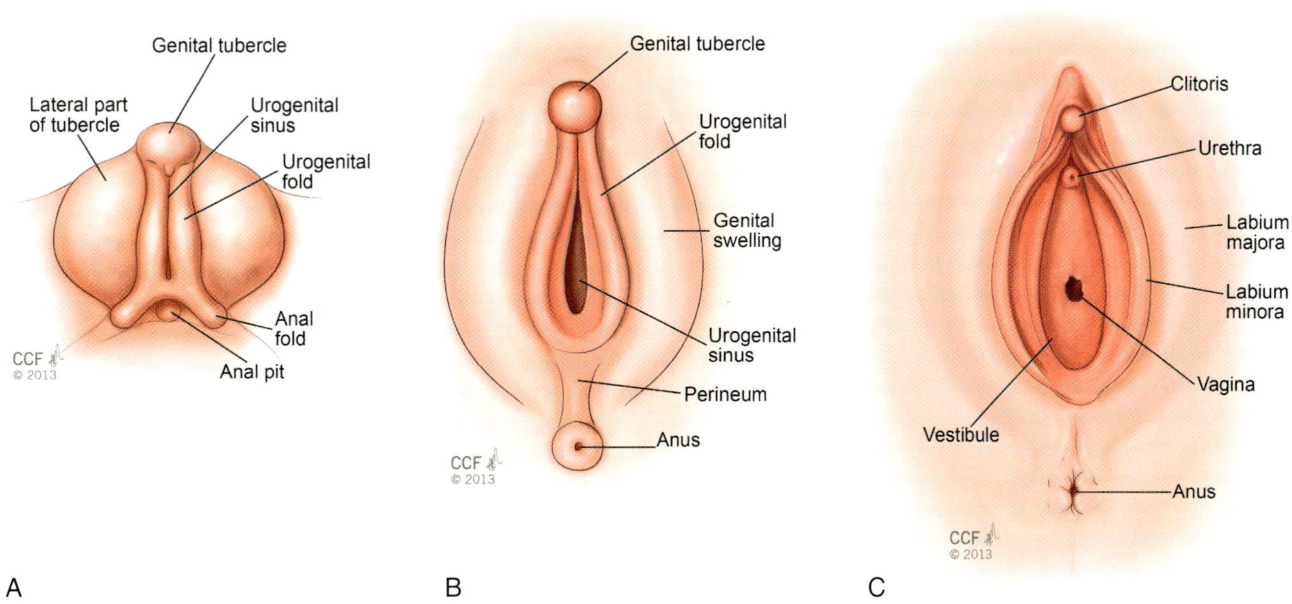

Fig. 2.9 **A**, Sexually indifferent stage of external genitalia development at approximately 4 to 5 weeks. **B**, At 20 weeks, sexual differentiation of the female external genitalia is evident. **C**, Newborn.

TABLE 2.3 Embryologic Origin and Female Derivative

Indifferent Structure	Female Derivative
Genital ridge	Ovary
Primordial germ cells	Ova
Sex cords	Follicular (granulosa) cells
Mesonephric tubules	Oophoron
	Paroophoron
Mesonephric ducts	Appendix of ovary
	Gartner's duct cyst
Paramesonephric ducts	Fallopian tubes
	Uterus
	Upper vagina
Definitive urogenital sinus (lower part)	Lower vagina
	Vulvar vestibule
Early urogenital sinus (upper part)	Urinary bladder
	Urethra
Genital tubercle	Clitoris
Genital folds	Labia minora
Genital swellings	Labial majora

TABLE 2.4 American Society of Reproductive Medicine Classification of Müllerian Anomalies

I. Hypoplasia/Agenesis	a. Vaginal
	b. Cervical
	c. Fundal
	d. Tubal
	e. Combined
II. Unicornuate	a. Communicating
	b. Noncommunicating
	c. No cavity
	d. No horn
III. Didelphus	
IV. Bicornuate	a. Complete
	b. Partial
V. Septate	a. Complete
	b. Partial
VI. Arcuate	
VII. Diethstilbestriol (DES)-related	

these disorders are beyond the scope of this chapter; however, treatments are often similar.

Classification. The classification of Müllerian anomalies helps with both the diagnosis and the comparison of outcomes after various treatment modalities. However, there is no single classification that encompasses all anomalies that have been reported in the literature.

Although the direct cause of the majority of these anomalies is not known, on the basis of our embryological knowledge the pathogenesis of many of these anomalies can be understood. On the basis of pathophysiology, Müllerian anomalies can be broadly classified as being related to (1) agenesis, (2) vertical fusion defects, or (3) lateral fusion defects. Compared with other anomalies, agenesis of the uterus and agenesis of the vagina are relatively common anomalies. Vertical fusion defects are usually the result of abnormal canalization of the vaginal plate and result in defects such as a transverse vaginal septum and imperforate hymen. Lateral fusion defects can be symmetrical or asymmetrical and include septum of the uterus and vagina, as well as unicornuate and bicornuate uteruses and related abnormalities.

There are endless variations to Müllerian and vaginal anomalies. It is impossible to note these variations effectively in any one classification system. Consequently, many investigators are still searching for that elusive classification system that can not only encompass all the anomalies noted in the vagina, cervix, uterus, and adnexa, but also translate into accurate comprehension and visualization of the defect by other colleagues.

The most accepted classification of uterine anomalies, published by the American Society of Reproductive Medicine (ASRM), places uterine anomalies into distinct groups based on anatomic configuration (Table 2.4). Because vaginal anomalies are not included in this classification, they must be described along with the uterine anomaly. This classification does not give insight into pathophysiology but is an effective way to communicate observations for purposes of treatment and prognosis.

Müllerian Agenesis (Mayer Rokitansky Kuster Hauser Syndrome). Müllerian agenesis (i.e., Mayer Rokitansky Kuster Hauser syndrome) was first described in 1829. Its incidence is reported to be 1 in every 5000 newborn females. The etiology of Müllerian agenesis remains unknown. It appears to be influenced by multifactorial inheritance, and rare familial cases have been reported. It does not appear to be transmitted in an autosomal dominant manner, because none of the female offspring of women with Müllerian agenesis (born via *in vitro* fertilization and surrogacy) have shown evidence of Müllerian agenesis. Because the vagina and associated uterine structures do not develop with this disorder, it is an ASRM class IA Müllerian anomaly. Patients typically present during their adolescent years with concerns of primary amenorrhea. As a cause of primary amenorrhea, Müllerian agenesis is second only to gonadal dysgenesis.

Patients with Müllerian agenesis will present with normal onset of puberty and appropriate secondary sexual characteristics, but apparently delayed menarche. They do not complain of cyclic pelvic pain, unlike patients with obstructive Müllerian anomalies. The external genitalia appear completely normal, with normal pubic hair growth and normally-sized labia minora, which is in contrast to patients with complete androgen insensitivity syndrome. Hymenal fringes may be evident, but the vaginal opening is absent. No pelvic masses suggestive of hematocolpos will be evident, which is in contrast to cases of complete transverse septum. Because these patients have a 46XX karyotype, normal ovaries will be present in the pelvis. Ovulation can be documented as a shift in basal body temperature. These patients' hormonal levels are normal, and their cycle length based on hormonal studies varies from 30 to 34 days. In addition, they may experience monthly pain (mittelschmerz) that is indicative of ovulation.

Müllerian agenesis is associated with renal and skeletal system anomalies. Renal abnormalities are noted in 40% of these patients. These include complete agenesis of a kidney, malposition of a kidney, and changes in renal structure. Skeletal abnormalities are noted in 12% of patients and include primarily spine defects and limb and rib defects. Patients with Müllerian agenesis should be actively assessed for these associated anomalies. Hearing difficulties have also been reported in patients with Müllerian agenesis. A higher rate of auditory defects has been noted in general in patients with Müllerian anomalies compared with those with normal Müllerian structures.

The diagnosis of Müllerian agenesis is confirmed via imaging techniques. Abdominal ultrasonography will demonstrate the lack of uterus and the existence of ovaries. The presence of a midline mass consistent with a blood collection usually indicates an obstructive Müllerian anomaly. The distinction between Müllerian agenesis and obstruction is extremely important, because an incorrect diagnosis can jeopardize appropriate management. With the advent of magnetic resonance imaging (MRI), laparoscopy is no longer considered necessary to make this diagnosis. Typical findings in the pelvis include portions of the fallopian tubes, normal ovaries, and usually small Müllerian remnants attached to the proximal portion of the fallopian tubes that may be solid or have functioning endometrial tissue. Direct communication with the radiologist about the differential diagnosis before imaging studies is important. On occasion, the unsuspecting radiologist may interpret the small uterine remnants as a uterus. Careful attention to the very small dimensions of this structure will alert the physician to this possibility. MRI is also important to evaluate coexisting anomalies of the urinary tract, such as renal agenesis and other renal malformations. It is critical to diagnose these before surgical treatment.

The diagnosis, usually made in early adolescence, must be explained to the patient with great sensitivity. At a time when being like her peers is extremely important, knowledge of this diagnosis can be psychologically devastating. Each patient must be reassured that her external genitalia appear normal, and that she will be able to have a normal sex life after the creation of a normally functioning vagina. Although usually not voiced, the inability to subsequently bear children is a major disappointment to teenagers. Fortunately, with assisted reproductive technology procedures including *in vitro* fertilization, surrogacy, and uterine transplantation (Brännström et al., 2015), having their own genetic child will be an option for many of these young women.

Receptor Abnormalities and Enzyme Deficiencies. These genetic disorders are secondary to enzyme deficiencies or defects in the hormone receptors of the sex steroid pathways. Because these affect sex steroid production during embryogenesis, development of the embryo and fetus can be greatly affected. Often affecting the embryo during the sexually indifferent stage, the absence of specific receptors or enzymes can completely change the hormonal environment, which leads to discrepancies between genotype and phenotype. The most common syndromes include complete androgen insensitivity syndrome, 5-alpha-reductase deficiency, 17-alpha-hydroxylase deficiency, vanishing testes syndrome, and absent testis determining factor.

Incomplete androgen insensitivity syndrome (partial testosterone resistance), 5-alpha-reductase deficiency, 17-alpha-hydroxylase deficiency, vanishing testes syndrome, and absent testis determining factor often have variable presentations, including ambiguous genitalia at birth, inappropriate virilization at puberty, and/or lack of pubertal development. These are rare, complex disorders that require the attention of a subspecialist for proper diagnosis.

Complete Androgen Insensitivity Syndrome. This is an x-linked recessive disorder in which there is a defect in the androgen receptor leading to testosterone resistance. This resistance leads to a failure of male sexual characteristic development. These individuals have a karyotype of XY and have a normal, functioning *SRY*. The testes develop normally during embryogenesis and produce normal levels of testosterone. However, because the receptor is defective, all downstream development dependent on testosterone does not occur. Specifically, the active development of the mesonephric ducts does not take place, leading to absence of the seminal vesicle, prostate, ductus deferens, epididymis, and maturation and descent of the testes. Because the embryo testis is normal, it produces MIS, also known as anti-Müllerian hormone, leading to active regression of the paramesonephric ducts. This prevents further development of the uterus, fallopian tubes, and upper vagina (see Fig. 2.6). These individuals are genetically male and have testes but are typically female in appearance. The testes are not fully developed, and often are located in the abdomen, inguinal canal, or labia. The external genitalia appear normal for a female infant at birth. At puberty, the testes make normal or high levels of testosterone, which is aromatized to estrogen in the cell, leading to normal female secondary sexual characteristics. At puberty, breast development occurs, but the areolas are pale, and the pubic and axillary hair is sparse. Similar to those with Müllerian agenesis, these patients often present with primary amenorrhea. The diagnosis of complete androgen insensitivity syndrome is made with physical examination and imaging demonstrating normal female external genitalia, absence of the upper vagina, uterus, ovaries, and fallopian tubes, high serum testosterone concentrations, and 46 XY karyotype. Please see Table 2.5 for the differences between complete androgen insensitivity syndrome and Müllerian agenesis. Because both disorders present without a vagina, the treatment options are the same. However, patients with complete androgen insensitivity syndrome should undergo surgical excision of the testes after puberty because of the increased risk of developing testicular cancer after age 25 years.

Treatment of Congenital Absence of the Vagina and Uterus

The first treatment goal for congenital absences of the vagina, including Müllerian agenesis and complete androgen insensitivity syndrome, is creation of a functional vagina to allow intercourse. Frank first proposed vaginal dilatation with use of a dilator as a means of creating a neovagina in 1938. Throughout the years, both nonsurgical and surgical methods to elongate the vagina have been developed. However, more

TABLE 2.5 Differences in Clinical Presentations of Müllerian Agenesis and Complete Androgen Insensitivity Syndrome

	Müllerian Agenesis	Complete Androgen Insensitivity Syndrome
Uterus	Absent	Absent
Ovaries	Present	Absent
Testes	Absent	Present (undescended)
Breast development	Normal	Normal
Vagina	Foreshortened	Foreshortened
Hormone assay	Normal estrogen	Normal or high male testosterone
Karyotype	XX	XY

recently, several comparative studies support the recommendation that dilation should be first-line treatment for vaginal agenesis (Herlin et al., 2018; Cheikhelard et al., 2018). The success of any technique depends in large part on the emotional maturity of the patient. Pretreatment counseling and continued support during treatment are important.

Vaginal Dilation. The simplicity and ease of vaginal dilation, as well as its low complication rate compared with surgical vaginoplasty, dictates its use as the initial form of therapy for most patients. The American College of Obstetrics and Gynecology released a committee opinion in 2018 that recommends nonsurgical management of vaginal agenesis as the first mode of treatment.

Frank's technique of dilation involves actively placing pressure with the dilators against the vaginal dimple (Fig. 2.10). The patient is not only in an awkward position, but the hand applying the pressure can become tired. In 1981, Ingram proposed the concept of passive dilation, where pressure is placed upon the dilator by sitting on a bicycle seat. Roberts reported a success rate of 92% in women who dilated the vagina via the Ingram technique for 20 minutes three times a day (2001). The average time to creation of a functional vagina was 11 months. This series demonstrated that an initial dimple smaller than 0.5 cm was all that was necessary to achieve adequate dilation. Failure of this technique was not related to length of vaginal dimple, but rather was more closely associated with the patient's youth. Failure of this technique was more common in patients younger than 18 years of age.

When the patient expresses a desire to proceed with therapy, she is shown the exact location of her vaginal dimple. The axis of dilator placement is also demonstrated (Fig. 2.11). The process is initiated by placement of the smallest dilator against the dimple. Pressure is kept upon the distal aspect of the dilator by sitting upon a stool while leaning slightly forward. When the dilator fits comfortably, she moves to the next size dilator. The patient is instructed to use this technique a minimum of 20 minutes a day but encouraged to dilate up to two to three times a day. In motivated patients, a functional vagina can be created in as little as 12 weeks. Counseling and psychological support are integral to successful treatment. Patients are requested to return to the office frequently to allow providers to monitor their progress, provide guidance, and answer questions. Intercourse may be attempted once the largest dilator fits comfortably.

Multiple types of graduated dilators made of various materials are present on the market, all of which are equivalent in achieving successful outcomes. Patients may stop and reinitiate the dilation at any time without any negative long-term sequelae. Patients are most often interested in initiating this therapy the summer before college, when they are mature enough and motivated to create the vagina. However, the timing of therapy is purely dependent on the patient's goals and desires. In a review of 245 cases, the mean age of starting treatment was 18 years of age, and the reported success rates were as high as 94.9%.

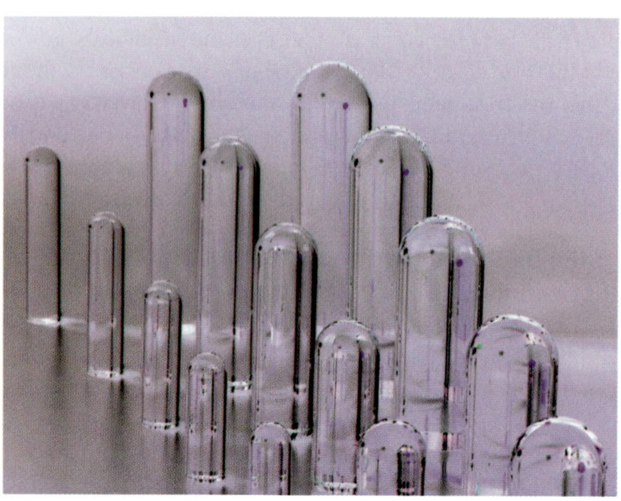

Fig. 2.10 Examples of vaginal dilators of different sizes.

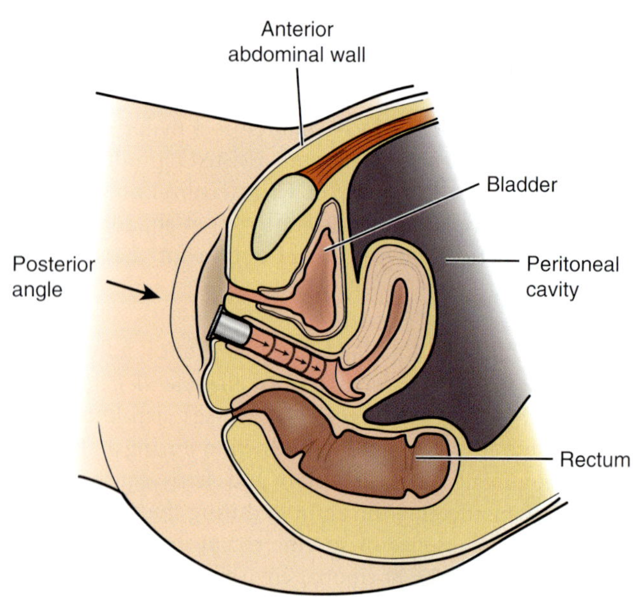

Fig. 2.11 Schematic drawing of angle of dilator placement. The patient is viewed in lithotomy position, and the axis is directed away from the bladder.

Surgical Options for Neovagina Creation

McIndoe procedure. The traditional surgical management of vaginal agenesis is to create a vaginal space, followed by placement of a lining to prevent stenosis. Multiple native tissue grafts and at least one synthetic graft have been used to line this cavity, with varying degrees of success in preventing subsequent stenosis of the neovagina (Table 2.6).

The most widely used surgical technique for creation of a neovagina is the McIndoe operation (Video 2.2). Traditionally, the first step of this procedure is procurement of the split-thickness skin graft by the plastic surgery team. This skin graft is sutured around a mold with 4-0 absorbable suture (Fig. 2.12). It is important that the mold is covered completely by the graft. Any sites that remain uncovered resulting from either a lack of sufficient tissue or a gaping hole in the suture line tend to result in the formation of granulation tissue. Thus, great care must be taken to obtain a sufficient amount of graft for this procedure.

The patient is placed in the dorsolithotomy position. A transverse incision is made in the vaginal vestibule, between the rectal and urethral openings (Fig. 2.13). In a patient who has not had prior surgery or radiation in the area, areolar tissue is now encountered. This tissue is easily dissected with either fingers or a Hagar dilator on either side of a median raphe (Fig. 2.14). The dissection is continued for at least the length of the mold, without entering the peritoneal cavity. By cutting the median raphe, the two channels are then connected. If the dissection is performed in this manner, minimal bleeding is encountered. Any bleeding sites must be controlled meticulously to avoid lifting of the graft from the newly created vaginal wall and subsequent nonadherence and necrosis.

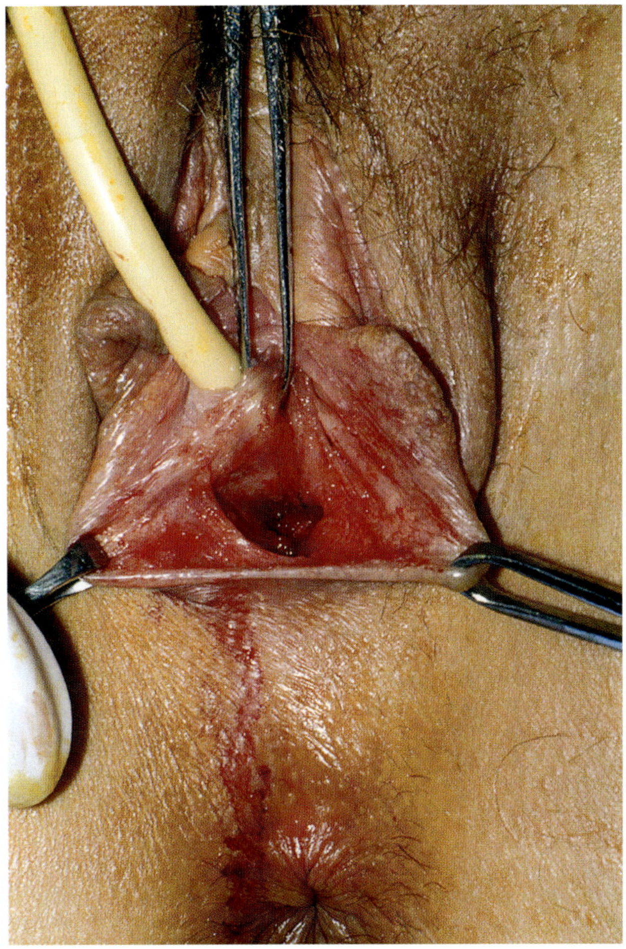

Fig. 2.13 The initial transverse cut was made on the fibrous tissue, and an initial space developed.

TABLE 2.6 Surgical Methods of Creating a Neovagina

Dissection of a perineal space	Split-thickness skin graft (McIndoe)
	Full-thickness skin graft
	Peritoneum (Davydov)
	Tissue engineering
	Muscle and skin flap
	Tissue expansion
Bowel vaginoplasty	Sigmoid colon
Vulvovaginal pouch	Williams vaginoplasty
Traction on retrohymeneal fovea	Vecchietti

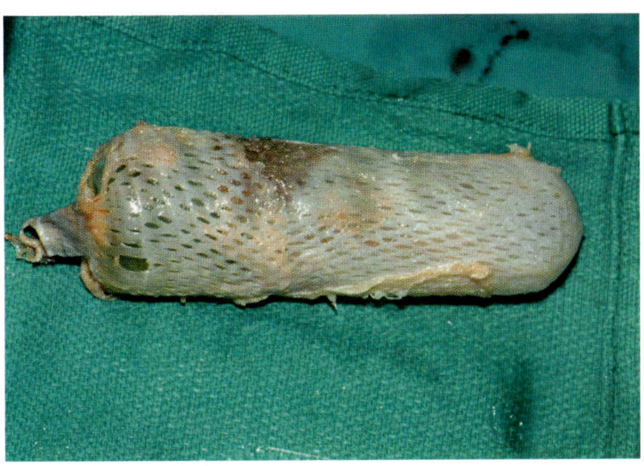

Fig. 2.12 Skin graft is sutured around a mold.

After creation of the vaginal space, the mold covered with the skin graft is placed inside the cavity (Fig. 2.15). At the introitus, the skin graft is attached with several separate 3-0 absorbable stitches. To hold the mold in place, several loose nonreactive sutures such as 2-0 silk are used to approximate the labia minora in the midline.

During the ensuing week, the patient is maintained on bed rest with broad-spectrum antibiotics, a low-residue diet, an indwelling catheter, and an agent to decrease bowel motility. Upon return to the operating room in one week, the mold is carefully removed. After the vaginal cavity is irrigated with warm saline, the graft site is carefully assessed for any signs of necrosis or underlying hematoma. Another soft mold is then reinserted and kept in place for the next 3 months, except during defecation and urination. Nighttime usage of the mold is recommended for the next 6 months. To prevent contracture of the vagina, the patient is instructed to reinsert the mold during extended times of sexual inactivity.

Difficulty in dissecting the space between the bladder and rectum and increased probability of bleeding and fistula formation

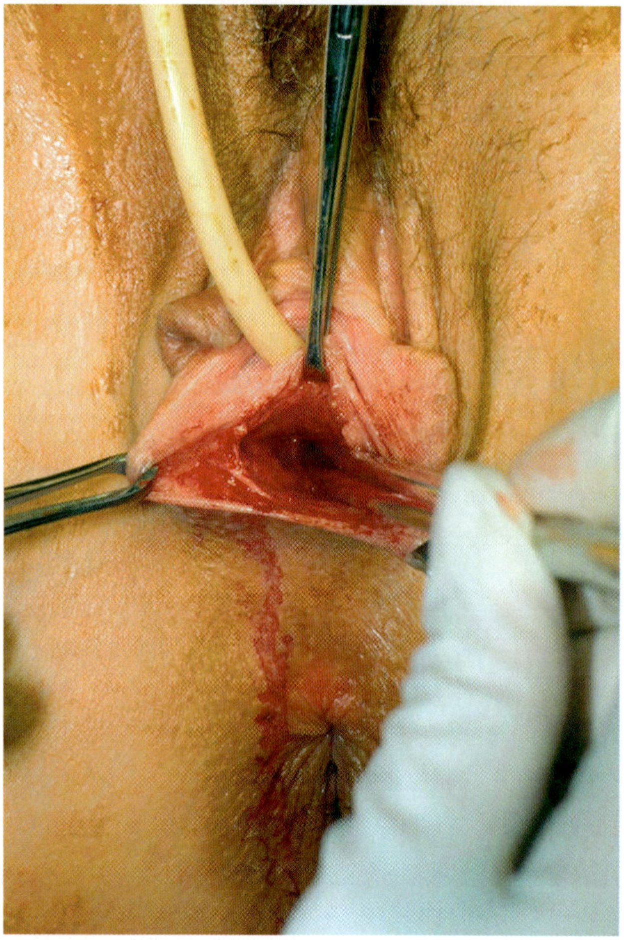

Fig. 2.14 Placement of Hagar dilator to create space for the graft. The direction of the Hagar dilators is posterior.

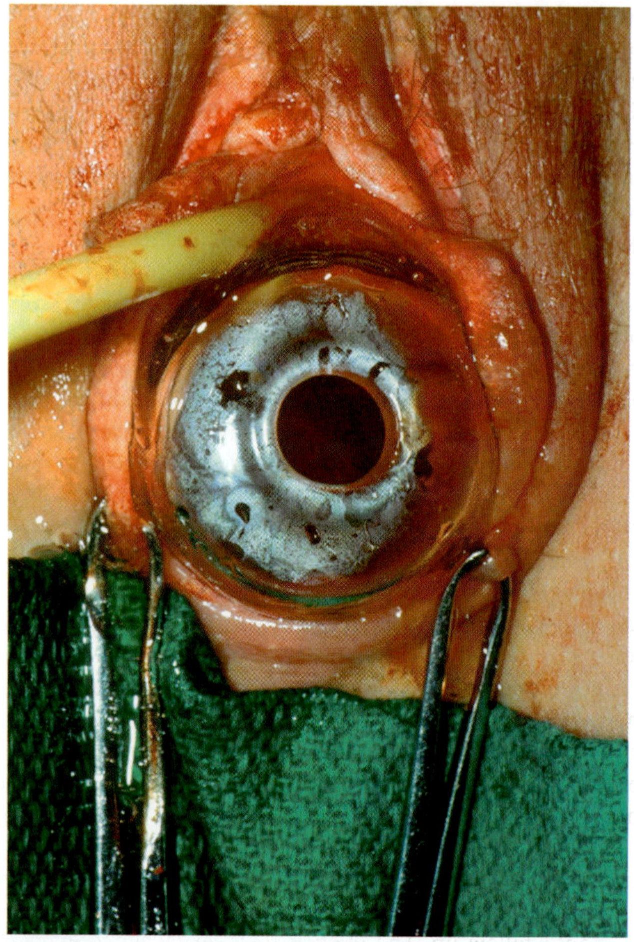

Fig. 2.15 The mold with the graft is placed in the space. Notice that the space to be created must accommodate the mold completely.

are encountered in the patient with a prior vaginoplasty procedure. Other problems that may be encountered include a narrow pubic arch, strong levator ani muscles, short perineum, prior hymenectomy, and a congenitally deep cul-de-sac. Surgical complications include postoperative infection and hemorrhage, failure of graft and formation of granulation tissue, and fistula formation. In a review of 58 studies in which a McIndoe procedure had been performed, the incidence of complications was low: intraoperative bladder or rectal perforation was observed in 1% to 4%, rectovaginal and vesicovaginal fistula formation in 1% to 3%, graft infection in 4%, and graft site infection in 5% of patients. Functional success was reported by 89.5% of these patients.

An 80% success rate has been reported with this procedure. Because success rates are highest in those patients who have not undergone prior vaginoplasty, patients must be counseled extensively before surgery regarding the need for prolonged use of the mold. Indeed, part of the presurgical assessment involves determination of patient maturity and motivation concerning use of dilators. Lack of compliance with postoperative use of dilators will lead to contracture and diminishment of vaginal length. Long-term data on the McIndoe procedure, although limited, consistently indicate an improvement in quality of life. In a long-term study by Klingele evaluating women who underwent a McIndoe procedure, 79% of patients reported improved quality of life, 91% remained sexually active, and 75% regularly achieved orgasm (2003). When Sabatucci and colleagues used autologous *in vitro* cultured vaginal tissue to line the newly created vaginal canal, the female sexual function index showed satisfactory sexual function compared with the general population and an improvement in the quality of life (2019).

The newly created vagina must be inspected at the time of the pelvic examination. Human papillomavirus infections have been reported on the neovaginal and vulvar tissues of women with vaginal agenesis. Transformation to squamous cell carcinoma from skin graft has been described.

Vecchietti procedure. Vecchietti described this method of creating a neovagina in 1965. Similar to vaginal dilation, this method avoids the use of a graft. The Vecchietti procedure is a one-step procedure in which a neovagina is created in approximately 7 days by continuous pressure on the vaginal dimple using an external acrylic "olive" that is connected by retroperitoneal sutures to a spring tension device on the lower abdomen. Although the original description of the Vecchietti procedure used laparotomy, this technique is currently performed laparoscopically (Video 2.3).

The first step in this procedure is to use a sharp ligature carrier (similar to a Stamey needle) to insert one end of a number 2 polyglycolic acid suture through the retrohymenal dimple into the peritoneal cavity between the bladder and the rectum under laparoscopic guidance. The other end of this suture is placed through a stent or "segmented dummy" (Brucker et al., 2008). The next step is to use a curved blunt ligature carrier to burrow retroperitoneally from a lateral suprapubic laparoscopic port site to the peritoneal fold between the bladder and the uterine remnant. The end of the suture introduced with the sharp ligature carrier is placed through the eye of this curved ligature carrier and pulled retroperitoneally back through the abdominal wall port site incision. This procedure is repeated on the opposite side with the other end of the suture. After the laparoscope is removed and the abdominal wall incisions are closed, the ends of the suture are attached to a suprapubic spring traction device located externally on the abdomen.

Postoperatively, constant traction is applied to the stent by daily readjustment of the tension of the sutures and traction device. The neovagina lengthens by 1 to 2 cm per day, such that a 10- to 12-cm vagina is created in 4 to 5 days. After creation of the vagina, the stent is removed, and the patient is sent home with a vaginal mold in place. After surgery, it is important to initiate regular sexual intercourse or routinely use dilators to maintain vaginal length.

Rall and colleagues report on the anatomic and functional success of 240 patients who underwent this procedure. All patients had a vaginal length measuring from 6 to 12 cm at 11-month follow-up. The median total sexual function index was 30, which was similar to controls. With the exception of the formation of granulation tissue in four patients, there were no complications.

Peritoneal graft: Davydov procedure. Use of the peritoneum to line the newly created vaginal space was popularized by Davydov, a Russian gynecologist, and was first described in the United States by Rothman in 1972. In the original description, a laparotomy is performed after creation of the vaginal space, as described for the McIndoe operation.

A cut is made on the peritoneum overlying the new vagina. Long sutures are applied to the anterior posterior and lateral sides of this peritoneum. The sutures are then pulled down through the vaginal space, thus pulling the peritoneum to the introitus. The edge of the peritoneum is then stitched to the mucosa of the introitus. Closing the peritoneum on the abdominal side forms the top of the vagina. Several investigators have also described the laparoscopic modification of this procedure. This procedure may have several advantages compared with the traditional McIndoe. The most significant advantage is the avoidance of donor site morbidity or cosmetic compromise that is typically associated with the McIndoe procedure. Additionally, there is no unappealing hair growth or risk of graft rejection with the Davydov procedure.

In Davydov's first reported series in 1980, sexual intercourse was initiated within several weeks of surgery in all but one of his 30 patients. On follow-up, the length of the vagina was noted to be 8 to 11 cm. Fedele et al. (2010) published a report on a series of 30 patients who underwent the laparoscopic modification of this procedure. The mean length of the neovagina was 8 cm at 6 months after surgery. Functional success was reported by 96% of patients who were sexually active. Complications of the Davydov technique can include damage to the bladder, rectum, and ureters. Thus, the patient can be at risk of fistula formation. Although in this series there were no severe complications, there is report of a rectovaginal fistula 18 months after the surgery in another series (Fedele et al., 2010). Previous pelvic surgery and adhesions may be a relative contraindication to this technique.

Other reconstruction options

Muscle and skin flap. These approaches are not procedures of choice for women with congenital absence of the vagina. However, they may be used for those who require vaginal reconstruction after exposure to radiation or multiple surgical procedures. The advantage of using a full-thickness skin flap is that it avoids the problem of contracture encountered with split-thickness grafts.

The use of gracilis myocutaneous flaps or rectus abdominus myocutaneous flaps for vaginal reconstruction has been reported. These approaches have been associated with a conspicuous scar and a higher failure rate. An alternative approach, introduced by Wee and Joseph in Singapore, demonstrated flaps that maintained good blood supply and innervation (1989). Known as a "pudendal–thigh flap vaginoplasty," this technique has been particularly successful in patients with vulvar anomalies. In a study by Monstrey et al. (2001) of patients with Müllerian agenesis, 100% of these procedures resulted in the creation of a functional vagina.

The patient's own labia majora and labia minora have also been used to create a vagina. Tissue expansion has also been advocated to create labiovaginal flaps, which are then used to line the neovagina. Other modifications of this procedure have been reported.

Bowel vaginoplasty. Similar to muscle and skin flap vaginoplasties, bowel vaginoplasty is not the procedure of choice in women with congenital absence of the vagina. However, this technique can be used for vaginal reconstruction in patients who have undergone pelvic radiation or in cases of previously failed vaginoplasty procedures. For this procedure, also known as a colocolpopoiesis, a portion of large bowel or sigmoid colon with its preserved vascular pedicle is sutured into the neovagina. Continuous use of dilators is not considered necessary, although constriction has been noted when ileum has been used. Success rates of up to 90% have been reported, but reported complications include profuse vaginal discharge, prolapse, introital stenosis, bowel obstruction, and colitis. Finally, there is a report of a mucinous adenocarcinoma arising in a neovagina lined with the sigmoid colon. A laparoscopic modification of this procedure has also been described. Given the increased complication rate, it seems appropriate to reserve this treatment modality for complex situations where a prior vaginoplasty technique has failed or when there are multiple urogenital malformations.

Longitudinal Vaginal Septum

A longitudinal vaginal septum is an example of a lateral fusion defect and is typically associated with uterine anomalies such as septate uterus and uterus didelphyis. The septum that divides the vagina can be either nonobstructing or obstructing. A nonobstructing vaginal septum is often asymptomatic and discovered at the time of a pelvic examination or childbirth. A woman with an obstructing vaginal septum often presents with increasingly severe dysmenorrhea and a unilateral vaginal mass.

Nonobstructing Longitudinal Vaginal Septum. Nonobstructing longitudinal vaginal septa account for 12% of malformations of the vagina. Although most are asymptomatic, some patients complain of continued vaginal bleeding despite placement of tampon, difficulty removing a tampon, or dyspareunia. The septum may be complete or partial and can exist in any portion of the vagina (Fig. 2.16). The communication can be extremely small, and a septum can easily be missed during physical examination, especially if there is a dominant vaginal canal. Once the diagnosis is made, both the uterus and renal anatomy should be assessed for associated anomalies. In one study by Haddad et al. (1997), 60% of patients with longitudinal vaginal septa were found to have a bicornuate uterus. Other investigators have noted a predominance of didelphic uteri in such cases.

A longitudinal vaginal septum should be removed in patients with complaints of dyspareunia and those who desire to be able to effectively use a tampon. In cases of didelphic uteri, removal of the septum may be necessary to allow sufficient access to each cervix for Pap smears. Some obstetricians advocate removal of a longitudinal vaginal septum before delivery to avoid potential dystocia and laceration of the septum. The number of patients with vaginal septa who have had successful vaginal deliveries remains unknown. However, emergent resection of a vaginal septum at the time of delivery to resolve dystocia has been reported. It seems reasonable to remove a thick longitudinal septum before pregnancy, or before delivery if discovered during pregnancy.

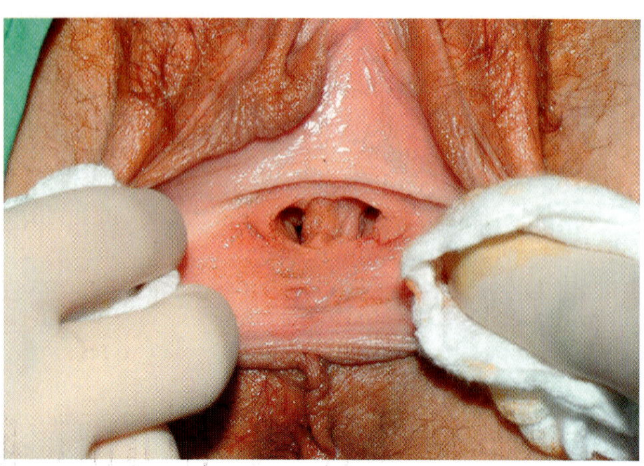

Fig. 2.16 Nonobstructing longitudinal vaginal septum.

The goal of surgery is to remove of a wedge of tissue without damaging the cervix, bladder, or rectum. A Foley catheter is placed in the bladder. Because longitudinal vaginal septa are well vascularized, the anterior border of the septum, followed by the posterior border, are removed using unipolar electrosurgery. Care must be taken not to remove the septum too close to the vaginal wall, as this will leave larger mucosa defects. The edges of these mucosal defects are reapproximated with 2-0 absorbable suture. Postoperative use of a vaginal mold is not necessary.

Obstructing Longitudinal Vaginal Septum. Women with an obstructing longitudinal septum usually present with normal-onset menarche and increasingly severe dysmenorrhea. These patients are most likely to have a didelphic uterus. One of the uteri has a patent outlet, while the other is obstructed (Fig. 2.17). If the obstruction is low in the vagina, eventually a bulge may be noted upon examination of the lower canal. However, a higher obstruction may be completely missed with just visual inspection, which is frequently the case in an adolescent. Digital examination may reveal a tense bulge in the vaginal wall (Fig. 2.18). In many instances the bulge is toward the anterior portion of the vagina between the twelve o'clock to three o'clock positions or the nine o'clock to twelve o'clock positions owing to the rotation of the two cervices.

Ultrasonography of the pelvis will usually show a pelvic mass, which can be misleading unless a vaginal septum is considered in the differential diagnosis. MRI is the best imaging mode for definitively diagnosing this abnormality. Like other Müllerian anomalies, a longitudinal vaginal septum is associated with renal abnormalities, including absent kidneys, pelvic kidneys, and duplicate ureters.

Some longitudinal septa will be found to be only partially obstructing, and a small opening in the septum can be found during menses with close inspection. Symptoms may vary from irregular and prolonged bleeding to profuse vaginal discharge.

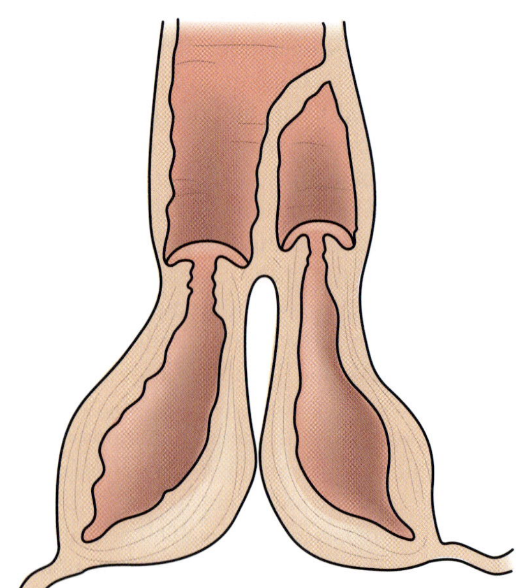

Fig. 2.17 Schematic of obstructing longitudinal septum.

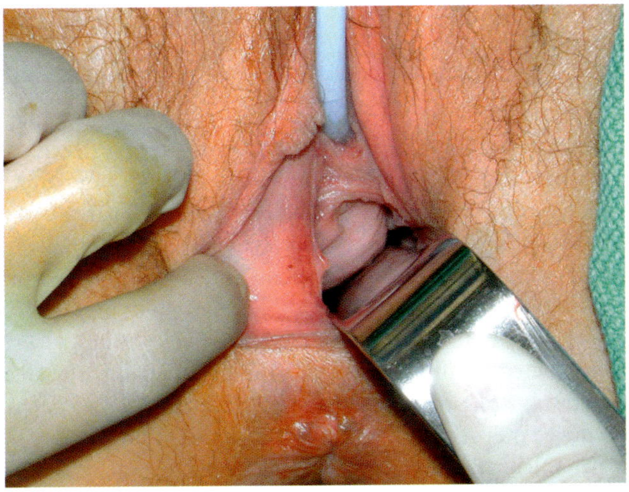

Fig. 2.18 An obstructing longitudinal septum usually presents as a bulge in the vagina.

Occasionally the pinpoint opening provides a pathway for organisms to access the obstructed vagina, leading to pelvic infection and pyocolpos. Physical examination is unlikely to reveal a tense bulge, but a slight fullness may sometimes be appreciated in the paravaginal area.

Accurate delineation of anatomy is a prerequisite for surgical excision of a noncommunicating longitudinal vaginal septum. The first step is to place a needle into the bulging vaginal wall to identify the correct plane of dissection. Once blood extrudes from the needle, the adjacent tissue is incised with electrosurgery to gain access into the obstructed vagina. Allis clamps are placed on the edges of this incision, and the cavity is assessed. When removing the medial border of this septum, care must be taken to avoid damaging the urethra. The septum should be removed in its entirety to allow easily access the second cervix for Pap smears. The raw mucosal edges are approximated with 2-0 absorbable suture. Use of a vaginal mold after surgery is not necessary because it would be impossible for the patient to place the stent in the correct position consistently. In difficult cases, use of either a resectoscope or hysteroscope to remove a longitudinal vaginal septum has been described.

The previously hidden cervix and obstructed vaginal canal will often appear abnormal. The cervix is usually flush with the vaginal fornix and often appears erythematous and glandular. Histologically, the obstructed vaginal canal and septum on its obstructed side will have columnar epithelium and glandular crypts. Some patients may complain of profuse vaginal discharge after removal of the septum. Metaplastic transformation of the vaginal mucosa to mature squamous epithelium can take years.

Simultaneous laparoscopy during removal of a vaginal septum is not recommended unless the diagnosis is unclear on MRI or imaging studies indicate concomitant pelvic masses. As in all cases of obstructive Müllerian anomalies, endometriosis is frequently encountered, even if the septum is only partially obstructing. With the possible exception of endometriomas, excision of the endometriosis is not recommended, because these lesions will regress after removal of the obstruction. The obstetric outcome of such patients is similar to that reported for patients with simple uterine didelphys. Pregnancy rates of 87% and live birth rates of 77% have been reported.

Transverse Vaginal Septum

Transverse vaginal septum results when there is failure of fusion and/or canalization of the urogenital sinus and paramesonephric ducts. The incidence of transverse vaginal septum appears to be between 1 in 21,000 to 1 in 72,000. A transverse vaginal septum may be located in the upper (46%), middle (40%), or lower (14%) third of the vagina. A transverse vaginal septum may be complete or incomplete and varies in thickness (Fig. 2.19 and 2.20).

Patients with a complete transverse vaginal septum generally present with a complaint of primary amenorrhea in early- to midpuberty. Pelvic pain is a common, but not universal, presenting complaint. Patients with high transverse vaginal septa are most likely to experience pelvic pain, and the pain will manifest earlier than in patients with septa located lower in the vagina. This is believed to be secondary to decreased space for the hematocolpos that ensues after initiation of menses. Patients with an incomplete transverse vaginal septum may complain of profuse vaginal discharge, dyspareunia, inability to insert tampon, or tearing during intercourse with resultant bleeding. If asymptomatic, it may not be discovered until a routine gynecologic examination. Very rarely a transverse vaginal septum may be detected in an infant or young child. In such instances, a mucocolpos can present as an abdominal mass. If large enough, this mass may cause ureteral obstruction with secondary hydronephrosis. Compression of the vena cava and cardiopulmonary failure has also been reported.

Manual and speculum examination provide the most important information for diagnosis of a transverse vaginal septum. If the septum is very low, a vaginal opening may not be appreciated on evaluation of the external genitalia. A low transverse vaginal septum can usually be differentiated from an imperforate hymen by visual inspection. By increasing intraabdominal pressure and increasing the bulge of the imperforate hymen, the

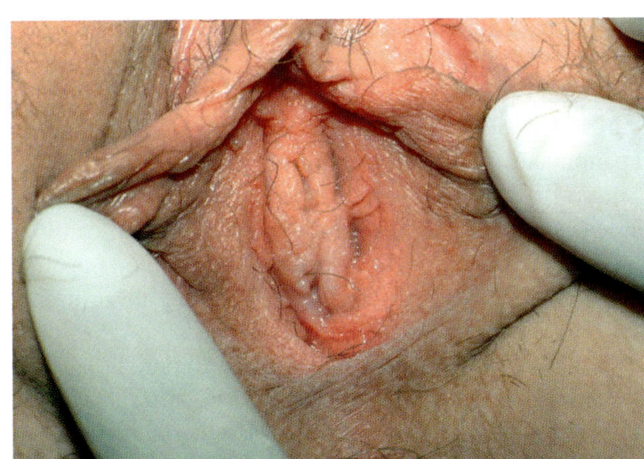

Fig. 2.19 Complete transverse septum. Notice that there is no bulge with a Valsalva maneuver that would be seen with an imperforate hymen.

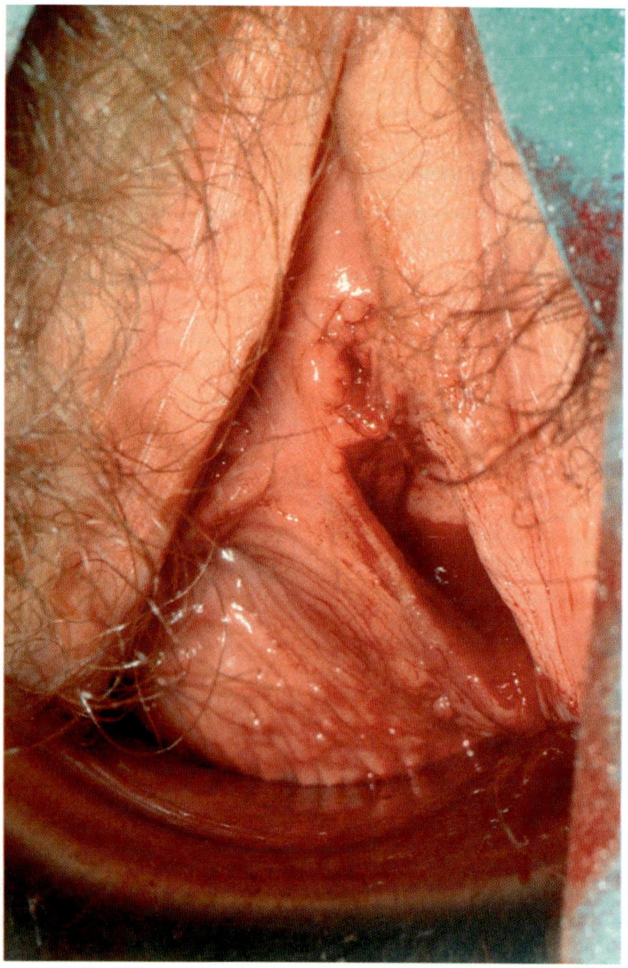

Fig. 2.20 Partial transverse septum.

Valsalva maneuver may further assist in this differentiation. If an opening to the vagina is noted, a manual or speculum examination may reveal a higher location of the septum. A rectal examination is very helpful in detecting a hematocolpos because the bulge is readily palpable.

Transperineal and transabdominal ultrasonography can sometimes diagnose and determine the thickness of a transverse vaginal septum. However, in most cases an MRI of the pelvis will be required to differentiate a transverse vaginal septum from other Müllerian anomalies such as cervical agenesis. These patients should also be evaluated for associated anomalies, including aortic coarctation, atrial septal defects, urinary tract anomalies, and malformations of the lumbar spine.

Surgical removal of a transverse vaginal septum is recommended as soon as practical after diagnosis to avoid continued retrograde menstruation. Endometriosis is common in patients with a transverse vaginal septum. However, removal of endometriosis lesions is not recommended, because relief of the obstruction leads to their spontaneous resolution. Delay in detection or treatment of a transverse vaginal septum may impair fertility secondary to irreversible pelvic adhesions, hematosalpingies, and endometriosis. In one long-term follow-up study by Rock et al. of 19 patients with transverse septa, 47% became pregnant (1982). However, a small study in Finland by Joki-Erkkila and Heinonen showed a significantly higher live-birth rate in women who had undergone very early diagnosis and management of their transverse vaginal septa (2003).

The unfortunate consequence of very early surgical management is an increased rate of vaginal stenosis after surgical repair. This is most likely because of inconsistent use of vaginal dilators by young adolescents, which are a necessary part of treatment of a thick vaginal septum (see later). An alternative to early surgery for very young patients is using depot medroxyprogesterone to suppress monthly endometrial shedding, thereby allowing surgery to be postponed. The young girl can be instructed to dilate the distal vagina to stretch the distal vaginal mucosa, potentially decreasing the need for a graft and helping to prepare her for postoperative use of the dilator.

The thickness and location of the septum will determine the best approach to surgery. Thin, low transverse vaginal septa are much easier to repair than thick, usually high septa. Transverse septa that are thin and low in the vagina can usually be excised without difficulty. If a slight bulge cannot be appreciated on visual examination, an angiocath needle is placed through the septum (Fig. 2.21). With return of thick blood through the angiocath, the plane of dissection becomes clear. Access is gained into the upper vaginal cavity by perforating the transverse septum with unipolar electrosurgery or scissors (Fig. 2.22). Concomitant pelvic ultrasound can also assist with correct axis of incision. The septum is excised in its entirety, and the upper vaginal mucosa is reapproximated to the lower vaginal mucosa using 2-0 absorbable suture (Fig. 2.23). In most instances, to prevent stenosis of the vagina continual use of a mold is recommended for several weeks after surgery.

Managing thick transverse septa can be quite challenging. Before surgery, the patient must be prepared for prolonged use of a mold and possible split-thickness skin graft to line the vagina. The main concern during the surgery is rectal injury; therefore, one can consider a mechanical bowel preparation or

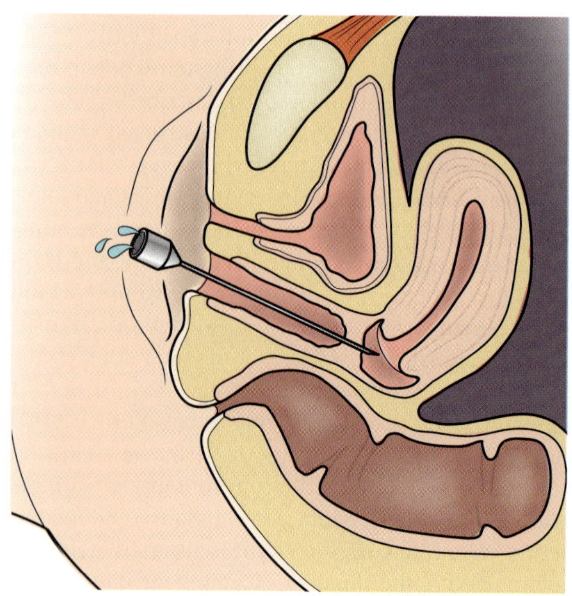

Fig. 2.21 Placement of angiocath into the transverse septum.

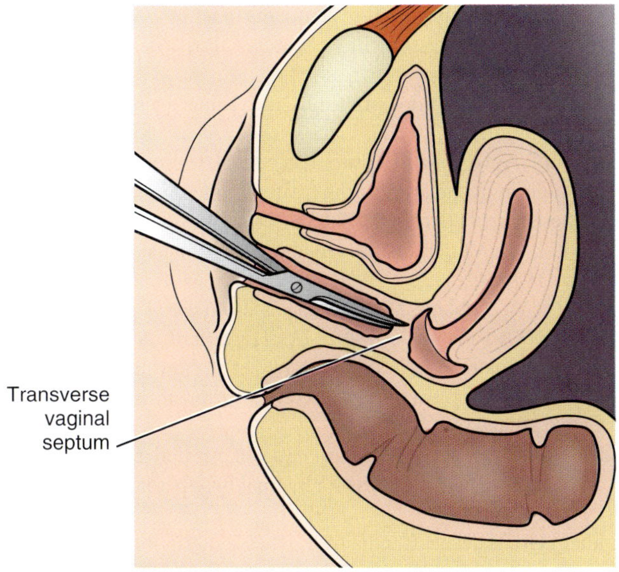

Fig. 2.22 Angle of incision into septum.

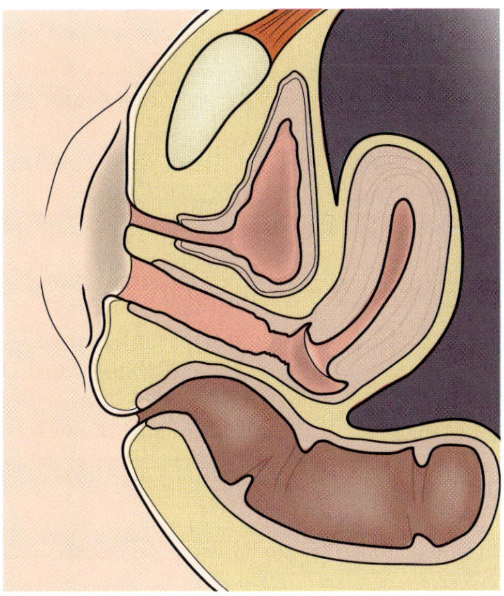

Fig. 2.23 Reapproximation of distal and proximal vagina mucosa after excision of the septum.

preoperative enema. During surgery, a bulge will not be seen in the presence of a thick transverse septum. The correct angle of dissection can be determined by inserting an angiocath needle into the hematocolpos under ultrasound guidance. In difficult cases, the septum can be approached transfundally via the uterus using laparoscopy or laparotomy.

The dissection is carried out taking care to protect the bladder and rectum. A Foley catheter is placed into the bladder. As the loose areolar tissue is being dissected, the rectum is frequently examined to ensure appropriate angle of dissection. If there is inadvertent entry into the bladder or the rectum, the procedure should be stopped and completed at a future date. After the cervix is visualized the goal is to reapproximate the upper vaginal epithelial tissue to the lower vaginal epithelium.

If a thick septum is completely incised, the distance between the vaginal mucosa of the proximal and distal portions of the vagina may be so great that the edges cannot be reapproximated without tension. For this reason, a Z-plasty technique, as first described by Garcia (1967), should be considered for correction of thick transverse vaginal septa or when the vagina is short. For this technique, four lower mucosal flaps are created by making oblique crossed incisions through the vaginal tissue on the perineal side of the transverse septum, taking great care to avoid injuring either the bladder or the rectum. Four upper mucosal flaps are created by making oblique crossed incisions through the vaginal tissue on the hematocolpos side of the transverse septum. The upper and lower mucosal flaps are separated by sharp and blunt dissection and sutured together at their free edges to form a continuous Z-plasty. Excellent results have been noted by Wierrani et al. (2003) in 13 patients who underwent this procedure. A vaginal mold must be used for 5 to 8 weeks after the procedure to avoid vaginal stenosis. If the patient is not sexually active, a dilator should be used at night for 6 to 8 additional months. The patient should be instructed in self-examination and should return if she notices any signs of early stenosis. In cases of a thick septum where a Z-plasty technique is not used, a skin graft may be required. The technique used is similar to that described for the McIndoe procedure. Prolonged use of a mold is required postoperatively.

Anomalies of the Hymen

Hymenal anomalies are derived from the incomplete degeneration of the hymen at birth. There are several variants, including imperforate, microperforate, septate, and cribriform. Imperforate hymen is the most common congenital anomaly of the female reproductive tract, occurring in 1/1000 women. Females present either at birth with a bulging hymen secondary to mucocolpos or at menarche with cyclic pelvic pain and hematocolpos. Distension of the vagina may lead to additional symptoms of a hymenal membrane with bluish discoloration, and defecatory and voiding dysfunction. Sometimes an imperforate hymen is discovered during a well-child check at the pediatrician's office.

Repair of the imperforate hymen is best undertaken after the tissue has undergone estrogenic stimulation. Therefore the ideal time is as a neonate (because of maternal estrogenic effects) or in the postpubertal/premenarchal girl. Repair of the imperforate hymen is not recommended between these times because of lack of estrogen in the pediatric vagina.

Under anesthesia, an incision is made in the imperforate hymen. This can be a stellate or elliptical incision. The borders of the incision should approximate the hymenal ring. Excess tissue is excised with electrocautery to create a normal-sized orifice, and the vaginal epithelium is sutured to the hymenal ring using absorbable suture (Video 2.4).

SUMMARY

Anomalies of the genitourinary tract are common, and basic knowledge of the embryology of this system is necessary for diagnosis and successful treatment of these patients. A careful history, physical examination, and imaging (most often MRI) are critical to make the correct diagnosis and subsequently offer appropriate treatment. Because of the close embryologic development of the urinary and genital systems, patients with congenital anomalies of the genital tract must also be evaluated for other anomalies of the urinary tract, such as renal anomalies. Management is based on the type of anomaly. Although conservative management with vaginal dilation for patients with congenital absence of the vagina is first-line, surgical treatment may be required for these patients. Surgical management is often most appropriate for those with other types of Müllerian anomalies such as vaginal septum and imperforate hymen.

BIBLIOGRAPHY

Acién P. Reproductive performance of women with uterine malformations. *Hum Reprod.* 1993;8:122.

Acién P. Incidence of Mullerian defects in fertile and infertile women. *Hum Reprod.* 1997;12:1372.

Acién P, Acién M, Sánchez-Ferrer M. Complex malformations of the female genital tract. New types and revision of classification. *Hum Reprod.* 2004;19:2377.

Acién P, Acién MI. The history of female genital tract malformation classifications and proposal of an updated system. *Hum Reprod Update.* 2011;17:693.

Aittomäki K, Eroila H, Kajanoja P. A population-based study of the incidence of Müllerian aplasia in Finland. *Fertil Steril.* 2001;76:624.

Akle CA, Adinolfi M, Welsh KI, et al. Immunogenicity of human amniotic epithelial cells after transplantation into volunteers. *Lancet.* 1981;2:1003.

Alessandrescu D, Peltecu GC, Buhimschi CS, Buhimschi IA. Neocolpopoiesis with split-thickness skin graft as a surgical treatment of vaginal agenesis: retrospective review of 201 cases. *Am J Obstet Gynecol.* 1996;175:131.

American College of Obstetrics and, Gynecology. ACOG Committee Opinion. No. 728: Müllerian agenesis: diagnosis, management, and treatment. *Obstet Gynecol.* 2018;131:e35.

American Fertility Society. Classifications of adnexal adhesions, distal tubal occlusion, tubal occlusion secondary to tubal ligation, tubal pregnancies, Mullerian anomalies, and intrauterine adhesions. *Fertil Steril.* 1988;49:944.

Ashworth MF, Morton KE, Dewhurst J, et al. Vaginoplasty using amnion. *Obstet Gynecol.* 1986;67:443.

Baltzer J, Zander J. Primary squamous cell carcinoma of the neovagina. *Gynecol Oncol.* 1989;35:99.

Belloli G, Campobasso P, Musi L. Labial skin-flap vaginoplasty using tissue expanders. *Pediatr Surg Int.* 1997;12:168.

Borruto F, Chasen ST, Chervenak FA, Fedele L. The Vecchietti procedure for surgical treatment of vaginal agenesis: comparison of laparoscopy and laparotomy. *Int J Gynaecol Obstet.* 1999;64:153.

Borruto F. Mayer-Rokitansky-Kuster syndrome: Vecchietti's personal series. *Clin Exp Obstet Gynecol.* 1992;19:273.

Brännström M, Johannesson L, Bokström H, et al. Livebirth after uterus transplantation. *Lancet.* 2015;385(9968):607-616.

Brucker SY, Gegusch M, Zubke W, et al. Neovagina creation in vaginal agenesis: development of a new laparoscopic Vecchietti-based procedure and optimized instruments in a prospective comparative interventional study in 101 patients. *Fertil Steril.* 2008; 90:1940.

Buss JG, Lee RA. McIndoe procedure for vaginal agenesis: Results and complications. *Mayo Clin Proc.* 1989;64:758.

Bugmann P, Amaudruz M, Hanquinet S, et al. Uterocervicoplasty with a bladder mucosa layer for the treatment of complete cervical agenesis. *Fertil Steril.* 2002;77:831.

Buttram Jr VC. Mullerian anomalies and their management. *Fertil Steril.* 1983;40:159.

Buttram Jr VC, Gibbons WE. Müllerian anomalies: a proposed classification. (An analysis of 144 cases). *Fertil Steril.* 1979;32:40.

Byrne J, Nussbaum-Blask A, Taylor WS, et al. Prevalence of Müllerian duct anomalies detected at ultrasound. *Am J Med Genet.* 2000;94:9.

Callens N, De Cuypere G, De Sutter P, et al. An update on surgical and nonsurgical treatments for vaginal hypoplasia. *Hum Reprod Update.* 2014;20:775.

Candiani GB, Fedele L, Candiani M. Double uterus, blind hemivagina, and ipsilateral renal agenesis: 36 cases and long-term follow-up. *Obstet Gynecol.* 1997;90:26.

Carey MP, Steinberg LH. Vaginal dystocia in a patient with a double uterus and a longitudinal vaginal septum. *Aust N Z J Obstet Gynaecol.* 1989;29:74.

Carlson BM. *Human Embryology and Developmental Biology.* 4th ed. Philadelphia: Mosby, Inc.; 2009.

Casey AC, Laufer MR. Cervical agenesis: septic death after surgery. *Obstet Gynecol.* 1997;90:706.

Chatwani A, Nyirjesy P, Harmanli OH, Grody MH. Creation of neovagina by laparoscopic vecchietti operation. *J Laparoendosc Adv Surg Tech A.* 1999;9:425.

Cheikhelard A, Bidet M, Baptiste A, et al. Surgery is not superior to dilation for the management of vaginal agenesis in Mayer-Rokitansky-Kuster-Hauser syndrome: a multicenter comparative observational study in 131 patients. *Am J Obstet Gynecol.* 2018;219(3)281.

Chudacoff RM, Alexander J, Alvero R, Segars JH. Tissue expansion vaginoplasty for treatment of congenital vaginal agenesis. *Obstet Gynecol.* 1996;87:865.

Costa EM, Mendonca BB, Inacio M, et al. Management of ambiguous genitalia in pseudohermaphrodites: new perspectives on vaginal dilation. *Fertil Steril.* 1997;67:229.

Counseller VS, Flor FS. Congenital absence of the vagina. *Surg Clin North Am.* 1957;37:1107.

Darai E, Soriano D, Thoury A, Bouillot JL. Neovagina construction by combined laparoscopic-perineal sigmoid colpoplasty in a patient with rokitansky syndrome. *J Am Assoc Gynecol Laparosc.* 2002;9:204.

Davydov SN. 12-year experience with colpopoiesis using the peritoneum. *Gynakologe.* 1980;13:120.

Davydov SN. Colpopoeisis from the peritoneum of the uterorectal space. *Akush Ginekol (Mosk).* 1969;45:55.

Deffarges JV, Haddad B, Musset R, Paniel BJ. Utero-vaginal anastomosis in women with uterine cervix atresia: long-term follow-up and reproductive performance. A study of 18 cases. *Hum Reprod.* 2001;16:1722.

Dhall K. Amnion graft for treatment of congenital absence of the vagina. *Br J Obstet Gynaecol.* 1984;91:279.

Edmonds DK. Congenital malformations of the genital tract. *Obstet Gynecol Clin North Am.* 2000;27:49.

Edmonds DK. Diagnosis, clinical presentation and management of cervical agenesis. In: Gidwani G, Falcone T, eds. *Congenital*

Malformations of the Female Genital Tract: Diagnosis and Management. 1st ed. Philadelphia: Lippincott Williams & Wilkins; 1999.

Edmonds DK, Rose GL, Lipton MG, Quek J. Mayer Rokitansky-Kuster-Hauser syndrome: review of 245 consecutive cases managed by a multidisciplinary approach with vaginal dilators. *Fertil Steril*. 2012;97:686.

Falcone T, Gidwani G, Paraiso M, et al. Anatomic variation in the rudimentary horns of a unicornuate uterus: implications for laparoscopic surgery. *Hum Reprod*. 1997;12:263.

Falcone T, Hemmings R, Kalife R. Laparoscopic management of a unicornuate uterus with a rudimentary horn. *J Gynecol Surg*. 1995;11:105.

Fedele L, Bianchi S, Zanconato G, Raffaelli R. Laparoscopic creation of a neovagina in patients with Rokitansky syndrome: analysis of 52 cases. *Fertil Steril*. 2000;74:384.

Fedele L, Frontino G, Restelli E, et al. Creation of a neovagina by Davidov's laparoscopic modified technique in patients with Rokitansky syndrome. *Am J Obstet Gynecol*. 2010;202:33.

Fliegner JR. A simple surgical cure for congenital absence of the vagina. *Aust N Z J Surg*. 1986;56:505.

Frank RT. The formation of an artificial vagina without operation. *Am J Obstet Gynecol*. 1938;35:1053.

Fraser IS, Baird DT, Hobson BM, et al. Cyclical ovarian function in women with congenital absence of the uterus and vagina. *J Clin Endocrinol Metab*. 1973;36:634.

Fujimoto VY, Miller JH, Klein NA, Soules MR. Congenital cervical atresia: report of seven cases and review of the literature. *Am J Obstet Gynecol*. 1997;177:1419.

Garcia RF. Z-plasty for correction of congenital transverse vaginal septum. *Am J Obstet Gynecol*. 1967;99:1164.

Gidwani G, Falcone T. *Congenital Malformations of the Female Genital Tract: Diagnosis and Management*. Philadelphia: Lippincott Williams & Wilkins; 1999.

Gosling JA. Anatomy. In: Stanton SL, ed. *Clinical Gynecologic Urology*. St Louis: Mosby; 1984.

Gosling JA, Dixon J, Humpherson JR. *Functional Anatomy of the Urinary Tract*. London: Gower; 1982.

Griffen JE, Creighton E, Madden JD, et al. Congenital absence of the vagina: the Mayer Rokitansky Kuster Hauser syndrome. *Ann Intern Med*. 1976;85:224.

Grimbizis GF, Camus M, Tarlatzis BC, et al. Clinical implications of uterine malformations and hysteroscopic treatment results. *Hum Reprod Update*. 2001;7:161.

Haddad B, Louis-Sylvestre C, Poitout P, Paniel BJ. Longitudinal vaginal septum: a retrospective study of 202 cases. *Eur J Obstet Gynecol Reprod Biol*. 1997;74:197.

Heinonen PK. Clinical implications of the didelphic uterus: long-term follow-up of 49 cases. *Eur J Obstet Gynecol Reprod Biol*. 2000;91:183.

Heinonen PK. Longitudinal vaginal septum. *Eur J Obstet Gynecol Reprod Biol*. 1982;13:253.

Herlin M, Bay Bjørn AM, Jørgensen LK, et al. Treatment of vaginal agenesis in Mayer-Rokitansky-Kuster-Hauser syndrome in Denmark: a nationwide comparative study of anatomical outcome and complications. *Fertil Steril*. 2018;110(4):746.

Hilton P. The mechanism of continence. In: Stanton SL, Tanagho EA, eds. *Surgery of Female Incontinence*. 2nd ed. New York: Springer-Verlag; 1986.

Hiroi H, Yasugi T, Matsumoto K, et al. Mucinous adenocarcinoma arising in a neovagina using the sigmoid colon thirty years after operation: a case report. *J Surg Oncol*. 2001;77:61.

Hojsgaard A, Villadsen I. McIndoe procedure for congenital vaginal agenesis: complications and results. *Br J Plastic Surg*. 1995;48:97.

Hopkins MP, Morley GW. Squamous cell carcinoma of the neovagina. *Obstet Gynecol*. 1987;69:525.

Hovsepian DM, Auyeung A, Ratts VS. A combined surgical and radiologic technique for creating a functional neo-endocervical canal in a case of partial congenital cervical atresia. *Fertil Steril*. 1999;71:158.

Hurst BS, Rock JA. Preoperative dilatation to facilitate repair of the high transverse vaginal septum. *Fertil Steril*. 1992;57:1351.

Ingram JM. The bicycle seat stool in the treatment of vaginal agenesis and stenosis: a preliminary report. *Am J Obstet Gynecol*. 1981;140:867.

Jackson ND, Rosenblatt PL. Use of Interceed absorbable adhesion barrier for vaginoplasty. *Obstet Gynecol*. 1994;84:1048.

Jacob JH, Griffin WT. Surgical reconstruction of the congenitally atretic cervix: two cases. *Obstet Gynecol Surv*. 1989;44:556.

Jayasinghe Y, Rane A, Stalewski H, Grover S. The presentation and early diagnosis of the rudimentary uterine horn. *Obstet Gynecol*. 2005;105:1456.

Joki-Erkkila MM, Heinonen PK. Presenting and long-term clinical implications and fecundity in females with obstructing vaginal malformations. *J Pediatr Adolesc Gynecol*. 2003;16:307.

Jones Jr HW. Reproductive impairment and the malformed uterus. *Fertil Steril*. 1981;36:137.

Joseph VT. Pudendal-thigh flap vaginoplasty in the reconstruction of genital anomalies. *J Pediatr Surg*. 1997;32:62.

Kaloo P, Cooper M. Laparoscopic-assisted Vecchietti procedure for creation of a neovagina: an analysis of five cases. *Aust N Z J Obstet Gynaecol*. 2002;42:307.

Klingele CJ, Gebhart JB, Croak AJ, et al. McIndoe procedure for vaginal agenesis: long-term outcome and effect on quality of life. *Am J Obstet Gynecol*. 2003;189:1569.

Krysiewicz S. Infertility in women: diagnostic evaluation with hysterosalpingography and other imaging techniques. *AJR Am J Roentgenol*. 1992;159:253.

Langman J. *Medical Embryology*. Baltimore: Williams & Wilkins; 1976.

Letterie GS. Combined congenital absence of the vagina and cervix. diagnosis with magnetic resonance imaging and surgical management. *Gynecol Obstet Invest*. 1998;46:65.

Letterie GS, Vauss N. Mullerian tract abnormalities and associated auditory defects. *J Reprod Med*. 1991;36:765.

Lodi A. Contributo clinico stastico sulle malformazioni della vagina osservate mella. clinica obstetricia e ginecologia di milano dal 1906 al 1950. *Ann Obstet Gynecol Med Perinatol*. 1951;73:1246.

Maizels M. Normal development of the urinary tract. In: Walsh PC, Gittes RF, Perlmutter AD, Stamey TA, eds. *Campbell's Urology*. 5th ed. Philadelphia: WB Saunders; 1986.

Markham SM, Parmley TH, Murphy AA, et al. Cervical agenesis combined with vaginal agenesis diagnosed by magnetic resonance imaging. *Fertil Steril*. 1987;48:143.

McCraw JB, Massey FM, Shanklin KD, Horton CE. Vaginal reconstruction with gracilis myocutaneous flaps. *Plast Reconstr Surg*. 1976;58:176.

Mobus VJ, Kortenhorn K, Kreienberg R, Friedberg V. Long-term results after operative correction of vaginal aplasia. *Am J Obstet Gynecol*. 1996;175:617.

Monstrey S, Blondeel P, Van Landuyt K, et al. The versatility of the pudendal thigh fasciocutaneous flap used as an island flap. *Plast Reconstr Surg*. 2001;107:719.

Montevecchi L, Valle RF. Resectoscopic treatment of complete longitudinal vaginal septum. *Int J Gynaecol Obstet.* 2004;84:65.

Motoyama S, Laoag-Fernandez JB, Mochizuki S, et al. Vaginoplasty with Interceed absorbable adhesion barrier for complete squamous epithelialization in vaginal agenesis. *Am J Obstet Gynecol.* 2003;188:1260.

Muckle CW. Developmental abnormalities of the female reproductive organs. In: Sciarra JJ, ed. *Gynecology and Obstetrics.* Vol 1. Hagerstown: Harper & Row; 1981.

O'Leary JL, O'Leary JA. Rudimentary horn pregnancies. *Obstet Gynecol.* 1963;22:371.

Oppelt P, Renner S, Brucker S. The VCUAM classification: a new classification for genital malformations. *Fertil Steril.* 2005;84:1493.

Ota H, Tanaka J, Murakami M, et al. Laparoscopy-assisted ruge procedure for the creation of a neovagina in a patient with Mayer-Rokitansky-Kuster-Hauser syndrome. *Fertil Steril.* 2000;73:641.

Parsons JK, Gearhart SL, Gearhart JP. Vaginal reconstruction utilizing sigmoid colon: complications and long-term results. *J Pediatr Surg.* 2002;37:629.

Patton PE. Anatomic uterine defects. *Clin Obstet Gynecol.* 1994;37:705.

Petrozza JC, Gray MR, Davis AJ, Reindollar RH. Congenital absence of the uterus and vagina is not commonly transmitted as a dominant genetic trait: outcomes of surrogate pregnancies. *Fertil Steril.* 1997;67:387.

Poland ML, Evans TN. Psychologic aspects of vaginal agenesis. *J Reprod Med.* 1985;30:340.

Pui MH. Imaging diagnosis of congenital uterine malformation. *Comput Med Imaging Graph.* 2004;28:425.

Rall K, Schickner MC, Barresi G, et al. Laparoscopically assisted neovaginoplasty in vaginal agenesis: a long-term outcome study in 240 patients. *J Pediat Gynecol.* 2014;27:379.

Rangaswamy M, Machado NO, Kaur S, Machado L. Laparoscopic vaginoplasty: using a sliding peritoneal flap for correction of complete vaginal agenesis. *Eur J Obstet Gynecol Reprod Biol.* 2001;98:244.

Ratnamm SS. Vaginal atresia. In: Ratnamm SS, Soon-Chyem N, Sen DK, eds. *Contributions to Obstetrics and Gynecology*. Singapore: Longman Singapore Publishers; 1991.

Reindollar RH, Byrd JR, McDonough PG. Delayed sexual development: a study of 252 patients. *Am J Obstet Gynecol.* 1981;140:371.

Reinhold C, Hricak H, Forstner R, et al. Primary amenorrhea: evaluation with MR imaging. *Radiology.* 1997;203:383.

Roberts CP, Haber MJ, Rock JA. Vaginal creation for Mullerian agenesis. *Am J Obstet Gynecol.* 2001;185:1349.

Robson MC, Krizek TJ. The effect of human amniotic membranes on the bacteria population of infected rat burns. *Ann Surg.* 1973;177:144.

Robson S, Oliver GD. Management of vaginal agenesis: review of 10 years practice at a tertiary referral centre. *Aust N Z J Obstet Gynaecol.* 2000;40:430.

Rock J, Breech L. Surgery for anomalies of the Mullerian ducts. In: Rock JA, Jones HW, III, eds. *TeLinde's Operative Gynecology.* 9th ed. Philadelphia: Lippincott Williams & Wilkins; 2003.

Rock JA, Carpenter SE, Wheeless CR, Jones III HWJ. The clinical management of maldevelopment of the uterine cervix. *J Pelv Surg* 1995;1:129.

Rock JA, Zacur HA, Dlugi AM, et al. Pregnancy success following surgical correction of imperforate hymen and complete transverse vaginal septum. *Obstet Gynecol.* 1982;59:448.

Romao RL, Salle JL, Wherrett DK. Update on the management of disorders of sex development. *Pediatr Clin North Am.* 2012;59:853.

Rothman D. The use of peritoneum in the construction of a vagina. *Obstet Gynecol.* 1972;40:835.

Sabatucci I, Palaia I, Marchese C, et al. Treatment of the Mayer-Rokitansky-Kuster-Hauser syndrome with autologous in vitro cultured vaginal tissue: descriptive study of long-term results and patient outcomes. *BJOG.* 2019;126(1):123.

Sadler TW. *Langman's Medical Embryology.* 11th ed. Baltimore: Lippincott Williams & Wilkins; 2010.

Sanfilippo JS, Wakim NG, Schikler KN, Yussman MA. Endometriosis in association with uterine anomaly. *Am J Obstet Gynecol.* 1986;154:39.

Saravelos SH, Cocksedge KA, Li TC. Prevalence and diagnosis of congenital uterine anomalies in women with reproductive failure: a critical appraisal. *Hum Reprod Update.* 2008;14:415.

Shapiro E, Huang H, Wu XR. New concepts on the development of the vagina. *Adv Exp Med Bio.* 2004;545:173.

Snyder HM. Anomalies of the ureter. In: Gillenwater JY, Grayhack JT, Howards SS, Duckett JW, eds. *Adult and Pediatric Urology*. Vol 2. Chicago: Mosby; 1987.

Song R, Wang X, Zhou G. Reconstruction of the vagina with sensory function. *Clin Plast Surg.* 1982;9:105.

Soong YK, Chang FH, Lai YM, et al. Results of modified laparoscopically assisted neovaginoplasty in 18 patients with congenital absence of vagina. *Hum Reprod.* 1996;11:200.

Stassart JP, Nagel TC, Prem KA, Phipps WR. Uterus didelphys, obstructed hemivagina, and ipsilateral renal agenesis: the University of Minnesota experience. *Fertil Steril.* 1992;57:756.

Stenchever MA, Droegemueller W, Herbst AL, Mishell DR, eds. *Comprehensive Gynecology*. 4th ed. Philadelphia: Mosby, Inc.; 2001.

Strubbe EH, Cremers CW, Dikkers FG, Willemsen WN. Hearing loss and the Mayer-Rokitansky-Kuster-Hauser syndrome. *Am J Otol.* 1994;15:431.

Syed HA, Malone PS, Hitchcock RJ. Diversion colitis in children with colovaginoplasty. *BJU Int.* 2001;87:857.

Soong YK, Chang FH, Lai YM, et al. Results of modified laparoscopically assisted neovaginoplasty in 18 patients with congenital absence of vagina. *Hum Reprod.* 1996;11:200.

Templeman CL, Hertweck SP, Levine RL, Reich H. Use of laparoscopically mobilized peritoneum in the creation of a neovagina. *Fertil Steril.* 2000;74:589.

Toaff ME, Lev-Toaff AS, Toaff R. Communicating uteri: review and classification with introduction of two previously unreported types. *Fertil Steril.* 1984;41:661.

Tobin GR, Day TG. Vaginal and pelvic reconstruction with distally based rectus abdominis myocutaneous flaps. *Plast Reconstr Surg.* 1988;81:62.

Tsai EM, Chiang PH, Hsu SC, et al. Hysteroscopic resection of vaginal septum in an adolescent virgin with obstructed hemivagina. *Hum Reprod.* 1998;13:1500.

Vechietti G. Neovagina nella sindrome di Rokitansky Kuster-Hauser. *Attual Obstet Gynecol.* 1965;11:131.

Veronikis DK, McClure GB, Nichols DH. The Vecchietti operation for constructing a neovagina: Indications, instrumentation, and techniques. *Obstet Gynecol.* 1997;90:301.

Verp MS, Simpson JL. Abnormal sexual differentiation and neoplasia. *Cancer Genet Cytogenet.* 1987;25:191.

Walters MD, Karram MM, eds. *Urogynecology and Reconstructive Pelvic Surgery*. 3rd ed. Philadelphia: Mosby, Inc.; 2007.

Wee JT, Joseph VT. A new technique of vaginal reconstruction using neurovascular pudendal-thigh flaps: a preliminary report. *Plast Reconstr Surg.* 1989;83:701.

Weijenborg PT, ter Kuile MM. The effect of a group programme on women with the Mayer-Rokitansky-Kuster-Hauser syndrome. *BJOG.* 2000;107:365.

Wierrani F, Bodner K, Spangler B, Grunberger W. "Z"-plasty of the transverse vaginal septum using Garcia's procedure and the Grunberger modification. *Fertil Steril.* 2003;79:608.

Willemsen WN. Renal—skeletal—ear- and facial-anomalies in combination with the Mayer—Rokitansky—Kuster (MRK) syndrome. *Eur J Obstet Gynecol Reprod Biol.* 1982;14:121.

3

Neurophysiology and Pharmacology of the Lower Urinary Tract

W. Thomas Gregory and Ian C. Fields

CHAPTER OUTLINE

INTRODUCTION

The two functions of the lower urinary tract are the storage of urine within the bladder and the timely expulsion of urine from the urethra. The precise neurologic pathways and neurophysiologic mechanisms that control these functions of storage and micturition are complex and not completely understood, with our understanding of many of these pathways adapted from animal models. Understanding the interaction of the autonomic nervous system, the peripheral nervous system, and the central nervous system (CNS) in lower urinary tract function is critical to patient care, as modulating those interactions is key to treatment of many lower urinary tract disorders. This chapter reviews the normal function and neurologic control of, and introduces clinical pharmacology concepts regarding, the lower urinary tract in women.

GENERAL NERVOUS SYSTEM ARRANGEMENTS

Neurons within the nervous system propagate signals via action potentials, an electrical event. This electrical event results in a chemical event at junctions with other nerves or end organs, relying on chemicals known as neurotransmitters. These neurotransmitters are selectively released from a nerve terminal by an action potential and interact with a specific receptor on an adjacent structure to elicit a specific physiologic response. These chemical events at the synapses can be excitatory or inhibitory.

The nervous system is arranged into the central and the peripheral systems. The CNS includes the brain and spinal cord. Within the brain and spinal cord, nerve cell bodies are arranged in groups of various sizes and shapes called nuclei. Fibers with a common origin and destination are called a tract. Synaptic relationships in the CNS are very complex, with contacts occurring between axons and cell bodies, axons and dendrites, cell body and cell body, or dendrite and dendrite.

Twelve pairs of cranial and 31 pairs of spinal nerves with their ganglia compose the peripheral nervous system. Synaptic relationships in the peripheral nervous system involve only neuron–neuron or neuron–effector interactions. The somatic component of the peripheral system innervates skeletal muscle and receives somatic sensory input.

The autonomic division innervates cardiac muscle, smooth muscle, and glands. The autonomic nervous system consists, in part, of general visceral efferent fibers, supplying the smooth muscle of viscera. Afferent fibers are closely associated with the autonomic efferents, and both the motor and sensory visceral neural activities ordinarily function at a subconscious level. Unlike the somatic motor system, the peripheral efferent autonomic fibers reach the effector organ by at least a two-neuron chain, constituting a preganglionic and a postganglionic neuron. Fibers arising from neurons of the intermediolateral cell column of the 12 thoracic and first two lumbar segments of the spinal cord constitute the sympathetic division (thoracolumbar) of the autonomic nervous system. The parasympathetic division (craniosacral) consists of fibers arising from the neurons of the second through the fourth intermediolateral cell column sacral segments and from cranial outflows.

Sympathetic nerves to the pelvic cavity originate in cord levels T10 to L2 (Fig. 3.1). Generally, their two-neuron chain consists of short preganglionic fibers and long postganglionic

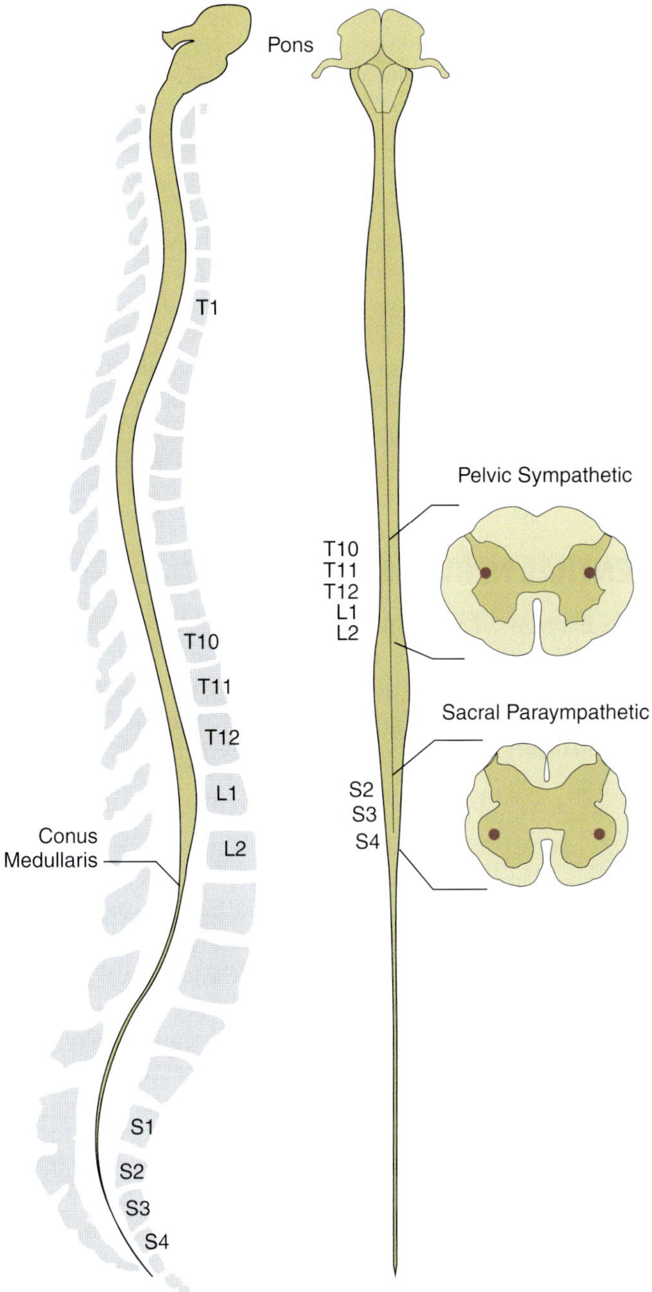

Fig. 3.1 Relationship of bony vertebral segments and relative locations of pelvic sympathetic and parasympathetic neurons, including cross-sectional views of the spinal cord. Note that the neuronal cell bodies do not exactly correlate with the bony spine. For example, sacral neuronal cell bodies are actually located at the rostral bony lumbar levels, with their projections traversing through the conus medullaris and cauda equina.

fibers. Some preganglionic axons pass via white rami communicantes to the paravertebral sympathetic chain, synapse, and pass by gray rami communicantes to the skeletal nerves. These constitute the paravertebral sympathetics, and they generally follow the segmental nerves to somatic structures. The other preganglionic sympathetic axons pass directly through the paravertebral ganglia to the prevertebral ganglia located at roots of arteries, for which they are named (e.g., lumbar splanchnic nerves terminate in inferior mesenteric and hypogastric ganglia). After synapsing in these ganglia, the postganglionic nerves travel through the right or left hypogastric nerve to join the pelvic plexus and follow the visceral arteries to the organs of the lower abdomen and pelvis. These constitute the prevertebral sympathetics. In addition to these two pathways, preganglionic sympathetic fibers may also ascend or descend within the paravertebral ganglia chain before synapsing or passing through to the prevertebral ganglia.

Pelvic parasympathetic system preganglionic fibers originate in spinal segments S2 through S4. The long preganglionic fibers travel through the pelvic nerve to join the hypogastric nerve in forming the pelvic plexus. These fibers continue to ganglia located within or very near the organs that they supply, thus having very short postganglionic fibers and much longer preganglionic fibers.

SENSORY INNERVATION

There are varying sizes and types of nerves. They are classified generally by size and myelination (Table 3.1) The largest, myelinated, fast-conducting Aα sensory nerves convey touch, or proprioception, within skeletal muscles. The smallest, nonmyelinated C nerve fibers are slow-conducting nerves that convey pain and temperature on the sensory side or act as postganglionic autonomic nerves on the motor side. The bladder afferent nerves are largely C fibers at birth, until maturation changes the afferents to Aδ (lightly myelinated, small) fibers. It is now appreciated that bladder insults, such as obstruction, bladder inflammation, or spinal cord disease, affecting pathways involved in lower urinary tract function can lead to neuroplastic changes in which some afferents again become C fibers as the bladder's response to the insults. Understanding the anatomy and physiology of the basic reflex pathways and central voluntary control involved in lower urinary tract function is necessary but appreciating the dynamic ability of the neurons to modify these pathways will provide important insights into evaluation of novel therapies.

The sensory innervation of the lower urinary tract is intricate and complex. A urothelial and suburothelial network has

TABLE 3.1 Afferent Nerve Fiber Types

Fiber Type	Location	Function	Role in Normal Bladder Function
Aα (myelinated)	Skeletal muscle	Proprioception	None
Aβ (myelinated)	Cutaneous	Mechanoreceptor	None
Aδ (finely myelinated axons)	Smooth muscle (detrusor)	Touch/pressure	Bladder fullness and wall tension
C (unmyelinated axons)	Mucosa (urothelium)	Nociception	Nociception

been described. Interactions involve cell-to-cell communication as well as neural pathways. The sensory nerves are denser in the urethra and trigone and sparser in the dome of the bladder. The afferent axons join their respective efferent nerves in the paths for the autonomic and somatic neural pathways. Controversy exists concerning where the major afferent supply travels. Some claim that the majority of afferent nerves travel with the hypogastric nerve to the thoracolumbar region of the spinal cord, while others state that they travel through the pelvic nerve and enter at the sacral levels. A specific nucleus, Gert's nucleus, is located ventrolateral to the dorsal horn cells of S1 to S2 and receives Aδ input from the bladder. Ascending projections from here reach to the periaqueductal gray (PAG) area in the mesencephalon. Both Aδ and unmyelinated C fibers provide the majority of this sensory innervation. Detrusor proprioceptive endings (Aδ fibers) exist as nerve endings in collagen bundles. They are stimulated by stretch or contraction and are responsible for the feeling of bladder fullness. Pain and temperature nerve endings (C fibers) are free in bladder mucosa and submucosa.

Afferent nerves are influenced by transient receptor potentials (TRPs), transmembrane cation channels that influence cytosolic ion concentration, mainly calcium and magnesium, as well as affecting other intracellular pathways. These channels have been divided into six subfamilies, with each subfamily having several unique channels. These channels are affected by many different stimuli (both chemical and physical) and play a major role in afferent activity, including detection and integration of noxious stimuli. They achieve this by a dual mechanism whereby their intracellular actions (cation concentrations) are combined with a second mechanism of influencing neurotransmitter release. Activation of C fibers plays a major role in bladder inflammation and overactivity and in conditions where C fiber neuroplastic changes have taken place. Purinergic receptor stimulation (chemical, C fiber) in an animal model enhances the spinal neuronal activity already seen with intravesical filling (Aδ physical stretch), and intravesical adenosine triphosphate (ATP) has been shown to stimulate detrusor overactivity. Purinergic signaling is also involved in the voiding reflex, as studies have shown that altered purinergic receptor expression is found in patients with detrusor overactivity.

Other neurotransmitters involved with bladder sensation include ATP, adenosine, nitric oxide (NO), vasoactive intestinal polypeptide, substance P, and pituitary adenylate cyclase–activating peptide. Some of these act simply as neurotransmitters, but others like NO are also released from the urothelium and act as modulators and messengers. The complex interactions of these neurotransmitters are still being investigated, but their role in conditions involving bladder pain may help influence future therapies (Fig. 3.2).

CENTRAL NERVOUS SYSTEM MODULATION

CNS neurons affecting bladder function may be spinal or supraspinal, with extensive dendritic communications. The chief excitatory neurotransmitter in the CNS is glutamate, frequently acting on *n*-methyl-D-aspartate receptors. The chief inhibitory CNS neurotransmitters are γ-aminobutyric acid (GABA) and glycine.

The detrusor and the periurethral striated muscle mechanisms have separate cortical and other higher-center regulation pathways. The higher centers chiefly affect the brainstem for the detrusor, whereas they act on the sacral cord for the periurethral mechanisms. The brain pathways known to be associated with bladder and pelvic floor activity include cortical pathways originating in the precentral gyrus, lateral prefrontal cortex, and anterior cingulate gyrus (ACG). Subcortical pathways originate in basal ganglia, brainstem raphe nuclei, locus ceruleus,

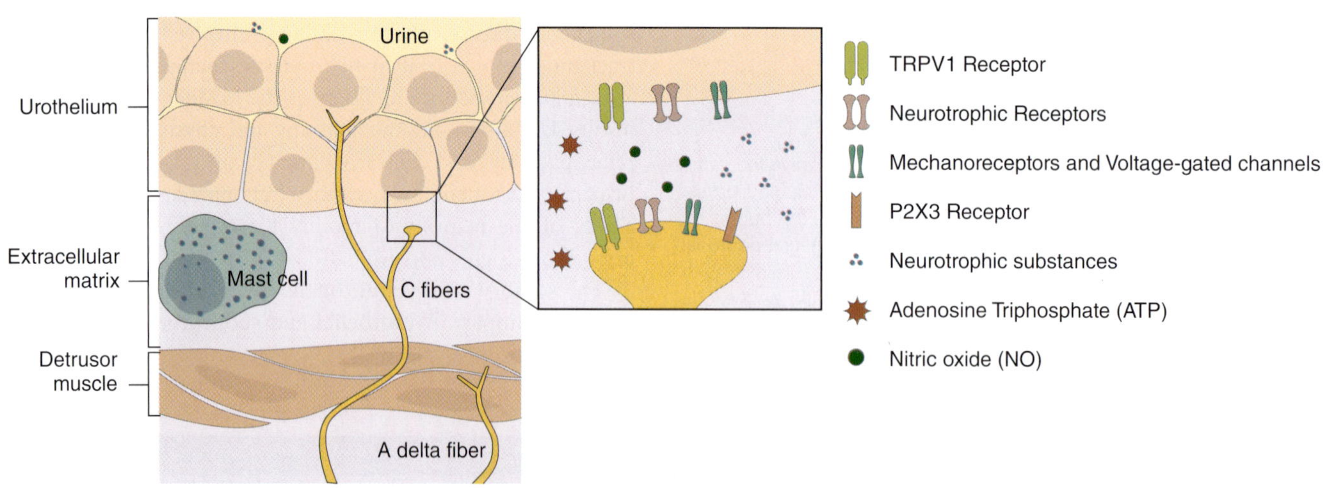

Fig. 3.2 Afferent signaling in the bladder wall. The urothelium "network," as well as the Aδ and C fibers, play roles and communicate. Receptors such as TRPV1 and other neurotrophic and mechanoreceptors respond to potential neurotrophins in the surrounding matrix. Neurotrophins may be produced by mast cells, detrusor cells, or the urothelium itself, which perpetuate the stimulation and contraction of the detrusor muscle (via purinergic receptors; see Fig. 3.6). The afferent fibers can also demonstrate maladaptive neuroplasticity and increase production of receptors, leading to hypersensitivity.

hypothalamus, and the midbrain PAG, and affect the brainstem, specifically the pontine micturition center (PMC), and lateral pons. Extensive communication takes place with all these structures to control storage and voiding.

Cortical and Subcortical Pathways

The brainstem's importance in lower urinary tract function has been known since 1921, when Barrington ablated this area in cats and produced permanent urinary retention. He demonstrated that the middle pons was the brain level from which bladder motor tone arises. This region in the pons has been called the pontine micturition center or the M region. Stimulation results in a decrease in urethral pressure and silence of pelvic floor electromyographic signal, followed by a rise in detrusor pressure (Fig. 3.3). Tracing studies reveal direct projections from the M region to the intermediolateral cell column of the sacral cord and the parasympathetic preganglionic bladder motor neurons. Other projections are to sacral cord interneurons that activate GABA inhibition of Onuf's nucleus neurons, resulting in relaxation of urethral skeletal muscle. The detrusor motor nuclei in the pons receive input from basal ganglia and coordinating afferents from the cerebellum and the PAG. The PAG then communicates with the M region to stimulate micturition. In addition to these important supraspinal tracts, there is evidence that spinal reflexes may also facilitate voiding. Electrical stimulation of urethral afferents can stimulate detrusor activity in spinal cord patients. This reflex has been postulated to augment bladder emptying by being activated when urine enters the urethra. Table 3.2 summarizes several important regions in the CNS involved in urine storage and voiding.

Stimulation of the same level of the pons at a more lateral position, the L region, results in contraction of the urethral sphincter by fibers originating from Onuf's nucleus (neuronal cell bodies for the urethral sphincter and other pelvic floor muscles located in the lateral aspect of the anterior horn of the gray matter of the sacral spinal cord from S2 to S4). Direct cortical relay to the L region gives voluntary micturition control. These brainstem activities, which are important for continence (L region) and micturition (M region) in adults, are replaced by reemerging pathologic primitive reflexes in disease states. Most important in this respect is the C fiber–mediated reflex that emerges following disconnection from pontine regulatory influences as a consequence of spinal cord disease. These effects are mediated by sensory neurotransmitters that are prompted

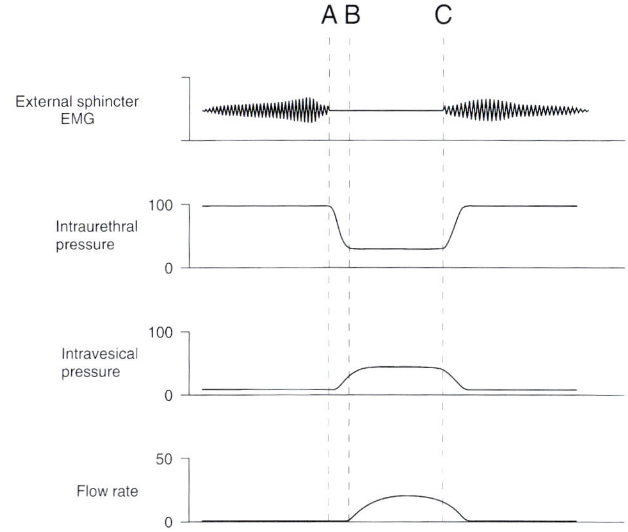

Fig. 3.3 Urodynamic representation of normal female micturition. **A**, Voluntary initiation of voiding with relaxation of external urethral sphincter and pelvic floor muscles and associated decrease in urethral pressure. **B**, Detrusor contraction occurs with increase in intravesical pressure; intraurethral pressure equals intravesical pressure, and urine flow is initiated. **C**, Voluntary termination of voiding. *EMG,* electromyography. (From Walters MD. Mechanisms of continence and voiding, with International Continence Society classification of dysfunction. *Obstet Gynecol Clin North Am.* 1989;16:773. With permission.)

TABLE 3.2 Selected Central Nervous System Structures Involved in Bladder Storage and Voiding

Structure	Location/Function
PAG	• Located in the midbrain and known for its role in pain modulation
	• Receives input from the distension receptors in the bladder via fibers ascending from Gert's nucleus
	• Relays neural signal to regions in the cerebral cortex, anterior cingulate gyrus, and prefrontal cortex and regulates output from these centers to the M region of the PMC
PMC	• Located in the dorsal pons; axons from the PMC synapse in the intermediolateral cell column on parasympathetic preganglionic motor neurons, which innervate the postganglionic neurons in the bladder wall
	• Activation of this pathway results in contraction of the bladder detrusor muscle
	• Facilitates external urethral sphincter relaxation by making contact with inhibitory sacral interneurons (via the neurotransmitters GABA and glycine), which project to motor neurons of the external urethral sphincter located in Onuf's nucleus to stimulate relaxation
Onuf's nucleus	• Neuronal cell bodies for the urethral sphincter and for the distal periurethral striated muscles and pelvic floor muscles
	• Found in the lateral aspect of the anterior horn of the gray matter of the sacral spinal cord from S2 to S4
	• Gives rise to the pudendal nerve
Gert's nucleus	• Located ventrolateral to the dorsal horn cells of S1-S2
	• Received Aδ input from the bladder
	• Projects to the PAG
Anterior cingulate gyrus/cortex	• Surrounds frontal corpus callosum
	• Abnormally activated in urgency incontinence

PAG, Periaqueductal gray; *PMC,* pontine micturition center; *GABA,* γ-aminobutyric acid.

to appear by nerve growth factors. Similar development of C fiber–afferentation is seen with bladder outlet obstruction and with bladder inflammatory states. In addition, with spinal cord injury it appears that the C fibers become sensitized to mechanical distension, a role reserved for Aδ fibers in the normal bladder. This leads to further activation of primitive, ineffective voiding reflexes, which are also modulated by TRP channels acting on the sensory side.

The basal ganglia are associated with the production of dopamine, one of the catecholamine neurotransmitters that is largely inhibitory to bladder activity. Nearly 75% of patients with decreased dopamine resulting from Parkinson disease have slowness of movement, gait disturbance, and tremor, as well as bladder overactivity. Serotonin (5-HT; from the raphe nuclei) acts to inhibit reflex bladder and pelvic nerve activity by suppressing afferent bladder information. The sympathetic autonomic nuclei and the sphincter motor nuclei also receive a serotonergic input from the raphe nucleus. Fibers from the raphe nuclei of the reticular formation may moderate responsiveness to different phases of the sleep–wake cycle or emotional states.

The locus ceruleus is the brainstem's CNS container of norepinephrine cell bodies. Norepinephrine acts to tonically facilitate continence-related reflexes.

The hypothalamus and midbrain PAG are activated during micturition. The anterior hypothalamus and PAG project to the pons M region and can induce bladder contraction via pontine parasympathetic pathways, whereas the posterior hypothalamus has sympathetic inhibitory pathways. The hypothalamus function, although poorly delineated, is known to involve β-endorphin neurotransmitters. Interneurons in the lumbosacral cord project strongly to the PAG, which in turn projects to the pons M region, thus making the PAG an important component in bladder reflex activities.

Pudendal cortical pathways affect periurethral striated muscle innervation by direct descending paths. At this level, the pudendal motor nuclei act as described to affect lower urinary tract skeletal muscle activity.

The limbic system in the temporal lobes exerts controls affecting all autonomic functions and is a favored site for epileptiform activity. Enkephalin is a notable neurotransmitter here as well as in the reticular formation. The cerebellum, where GABA is prominent along with standard neurotransmitters, regulates muscle tone and coordinates movement. Disease in this area produces spontaneous, high-amplitude detrusor overactivity.

The ACG and the prefrontal cortex have rich communications with the brainstem areas concerned with lower urinary tract function. Imaging studies show increased activity of the ACG during filling and voiding. It projects heavily to the PAG, which in turn connects to the M region in the pons. Depending on the area affected within the ACG, lesions may lead to bladder overactivity. The prefrontal cortex is thought to play a major role in volitional voiding and deciding the social appropriateness of voiding. Lesions here lead to inappropriate bladder overactivity and voiding.

There has been increased interest in neural circuits, as opposed to isolated centers of cortical brain activity, as they relate to the process of bladder filling, storage, and voiding. This has led to a number of studies intended to better characterize the connectivity to support the integrity of these circuits as they relate to bladder function. Functional MRI studies in continent women demonstrate activation of a large number of brain regions that change significantly between full versus empty bladder in regions including the medial frontal gyrus, posterior cingulate, inferolateral temporal and postcentral gyrus, amygdala, and caudate. In women with incontinence, very few regions show different levels of activation when the bladder is full versus when it is empty. The changes in functional connectivity when the bladder is full suggest that there is a central process responsible for control in the full bladder state, and that this relies on how brain systems are functionally integrated.

Spinal Cord

By adolescence, disparity in growth of the spinal cord and the vertebral column leads to the cord terminating around the first lumbar vertebra (Fig. 3.1). The adult conus medullaris is quite short and contains the entire S1 to S5 segment. Because the spinal cord terminates well above the respective segmental foramina, the cauda equina describes the terminal ventral and dorsal nerve roots as they travel through the spinal canal to exit. The cauda equina is subject to various spinal pathologies, including lumbar disc disease, trauma, tethered cord, and spinal stenosis. Although the thoracolumbar levels are important in sympathetic autonomic influence of the lower urinary tract, the conus medullaris has greater significance, because autonomic detrusor nuclei and pudendal somatic nuclei are housed in the intermediolateral and ventromedial anterior gray matter, respectively. The conus medullaris also houses neurons involved with defecation and sexual function, with relays for cortical separation of these visceral functions (encephalization) developing after birth.

BLADDER FILLING AND STORAGE

The autonomic nervous system controls the lower urinary tract by its actions on the ganglia, detrusor muscle, and smooth muscle of the trigone and urethra. The storage of urine in the bladder relies strongly on activation of sympathetic activity and inhibition of parasympathetic activity. The main neural pathways involved in bladder filling and voiding are summarized in Fig. 3.4 and 3.5.

Three sympathetic neural responses to afferent pelvic nerve firing associated with increasing bladder volume have been demonstrated experimentally: (1) β-receptor–mediated relaxation of the detrusor musculature; (2) α-receptor–mediated increase in urethral smooth muscle activity and urethral pressure; and (3) inhibition of ganglionic transmission in the pelvic (vesical) ganglia, which, in effect, inhibits sacral parasympathetic outflow to the bladder. These actions are illustrated in (Fig. 3.4).

Somatic activation of the lower urinary tract outlet is regulated by afferent pelvic nerve spinal reflexes that keep tonic resistance to the urethra so that urethral pressure is greater than detrusor pressure. Cortical tracts to the urethra and tracts involving the L region of the pons also take part in the voluntary assistance to storage.

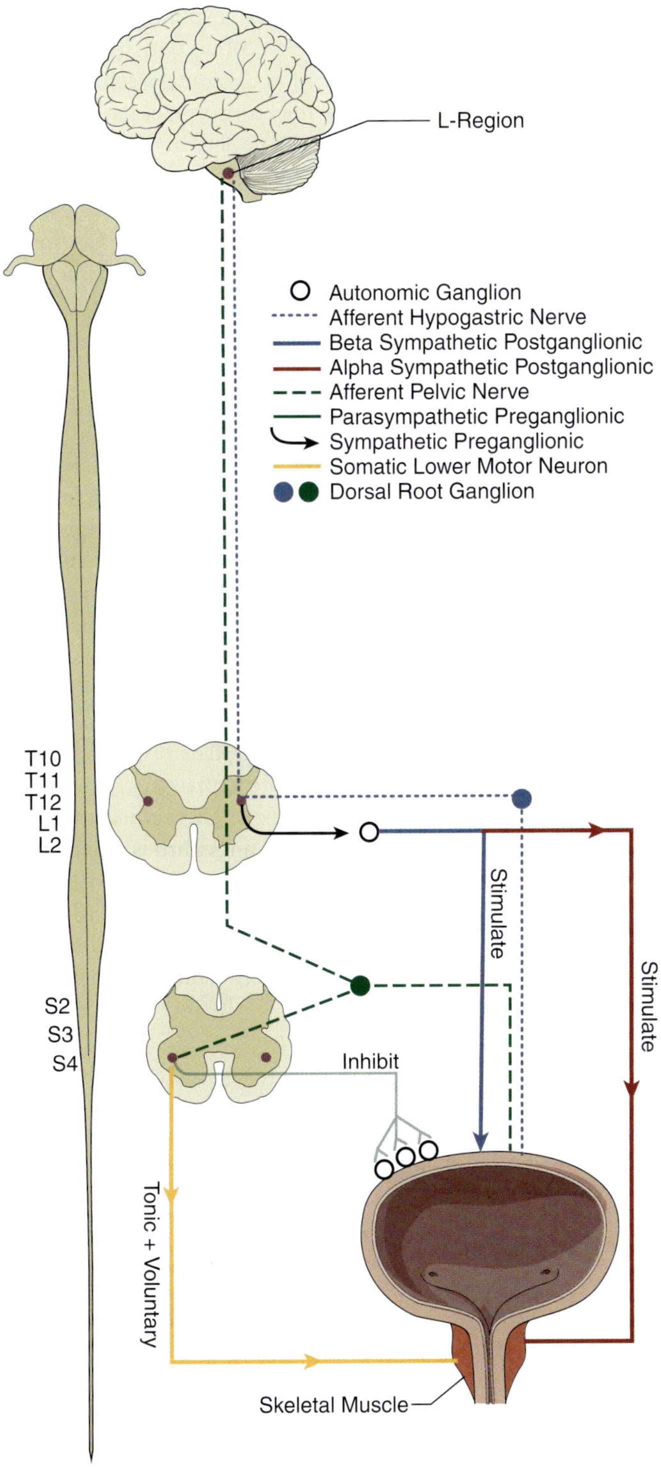

Fig. 3.4 Summary of major neurologic pathways involved in bladder storage. Bladder distention results in afferent pelvic nerve discharge. After synapse in the pudendal nucleus, efferent pudendal nerve impulses result in contraction of the external urethral sphincter. At the same time, afferent sympathetic discharges traverse the hypogastric nerve and further ascend to the L region in the pons. After synapse in sympathetic nuclei, efferent firing causes (1) inhibition of transmission of postganglionic parasympathetic neuron, which inhibits detrusor contraction, and (2) increased tone at the bladder neck. The net effect is that urethral pressure remains greater than detrusor pressure, facilitating urine storage.

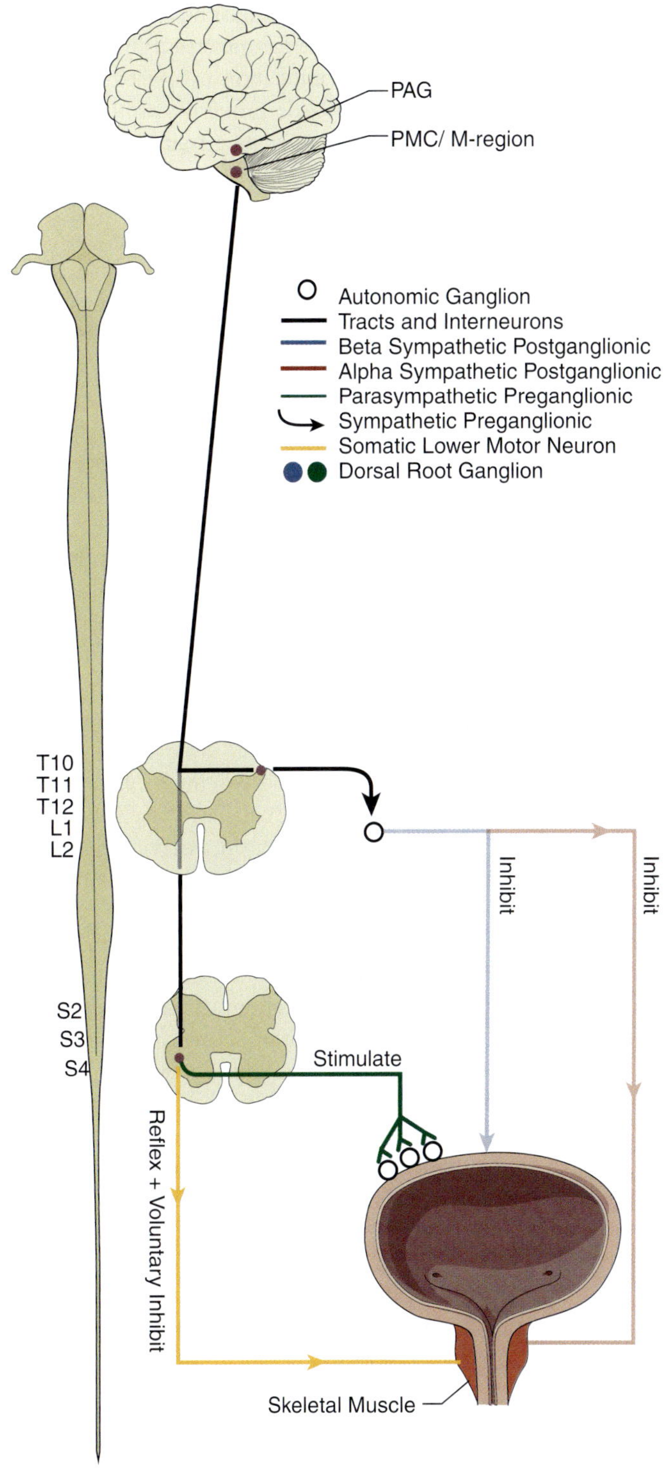

Fig. 3.5 Summary of major neurologic pathways involved in voiding. Descending efferent pathways from the pontine micturition center cause (1) inhibition of pudendal firing, which relaxes the external sphincter, (2) inhibition of sympathetic firing, which opens the bladder neck and permits postganglionic parasympathetic transmission, and (3) pelvic parasympathetic firing, which causes detrusor contraction. The net result is that relaxation of the external sphincter causes a decrease in urethral pressure, followed by detrusor contraction, and voiding ensues. The interneurons and ascending tracts provide feedback until voiding is complete. *PAG,* Periaqueductal gray; *PMC,* pontine micturition center.

During physiologic bladder filling, little or no increase in intravesical pressure is observed, despite large increases in urine volume. This process, called accommodation, is caused primarily by the passive elastic and viscoelastic properties of the smooth muscle and connective tissue of the bladder wall. During filling, muscle bundles in the bladder wall undergo reorganization, and the muscle cells elongate to up to four times their original length. As bladder filling progresses, at a certain bladder wall tension, a desire to void is felt, although it has not been determined where this sensation is processed in the brain. Mechanoreceptors in the bladder wall are activated (Aδ fibers), and action potentials run with afferents following parasympathetic pelvic nerves to the spinal cord at the S2 to S4 and with afferents following sympathetic nerves to the thoracolumbar cord. As filling increases to a critical intravesical pressure, or with rapid bladder filling, detrusor muscle contractility is inhibited, and urethral sphincter muscle activity is enhanced by activation of a spinal sympathetic reflex.

The sympathetic preganglionic fibers from the thoracolumbar spine synapse in the paravertebral or prevertebral sympathetic pathways. Preganglionic neurons reach the inferior mesenteric ganglia by the lumbar splanchnic nerves. After synapse they continue as postganglionic nerves through the hypogastric nerves to the presacral fascia, across the upper posterior lateral pelvic wall, within 1 to 2 cm of the ureter.

After these fibers join the pelvic nerves, the pelvic plexus is formed, running medial to the internal iliac vessels overlying the anterior lateral lower rectum near the anorectal junction. The plexus spreads in the lateral wall of the upper one third of the vagina beneath the uterine artery, medial to the ureter and 2 cm inferolateral to the cervix. Within the vesicovaginal space, the plexus supplies the upper vagina, bladder, proximal urethra, and lower ureter. Sympathetic preganglionic neurons generally use the acetylcholine neurotransmitter acting on nicotinic receptors. The sympathetic postganglionic fibers are primarily noradrenergic, with norepinephrine being the chief neurotransmitter. Norepinephrine stimulation of β3-adrenergic receptors located in the bladder body causes relaxation of the smooth muscle. Stimulation of α_1 receptors in bladder base and urethral smooth muscle by norepinephrine causes muscle contraction. In addition, norepinephrine also acts as a neurotransmitter at the parasympathetic ganglia, and α-adrenergic receptors, when stimulated, depress parasympathetic pelvic ganglion transmission by suppression of presynaptic cholinergic neurotransmitter release.

Thus, sympathetic relaxation of detrusor body smooth muscle, contraction of bladder base and urethral smooth muscle, and depression of parasympathetic ganglionic transmission all act to promote urine storage.

VOIDING

Voiding is largely a parasympathetic event. Fig. 3.5 presents a summary of the major neurologic pathways involved in voiding.

Normal voiding is a voluntary act involving reflex-coordinated relaxation of the urethra and sustained contraction of the bladder until emptying is complete. In healthy women, the micturition reflex is probably not a simple segmental sacral reflex, but rather is modulated supraspinally in the PMC. Voluntary control of the micturition reflex is mediated by connections between the prefrontal cerebral cortex and the pons. Voluntary control of the external urethral sphincter is via the corticospinal pathway connecting the frontal cortex with Onuf's nucleus in the ventral horn of the sacral spinal cord. Under normal circumstances, voiding is likely controlled voluntarily by complex interactions among cortical areas (prefrontal cortex), subcortical areas (thalamus, hypothalamus, basal ganglia, and limbic system), and the brainstem (mesencephalic-pontine-medullary reticular formation).

With filling to bladder capacity, stimuli from the bladder cause afferent discharges that traverse pathways in the spinal cord to synapse largely in the PAG. Voiding is initiated voluntarily or when the bladder volume is so large that it is no longer possible to suppress micturition. To initiate voiding, the external urethral sphincter relaxes voluntarily via inhibition of somatic motor neurons from the ventral horn. Efferent impulses from the PMC run in the descending tracts to inhibit pudendal firing (relaxing the external sphincter) and to stimulate parasympathetic neurons at levels S2 to S4, causing detrusor contraction. During voiding, sympathetic efferents are inhibited, which opens the bladder neck and permits postganglionic parasympathetic transmission. The micturition reflex depends upon activation of glutamate receptors and is modulated by serotonergic and noradrenergic systems of brainstem that tend to support storage reflexes. Fight-or-flight situations affect micturition via 5-hydroxytryptamine (5-HT) and norepinephrine modulation. Aδ afferents, activated by stretch, travel to the PAG to constitute a spinobulbospinal reflex. The efferent arm from the PMC activates sacral parasympathetic neurons that travel to the pelvic nerve, with acetylcholine neurotransmitters acting on M_2 and M_3 receptors, and via interneuron GABA activity inhibiting Onuf's nucleus.

Intravesical pressure is increased by a highly controlled coordinated contraction of the bulk of the detrusor muscle. Descent and funneling of the bladder neck and proximal urethra occur, and urine flow begins. Afferent feedback from the urethra to the spinal cord when urine enters the proximal urethra further augments bladder contraction to complete emptying.

Brainstem modulation of the micturition reflex allows for a detrusor contraction long enough to completely evacuate intravesical contents. With voluntary termination of voiding or with the stop test, the striated muscles of the urethra and pelvic floor contract to elevate the bladder base, increase intraurethral pressure, and empty the urethra of urine. The detrusor muscle is reflexively inhibited, and intravesical pressure returns to normal.

The parasympathetic preganglionic fibers arise from nerve roots S3 and S4 and, occasionally, S2, with the cell bodies being in the sacral cord, the conus medullaris. These fibers emerge from the piriformis muscle overlying the sacral foramina and enter the presacral fascia near the ischial spine at the posterior layer of the hypogastric sheath forming the pelvic nerve, where they then contribute to the already described pelvic plexus. The pelvic plexus has freely interconnected nerves in the pelvic fascia that supply the rectum, genitalia, and lower urinary tract. The parasympathetic fibers to the urinary tract terminate in ganglia located within the wall of the bladder, a location quite vulnerable to end-organ disease, such as overstretch, infection, or fibrosis. At the ganglia, excitatory transmission occurs from activation of nicotinic receptors, with some ganglionic cells having secondary muscarinic receptors. Multiple neuropeptide agents also function at these ganglia, including those that modulate adrenergic, purinergic, and peptidergic activity.

At the detrusor muscle, postganglionic parasympathetic detrusor nerve fibers release one of two neurotransmitters. The chief neurotransmitter is cholinergic, with muscarinic receptors, and a second major neurotransmitter is noncholinergic and nonadrenergic. ATP is a major mediator of these noncholinergic, nonadrenergic contractions.

Muscarinic receptors are present in the CNS, eye lacrimal glands, salivary glands, heart, gallbladder, stomach, and colon. Five types ($M_{1–5}$) have been identified. In detrusor muscle, M_2 and M_3 predominate. Although there are more detrusor M_2 receptors, the M_3 receptors have a more direct positive impact on detrusor contractions (Fig. 3.6). Generalized inhibition of these receptors can lead to dry mouth, slowed gastrointestinal motility, blurred vision, increased heart rate, heat intolerance, sedation with reductions in memory and attention, delirium, drowsiness, fatigue, and impairment of other cognitive functions. Theoretically, anticholinergic medications more selective for M_3 receptors should have more therapeutic effects against bladder overactivity with fewer side effects; this has yet to be clearly demonstrated in clinical trials.

Cholinergic receptors are more present in the body than in the base of the bladder, whereas adrenergic and neuropeptide receptors are more prevalent in the base of the bladder. Neuropeptide modulators include vasoactive intestinal polypeptide and substance P. Histaminic and purinergic receptors may also be present in detrusor smooth muscle.

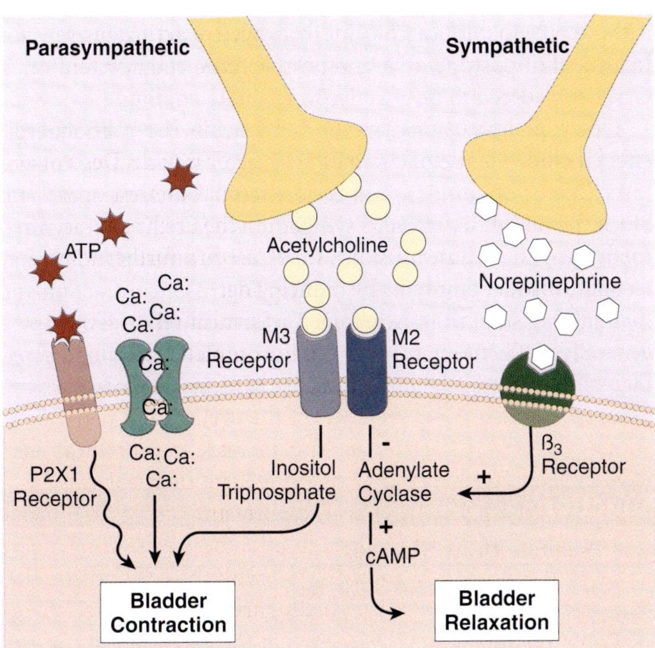

Fig. 3.6 Muscarinic and β-3 receptor involvement in detrusor contraction and relaxation. Acetylcholine from parasympathetic fibers interacts with M3 receptors, leading to detrusor contraction. When acetylcholine interacts with M2 receptors, adenylate cyclase activity is inhibited, which decreases bladder relaxation facilitated by stimulation of β-3 receptors, which produce the opposite effect. In pathologic situations, adenosine triphosphate can stimulate purinergic receptors and lead to detrusor contractions. *ATP,* Adenosine triphosphate.

INNERVATION OF LOWER URINARY TRACT OUTLET

Smooth Muscle of Trigone and Urethra

The innervation of the trigone smooth muscle fibers is an almost exclusively adrenergic innervation, with chiefly α_1 receptors. Cholinergic development in the bladder is present at birth, whereas adrenergic development occurs later.

The proximal urethral smooth muscle is rich in α-adrenergic receptors responsive to norepinephrine neurotransmitter. Acetylcholine, substance P, vasoactive intestinal polypeptide, and histamine are all additional potential transmitters in the urethra. NO is prominent in the parasympathetic postganglionic innervation of the urethra, and exogenous NO or parasympathetic nerve stimulation relaxes urethral smooth muscle.

Skeletal Muscle of Lower Urinary Tract: Somatic Innervation

In the lower urinary tract, the somatic system involves skeletal muscle in the lower urinary tract outlet. Neurons from Onuf's nucleus gives rise to the pudendal nerve, which is classically thought to provide the efferent innervation of the striated sphincter. 5-HT and norepinephrine enhance the effects of glutamate, the primary excitatory neurotransmitter for pudendal motor neurons. This is the proposed mechanism of action of duloxetine (a 5-HT–norepinephrine reuptake inhibitor) in treating stress incontinence. The pudendal nerve, using acetylcholine, activates nicotinic cholinergic receptors to contract the rhabdosphincter. The α motor neurons of Onuf's nucleus are unique in many ways: neuronal cell body size, location, and resistance to polio and amyotrophic lateral sclerosis.

The exact neuropathways supplying the urethral sphincter skeletal muscle are controversial. The proximal intramural component of the striated urogenital sphincter muscle (urethral sphincter, rhabdosphincter) is variably innervated by somatic efferent branches of the pelvic nerves, a component of the pelvic plexus. However, the more distal periurethral striated muscles (compressor urethrae and urethrovaginal sphincter) are innervated by the pudendal nerve, as is the skeletal muscle of the external anal sphincter and perineal muscles.

Typically, somatic motor activity regulates skeletal muscle contraction by spinal reflexes, with the afferent arm of the reflex originating in muscle spindles, synapses taking place in the spinal cord, and the efferent arm originating in anterior horn cells with the axon going to the muscle. Unlike typical somatic reflex pathways that are regulated by sensory nerves from muscle spindles, the afferent regulation of the urethral sphincter somatic reflex is different, because urethral skeletal muscle has no spindles.

The urethral sphincter muscle is an integral part of the urethral wall and is made up of all slow-twitch (type 1) fibers. The periurethral muscles (compressor urethrae and urethrovaginal sphincter) are composed of mostly slow-twitch fibers with a variable concentration of fast-twitch (type 2) fibers. These fibers combine to provide constant tonus, with emergency reflex activity mainly in the distal half of the urethra.

The segmental spinal reflex response leading to pudendal nerve function involves several spinal cord segments. Afferent fibers involved in the reflex have both segmental and supraspinal routing. This dual routing explains the bimodal response of pudendal motor neurons when pudendal sensory nerves are stimulated, and it differs from stimulation of pelvic detrusor afferents.

The neurotransmitter at the periurethral skeletal neuromuscular junction is acetylcholine, and the receptors are nicotinic type. The intimate adherence of the neuromuscular junction to the striated muscle fibers conveys a resistance to blockade by neuromuscular blocking agents.

CLINICAL PHARMACOLOGY OF THE LOWER URINARY TRACT

Thorough understanding of the neurologic control of the urinary bladder and its outlet allows one to intelligently use pharmacologic agents to manage many types of lower urinary tract dysfunction. More specific guidelines for pharmacologic treatments of various lower urinary tract complaints and reviews of the clinical studies using these agents are found in other chapters.

Most pharmacologic agents produce their effects by combining with cell receptors. The drug–receptor interaction initiates a series of biochemical and physiologic changes that characterize the effects produced by the agent. In general, drugs alter lower urinary tract function by affecting synthesis, transport, storage, and release of the neurotransmitter; the combination of the neurotransmitter with postjunctional receptors; or the inactivation, degradation, or reuptake of the neurotransmitter. The pharmacologic effects on other organ systems are responsible for many of the unwanted side effects of these agents. Clinically, pharmacologic agents can be grouped into those that facilitate bladder emptying and those that facilitate urine storage (Table 3.3). Patients with disorders of bladder emptying have voiding dysfunction; theoretically, drugs that improve bladder emptying would do so by increasing bladder contractility or by decreasing outlet resistance. Patients with disorders of urine storage often present with urinary frequency, urgency, or urinary incontinence (stress and/or urgency). Agents that facilitate urine storage act by inhibiting bladder contractility—thereby increasing bladder capacity—by increasing outlet resistance or by reducing sensation or afferent input necessary to trigger voiding. The most effective and commonly used agents act on either the parasympathetic or sympathetic systems.

THERAPY TO FACILITATE BLADDER EMPTYING

Increasing Intravesical Pressure

A major portion of the final common pathway in a physiologic bladder contraction is stimulation of the muscarinic receptor sites at the postganglionic, parasympathetic neuromuscular junction. Parasympathetic nerve stimulation causes the release of acetylcholine at postsynaptic, parasympathetic receptor sites. Acetylcholine release produces muscarinic and nicotinic effects; one of the muscarinic effects is contraction of the detrusor muscle and relaxation of the trigone. Acetylcholine itself cannot be used for therapeutic purposes because of actions at central and ganglionic levels and because of its rapid hydrolysis by acetylcholinesterase and nonspecific cholinesterase. Bethanechol chloride exhibits a selective acetylcholine-like action on the urinary bladder and gut, with little or no action at therapeutic dosages on ganglia or the cardiovascular system. Bethanechol chloride is cholinesterase-resistant and causes a contraction of smooth muscle from the bladder, bladder neck, and urethra, thus preventing coordinated and complete bladder emptying. Although bethanechol chloride had been used extensively for treatment of postoperative and postpartum urinary retention, it is not considered to be effective to facilitate voiding.

Other pharmacologic methods of achieving a cholinergic effect include the use of cholinesterase agents, dopamine antagonists (metoclopramide), and α-adrenergic blocking agents (to block the inhibitory effect of sympathetics on pelvic parasympathetic ganglionic transmission). In addition, prostaglandins may facilitate bladder emptying by inducing detrusor contraction and maintaining smooth muscle tone. Unfortunately, drug therapy is generally ineffective in causing detrusor contraction and improving voiding, especially in the presence of neurogenic disease.

TABLE 3.3 Drug Effects on Lower Urinary Tract Function

Therapy to Facilitate Bladder Emptying	Therapy to Facilitate Urine Storage
Increasing intravesical pressure/bladder contractility	Inhibiting bladder contractility/increasing bladder capacity
Parasympathomimetic agents, prostaglandins, blockers of inhibition, α-adrenergic antagonists, opioid antagonists	Antimuscarinic agents, anticholinergic agents, β-adrenergic agonists, prostaglandin inhibitors, tricyclic antidepressants, botulinum A toxin, potassium channel openers
Decreasing outlet resistance at the level of the smooth sphincter	Increasing outlet resistance
β-adrenergic agonists, α-adrenergic antagonists	α-adrenergic agonists, tricyclic antidepressants, SNRI, β-adrenergic antagonists, estrogen, β-adrenergic agonists
At the level of the striated sphincter	Afferent nerve inhibitors/decreasing sensory input
Skeletal muscle relaxants, centrally acting relaxants, botulinum A toxin, dantrolene, baclofen, α-adrenergic antagonists	Botulinum A toxin, local anesthetics, dimethyl sulfoxide, vanilloid receptor agonists

SNRI, Serotonin–norepinephrine reuptake inhibitor.

Decreasing Outlet Resistance

The lower urinary tract has α- and β-adrenergic receptor sites, the functions of which have been discussed. Facilitation of bladder emptying could be achieved by the use of α-adrenergic antagonists, which decrease outlet resistance by smooth muscle relaxation of the bladder neck and proximal urethra. Some investigators have suggested that these agents may also affect striated sphincter tone. α-sympathetic blocking agents have thus been used to treat both smooth sphincter dyssynergia and detrusor-striated sphincter dyssynergia.

Botulinum A toxin, a substance that inhibits acetylcholine release from cholinergic nerve terminals, is a presynaptic neuromuscular blocking agent that induces selective and reversible muscle weakness for up to several months when injected intramuscularly in minute quantities. Other potential indications for botulinum A toxin include detrusor-sphincter dyssynergia, motor and sensory urgency, and certain pain disorders. Botulinum A toxin appears to be effective to treat detrusor-sphincter dyssynergia when injected either transurethrally or transperineally into the external urethral sphincter.

THERAPY TO FACILITATE URINE STORAGE

Decreasing Bladder Contractility

Overactivity of the bladder during filling may present as involuntary detrusor contractions, decreased bladder compliance, and/or urgency with or without incontinence. The treatments of detrusor overactivity are discussed thoroughly in Chapters 31 and 32. Pharmacologic agents used to treat detrusor overactivity are directed toward inhibiting bladder contractility or decreasing sensory input during filling. Atropine and atropine-like agents depress detrusor overactivity of any cause by inhibiting muscarinic cholinergic receptor sites. Currently available anticholinergic agents include oxybutynin, tolterodine, fesoterodine, trospium chloride, solifenacin, and darifenacin. Direct instillation into the bladder has also been described. Efficacy for the treatment of overactive bladder is similar among these agents, although their side effect profiles may differ somewhat. This is likely owing, at least in part, to their differing selectivity for muscarinic receptor subtypes, and thus they have different effects on the body in addition to their actions on the bladder. Oxybutynin has moderate selectivity for M_3 over M_2, M_4, and M_5 receptors but greater affinity for M_3 and M_1 receptors. Tolterodine, fesoterodine, and trospium chloride have only modest selectivity for one type of muscarinic receptor compared with another. Solifenacin, like oxybutynin, is more selective for M_1 and M_3 receptors over other types, and darifenacin shows the highest selectivity for M_3 receptors. The impact of these differences in receptor selectivity is probably responsible for some of the differences between drugs in rates of dry mouth, slowed gastrointestinal motility, blurred vision, heart rate changes, and sedation.

Patients can also have reductions in memory and attention, delirium, drowsiness, and fatigue, and these changes are partially attributed to the drug's relative ability to cross the blood–brain barrier. Blood–brain barrier permeability increases with age, stress, and certain diseases. All five receptor subtypes are expressed in the brain. M_1 is predominant in the forebrain and hippocampus (working memory and inhibition), M_2 affects flexibility and memory, and M_3 and M_5 affect learning. Darifenacin is more selective for M_3 and least likely to block M_1. Oxybutynin has small molecular weight, high lipophilicity, and neutral polarity, making it more likely to cross the barrier than larger, less lipophilic, polarized drugs, such as darifenacin, tolterodine, and trospium. Trospium is a quaternary amine that is also less lipophilic and less likely to cross the blood–brain barrier in patients where CNS side effects are of concern.

Tricyclic antidepressants, particularly imipramine hydrochloride, have prominent systemic anticholinergic effects, weak antimuscarinic effects on bladder smooth muscle, antihistaminic effects, and local anesthetic properties. Imipramine also appears to increase bladder outlet resistance by a peripheral blockade of noradrenaline uptake. Thus, it may be effective for the treatment of urine storage disorders by both decreasing bladder contractility and increasing outlet resistance.

Injections of botulinum A toxin into the detrusor muscle were first tested to treat neurogenic detrusor overactivity in spinal cord–injured patients and in children with myelomeningocele. Excellent results from injecting this agent into the detrusor in the context of neurogenic detrusor overactivity led to an expansion of this treatment to incontinence owing to idiopathic detrusor overactivity. Dosages from 100 to 200 units of onabotulinum toxin A are used, and treatment can be individualized.

Several intravesical treatment options to treat neurogenic detrusor overactivity have been attempted. These treatments either act on the afferent arc of the reflex, such as local anesthetics or vanilloid, or on the efferent cholinergic transmission to the detrusor muscle, such as intravesical oxybutynin or botulinum-A toxin. TRP vanilloid receptor agonists reduce sensation or afferent input that is necessary to trigger micturition. These drugs include capsaicin and resiniferatoxin (RTX). RTX is a pungent substance from a cactus that is 1000 times more potent than capsaicin in interacting with vanilloid receptors to excite and then desensitize afferent nerves, particularly C fiber or bladder afferents, and is much less painful than capsaicin for bladder injection. These drugs might raise the volume threshold for micturition and are potentially useful for pain disorders and overactive bladder, with or without urgency incontinence. Clinical application of these substances has been limited. Capsaicin has proven too painful for patient use, and problems with manufacturing RTX have not been overcome.

Other drugs that have been used to decrease bladder contractility include prostaglandin inhibitors and dimethyl sulfoxide. The overall clinical response has generally been small with these agents.

Promoting Bladder Storage

The β-adrenergic agonists offer an alternative solution to bladder overactivity. Rather than act on the contractility (acetylcholine receptors) side of the bladder by blocking receptors, and therefore contractions, β3 agonists promote urine storage by stimulating their receptors. Mirabegron, a β3 agonist, has been shown to be efficacious, with a different side-effect profile compared with anticholinergics, and is now approved for use in the United States.

Increasing Outlet Resistance

Because of the preponderance of α-adrenergic receptor sites in the bladder neck and proximal urethra, α-adrenergic agonists (such as pseudoephedrine and phenylephrine) have been used to produce urethral smooth muscle contraction, thereby increasing resting urethral pressure and resistance to outflow.

Duloxetine is a potent and balanced dual 5-HT–norepinephrine reuptake inhibitor that potentiates the physiologic actions of endogenous 5-HT and norepinephrine (by inhibiting the reuptake of these neurotransmitters in the presynaptic element), thereby enhancing the CNS continence control mechanisms. Duloxetine is believed to stimulate pudendal nerve motor output resulting from increased levels of 5-HT and norepinephrine in the pudendal motor nucleus. This appears to improve urethral closure pressure and urethral resistance. Although approved in Europe, duloxetine was withdrawn from further study in the United States.

Estrogens affect adrenergic nerves by influencing excitability, neuronal influences on the muscle, receptor density and sensitivity, and transmitter metabolism. The clinical use of estrogen is discussed in Chapter 10.

BIBLIOGRAPHY

Andrew J, Nathan PW. Lesions on the anterior frontal lobes and disturbances of micturation and defaecation. *Brain*. 1964;87:233.

Athwal BS, Berkley KJ, Hussain I, et al. Brain responses to changes in bladder volume and urge to void in healthy men. *Brain*. 2001;124:369.

Bacsu CD, Chan L, Tse V. Diagnosing detrusor sphincter dyssynergia in the neurological patient. *BJU Int*. 2012;109(suppl 3):31.

Barrington FJ. The nervous mechanism of micturition. *Q J Exp Physiol*. 1914;8:33.

Barrington FJ. The relation of the hind-brain to micturition. *Brain*. 1921;44:23.

Beck RP. Neuropharmacology of the lower urinary tract in women. *Obstet Gynecol Clin North Am*. 1989;16:753.

Bennett BC, Kruse MN, Roppolo JR, et al. Neural control of urethral outlet activity in vivo: role of nitric oxide. *J Urol*. 1995;153:2004.

Blaivas JG. The neurophysiology of micturition: a clinical study of 550 patients. *J Urol*. 1982;127:958.

Blaivas JG. Pathophysiology of lower urinary tract dysfunction. *Urol Clin North Am*. 1985;12:216.

Bradley WE. Cerebro-cortical innervation of the urinary bladder. *Tohoku J Exp Med*. 1980;131:7.

Bradley WE, Timm GW, Scott FB. Innervation of the detrusor muscle and urethra. *Urol Clin North Am*. 1974;1:3.

Burnstock G, Dumsday B, Smythe A. Atropine resistant excitation of the urinary bladder: the possibility of transmission via nerves releasing a purine nucleotide. *Br J Pharmacol*. 1972;44:451.

Cameron AP, Clemens JQ, Latini JM, McGuire EJ. Combination drug therapy improves compliance of the neurogenic bladder. *J Urol*. 2009;182:1062.

Cardozo L, Drutz HP, Baygani SK, Bump RC. Pharmacological treatment of women awaiting surgery for stress urinary incontinence. *Obstet Gynecol*. 2004;104:511.

Chancellor MB, de Groat WC. Intravesical capsaicin and resiniferatoxin therapy: spicing up ways to treat the overactive bladder. *J Urol*. 1999;162:3.

Cruz F. Mechanisms involved in new therapies for overactive bladder. *Urology*. 2004;63:65.

de Groat WC, Griffiths D, Yoshimura N. Neural control of the lower urinary tract. *Compr Physiol*. 2015;5:327.

de Groat WC. Integrative control of the lower urinary tract: preclinical perspective. *Br J Pharmacol*. 2006;147(suppl 2):S25.

de Groat WC, Booth AM, Krier J, et al. Neural control of the urinary bladder and large intestine. In: Brooks CM, Koizumi K, Sato A, eds. *Integrative Functions of the Autonomic Nervous System*. North Holland: Elsevier, Amsterdam, Biomedical Press; 1979.

de Groat WC, Lalley PM. Reflex firing in the lumbar sympathetic outflow to activation of vesical afferent fibres. *J Physiol*. 1972;226:289.

de Groat WC, Ryall RW. Recurrent inhibition in sacral parasympathetic pathways to the bladder. *J Physiol*. 1968;196:579.

de Groat WC, Saum WR. Sympathetic inhibition of the urinary bladder and of pelvic ganglionic transmission in the cat. *J Physiol*. 1972; 220:297.

de Groat WC, Theobald RJ. Reflex activation of sympathetic pathways to vesical smooth muscle and parasympathetic ganglia by electrical stimulation of vesical afferents. *J Physiol*. 1976;259:223.

de Groat WC, Yoshimura N. Pharmacology of the lower urinary tract. *Ann Rev Pharmacol Toxicol*. 2001;41:691.

Downie JW, Armour JA. Relation of afferent nerve activity in the pelvic plexus with pressure, length, and wall strain in the urinary bladder of the cat. *Soc Neurosci Abstr*. 1982;8:858.

Duffau H, Capelle L. Incontinence after brain glioma surgery: new insights into the cortical control of micturition and continence. Case report. *J Neurosurg*. 2005;102:148.

Edvardsen P. Changes in urinary-bladder motility following lesions in the nervous system in cats. *Acta Neurol Scand*. 1966;42:25.

Elbadawi A. Neuromorphologic basis of vesicourethral function. I. Histochemistry, ultrastructure, and function of intrinsic nerves of the bladder and urethra. *Neurourol Urodyn*. 1982;1:3.

Elbadawi A. Autonomic muscular innervation of the vesical outlet and its role in micturition. In Hinman Jr F, ed. *Benign Prostatic Hypertrophy*. New York: Springer-Verlag; 1983:330.

Finkbeiner A, Welch L, Bissada N. Uropharmacology. IX. Direct acting smooth muscle stimulants and depressants. *Urology*. 1978;12:128.

Fletcher TF, Bradley WE. Neuroanatomy of the bladder-urethra. *J Urol*. 1978;119:153.

Floyd K, Hick VE, Morrison JF. Mechanosensitive afferent units in the hypogastric nerve of the cat. *J Physiol*. 1976;259:457.

Fowler CJ, Griffiths D, de Groat WC. The neural control of micturition. *Nat Rev*. 2008;9:453.

Fowler CJ, Auerbach S, Ginsberg D, et al. OnabotulinumtoxinA improves health-related quality of life in patients with urinary incontinence due to idiopathic overactive bladder: a 36-week, double-blind, placebo-controlled, randomized, dose-ranging trial. *Eur Urol*. 2012;62:148.

Furuta A, Suzuki Y, Hayashi N, et al. Transient receptor potential A1 receptor-mediated neural cross-talk and afferent sensitization induced by oxidative stress: implication for the pathogenesis of interstitial cystitis/bladder pain syndrome. *Int J Urol*. 2012;19:429.

Gibson A. The influence of endocrine hormones on the autonomic nervous system. *J Auton Pharmacol*. 1981;1:331.

Gosling JA, Dixon JS. The structure and innervation of smooth muscle in the wall of the bladder neck and proximal urethra. *Br J Urol*. 1975;47:549.

Gosling JA, Dixon JS, Critchley HO. A comparative study of the human external sphincter and periurethral levator ani muscles. *Br J Urol*. 1981;53:35.

Griffiths D, Derbyshire S, Stenger A, Resnick N. Brain control of normal and overactive bladder. *J Urol*. 2005;174:1862.

Holstege G. Micturition and the soul. *J Comp Neurol.* 2005;493:15.
Holstege G, Kuypers HG, Boer RC. Anatomical evidence for direct brain stem projections to the somatic motoneuronal cell groups and autonomic preganglionic cell groups in cat spinal cord. *Brain Res.* 1979;171:329.
Huang YH, Bih LI, Chen GD, et al. Autonomic dysreflexia during urodynamic examinations in patients with suprasacral spinal cord injury. *Arch Phys Med Rehabil.* 2011;92:1450.
Ikeda Y, Zabbarova IV, Birder LA, et al. Botulinum neurotoxin serotype A suppresses neurotransmitter release from afferent as well as efferent nerves in the urinary bladder. *Eur Urol.* 2012;62:1157.
Ioanid CP, Noica N, Pop T. Incidence and diagnostic aspects of the bladder disorders in diabetics. *Eur Urol.* 1981;7:211.
Ikeda Y, Zabbarova I, Birder L, et al. Botulinum neurotoxin serotype A suppresses neurotransmitter release from afferent as well as efferent nerves in the urinary bladder. *Eur Urol.* 2012;62(6):1157.
Jünemann K, Thüroff J. Innervation. In: Brubaker LT, Saclarides TJ, eds. *The Female Pelvic Floor: Disorders of Function and Support.* Philadelphia: F.A. Davis; 1996.
Kanai A, Andersson KE. Bladder afferent signaling: recent findings. *J Urol.* 2010;183:1288.
Keast JR, Kawatani M, De Groat WC. Sympathetic modulation of cholinergic transmission in cat vesical ganglia is mediated by alpha 1- and alpha 2-adrenoceptors. *Am J Physiol.* 1990;258:R44.
Kelin LA. Urge incontinence can be a disease of bladder sensors. *J Urol.* 1988;139:1010.
Khanna OP. Vesicourethral smooth muscle: function and relation to structure. *Urology.* 1981;18:211.
Kumar V, Chapple CR, Surprenant AM, Chess-Williams R. Enhances adenosine triphosphate release from the urothelium of patients with painful bladder syndrome: a possible pathophysiological explanation. *J Urol.* 2007;178(4 Pt 1):1533.
Leippold T, Reitz A, Schurch B. Botulinum toxin as a new therapy option for voiding disorders: current state of the art. *Eur Urol.* 2003;44:165.
Lensch E, Jost WH. Autonomic disorders in multiple sclerosis. *Autoimmune Dis.* 2011;2011:803841.
Mahoney DT, Laberte RO, Blais DJ. Integral storage and voiding reflexes: neurophysiologic concept of continence and micturition. *Urology.* 1977;10:95.
McGuire EJ. Experimental observations on the integration of bladder and urethral function. *Invest Urol.* 1978;15:303.
McGuire EJ. The innervation and function of the lower urinary tract. *J Neurosurg.* 1986;65:278.
McGuire EJ, Woodside JR, Borden TA, Weiss RM. Prognostic value of urodynamic testing in myelodysplastic patients. *J Urol.* 1981;126:205.
Morrison J, Steers WD, Brading A, et al. Neurophysiology and neuropharmacology. In: *The 3rd International Consultation on Incontinence.* Paris: Health Publication Ltd; 2005.
Mundy AP. Clinical physiology of the bladder, urethra and pelvic floor. In: Mundy AP, Stephenson TP, Wein AJ, eds. *Urodynamics: Principles, Practice and Application.* New York: Churchill Livingstone; 1984.
Munoz A, Smith CP, Boone TB, Somogyi GT. Overactive and underactive bladder dysfunction is reflected by alterations in urothelial ATP and NO release. *Neurochem Int.* 2011;58:295.
Nakamura T, Yoshimura M, Shinnick-Gallagher P, et al. Alpha 2 and alpha 1-adrenoceptors mediate opposing actions on parasympathetic neurons. *Brain Res.* 1984;323:349.
Nardos R, Gregory WT, Krisky C, et al. Examining mechanisms of brain control of bladder function with resting state functional connectivity MRI. *Neurourol Urodyn.* 2014;33:493.
Nardos R, Karstens L, Carpenter S, et al. Abnormal functional connectivity in women with urgency urinary incontinence: Can we predict disease presence and severity in individual women using Rs-fcMRI. *Neurourol Urodyn.* 2015;35(5):564.
Nilius B. Transient receptor potential (TRP) cation channels: rewarding unique proteins. *Bull Mem Acad R Med Belg.* 2007;162:244.
Ohlstein EH, von Keitz A, Michel MC, et al. A multicenter, double-blind, randomized, placebo-controlled trial of the β3-adrenoceptor agonist solabegron for overactive bladder. *Eur Urol.* 2012;62:834.
Pernow B. Substance P. *Pharmacol Rev.* 1983;35:85.
Raezer D, Wein AJ, Jacobowitz D, et al. Autonomic innervation of canine urinary bladder: cholinergic and adrenergic contributions and interaction of sympathetic and parasympathetic systems in bladder function. *Urology.* 1973;2:211.
Reitz A, Schurch B. Intravesical therapy options for neurogenic detrusor overactivity. *Spinal Cord.* 2004;42:267.
Reitz A, Stöhrer M, Kramer G, et al. European experience of 200 cases treated with botulinum-A toxin injections into the detrusor muscle for urinary incontinence due to neurogenic detrusor overactivity, *Eur Urol.* 2004;45:510.
Sakakibara R, Hattori T, Yasuda K, Yamanishi T. Micturition disturbance in acute transverse myelitis. *Spinal Cord.* 1996;34:481.
Shapiro E. Clinical implications of genitourinary embryology. *Curr Opin Urol.* 2009;19:427.
Shergill IS, Arya M, Hamid R, et al. The importance of autonomic dysreflexia to the urologist. *BJU Int.* 2004;93:923.
Sillen U. Central neurotransmitter mechanisms involved in the control of urinary bladder function. *Scand J Urol Nephrol.* 1980;58:1.
Sirls LT, Zimmern PE, Leach GE. Role of limited evaluation and aggressive medical management in multiple sclerosis: a review of 113 patients. *J Urol.* 1994;151:946.
Steers WD. Physiology and pharmacology of the bladder and urethra. In: Walsh PC, Retik AB, Vaughan ED, et al. *Campbell's Urology.* 7th ed. Philadelphia: WB Saunders; 1998.
Steers WD, Creedon D, Tuttle JB. Immunity to NGF prevents afferent plasticity following hypertrophy of the urinary bladder. *J Urol.* 1996;155:378.
Stohrer M, Schurch B, Kramer G, Schmid D. Botulinum A toxin detrusor injections in the treatment of detrusor hyperreflexia. *J Urol.* 2000;163:244A.
Swash M. Innervation of the bladder, urethra and pelvic floor. In: Drive JO, Hilton P, Stanton SL, eds. *Micturition.* London: Springer-Verlag; 1990.
Tadic SD, Tannenbaum C., Resnick NM, Griffiths D. Brain responses to bladder filling in older women without urgency incontinence. *Neurourol Urodyn.* 2013;32:435.
Tanagho EA, Miller ER. Initiation of voiding. *Br J Urol.* 1970;42:175.
Thor KB. Targeting serotonin and norepinephrine receptors in stress urinary incontinence. *Int J Gynaecol Obstet.* 2004;86(suppl 1):S38.
Todorova A, Vonderheid-Guth B, Dimpfel W. Effects of tolterodine, trospium chloride, and oxybutynin on the central nervous system. *J Clin Pharmacol.* 2001;41:636.
Tulloch AG. Sympathetic activity of internal urethral sphincter in empty and partially filled bladder. *Urology.* 1975;5:353.
Tyagi P, Tyagi V, Chancellor M. Mirabegron: a safety review. *Expert Opin Drug Saf.* 2011;10:287.
Uvelius B, Gabella G. Relation between cell length and force production in urinary bladder smooth muscle. *Acta Physiol Scand.* 1980;110:357.
van Kerrebroeck P, Abrams P, Lange R, et al. Duloxetine versus placebo in the treatment of European and Canadian women with stress urinary incontinence. *BJOG.* 2004;111:249.

Venkatachalam K, Montell C. TRP channels. *Annu Rev Biochem.* 2007;76:387.

Veselá R, Asklund H, Aronsson P, et al. Coupled nitric oxide and autonomic receptor functional responses in the normal and inflamed urinary bladder of the rat. *Physiol Res.* 2012;61:371.

Walters MD. Mechanisms of continence and voiding, with International Continence Society classification of dysfunction. *Obstet Gynecol Clin North Am.* 1989;16:773.

Wang P, Luthin GR, Ruggieri MR. Muscarinic acetylcholine receptor sub-types mediating urinary bladder contractility and coupling to GTP binding proteins. *J Pharmacol Exp Ther.* 1995;273:959.

Wein AJ. Pharmacology of incontinence. *Urol Clin North Am.* 1995;22:557.

Wein AJ, Arsdalen KV, Levin RM. Pharmacologic therapy. In: Krane RJ, Siroky MB, eds. *Clinical Neurourology*. 2nd ed. Boston: Little Brown & Co; 1991.

Wein AJ, Barrett DM. *Voiding Function and Dysfunction*. Chicago: Mosby; 1988.

Winter DL. Receptor characteristics and conduction velocities in bladder efferents. *J Psychiatr Res.* 1971;8:225.

4

Physiology of the Pelvic Muscles, Vagina, and Anorectum

Megan R. Routzong, Rebecca Shaffer, and Pamela A. Moalli

CHAPTER OUTLINE

PELVIC FLOOR

Anatomy and Composition

The pelvic floor is a highly complex, heterogeneous structure that supports the pelvic organs. In certain cases, such as childbirth, substantial stretch and accommodation of the pelvic floor must occur. Although the precise physiology by which the pelvic floor provides support to the vagina is not understood, it is known to comprise a combination of striated muscles, connective tissues, and bones. Together, this support mechanism serves to maintain the location and orientation of the uterus, vagina, bladder, urethra, and anorectum in the pelvis while allowing appropriate motion for physiological functions, such as defecation (Rostaminia et al., 2020b).

Pelvic floor muscles are largely composed of striated muscle. The predominant muscle group is the levator ani, but the pelvic floor includes superficial muscles (bulbocavernosus, ischiocavernosus, and deep and superficial transverse perinei) that lie inferiorly and the coccygeus that lies posteriorly and superiorly to the levator ani (Fig. 4.1). The pelvic floor extends anteriorly to the pubis, laterally to the arcus tendineus levator ani (ATLA), and posteriorly to the sacrum and coccyx via the anococcygeal raphe (or levator plate).

The levator ani have historically been defined as being composed of three muscles; the iliococcygeus, pubococcygeus, and puborectalis (Smith, 1923) (see Chapter 1). Using these terms, the iliococcygeus is the most superior, posterior, and lateral of the levator ani, while the puborectalis is the most inferior and medial, although the literature contains a large variety of terms for the same pelvic floor muscles, some of which may imply incorrect origin-insertion pairs (Kearney et al., 2004). This led Lawson (1974) to use the term "pubovisceral muscle" as a replacement for the terms puborectalis and pubococcygeus, as the latter imply that muscle fibers connect the pubis and coccyx directly, whereas the former is thought to be more representative of actual origin-insertion pairs (Kearney et al., 2004). The pubovisceral muscle includes any muscle that originates at the pubis and inserts into or acts as a sling to support pelvic viscera (Wall, 1993). However, using the term "pubovisceral" has resulted in its own confusion, as studies have equated it the pubococcygeus [as suggested by Kearney et al. (2004)], the puborectalis, or both. Additionally, there is variation in which muscles define the levator ani. Although Smith (1923) used the terms iliococcygeus, pubococcygeus, and puborectalis, Lawson (1974) referred to the pubovisceral (including the puborectalis), iliococcygeus, and coccygeus muscles. Lawson (1974) substituted "puborectalis" for "puboanal sphincteric sling" to emphasize that some muscle fibers insert into the external anal sphincter. Kearney et al. (2004) suggested using "puborectalis" instead, although they agreed on the puboanalis' origin-insertion pairs.

To remain consistent with previous literature, and based on our own studies, we suggest defining the levator ani as the pubovisceral and iliococcygeus muscles, where the pubovisceralis is composed of the puborectalis, puboanalis, puboperinealis, and pubovaginalis. However, it is worth noting that the term "pubovisceral muscle" is not officially recognized by *Terminologia Anatomica* (see Chapter 1).

The pubovisceral muscle attaches bilaterally to the pubic bone just lateral to midline. This bilateral attachment creates the levator hiatus—an opening where the urethra, vagina, and rectum pass through the pelvic floor. The puborectalis attaches at the pubic bone, and the left and right portions meet behind the rectum, forming a sling observed anatomically as the anorectal angle. The puboanalis, puboperinealis, and pubovaginalis

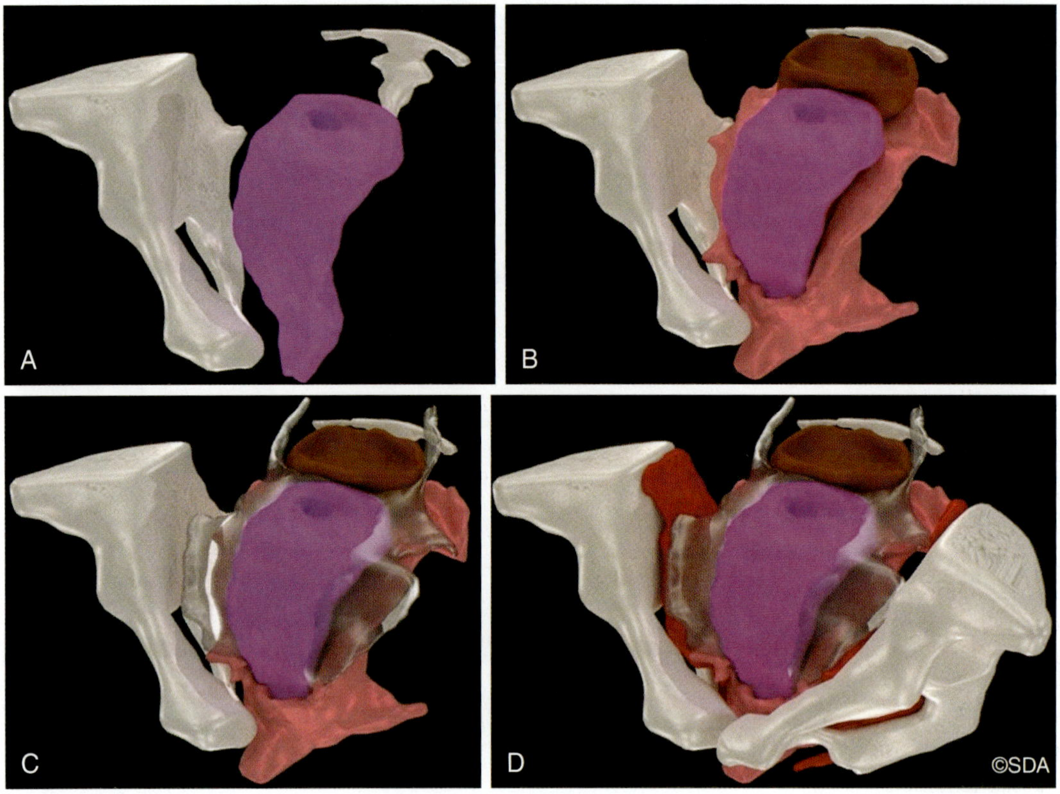

Fig. 4.1 Digital illustrations from magnetic resonance image segmentations demonstrating normal vaginal support. **A**, Depicts a normally supported vagina (*purple*) with an inferior portion of the right bony pelvis and coccyx (*white*); **B**, with the addition of the rectum (*brown*) and pelvic floor muscles (coccygeus superiorly, then the levator ani, and the superficial perineal muscles inferiorly) (*pink*); **C**, level I (inferior) and level II (superior) connective tissue support added (*transparent, gray*); **D**, left-sided bony pelvis (*white*) and obturator muscles (*red*) added.

insert into the intersphincteric groove, perineal body, and vagina, respectively. The iliococcygeus originates from a connective tissue condensation (the ATLA) of the lateral pelvis and attaches to the coccyx. The left and right sections of the levator ani coalesce along a midsagittal, posterior line between the sacrum and coccyx, forming the levator plate upon which the upper two-thirds of the vagina, uterus, and rectum rest nearly horizontally. The levator plate is also called the anococcygeal raphe, but should not be confused with the more superficial anococcygeal ligament that runs directly between the external anal sphincter and coccyx. As the levator ani muscles contract, they squeeze the structures within the levator hiatus by pulling them toward the pubic rami, which generates pressure in those organs by reducing available space.

In humans, the nervous system is divided in two (see Chapter 3). The central nervous system (CNS) includes the brain and spinal cord, whereas the peripheral nervous system (PNS) comprises the somatic and autonomic nervous systems. Somatic nerves primarily innervate striated muscle and allow execution of voluntary actions. Conversely, the autonomic nervous system underlies baseline, homeostatic functions that occur without conscious thought. This includes innervation of the smooth muscle of visceral organs and glandular functions. Somatic innervation to the levator ani is provided by efferent (motor) nerves arising primarily from the nerve to the levator ani (originating from spinal cord levels S2–S4), which innervates the superior portion of the levator ani, and to a lesser extent from the pudendal nerve (also from S2–S4), innervating the inferior portion. The levator ani maintain a baseline contractile tone that preserves the orientation of the pelvic organs (Parks et al., 1962; Parks et al., 1966). This constant tone relies on proprioceptive afferent input processed by the dorsal root ganglia in the spine and afferent sensory nerves. Humans can voluntarily increase pelvic muscle contractions, but the muscles rapidly fatigue, and tone returns to baseline after roughly 1 minute (Parks et al., 1962).

Smooth muscle fibers are primarily contained within viscera, allowing for stretch during filling and evacuation of visceral contents in combination with autonomic reflexes. Connective tissue contains varying amounts of smooth muscle cells. Many components of the pelvic floor are altered by menopause or prolapse, including smooth muscle cells. Ozdegirmenci et al. (2005) determined via computational analyses that the predicted ratio of smooth muscle cells in the round ligament is decreased in women with prolapse.

In orthopedic terminology, ligaments are dense connective tissues bridging bone to bone, whereas tendons are connections between muscle and bone. Within the abdomen and pelvis, the term "ligament" is used more variably. It may refer to a fold of peritoneum formed during embryonic development, like the hepatoduodenal ligament, which contains the portal triad (the hepatic artery, portal vein, and common bile duct). In the pelvis, ligaments usually refer to connective tissue suspensions tethering the viscera to the pelvic sidewall and bony pelvis. Connective tissue condensations that provide support to the vagina and uterus include the cardinal-uterosacral ligament complex and the paravaginal attachments to the arcus tendineus fasciae pelvis (ATFP). This is collectively known as the endopelvic fascia.

The endopelvic fascia is a continuation of the web of connective tissue originating at the level of the uterine artery's insertion at the uterus and extending bilaterally to the pelvic sidewalls and caudally to suspend the cervix and vagina, periodically solidifying into ligaments. Close to the uterus and cervix, it is termed the parametrium, and at the level of the external cervical os it becomes the paracolpium (DeLancey, 1993). These connective tissue attachments have been organized into a conceptual framework of levels corresponding to different anatomic sites on the vagina (DeLancey, 1992; DeLancey, 1994) (see Fig. 1.15). Level I refers to the support of the vagina at its apex provided by the cardinal and uterosacral ligaments. Level II is the lateral support of the midportion of the vagina where the endopelvic fascia coalesces with the ATFP on either side. More distally, the vagina attaches to the arcus tendineus fascia rectovaginalis. Level III support for the distal vagina is provided by the perineal body, the perineal membrane, and the superficial muscles. The transverse perinei and bulbocavernosus intersect at the perineal body, which is composed of multiple layers with varying fiber orientations (Larson et al., 2010; Shafik et al., 2007). Injury at different levels of vaginal support will cause distinct anatomic defects.

Connective tissue is composed of collagen, elastin, proteoglycans, and the extracellular matrix (ECM) acting as a scaffold for the other components. Collagen provides tensile strength, which is the stress a material can undergo before breaking while being pulled. Elastin provides resilience, or elasticity, which is a tissue's ability to snap back into place after being deformed. Proteoglycans are extracellular proteins that are vital for cell-to-cell connections or connections between cells and the ECM. Small proteoglycans (decorin, fibromodulin, biglycan, luminican, and chondroadherin) bind with glycosaminoglycans to form complexes in the ECM and resist compression by restricting the motion of water molecules (Abramowitch et al., 2009). Other proteoglycans, including fibronectin, vitronectin, and laminin, serve to create cell-to-cell bindings (Tinelli et al., 2010). Connective tissue composition is dynamic, with production and degradation of collagens occurring as the tissue endlessly remodels in response to stresses, aging, and injury. Tissue breakdown occurs through the enzymatic activity of acid cathepsins and matrix metalloproteinases (MMPs), which break down collagen fiber cross-links and lead to cleavage of the collagen fibers themselves, respectively (Burleigh et al., 1974).

Of the 19 known types of collagens, types I and III are found most commonly in epithelial tissues (Jackson et al., 1996). Type I is the most common throughout the body. It forms large fibers and is a main contributor to tensile strength, although types II and III also form strong fibers that resist tension. Type III fibers are smaller than type I fibers and are found more frequently in tissues that require flexibility, such as blood vessel walls (Moalli et al., 2004). Type IV collagen assembles into a network configuration instead of distinct fibers and helps form the basement membrane beneath fibers (Tinelli et al., 2010). Type V collagen forms small fibrils, is frequently found in wound healing, and likely directs fibrillogenesis. Heterogeneous fibrils are formed when type I collagen copolymerizes with type III or V collagen. As the proportion of type III and IV collagens increases relative to type I collagens, tissues become weaker. Hormones may influence the balance of collagen types within the tissues. After menopause, if hormone therapy is not initiated, the amount of type I collagen decreases by 75% (compared with premenopausal women), and the ratio of type I to type III/V collagen decreases in the ATFP (Moalli et al., 2004). Thus, after menopause, there is an increased amount of type III and V collagens in human connective tissue. Changes in collagen composition are also likely to be associated with pelvic organ prolapse. Jackson et al. (1996) found that total collagen content and collagen solubility were decreased in premenopausal women with prolapse compared with controls. They also found that MMP and cathepsin activity increased in prolapse patients, leading to more rapid turnover of collagen (Jackson et al., 1996). Overall, the changes in collagen found in women with prolapse likely decrease the tensile strength of the tissue, a risk factor for prolapse.

Function and Biomechanical Properties

In nonhuman mammalian species, especially quadrupeds, the levator ani primarily control tail movement, and the connective tissues alone act as the primary support (Abramowitch et al., 2009). For example, the rat has connective tissue attaching the upper vagina to the spine, similar to the human uterosacral ligaments; paravaginal attachments from the lateral vagina to the dense connective tissue, similar to the ATFP; and attachments connecting the distal vagina to the anterior surface of the ischiopubic rami, emulating level III support (Moalli et al., 2005). Although the connective tissues are similar, the pelvic floor muscles differ considerably. In humans, portions of the pubovisceral muscle attach directly to the vagina and rectum, whereas in rodents these attachments are provided by loose connective tissues. Anatomical differences should be considered when choosing appropriate animal models for research studies.

In humans, because of the adoption of an upright posture, the levator ani and connective tissues work together to support the pelvic organs. When pelvic floor muscles contract at baseline, the tension experienced by supportive ligaments is reduced. If the muscles are damaged, as may occur with vaginal birth, or if those muscles are compromised because of nerve damage, then the shelf supporting the pelvic organs may sag. This may cause organs to change orientation or descend through the urogenital hiatus (the opening in the levator ani anterior to the perineal body where the urethra and vagina pass through the pelvic floor), and can cause excessive straining of connective tissues attached to those organs. Vaginal birth likely serves as an instigating event for damage, but progressive muscle deterioration may also occur as women age. Some suspect that pudendal nerve trauma (i.e., stretch during childbirth) may play a role, although this is a point of contention, as some studies suggest that most nerve injury that occurs with vaginal birth resolves (Allen et al., 1990), whereas others show worsening neuropathy and organ function over time (Snooks et al., 1990). Other risks include chronic increased intraabdominal pressure or repetitive high-pressure straining, as occurs in patients with obesity, chronic cough conditions, chronic obstructive pulmonary disease, habitual heavy lifting, or chronic constipation.

Recent work has sought to elucidate the biomechanical properties of the pelvic floor, which supports the pelvic organs against the effects of gravity and increased intraabdominal pressure. The biomechanical parameter of deformation, a general term for the change in size or configuration of a material due external forces or changes in temperature, is applicable to this discussion. Deformation can be referred to more specifically as strain or stretch, where a state of no deformation is indicated by a strain of 0 and a stretch of 1, and stretch can be converted to strain by subtracting 1. Forces may be tensile, applied by pulling; compressive, applied by pushing; shear, applied by sliding; or torsion, applied by twisting. Ligaments typically exhibit viscoelastic behavior—the ability to initially resist strain, then stretch, and then regain their previous configuration once forces are removed—because they contain water, collagen, and elastin. Water aids with resisting compression, collagen with resisting tension, and elastin with the recovery of the tissue after deformation. When a tissue undergoes excessive strain, meaning the yield strength (the stress value at the yield point) and the elastic, or linear, region of the stress-strain curve are surpassed, it experiences microdamage that may cause loss of this recoil ability and permanent deformation (Fig. 4.2). If the tissue is stretched even further, it will suffer structural failure and rupture. Collagen remodels in damaged ligaments as they heal. After healing, the ligament composition does not perfectly resemble that of the ligament before injury; the ligament is frequently stiffer and may be permanently elongated, both of which contribute to the loss of its recoil ability and increased susceptibility to future injury (Tinelli et al., 2010).

Biomechanical properties may be structural or mechanical, as described by Abramowitch et al. (2009). Both describe how tissues respond to an applied load; but structural properties are dependent on the size of the tissue sample tested. Thus, a larger sample generally performs better. One common mechanical test is a uniaxial, tensile load to failure test (Fig. 4.3; Abramowitch et al., 2009). In this test, one edge of a tissue is rigidly fixed to the base of the mechanical testing system, while the other end is connected to a movable arm containing a load cell. The arm displaces that end of the tissue until it fails, while the system generates a load-elongation curve. The linear stiffness of the tissue is the slope of the linear portion of this curve. In contrast, mechanical properties describe tissue behavior independent of size. These properties can also be obtained from a load to failure test by converting the forces and elongations to stresses and strains, respectively, resulting in a stress-strain curve (Fig. 4.4; Abramowitch et al., 2009). Stress is calculated by dividing the applied force by the tissue's cross-sectional area, whereas strain is the change in length of the sample divided by its original length. The tangent modulus (called the elastic modulus or Young's modulus when describing the linear region) is the slope of this stress-strain curve. The tensile strength of the tissue is the maximal stress it can support before rupture and corresponds with the ultimate strain—the maximal strain it can support. As these properties are calculated per unit area, they offer a more direct measurement of the composition of the tissue and the results are more generalizable.

Biomechanical properties of a tissue can differ depending on the axis in which the sample is stretched, termed anisotropy. This is common in biological tissues, as there are preferred collagen alignments. For example, tendons and ligaments are

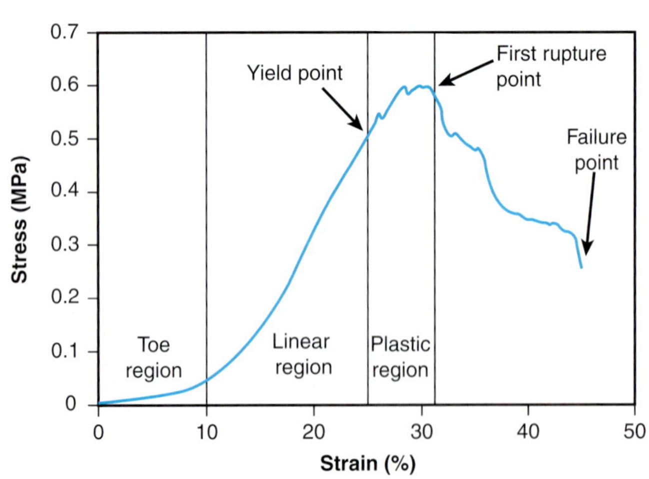

Fig. 4.2 Example of a typical stress-strain curve for tensile testing of a biological soft tissue, with points and regions of interest labeled. (From Gaur P, Chawla A, Verma K, et al. Characterisation of human diaphragm at high strain rate loading. *J Mech Behav Biomed Mater.* 2016;60:603. With permission.)

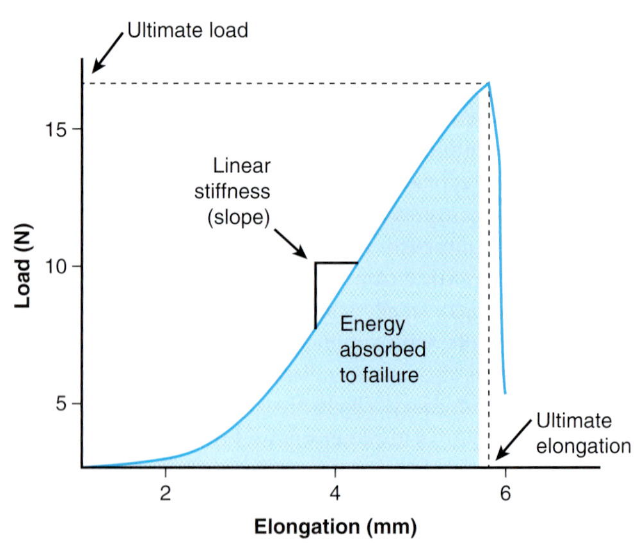

Fig. 4.3 Structural properties are frequently measured using a uniaxial load-elongation test to failure, resulting in a load-elongation curve for the tissue complex. (Modified from Abramowitch SD, Feola A, Jallah Z, Moalli P. Tissue mechanics, animal models, and pelvic organ prolapse: a review. *Eur J Obstet Gynecol Reprod Biol.* 2009;144(suppl 1):S146. With permission.)

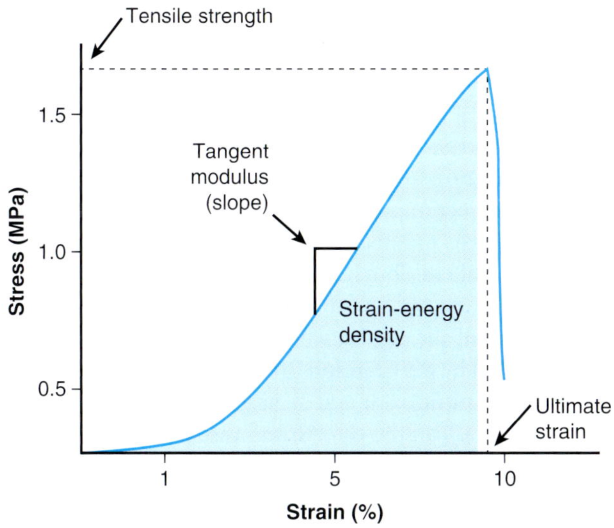

Fig. 4.4 Mechanical properties are frequently measured using the uniaxial tensile test to failure, resulting in a stress-strain curve. (Modified from Abramowitch SD, Feola A, Jallah Z, Moalli P. Tissue mechanics, animal models, and pelvic organ prolapse: a review. *Eur J Obstet Gynecol Reprod Biol.* 2009;144(suppl 1):S146. With permission.)

considered transversely isotropic, a type of anisotropy, as collagen is predominantly aligned along one axis. These tissues will behave differently if pulled perpendicularly versus in parallel to that collagen alignment. Using the uniaxial tensile test example, when pulling parallel to collagen fibers, collagen is the dominant contribution to the measured mechanical properties. If pulling perpendicularly, the ground substance (for connective tissues) or the tissue between collagen fibers is the main contribution.

Stretch must occur during childbirth. After the fetal head descends through the cervix and into the vagina, it must pass through the urogenital hiatus. The bones of the fetal skull differentially deform based on whether the fetus is preterm or at term, the shape of the mother's pelvis, and expulsive labor forces, but the head still must narrow and elongate as molding occurs during the second stage of labor (Ami et al., 2019). The average suboccipitobregmatic diameter, the smallest aspect of the presenting fetal head, is roughly 9.2 cm (Pu et al., 2011) after molding. The average frontooccipital diameter, the longest distance between the occipital and frontal bones, is 10.3 cm at the initiation of the second stage of labor, 10.8 cm once expulsion begins, and 11.2 cm at crowning (Bamberg et al., 2016). The urogenital hiatus is approximately 2.5 cm transversely between medial borders in an average nonpregnant woman without prolapse (DeLancey & Hurd, 1998). It must rapidly dilate during delivery, similar to the dilation of the cervix but over a much shorter time frame. Brooks et al. (1995) determined that the maximum stretch ratio, another term for stretch, before muscle undergoes structural failure with subsequent rupture of muscle fibers, is 1.5. Several finite element simulations of vaginal delivery have been created to predict the stretch in maternal soft tissues, specifically at the pubovisceral muscle enthesis and perineal body, two common sites of injury during vaginal delivery that have been linked with the later development of pelvic floor disorders, such as pelvic organ prolapse. These models predicted maximum stretch ratios of maternal soft tissues that surpass this 1.5× threshold, with values ranging from 1.6 to 4.1 (Li et al., 2010; Parente et al., 2008; Routzong et al., 2019). Thus, it is likely that most vaginal deliveries lead to some degree of stretch injury. Although, owing to tissue remodeling during pregnancy, it is also likely that this 1.5× stretch injury threshold may be higher in women at term. Further investigation is required, but Alperin et al. (2016) found, using a rat model, that remodeling of the pelvic floor resulted in increased muscle stiffness in pregnancy, a plausible mechanism for protecting pelvic floor tissues from injury during delivery.

Compared with other medical fields, such as orthopedic surgery, female pelvic medicine and reconstructive surgery research is still in its infancy. We are only beginning to understand the effect of childbirth injuries, chronic pressure, chronic constipation or cough, or other trauma to the pelvic floor. We poorly understand pelvic floor tissue healing and repair and how variations in healing may predispose women to pelvic floor disorders later in life. In the future, it will be critical to improve our knowledge of these components if we are to elucidate the mechanisms of pelvic organ prolapse and to improve the longevity and specificity of our surgical corrections.

VAGINA

Anatomy and Composition

The vagina is made of muscle and connective tissues and is richly vascular. It is a fibromuscular tube extending from the cervix to the perineum. Vaginal layers include an epithelial surface, the lamina propria, muscularis, and adventitia, whereas its surface is lined with nonkeratinizing stratified squamous epithelial cells. Histologically, there are four main epithelial layers: (1) most superficially, nonkeratinized cells with small, pyknotic nuclei; (2) an intermediate glycogen-containing cellular layer; (3) proliferating parabasal cells; and (4) the basal epithelial layer (Forsberg, 1995). Adjacent to the epithelium is the lamina propria, or subepithelium, a layer of dense connective tissue composed of collagen and elastin. Next is the muscularis, composed of smooth muscle cells with blood vessels intercalated between smooth muscle bundles. The smooth muscle has a circular configuration in its inner layer and a longitudinal orientation in its outer layer (Siddique, 2003). Lastly, the adventitia is made of loose connective tissue, containing collagen, elastin, and additional smooth muscle and vasculature. The connective tissue composition here includes 84% collagen and 13% elastin (Abramowitch et al., 2009; Moalli et al., 2004). The vagina and the endopelvic fascia have very similar collagen configurations (Keane et al., 1997), so clinically obtained vaginal biopsies may allow extrapolation to the collagen composition of the endopelvic fascia.

Embryology and Innervation (see also Chapter 2)

The innervation between the proximal and distal vagina differs, beginning early in embryogenesis. The distal two-thirds of the vagina arise from an outgrowth of the endoderm of the urogenital sinus, the paired sinovaginal bulbs. The proximal third of the vagina, the cervix, and the uterus arise from the uterovaginal primordium, which results from fusion of the paramesonephric ducts in the midline. The solid sinovaginal bulbs fuse together, grow cephalad, and then fuse with the uterovaginal primordium. This structure then canalizes to form the vagina. Reflecting differential embryologic origins, innervation to the upper vagina is via the inferior hypogastric nerve plexus, whereas innervation to the lower vagina and skin is from the pudendal nerve. The spinal origin of these nerves is the sacral levels S2 to S4 (Siddique, 2003).

Important to note is the convergence of sensory input from the pelvis at the level of the spinal cord and brain. Although afferent sensations are tracked independently from various end organs, there is dynamic processing of the inputs centrally, so pathophysiology from one organ may affect others. This explains the expression of several pelvic pain syndromes within one individual, such as endometriosis, interstitial cystitis, irritable bowel syndrome, and fibromyalgia. There may also be overlap of sensory nerve fibers within the pelvic nerve plexus.

Orientation and Structural Support

The epithelium contributes little to the structural integrity of the vagina, which is instead supplied by deeper layers of connective tissue and smooth muscle, whereas the levator ani and connective tissues provide external support (DeLancey, 1992; Moalli et al., 2004). In the midsagittal plane, the vagina contains a convex angle; the uppermost portion is nearly horizontal as it rests on top of the levator ani, and the distal portion descends more vertically. The angle occurs as the vagina descends through the levator hiatus and is caused, in part, by contraction of the levator ani at baseline. Funt et al. (1978) found this angle to be 130 degrees on average in the supine position on x-ray vaginogram, and others noted that it can be influenced by pregnancy and hysterectomy (Lee et al., 2019; Oliphant et al., 2018). If this angle is lost owing to lack of puborectalis muscle tone or compromised connective tissues, the urogenital hiatus will widen, and the risk of prolapse and herniation through that hiatus will increase (Nichols et al., 1970). A 20% larger urogenital hiatus before development of prolapse symptoms and a four times larger increase in hiatus size over a 5-year period was noted in women who developed pelvic organ prolapse compared with controls (Handa et al., 2019). This has practical effects when considering the approach for a prolapse repair. Any repair that changes the vaginal angle may circumvent this normal anatomic support. Postoperative angles were measured after abdominal sacrocolpopexy with Burch colposuspension (137–149 degrees) and sacrospinous ligament fixation (215–220 degrees) (Rane et al., 2004; Sze et al., 2001). In these cases, it is worth noting that the normal anatomy has already been disrupted, leading to the prolapse. However, based on imaging studies, it seems that sacrocolpopexy restores the normal vaginal angle better than sacrospinous ligament fixation.

Because of its attachments to the ATFP and arcus tendineus rectovaginalis, the midvagina in axial cross-section for a woman with normal support often has an "H" or a "W" configuration. This has been confirmed on magnetic resonance imaging, although more robust characterization of vaginal configuration and variation is required (Fielding et al., 1996; Barnhart et al., 2004).

Function

Normal vaginal functions include response to hormonal stimulation, lubrication and stretching during sexual activity, immunologic protection against infectious diseases, mechanical support of pelvic organs, and remodeling and stretching to allow for vaginal childbirth.

One consequence of sexual excitation is genital congestion in the lower third of the vagina, which is a reflexive autonomic response regulated by the CNS and PNS. The major neurotransmitters involved are nitric oxide and cyclic guanosine monophosphate (cGMP), which act on the clitoris, and vasoactive intestinal polypeptide (VIP), which affects the vagina (Castiglione et al., 2013). With this reflexive response, the genitals become engorged, and lubrication increases. This is partly mediated by increased vascular flow and capillary permeability and is dependent on estrogen. Both cGMP and cyclic adenosine monophosphate (cAMP) aid in the regulation of vaginal smooth muscle tone, the loss of which allows for engorgement during sexual arousal (Pace et al., 2011). Inhibition of phosphodiesterase type 5, which degrades cGMP, enhances the relaxation of the clitoris and vagina, which can also be relaxed by VIP with a concomitant increase in cAMP (Castiglione et al., 2013). After menopause, paravaginal vasodilation is compromised because of a decrease in the number of estrogen receptors on the vascular endothelium, which may lead to deficits in the genital congestion response (Basson, 2009). Hormone therapy decreases autonomic and sensory vaginal innervation density in postmenopausal women, corresponding with reduced VIP immunoreactivity, which may explain how hormone therapy reduces vaginal pain and discomfort (Griebling et al., 2012).

Before menarche, the vaginal epithelium is thin, and the vaginal pH is high (>4.7) (Fig. 4.5). As the ovaries initiate endogenous estrogen production, the epithelium thickens. The vagina maintains an acidic pH (<4.5) once menstruation begins (Muhleisen & Herbst-Kralovetz, 2016). This pH level is thought to be established as the naturally predominant *Lactobacillus* bacteria ferment glycogen in the epithelium, converting it into antimicrobial lactic acid that protects against infection and adverse pregnancy outcomes (Mirmonsef et al., 2016; O'Hanlon et al., 2019; Fettweis et al., 2012). Sjoberg et al. (1988) collected vaginal biopsies from women throughout the menstrual cycle and found that the epithelium thickens, and the superficial epithelial cells mature when circulating estrogen levels are high. With high progesterone levels, superficial cell layers are shed, and the basal portion of the epithelium is more quiescent. At the time of ovulation, the epithelium is maximally thickened and mature. After menopause, serum estrogen levels decrease, and estrogen receptors are downregulated. The ratio of epithelial intermediate and parabasal cells increases, with few superficial basal cells observed. There is less vaginal blood flow, reduced elasticity, and a decrease in normal vaginal secretions. The microbiome is altered in this new milieu, with the disappearance of lactobacilli and emergence of rectal bacteria. The latter increase susceptibility to urinary tract infections, which occur more frequently after menopause, likely by altering

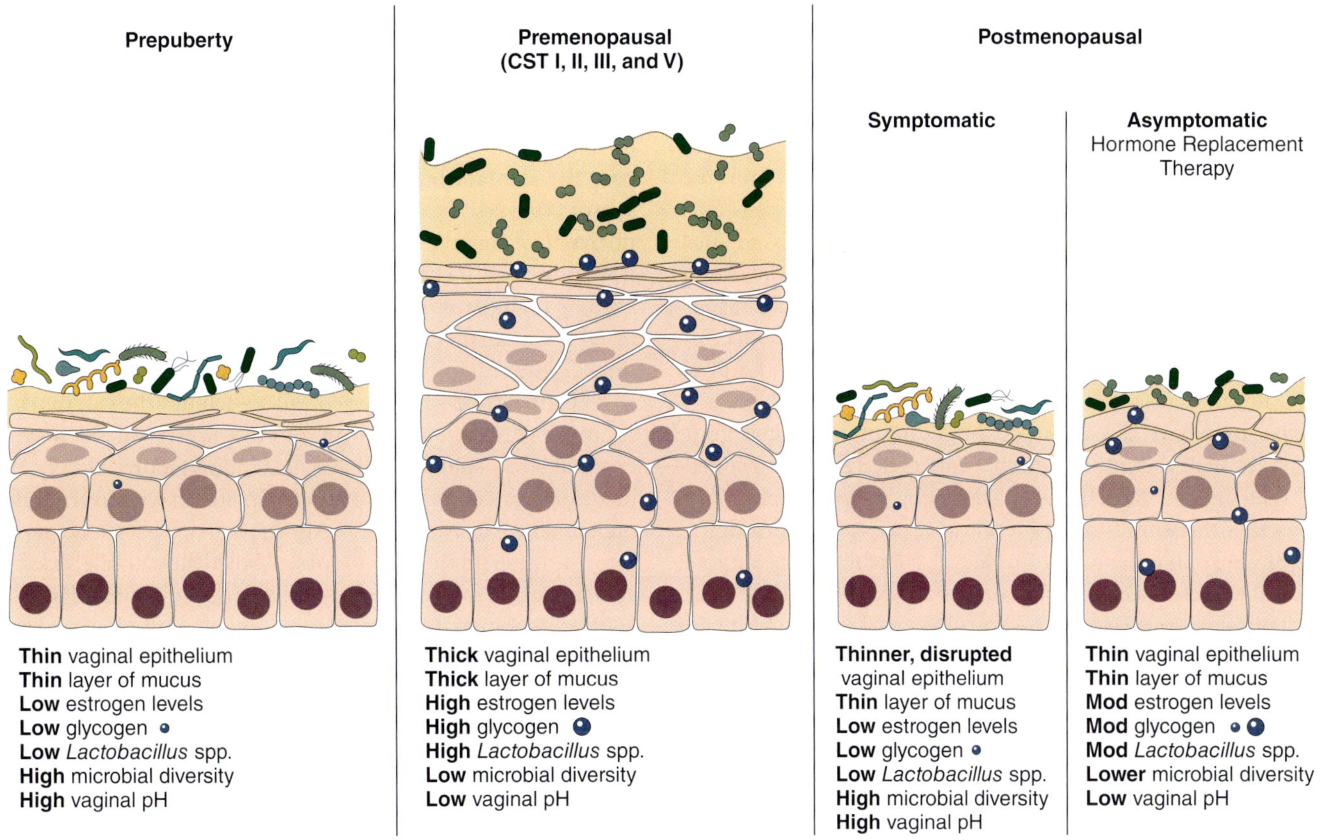

Fig. 4.5 Visualization of changes in the vaginal microbiome and corresponding hormonal and microanatomical features across the female lifespan. (From Muhleisen AL, Herbst-Kralovetz MM. Menopause and the vaginal microbiome. *Maturitas.* 2016;91:42. With permission.)

endogenous bladder flora. Estrogen receptors are restored, and vaginal lactobacilli return, if hormone therapy, particularly estrogen, is administered (Muhleisen & Herbst-Kralovetz, 2016; Basson, 2009). The frequency of urinary tract infections may also be reduced through the restoration of vaginal flora with lactobacilli using probiotics—an alternative for postmenopausal women unable to use estrogen (Caretto et al., 2017).

One critical function of the vagina is to stretch during vaginal delivery. However, vaginal parturition is a major risk factor for the development of pelvic floor disorders, although researchers are attempting to elucidate this disease mechanism. Throughout the body, elastin is generally a stable, permanent, but nonrenewable tissue component. Remarkably, in the vagina, elastin is degraded during labor and resynthesized after childbirth. Rodent models of pelvic organ prolapse were developed in which proteins important for elastin fiber assembly were genetically knocked out, including null mutations in the genes encoding lysyl oxidase-like-1, as reported by Liu et al. (2006) and Lee et al. (2008), and fibulin-5, as reported by Drewes et al. (2007). These rodent models show that pelvic organ prolapse is associated with pregnancy. Budatha et al. (2011) revealed that fibulin-5 downregulates MMP-9 activity, maintaining vaginal wall integrity and preventing pelvic organ prolapse. Vaginal fibulin-5 not only protects against parturition- and elastase-induced prolapse but is critical during development to establish baseline pelvic organ support (Chin et al., 2016).

Biomechanical Properties and Histology

Vaginal biomechanical properties demonstrate anisotropy, which often requires planar biaxial tensile testing (where thin, flat tissue samples are pulled in two directions simultaneously) to fully describe its complex mechanical behavior—as vaginal tissue behaves differently when stretched longitudinally versus circumferentially. This is seen in the disproportional circumferential stretch required for vaginal parturition compared with its moderate lengthening. In rat vaginal tissue, this anisotropic behavior is influenced not only by collagen and smooth muscle fiber orientation, but also by the innervation of the tissue (Huntington et al., 2019).

Jean-Charles et al. (2010) and Martins et al. (2013) demonstrated with uniaxial tensile testing that anterior vaginal wall tissue from women with prolapse is significantly stiffer than cadaveric samples from women without prolapse. To rule out the effects of age and menopause, Lei et al. (2007) tested pre- and postmenopausal tissues from women with and without prolapse. Prolapse samples on average had shorter lengths of maximum elongation and fracture and increased elastic moduli, supporting that connective tissues of women with prolapse have decreased elasticity and increased stiffness. Thus, independent of menopause, prolapse itself is associated with changes in vaginal composition. Badiou et al. (2008) found a decreased amount of smooth muscle cells in biopsies from the anterior vaginal wall of women with prolapse versus controls. These women have a greater fraction of collagen and ECM within the vaginal muscularis. In addition, the normally tightly organized smooth muscle bundles were less dense and less rigidly structured. Kerkhof et al. (2014) evaluated histological and biochemical features of the anterior vaginal wall of premenopausal women with and without prolapse and found no significant differences but noted an increase in smooth muscle cells and pyridinoline collagen cross-links in the prolapsed tissue sites compared with the nonprolapsed tissue sites of the same women. This suggests that changes between the vaginas of women with and without prolapse are not a systemic defect in tissue composition but are, more likely, an effect of the prolapse, not the cause.

This may have direct clinical implications to vaginal graft materials, such as synthetic mesh. Feola et al. (2013) implanted different meshes into rhesus macaques by sacrocolpopexy and found that the stiffest meshes resulted in the greatest deterioration of vaginal mechanical properties. This highlights the importance of understanding vaginal and mesh/graft structure, their mechanical properties, and how they interact *in vivo*, which will be critical as next-generation graft materials are developed.

ANORECTUM

Anatomy and Composition

The rectum and anus are the terminal portions of the gastrointestinal tract. The rectum, in order from its inner to outer layer, is composed of a mucosal surface, submucosal layer, muscularis, and serosal layer (Fig. 4.6). The muscular layer is composed of an inner circular layer of smooth muscle fibers and an outer longitudinal layer. The rectum, like the entire gastrointestinal tract, includes a network of intrinsic neurons, located in the submucosa (submucosal, or Meissner's, plexus) and between the circular and longitudinal muscle layers (myenteric, or Auerbach's, plexus). The rectal mucosal surface and proximal anus are lined with columnar epithelium until the dentate or pectinate line, where the epithelium transitions to squamous epithelium at roughly the midpoint of the anal canal (Irving & Catchpole, 1992). The distal anus past the dentate line is called the anoderm and has many sensory nerves that allow for determination of tactile and nociceptive signals. This area is important for continence, as it helps determine the composition (solid, liquid, or gas) of a bolus passing from the rectum. The termination of the anal canal is the anal verge, where the anal epithelium changes to the keratinized epithelium of the perianal skin.

The anal canal sphincter complex includes the internal anal sphincter (IAS), composed of smooth muscle fibers, and the external anal sphincter (EAS), extending more distally and made of striated muscle. It may also include a component of the puboanalis, which is composed of striated muscle and inserts into the intersphincteric groove. Above the dentate line, the anal mucosa is folded into the columns of Morgagni (Haubrich, 2002), which may contribute to the baseline coaptation of the anal canal, and the anal vascular cushions in the submucosa, which provide a final passive seal for the anal canal when engorged with blood (Lestar et al., 1992).

Anal continence is complex, requiring coordination of multiple muscle types. The IAS is the final extension of the rectal circular smooth muscle and is under autonomic control. It is wrapped proximally by the puborectalis and distally by the EAS. The EAS is innervated by the inferior hemorrhoidal branch of the pudendal nerve; thus, it is under volitional control. A portion of the EAS anteriorly fuses with the perineal body and the transverse perinei muscle bodies (Raizada et al., 2011). The EAS and IAS provide the resting pressure of the anal canal. Historically, it was found that the IAS contributed to up to 85% of the resting pressure; thus, it is a major component of baseline fecal

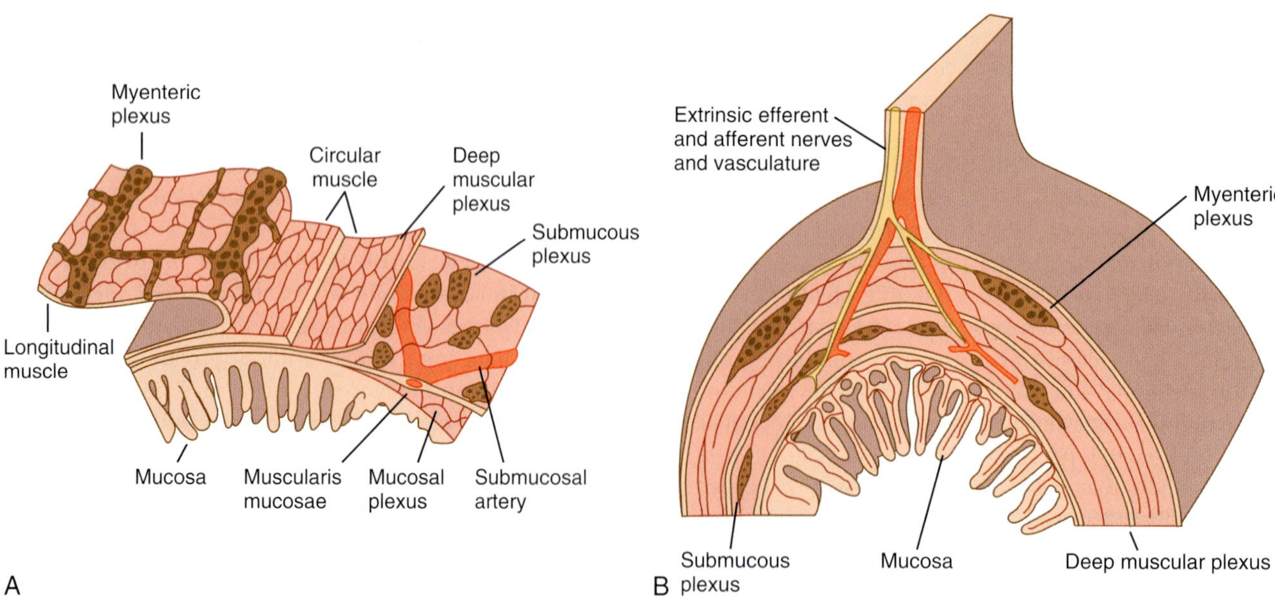

Fig. 4.6 Layers of intestinal wall showing the locations of the submucosal and myenteric nerve plexuses: **A**, three-dimensional representation and **B**, cross-sectional representation. (From Kandel ER, Schwartz JH, Jessell TM. *Principles of Neural Science*. 4th ed. New York: McGraw-Hill; 2000. With permission.)

continence (Frenckner & Euler, 1975). With improved measurements and the ability to perform manometry with concurrent endoanal ultrasound, the anatomy of the canal has been more precisely determined. Wong et al. (1998) took measurements in an upright position and showed that the EAS may play a major role in baseline pressure. Using cadaveric specimens, Stewart et al. (2018) found that the EAS is made of long, striated muscle fibers affording rapid contraction without decreased force and a physiological cross-sectional area (a measure of isometric force generating capacity) in the intermediate range. The EAS can be further recruited via voluntary control, increasing pressure and improving maintenance of continence when rectal filling occurs, which abates feelings of urgency while awaiting a socially acceptable time to defecate.

The puborectalis suspends the rectum anteriorly toward the pubis. Contraction via baseline muscle tone helps form an anorectal angle of 90 degrees, which is thought to contribute to baseline fecal continence (Palit et al., 2012). With voluntary squeeze, the anorectal angle narrows and moves ventrally and cranially, deferring defecation. In asymptomatic women, Tirumanisetty et al. (2018) found the anorectal angle to be 100 degrees at rest, 70 degrees during squeeze, and 120 degrees during defecation, and to be influenced by age, body mass index, and parity. Using magnetic resonance imaging, three-dimensional endoanal ultrasound, and high-definition anal manometry, Raizada et al. (2011) found that the proximal anal sphincter mechanism includes some voluntary control supplied by the puborectalis muscle. Upon voluntary squeeze in humans, pressure increases asymmetrically, with the strongest pressures at the anterior and most distal portions of the anal canal. A portion of the puborectalis was found to occlude the cranial portion of the anal sphincter, just as the EAS contracts the distal portion (Raizada et al., 2011). In addition to its effects on the anorectal angle, the puborectalis likely contributes to continence as part of the anal sphincter mechanism. The exact influence of the EAS versus the puborectalis on continence has yet to be determined.

A clinical example of a malfunctioning anal sphincter mechanism is in obstructed defecation, which results from functional disorders (i.e., pelvic floor dyssynergia or anismus) or structural disorders (i.e., pelvic floor anatomical defects). In these functional disorders, there is paradoxical contraction of the anal sphincter complex or an inability to coordinate the abdominal, rectal, and pelvic floor muscles with defecatory attempts. Dyssynergia is implicated in the etiology of up to 50% of patients with chronic constipation (Rao, 2001). Dailianas et al. (2000) found that abnormal contractions of the puborectalis and EAS contributed to dyssynergic defecation. Meanwhile, rectal support defects have been associated with obstructed defecation symptoms (Rostaminia et al., 2020a). In conclusion, proper function and support of these striated muscles is necessary for normal defecation, with the ability to recruit and then relax muscles on demand.

Innervation

Intrinsic Enteric Nervous System. The normal colorectal function is dependent on proper innervation of the bowel. As formerly discussed, the nervous system can be divided into the CNS and PNS, but the gastrointestinal tract contains another distinct and separate component of the nervous system, the enteric nervous system (ENS). Most colon nerve control is supplied by the ENS with a network of ganglia in the gut wall controlling basic functions, such as peristalsis or secretory reflexes (see Fig. 4.6). In this intrinsic enteric nerve plexus, neuronal cell bodies are located in the muscularis of the bowel wall and can control intestinal functions even when separated from the CNS. Though, in normal physiology, the ENS is not autonomous, but an integrated system in which reflexes—both local and those controlled through the sympathetic ganglia, the gut, and the CNS—and central control systems interact (Furness et al., 2014). There are roughly 200 to 600 million neurons in the ENS, modulating and propagating signals along the length of the bowel through the release of neurotransmitters.

There are two major examples of clinical diseases that affect the ENS ganglia. The first is Hirschsprung disease, a congenital disease resulting from incomplete migration of neural crest cells during development. This leads to no identifiable ganglion cells in the myenteric plexus for a portion of the intestinal tract, typically in the colon. Disease sequelae include chronic constipation and proximal dilation of the colon, called congenital megarectum, owing to the contracted distal aganglionic section. Rectal wall biopsies confirm an absence of neuronal ganglia. The second is seen in patients with Chagas disease, a tropical parasitic infection. When the disease becomes chronic, there is a decrease in the number of ganglionic cells found in the myenteric plexus. The ganglia normally contain nitric oxide–producing ENS neurons, which allow IAS inhibition, resulting in defecation. For both of these conditions, the IAS is unable to relax, resulting in continued tonic contraction and failure to pass rectal bolus contents; ballooning of the rectal wall eventually occurs and may result in a megarectum state.

Sympathetic Control. The intrinsic ENS interacts with the somatic and autonomic nervous systems. Extrinsic nerve supply to the bowel is supplied by the autonomic nervous system—the sympathetic and parasympathetic systems. The extrinsic inputs modulate the actions of the intrinsic system, but the intrinsic system maintains predominant control of bowel function. These extrinsic nerves directly innervate enteric smooth muscle and may also innervate the ENS ganglia.

As formerly discussed in this book, the autonomic motor system's ability to affect distant targets involves a chain of neural connections. In contrast to the somatic motor system, which innervates striated muscle, in the somatic system a neuronal cell body is typically located within the CNS, and a single, very long axon travels through the body before synapsing on its end target, the muscle. The autonomic system has an intervening synapse somewhere along its pathway; thus, it has, at minimum, a two-neuron chain. The term *efferent* describes pathways traveling away from the CNS, typically descending toward a target and carrying information regarding motor effects. Afferent describes ascending pathways traveling from the end organ back toward the CNS, typically transmitting sensory information from the target. For efferent autonomic nerves traveling toward a target organ, the first neuron usually has its neuronal cell body in the

CNS and synapses onto the cell body of a subsequent neuron in an autonomic ganglion. Axons of central neurons traveling toward ganglia are called preganglionic fibers, and axons traveling from ganglionic cell bodies are called postganglionic fibers. The postganglionic fibers can synapse onto the final target or another intervening cell.

Sympathetic neurons have cell bodies in the intermediolateral region of the spinal cord (Fig. 4.7). Axons exit the spinal cord via the ventral root, briefly run with the somatic motor nerves in the spinal nerve, then enter the sympathetic nerve trunks, which run along each side of the spinal cord and contain periodic ganglia in a paravertebral chain. The connections between the spinal nerve and paravertebral chains are called white myelinated rami. Each preganglionic axon then synapses with multiple postsynaptic cell bodies in different ganglia. Postganglionic axons leave the sympathetic chain via gray unmyelinated rami and travel in large bundles along spinal nerves projecting to targets throughout the body. Pelvic sympathetic nerve supply comes from the T5 to L2 spinal cord levels.

In the colorectal system, some sympathetic preganglionic fibers leave the spinal cord, travel through the paravertebral chain without forming a synapse, follow branches of the splanchnic nerve, then synapse into postsynaptic cell bodies within the prevertebral ganglia. These ganglia are located slightly away from the spinal cord and include the celiac, superior mesenteric, and inferior mesenteric ganglia (Kandel et al., 2000). In the rectum, sympathetic nerve supply contributes to smooth muscle relaxation and IAS contraction (Wester & Brubaker, 1998).

Parasympathetic Control. In the parasympathetic system, cell bodies are in specific nuclei in the brainstem and in sacral segments S2 to S4 of the spinal cord. Unlike sympathetic ganglia, the parasympathetic system has very long preganglionic nerves and short postganglionic connections, such that the ganglia are usually located within the wall of the target organ. Thus, the relay point in these connections is located in the periphery of the body. This has practical importance for pathologic conditions. For example, if urinary retention occurs, the bladder wall may stretch and could irreversibly damage the parasympathetic neural connections in the visceral wall. In the rectum, parasympathetic nerve supply activates smooth muscle, leading to rectal contraction and IAS relaxation (Wester & Brubaker, 1998). These actions, in addition to those that are intrinsically-mediated, are necessary for defecation.

The parasympathetic nerve supply for the upper colon arises from the vagus nerve, and for the distal colon and rectum arises from the sacral nerve plexus. The innervation from the vagus nerve travels along the course of the superior mesenteric artery, and innervation of the sacral nerve plexus parallels the course of the inferior mesenteric artery. The dorsal vagal nucleus is in the brainstem and contains parasympathetic neuronal cell bodies; preganglionic fibers then project via an association with cranial nerve X before synapsing in ganglia associated with thoracic and abdominal targets, including the upper gastrointestinal tract. Where the sacral nerve arises in segments S2 to S4 of the spinal cord, the parasympathetic preganglionic cell bodies also lie in the intermediolateral column and exit the ventral roots of the cord parallel to the sympathetic fibers. The parasympathetic nerves then travel in the pelvic nerve toward the pelvic ganglion nerve plexus (Kandel et al., 2000).

Extrinsic Afferents. Sensory afferent information from the bowel is communicated directly to the spinal cord via sensory nerves that travel through posterior sacral nerve roots to levels S2 to S4 and pass through two major neural pathways: (1) originating from the lumbar splanchnic/colonic nerves and (2) traveling via the pelvic/rectal nerves. Like most visceral afferents, rectal afferents are polymodal (can be activated by different stimulus modalities). The

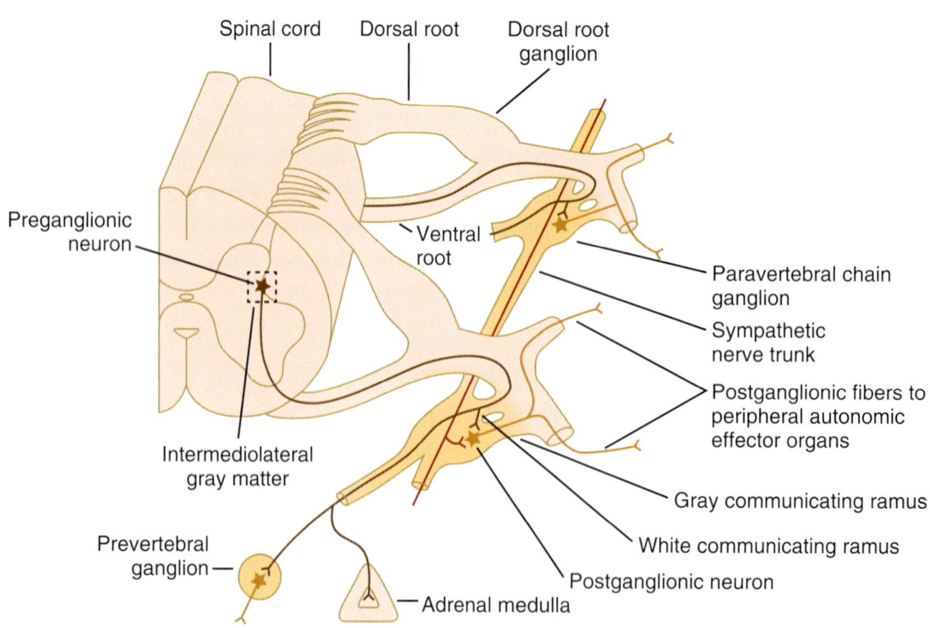

Fig. 4.7 Pictorial representation of the sympathetic preganglionic and postganglionic axons. (From Kandel ER, Schwartz JH, Jessell TM. *Principles of Neural Science.* 4th ed. New York: McGraw-Hill; 2000. With permission.)

best-characterized afferents are mechanosensitive and respond to distention of the colon, conveying a sense of fullness or urgency. Afferents can also respond to chemical signals, such as inflammatory cytokines, which may contribute to tenesmus or frustrated defecation attempts. The afferents likely communicate information when the colonic wall contracts, which may initiate the visceral pain sensations experienced as colonic spasms or "colicky pain."

Clinically, the importance of balancing excitatory and inhibitory influences can be highlighted by the example of patients with spinal cord injuries (SCIs) who develop neurogenic bowel symptoms. For these patients, constipation is a prevalent problem, likely resulting from inadequate sensory afferent input. They may also experience fecal impaction and lack of control when a bowel movement arrives, resulting in fecal incontinence. Here, inhibitory control is inadequate. One rare and extreme treatment involves a posterior sacral rhizotomy, in which the posterior nerve roots at the S2 to S4 levels are ligated to decrease irritative or spastic sensations from reaching the spinal cord via the normal reflex arc (Ebert, 2012). Reflexive defecation can no longer occur, but it improves control for patients, as the risk of incontinence is much lower once the spastic activity is truncated. Manual rectal stimulation or anterior sacral nerve root electrical stimulators must be used to initiate the defecatory sequence after this treatment.

Defecation and Continence

Normal control of defecation is a combination of reflexive action and voluntary control. The act of defecation consists of four phases: (1) antegrade stool transit by colonic propulsion, (2) storage of stool in the rectum until defecation, (3) passage of stool, and (4) defecation resolution (Palit et al., 2012). Defecation involves the interaction of enteric neurologic control, stool composition and consistency, spinal reflexes, and voluntary control established at toilet training.

The ENS is responsible for most bowel actions. Peristalsis involves the sequential contraction of adjacent segments of the bowel wall. During contraction, smooth muscle fibers shorten, and waste contents progress in the direction of a propagating wave if not impeded by a downstream obstruction. Obstructions typically present as functional rather than structural. Functional obstructions include retained fecal matter or contracted colon segments. Normal peristaltic movement is accompanied by the maintenance of a low intraluminal pressure (Brookes et al., 2009). However, if obstruction occurs and resistance is met, pressure in the segment increases, the smooth muscle does not shorten, and the contents do not advance.

Once food and waste pass into the large intestine, colonic contractions may move contents either antegrade toward the rectum (aboral) or retrograde toward the mouth (oral). Within the colon there is a mix of antegrade and retrograde contractions, with the balance normally toward antegrade such that there is net forward propulsion of colonic contents. Unlike more proximal areas of the gastrointestinal tract, the colon does not exhibit stereotypic patterns of motor activity, with many contractions leading only to segmentation or transit over short distances (i.e., nonpropagating waves). However, occasional powerful contractions originate in the proximal colon and migrate distally, typically resulting in defecation. These enterically controlled propagating waves are termed mass movements or giant migrating contractions, first described in the intestines of cats by Cannon (1902). There appears to be a circadian rhythm for peristalsis, with propagating and nonpropagating waves occurring less frequently at night (Brookes et al., 2009; Rao et al., 2004). Healthy individuals demonstrate minimal colonic activity at night, and changes in biological rhythms have been associated with gastrointestinal symptoms, such as diarrhea and constipation, supporting that the circadian rhythm and its disturbance influence gastrointestinal and colon physiology (Hoogerwerf, 2009).

In the rectum, like the colon, enterically controlled periodic contractions seem to be the dominant motor activity (Orkin et al., 1989). Auwerda et al. (2001) studied the circadian rhythm of these "rectal motor complexes" and noted a dramatic reduction during sleep and increases during daily ambulant activities. Rao et al. (2004) found 5% of contractions to be antegrade and 14% to 36% to be retrograde. The remaining contractions either propagated bidirectionally or did not move rectal contents (Rao & Welcher, 1996). It is thought that nonpropagating and retrograde contractions enable the rectum to store stool rather than continuing to move it antegrade.

In addition to smooth muscle cells, a population of cells known as the interstitial cells of Cajal (ICCs) help to control peristalsis and act as "intrinsic pacemakers" (Brookes et al., 2009). ICCs are mesenchymal cells formed from the same common precursor stem cells as the smooth muscle cells, though, in contrast to smooth muscle, ICCs have few contractile elements and generate spontaneous electrical activity when isolated (Mostafa et al., 2010). They contain c-KIT, a tyrosine kinase that preferentially influences ICCs over smooth muscle cells. ICCs have unique properties that lead to rhythmic changes in their membrane potentials, which are rapidly and passively conducted and spread to neighboring smooth muscle cells. Some evidence suggests direct activation of ICCs by sympathetic extrinsic nerves. ICC activation results in wave patterns with unique frequencies for different areas of the gastrointestinal tract. For example, the actions of the ICCs lead to the propagation of slow (Smith et al., 1987b) and faster waves that propagate toward the rectum (Smith et al., 1987a). The slow waves (oscillating 3–6 times/min) were first observed to originate from ICCs near the submucosal border in the canine gut, and fast waves (15–20 waves/min) were found to originate from ICCs near the myenteric border. Although ICCs only make up about 5% of the cells present in the tunica muscularis of the gastrointestinal tract, they significantly influence gastrointestinal physiology and motility (Mostafa et al., 2010).

Hormones, neurotransmitters, and other stimuli can alter the amplitude of the slow waves triggered by the ICCs. If the amplitude exceeds a predetermined threshold, then depolarization occurs, and superimposed spikes of action potentials are triggered. These action potentials are associated with calcium increases in adjacent smooth muscle cells, leading to contractions. Current evidence suggests that the ICC network ensures rapid spread of electrical signals; thus, it coordinates the effector (smooth muscle) cells within functional units of the gastrointestinal tract. This network also translates neuronal signals; thus, it is an important intermediary. Numerous gastrointestinal disorders have been linked with changes in the quantity, structure, and/or density of ICCs. For example, reduction in the number of ICCs leads to decreased smooth muscle cell contractility and reduced intestinal transit, a type of chronic constipation, and could play a role in other colorectal disorders (Mostafa et al., 2010).

Colonic peristalsis was traditionally measured using colonic manometry with sensors spaced along the gastrointestinal tract to record pressure changes. Newer techniques include 24-hour spatiotemporal manometry and allow for improved spatial resolution, with closer sensors and correlation of pressure changes with specific events, such as defecation (Dinning et al., 2008).

Gastrointestinal transit time affects stool volume and consistency (Palit et al., 2012). In the bowel, various circulating hormones such as somatostatin, menstrual hormones, and humoral factors such as substance P, VIP, and cholecystokinin may affect gastrointestinal motility. They act on the intrinsic enteric nerve plexus to regulate contractility. As waste progresses through the length of the intestinal tract, its content typically becomes more viscous because of water loss as it is absorbed through the bowel wall. There is also a complex interaction between the composition of stool and the bowel. For example, stool with a high osmotic load, as seen in patients with lactose intolerance, experiences more rapid colonic transit than stool with other compositions (Rao, 2004).

Reflexes play a role in normal physiologic function. Defecation can be initiated by the gastrocolic reflex, in which stretching of the stomach leads to increased gastrointestinal peristalsis. Other important reflexes for defecation include the rectosphincteric inhibitory reflex or the rectoanal inhibitory reflex (RAIR), where distention of the rectum with solid stool or gas leads to IAS relaxation. In infants and "spinalized" individuals, this leads to evacuation. To counteract the RAIR, humans learn to voluntarily contract the EAS and delay defecation. The RAIR is largely enterically controlled, although there is an element of parasympathetic control contributing to IAS relaxation. A decrease of at least 10% in the resting anal pressure (as measured by anorectal manometry) is considered normal relaxation (Dailianas et al., 2000).

Voluntary control of defecation is instilled by toilet training and allows individuals to suppress defecation until it is socially acceptable (i.e., using a toilet). Voluntary relaxation of the pelvic floor muscles is then necessary to initiate defecation. Defecation can only occur when the puborectalis and EAS relax. In addition, humans voluntarily increase intraabdominal pressure to complete the defecatory process, typically by tensing the abdominal musculature.

During voluntary suppression of defecation, distention of the rectum occurs, which is termed accommodation and is critical for the storage capacity of the rectum. In studies in guinea pigs and mice, a population of mechanosensitive afferent nerves activated by low levels of stretch (i.e., small changes in the amount of distension or small muscular contractions) was identified in the rectum (Lynn et al., 2003). It is hypothesized that this nerve population is vital for rectal accommodation and provides the majority of afferent synaptic input to the sacral parasympathetic nucleus (Yamanouchi et al., 2002). It has been shown that the rectum may accommodate stool volumes of up to 400 mL (Irving & Catchpole, 1992).

The next step in the regulation of defecation and the maintenance of continence is sampling, a term originated by Duthie and Bennett (1963) that describes the relaxation of the cephalic portion of the anal sphincter after distension of the rectum, which allows the pressure between the rectum and the anal canal to equilibrate. As the pressures equalize, the rectal contents come into contact with the anal mucosa and the very sensitive anoderm, only allowing voluntary release of those contents when appropriate. Miller et al. (1988) measured a thermal temperature gradient via a transrectal thermal electrode between the rectum and the upper, middle, and lower portions of the anal canal. By measuring pressure within the rectum and the middle of the anal canal, they determined that the anal sphincter relaxed, and pressures equalized approximately seven times hourly. The importance of sampling has been shown in patients with fecal incontinence with decreased sensory discrimination in the anal canal and decreased ability to determine temperature differentials between the rectum and the anal canal (Miller et al., 1988).

In summary, when a waste bolus moves into the rectum, the rectum distends, the IAS relaxes, the puborectalis and EAS voluntarily relax, and the abdominal musculature is recruited to further increase intraabdominal pressure. After defecation, final reflexes include the closing or postdefecation reflex, which engages after the rectum is emptied, when the pelvic floor muscles contract and are elevated to their baseline positions, restoring continence (Parks et al., 1966).

Neurologic Abnormalities

Neurologic abnormalities may occur in the CNS or PNS. The effects of SCIs frequently include bowel and bladder function abnormalities, as population studies show that 27% to 62% of SCI patients have colorectal problems (Ebert, 2012). Other central neurologic diseases that affect colorectal function include multiple sclerosis and Parkinson disease.

For those with spinal cord lesions at the level of the sacral nerves, deficits typically result in constipation because of slower colonic transit time in the sigmoid colon, allowing for extended absorption of water and more viscous stool. These patients have decreased rectal compliance; however, digital stimulation of the anorectum can trigger defecation, as other colonic reflex arcs remain functional (Gutman & Ellerkmann, 2003). Patients with lesions above the sacrum are at risk of fecal incontinence, as they cannot feel or voluntarily activate the EAS.

Patients with SCIs above the level of S2 to S4 must develop alternative methods for increasing intraabdominal pressure. Those with SCIs above the level of T5 recruit contraction of the intercostal muscles and diaphragm; patients with SCIs at the level of the cervical spine exclusively contract the diaphragm (Ebert, 2012). However, this still requires stabilization of the abdominal wall so that it will not balloon outward as pressure increases. This is the issue that affects many patients with SCIs, as they must rely only on colonic mechanisms for defecation.

Lower spinal cord lesions [i.e., at the level of the sacral nerves (S2–S4)] will affect parasympathetic control of the bowel and may cause constipation and incontinence. Constipation may arise because of decreased motility of the descending colon. Problems with defecation because of decreased rectal sensation, increased rectal distention, and decreased rectal tone may lead to fecal incontinence (Gutman & Ellerkmann, 2003).

SUMMARY

The pelvic floor is a complex system of interconnected muscles and connective tissues that support the pelvic organs by maintaining their location and orientation within the pelvis and allowing appropriate motion and deformation when needed to carry out physiological functions. The vagina must respond to hormonal stimulation, lubricate and stretch during sexual activity, provide immunologic protection against infectious diseases, support the pelvic organs mechanically, and remodel and stretch extensively during vaginal delivery. The rectum and anus are the distal portions of the gastrointestinal tract where continence is maintained by the anal canal sphincter complex, consisting of the internal anal sphincter (composed of smooth muscle) and the external anal sphincter (composed of striated muscle). Injury or changes attributed to age and/or menopause may result in reduced functionality of the pelvic floor, vagina, and/or anorectum, which, in many cases, results in the development of pelvic floor disorders.

BIBLIOGRAPHY

Abramowitch SD, Feola A, Jallah Z, Moalli P. Tissue mechanics, animal models, and pelvic organ prolapse: a review. *Eur J Obstet Gynecol Reprod Biol.* 2009;144(suppl 1):S146.

Allen RE, Hosker GL, Smith ARB, Warrell DW. Pelvic floor damage and childbirth: a neurophysiological study. *BJOG.* 1990;97:770.

Alperin M, Kaddis T, Pichika R, et al. Pregnancy-induced adaptations in intramuscular extracellular matrix of rat pelvic floor muscles. *Am J Obstet Gynecol.* 2016;215:210.

Ami O, Maran JC, Gabor P, et al. Three-dimensional magnetic resonance imaging of fetal head molding and brain shape changes during the second stage of labor. *PLoS One.* 2019;14(5):e0215721.

Auwerda JJA, Bac DJ, Schouten WR. Circadian rhythm of rectal motor complexes. *Dis Colon Rectum.* 2001;44(9):1328.

Badiou W, Granier G, Bousquet PJ, et al. Comparative histological analysis of anterior vaginal wall in women with pelvic organ prolapse or control subjects. A pilot study. *Int Urogynecol J.* 2008;19:723.

Bamberg C, Deprest J, Sindhwani N, et al. Evaluating fetal head dimension changes during labor using open magnetic resonance imaging. *J Perinat Med.* 2016;45:305.

Barnhart KT, Scott E, Malamud D. Lesson learned and dispelled myths: three-dimensional imaging of the human vagina. *Fertil Steril.* 2004;81:1383.

Basson R. Pharmacotherapy for women's sexual dysfunction. *Expert Opin Pharmacother.* 2009;10:1631.

Brookes SJ, Dinning PG, Gladman MA. Neuroanatomy and physiology of colorectal function and defecation: from basic science to human clinical studies. *Neurogastroenterol Motil.* 2009;21(suppl 2):9.

Brooks SV, Zerba E, Faulkner JA. Injury to muscle fibres after single stretches of passive and maximally stimulated muscles in mice. *J Physiol.* 1995;488(Pt 2):459.

Budatha M, Roshanravan S, Zheng Q, et al. Extracellular matrix proteases contribute to progression of pelvic organ prolapse in mice and humans. *J Clin Invest.* 2011;121:2048.

Burleigh MC, Barrett AJ, Lazarus GS. Cathepsin b1. A lysosomal enzyme that degrades native collagen. *Biochem J.* 1974;137:387.

Cannon WB. The movements of the intestines studied by means of the röntgen rays. *J Med Res.* 1902;7:72.

Caretto M, Giannini A, Russo E, Simoncini T. Preventing urinary tract infections after menopause without antibiotics. *Maturitas.* 2017;99:43.

Castiglione F, Bergamini A, Russo A, et al. Inhibition of phosphodiesterase 4 enhances clitoral and vaginal blood flow responses to dorsal clitoral nerve stimulation or PGE1 in anesthetized female rats. *J Sex Med.* 2013;10:939.

Chaudhry Z, Tarnay C. Descending perineum syndrome: a review of the presentation, diagnosis, and management. *Int Urogynecol J.* 2016;27:1149.

Chin K, Wieslander C, Shi H, et al. Pelvic organ support in animals with partial loss of fibulin-5 in the vaginal wall. *PLoS One.* 2016;11:4.

Dailianas A, Skandalis N, Rimikis MN, et al. Pelvic floor study in patients with obstructive defecation: influence of biofeedback. *J Clin Gastroenterol.* 2000;30:176.

DeLancey JO. Anatomic aspects of vaginal eversion after hysterectomy. *Am J Obstet Gynecol.* 1992;166:1717.

DeLancey JO. Anatomy and biomechanics of genital prolapse. *Clin Obstet Gynecol.* 1993;36:897.

DeLancey JO. The anatomy of the pelvic floor. *Curr Opin Obstet Gynecol.* 1994;6:313.

DeLancey JOL, Hurd WW. Size of the urogenital hiatus in the levator ani muscles in normal women and women with pelvic organ prolapse. *Obstet Gynecol.* 1998;91:364.

Dinning PG, Szczesniak MM, Cook IJ. Twenty-four hour spatiotemporal mapping of colonic propagating sequences provides pathophysiological insight into constipation. *Neurogastroenterol Motil.* 2008;20:1017.

Drewes PG, Yanagisawa H, Starcher B, et al. Pelvic organ prolapse in fibulin-5 knockout mice: pregnancy-induced changes in elastic fiber homeostasis in mouse vagina. *Am J Pathol.* 2007;170:578.

Duthie HL, Bennett RC. The relation of sensation in the anal canal to the functional anal sphincter: a possible factor in anal continence. *Gut.* 1963;4:179.

Ebert E. Gastrointestinal involvement in spinal cord injury: a clinical perspective. *J Gastrointestin Liver Dis.* 2012;21:75.

Feola A, Abramowitch S, Jallah Z, et al. Deterioration in biomechanical properties of the vagina following implantation of a high-stiffness prolapse mesh. *BJOG.* 2013;120:224.

Fettweis JM, Serrano MG, Girerd PH, et al. A new era of the vaginal microbiome: advances using next-generation sequencing. *Chem Biodivers.* 2012;9:965.

Fielding JR, Versi E, Mulkern RV, et al. MR imaging of the female pelvic floor in the supine and upright positions. *J Magn Reson Imaging.* 1996;6:961.

Forsberg JG. A morphologist's approach to the vagina–age-related changes and estrogen sensitivity. *Maturitas.* 1995;22:S7.

Frenckner B, Euler CV. Influence of pudendal block on the function of the anal sphincters. *Gut.* 1975;16:482.

Funt MI, Thompson JD, Birch H. Normal vaginal axis. *South Med J.* 1978;71:1534.

Furness JB, Callaghan BP, Rivera LR, Cho HJ. The enteric nervous system and gastrointestinal innervation: integrated local and central control. *Adv Exp Med Biol.* 2014;817:39.

Gaur P, Chawla A, Verma K, et al. Characterisation of human diaphragm at high strain rate loading. *J Mech Behav Biomed Mater.* 2016;60:603.

Griebling TL, Liao Z, Smith PG. Systemic and topical hormone therapies reduce vaginal innervation density in postmenopausal women. *Menopause.* 2012;19:630.

Gutman RE, Ellerkmann RM. Colo-rectal-anal pathophysiology and pharmacology. *J Pelvic Med Surg.* 2003;9:149.

Handa VL, Blomquist JL, Carroll M, et al. Longitudinal changes in the genital hiatus preceding the development of pelvic organ prolapse. *Am J Epidemiol.* 2019;188:2196.

Haubrich WS. Morgagni of the foramen and columns of Morgagni. *Gastroenterology.* 2002;123:424.

Hoogerwerf WA. Role of biological rhythms in gastrointestinal health and disease. *Rev Endocr Metab Dis.* 2009;10:293.

Huntington A, Rizzuto E, Abramowitch S, et al. Anisotropy of the passive and active rat vagina under biaxial loading. *Ann Biomed Eng.* 2019;47:272.

Irving MH, Catchpole B. ABC of colorectal diseases. Anatomy and physiology of the colon. rectum, and anus. *BMJ.* 1992;304:1106.

Jackson SR, Avery NC, Tarlton JF, et al. Changes in metabolism of collagen in genitourinary prolapse. *Lancet.* 1996;347:1658.

Jean-Charles C, Rubod C, Brieu M, et al. Biomechanical properties of prolapsed or non-prolapsed vaginal tissue: impact on genital prolapse surgery. *Int Urogynecol J.* 2010;21:1535.

Kandel ER, Schwartz JH, Jessell TM. *Principles of Neural Science.* 4th ed. New York: McGraw-Hill; 2000.

Keane DP, Sims TJ, Abrams P, Bailey AJ. Analysis of collagen status in premenopausal nulliparous women with genuine stress incontinence. *Br J Obstet Gynaecol.* 1997;104:994.

Kearney R, Sawhney R, DeLancey JOL. Levator ani muscle anatomy evaluated by origin-insertion pairs. *Obstet Gynecol.* 2004;104:168.

Kerkhof MH, Ruiz-Zapata AM, Bril H, et al. Changes in tissue composition of the vaginal wall of premenopausal women with prolapse. *Am J Obstet Gynecol.* 2014;210:168.

Larson KA, Yousuf A, Lewicky-Gaupp C, et al. Perineal body anatomy in living women: 3-dimensional analysis using thin-slice magnetic resonance imaging. *Am J Obstet Gynecol.* 2010;203:494.e15.

Lawson JON. Pelvic anatomy. I. Pelvic floor muscles. *Ann R Coll Surg Engl.* 1974;54:244.

Lee DD, Siegelman ES, Chua WY, et al. Comparison of vaginal axis in women who have undergone hysterectomy versus women with an intact uterus. *Female Pelvic Med Reconstr Surg.* 2019;25:313.

Lee UJ, Gustilo-Ashby AM, Daneshgari F, et al. Lower urogenital tract anatomical and functional phenotype in lysyl oxidase like-1 knockout mice resembles female pelvic floor dysfunction in humans. *Am J Physio Renal Physiol.* 2008;295:F545.

Lei L, Song Y, Chen R. Biomechanical properties of prolapsed vaginal tissue in pre- and postmenopausal women. *Int Urogynecol J.* 2007;18:603.

Lestar B, Penninck F, Rigauts H, Kerremans R. The internal anal sphincter can not close the anal canal completely. *Int J Colorectal Dis.* 1992;7:159.

Li X, Kruger JA, Nash MP, Nielsen PMF. Modeling childbirth: elucidating the mechanisms of labor. *WIRES Syst Biol Med.* 2010;2:4:460.

Liu X, Zhao Y, Pawlyk B, et al. Failure of elastic fiber homeostasis leads to pelvic floor disorders. *Am J Pathol.* 2006;68:519.

Lynn PA, Olsson C, Zagorodnyuk V, et al. Rectal intraganglionic laminar endings are transduction sites of extrinsic mechanoreceptors in the guinea pig rectum. *Gastroenterology.* 2003;125:786.

Martins P, Silva-Filho L, Rodrigues Maciel da Fonseca AM, et al. Biomechanical properties of vaginal tissue in women with pelvic organ prolapse. *Gynecol Obstet Invest.* 2013;75:85.

Miller R, Bartolo DC, Roe A, et al. Anal sensation and the continence mechanism. *Dis Colon Rectum.* 1988;31:433.

Miller R, Lewis GT, Bartolo DCC, et al. Sensory discrimination and dynamic activity in the anorectum – evidence using a new ambulatory technique. *Br J Surg.* 1988;75:1003.

Mirmonsef P, Hotton AL, Gilbert D, et al. Glycogen levels in undiluted genital fluid and their relationship to vaginal pH, estrogen, and progesterone. *PLoS One.* 2016;11(4):e0153553.

Moalli PA, Howden NS, Lowder JL, et al. A rat model to study the structural properties of the vagina and its supportive tissues. *Am J Obstet Gynecol.* 2005;192:80.

Moalli PA, Talarico LC, Sung VW, et al. Impact of menopause on collagen subtypes in the arcus tendineous fasciae pelvis. *Am J Obstet Gynecol.* 2004;190:620.

Mostafa RM, Moustafa YM, Hamdy H. Interstitial cells of Cajal, the Maestro in health and disease. *World J Gastroenterol.* 2010;16:3239.

Muhleisen AL, Herbst-Kralovetz MM. Menopause and the vaginal microbiome. *Maturitas.* 2016;91:42.

Nichols DH, Milley PS, Randall CL. Significance of restoration of normal vaginal depth and axis. *Obstet Gynecol.* 1970;36:251.

O'Hanlon DE, Come RA, Moench TR. Vaginal pH measured in vivo: lactobacilli determine pH and lactic acid concentration. *BMC Microbiol.* 2019;19:13.

Oliphant S, Canavan T, Palcsey S, et al. Pregnancy and parturition negatively impact vaginal angle and alter expression of vaginal MMP-9. *Am J Obstet Gynecol.* 2018;218:242.

Orkin BA, Hanson RB, Kelly KA. The rectal motor complex. *Neurogastroenterol Motil.* 1989;1:5.

Ozdegirmenci O, Karslioglu Y, Dede S, et al. Smooth muscle fraction of the round ligament in women with pelvic organ prolapse: a computer-based morphometric analysis. *Int Urogynecol J.* 2005;16:39.

Pace G, Palumbo P, Miconi G, et al. PDE-5 and NOS II mRNA expression in menopausal women: a molecular biology study. *World J Urol.* 2011;29:243.

Palit S, Lunniss PJ, Scott SM. The physiology of human defecation. *Dig Dis Sci.* 2012;57:1445.

Parente MPL, Jorge RMN, Mascarrenhas T, et al. Deformation of the pelvic floor muscles during a vaginal delivery. *Int Urogynecol J.* 2008;19:65.

Parks AG, Porter NH, Hardcastle J. The syndrome of the descending perineum. *Proc R Soc Med.* 1966;59:477.

Parks AG, Porter NH, Melzak J. Experimental study of the reflex mechanism controlling the muscles of the pelvic floor. *Dis Colon Rectum.* 1962;5:407.

Pu F, Xu L, Li D, et al. Effect of different labor forces on fetal skull molding. *Med Eng Phys.* 2011;33:620.

Raizada V, Bhargava V, Karsten A, Mittal RK. Functional morphology of anal sphincter complex unveiled by high definition anal manometery and three dimensional ultrasound imaging. *Neurogastroenterol Motil.* 2011;23:1013.

Rane A, Lim YN, Withey G, Muller R. Magnetic resonance imaging findings following three different vaginal vault prolapse repair procedures: a randomised study. *Aust N Z J Obstet Gynaecol.* 2004;44:135.

Rao SS. Dyssynergic defecation. *Gastroenterol Clin North Am.* 2001;30:97.

Rao SS. Pathophysiology of adult fecal incontinence. *Gastroenterology.* 2004;126:S14.

Rao SS, Sadeghi P, Beaty J, Kavlock R. Ambulatory 24-hour colonic manometry in slow-transit constipation. *Am J Gastroenterol.* 2004;99:2405.

Rao SS, Welcher K. Periodic rectal motor activity: the intrinsic colonic gatekeeper? *Am J Gastroenterol.* 1996;91:890.

Rostaminia G, Abramowitch S, Chang C, Goldberg RP. Descent and hypermobility of the rectum in women with obstructed defecation symptoms. *Int Urogynecol J.* 2020a;31:337.

Rostaminia G, Routzong M, Chang C, et al. Motion of the vaginal apex during strain and defecation. *Int Urogynecol J.* 2020b;31:391.
Routzong MR, Moalli PA, Maiti S, et al. Novel simulations to determine the impact of superficial perineal structures on vaginal delivery. *Interface Focus.* 2019;9:0011.
Shafik AA, El Sibai O, Shafik AA, Shafik IA. A novel concept for the surgical anatomy of the perineal body. *Dis Colon Rectum.* 2007;50:2120.
Siddique SA. Vaginal anatomy and physiology. *J Pelvic Med Surg.* 2003;9:263.
Sjoberg I, Cajander S, Rylander E. Morphometric characteristics of the vaginal epithelium during the menstrual cycle. *Gynecol Obstet Invest.* 1988;26:136.
Smith TK, Reed JB, Sanders KM. Origin and propagation of electrical slow waves in circular muscle of canine proximal colon. *Am J Physiol.* 1987a;252:C215.
Smith TK, Reed JB, Sanders KM. Interaction of two electrical pacemakers in muscularis of canine proximal colon. *Am J Physiol.* 1987b;252:C290.
Smith WC. The levator ani muscle; Its structure in man, and its comparative relationships. *Anat Rec.* 1923;26:175.
Snooks SJ, Swash M, Mathers SE, Henry MM. Effect of vaginal delivery on the pelvic floor: a 5-year follow-up. *Br J Surg.* 1990;77:1358.
Stewart AM, Cook MS, Dyer KY, Alperin M. Structure–function relationship of the human external anal sphincter. *Int Urogynecol J.* 2018;29:673.
Sze EH, Meranus J, Kohli N, et al. Vaginal configuration on MRI after abdominal sacrocolpopexy and sacrospinous ligament suspension. *Int Urogynecol J Pelvic Floor Dysfunct.* 2001;12:375.
Tinelli A, Malvasi A, Rahimi S, et al. Age-related pelvic floor modifications and prolapse risk factors in postmenopausal women. *Menopause.* 2010;17:204.
Tirumanisetty P, Prichard D, Fletcher JG, et al. Normal values for assessment of anal sphincter morphology, anorectal motion, and pelvic organ prolapse with MRI in healthy women. *Neurogastroenterol Motil.* 2018;30:e13314.
Wall LL. The muscles of the pelvic floor. *Clin Obstet Gynecol.* 1993;36:910.
Wester C, Brubaker L. Normal pelvic floor physiology. *Obstet Gynecol Clin North Am.* 1998;25:707.
Wong RF, Bonapace Jr ES, Chung CY, et al. Simultaneous endoluminal sonography and manometry to assess anal sphincter complex in normal subjects. *Dig Dis Sci.* 1998;43:2363.
Yamanouchi M, Shimatani H, Kadowaki M, et al. Integrative control of rectoanal reflex in guinea pigs through lumbar colonic nerves. *Am J Physiol Gastrointest Liver Physiol.* 2002;283:G148.

5

Pathophysiology of Pelvic Floor Disorders

Danielle Patterson and Victoria L. Handa

CHAPTER OUTLINE

INTRODUCTION

This chapter addresses the pathophysiology of stress urinary incontinence, pelvic organ prolapse, and fecal incontinence (FI). As Fig. 5.1 depicts, overlap of pelvic floor disorders in women suggests that there may be common risk factors or a common pathophysiology to these disorders. Pathophysiologic pathways involved in urgency urinary incontinence and overactive bladder are described in Chapter 31.

STRESS URINARY INCONTINENCE

Urinary incontinence is defined by the International Continence Society as the unintentional, accidental loss of urine. Stress urinary incontinence (SUI) is the complaint of any involuntary loss of urine on effort or physical exertion or on sneezing or coughing (Haylen et al., 2010).

Continence is dependent on the integrated function between pelvic floor muscles, fascia, and nerves. Failure of one without compensation from the others leads to incontinence. This section reviews the anatomy and physiology of continence, the pathophysiology of SUI, and the impact of childbirth on SUI.

Elements of Urinary Continence

To maintain continence, the urethral pressure must be greater than the intravesical pressure at rest and under stress conditions. This sounds simple but involves a complex interplay of neurologic, muscular, and connective tissue supports to function.

Connective Tissue. Studies have shown that both collagen and elastin play a role in urinary continence in women. Keane et al. (1997) found that nulliparous women with SUI have significantly less collagen than controls and have a decreased ratio of type I to type III collagen. A study by Skorupski et al. (2006) found a mutated type I collagen gene more frequently in women with SUI. Genes involved in elastin metabolism are differently expressed in periurethral vaginal tissue from women with SUI than controls. Elastin remodeling may be important in the molecular etiology of SUI (Chen et al., 2006). There may also be a hormonal component to these changes in elastin metabolism.

Another study by Chen et al. (2007) showed that, during the secretory phase, elastolytic activity is increased in pelvic tissues from women with SUI compared with controls, and that this is mediated through an increase in neutrophil elastase and a concurrent decrease in alpha-1 antitrypsin expression. Pantatosakis et al. (2016) showed that expression of estrogen-β, elastin, decorin, fibromodulin, and vasoactive intestinal peptide are all significantly lower in women with SUI versus controls. They theorized that estrogen receptor β–dependent remodeling of the extracellular matrix of vaginal tissue is a cause of SUI. These studies show that further research is needed in this area to elucidate causes of urinary incontinence.

Bladder. The bladder wall is composed of smooth muscle and connective tissue. During bladder filling, the bladder accommodates to the increasing urine volume with little to no increase in intravesical pressure. This is mediated by activation of a spinal sympathetic reflex pathway that inhibits parasympathetic ganglionic transmission and stimulation of β-adrenergic receptors in the bladder body, thus relaxing detrusor contraction.

Urethra. The urethra is supported inferiorly by the anterior vaginal wall and laterally by the pubourethral ligaments that attach to the levator ani. These ligaments have been described

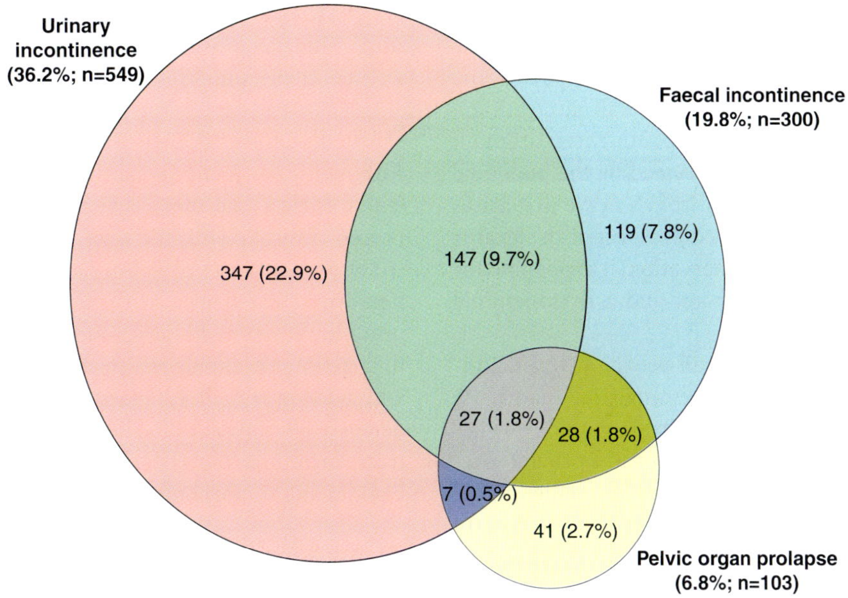

Fig. 5.1 Venn diagram showing the prevalence and concurrence of pelvic floor disorders in 1517 older women in a community setting in Australia. (From Zeleke BM, Bell RJ, Bilah B, Davis SR. Symptomatic pelvic floor disorders in community-dwelling older Australian women. *Maturitas*. 2016;85:34. with permission.)

on magnetic resonance imaging, but their existence is still controversial (Klutke & Siegel, 1995; Kirschner-Hermanns et al., 1993; Aronson et al., 1995). The support provided by the anterior vagina has been likened to a hammock (Fig. 5.2) (DeLancey, 1994). The anterior vagina is laterally attached to the arcus tendineous fasciae pelvis (ATFP), which is a condensation of fascia arising from the levator ani muscles. The ATFP is also the attachment point between the levator ani and obturator internus muscles. The importance of the vaginal "hammock" is discussed in the sections that follow.

The female urethra is 3.5 to 4.5 cm in length. At least two-thirds of this is above the levator ani. Additional contributions to continence are made by the urethral smooth muscle and vascular coaptation. Smooth muscles at the intramural portion of the urethra aid in continence. Longitudinal and circular smooth muscle runs the length of the urethra and surrounds a vascular plexus, which aids in urethral coaptation. The role of the longitudinal smooth muscle is less clear.

The urethra is a pliable structure that must be sealed or coapted completely to maintain continence. Zinner et al. (1980, 1983) showed using mechanical models that there is higher resistance to water flow with a softer lumen and lubricating filler in the outflow tube. Studies rarely address urethral softness or mucosal seal when investigating incontinence. When surgery or radiation cause a stiff urethra, urethral closure is poor. The effects of surgery or radiation may be related to changes in the vascular plexus affecting coaptation, or to changes in the muscles or nerves. More study in this area is needed to delineate the role of urethral softness.

There are three muscles that compose the female urethral sphincter: the rhabdosphincter, the compressor urethrae, and the urethrovaginal sphincter. The rhabdosphincter is the most analogous to the anal sphincter, a circular striated muscle that encompasses the urethral lumen. The compressor urethrae and urethrovaginal sphincter are striated muscles that arch over the

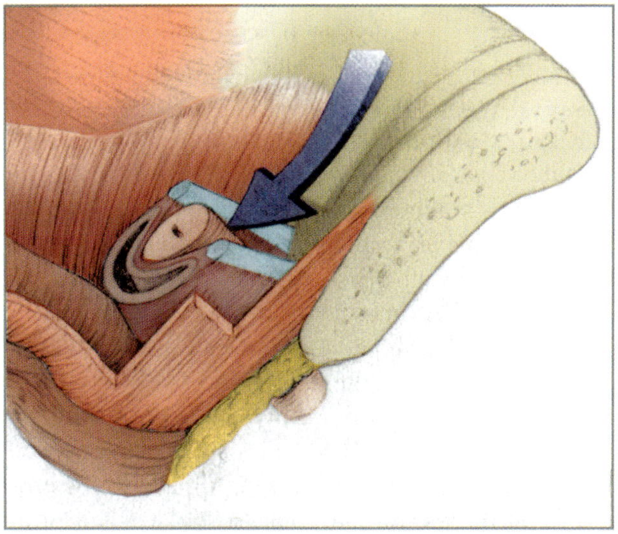

Fig. 5.2 Hammock hypothesis for stress continence. Lateral view of pelvic floor with urethra, vagina, and fascial tissues at level of bladder neck, indicating compression of the urethra by downward force (*arrow*) against supportive tissues (levator ani muscles and vaginal hammock suspended by attachments to the arcus tendineous fasciae pelvis), indicating influence of abdominal pressure on urethra. (From DeLancey JOL. Structural support of the urethra as it relates to stress urinary incontinence: the hammock hypothesis. *Am J Obstet Gynecol*. 1994;170:1713. With permission.)

urethral lumen and exert downward pressure on the urethra against the anterior vaginal wall with contraction. All three muscles are innervated by branches of the pudendal nerve (S2–S4).

Levator Ani. The iliococcygeus, pubococcygeus, and puborectalis muscles together make up the levator ani. The pubococcygeus has three components: the puboperineus, pubovaginalis, and puboanalis. The pubococcygeus and puborectalis muscles close the urogenital hiatus with contraction to compress the urethra, vagina, and rectum. This augments the support of the pubourethral ligament and anterior vaginal wall in creating a firm support for the urethra to maintain continence. Although the urethral sphincter muscles are innervated by the pudendal nerve, these muscles are all innervated from a nerve that arises from S2 to S4 and travels along the medial aspect of the levator muscles. Because of their separate innervation, it is possible for a woman to have functional levator ani and a dysfunctional urethral sphincter.

The levator ani provide support to all pelvic organs including the urethra. As they pass through the urogenital hiatus, the urethra, vagina, and anus are supported by the tonic contractions of the levator ani muscles. The levator ani provide urethral support that is distinct from and in addition to the vaginal "hammock." Both anterior vaginal wall support and levator ani support of the urethra are important in maintaining continence. Many authors have concluded that continence during increased intraabdominal pressure depends on maintaining the proximal urethra in a retropubic position (Jeffcoate & Roberts, 1952; Hodgkinson, 1953; Enhorning, 1961). A stable anterior vaginal wall attached to the ATFP with tonic contraction of the levator ani prevents urethral and bladder neck descent and contributes to urethral compression with straining. This theory of the importance of the retropubic urethra is supported by the success of retropubic operations for the correction of SUI (i.e., Burch and Marshall–Marchetti–Krantz urethropexies). This theory, however, is challenged by the fact that midurethral slings are successful and yet do not modify the position of the proximal urethra. They work by providing a stable suburethral support for effective urethral closure.

The pubourethral ligaments are the lateral fascial and muscular attachments of the urethra to the levator ani. These ligaments likely also contribute to continence. They are distinct from the pubovesical muscles, which arise from the ATFP and insert on the urethra.

The levator ani, together with the striated periurethral muscles (rhabdosphincter, compressor urethrae, and urethrovaginal sphincter) have two roles in maintaining continence. Slow-twitch fibers provide resting urethral tone, and fast-twitch fibers provide rapid contraction in response to increased intraabdominal pressure. With rapid increases in intraabdominal pressure there are reflex as well as voluntary increases in periurethral striated muscle contraction to augment urethral pressure. This occurs predominantly in the mid- and distal urethra. In fact, urethral pressure spikes have been shown to precede intravesical pressure spikes during cough in continent women (Constantinou & Govan, 1982). Lund et al. (1959) used cinefluorography to study what happens when a woman is asked to interrupt her urine stream. The voluntary musculature immediately interrupts the urine stream in the midurethra owing to the periurethral striated muscle contraction against a stable suburethral base (anterior vaginal wall) and levator plate. The urine distal to the contracted area is voided, and the urine proximal flows back into the bladder. The bladder is then seen to rise cephalad owing to the effect of levator contraction on the position of the anterior vaginal wall and bladder. This is representative of fast-twitch muscle contraction. This demonstrates that normal urinary continence in women involves multiple interconnected mechanisms.

Neurophysiologic Considerations

Although stress incontinence is thought of as an anatomic problem, it is clear that there is also a neurologic basis for SUI. This is seen clinically with the treatment of SUI with duloxetine. A study by Kenton et al. (2011) also showed that SUI may be a neuromuscular defect, as continent women had better motor unit recruitment with larger-amplitude, longer-duration motor unit action potentials on electromyography testing compared with women with SUI, suggesting better urethral innervation. A detailed description of the neurophysiology of the lower urinary tract, including the efferent and afferent pathways related to bladder and urethral function, is included in Chapter 3.

Coordinating Reflexes. There is evidence that female urinary incontinence is not just a structural abnormality, but also results from neuromuscular dysfunction. An example of this coordination is the guarding reflex, which maintains continence with progressive bladder distension. With bladder filling, stretch receptors in the detrusor send afferent signals to the spinal cord, activating pudendal somatic efferent stimulation. The afferent stimulation increases with increasing bladder volume. At the same time, the efferent stimulation to the external urethral sphincter increases to maintain continence via augmented sphincter and urethral smooth muscle tone. Another sacral reflex is the activation of the pelvic floor muscles immediately before increased abdominal pressure, leading to a measurable rise in urethral pressure.

Mechanisms of Female Urinary Continence and Incontinence

Historical Insights. Theories of female urinary incontinence historically were based on two ideas: urethral support defects or a dysfunctional urethral sphincter. Victor Bonney examined female urinary incontinence in 1923 and proposed that incontinence was associated with a loss of distal anterior vaginal wall support. In the 1930s Stevens and Smith developed a new theory about the importance of urethral sphincter function over anterior vaginal wall support in maintaining continence based on their work using bead-chain cystography (Stevens & Smith, 1937). Other prominent surgeons of the time echoed this thought with the idea that incontinence could come from an increase in expulsive force, a decrease in urethral resistance, or a combination of both (Barnes, 1940). In the 1980s, Hilton and Stanton determined that deficient pressure transmission ratios were noted in incontinent subjects and not in continent controls and concluded that this is the main cause of SUI. They also found that subjects with SUI had lower total urethral length and lower maximum urethral pressure, and that these factors decreased with increasing severity of incontinence (Hilton & Stanton, 1983). They did not, however, correlate pressure transmission ratios to urethral mobility or determine if the deficient pressure transmission results from urethral hypermobility, abnormal reflex urethral muscle contraction, or other factors.

In the mid-1900s, research on SUI using bead-chain cystourethrograms contributed to the idea that a posterior urethrovesical (PUV) angle between 90 and 100 degrees is essential to maintaining continence, and it was suggested that abnormal PUV angles were always associated with SUI (Green, 1962; Hodgkinson, 1953). However, this theory was later rejected when the reliability of bead-chain cystourethrography in the diagnosis of SUI was found to be poor (Fantl et al., 1981).

Work in the 1960s cast doubt on the theory that the urethra is an abdominal organ and that loss of position causes urinary incontinence (Greenwald et al., 1967). This work placed more support on the argument of urethral sphincter function in the maintenance of continence. Later research focused on pudendal nerve dysfunction as a plausible cause of stress incontinence. Indeed, it was shown that pudendal terminal motor latency is delayed in women with urinary incontinence. Smith et al. (1989) confirmed this by demonstrating that partial denervation of pelvic floor muscles with subsequent reinnervation is a normal part of aging and is increased with childbirth. In fact, women with urinary incontinence, FI, and pelvic organ prolapse all have significantly greater denervation of the pelvic floor than asymptomatic women.

Rather than seeing this as evidence that urinary incontinence may arise from multiple mechanisms (e.g., neuromuscular dysfunction and defective support), one or two mechanisms have typically been seen as prevailing theories on the cause of SUI in women. The Agency for Health Care Policy and Research published a monograph in 1992 that popularized the term "intrinsic sphincter deficiency" (ISD). This was described as a subset of SUI defined as loss of sphincter function, possibly as a result of neuromuscular injury. There is not, however, a clear pathophysiologic mechanism to explain ISD, and it remains a clinical diagnosis.

Lastly, in the 1980s work by Blaivas and Olsson defined urinary incontinence by type in an effort to predict treatment outcome. They divided urinary incontinence into five types based on fluoroscopic urodynamic testing (Blaivas & Olsson, 1988). These classifications, however, did not define the cause of support loss or sphincteric loss or the extent to which each of those contributed to dysfunction. Treatments then did not stem from precise correction of the continence anatomy, and this classification system has fallen out of use.

Unifying Theories on the Causes of Urinary Incontinence. As noted, over the past 100 years anatomists, physiologists, and clinicians have struggled to identify the cause of SUI, and no single mechanism appears to explain this condition. More recently, two theories emerged to explain a more comprehensive view of SUI that accounts for many of the varied observations described previously.

Petros and Ulmsten's Integral Theory arose at the time of the development of the tension-free midurethral sling for the treatment of SUI. It stated that "stress and urge incontinence both arise from the same anatomic defect, a lax vagina" (Petros & Ulmsten, 1990). The Integral Theory, based on the authors' understanding of pelvic anatomy, described the vagina as having two anatomic regions, with the pubourethral ligament in between them to act as a fulcrum. These regions function together to maintain urinary continence and normal bladder sensation by transmitting voluntary and involuntary muscle contractions involved in bladder neck and urethral closure. The vaginal segments also support hypothesized stretch receptors in the proximal urethra and trigone. The pubourethral ligament, in their theory, is hypothesized to extend from the midurethra to the symphysis pubis. The Integral Theory describes three urethral closure mechanisms. The two normal closure mechanisms are at the urethra and bladder neck. The third is the recruitment of the pelvic floor muscles, should the first two mechanisms fail. The urethral closure mechanism is located in the vaginal segment between the urethral meatus and the pubourethral ligament (the hammock) and is oriented vertically. The second urethral closure mechanism is located in the vaginal segment between the pubourethral ligament and the bladder neck (the supralevator vagina) and is horizontal. In this theory, the pubococcygeus and external urethral sphincter muscles contract at the hammock portion of the vagina to facilitate urethral closure. This pulls the hammock portion of the vagina ventrally. (It should be noted that this "hammock" is not the same structure described in the hammock hypothesis described later.) Part of the supralevator vagina lies in the "zone of critical elasticity," which is below the proposed stretch receptors at the bladder base. This area of the supralevator vagina is pulled back and downward with levator contraction, thus closing the bladder neck. If the "zone of elasticity" does not adequately support the stretch receptors, this leads to symptomatic detrusor overactivity. The complicated and complex anatomic relationships proposed in the integral theory make this difficult to understand and apply.

The hammock hypothesis was introduced by DeLancey in 1994 (Fig. 5.2). In this hypothesis the anterior vagina provides support to the urethra and bladder through its attachment to the levator ani muscles and the ATFP. This support causes urethral compression during increased intraabdominal pressure. It also provides a base for the striated urethral sphincter muscles to exert compression. This hypothesis does not include the need for an intraabdominal urethral position. However, it also emphasizes the importance of the levator ani in maintenance of continence. The hammock hypothesis does not attempt to explain detrusor overactivity like the Integral Theory. It does attempt to merge the support versus sphincter debate with the statement that urinary continence is "most likely related to a combination of independent factors" (DeLancey, 1994).

Impact of Childbirth on Urinary Incontinence

It is clear that increased parity is related to increased prevalence of urinary incontinence. In the 2005 to 2006 National Health and Nutrition Examination Survey, 6.5% of nulliparous women and 24% of women with three or more children reported urinary incontinence. Some 25% to 75% of all pregnant women report symptoms of SUI during pregnancy. Primiparous women have three times higher prevalence of SUI than their nulligravid counterparts (Hansen et al., 2012).

It is less clear whether pregnancy itself or vaginal delivery is the cause of SUI in most women. Given that occasional urinary incontinence is very common, it may be better to evaluate the impact of delivery on clinically significant incontinence. A large Norwegian study found that women who delivered vaginally had a 2.2-fold increased risk of moderate to severe urinary incontinence compared with those who delivered via cesarean section (Rortveit et al., 2003). In a retrospective cohort study of parous women 5 to 10 years after delivery, the odds of bothersome SUI doubled with at least one vaginal birth compared with women who delivered only via cesarean section (Handa et al., 2011). Additionally, operative vaginal birth has been associated with increased rates of SUI (Handa et al., 2012). Women who deliver vaginally have three times the odds, and women with operative delivery 20 times the odds, of having surgery for SUI than women who deliver via cesarean section (Leijonhufvud et al., 2011).

The term breech trial assessed the differences in pelvic floor symptoms between women with planned elective cesarean delivery and planned vaginal birth at 3 months postpartum. Women in the planned cesarean delivery group reported less urinary incontinence than those in the planned vaginal delivery group (4.5% vs. 7.3%). These findings were limited because of the number of women in the planned vaginal delivery group who ultimately delivered by cesarean section (Hannah et al., 2002).

Note that, although these studies show an increase in bothersome urinary incontinence with vaginal over cesarean delivery, the protective effect of cesarean delivery and nulliparity decreases with time. By age 50 to 60 years, the rates of urinary incontinence in women are the same regardless of mode of delivery.

PELVIC ORGAN PROLAPSE

Elements of Support

The pelvic viscera are supported by a system of muscles and connective tissue. The anatomy of pelvic organ support is described in Chapter 1.

Levator Ani Muscle. As previously described, a critical component of uterovaginal support is the levator ani muscle complex, comprising the iliococcygeus, pubococcygeus, and puborectalis muscles. The urethra, vagina, and rectum pass through the levator hiatus, a space between these paired muscles. Posterior to the rectum is the levator plate, which extends from the levator hiatus to the coccyx.

The levator muscles are unique skeletal muscles, in that they maintain tone in the absence of voluntary contraction (Corton & DeLancey, 2019). The resting tone of the pubococcygeus muscle maintains closure of the urogenital hiatus. In addition, levator tone maintains a relatively horizontal position of the levator plate, which then forms a platform that supports the uterus, proximal vagina, and rectum.

Connective Tissue. The uterosacral and cardinal ligaments support the proximal vagina and uterus by pulling the vaginal apex and cervix toward the sacrum, thus positioning these organs over the levator plate and allowing these organs to be supported by the levator ani muscle (Corton & DeLancey, 2019). Prolapse is hypothesized to occur if the vagina and uterus are instead positioned over the levator hiatus, such as might happen with hiatal widening or disruption of the uterosacral ligaments. In that situation, the pelvic organs are not supported by the levator ani muscle complex. As the organs descend into the levator hiatus, the support provided by attachments of the uterosacral and cardinal ligaments eventually becomes insufficient and fails over time. This hypothesis was advanced by Norton (1993), who likened the support of the pelvic organs to a boat at the dock (Fig. 5.3), in which the ligaments serve as the "lines" tethering the ship to the dock. According to this analogy, the uterosacral and cardinal ligaments hold the "ship" (vagina and uterus) in position, but they are not sufficient to support the ship if the water (analogous to the intact and functional levator ani muscle complex) is withdrawn.

In addition to the role of the uterosacral ligament in maintaining the position of the vaginal apex, several studies have suggested a role for connective tissue quality. Specifically, defects in connective tissue remodeling and homeostasis have been implicated in animal models of prolapse. Murine knockout models

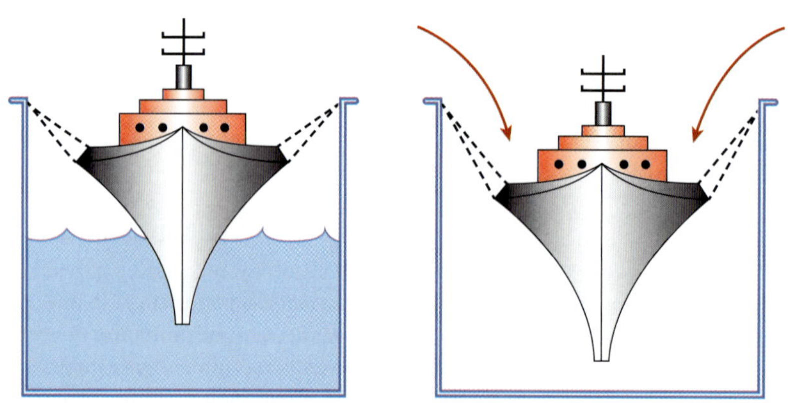

Fig. 5.3 The "boat in dry-dock" analogy. The first figure shows a boat (analogous to the uterus and vaginal apex) supported by the water (analogous to the support provided by the normal levator plate). The lines (analogous to the uterosacral-cardinal ligament complex) maintain the position of the boat but do not provide support. The second figure shows that, if the water (levator plate) does not provide the needed support, the demands on the lines (ligaments) will ultimately exceed their capacity to provide support. (Modified from Bo K, ed. Evidence Based Physical Therapy for the Pelvic Floor. 2nd ed. New York: Elsevier Ltd.; 2015. With permission.)

with genetically engineered deficiencies in proteins responsible for collagen and elastin remodeling have been shown to develop prolapse, either spontaneously or after parturition. For example, fibulin-5 and lysyl oxidases are required for normal elastic fiber synthesis; mice deficient in the gene encoding fibulin-5 develop spontaneous prolapse (Wieslander et al., 2006), whereas *LOXL-1* knockout mice (Boraziani et al., 2019) typically develop prolapse only after a traumatic event (such as vaginal delivery or simulated delivery via vaginal distension). The mechanism for the latter may be impaired recovery and repair. These models raise the possibility that interventions to improve connective tissue repair (such as regenerative medicine and stem cell transplantation) could potentially facilitate effective repair after pregnancy and delivery (Pathi et al., 2012; Gräs et al., 2017). Also, there is some evidence for genetic polymorphisms in human women with prolapse: a systematic review by Ward et al. (2014) suggested that variants of the collagen type 3 alpha 1 (*COL3A1*) gene may be associated with prolapse in some populations.

Mechanisms of Injury

Levator Ani Muscle Avulsion. Levator ani muscle avulsion (detachment from the bony pelvis) can be palpated on physical examination and was observed by gynecologists as early as the 1940s (Gainey, 1943). This observation was largely overlooked until the advent of high-resolution imaging, such as three-dimensional ultrasound and magnetic resonance imaging. These techniques have demonstrated levator avulsions in 15% to 30% of women after vaginal childbirth (DeLancey et al., 2003; Caudwell-Hall et al., 2017; Dietz & Lanzarone, 2005).

Levator ani muscle detachment is likely a complication of excessive stretching of the levator during the passage of the fetal head. This theory is supported by a biomechanical computer simulation of the descent of fetal head through the levator hiatus (Lien et al., 2004). As the fetal head descends, the levator ani muscle complex must stretch to accommodate the diameter of the presenting part. This model predicts that the demand for muscle stretching is greatest for the medial pubococcygeus muscle, which is required to stretch to more than three times its resting length to accommodate the fetal head. Thus, the medial levator ani muscles are at greatest risk for injury during parturition. Indeed, this conclusion is consistent with magnetic resonance imaging (Fig. 5.4) and three-dimensional ultrasound imaging (Fig. 5.5), which can be used to demonstrate detachment of the pubococcygeus muscle after vaginal delivery (DeLancey et al., 2003; Caudwell-Hall et al., 2017; Dietz & Lanzarone, 2005).

Evaluation for levator ani muscle avulsion is not part of contemporary clinical practice and yet, in the research setting, avulsion is strongly associated with pelvic organ prolapse. For example, in a study of 453 women an average of 11 years after vaginal delivery (Handa et al., 2019a), levator avulsion more than doubled the odds for prolapse beyond the hymen. Also, studies comparing women presenting for treatment of prolapse and controls without prolapse have found that women with prolapse are two to four times more likely to demonstrate levator avulsions (Dietz & Simpson, 2008; DeLancey et al., 2007).

Levator Muscle Function. Levator ani strength is reduced after vaginal childbirth compared with cesarean delivery (Friedman et al., 2012). Among vaginally parous women, levator ani avulsion is further associated with poor muscle strength (Handa et al., 2020). The strength of the levator muscle plays an important role in pelvic organ support. Weakening of the levator ani muscle complex, as measured during voluntary contraction, is associated with uterovaginal prolapse (Borello-France et al., 2007; Blomquist et al., 2020; DeLancey et al., 2007; Diez-Itza et al., 2011). A role for muscle strength in the development of prolapse is further suggested by studies that demonstrate improved pelvic organ support and reduction of prolapse symptoms after pelvic floor muscle training (Li et al., 2016).

Levator Hiatus Size. The width of the levator hiatus is strongly and significantly associated with prolapse (Handa et al., 2019b). In a study of vaginally parous women an average of 11 years after delivery, prolapse beyond the hymen was observed among only 11% of women with a levator hiatus less than 20 cm^2 and in almost 50% of women with a hiatus greater than 35 cm^2. The odds for prolapse increased 50% for each 5 cm^2 increase in hiatus area.

Impact of Childbirth on Pelvic Organ Prolapse

As discussed in Chapter 6, nulliparous women are at significantly lower risk of prolapse compared with parous women. This was reported more than 20 years ago by Mant et al. (1997), who found that parity was strongly associated with surgery for prolapse. Also, among a study of 487 Swedish women, Samuelsson et al. (1999) found that prolapse on examination was associated with parity. Among parous women, prolapse is strongly associated with vaginal versus cesarean childbirth (Handa et al., 2011). The odds of prolapse are highest for women who have experienced at least one operative vaginal birth.

There are several reasons why vaginal delivery may lead to prolapse later in life. The impact of levator ani muscle avulsion has been discussed previously. But pregnancy and childbirth may have other impacts on pelvic organ support. One potential contributor may be antepartum maternal adaptations that are thought to prepare the pelvic floor for the events of parturition.

In humans, these maternal adaptations are evidenced by a deterioration in pelvic organ support during normal pregnancy (Oliphant et al., 2014). For example, mild pelvic organ prolapse is more common among pregnant nulliparous women compared with nonpregnant nulligravid controls (O'Boyle et al., 2002). In the rat, levator muscle fibers lengthen during pregnancy (Alperin et al., 2015). Also, smooth muscle cells demonstrate noncontractile phenotypes during pregnancy, and collagen becomes more loosely packed (Daucher et al., 2007). These changes result in increased vaginal distensibility, presumably to facilitate stretching during labor and delivery (Alperin et al., 2010). Elastin homeostasis is also impacted during pregnancy: in fibulin-5-deficient mice, a model for impaired elastic fiber synthesis, vaginal distension induces pelvic organ prolapse (Rahn et al., 2008). These findings suggest that disruption of the normal mechanisms for elastin homeostasis may contribute to the development of prolapse postpartum.

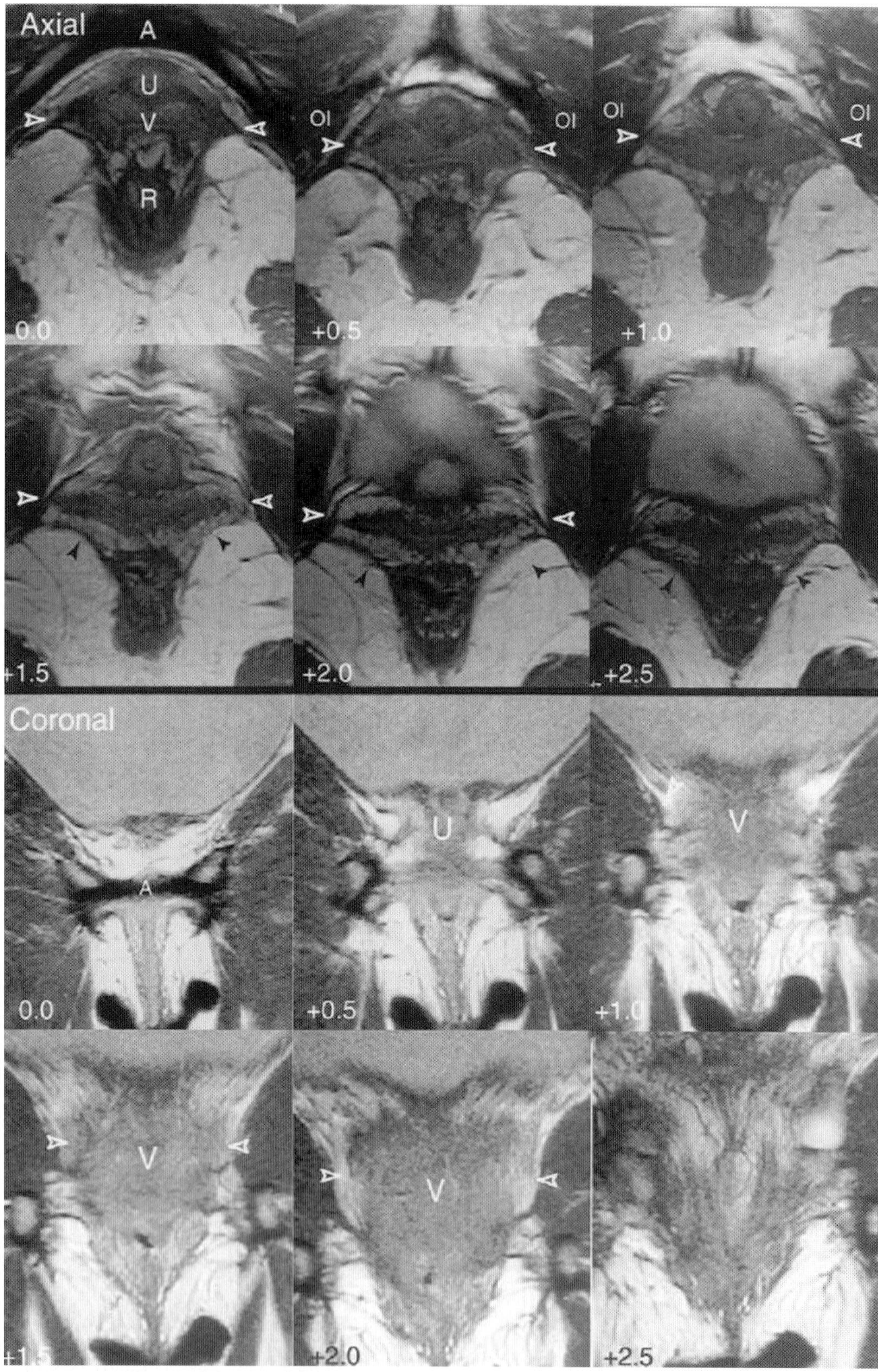

Fig. 5.4 Axial and coronal images of a 38-year-old incontinent primiparous woman. The area where the pubovisceral (pubococcygeus) portion of the levator ani muscle is missing (*open arrowhead*) between the urethra *(U)*, vagina *(V)*, rectum *(R)*, and obturator internus *(OI)* muscle is shown. The vagina protrudes laterally into the defects to lie close to the obturator internus muscle. *A*, Arcuate pubic ligament. (From DeLancey JO, Kearney R, Chou Q, et al. The appearance of levator ani muscle abnormalities in magnetic resonance images after vaginal delivery. *Obstet Gynecol.* 2003;101:46. With permission.)

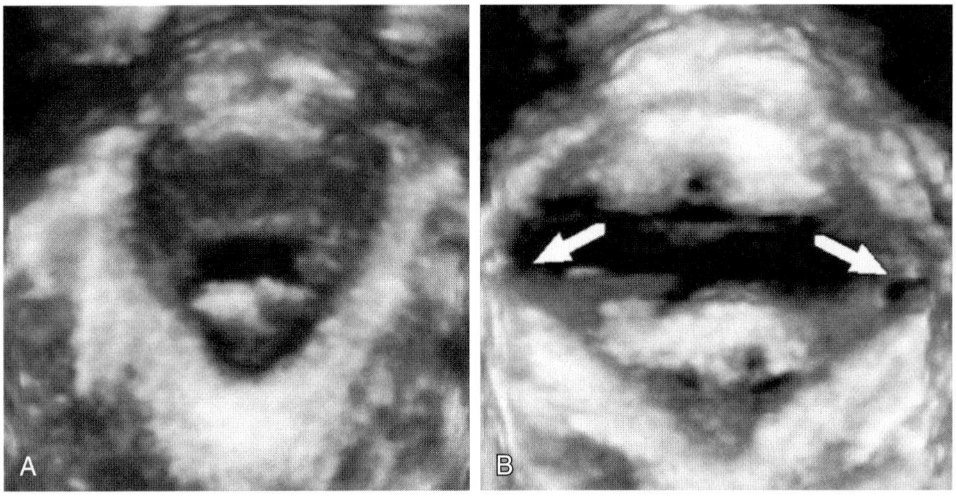

Fig. 5.5 Axial-rendered volume representation of the puborectalis–pubococcygeus complex on three-dimensional pelvic floor ultrasound at 38 weeks' gestation (**A**) and 4 months postpartum (**B**). Both images were obtained on Valsalva maneuver. The *arrows* indicate a bilateral avulsion injury, which was associated with markedly increased pelvic organ descent. (From Dietz HP, Lanzarone V. Levator trauma after vaginal delivery. *Obstet Gynecol.* 2005;106:707. With permission.)

It has been hypothesized that inadequate pelvic floor adaptation during pregnancy could predispose a woman to levator ani avulsion during delivery: if the levator ani muscle is not sufficiently distensible, avulsion may be the inevitable result. This theory was tested by a randomized trial of a device designed to mechanically stretch the levator ani muscle during the last month of pregnancy, the EPI-No birth trainer (Kamisan Atan et al., 2016). Levator avulsions were observed in 12% of women assigned to use the trainer versus 15% of controls (P = .39). This study suggests that mechanical stretching of the levator muscle may not be an effective prevention strategy.

FECAL INCONTINENCE

FI, as defined by the Rome IV criteria, is the uncontrolled passage of solid or liquid stool. Anal incontinence also includes the uncontrolled passage of gas. There is no distinction made based on the presumed mechanism for the incontinence: functional, structural, or neurologic. Indeed, emerging evidence supports that there are multiple factors that contribute to FI, and that effective treatment need not be based on the presumed etiology. More information on the epidemiology of FI and its impact on quality of life is found in Chapters 6 and 27.

Anatomy and Physiology

The ability to maintain fecal continence is dependent on many factors, including an intact anal sphincter mechanism, a compliant rectal reservoir, efficient evacuation, appropriate stool volume and consistency, adequate intestinal motility, sufficient pelvic floor structural integrity, intact innervation, intact cortical awareness, intact cognition, and ready access to toileting facilities. FI occurs when one or more of these mechanisms are impaired and the others cannot compensate. Thus, FI is usually a result of multiple factors, and not just one of these mechanisms.

Dysfunction leading to FI can be classified as suprasphincteric or sphincteric. Suprasphincteric dysfunction involves stool consistency and volume, rectal compliance and motility, the rectoanal inhibitory reflex (RAIR), and rectal sensation. Chronic liquid stools and abnormal rectal compliance also lead to FI. This mechanism of FI is common in patients with conditions such as ulcerative colitis and radiation proctitis. These patients have decreased rectal compliance such that smaller volumes of stool cause urgency, which often leads to incontinence (Zorcolo & Bartolo, 2007).

The RAIR enables the contents of the rectum to come in contact with the upper anal canal epithelium for sampling. In this reflex, the presence of stool leads to relaxation of the internal anal sphincter (IAS), whereas the external anal sphincter (EAS) contracts to maintain continence. This sampling happens several times an hour and allows distinction between solid, liquid, and gas to allow storage of bowel contents or expulsion when appropriate (Miller et al., 1988). If the sampling mechanism is defective, and sphincter tone is poor, the patient may be unaware of impending incontinence (Zorcolo & Bartolo, 2007).

Rectal sensation is critical to normal evacuation and continence. Both rectal hyposensitivity and hypersensitivity can lead to FI (Chan et al., 2005a; Gladman et al., 2006). The rectum does not have its own proprioceptors; instead, rectal sensation comes from the levator muscles and anal sphincters, which are innervated by the pudendal nerve. A cause of FI in patients with an intact anal sphincter is disturbed sensation and impaired evacuation of the rectum attributed to pudendal neuropathy (Hancke & Schurholz, 1987; Lubowski & Nichols, 1988).

Animal models suggest that FI may result from damage to peripheral nerves, including the pudendal, pelvic, or inferior rectal nerves (Evers et al., 2017). van Meegdenburg et al. (2015) found that voluntary anal sphincter contraction is significantly weaker in patients with pudendal neuropathy. This most likely results in fecal urgency incontinence. Additionally, pudendal neuropathy is often cited as a risk factor for persistent FI after sphincteroplasty (Gilliland et al., 1998).

Rectal hyposensitivity is associated with medical conditions such as dementia, stroke, and encephalopathy, which alter mental status. Sensory neuropathies contributing to FI may also be associated with conditions including diabetes, spina bifida, and meningocele (Zorcolo & Bartolo, 2007). Pelvic nerve injury, as well as abnormal toilet behavior, are also thought to lead to rectal hyposensitivity (Gladman et al., 2006). Rectal hyposensitivity may be associated with poor evacuation and constipation but may also be a cause of passive FI. Moreover, the decreased rectal sensation and poor motility associated with constipation can lead to impaction and overflow incontinence (Sun et al., 1990).

Rectal hypersensitivity is also associated with FI and may be caused by impaired relaxation of the rectum. Other proposed mechanisms of hypersensitivity include sensitization of the extrinsic peripheral pathways, central afferent mechanisms, or low-grade inflammation (Lembo 1994; Mayer & Gebhart, 1994; Spiller et al., 2000). Rectal hypersensitivity is also an independent trigger for fecal urgency. It has been noted that, when sphincteric dysfunction coexists with rectal hypersensitivity, patients have increased frequency of stool, fecal urgency, and incontinence compared with those with isolated sphincter dysfunction (Chan et al., 2005b).

In addition to these suprasphincteric causes of FI, dysfunction of the anal sphincter itself also contributes to this condition. Sphincteric dysfunction can involve the IAS or the EAS. The IAS is made of circular smooth muscle and is under continuous contraction until defecation. With age, the resting tone of the IAS decreases with the gradual degradation of the muscle fibers (Eckadt & Elmer, 1991). Structural damage to the IAS can occur with anal surgery, anorectal trauma, or childbirth. The incidence of sphincter disruption at the time of childbirth is as high as 15% in some populations, and ultrasound suggests that subclinical damage to the IAS may complicate up to 35% of vaginal deliveries (Sultan et al., 1993). Passive FI may occur in these cases if the EAS contraction cannot overcome the low IAS tone.

The EAS, unlike other skeletal muscle, maintains a continuous resting tone (Floyd & Walls, 1953). The normal response of the EAS to stimuli such as increased intraabdominal pressure or rectal distention is increased contraction to allow time for rectal accommodation. The ability to voluntarily increase tone lasts about 40 to 60 seconds, which is usually sufficient to allow for accommodation (Schuster et al., 1965). If the sphincter cannot voluntarily contract for this long, FI can occur. The most common cause of damage to the EAS is vaginal delivery.

Impact of Childbirth on Fecal Incontinence

Laceration of the anal sphincter occurs in 2% to 16% of vaginal deliveries (Lowder et al., 2007; Ritcher et al., 2002). Many studies have shown a significant risk of FI after obstetric anal sphincter laceration, despite recognition and repair at the time of delivery. In the Childbirth and Pelvic Symptoms study conducted in 2006 by the Pelvic Floor Disorders Network, FI was observed 6 months after delivery among 17% of women with an obstetric anal sphincter laceration, compared with only 8% of women who delivered vaginally without a sphincter laceration. FI is similar between women who delivered by cesarean and those who deliver vaginally without a sphincter laceration (Borello-France et al., 2006; Evers et al., 2012). The risk of FI associated with obstetrical trauma has been found to persist to at least 10 years postpartum (Evers et al., 2012), but does appear to decline with age. By 30 years postpartum, the reported prevalence of FI is not associated with delivery type (Nygaard et al., 1997).

Few studies have compared the risk of FI associated with third- versus fourth-degree anal sphincter lacerations. It has been hypothesized that trauma to the IAS, presumably more common with fourth-degree laceration, may not be effectively addressed by conventional repairs. Given that the function of the internal sphincter is to maintain passive continence, repair of this would theoretically decrease FI. Indeed, a retrospective single site study showed a 10-fold greater incidence of worse bowel control after delivery than before delivery in those with fourth-degree lacerations (30.6%) versus those with third-degree lacerations (3.6%) (Fenner et al., 2003). This was confirmed in another study by the Pelvic Floor Disorders Network that found two-fold greater odds of FI after fourth-degree compared with third-degree laceration (Burgio et al., 2007). Two small European cohort studies addressed the feasibility and effectiveness of repair of the IAS at delivery. In a British study, investigators were unable to identify 40% of the torn internal sphincters, and 33% of the repairs failed (Sultan et al., 1999). In contrast, in a Norwegian study investigators were able to identify and repair all but one torn internal sphincter (6% missed), and only two (16%) of these repairs failed. After a median follow-up of 34 months, only two (7%) subjects reported incontinence of solid or liquid stool (Kairaluoma et al., 2004). These data are promising but should be confirmed in larger controlled trials.

Third- and fourth-degree anal sphincter lacerations may recur in 7.5% to 10% of subsequent vaginal deliveries (McKenna et al., 2003). This has led some physicians to recommend cesarean section for all subsequent deliveries after a third- or fourth-degree laceration. However, the effect of subsequent vaginal delivery on FI in women with previous third-degree lacerations has not been definitively established. The impact of subsequent delivery may depend on whether sphincter laceration recurs. Three small, prospective, European studies have reported differing results with respect to FI after subsequent vaginal delivery (Pollack et al., 2004; Fornell et al., 2005; Tetzschner et al., 1996). More data are needed to make recommendations regarding delivery mode for subsequent pregnancy after third-degree anal sphincter lacerations. This may depend, in part, on continued symptoms of FI.

In contrast, data are more consistent regarding subsequent delivery after fourth-degree anal sphincter lacerations. In a Swiss study, women with one or more vaginal deliveries after fourth-degree laceration were more likely to have FI (28% vs. 22%) than those with no subsequent vaginal deliveries (Sangalli et al., 2000). Another US study of women who had experienced fourth-degree laceration found that, although rates of FI were similar in all women, the severity of incontinence was worse in women with at least two subsequent vaginal deliveries versus one or no subsequent deliveries (11%, 0%, and 0%, respectively) (Sze, 2005). It appears from these data that vaginal delivery after fourth-degree anal sphincter laceration may worsen FI. It may be beneficial to consider elective cesarean delivery in these women, especially those with continued symptoms of FI.

BIBLIOGRAPHY

Stress Urinary Incontinence

Aronson MP, Bates SM, Jacoby AF, et al. Periurethral and paravaginal anatomy: an endovaginal magnetic resonance imaging study. *Am J Obstet Gynecol.* 1995;173:1702.

Barnes A. A method of evaluating the stress of urinary incontinence. *Am J Obstet Gynecol.* 1940;40:381.

Blaivas JG, Olsson CA. Stress incontinence: classification and surgical approach. *J Urol.* 1988;139:727.

Chen B, Wen Y, Xu X, Polan ML. The role of neutrophil elastase in elastin metabolism of pelvic tissues from women with stress urinary incontinence. *Neurourol Urodyn.* 2007;26:274.

Chen B, Wen Y, Zhang Z, et al. Microarray analysis of differentially expressed genes in vaginal tissues from women with stress urinary incontinence compared with asymptomatic women. *Hum Reprod.* 2006;21:22.

Constantinou CD, Govan DE. Spinal distribution and timing of transmitted and reflexly generated urethral pressures in healthy women. *J Urol.* 1982;127:964.

DeLancey JOL. Structural support of the urethra as it relates to stress urinary incontinence: the hammock hypothesis. *Am J Obstet Gynecol.* 1994;170:1713.

Enhorning G. Simultaneous recording of intravesical and intraurethral pressure. *Acta Chir Scand.* 1961;276:1.

Fantl JA, Hurt GW, Beachley MC, et al. Bead-chain cystourethrogram: an evaluation. *Obstet Gynecol.* 1981;58:237.

Green TH. Development of a plan for the diagnosis and treatment of urinary stress incontinence. *Am J Obstet Gynecol.* 1962;83:632.

Greenwald SW, Thonbury JR, Dunn LJ. Cystourethrography as a diagnostic aid in stress incontinence: an evaluation. *Obstet Gynecol.* 1967;29:324.

Handa VL, Blomquist JL, McDermott KC, et al. Pelvic floor disorders after vaginal birth: effect of episiotomy, perineal lacerations and operative birth. *Obstet Gynecol.* 2012;119:233.

Hannah ME, Hannah WJ, Hodnett ED, et al. Outcomes at 3 months after planned cesarean versus planned vaginal delivery for breech presentation at term: The International Randomized Term Breech Trial. *JAMA.* 2002;287:1822.

Hansen BB, Svare J, Viktrup L, et al. Urinary incontinence during pregnancy and 1 year after delivery in primiparous women compared with a control group of nulliparous women. *Neurourol Urodyn.* 2012;31:475.

Haylen BT, de Ridder D, Freeman RM, et al. An International Urogynecologic Association (IUGA)/International Continence Society (ICS) Joint Report on the Terminology for Female Pelvic Floor Dysfunction. *Neurourol Urodyn.* 2010;29:4.

Hilton P, Stanton SL. Urethral pressure measurement by microtransducer: the results in symptom-free women and in those with genuine stress incontinence. *Br J Obstet Gynecol.* 1983;90:919.

Hodgkinson CP. Relationships of the female urethra and bladder in urinary stress incontinence. *Am J Obstet Gynecol.* 1953;90:919.

Jeffcoate TN, Roberts H. Observations on stress incontinence of urine. *Am J Obstet Gynecol.* 1952;64:721.

Keane DP, Sims TJ, Abrams P, Bailey AJ. Analysis of collagen status in premenopausal nulliparous women with genuine stress incontinence. *BJOG.* 1997;104:994.

Kenton K, Mueller E, Brubaker L. Continent women have better urethral neuromuscular function than those with stress incontinence. *Int Urogynecol J.* 2011;22:1479.

Kirschner-Hermanns R, Wein B, Niehaus S, et al. The contribution of magnetic resonance imaging of the pelvic floor to the understanding of urinary incontinence. *Br J Urol.* 1993;72:715.

Klutke CG, Siegel CL. Functional female pelvic anatomy. *Urol Clin North Am.* 1995;22:487.

Leijonhufvud A, Lundholm C, Cnattingius S, et al. Risks of stress urinary incontinence and pelvic organ prolapse in relation to mode of childbirth. *Am J Obstet Gynecol.* 2011;204:70.

Lund CJ, Fullerton RE, Tristan TA. Cinefluorographic studies of the bladder and urethra in women. *Am J Obstet Gynecol.* 1959;78:706.

Pantatosakis E, Karandrea D, Liapis E, et al. Immunohistochemical expression of hormonal receptors, collagen, elastin and proteoglycans in genuine urinary incontinence. *Clin Exp Obstet Gynecol.* 2016;43:849.

Petros P, Ulmsten U. An integral theory of female urinary incontinence. *Acta Obstet Gynecol Scand Suppl.* 1990;153:7.

Rortveit G, Daltveit AK, Hannestad YS, Hunskaar S. Urinary incontinence after vaginal delivery or cesarean section. *N Engl J Med.* 2003;348:900.

Skorupski P, Krol J, Starega J, et al. An alpha-1 chain of type I collagen Sp1-finding site polymorphism in women suffering from stress urinary incontinence. *Am J Obstet Gynecol.* 2006;194:346.

Smith AR, Hosker GL, Warrell DW. The role of partial denervation of the pelvic floor in the aetiology of genitourinary prolapse and stress incontinence of urine. A neurophysiological study. *Br J Obstet Gynaecol.* 1989;96:24.

Stevens W, Smith S. Roetgenological examination of the female urethra. *J Urol.* 1937;37:194.

Zeleke BM, Bell RJ, Bilah B, Davis SR. Symptomatic pelvic floor disorders in community-dwelling older Australian women. *Maturitas.* 2016;85:34.

Zinner NR, Sterling AM, Ritter RC. Evaluation of inner urethral softness. *Urology.* 1983;22:446.

Zinner NR, Sterling AM, Ritter RC. Role of inner urethral softness in urinary incontinence. *Urology.* 1980;16:115.

Pelvic Organ Prolapse

Alperin M, Feola A, Duerr R, et al. Pregnancy- and delivery-induced biomechanical changes in rat vagina persist postpartum. *Int Urogynecol J.* 2010;21(9):1169.

Alperin M, Lawley DM, Esparza MC, Lieber RL. Pregnancy-induced adaptations in the intrinsic structure of rat pelvic floor muscles. *Am J Obstet Gynecol.* 2015;213(2):191.e1.

Blomquist JL, Carroll M, Muñoz A, Handa VL. Pelvic floor muscle strength and the incidence of pelvic floor disorders after vaginal and cesarean delivery. *Am J Obstet Gynecol.* 2020;222:62.e1.

Bo K, ed. *Evidence Based Physical Therapy for the Pelvic Floor.* 2nd ed. New York: Elsevier Ltd.; 2015.

Boraziani A, Couri BM, Kuang M, et al. Role of lysyl oxidase like 1 in regulation of postpartum connective tissue metabolism in the mouse vagina. *Biol Reprod.* 2019;101:916.

Borello-France DF, Handa VL, Brown MB, et al. Pelvic Floor Disorders Network. Pelvic-floor muscle function in women with pelvic organ prolapse. *Phys Ther.* 2007;87:399.

Caudwell-Hall J, Kamisan Atan I, Martin A, et al. Intrapartum predictors of maternal levator ani injury. *Acta Obstet Gynecol Scand.* 2017;96:426.

Corton MM, DeLancey JOL. Surgical anatomy of the female pelvis. In: Handa VL, Van Le L, eds. *Telinde's Operative Gynecology.* 12th ed. Philadelphia: Wolters Kluwer; 2019.

Daucher JA, Clark KA, Stolz DB, et al. Adaptations of the rat vagina in pregnancy to accommodate delivery. *Obstet Gynecol.* 2007;109:128.
DeLancey JO, Kearney R, Chou Q, et al. The appearance of levator ani muscle abnormalities in magnetic resonance images after vaginal delivery. *Obstet Gynecol.* 2003;101:46.
DeLancey JO, Morgan DM, Fenner DE, et al. Comparison of levator ani muscle defects and function in women with and without pelvic organ prolapse. *Obstet Gynecol.* 2007;109:295.
Dietz HP, Lanzarone V. Levator trauma after vaginal delivery. *Obstet Gynecol.* 2005;106:707.
Dietz HP, Simpson JM. Levator trauma is associated with pelvic organ prolapse. *BJOG.* 2008;115:979.
Diez-Itza I, Arrue M, Ibañez L, et al. Postpartum impairment of pelvic floor muscle function: factors involved and association with prolapse. *Int Urogynecol J.* 2011;22:1505.
Friedman S, Blomquist JL, Nugent JM, et al. Pelvic muscle strength after childbirth. *Obstet Gynecol.* 2012;120:1021.
Gainey HL. Post-partum observation of pelvic tissue damage. *Am J Obstet Gynecol.* 1943;46:457.
Gräs S, Tolstrup CK, Lose G. Regenerative medicine provides alternative strategies for the treatment of anal incontinence. *Int Urogynecol J.* 2017 Mar;28:341.
Handa VL, Blomquist JL, Knoepp LR, et al. Pelvic floor disorders 5-10 years after vaginal or cesarean childbirth. *Obstet Gynecol.* 2011;118:777.
Handa VL, Blomquist JL, Roem J, et al. Levator morphology and strength after obstetrical avulsion of the levator ani muscle. *Female Pelvic Med Reconstr Surg.* 2020;26:56.
Handa VL, Blomquist JL, Roem J, et al. Pelvic floor disorders after obstetrical avulsion of the levator ani muscle. *Female Pelvic Med Reconstr Surg.* 2019a;25:3.
Handa VL, Roem J, Blomquist JL, et al. Pelvic organ prolapse as a function of levator ani avulsion, hiatus size, and strength. *Am J Obstet Gynecol.* 2019b;221:41.e1.
Kamisan Atan I, Shek KL, Langer S, et al. Does the Epi-No(®) birth trainer prevent vaginal birth-related pelvic floor trauma? A multicentre prospective randomised controlled trial. *BJOG.* 2016;123:995.
Li C, Gong Y, Wang B. The efficacy of pelvic floor muscle training for pelvic organ prolapse: a systematic review and meta-analysis. *Int Urogynecol J.* 2016;27:981.
Lien KC, Mooney B, DeLancey JO, Ashton-Miller JA. Levator ani muscle stretch induced by simulated vaginal birth. *Obstet Gynecol.* 2004;103:31.
Mant J, Painter R, Vessey M. Epidemiology of genital prolapse: observations from the Oxford Family Planning Association Study. *Br J Obstet Gynaecol.* 1997;104:579.
Norton PA. Pelvic floor disorders: the role of fascia and ligaments. *Clin Obstet Gynecol.* 1993;36:926.
O'Boyle AL, Woodman PJ, O'Boyle JD, et al. Pelvic organ support in nulliparous pregnant and nonpregnant women: a case control study. *Am J Obstet Gynecol.* 2002;187:99.
Oliphant SS, Nygaard IE, Zong W, et al. Maternal adaptations in preparation for parturition predict uncomplicated spontaneous delivery outcome. *Am J Obstet Gynecol.* 2014;211:630.e1.
Pathi SD, Acevedo JF, Keller PW, et al. Recovery of the injured external anal sphincter after injection of local or intravenous mesenchymal stem cells. *Obstet Gynecol.* 2012;119:134.
Rahn DD, Acevedo JF, Word RA. Effect of vaginal distention on elastic fiber synthesis and matrix degradation in the vaginal wall: potential role in the pathogenesis of pelvic organ prolapse. *Am J Physiol Regul Integr Comp Physiol.* 2008;295:R1351.
Samuelsson EC, Victor FT, Tibblin G, Svärdsudd KF. Signs of genital prolapse in a Swedish population of women 20 to 59 years of age and possible related factors. *Am J Obstet Gynecol.* 1999;180:299.
Ward RM, Velez Edwards DR, Edwards T, et al. Genetic epidemiology of pelvic organ prolapse: a systematic review. *Am J Obstet Gynecol.* 2014;211:326.
Wieslander CK, Acevedo JF, Drewes PG, et al. Pelvic organ prolapse severity increases with age in fibulin-5 knockout mice. *Int Urogynecol J.* 2006;17:S371.

Fecal Incontinence

Borello-France D, Burgio KL, Richter HE. Fecal and urinary incontinence in primiparous women. *Obstet Gynecol.* 2006;108(4):863.
Burgio KL, Borello-France D, Ritcher HE, et al. Risk factors for fecal and urinary incontinence after childbirth: the childbirth and pelvic symptoms study. *Am J Gastroenterol.* 2007;102:1998.
Chan CL, Lunniss PJ, Wang D, et al. Rectal sensorimotor dysfunction in patients with urge faecal incontinence: evidence from prolonged manometric studies. *Gut.* 2005a;54:1263.
Chan CL, Scott SM, Williams NS, Lunniss PJ. Rectal hypersensitivity worsens stool frequency, urgency and lifestyle in patients with urge fecal incontinence. *Dis Colon Rectum.* 2005b;48:134.
Eckadt VF, Elmer T. Reliability of anal pressure measurements. *Dis Colon Rectum.* 1991;34:72.
Evers EM, Blomquist JL, McDermott KC, Handa VL. Obstetrical anal sphincter laceration and anal incontinence 5-10 years after childbirth. *Am J Obstet Gynecol.* 2012;207:425.e1.
Evers J, Jones JFX, O'Connell PR. Systematic review of animal models used in research of origins and treatments of fecal incontinence. *Dis Colon Rectum.* 2017;60:614.
Fenner DE, Genberg B, Brahma P, et al. Fecal and urinary incontinence after vaginal delivery with anal sphincter disruption in an obstetrics unit in the United States. *Am J Obstet Gynecol.* 2003;189:1543.
Floyd WF, Walls EW. Electromyography of the sphincter ani externus in man. *J Physiol.* 1953;122:599.
Fornell EU, Matthiesen L, Sjodhl R, et al. Obstetric anal sphincter injury ten year after: subjective and objective long term effect. *BJOG.* 2005;112:312.
Gilliland R, Altomare DF, Moreira Jr H, et al. Pudendal neuropathy is predictive of failure following anterior overlapping sphincteroplasty. *Dis Colon Rectum.* 1998;41:1516.
Gladman MD, Lunniss PJ, Scott SM, Swash M. Rectal hyposensitivity. *Am J Gastroeneterol.* 2006;101:1140.
Hancke E, Schurholz M. Impaired rectal sensation in idiopathic fecal incontinence. *Int J Colorectal Dis.* 1987;2:146.
Kairaluoma MV, Raivio P, Aarnio MT, Kellokumpu IH. Immediate repair of obstetric anal sphincter rupture: medium-term outcome of the overlap technique. *Dis Colon Rectum.* 2004;47:1358.
Lowder JL, Burrows LJ, Krohn MA, Weber AM. Risk factors for primary and subsequent anal sphincter lacerations: a comparison of cohorts by parity and prior mode of delivery. *Am J Obstet Gynecol.* 2007;196:344.e1.
Lubowski DZ, Nichols RJ. Faecal incontinence associated with reduced pelvic sensation. *Br J Surg.* 1988;75:1086.
Mayer EA, Gebhart GF. Basic and clinical aspects of visceral hyperalgesia. *Gastroenterology.* 1994;107:271.
McKenna DS, Ester JB, Fischer JR. Elective cesarean delivery for women with a previous anal sphincter rupture. *Am J Obstet Gynecol.* 2003;189:1251.
Miller R, Lewis GT, Bartolo DCC, et al. Sensory discrimination and dynamic activity in the anorectum: evidence using a new ambulatory technique. *Br J Surg.* 1988;75:1003.

Nygaard IE, Rao SS, Dawson JD. Anal incontinence after anal sphincter disruption: a 30-year retrospective cohort study. *Obstet Gynecol.* 1997;89:896.

Pollack J, Nordenstam J, Brismar S, et al. Anal incontinence after vaginal delivery: a five year prospective cohort study. *Obstet Gynecol.* 2004;104:1397.

Richter HE, Brumfield CG, Cliver SP, et al. Risk factors associated with anal sphincter tear: a comparison of primiparous patients, vaginal birth after cesarean deliveries, and patients with previous vaginal delivery. *Am J Obstet Gynecol.* 2002;187:1194.

Sangalli MR, Floris L, Faltin D, Weil A. Anal incontinence in women with third and fourth degree perineal tears and subsequent vaginal deliveries. *Aust N Z J Obstet Gynecol.* 2000;3:244.

Schuster MM, Hookman P, Hendrix TR, Mendeloff AI. Simultaneous manometric recording to internal and external anal sphincter reflexes. *Bull Johns Hopkins Hosp.* 1965;116:79.

Spiller RC, Jenkins D, Thornley JP, et al. Increased rectal mucosal enteroendocrine cells, T lymphocytes and increased gut permeability following acute Campylobacter enteritis and in post-dysenteric irritable bowel syndrome. *Gut.* 2000;47:804.

Sultan AH, Kamm MA, Hudson CN, et al. Anal-sphincter disruption during vaginal delivery. *N Engl J Med.* 1993;329:1905.

Sultan AH, Monga AK, Kumar D, Stanton SL. Primary repair of obstetric anal sphincter rupture using the overlap technique. *BJOG.* 1999;106:318.

Sun WM, Read NW, Miner PB. Relationship between rectal sensation and anal function in normal subjects and patients with faecal incontinence. *Gut.* 1990;31:1056.

Sze EHM. Prevalence and severity of anal incontinence in women with and without additional vaginal deliveries after a fourth-degree perineal laceration. *Dis Colon Rectum.* 2005;48:66.

Tetzschner T, Sørensen M, Lose G, Christiansen J. Anal and urinary incontinence in women with obstetric anal sphincter rupture. *BJOG.* 1996;103:1034.

van Meegdenburg MM, Heineman E, Broens PMA. Pudendal neuropathy alone results in urge incontinence rather than in complete fecal incontinence. *Dis Colon Rectum.* 2015;58:1186.

Zorcolo L, Bartolo DCC. Pathophysiology of faecal incontinence. In: Ratto C, Doglietto GB, eds. *Fecal Incontinence Diagnosis and Treatment.* Italy: Springer; 2007.

6

Epidemiology and Psychosocial Impact of Female Pelvic Floor Disorders

Vivian W. Sung and Catherine S. Bradley

CHAPTER OUTLINE

EPIDEMIOLOGY

Female pelvic floor disorders include urinary incontinence, pelvic organ prolapse, and anal incontinence, as well as emptying disorders of the lower urinary and gastrointestinal tracts. These conditions can have a significant impact on a woman's functioning and quality of life, and are associated with limitations that can negatively impact a woman's wellness and health. With the aging population, female pelvic floor disorders are a significant issue from both an individual and public health perspective. This chapter reviews the epidemiology of risk factors for and psychosocial impact of the three most prevalent pelvic floor disorders: urinary incontinence, pelvic organ prolapse, and anal incontinence.

Urinary Incontinence

In general, urinary incontinence can be characterized by the presence of specific symptoms, frequency of urine leakage, severity of leakage, degree of bother to the woman, and type of incontinence. Prevalence and incidence rates can vary widely depending on the definition used, as well as measurement and survey methods and population differences. Of note, although this chapter discusses the epidemiology of urinary incontinence, including urgency urinary incontinence, a more detailed discussion of the epidemiology and costs of overactive bladder, with and without incontinence, can be found in Chapter 31.

Prevalence. Prevalence rates reflect the total number of cases of disease in the population at a given time. For urinary incontinence, definitions used in the literature range from using the presence of leakage (yes/no) to using the frequency of leakage (daily, weekly, monthly, ever) to using symptom bother to determine prevalence. Different definitions can lead to variability in reported prevalence and incidence rates (Stewart et al., 2013).

A review of 21 studies by Thom et al. (1998) found the average prevalence of any incontinence for older women was 34%, and 12% for daily incontinence. For middle-aged and younger adults, the average prevalence of any incontinence was slightly lower, at 25%, in the same study. Nygaard et al. (2008) analyzed the National Health and Nutrition Examination Survey (NHANES) and used a more strict definition, defining incontinence as "at least weekly leakage or monthly leakage more than drops." Based on this definition, the authors reported a prevalence of 15.7%. Also using NHANES data, Markland et al. (2011) reported a prevalence of 51% when incontinence was defined as any positive response. Table 6.1 summarizes the prevalence of urinary incontinence based on age group and varying definitions.

Prevalence rates also vary based on symptom severity. Again using NHANES data, Minassian et al. (2008) reported that the prevalence of any urinary incontinence in women aged 50 to 59 years was 19.9% for "mild" incontinence, 16.5% for "moderate" incontinence, and 25% for "severe" incontinence. These prevalence rates remained stable from 2005 to 2010 (Wu et al., 2014). Variable prevalence rates were also seen in other age groups based on symptom severity.

The type of urinary incontinence is also important when considering the prevalence of the condition, in addition to age (Fig. 6.1). The prevalence of stress urinary incontinence ranges from 33% to 54%, of urgency urinary incontinence ranges from 12% to 16%, and of mixed urinary incontinence ranges from 19% to 50% in populations reporting any incontinence. Similar data are available from multiple countries documenting that these conditions are highly prevalent worldwide.

TABLE 6.1 Prevalence Rates and Definitions of Urinary Incontinence, by Age Group and Definition

Author	Definition Used	Prevalence (%)
All Ages		
Nygaard et al. (2008)	At least weekly leakage or monthly leakage more than drops	15.7
Markland et al. (2011)	Any leakage	51.1
Middle Ages		
Nygaard et al. (2008) (ages 40–59 years)	At least weekly leakage or monthly leakage more than drops	17.2
Waetjen et al. (2007) (ages 42–52 years)	At least monthly incontinence	46.7
Irwin et al. (2006) (ages 40–59 years)	Any urine loss	13.7
Older Ages		
Nygaard et al. (2008) (ages ≥60 years)	At least weekly leakage or monthly leakage more than drops	23.3–31.7
Irwin et al. (2006) (ages ≥60 years)	Any urine loss	20
Hagan et al. (2018) (ages 56–81 years)	Slight leakage	34
	Moderate leakage	45
	Severe leakage	21

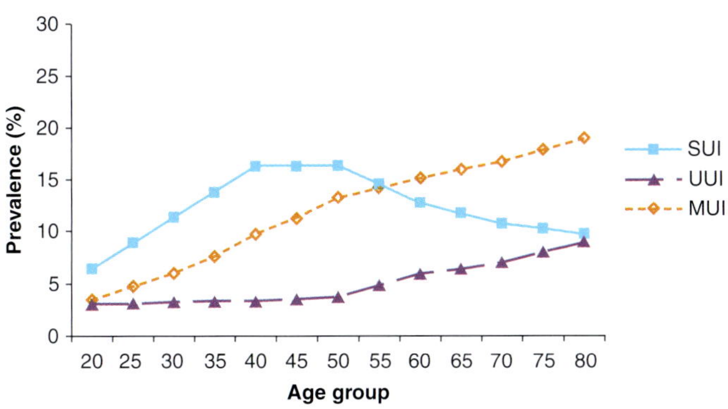

Fig. 6.1 Prevalence of urinary incontinence based on incontinence subtype and age group. *MUI*, Mixed urinary incontinence; *SUI*, stress urinary incontinence; *UUI*, urgency urinary incontinence. (Modified from Minassian VA, Bazi T, Stewart WF. Clinical epidemiological insights into urinary incontinence. *Int Urogynecol J*. 2017;28:689.)

Incidence, Remission, Improvement, and Progression. Urinary incontinence is a dynamic condition, and symptoms may wax and wane. Incidence rates reflect the number of new cases of disease in the population during a specified period of time. The average one-year incidence ranges from 6.9% to 11.1% in the United States in women younger than 55 years (Townsend et al., 2007; Waetjen et al., 2007). The rate is higher in older women, estimated to be 13.8% over 1 year in women 54 to 79 years of age. Reported 1-year remission rates range from 4.6% to 9.1% (Komesu et al., 2009; Lifford et al., 2008; Townsend et al., 2007). In one meta-analysis by Stewart et al. (2013), age-specific incidence was less than 2/1000 person-years in women younger than 40 years, 5/1000 person-years at age 50 years, and 3/1000 person-years at 60 to 65 years, but then increased in later decades in life. In a study by Hagan et al. (2018) that analyzed data from the Nurse's Health Study, the authors reported that most women reported persistence or progression of urinary incontinence symptoms over time, with few (3%–11%) reporting remission. Younger women and those with less severe symptoms were more likely to report remission or improvement over 10 years. In a follow-up study, Minassian et al. (2020) evaluated the natural history of urinary incontinence by subtype and found that most women with incident stress and urgency urinary incontinence continued to experience similar subtype symptoms over an 8-year time period. Women with more severe incident symptoms and obese women were more likely to have persistent symptoms or progress to mixed urinary incontinence over time. Only 4% to 12% reported resolution of their urinary incontinence over the time period.

Urinary Incontinence During Pregnancy and Postpartum. Stress urinary incontinence is common during pregnancy, with a prevalence ranging from 40% to 59%. In general, the severity may worsen throughout pregnancy. In postpartum women, stress urinary incontinence will resolve in many, and the prevalence is estimated to range from 15% to 30% (Milsom et al., 2017). In longitudinal studies, the cumulative incidence rate of urinary incontinence is estimated to be approximately 39% (Solans-Domenech et al., 2010). Up to 26% of women who report urinary incontinence during pregnancy will have persistent leakage in the postpartum period; the majority will have resolution. In a large cohort study by Handa et al. (2015), women were followed annually for up to 5 years after their first delivery. During follow-up, the incidence of bothersome stress urinary incontinence was 2.5/100 woman-years, and for overactive bladder it was 1.7/100 woman-years. Urinary incontinence was more common in the vaginal birth group compared to those who received cesarean section, but the differences lessened as time from childbirth increased. Blomquist et al. (2018) reported that, following spontaneous vaginal delivery, the 15-year cumulative incidence of stress incontinence was 34.3%, and of overactive bladder was 21.8%. Compared with spontaneous delivery, cesarean delivery was associated with a significantly lower risk of developing either condition during the time period.

Costs. The financial burden of urinary incontinence and overactive bladder syndrome is significant and includes direct and indirect costs. Direct costs include costs to the patient for routine care (absorbent products, laundry), medical visits, and treatments. Indirect costs include loss of productivity and costs of paid or unpaid caregivers, which are more difficult to measure (Table 6.2). Many studies support that the largest cost item associated with urinary incontinence for both community-dwelling women, as well as those in nursing homes, remains routine care and supplies, with only a minimal proportion of the costs going to evaluation and treatment. Although most studies evaluate the direct costs because of accessibility of data, the economic impact of indirect costs should not be underemphasized.

A study by Wilson et al. (2001) estimated that the annual direct cost of urinary incontinence for women was $12.4 billion (2001 US dollars), and the largest cost category was routine care (70% of costs), followed by nursing home admissions (14%), treatment (9%), complications (6%), and diagnosis and evaluation (1%). Medicare spending on incontinence treatment continues to increase dramatically. For Medicare beneficiaries aged 65 years and older, Thom et al. (2005) used multiple national databases and reported that the expenditures for inpatient and outpatient medical care doubled from $128 million in 1992 to $234 million in 1998. They also estimated that 23% of incontinent women missed an average of 28.7 hours of work because of inpatient and outpatient care associated with urinary incontinence treatment. A systematic review by Coyne et al. (2014) that focused on urgency urinary incontinence reported that the projected total cost including direct, indirect, and intangible costs would be $76.2 billion in 2015 and $82.6 billion in 2020 in the United States alone.

At the individual level, annual routine costs alone in 2005 were estimated to be $250 to $900 per woman (Subak et al., 2008). Direct costs for incontinence management increase significantly with greater incontinence frequency. Subak et al. (2012) evaluated the impact of incontinence improvement on incontinence-associated costs and found that the mean cost for an individual decreased by 23% for each decrease of seven incontinence episodes per week. Because most of the cost associated with incontinence care is out of pocket, patients assume great financial responsibility in managing this condition.

TABLE 6.2 Costs of Urinary Incontinence

Type of Cost	Examples
Direct Costs	
Diagnostic and evaluation costs	Physician consultation and evaluation, laboratory, diagnostic procedures
Treatment costs	Surgery, medication, pelvic/behavioral therapy
Routine care costs	Nursing labor, supplies, laundry
Rehabilitation costs	Nursing, supplies
Incontinence consequence costs	Skin breakdowns, urinary tract infections, falls, nursing home/assisted living care
Indirect Costs	
Costs of unpaid caregivers	Time, loss of work
Loss of productivity	Missed time from work for diagnosis/treatment, missed time from work because of morbidity

Pelvic Organ Prolapse

Similar to incontinence, definitions for pelvic organ prolapse are also variable. The International Continence Society defines prolapse as the descent of one or more of the anterior vaginal wall, posterior vaginal wall, and the apex of the vagina or vault. Most epidemiologic studies define prolapse based on either physical examination findings or patient symptom report.

Prevalence, Incidence, Remission, and Progression. Most population-based surveys define prolapse based solely on patient symptoms, commonly defined as an affirmative response to seeing/feeling a vaginal bulge. Using this definition, the prevalence of prolapse symptoms ranges from 2.9% to 8% in the United States (Bradley et al., 2005; Nygaard et al., 2008; Rortveit et al., 2007). These studies did not include physical examination information. Additional studies from the Women's Health Initiative (WHI) including US women aged 50 to 79 years found the prevalence of any degree of prolapse based on examination alone of grades 1 to 3 prolapse to be 41.1% (Handa et al., 2004; Hendrix et al., 2002). Table 6.3 presents the estimated prevalence of prolapse. Prevalence estimates based on examination findings alone are higher compared with those based on symptom reports alone.

Data are limited for the incidence and remission of pelvic organ prolapse. Based on the WHI data, the incidence of grades 1 to 3 prolapse is estimated to be 9.3/100 woman-years for cystocele, 5.7/100 woman-years for rectocele, and 1.5/100 woman-years for uterine prolapse. The remission rates are estimated to be up to 9%, with cystocele having higher remission rates than rectocele. Prolapse progression ranged from 1.9% for uterine prolapse, to 9.5% for cystocele, and 14% for rectocele. Older, parous women are more likely to develop new or progressive prolapse than to regress. Progression and resolution appear to be dependent on baseline severity of prolapse.

After pregnancy and delivery, 31% of women have stage 2 prolapse. After delivery, 14% to 15% of women have prolapse at

TABLE 6.3 Prevalence of Pelvic Organ Prolapse

Study	Definition of Prolapse	Prevalence
Swift et al. (2005)	Examination only	Stage 0 = 24% Stage 1 = 38% Stage 2 = 35% Stage 3 = 2%
Hendrix et al. (2002)	Examination only	Any prolapse = 41.1% Cystocele = 34.3% Uterine = 14.2% Rectocele = 18.6%
Handa et al. (2004)	Examination only	Cystocele = 24.6% Uterine = 3.8% Rectocele = 12.9%
Rortveit et al. (2007)	Symptoms only	5.70%
Nygaard et al. (2008)	Symptoms only	2.90%
Slieker-ten Hove et al. (2009)	Symptoms only	11.40%

or below the hymen, and 5% have this after cesarean delivery. In a longitudinal study by Handa et al. (2018), women were enrolled 5 to 10 years from their first delivery and followed annually for 4 to 9 years. The majority of women demonstrated worsening in pelvic support over time, and vaginal birth was associated with worse support 5 years from delivery and more rapid deterioration in apical support.

Costs. There are limited cost analysis data available for pelvic organ prolapse. In 1997, the direct cost of pelvic organ prolapse surgery was estimated to be $1.0 billion based on national average Medicare reimbursement. Physician services accounted for 29% of costs, and hospitalization accounted for 71% (Subak et al., 2001). A study using 2011 data from the Nationwide Inpatient Sample by Sanses et al. (2017) reported that the mean cost per admission for inpatient pelvic organ prolapse surgery was $9035. Higher costs were associated with longer length of stay, patient comorbidities, and public hospitals. It is predicted that the annual economic cost of pelvic organ prolapse surgeries will grow at twice the rate of population growth because of aging populations in the United States and Europe over the next decades (Cheon & Maher, 2013). There are few data on the indirect costs or direct patient costs of pelvic organ prolapse.

Anal Incontinence

Prevalence, Incidence, and Remission. Anal incontinence includes the involuntary passage of gas, mucus, liquid, or solid stool. The prevalence and epidemiology of anal incontinence have been poorly documented, and many women are too embarrassed to report the condition. Most epidemiologic studies focus on fecal incontinence (any involuntary leakage of stool). Depending on the definition and reporting methods used, the prevalence of fecal incontinence in US women ranges from 2.2% to 24%. When defined as any leakage in the past year, the prevalence is estimated to be approximately 24% (Varma et al., 2006). When defined as at least monthly leakage, the prevalence is estimated to be approximately 9% (Nygaard et al., 2008).

Whitehead et al. (2009) estimated the prevalence of different types and frequencies of fecal incontinence in noninstitutionalized US women using NHANES data. The overall prevalence of fecal incontinence within the past month was 8.9%, and increased with age from 2.6% in 20- to 29-year-old women to 15.3% in women aged 70 years and older. The most common type of incontinence was watery/liquid stool (>20%), followed by hard stool and normal stool (~9% for both). Some 51% of women reported leakage of gas in the past month, and 21% reported at least daily leakage of gas. A 2016 systematic review included 30 epidemiologic studies of fecal incontinence in community-based adults and reported a similar overall prevalence of fecal incontinence (liquid or solid stool incontinence occurring at least monthly) when identified during in-person or telephone surveys (8.3%–8.4%), but slightly higher prevalence when identified using mail surveys (11.2%–12.4%) (Sharma et al., 2016).

Data regarding the incidence, regression, and progression of anal incontinence are extremely limited. Markland et al. (2010) estimated the incidence and remission of fecal incontinence in Medicare beneficiaries. Defining fecal incontinence as any loss of bowel control during the previous year, the incidence rate at 4 years was approximately 18% in women, and the remission rate was 57%. The overall incidence rate for the development of more severe fecal incontinence, defined as monthly or greater incontinence, was 6.3%. A community-based study in women over 50 years of age reported new fecal incontinence (self-reported problems with stool leakage) over a 9-year period in 6.2% (Rey et al, 2010).

Anal Incontinence During Pregnancy and Postpartum. During pregnancy, up to 10% of women present with anal incontinence, and the cumulative incidence rate is estimated to be 10.3% (Solans-Domenech et al., 2010). Of the women reporting anal incontinence during pregnancy, 29.7% reported persistent anal incontinence postpartum. Six months postpartum, fecal incontinence (liquid or solid stool) occurs before labor in 8% of primiparous women who deliver via vaginal delivery or cesarean birth. This rate increases to 17% in those who have anal sphincter laceration at time of their vaginal delivery (Borello-France et al., 2006).

Costs. Mellgren et al. (1999) reported the average lifetime cost to be approximately $17,166 per patient for treatment, follow-up, physician evaluation, and protective materials in 1996, and average surgical costs were $8555 per procedure. Sung et al. (2007) estimated the hospital cost of inpatient surgery alone for female fecal incontinence to be $6000 per surgical admission in 2003, totaling $24.5 million spent on hospital costs for surgery alone that year. This estimate did not include direct costs of physician services or any indirect costs. Women undergoing treatment for fecal incontinence at a tertiary care clinic self-reported an average annual total cost of $4110 (median = $1594) related to their fecal incontinence, including direct and loss of productivity costs (Xu et al., 2012).

Coexisting Pelvic Floor Disorders

Pelvic floor disorders often coexist in the same woman, although rates of coexistence differ across studies. In a study of community-dwelling women aged 25 to 84 years, 23.7% reported symptoms of one or more pelvic floor disorders (stress urinary incontinence, overactive bladder, pelvic organ prolapse, or anal incontinence), and 50% to 80% of those women had symptoms of at least two disorders (Lawrence et al., 2008). In a racially-diverse cohort of middle-aged and older women, 34% reported symptoms of at least one pelvic floor disorder, and of those, 16% reported symptoms of more than one disorder (Rortveit et al., 2010; Fig. 6.2). A large national registry study of women 20 years after single vaginal or cesarean delivery found that almost half had symptoms of a pelvic floor disorder, and approximately one third of those women had symptoms of two or more disorders. (Gyhagen et al., 2015). Coexisting pelvic floor disorders increase with age and vaginal delivery and are associated with increased frustration related to symptoms.

Future Projections

It is projected that future demands for ambulatory care and surgical treatment for female pelvic floor disorders will increase.

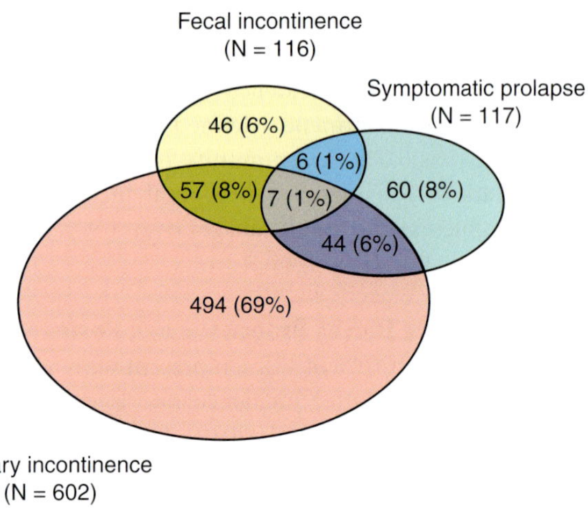

Fig. 6.2 Overlap of the prevalence of urinary incontinence (UI; weekly or more), symptomatic pelvic organ prolapse (POP), and fecal incontinence (FI; monthly or more) in 714 symptomatic women. (From Rortveit G, Subak LL, Thom DH, et al. Urinary incontinence, fecal incontinence and pelvic organ prolapse in a population-based, racially diverse cohort. *Female Pelvic Med Reconstr Surg*. 2010;16:278. With permission.)

Using NHANES prevalence rates and US Census Bureau projections, Wu et al. (2009) estimated that the number of American women with at least one pelvic floor disorder will increase from 28.1 million in 2010 to 43.8 million in 2050. During this time period, the number of women with urinary incontinence will increase 55% from 18.3 million to 28.4 million. Fecal incontinence will increase 59% from 10.6 million to 16.8 million, and the number of women with prolapse will increase 46% from 3.3 million to 4.9 million.

Similar studies suggest a 35% increase in demand for new-patient visits for pelvic floor disorders between 2010 and 2013 (Kirby et al., 2013) and an increase in pelvic floor surgeries. In fact, Wu et al. (2011) project that the total number of women who will undergo stress urinary incontinence surgery will increase almost 50% from 210,700 in 2010 to 310,050 in 2050. Similarly, the total number of women who will undergo prolapse surgery is predicted to increase from 166,000 in 2010 to 245,970 in 2050. These estimates assume that the rates of surgery remain unchanged.

CAUSES AND PREVENTION OF PELVIC FLOOR DISORDERS

Causes of pelvic floor disorders are multifactorial, and it is difficult to understand the relative importance of each factor for a specific individual or population. However, it is useful to appreciate the impact of each factor on the development of pelvic floor disorders to potentially aid in disease prevention.

Race

The role of race as a predisposing risk factor for pelvic floor disorders remains unclear. Although some studies report that White women are at increased risk for stress urinary incontinence (Fenner et al., 2008; Kim et al., 2005; Sze et al., 2002; Thom et al., 2006), symptomatic pelvic organ prolapse (Hendrix et al., 2002; Rortveit et al., 2007; Whitcomb et al., 2009), and fecal incontinence (Markland et al., 2010) this is not a consistent finding. Thom et al. (2006) specifically evaluated urinary incontinence prevalence among major racial and ethnic groups and found that the prevalence of all types of incontinence was highest in Hispanic women (36%), followed by White (30%), Black (25%), and Asian (19%) women. Fenner et al. (2008) also found that a significantly higher proportion of White women reported stress incontinence compared to Black women (39% vs. 25%). However, other studies found no difference in pelvic floor disorders among racial/ethnic groups (Nygaard et al., 2008). Large epidemiologic studies assessing fecal incontinence symptoms also found no difference by race (Whitehead et al., 2009; Ditah et al., 2014).

Most studies of pelvic floor disorders and race have been performed in predominantly White populations. Studies in a large, urban, racially diverse health system found the highest prevalence of stress urinary incontinence and overactive bladder in Hispanic women (Mckellar & Abraham, 2019a; Mckellar et al., 2019). Black women had similar rates of stress urinary incontinence but higher rates of overactive bladder than White women in this population. Differences in these results compared to other studies may have occurred because the urinary incontinence conditions were identified using diagnosis codes (suggesting a treatment-seeking component), rather than from epidemiologic surveys.

Differences in physiologic makeup may predispose some racial and ethnic groups to pelvic floor disorders. For example, magnetic resonance imaging measurements of bony architecture and soft tissue show that White women have a wider pelvic inlet, wider outlet, and shallower anteroposterior outlet than African-American women (Handa et al., 2008). When compared with White women, African-American women also demonstrated a 29% higher average urethral closure pressure during a maximum pelvic muscle contraction (Howard et al., 2000).

Age

There is a significant increase in the prevalence of pelvic floor disorders with age, increasing from 9.7% (95% confidence interval [CI], 7.8%–11.7%) in women aged 20 to 39 years, to 26.5% (95% CI, 23.0%–29.9%) in women aged 40 to 59 years, to 36.8% (95% CI, 32.0%–41.6%) in women aged 60 to 79 years, to 49.7% (95% CI, 40.3%–59.1%) in women aged 80 years or older ($P < .001$; Nygaard et al., 2008). For urinary incontinence, the prevalence increases from 17% to 32% for women aged 40 to 59 years versus women over 80 years of age. The incidence of urinary incontinence also increases with age, and remission is more likely in younger women (Hagan et al., 2018). Ditah et al. (2014) reported that, for anal incontinence, the prevalence increases from 2.9% at ages 20 to 30 years to 16.2% in people aged 70 years or older.

Familial and Genetic Linkage

Epidemiologic evidence suggests that family history of prolapse is a risk factor for disease, and a meta-analysis including eight studies with over 1000 prolapse patients showed that women with prolapse are more likely to have family members with the same condition when compared with controls (Lince et al., 2012). Family-based studies have shown there is an autosomal dominant inheritance of pelvic floor disorders. In addition, candidate gene studies, expression studies, and linkage studies have all been suggestive of a genetic contribution to pelvic organ prolapse (Allen-Brady et al., 2011).

Candidate gene studies have focused on collagen and elastin biosynthesis, extracellular matrix metabolism, and hormone receptors. For example, it is understood that collagen is one of the main constituents of the connective tissue in the pelvic floor, with type I collagen being well organized and type III collagen being common in loose areolar tissue. It is unclear if changes in collagen types I and III content in pelvic support tissues are associated with pelvic organ prolapse, with some studies finding higher levels of type III collagen in women with prolapse and others finding no difference or lower levels (Gong et al., 2019). Other research suggests that changes to the morphology and structure of collagen fibrils occur in women with pelvic organ prolapse. A meta-analysis of genetic epidemiology studies identified associations between a collagen type 3 alpha 1 genetic polymorphism and pelvic organ prolapse (Ward et al., 2014).

Childbirth

Perhaps secondary to increased abdominal pressure and/or connective tissue changes, pregnancy itself has been shown to be a risk factor for pelvic floor disorders. However, the major inciting factor for pelvic floor disorders in parous women is likely childbirth. Nygaard et al. (2008) reported that the proportion of women reporting at least one pelvic floor disorder increased incrementally with parity, at 12.8%, 18.4%, 24.6%, and 32.4% for 0, 1, 2, and 3 or more deliveries, respectively ($P < .001$). A Swedish nationwide matched cohort study of women 20 years after a single vaginal or cesarean delivery found that cesarean in comparison to vaginal delivery was associated with a 30% and 92% reduction in the prevalence of urinary incontinence and pelvic organ prolapse symptoms, respectively (Akervall et al. 2020; Gyhagen et al. 2019).

To further evaluate the association between pelvic floor disorders and mode of delivery, Handa et al. (2012) conducted a longitudinal cohort study following women for 5 to 10 years from first delivery. When compared with cesarean delivery without labor, spontaneous vaginal birth was associated with higher odds of stress incontinence (odds ratio [OR] 2.9 [95% CI, 1.5–5.5]) and prolapse at or beyond the hymen (OR 5.6 [95% CI, 2.2–14.7]). Operative vaginal deliveries and perineal lacerations have also been associated with pelvic floor disorders. In the same cohort study, women who suffered anal sphincter laceration during vaginal delivery were most likely to report anal incontinence 5 to 10 years after first delivery compared with women who had vaginal delivery without sphincter laceration and cesarean delivery without labor (Evers et al., 2012). Anal incontinence was similar between women who delivered by cesarean section and those who delivered vaginally without sphincter laceration.

The pathophysiologic mechanisms linking childbirth and later pelvic floor disorders are described in detail in Chapter 5.

Constipation

Constipation and straining associated with constipation have been associated with pelvic floor disorders. In a meta-analysis of 16 observational studies Lian et al. (2019) identified a significant association between constipation and urinary incontinence in women (OR 2.46, 95% CI 1.79–3.38). Constipation is also more common in women with pelvic organ prolapse compared to women without prolapse (Arya et al., 2005), and many providers may counsel patients to avoid constipation and related straining at stool to reduce the risk of prolapse. However, whether the associations between constipation and urinary incontinence and prolapse are causal remains unproven.

Obesity

Increased body mass index (BMI) is a risk factor for pelvic floor disorders. Many studies have shown that obesity is a risk factor for urinary incontinence. In addition, several studies have shown that both stress and urgency incontinence improve when patients lose weight through lifestyle changes and/or bariatric surgery (Greer et al., 2008; Subak et al., 2015). In a clinical trial of women randomized to an active weight loss program compared to educational materials, weight loss was associated with improvements in incontinence episodes among overweight and obese women (Subak et al., 2009).

A cross-sectional study of postmenopausal women who enrolled in the WHI Hormone Therapy Clinical Trial found an increased risk of prolapse in women with a BMI of 25 or higher (Hendrix et al., 2002). To further understand the longitudinal effects of obesity on prolapse, Kudish et al. (2009) performed a secondary analysis of the WHI data to evaluate the relationship between change in weight and prolapse progression/regression in postmenopausal women during a 5-year period. They found being overweight or obese was highly associated with the progression of prolapse when compared to women with a healthy BMI. However, weight loss was not associated with prolapse regression.

Obesity was not associated with fecal incontinence in a large epidemiologic study after adjusting for other factors (Ditah et al., 2014), but Richter et al. (2005) found prevalence rates of anal incontinence to be high among morbidly obese women compared with the general population. In addition, bariatric surgery in morbidly obese women was associated with a decrease in fecal incontinence (solid or liquid stool) from 19.4% to 9.1% at 6 months and 8.6% at 12 months ($P = .018$; 95% CI, 2.1–19.4) (Burgio et al., 2007). Obesity also increases the risk of anal incontinence 1 year postpartum in women with anal sphincter laceration (Gommesen et al., 2020).

Smoking

Several studies suggest a positive association between smoking and urinary incontinence. A large population-based study, the Norwegian Epidemiology of Incontinence in the County of Nord-Trøndelag (EPINCONT) study, investigated the association between modifiable lifestyle factors such as smoking and urinary incontinence. In this study both former and current smoking was associated with incontinence, limited to those women who smoked 20 cigarettes a day or who had a 15–pack-year history, suggesting a dose-response relationship (Hannestad et al., 2003). The EPINCONT study found that the effect of smoking on incontinence was reduced after adjusting for coughing and dyspnea; however, there was a persistent effect from smoking not mediated by airway disorders.

Menopause/Hormone Replacement Therapy

The female genital tract and the lower urinary tract arise from the same embryologic origin and thus are both sensitive to the effects of sex hormones. Transition to a hypoestrogenic state during menopause leads to changes in the vaginal and urethral mucosa. This could theoretically impact the development of incontinence. Sherburn et al. (2001) reported on a population-based cohort of women who experienced menopausal transition and found no association with the development of urinary incontinence. This is consistent with other epidemiologic studies that have not found an association between the onset of menopause and an increase in urinary incontinence. It is possible that the effects of a hypoestrogenic state may not be apparent in the first few years. In addition, menopause is associated with age, making it difficult to separate any independent effects of hormonal changes and aging.

Although systemic vaginal estrogen was in the past often promoted as beneficial for lower urinary tract symptoms, in the last 20 years the role of estrogen has become less clear. In the Heart & Estrogen/Progestin Replacement Study, exogenous estrogen and progesterone were associated with worsening incontinence (39% vs. 27%, $P = .001$). This was evident by 4 months of treatment and true for both urgency and stress incontinence symptoms (Grady et al., 2001). Similarly, in the WHI, Hendrix et al. (2005) found that exogenous hormone therapy increased the risk of all types of urinary incontinence at 1 year in women who were continent at baseline. This risk was highest for stress incontinence (estrogen and progesterone: relative risk [RR], 1.87 [95% CI, 1.61–2.18]; estrogen alone: RR, 2.15 [95% CI, 1.77–2.62]), followed by mixed incontinence (estrogen and progesterone: RR, 1.49 [95% CI, 1.10–2.01]; estrogen alone: RR, 1.79 [95% CI, 1.26–2.53]). They also found that menopausal hormone therapy worsened the severity of incontinence among symptomatic women after 1 year.

Research on the treatment of overactive bladder with vaginal estrogen has had conflicting results. Two trials (one comparing vaginal estradiol ring with oral oxybutynin and one comparing vaginal estradiol cream with oral tolterodine) found that vaginal estrogen and the oral medications resulted in similar improvements in overactive bladder symptoms (Ellington et al., 2016; Nelken et al., 2011). However, other trials compared tolterodine alone to tolterodine plus vaginal estrogen and found no or limited improvement from the addition of vaginal estrogen (Serati et al., 2009; Tseng et al., 2009). The Cochrane Incontinence Review Group summarized all studies up to June 2012 (Cody et al., 2012) and concluded that urinary incontinence may be improved with the use of local estrogen treatment, although long-term effects are unknown. Conversely, systemic hormone replacement therapy using conjugated equine estrogen may worsen incontinence. There are too few data to reliably address other aspects of estrogen therapy, such as estrogen type and dose, and no direct evidence comparing routes of administration.

PSYCHOSOCIAL IMPACT OF PELVIC FLOOR DISORDERS

Our women's problems have been shoved under the rug for so many years. And that's what I did for a long time too because I was so embarrassed.

Anonymous Patient, 2008

The societal and personal burdens of pelvic floor disorders and their associated treatments lie in their major impact on quality of life and functioning. Pelvic floor disorders can have a negative impact on a woman's physical, social, emotional, and sexual function. Fig. 6.3 shows an abbreviated framework of the effects of urinary incontinence on a woman's life. These conditions can interfere with both participation in and satisfaction with physical and social activities. Women may restrict or completely eliminate activities outside of the home. At the most severe end, women may become increasingly isolated and homebound. These themes are consistent for pelvic organ prolapse and fecal incontinence as well (Sung et al., 2014a; Sung et al., 2014b).

Many women may still do physical functions and activities, particularly those associated with responsibility. However, they may limit their extent of participation (for example, they may not exercise or participate as long as they would like). Studies have shown that incontinence is a barrier to physical activities (Nygaard et al., 2005) and that treatment is associated with improvements in both physical functioning and physical activity levels (Sung et al., 2012).

In addition to restricting their activities, many women develop coping and adaptive methods to minimize the impact of these conditions (Wren et al., 2006). This may include extensive preparation before certain activities (for example, voiding multiple times, bathroom mapping, wearing protection, and donning extra clothes before exercise) or other dietary and behavioral changes (for example, restricting fluid intake before certain activities).

Sexual function is also negatively impacted by these conditions. Incontinence and prolapse may be a direct cause of sexual dysfunction because of physical discomfort, or these conditions may cause embarrassment that leads to avoidance of intimacy and sexual relations. Treatment has been associated with improvements in sexual function, but not all studies demonstrate significant improvement.

In elderly women, these disorders, particularly urinary or anal incontinence, may lead to such disability and dependency that caregivers are no longer able to provide the necessary care. Therefore incontinence is a major factor leading to the institutionalization of elderly patients.

Ultimately, how pelvic floor disorders impact a woman's life depends on multiple factors, including the severity of symptoms, the individual's coping mechanisms, and a host of external mediators. However, it is clear that these conditions can have far-reaching effects on a woman's functioning and quality of life.

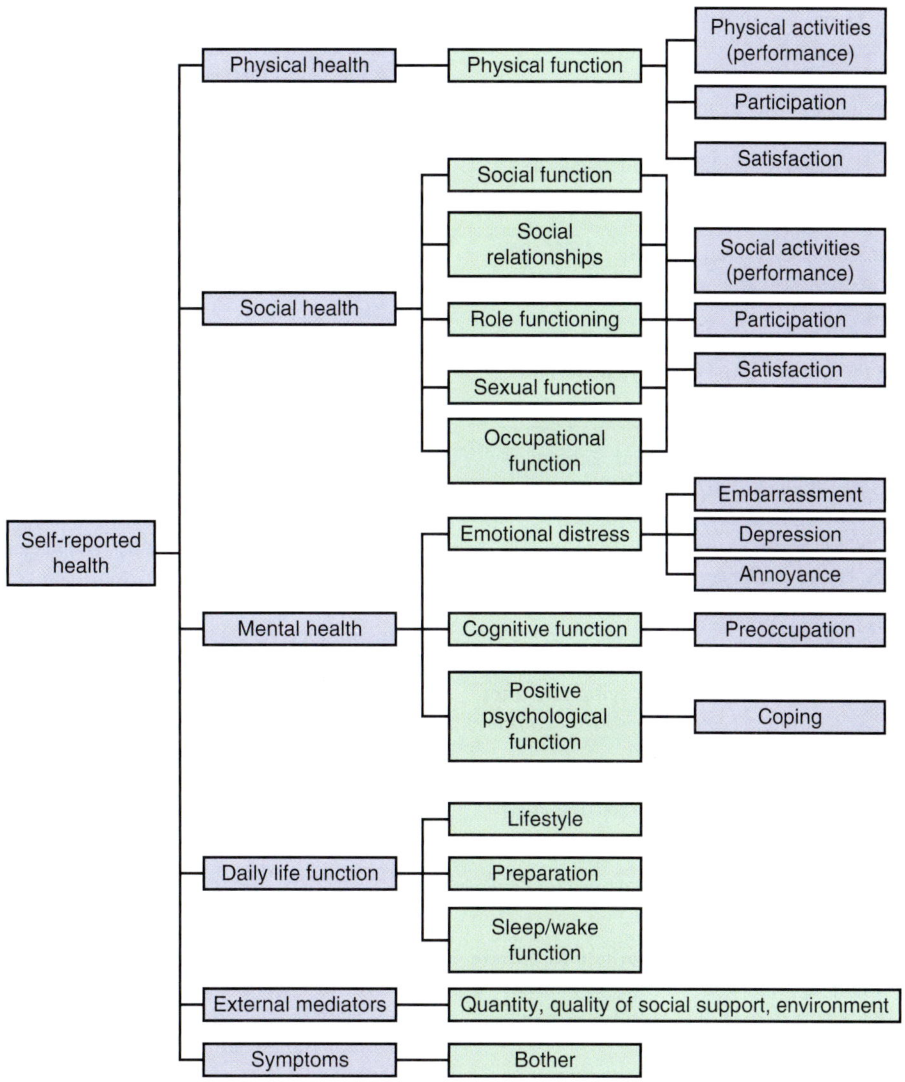

Fig. 6.3 Conceptual framework for impact of incontinence on a woman's life. (Modified from Sung VW, Rogers R, Williams DA, Clark MA. Content validation of the Patient-Reported Outcomes Measurement Information System (PROMIS) framework in women with urinary incontinence. *Neurourol Urodyn.* 2011;30:503.)

BIBLIOGRAPHY

Akervall S, Othman JA, Molin M, Gyhagen M. Symptomatic pelvic organ prolapse in middle-aged women: a national matched cohort study on the influence of childbirth. *Am J Obstet Gynecol.* 2020;222:356.e1.

Allen-Brady K, Cannon-Albright L, Farnham JM, et al. Identification of six loci associated with pelvic organ prolapse using genome-wide association analysis. *Obstet Gynecol.* 2011;118:1345.

Arya LA, Novi JM, Shaunik A, et al. Pelvic organ prolapse, constipation, and dietary fiber intake in women: a case-control study. *Am J Obstet Gynecol.* 2005;192:1687.

Barber MD, Kuchibhatla MN, Pieper CF, Bump RC. Psychometric evaluation of 2 comprehensive condition-specific quality of life instruments for women with pelvic floor disorders. *Am J Obstet Gynecol.* 2001;185:1388.

Blandon RE, Bharucha AE, Melton LJ III, et al. Risk factors for pelvic floor repair after hysterectomy. *Obstet Gynecol.* 2009;113:601.

Blomquist JL, Munoz A, Carroll M, Handa VL. Association of delivery mode with pelvic floor disorders after childbirth. *JAMA.* 2018;320:2438.

Bø K. Urinary incontinence, pelvic floor dysfunction, exercise and sport. *Sports Med.* 2004;34:451.

Borello-France D, Burgio KL, Richter HE, et al. Fecal and urinary incontinence in primiparous women. *Obstet Gynecol.* 2006;108:863.

Bradley CS, Nygaard IE. Vaginal wall descensus and pelvic floor symptoms in older women. *Obstet Gynecol.* 2005;106:759.

Bradley CS, Zimmerman MB, Qi Y, Nygaard IE. Natural history of pelvic organ prolapse in postmenopausal women. *Obstet Gynecol.* 2007;109:848.

Brown JS, Grady D, Ouslander JG, et al. Prevalence of urinary incontinence and associated risk factors in postmenopausal women. Heart & Estrogen/Progestin Replacement Study (HERS) Research Group. *Obstet Gynecol.* 1999;94:66.

Brown JS, Seeley DG, Fong J, et al. Urinary incontinence in older women: who is at risk? Study of Osteoporotic Fractures Research Group. *Obstet Gynecol.* 1996;87:715.

Burgio KL, Richter HE, Clements RH, et al. Changes in urinary and fecal incontinence symptoms with weight loss surgery in morbidly obese women, *Obstet Gynecol.* 2007;110:1034.

Cardozo L, Khoury S, Wein AJ, eds. *Incontinence: 4th International Consultation on Incontinence*. Paris, France: Health Publication Ltd; 2009:35.

Cheon C, Maher C. Economics of pelvic organ prolapse surgery. *Int Urogynecol J.* 2013;24:1873.

Chiaffarino F, Chatenoud L, Dindelli M, et al. Reproductive factors, family history, occupation and risk of urogenital prolapse. *Eur J Obstet Gynecol Reprod Biol.* 1999;82:63.

Cody JD, Jacobs ML, Richardson K, et al. Oestrogen therapy for urinary incontinence in post-menopausal women. *Cochrane Database Syst Rev.* 2012;10:CD001405.

Coyne KS, Wein A, Nicholson S, et al. Economic burden of urgency urinary incontinence in the United States: a systematic review. *J Manag Care Pharm.* 2014;20:130.

DeLancey JO, Morgan DM, Fenner DE, et al. Comparison of levator ani muscle defects and function in women with and without pelvic organ prolapse. *Obstet Gynecol.* 2007;109:295.

Dietz HP, Simpson JM. Levator trauma is associated with pelvic organ prolapse. *BJOG.* 2008;115:979.

Ditah I, Devaki P, Luma HN, et al. Prevalence, trends, and risk factors for fecal incontinence in United States adults, 2005-2010. *Clin Gastroenterol Hepatol.* 2014;12:636.

Ellington DR, Szychowski JM, Malek JM, et al. Combined tolterodine and vaginal estradiol cream for overactive bladder symptoms after randomized single-therapy treatment. *Female Pelvic Med Reconstr Surg.* 2016;22:254.

Evers EC, Blomquist JL, McDermott KC, Handa VL. Obstetrical anal sphincter laceration and anal incontinence 5-10 years after childbirth. *Am J Obstet Gynecol.* 2012;207:425.e1.

Fenner DE, Trowbridge ER, Patel DA, et al. Establishing the prevalence of incontinence study: racial differences in women's patterns of urinary incontinence. *J Urol.* 2008;179:1455.

Gommesen D, Nohr EA, Qvist N, Rasch V. Obstetric perineal ruptures-risk of anal incontinence among primiparous women 12 months postpartum: a prospective cohort study. *Am J Obstet Gynecol.* 2020;222(2):165.e1.

Gong R, Xia Z. Collagen changes in pelvic support tissues in women with pelvic organ prolapse. *Eur J Obstet Gynecol Reprod Biol.* 2019;234:185.

Grady D, Brown JS, Vittinghoff E, et al. Postmenopausal hormones and incontinence: the heart and estrogen/progestin replacement study. *Obstet Gynecol.* 2001;97:116.

Greer WJ, Richter HE, Bartolucci AA, et al. Obesity and pelvic floor disorders: a systematic review. *Obstet Gynecol.* 2008;112:341.

Gyhagen M, Akervall S, Milsom I. Clustering of pelvic floor disorders 20 years after one vaginal or one cesarean birth. *Int Urogynecol J.* 2015;26:1115.

Gyhagen M, Akervall S, Molin M, Milsom I. The effect of childbirth on urinary incontinence: a matched cohort study in women aged 40-64 years. *Am J Obstet Gynecol.* 2019;221:322.e1.

Hagan KA, Erekson E, Austin A, et al. A prospective study of the natural history of urinary incontinence in women. *Am J Obstet Gynecol.* 2018;218:502.e1.

Handa VL, Blomquist JL, Knoepp LR, et al. Pelvic floor disorders 5–10 years after vaginal or Cesarean childbirth. *Obstet Gynecol.* 2011;118:777.

Handa VL, Blomquist JL, McDermott KC, et al. Pelvic floor disorders after vaginal birth: effect of episiotomy, perineal laceration, and operative birth. *Obstet Gynecol.* 2012;119:233.

Handa VL, Blomquist JL, Roem J, Munoz A. Longitudinal study of quantitative changes in pelvic organ support among parous women. *Am J Obstet Gynecol.* 2018;218:320.

Handa VL, Garrett E, Hendrix S, et al. Progression and remission of pelvic organ prolapse: a longitudinal study of menopausal women. *Am J Obstet Gynecol.* 2004;190:27.

Handa VL, Lockhart ME, Fielding JR, et al. Racial differences in pelvic anatomy by magnetic resonance imaging. *Obstet Gynecol.* 2008;111:914.

Handa VL, Pierce CB, Munoz A, Blomquist JL. Longitudinal changes in overactive bladder and stress incontinence among parous women. *Neurourol Urodyn.* 2015;34:356.

Hannestad YS, Rortveit G, Daltveit AK. Are smoking and other lifestyle factors associated with female urinary incontinence? The Norwegian EPINCONT study. *BJOG.* 2003;110:247.

Hendrix SL, Clark A, Nygaard I, et al. Pelvic organ prolapse in the Women's Health Initiative: gravity and gravidity. *Am J Obstet Gynecol.* 2002;186:1160.

Hendrix SL, Cochrane BB, Nygaard IE, et al. Effects of estrogen with and without progestin on urinary incontinence. *JAMA.* 2005;293:935.

Howard D, Delancey JO, Tunn R, et al. Racial differences in the structure and function of the stress urinary continence mechanism. *Obstet Gynecol.* 2000;95:713.

Irwin DE, Kopp ZS, Agatep B, et al. Worldwide prevalence estimates of lower urinary tract symptoms, overactive bladder, urinary incontinence and bladder outlet obstruction. *BJU Int.* 2011;108:1132.

Irwin DE, Milsom I, Hunskaar S, et al. Population-based survey of urinary incontinence, overactive bladder, and other lower urinary tract symptoms in five countries: results of the EPIC study. *Eur Urol.* 2006;50:1306.

Irwin DE, Mungapen L, Milsom I, et al. The economic impact of overactive bladder syndrome in six western countries. *BJU Int.* 2009;103:202.

Jelovsek JE, Walters MD, Paraiso MF, Barber MD. Functional bowel disorders and pelvic organ prolapse: a case-control study. *Female Pelvic Med Reconstr Surg.* 2010;16:209.

Kim S, Harvey MA, Johnston S. Review of the epidemiology and pathophysiology of pelvic floor dysfunction: do racial differences matter? *J Obstet Gynaecol Can.* 2005;27:251.

Kirby AC, Luber KM, Menefee SA. An update on the current and future demand for care of pelvic floor disorders in the United States. *Am J Obstet Gynecol.* 2013;209:584.e1.

Komesu YM, Rogers RG, Schrader RM, Lewis CM. Incidence and remission of urinary incontinence in a community-based population of women ≥50 years. *Int Urogynecol J Pelvic Floor Dysfunct.* 2009;20:581.

Kruger JA, Dietz HP, Murphy BA. Pelvic floor function in elite nulliparous athletes. *Ultrasound Obstet Gynecol.* 2007;30:81.

Kudish BI, Iglesia CB, Sokol RJ, et al. Effect of weight change on natural history of pelvic organ prolapse. *Obstet Gynecol.* 2009;113:81.

Lawrence JM, Lukacz ES, Nager CW, et al. Prevalence and co-occurrence of pelvic floor disorders in community-dwelling women. *Obstet Gynecol.* 2008;111:678.

Lian WQ, Li FJ, Huang HX, et al. Constipation and risk of urinary incontinence in women: a meta-analysis. *Int Urogynecol J.* 2019;30:1629.

Lifford KL, Townsend MK, Curhan GC, et al. The epidemiology of urinary incontinence in older women: incidence, progression, and remission. *J Am Geriatr Soc.* 2008;56:1191.

Lince SL, van Kempen LC, Vierhout ME, Kluivers KB. A systematic review of clinical studies on hereditary factors in pelvic organ prolapse. *Int Urogynecol J.* 2012;23:1327.

Liu X, Zhao Y, Pawlyk B, et al. Failure of elastic fiber homeostasis leads to pelvic floor disorders. *Am J Pathol.* 2006;168:519.

Lubowski DZ, Swash M, Nicholls RJ, et al. Increase in pudendal nerve terminal motor latency with defaecation straining. *Br J Surg.* 1988;75:1095.

Markland AD, Goode PS, Burgio KL, et al. Incidence and risk factors for fecal incontinence in black and white older adults: a population-based study. *J Am Geriatr Soc.* 2010;58:1341.

Markland AD, Richter HE, Fwu C, et al. Prevalence and trends of urinary incontinence in adults in the United States, 2001 to 2008. *J Urol.* 2011;186:589.

Mckellar K, Abraham N. Prevalence, risk factors, and treatment for women with stress urinary incontinence in a racially and ethnically diverse population. *Neurourol Urodyn.* 2019;38:934.

Mckellar K, Bellina E, Schoenbauma E, Abraham N. Prevalence, risk factors, and treatment for overactive bladder in a racially diverse population. *Urology.* 2019;126:70.

McLennan MT, Harris JK, Kariuki B, et al. Family history as a risk factor for pelvic organ prolapse. *Int Urogynecol J Pelvic Floor Dysfunct.* 2008;19:1063.

Mellgren A, Jensen LL, Zetterstrom JP, et al. Long-term cost of fecal incontinence secondary to obstetric injuries. *Dis Colon Rectum.* 1999;42:857.

Melville JL, Katon W, Delaney K, et al. Urinary incontinence in US women. *Arch Intern Med.* 2005;165:537.

Milsom I, Altman D, Cartwright R, et al. Chapter 1: Epidemiology of urinary (UI) and other lower urinary tract symptoms (LUTS), pelvic organ prolapse (POP) and anal incontinence (AI). In: Abrams P, Cardozo L, Wagg A, Wein A, eds. *Incontinence.* 6th ed. ICS/ICUD; 2017.

Minassian VA, Bazi T, Stewart WF. Clinical epidemiological insights into urinary incontinence. *Int Urogynecol J.* 2017;28:689.

Minassian VA, Hagan KA, Erekson E, et al. The natural history of urinary incontinence subtypes in the Nurses' Health Studies. *Am J Obstet Gynecol.* 2020;222:163.

Minassian VA, Stewart WF, Wood GC. Urinary incontinence in women: variation in prevalence estimates and risk factors. *Obstet Gynecol.* 2008;111:324.

Moalli PA, Jones Ivy S, Meyn LA, Zyczynski HM. Risk factors associated with pelvic floor disorders in women undergoing surgical repair. *Obstet Gynecol.* 2003;101:869.

Nelken RS, Ozel BZ, Leegant AR, et al. Randomized trial of estradiol vaginal ring versus oral oxybutynin for the treatment of overactive bladder. *Menopause.* 2011;18:962.

Norton P, Allen-Brady K, Cannon-Albright L. Significant linkage evidence of a predisposition gene for pelvic floor disorders on chromosome 9. *J Pelvic Med Surg.* 2008;14:219.

Norton P, Boyd C, Deak S. Abnormal collagen ratios in women with genitourinary prolapse. *Neurourol Urodyn.* 1992;11:2.

Nygaard I, Barber MD, Burgio KL, et al. Prevalence of symptomatic pelvic floor disorders in US women. *JAMA.* 2008;300:1311.

Nygaard I, Girts T, Fultz NH, et al. Is urinary incontinence a barrier to exercise in women? *Obstet Gynecol.* 2005;106:307.

Rey E, Choung RS, Schleck CD, et al. Onset and risk factors for fecal incontinence in a US community. *Am J Gastroenterol.* 2010;105:412.

Richter HE, Burgio KL, Brubaker L, et al. Factors associated with incontinence frequency in a surgical cohort of stress incontinent women. *Am J Obstet Gynecol.* 2005;193:2088.

Richter HE, Burgio KL, Clements RH, et al. Urinary and anal incontinence in morbidly obese women considering weight loss surgery. *Obstet Gynecol.* 2005;106:1272.

Robinson D, Cardozo L. Estrogens and the lower urinary tract. *Neurourol Urodyn.* 2011;30:754.

Rogers RG, Kammerer-Doak D, Villarreal A, et al. A new instrument to measure sexual function in women with urinary incontinence or pelvic organ prolapse. *Am J Obstet Gynecol.* 2001;184:552.

Rortveit G, Brown JS, Thom DH, et al. Symptomatic pelvic organ prolapse: prevalence and risk factors in a population-based, racially diverse cohort. *Obstet Gynecol.* 2007;109:1396.

Rortveit G, Subak LL, Thom DH, et al. Urinary incontinence, fecal incontinence and pelvic organ prolapse in a population-based, racially diverse cohort. *Female Pelvic Med Reconstr Surg.* 2010;16:278.

Sanses VDT, Schiltz NK, Richter HE, Koroukian SM. Trends and factors influencing prolapse surgical costs and length of stay in the U.S. *Female Pelvic Med Reconstr Surg.* 2017;22:103.

Schaffer JI, Wai CY, Boreham MK. Etiology of pelvic organ prolapse. *Clin Obstet Gynecol.* 2005;48:639.

Serati M, Salvatore S, Uccella S, et al. Is there a synergistic effect of topical oestrogens when administered with antimuscarinics in the treatment of symptomatic detrusor overactivity? *Eur Urol.* 2009;55:713.

Sharma A, Yuan L, Marshall RJ, et al. Systematic review of the prevalence of fecal incontinence. *Br J Surg.* 2016;103(12):1589.

Sherburn M, Guthrie JR, Dudley EC, et al. Is incontinence associated with menopause? *Obstet Gynecol.* 2001;98:628.

Shumaker SA, Wyman JF, Uebersax JS, et al. Health-related quality of life measures for women with urinary incontinence: the incontinence impact questionnaire and the urogenital distress inventory. Continence Program in Women (CPW) Research Group. *Qual Life Res.* 1994;3:291.

Slieker-ten Hove MC, Pool-Goudzwaard AL, Eijkemans MJ, et al. Pelvic floor muscle function in a general female population in relation with age and parity and the relation between voluntary and involuntary contractions of the pelvic floor musculature. *Int Urogynecol J Pelvic Floor Dysfunct.* 2009;20:1497.

Snooks SJ, Barnes PR, Swash M, et al. Damage to the innervation of the pelvic floor musculature in chronic constipation. *Gastroenterology.* 1985;89:977.

Solans-Domenech M, Sanchez E, Espuna-Pons M. Urinary and anal incontinence during pregnancy and postpartum: incidence, severity, and risk factors. *Obstet Gynecol.* 2010;115:618.

Spence-Jones C, Kamm MA, Henry MM, et al. Bowel dysfunction: a pathogenic factor in uterovaginal prolapse and urinary stress incontinence. *BJOG.* 1994;101:147.

Steers WD, Lee KS. Depression and incontinence. *World J Urol.* 2001;19:351.

Stewart WF, Hirsh AG, Kirchner HL, et al. Urinary incontinence incidence: quantitative meta-analysis of factors that explain variation. *J Urol.* 2013;191:996.

Subak LL, Brubaker L, Chai TC, et al. High costs of urinary incontinence among women electing surgery to treat stress incontinence. *Obstet Gynecol.* 2008;111:899.

Subak LL, King WC, Belle SH, et al. Urinary incontinence before and after bariatric surgery. *JAMA Intern Med.* 2015;175;1378.

Subak LL, Marinilli Pinto A, Wing RR, et al. Decrease in urinary incontinence management costs in women enrolled in a clinical trial of weight loss to treat urinary incontinence. *Obstet Gynecol.* 2012;120:277.

Subak LL, Waetjen LE, van den Eeden S, et al. Cost of pelvic organ prolapse surgery in the United States. *Obstet Gynecol.* 2001;98:646.

Subak LL, Wing R, West DS, et al. Weight loss to treat urinary incontinence in overweight and obese women. *N Engl J Med.* 2009;360:481.

Sung VW, Kassis N, Raker CA. Improvements in physical activity and functioning after undergoing midurethral sling procedure for urinary incontinence. *Obstet Gynecol.* 2012;120:573.

Sung VW, Rogers ML, Myers DL, et al. National trends and costs of surgical treatment for female fecal incontinence. *Am J Obstet Gynecol.* 2007;197:652.e1.

Sung VW, Rogers R, Williams DA, Clark MA. Content validation of the Patient-Reported Outcomes Measurement Information System (PROMIS) framework in women with urinary incontinence. *Neurourol Urodyn.* 2011;30:503.

Sung VW, Rogers RG, Barber MD, Clark MA. Conceptual framework for patient-important outcomes for pelvic organ prolapse. *Neurourol Urodyn.* 2014a;33:414.

Sung VW, Rogers RG, Bann CM, et al. Symptom outcomes important to women with anal incontinence: a conceptual framework. *Obstet Gynecol.* 2014b;123:1023.

Swift SE, Tate SB, Nicholas J. Correlation of symptoms with degree of pelvic organ support in a general population of women: what is pelvic organ prolapse? *Am J Obstet Gynecol.* 2003;189:372.

Swift S, Woodman P, O'Boyle A, et al. Pelvic Organ Support Study (POSST): the distribution, clinical definition, and epidemiologic condition of pelvic organ support defects. *Am J Obstet Gynecol.* 2005;192:795.

Sze EH, Jones WP, Ferguson JL, et al. Prevalence of urinary incontinence symptoms among black, white, and Hispanic women. *Obstet Gynecol.* 2002;99:572.

Thom DH, Brown JS. Reproductive and hormonal risk factors for urinary incontinence in later life: a review of the clinical and epidemiologic literature. *J Am Geriatr Soc.* 1998;46:1411.

Thom DH, van den Eeden SK, Ragins AI, et al. Differences in prevalence of urinary incontinence by race/ethnicity. *J Urol.* 2006;175:259.

Thom DH, Nygaard IE, Calhoun EA. Urologic diseases in America project: urinary incontinence in women-national trends in hospitalizations, office visits, treatment and economic impact. *J Urol.* 2005;173:1295.

Townsend MK, Danforth KN, Lifford KL, et al. Incidence and remission of urinary incontinence in middle-aged women. *Am J Obstet Gynecol.* 2007;197:167.e1.

Townsend MK, Danforth KN, Rosner B, et al. Physical activity and incident urinary incontinence in middle-aged women. *J Urol.* 2008;179:1012.

Tseng LH, Wang AC, Chang YL, et al. Randomized comparison of tolterodine with vaginal estrogen cream versus tolterodine alone for the treatment of postmenopausal women with overactive bladder syndrome. *Neurourol Urodyn.* 2009;28:47.

Varma MG, Brown JS, Creasman JM, et al. Fecal incontinence in females older than aged 40 years: who is at risk? *Dis Colon Rectum.* 2006;49:841.

Waetjen LE, Liao S, Johnson WO, et al. Factors associated with prevalent and incident urinary incontinence in a cohort of midlife women: a longitudinal analysis of data: study of women's health across the nation. *Am J Epidemiol.* 2007;165:309.

Ward RM, Velez Edwards DR, Edwards T, et al. Genetic epidemiology of pelvic organ prolapse: a systematic review. *Am J Obstet Gynecol.* 2014;211:326.

Weber AM, Walters MD, Ballard LA, et al. Posterior vaginal prolapse and bowel function. *Am J Obstet Gynecol.* 1998;179:1446.

Whitcomb EL, Rortveit G, Brown JS, et al. Racial differences in pelvic organ prolapse. *Obstet Gynecol.* 2009;114:1271.

Whitehead WE, Borrud L, Goode PS, et al. Fecal incontinence in US adults: epidemiology and risk factors, *Gastroenterology.* 2009;137:512.e1.

Wilson L, Brown JS, Shin GP, et al. Annual direct cost of urinary incontinence. *Obstet Gynecol.* 2001;98:398.

Woodman PJ, Swift SE, O'Boyle AL, et al. Prevalence of severe pelvic organ prolapse in relation to job description and socioeconomic status: a multicenter cross-sectional study. *Int Urogynecol J Pelvic Floor Dysfunct.* 2006;17:340.

Wren PA, Janz NK, Brubaker L, et al. Development of the Measure of Adaptations for Pelvic Symptoms (MAPS): the importance of incorporating the female patient's voice. *Appl Res Qual Life.* 2006;1:239.

Wu JM, Hundley AF, Fulton RG, Myers ER. Forecasting the prevalence of pelvic floor disorders in U.S. women: 2010–2050. *Obstet Gynecol.* 2009;114:1278.

Wu JM, Kawasaki A, Hundley AF, et al. Predicting the number of women who will undergo incontinence and prolapse surgery, 2010 to 2050. *Am J Obstet Gynecol.* 2011;205:230.e1.

Wu JM, Vaughan CP, Goode PS, et al. Prevalence and trends of symptomatic pelvic floor disorders in U.S. women. *Obstet Gynecol.* 2014;123:141.

Wu JM, Visco AG, Grass EA, et al. Comprehensive analysis of LAMC1 genetic variants in advanced pelvic organ prolapse. *Am J Obstet Gynecol.* 2012;206:447.e1.

Xu S, Menees SB, Zochowski MK, Fenner DE. Economic cost of fecal incontinence. *Dis Colon Rectum.* 2012;55:586.

7

Synthetic Mesh and Biologic Grafts: Properties and Biomechanics

Katrina M. Knight, Brittany R. Egnot, and Pamela A. Moalli

CHAPTER OUTLINE

INTRODUCTION

The female pelvis is comprised of a complex, interconnected network of connective tissues and muscles that collectively work together to provide support to the pelvic organs. The vagina also provides support to the pelvic organs by supporting the urethra and bladder anteriorly, the uterus apically, and the rectum posteriorly. In the event that support to the pelvic organs is lost, via damage to or abnormalities in the connective tissues, muscles, and/or vagina, the pelvic organs unnaturally descend from their normal anatomic position into the vaginal canal, resulting in pelvic organ prolapse (POP).

To surgically restore support to the pelvic organs, a native tissue repair can be performed in which a patient's own connective tissues and muscles are used. Given that the integrity of the existing connective tissues and muscles are likely compromised in women with prolapse, it is perhaps not surprising that native tissue repairs are associated with high failure rates: 40% by 2 years and 70% by 5 years (Barber et al., 2014; Jelovsek et al., 2018). As a result, surgeons began to use synthetic meshes and biologic grafts to reinforce repairs and improve patient outcomes.

The methods by which synthetic meshes and biologic grafts restore support to the pelvic organs vary. Synthetic meshes are permanent—they are designed to last for the lifetime of the patient. Support is therefore dependent on the strength of the synthetic mesh and how well the mesh integrates with the host tissue. Chemically crosslinked biologic materials were intended to act similarly to permanent materials with modifications designed to prevent host degradation. Unfortunately, these products were associated with similar or increased rates of complications relative to synthetic meshes. More recently, biologic grafts have been designed to intentionally degrade over time and to facilitate the rebuilding of damaged or compromised tissues; hence, biologic grafts act as an initial reinforcement, and following degradation and then repair by host immune cells, support is provided by the newly formed tissue.

Since the introduction of the first transvaginal prolapse mesh "kit" in 2002 (US Food and Drug Administration [FDA], 2011), synthetic meshes have been widely used in the surgical repair of prolapse. The increased use of mesh was also paralleled with a surge in the number of complications reported, which led the FDA to issue two consecutive public health notifications (PHNs) in 2008 and 2011 warning of complications associated with transvaginal meshes and upgrading them from Class II to Class III devices in 2018. As Class III devices, industry was now required to perform small clinical trials before bringing new products to the market. In 2019, the FDA mandated that manufacturers of transvaginal prolapse meshes stop the sale and distribution of their products, citing a failure to demonstrate reasonable assurance of safety and effectiveness. This series of events has prompted surgeons and their patients to reconsider the use of biologic grafts in prolapse and incontinence surgeries. Fortunately, mechanistic studies to define the mechanism of mesh and biologic graft complications have increased over the past 10 years and have identified factors contributing to complications.

The overall goal of this chapter is to provide the reader with a review of basic science and clinical studies that have aided our understanding of how the properties and mechanics of synthetic meshes and biologic grafts impact the host response, and how these factors may contribute to complications.

SYNTHETIC MESHES

Overview of Synthetic Meshes

The use of synthetic meshes for the treatment of POP dates back to the 1970s (Fig. 7.1). During that time, there were no FDA-approved meshes for the abdominal repair of prolapse (sacrocolpopexy). The meshes used in sacrocolpopexy were the same as those approved for hernia repair. In the 1990s, gynecologists began cutting hernia mesh products into the desired shape and utilizing these modified meshes for the transvaginal repair of prolapse and surgical treatment of stress urinary incontinence (SUI). Given the surgical demand for a mesh product in the urogynecology space, companies started remarketing their hernia products and developing products targeted for stress urinary incontinence (SUI) and prolapse.

In 1998, tension-free vaginal tape (TVT; Ethicon, Somerville, NJ, United States) was developed as one of the first commercially marketed "kits" to treat SUI. Unlike previous SUI products, TVT was placed under the midurethra, and the surgery could be performed under intravenous sedation instead of general anesthesia. The product was an immediate success, leading to a competitive market with multiple manufacturers introducing their own versions of the midurethral sling (Table 7.1). The products were all polypropylene but differed in their weight, pore size, knit patterns, mesh thickness, etc.

Based on the success of midurethral slings, transvaginal prolapse mesh kits based on a similar concept were introduced to the market. The first preconfigured mesh for prolapse repair, cleared by the FDA in 2002, was Prolift (Ethicon, Somerville, NJ, United States), a transvaginal mesh kit utilizing the prolapse

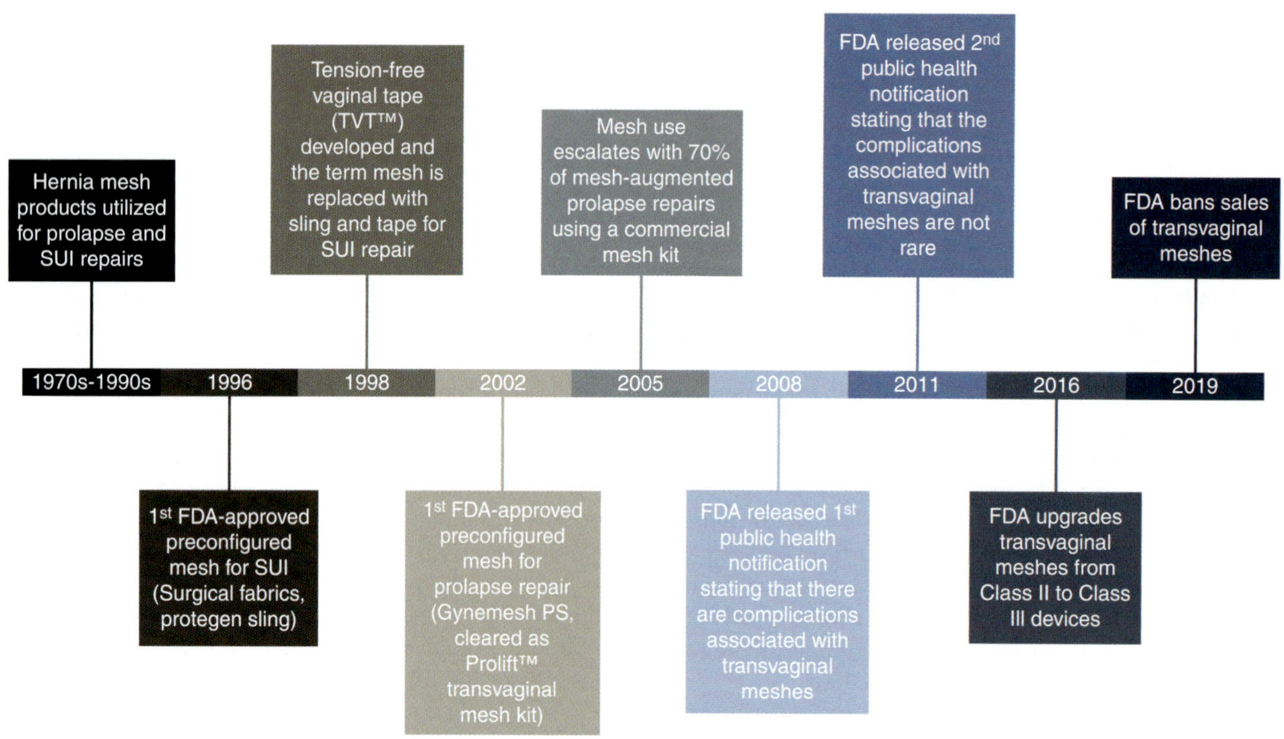

Fig. 7.1 Timeline of mesh product development and usage, from conception to present day. *FDA*, US Food and Drug Administration; *SUI*, stress urinary incontinence.

TABLE 7.1 Comparison of Weight, Pore Size, and Mesh Thickness as Reported by the Manufacturers of Various Slings

Sling	Weight (g/m²)	Pore Size (μm)	Mesh Thickness (mm)
American Medical Systems SPARC/Monarc	110	1000	0.66
Bard Uretex	81	1160	0.62
Boston Scientific Advantage/Obtryx	100	1182	0.66
Caldera T-sling	140	698	0.48
Gynecare TVT/TVT-O	100	1379	0.63
Coloplast Aris (Mentor Aris)	70	374	0.27

(From Moalli PA, Papas N, Menefee S, et al. Tensile properties of five commonly used mid-urethral slings relative to the TVT™. *Int Urogynecol J Pelvic Floor Dysfunct.* 2008;19:655.)

mesh Gynemesh PS, which had been renamed from the hernia mesh Prolene Soft. These kits offered the potential of a procedure to repair prolapse that was technically easier relative to sacrocolpopexy and had a shorter operation time. As a result, the use of transvaginal meshes escalated in prolapse surgery such that, by 2005, mesh kits were being used in over 70% of mesh-augmented prolapse repairs, and by 2010 over one-third of the 300,000 prolapse surgeries performed annually used mesh (both transvaginal and sacrocolpopexy) (FDA, 2011).

Companies were originally able to remarket their hernia products for POP and SUI as 510K devices because hernia products were in existence before the 1976 Medical Device Amendments Act. Using this mechanism, companies were able to avoid costly premarket testing of new devices. Unfortunately, this resulted in the use of products that were not specifically designed for the unique soft tissues and loading conditions within the female pelvis. Not surprisingly, the accelerated use of mesh was also paralleled by an increase in the number of complications, with pain and mesh exposure through the vaginal epithelium the most commonly reported symptoms (FDA, 2011). As a result, the FDA released the first PHN in 2008 warning of complications associated with transvaginal meshes, and in 2011 released an updated notification stating that these complications are not rare, occurring in approximately 20% of cases (FDA, 2011). Following this PHN, public and clinical views on the use of mesh in prolapse surgeries shifted. Specifically, the use of synthetic meshes in the transvaginal repair of prolapse declined, whereas there was no change reported for the use of synthetic mesh in transabdominal or suburethral sling procedures (Clemons et al., 2013). Rac (2017) reported a three-fold increase in mesh sling revision surgeries at tertiary academic medical centers in the United States from 2007 to 2013. The continued rise of complications resulted in the FDA reclassifying transvaginal meshes for POP from Class II to Class III devices in 2016, and ultimately led to the halt of the sale and distribution of the devices in 2019. In time, other countries, including the United Kingdom, Ireland, Australia, and New Zealand, issued similar orders for cessation of all use of polypropylene mesh products in surgeries. Although not as severe, synthetic meshes used in sacrocolpopexy are also associated with complications, at a rate of approximately 10.5% over 7 years, and this rate increases with time (Nygaard et al., 2013). The pathogenesis of mesh complications is unclear; however, research studies suggest that mesh textile properties, mesh structural properties, and the mechanical behavior of mesh are all contributing factors.

Textile Properties and Implications for the Host Response

Pore size and porosity, mesh weight, knit pattern, and filament type are all key textile properties that can significantly impact the host response. In the following sections, each of these textile properties and the studies that have shed light on their role in the host response will be discussed. Important studies performed in humans and in animal models in both the abdominal hernia and urogynecology literature will also be discussed.

Filament Type. Synthetic meshes are manufactured from individual fibers that are either monofilament or multifilament. As the name implies, a multifilament fiber consists of multiple filaments that are either braided or interwoven to create one fiber. Relative to monofilament fibers, the surface area of multifilament fibers is increased by a factor of at least 1.57 (Klinge et al., 2002a), and the increased surface area likely provides more area for bacteria to adhere and proliferate. Furthermore, multifilament fibers potentially have spaces less than 10 μm in diameter within the fibers themselves (as a result of the braided or interwoven filaments) that allow for the passage of bacteria but limit the passage of macrophages or neutrophils (Amid, 1997). These spaces consequently act as a harbor for bacterial proliferation (Iglesia et al., 1997). Indeed, synthetic meshes with multifilament fibers are associated with higher bacterial colonization (Engelsman et al., 2010). Consequently, current meshes are manufactured from monofilament fibers, and multifilament fibers are avoided.

Knit Pattern. The knit pattern describes the way that the fibers are combined during the manufacturing process of the mesh, and governs the behavior of the mesh. Knitting and weaving are two of the most common knit patterns. To knit a mesh, a single fiber is continually looped into a warp-lock, interlock, or circular knit style. Conversely, a woven mesh is constructed from the interlacing of two sets of fibers that run perpendicular to one another. Relative to knitted meshes, woven meshes have superior shape memory and mechanical strength. However, they conform poorly to underlying tissues/structures and are susceptible to fraying when cut (Cosson et al., 2003). Knitted meshes, on the other hand, have increased flexibility, which affords them high conformity to underlying tissues/structures and greater porosity than woven meshes. The larger pores of knitted meshes reduce the risk of infection (Chen et al., 2007; Cobb et al., 2009; Wohlrab et al., 2009), which will be discussed in more detail in the next section. Given these advantages, knitting is the preferred manufacturing technique for current urogynecologic meshes.

Pore Size and Porosity. Pore size and porosity (the amount of void space relative to the total area of the mesh) are key textile properties that can significantly influence the host response to mesh. As alluded to in the previous section, large pores decrease the risk of bacterial colonization and increase vascular penetration relative to small pores. Additionally, large pores allow for the ingrowth of tissue, which can improve the mechanical integrity of the resulting mesh-tissue complex (Patel et al., 2012). Similar to the small pores within multifilament fibers, mesh pores smaller than 10 μm are also conducive to bacterial proliferation and persistent infection (Amid, 1997). Furthermore, small-pore, low-porosity meshes are associated with increased inflammation, fibrous tissue deposition, and potential for adhesion relative to large-pore, high-porosity meshes (Greca et al., 2001; Klinge et al., 2002c; Conze et al., 2004; Greca et al., 2008; Orenstein et al., 2012). Small-pore meshes are also at an increased risk of undergoing "bridging fibrosis."

Bridging fibrosis is a phenomenon that occurs when the perifiber inflammatory reaction around a single fiber merges or "bridges" with a neighboring fiber (or fibers in the case of a mesh knot), which results in the formation of a continuous fibrotic response or encapsulation of the mesh. This phenomenon is associated with an increase in pain, which is likely a result of tension on the surrounding tissues because of contraction of the myofibroblasts present in the capsule (Rudolph et al., 1981; Tomasek et al., 2002; Desmouliere et al., 2005; Hinz, 2007; Duffield et al., 2013). In addition to pore size, the thickness of the fibrous capsule is likely dependent on the polymer; more specifically in regards to how the tissue interacts with the surface of the fiber and the hydrophobicity of the polymer (Klinge et al., 2002d). For polypropylene, 1 mm has been identified as the minimum pore diameter required to allow for adequate tissue ingrowth and to prevent bridging fibrosis (Klinge et al., 2002c; Klinge and Klosterhalfen, 2012). However, it is important to note that 1 mm is specific to polypropylene meshes and hernia repair. The minimum pore diameter likely changes with the polymer (e.g., 630 μm is the minimal diameter for co-PVDF, a blend of polyvinylidene fluoride and hexafluorpropylene (Conze et al., 2008)) and for meshes implanted in the vagina, given that the host response to mesh is more robust in the vagina relative to the abdomen (Pierce et al., 2009; Feola et al., 2015).

Mesh Weight and Surface Area. In addition to filament type, knit pattern, and pore size, urogynecologic meshes are also classified into different categories based on weight, defined by the specific gravity (g/m^2), as lightweight (<45 g/m^2) or heavyweight (>45 g/m^2). In general, lightweight meshes tend to have larger pores, higher porosity, and decreased stiffness relative to heavyweight meshes. Consequently, lightweight meshes typically have improved biocompatibility compared with heavyweight meshes (Patel et al., 2012). Specifically, heavyweight meshes are associated with increased apoptotic cells surrounding mesh fibers, a more pronounced and prolonged inflammatory response, and a higher turnover of the tissues surrounding the mesh fibers after 1 year of implantation (Klinge et al., 2002b; Rosch et al., 2003; Costello et al., 2007; Novitsky et al., 2008; Liang et al., 2013; Brown et al., 2015; Nolfi et al., 2016). Lightweight meshes, on the other hand, tend to have a reduced amount of fibrosis and inflammation, a higher potential for tissue incorporation within the mesh pores, and reduced potential for adhesion and pain (Klinge et al., 1998a; Klinge et al., 1998b; Klinge et al., 2002c; Klinge et al., 2002b; Conze et al., 2004; O'Dwyer et al., 2005). Collectively, these results suggest that lightweight meshes are clinically more beneficial than heavyweight meshes, and it is for this reason that companies made the switch from producing heavyweight meshes to producing lightweight meshes, which is the current standard.

It is generally understood that lightweight meshes are more biocompatible than heavyweight meshes. However, contrasting results were observed in a study conducted by Weyhe et al. 2006 comparing a heavyweight (large-pore, knitted) and lightweight (small-pore, woven) polypropylene mesh implanted in the abdomen of rats. The heavyweight mesh was associated with a reduced fibrotic reaction, improved tissue integration, and significantly fewer macrophages at the implant surface than the lightweight mesh (Weyhe et al., 2006). These results suggest that pore size is more important than mesh weight, and corroborate that knitted meshes are associated with a more favorable host response than woven meshes. However, it is important for the reader to keep in mind that mesh weight, pore size, and stiffness are interconnected, and that changing one property will affect the others. Thus, it is difficult to attribute the host response to a single factor, and it is vital that all aspects of urogynecologic meshes are considered when evaluating their biocompatibility. Moreover, as detailed below, the geometry of a mesh often changes according to the direction of loading. Indeed, wide-pored meshes with unstable geometries can be substantially smaller-pored and stiffer when loaded *in vivo*. It is therefore important to consider multiple factors when choosing a mesh.

Surface area, a measure of the amount of material that is in contact with the tissue, is another factor that can impact the host response to mesh (Leveen & Barberio, 1949; Conze et al., 2004). Similar to heavyweight meshes, meshes with a larger surface area yield a strong and more active inflammatory response compared with meshes with a smaller area of contact with the host tissue (Klosterhalfen et al., 1998; Cosson et al., 2003). Surface area is particularly problematic for multifilament meshes, as the surface area is increased by approximately 50% compared with monofilament meshes, thereby providing a greater surface for bacterial adherence and proliferation (Klinge et al., 2002a).

Structural Properties and Implications for the Host Response

In the next few sections, the mechanics of meshes will be reviewed, with an emphasis placed on understanding the difference between structural and mechanical properties, the tests used to determine the structural properties of mesh, and the implications of structural properties for the host response.

Structural Versus Mechanical Properties. Structural and mechanical properties are two distinct properties that are evaluated through mechanical testing. Although these properties are related, the interpretation of structural and mechanical properties differs drastically. Structural properties describe how an applied force or deformation affects a material/device or collection of materials/devices (e.g., synthetic mesh). These properties are dependent on the type of material, the amount of material, the shape of the material, the direction of the applied force, and how the material is constrained and/or connected to other materials. Mechanical properties describe how an applied force or deformation affects a single material, and the response to the applied force or deformation is a result of the atomic and molecular interactions within the material (e.g., a single strand of polypropylene). Unlike structural properties, mechanical properties are not dependent on the size and shape of the material. For example, the structural properties of a large steel rod will be higher than that of a small steel rod; however, the mechanical properties will be the same because the rods are composed of the same material, steel.

Within the urogynecology literature, the following structural properties are commonly reported for meshes; ultimate load, ultimate elongation, relative elongation, stiffness, and energy absorbed. The ultimate load is the maximum amount of force that a mesh can withstand before failure, in which failure is defined as the permanent destruction of the mesh. The maximum change in length of the mesh before failure is defined as the ultimate elongation. Similarly, relative elongation is the maximum change in length of the mesh before failure, normalized to the initial length of the mesh. Stiffness describes the ability of the mesh to resist deformation and is the most commonly used term to describe urogynecologic meshes. Energy absorbed is the amount of energy that is required to bring a mesh to failure (i.e., it is a measure of toughness). As alluded to previously, the structural properties are dependent on the size and shape of the structure (i.e., mesh) being tested, whereas the mechanical properties are independent of size and shape.

In the urogynecology literature, stress, strain, tangent modulus/Young's modulus, and strain energy density are often inappropriately reported when describing the properties of mesh. Synthetic meshes are discontinuous structures (i.e., they are filled with void spaces), and they cannot be treated as a continuum, which is a requirement of mechanical tensile tests. Thus, the size and shape of the mesh will dictate the properties, and only structural properties (e.g., load, elongation, stiffness, and energy absorbed) or normalized structural properties (e.g., relative elongation) should be reported for meshes. For additional information regarding mechanical properties, the interested reader should refer to Knight and Moalli (2016).

Mechanical Tests Used to Determine Structural Properties. The structural properties of synthetic mesh are often determined using the same mechanical tests that are used to assess the properties of vaginal tissue. However, the applicability of the testing method, the experimental protocol, and the interpretation of the results will differ for mesh as a result of the structural differences between synthetic mesh and vaginal tissue. Synthetic meshes are highly porous, discontinuous materials, whereas vaginal tissues are continuous materials, meaning there is material at every location within the tissue, and the material is interconnected. It is important to note that the continuity of vaginal tissue is assumed at the fiber level. As stated above, the porous and discontinuous architecture of synthetic meshes restricts the use of mechanical testing that is only applicable to continuous materials. Additionally, the knit pattern restricts the type of testing that can be performed on synthetic meshes. Samples are often cut into a particular shape for a given mechanical test. Depending on the shape, cutting a synthetic mesh could disrupt the knit pattern and alter the mechanical behavior of the mesh, which will also impact the structural properties of the mesh. Lastly, the process of knitting a mesh creates interlaced fibers, which produces nonuniform and local deformations throughout the mesh structure. It is therefore important that the assumptions of a particular mechanical test and the interpretation of the results are thoroughly understood before performing any mechanical test on synthetic meshes.

Uniaxial Tensile Test. The uniaxial tensile test is one of the mechanical tests that is most commonly used within the urogynecology field to evaluate the structural properties of synthetic meshes. As the name implies, a uniaxial tensile test involves loading mesh along one direction (typically the primary axis of the mesh) to measure the response of the mesh to the applied load. Unidirectional loading is similar to the loading conditions experienced by mesh implanted via a sacrocolpopexy. Specifically, mesh is clamped on opposing ends and is loaded at a constant rate until it fails, referred to as a "load to failure" test (Fig. 7.2A). The load and elongation are recorded and then used to create a load-elongation curve, which typically has a toe region (large amount of elongation with small changes in force) followed by a linear region (the relationship between load and elongation is relatively linear) and then a failure region (permanent damage to the mesh has occurred) (Fig. 7.2B). The load-elongation curve is then used to determine the structural properties: ultimate load, ultimate elongation, stiffness, and energy absorbed (Fig. 7.2C). For bilinear curves, the stiffness is often reported as low or high. The interested reader should refer to Knight and Moalli (2016) for a more in-depth explanation of the methodology and caveats to uniaxial tensile testing.

Ball-Burst Test. The structural properties of synthetic mesh can also be obtained using ball-burst testing, which is also referred to as biaxial tensiometry. During ball-burst testing, a piece of mesh (typically square or circular) is securely sandwiched between two clamps (typically circular), and a steel ball head is pushed through the mesh at a constant rate until rupture (failure) (Fig. 7.3A). Similar to uniaxial tensile testing, the load and displacement are recorded and used to generate a load-extension curve, which has the characteristic toe, linear, and failure regions. The load-extension curve is then used to determine the ultimate load, ultimate extension, stiffness, and energy absorbed (Fig. 7.3B). The interested reader should refer to Knight and Moalli (2016) for a more in-depth explanation of the methodology and caveats to ball-burst testing.

Structural Properties. To date, all synthetic meshes are type I polypropylene (pore size >75 μm) meshes. They are knitted, have wide pores (most >1 mm, porosity >55%), and are lightweight (<45 g/m^2). However, the size and shape of the pores, as well as the knit pattern for each mesh, are distinct (Fig. 7.4), which contributes to the differing structural properties of the mesh. The structural and textile properties are not independent of one another, as the stiffness, ultimate load, and energy absorbed, as determined by ball-burst testing, are shown to correlate with specific weight and porosity (Feola et al., 2013). When comparing the structural properties of synthetic meshes, it is important to note that the structural properties obtained from a ball-burst test are higher than those obtained from a uniaxial test (Table 7.2). This is a direct result of the boundary conditions imposed on the mesh. During a ball-burst test, the mesh is constrained along the entire perimeter, and the testing area of the mesh is small, which artificially increases the stiffness of the mesh. It is therefore important that the testing method used is considered when comparing the structural properties of different meshes.

The structural properties of slings obtained via uniaxial tensile testing also differ (Table 7.3) (Moalli et al., 2008). Similar to

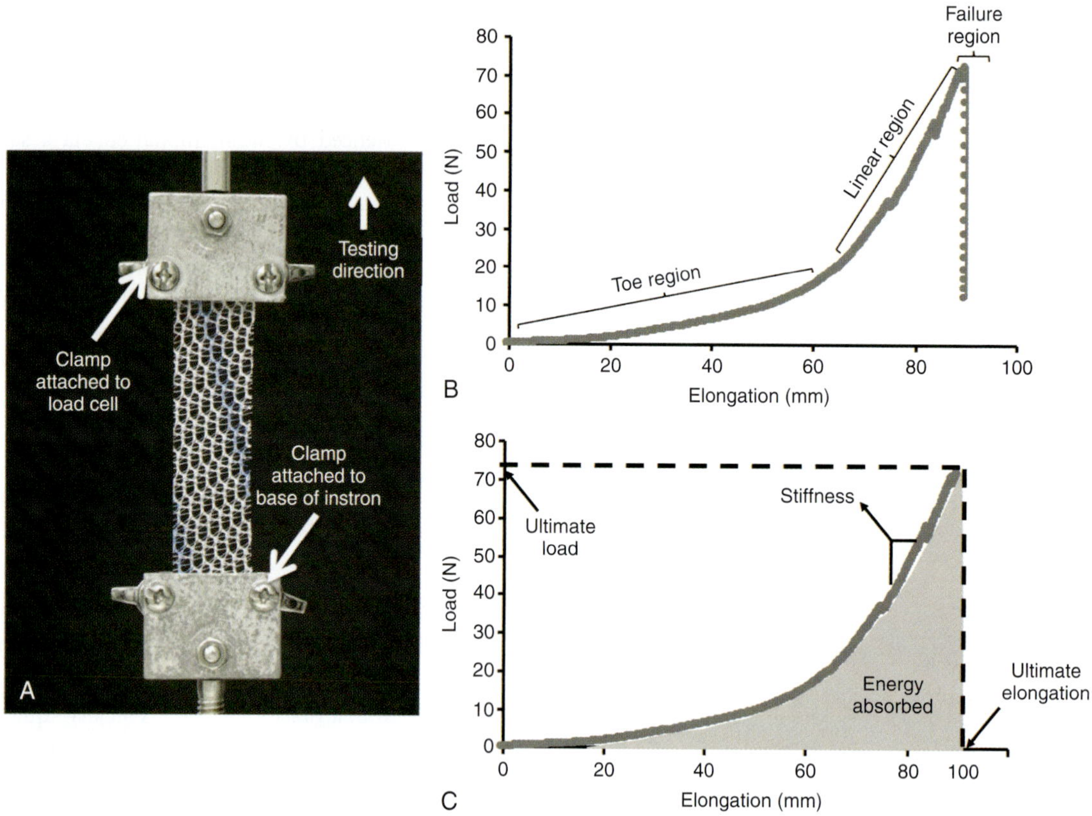

Fig. 7.2 Synthetic mesh clamped on opposing ends and attached to a uniaxial tensile testing machine (**A**). An example load-elongation curve following a uniaxial tensile test to failure demonstrating the characteristic toe, linear, and failure regions (**B**) and the resulting structural properties ultimate load, ultimate elongation, stiffness, and energy absorbed (**C**).

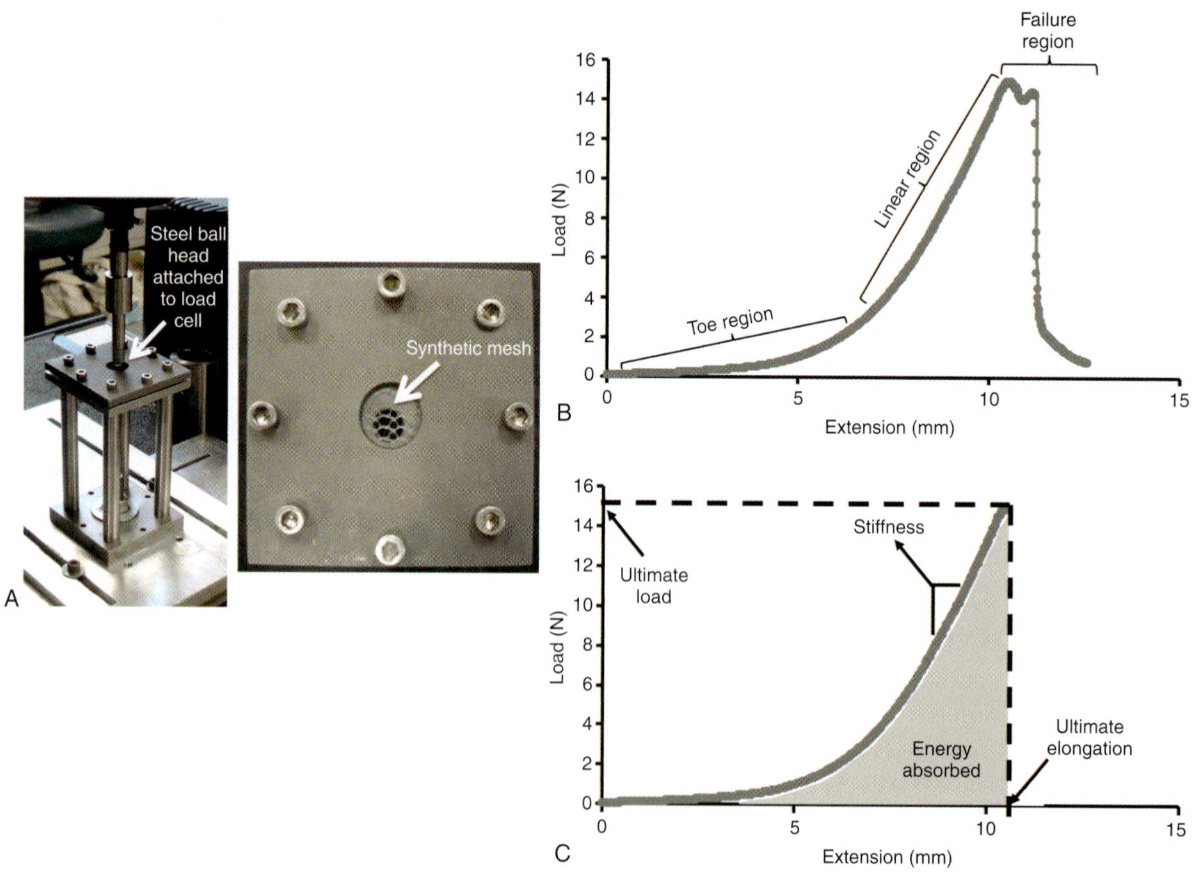

Fig. 7.3 Synthetic mesh sandwiched between two clamps and attached to a ball-burst testing machine (**A**). An example load-elongation curve following a ball-burst test to failure demonstrating the characteristic toe, linear, and failure regions (**B**) and the resulting structural properties ultimate load, ultimate elongation, stiffness, and energy absorbed (**C**).

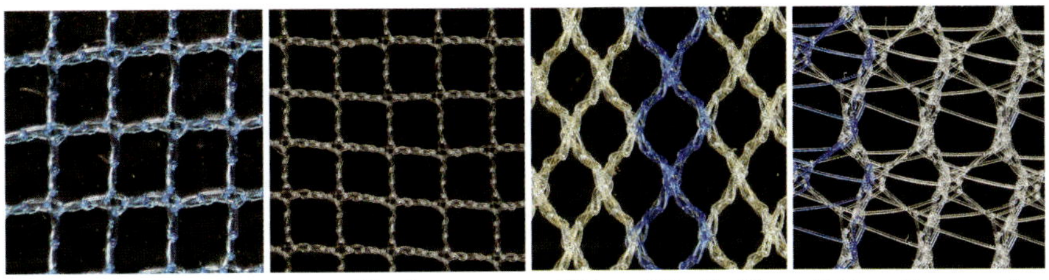

Fig. 7.4 Close-up images of four synthetic meshes (10 mm × 10 mm) with differing pore sizes and shapes.

TABLE 7.2 Comparison of Stiffness and Load at Failure Obtained Via Uniaxial Tensile and Ball-Burst Testing of Various Meshes

	STRUCTURAL PROPERTIES VIA UNIAXIAL TENSILE TEST			STRUCTURAL PROPERTIES VIA BALL-BURST TEST	
Synthetic Mesh	**Low Stiffness (N/mm)**	**High Stiffness (N/mm)**	**Load at Mesh Failure (N)**	**Stiffness (N/mm)**	**Load at Mesh Failure (N)**
Boston Scientific Polyform	0.130 ± 0.01	1.42 ± 0.11	53.8 ± 4.8	28 ± 0.43	108 ± 5.7
Coloplast NovaSilk	0.072 ± 0.05	0.508 ± 0.09	19.6 ± 4.5	16 ± 5.5	54 ± 19
Ethicon Gynemesh PS (Prolift)	0.286 ± 0.02	1.37 ± 0.09	46.3 ± 2.6	28 ± 2.7	108 ± 8.6
Ethicon Ultrapro (Prolift + M)	0.009 ± 0.00	0.236 ± 0.02	7.83 ± 0.7	22 ± 2.8	76 ±12
Coloplast Restorelle (Mpathy Medical Smartmesh, Minimesh)	0.178 ± 0.03	0.592 ± 0.04	22.7 ± 1.8	11 ± 0.89	45 ± 3.8

For uniaxial tensile testing, the dimensions of the meshes were 75 mm × 15 mm, and the dimensions for ball-burst testing were 25 mm × 25 mm. Data are presented as mean ± standard deviation. Over the years, some synthetic meshes have undergone multiple name changes because of changes in ownership; previous names are given in parentheses.

(From Shepherd JP, Feola AJ, Abramowitch SD, Moalli PA. Uniaxial biomechanical properties of seven different vaginally implanted meshes for pelvic organ prolapse. *Int Urogynecol J Pelvic Floor Dysfunct.* 2012;23:613; Feola A, Barone W, Moalli P, Abramowitch S. Characterizing the ex vivo textile and structural properties of synthetic prolapse mesh products. *Int Urogynecol J Pelvic Floor Dysfunct.* 2013;24:559–564.)

TABLE 7.3 Structural Properties of Various Slings Obtained Via Uniaxial Tensile Testing

	STRUCTURAL PROPERTIES VIA UNIAXIAL TENSILE TEST			
Sling	**Low Stiffness (N/mm)**	**High Stiffness (N/mm)**	**Load at Sling Failure (N)**	**Relative Elongation at Sling Failure (%)**
American Medical Systems SPARC/Monarc	0.09 ± 0.03	1.7 ± 0.2	79.2 ± 5.5	115.2 ± 7.4
Bard Uretex	0.16 ± 0.07	1.2 ± 0.1	59.8 ± 5.1	92.3 ± 6.7
Boston Scientific Advantage/Obtryx	0.05 ± 0.03	1.9 ± 0.1	69.6 ± 8.3	107.3 ± 10.0
Caldera T-sling	1.2 ± 0.3	N/A	82.0 ± 15.0	105.9 ± 4.9
Gynecare TVT/TVT-O	0.09 ± 0.01	2.0 ± 0.3	73.5 ± 11.8	108.1 ± 4.5
Mentor Aris	1.5 ± 0.4	N/A	56.3 ± 7.0	42.7 ± 5.5

The length of slings were ~7.8 cm, and the aspect ratio (length to width) of the slings tested was 8, with the exception of the Boston Scientific sling, which had an aspect ratio of 3–3.5. Data are presented as mean ± standard deviation.

(From Moalli PA, Papas N, Menefee S, et al. Tensile properties of five commonly used mid-urethral slings relative to the TVT™. *Int Urogynecol J Pelvic Floor Dysfunct.* 2008;19:655.)

synthetic meshes, the differing structural properties occur as a result of the distinct knit pattern, as well as the size and shape of the pores within each device. It is important for the interested reader to note that uniaxial tensile testing is preferred over ball-burst testing to determine the structural properties of slings, given the dimensions (aspect ratio) of slings.

Stiffness and the Host Response. From a functional perspective, the ideal synthetic mesh should be strong and stiff enough to withstand and maintain its architectural geometry and structure in response to *in vivo* loads. As one can imagine, a mesh that is not strong enough could break (mesh failure), which would result in prolapse recurrence. Similarly, prolapse recurrence could occur if the mesh is not stiff enough and permanently elongates with tensioning and loading. It is also important that synthetic meshes are not so strong or so stiff that they impede normal physiologic function (e.g., the ability of the vagina to elongate, contract, etc.) or affect the normal structure of the vagina (e.g., vaginal thickness and smooth muscle morphology). Specifically, meshes that are too stiff can lead to stress shielding.

Stress shielding is a phenomenon that occurs when there are stiffness mismatches between two interconnected materials. The stiffer material bears the majority of physiologic loads, thereby "shielding" the less stiff material from experiencing the loads it normally experiences, which can lead to a maladaptive remodeling response, resulting in degeneration and atrophy (Huiskes et al., 1987; Goel et al., 1991; Yamamoto et al., 1993; Rumian et al., 2009). A classic example of stress shielding is the degeneration of the surrounding hip bone after the implantation of a stiff artificial joint. Studies have shown evidence of stress shielding within the urogynecology field. The implantation of synthetic meshes with varying amounts of stiffness onto nonhuman primate (rhesus macaque) vaginas via abdominal sacrocolpopexy negatively impacted the vagina. However, the stiffest mesh was associated with the greatest negative impact on the vagina. Stress shielding led to thinning of the vaginal smooth muscle (Fig. 7.5), degradation of collagen and elastin, and increased apoptosis in the area of the mesh fibers (Liang, et al., 2013). Ongoing tissue degradation was evidenced by an increase in active matrix metalloproteinases (MMPs) MMP-1, MMP-8, and MMP-13, and total MMP-2 and MMP-9 (Liang et al., 2015). Additionally, deterioration of the mechanical properties, particularly the ability of the vagina to contract, was significantly impaired with the implantation of the stiffest mesh. Collectively, these results suggest that stress shielding induced by the implantation of polypropylene mesh leads to vaginal degeneration and atrophy.

Characterization of the Ex Vivo Mechanical Behavior of Synthetic Meshes and Implications for the Host Response

The mechanical behavior of synthetic meshes is a broad term that describes how a mesh (i.e., the architectural geometry of the pores and the overall structure of the mesh) responds to various deformations, loads, and boundary conditions. Mechanical tests, as well as computational modeling, have played an instrumental role in providing insight into how mesh behavior may impact the host response to mesh.

Anisotropy. Synthetic meshes are typically designed by manufacturers such that there is an intended orientation in which the mesh should be implanted. For some urogynecologic and hernia meshes, the structural properties will vary depending on the direction in which the mesh is deformed or loaded, a phenomenon referred to as anisotropy (Saberski et al., 2011; Feola et al., 2014). UltraPro (marketed as Prolift+M by Ethicon, Somerville, NJ, United States) is an example of a mesh that is anisotropic. The structural stiffness of UltraPro when loaded perpendicular to the blue orientation lines (UltraPro perpendicular, the intended orientation of implantation) is 0.009 ± 0.002 N/mm, whereas the stiffness is orders of magnitude higher when UltraPro is loaded parallel to the blue orientation lines (UltraPro parallel, 0.258 ± 0.085 N/mm) (Feola et al., 2014). The implantation of UltraPro in the perpendicular orientation was associated with less of a negative impact on the nonhuman primate vagina compared with the parallel orientation, owing to the decreased stiffness (Jallah et al., 2016). Given the significant impact that stiffness can have on the host response to mesh, understanding the mechanical behavior of synthetic meshes, including anisotropy, would provide surgeons with a better understanding of mesh behavior before implantation. Such knowledge would

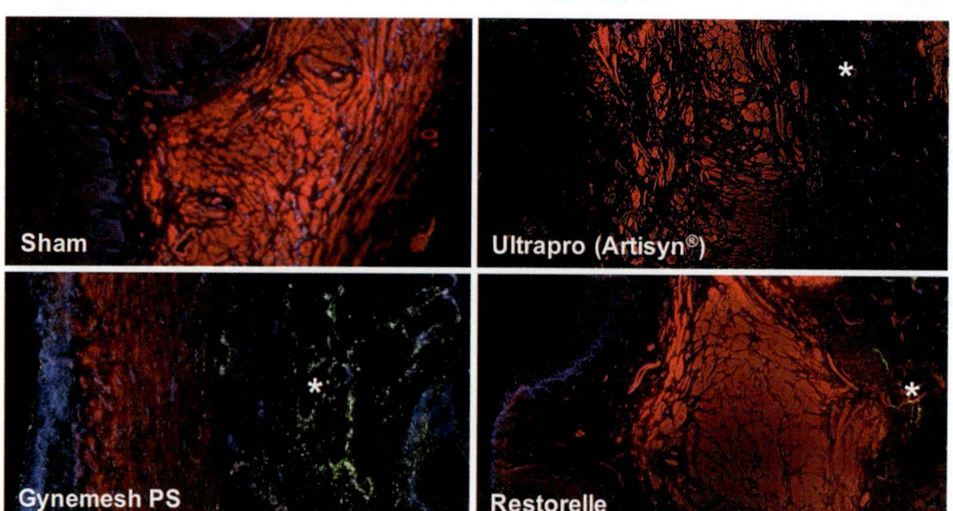

Fig. 7.5 Representative cross-sectional images of the nonhuman primate vagina without (sham) and with mesh implanted with the smooth muscle fluorescently labeled (*red signal*). Implanting the stiffest mesh Gynemesh PS onto the vagina resulted in significant thinning and disorganization of the smooth muscle. Additionally, there was an increased amount of apoptosis (*green signal*) surrounding the mesh fibers (*) of Gynemesh PS. *UltraPro is the same as Artisyn and Prolift + M.

also provide guidance on the appropriate direction of implantation, leading to improved outcomes for patients.

Pore Collapse via Tensile Loading. *Ex vivo* mechanical testing and computational modeling of synthetic meshes have demonstrated that the geometry of most meshes changes substantially when loaded. In regard to planar deformation, the pores collapse, and the porosity is significantly reduced for the majority of current synthetic meshes with uniaxial loading. This behavior is observed for both transvaginal and sacrocolpopexy meshes and occurs at loads that are well within the physiologic range. Otto et al. observed significant pore collapse associated with a loss of porosity within the arms of transvaginal meshes when elongated in response to relatively small loads (Otto et al., 2014). Similarly, Barone et al. (2019) observed that the pores in the arms of a transvaginal mesh, as well as those within the central body of the mesh (between the superior arms), are most susceptible to a reduction in pore size and a loss of porosity. Indeed, the arms and the central body of transvaginal meshes have been identified as problematic areas for patients experiencing mesh complications (e.g., mesh shrinkage/contraction, tenderness upon palpation of contracted mesh, pain, dyspareunia) (Feiner & Maher, 2010). Pore collapse, a reduction in porosity, and a complete loss in porosity (for some meshes) are also observed for sacrocolpopexy meshes (Barone et al., 2016). Regardless of the type of mesh (vaginal or abdominal), the degree of pore collapse is driven by the pore geometry, with square pore geometry being the most stable. The amount of pore collapse is also impacted by the degree to which the mesh is elongated or loaded, with increasing elongation and load resulting in increasing pore collapse (Fig. 7.6). Depending on the degree of pore collapse, the diameter of the pores can decrease to below 1 mm, which would make urogynecologic meshes more susceptible to poor tissue integration, bridging fibrosis, encapsulation, and pain. Clinically, mesh explants removed from patients experiencing mesh complications often exhibit mesh pore collapse with little to no tissue integration between the pores (Fig. 7.7). Collectively, these results and observations suggest that maintaining an open pore geometry is critical and future studies are needed to substantiate that pore collapse leads to mesh complications.

Permanent Elongation via Cyclic Loading. Synthetic meshes are intended to be implanted for the duration of a woman's life. As a result, meshes will undergo repetitive (i.e., cyclic) loading. Shepherd et al. (2012) and Jones et al. (2009) have found that synthetic meshes exposed to cyclic loads (0.5–15 N) within the physiologic range permanently elongate (i.e., the mesh does not return to the original length post cyclic loading). Slings also

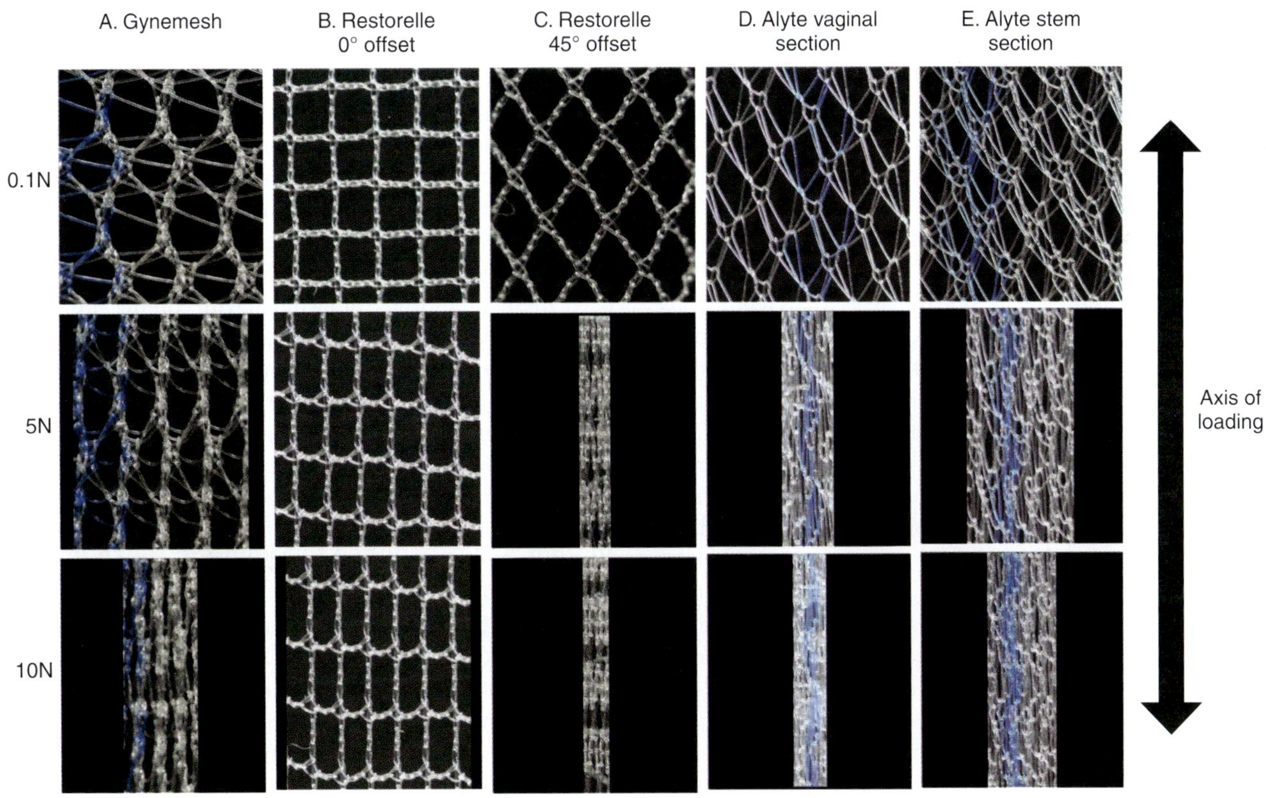

Fig. 7.6 Representative images of the midsection of Gynemesh (**A**), Restorelle 0-degree offset—the pores along the axis of loading are in the square configuration (**B**), Restorelle rotated 45-degrees offset—the pores along the axis of loading are in the diamond configuration (**C**), Alyte vaginal section (**D**), and Alyte stem section (**E**) at 0.1 N, 5 N, and 10 N. The degree of pore collapse increases with increasing load, with the square pore geometry (**B**) being the most stable. However, rotating the square pore mesh (**B**) by 45 degrees resulted in an unstable diamond pore configuration (**D**) in which the pores significantly collapse with loading. All images are 10 mm × 10 mm.

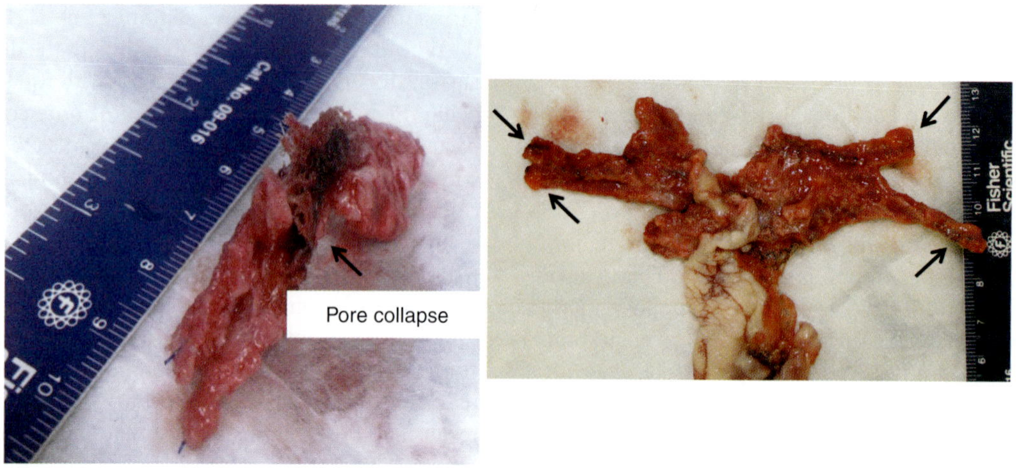

Fig. 7.7 Mesh explants removed from patients with exposures demonstrating little to no tissue incorporation in the area where the mesh pores have collapsed and the arms of the mesh (*black arrows*) have contracted into thin bands, which is also consistent with pore collapse.

demonstrate permanent elongation with cyclic loading (Moalli et al., 2008). The observed permanent elongation is likely a result of reorganization of the mesh or sling structure (e.g., the fibers are realigning), which can be particularly problematic in the initial stages of implantation when tissue has not grown into the pores of the mesh or sling. Clinically, a mesh that continually elongates could result in prolapse recurrence. The current trend of manufacturing meshes with decreased stiffness may make synthetic meshes more susceptible to permanent elongation. To date permanent elongation has not been associated with mesh complications but may lead a surgeon to tension a mesh more tightly so as to avoid mesh elongation and prolapse recurrence.

Boundary Conditions (Nonplanar Deformation). Surgeons use continuous and interrupted sutures to attach synthetic mesh to the vagina, sacrum, or the pelvic side wall (e.g., arcus tendineous or sacrospinous ligament). Mechanically, suture attachment points serve as boundaries, and boundary conditions impact the structural properties of a mesh when it is loaded or deformed. For example, the mesh is circumferentially constrained during ball-burst testing, which prevents the pores of the mesh from collapsing during testing. This is in contrast to uniaxial tensile testing, in which the mesh is clamped on opposing ends, and the mesh contracts in the perpendicular direction. The differing boundary conditions ultimately result in the structural properties for a single mesh being different (e.g., Restorelle uniaxial stiffness is 0.178 ± 0.03 N/mm, whereas the ball-burst stiffness is 11 ± 0.89 N/mm; see Table 7.2) (Shepherd et al., 2012; Feola et al., 2013).

Boundary conditions also impact how synthetic meshes respond to deformation and load. In a study conducted by Barone et al. (2015), boundary conditions were found to impact the surface curvature of a mesh (i.e., how much the mesh wrinkled/bunched or underwent nonplanar deformation). Specifically, three different boundary conditions were imposed on a low-stiffness mesh and a high-stiffness mesh: (1) mesh was completely clamped on both ends (representative of implanting mesh with continuous sutures), typical of a uniaxial tensile test; (2) mesh was clamped on one end, and two-point loads (i.e., two sutures) were applied on the opposing end, and; (3) two-point loads were applied on both ends of the mesh (Fig. 7.8A–C). The point loads are analogous to implanting mesh using interrupted sutures. The results of this study demonstrated that increasing the number of point loads from 0 to 4, as well as increasing the applied load, resulted in an increase in the amount of out-of-plane deformation (i.e., mesh curvature) which is visually apparent as mesh wrinkling/bunching (Fig. 7.8 D–I). In areas where the mesh wrinkles, there is a higher concentration of mesh, which could potentially increase the host foreign body response. Additionally, mesh wrinkling may result in the development of nonuniform stress distributions on the vagina. Collectively, these changes may increase the risk of mesh complications. Indeed, meshes removed from women with complications demonstrate mesh wrinkling (Fig. 7.9) (Svabik et al., 2011). Wrinkling of meshes with stiffness values that exceed those of the vagina reproduce a mesh exposure—one of the most common complications observed after implantation of synthetic mesh. Future studies are warranted to understand the mechanistic implications of mesh wrinkling.

In Vivo Host Response to Synthetic Mesh Implanted on the Vagina

Because of the ethical dilemmas surrounding the procurement and utilization of human tissues and subjects, much of the information to date regarding the host response to mesh has been obtained from the abdominal hernia literature and from animal models. However, research studies within the past two decades utilizing both animals and human specimens have begun to shed light on the vaginal host response to synthetic mesh. These studies have also aided our understanding of potential mechanisms of mesh complications. In the following sections, the findings from these human and animal studies will be reviewed, with a focus on basic science studies of the vagina.

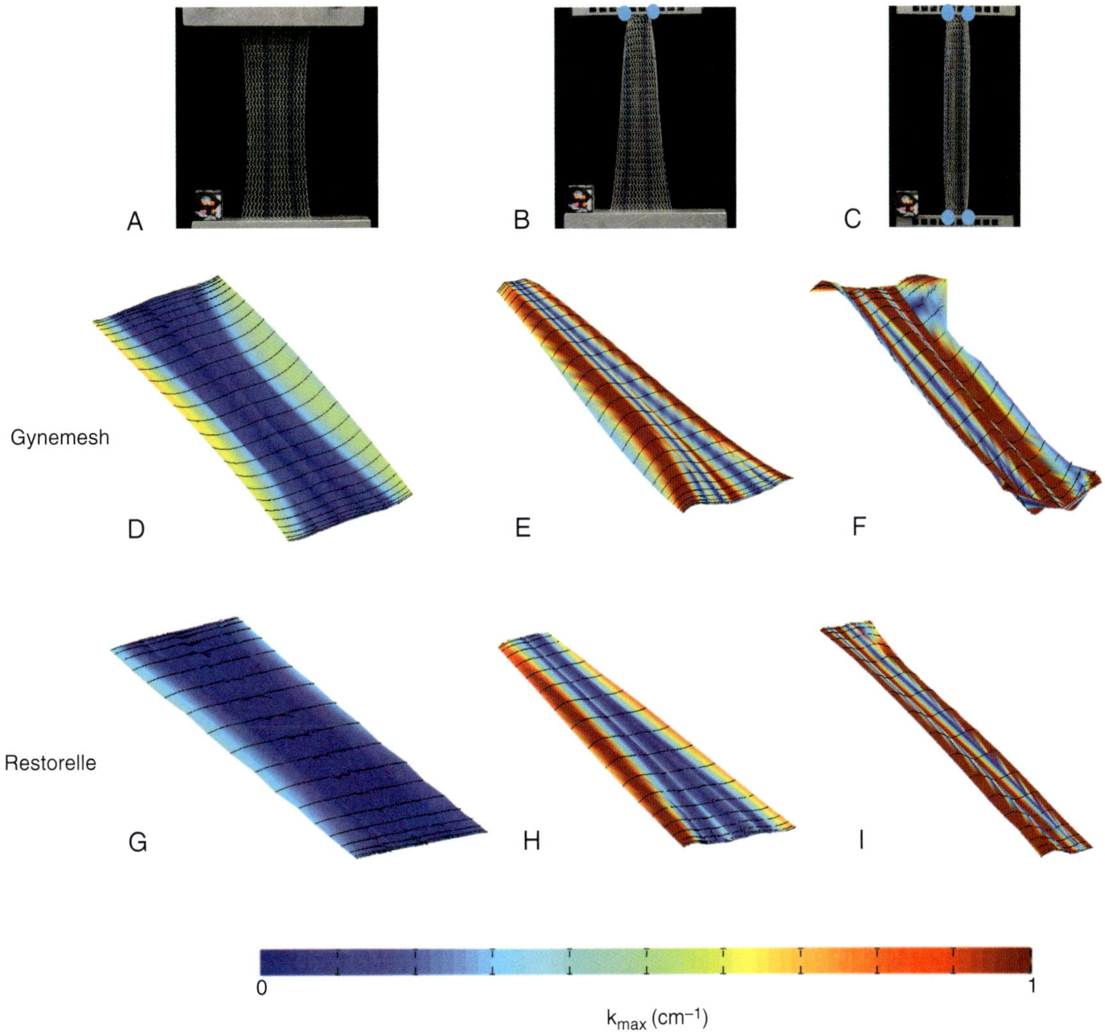

Fig. 7.8 Representative images of synthetic mesh depicting the following boundary conditions: **(A)** clamped on opposing ends, **(B)** one end clamped and two sutures on the opposing end, and **(C)** two sutures on opposing ends. *Blue dots* represent suture attachments. Increasing the amount of suture attachments resulted in increased mesh wrinkling (k_{max}) for both Gynemesh (**D–F**) and Restorelle (**G–I**), as shown in *red*.

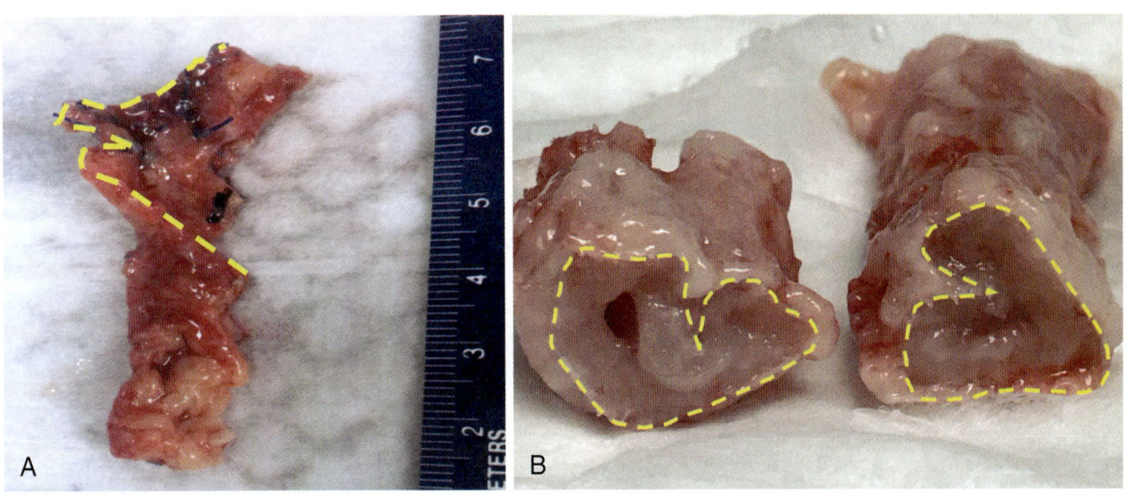

Fig. 7.9 Mesh explant removed from a patient for the indication of pain (**A**) and from the vagina of a rabbit following 12 weeks of mesh implantation (**B**). Mesh wrinkling is observed in both explants, as delineated by the *yellow outline*.

Macrophages and the Host Response to Synthetic Mesh. Once implanted in the body, synthetic meshes are perceived as foreign, which induces an innate immune response that involves a predominance of macrophages after the initial recruitment of neutrophils (Anderson, 2001; Anderson et al., 2008). Macrophages in particular have been identified as key immune cells that can directly impact the long-term functional outcomes of mesh (Brown et al., 2012a; Brown et al., 2012b). In response to various microenvironmental cues, macrophages differentiate into phenotypes that exist along a continuum from M1 (classically activated, proinflammatory) to M2 (antiinflammatory, homeostatic, wound healing), and these phenotypes have different functional properties and patterns of gene expression (Mills et al., 2000; Mantovani et al., 2004; Mosser & Edwards, 2008). Specifically, M1 macrophages are associated with a proinflammatory response that is characterized by the release of high levels of toxic reactive oxygen species, inducible nitric oxide synthase, and proinflammatory cytokines such as tumor necrosis factor (TNF)-α, interleukin (IL)-1β, and IL-6. M2 macrophages, in contrast, are associated with a constructive remodeling response characterized by cytokines and other molecules that promote tissue remodeling (e.g., high molecular weight IL-10, low molecular weight IL-12, and IL-23) (Mantovani et al., 2004; Mosser & Edwards, 2008; Brown & Badylak, 2013; Gundra et al., 2014). An excessive M1 macrophage response can result in damage to host tissue, whereas a prolonged M2 macrophage response can cause excessive tissue deposition and fibrosis (Murray & Wynn, 2011), suggesting that there is a balance between the M1 and M2 macrophage responses that will yield an optimal tissue response to mesh.

Human and Animal Studies. In studies conducted by Nolfi et al. (2016) and Tennyson et al. (2019), macrophages were the primary cell type surrounding the mesh fibers of explants removed from women undergoing mesh excision surgery for the indication of pain or mesh exposure (Fig. 7.10B). Tennyson et al. (2019) also observed a distinct population of T cells that was localized away from the mesh-tissue interface in a teardrop shape (Fig. 7.10C). Irrespective of the indication for removal, the mesh explants were associated with a high level of proremodeling (IL-4 and IL-10) and proinflammatory (TNF-alpha, IL-12p40p70, and IL-12p70) cytokines, as well as the proinflammatory chemokine CXCL10 and the proremodeling chemokine CCL17 (Nolfi et al., 2016). For the mesh explants removed for the indication of exposure, there was an increase in pro–MMP-9 (Nolfi et al., 2016) and $CD8^+$ cytotoxic T cells (Tennyson et al., 2019) relative to the mesh explants removed for pain, which is suggestive of tissue degradation. For the mesh explants removed for the indication of pain, there was a positive correlation between the proinflammatory cytokine IL-12p4p70 and the percentage of M2 macrophages and between transforming growth factor (TGF)-β and collagen type I. Furthermore, there were thicker (more mature) collagen fibers present within the mesh explants removed for pain compared with those removed for exposure. Together, these results suggest that increased mature collagen deposition and fibrosis are potential mechanisms of pain. The results from these two studies collectively provide evidence of an active and robust response that persists years after implantation. Moreover, differential macrophage activation likely contributes to different mechanisms of mesh exposure and pain.

Investigating the role of T regulatory (T_{reg}) cells in the host response to mesh explants and midurethral slings removed from patients for pain or exposure, Artsen et al. (2019) also observed T cells, specifically $CD8^+$ cytotoxic T cells and T_{reg} cells, localized around mesh fibers in a teardrop shape. In contrast to the macrophages, which immediately surrounded the mesh fibers, the T cells were in the "cap" of the teardrop. This response was found to persist years after mesh implantation. Relative to midurethral slings, prolapse mesh explants were associated with a higher concentration of T_{reg} cells, which is consistent with clinical findings of higher complication rates with prolapse mesh versus midurethral slings. However, there were no significant differences observed in the concentration of T_{reg} cells and the amount of TGF-β1 between patients with pain versus mesh exposure, or between patients with a midurethral sling versus prolapse mesh, which suggests that pain and mesh

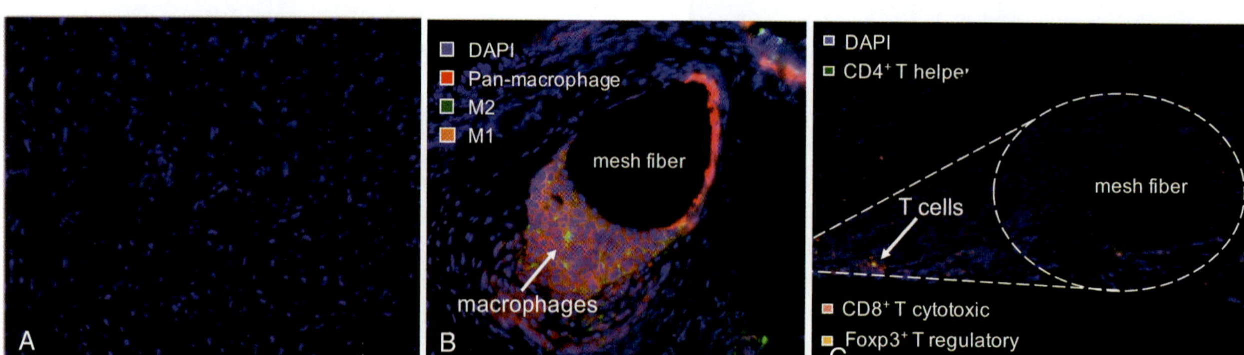

Fig. 7.10 Immunofluorescent micrographs of mesh explants removed from patients with complications. Macrophages (predominately M1) surround mesh fibers (**B**), whereas T cells localize away from mesh fibers (**C**). **A**, Mesh patient control tissue containing no macrophages or T cells. 4′, 6-diamidino-2-phenylindole (DAPI; *blue*): M1 proinflammatory macrophage marker CD88 (*orange*); M2 proremodeling macrophage marker CD206 (*green*, **B**); $CD4^+$ T helper (*green*, **C**); $CD8^+$ T cytotoxic (*red*); Foxp3+ T regulatory (*orange*). Original magnification, ×200.

exposure may exist on the same pathophysiologic spectrum. Furthermore, the concentration of T_{reg} cells and the amount of fibrosis were inversely correlated, suggesting an antifibrotic role for T_{reg} cells. The concentration of T_{reg} cells was also inversely correlated with TGF-β1, implicating TGF-β1 as a likely contributor to fibrosis. Collectively, these results highlight the protective role that T_{reg} cells play in the host response to mesh. In a recent study comparing characteristics of women with mesh complications who "respond" to removal measured by a reduction in symptoms versus "nonresponders" whose symptoms persist, responders were found to have higher concentrations of T_{reg} cells in the mesh area (Artsen et al., in press).

Similar to humans, M1 macrophages were the dominate cell type at the mesh-tissue interface following the implantation of polypropylene mesh via a sacrocolpopexy in nonhuman primates (rhesus macaques) (Brown et al., 2015). Additionally, the ratio of M2 to M1 macrophages was increased for the lighter-weight, higher-porosity mesh compared with the heavier-weight, lower-porosity mesh, and the percentage of M1 and M2 macrophages was positively correlated with mesh perimeter. These results, combined, provide a link between the number of mesh fibers (i.e., mesh burden) and the host response. Specifically, the host response is increased with decreasing pore size. Future studies are needed to characterize the T cell response to mesh in the nonhuman primate.

BIOLOGIC GRAFTS

Overview of Biologic Grafts

When describing grafts used in urogynecologic procedures, the term "biologic" refers to the content and source of the graft. Cellular or decellularized tissues, chemically altered extracellular matrix, and synthetic mesh modified with biomolecules can fit into the category of biologic. Use of biologic materials in SUI and POP repair long predates the emergence of synthetics, with the earliest recorded use being utilization of the gracilis muscle flap in 1907 as a suburethral sling (Schultheiss et al., 2000). Later use of biologics in SUI repair include the Aldridge procedure reported in 1942 (Aldridge, 1942) and the rectus fascia sling described in 1978 (McGuire & Lytton, 1978). These procedures were limited by longer operating times and donor site morbidity, leading to the development of synthetic materials. However, increased adverse event reports from patients undergoing SUI/POP repair with synthetic mesh has led to a resurgence of interest in biologic-derived grafts as alternatives. Conceptually, the biomechanical, molecular, and immunologic properties of human- and animal-derived materials should better facilitate their integration into host tissue and promote regeneration of normal architecture. However, the *in vivo* performance of these materials has proved to be highly variable, and more research is needed to characterize the host response to these materials and the clinical implications.

Different frameworks can be used to classify biomaterial grafts used in SUI/POP repair: for example, autologous versus allograft, regenerative versus permanent, homogeneous versus composite, and cellular versus acellular are commonly used. However, biologic grafts can be divided into three main categories: autografts, allografts, and xenografts (Fig. 7.11). Autografts used in SUI repair are most commonly permanent, homogeneous tissue flaps taken from the rectus abdominis fascia or fascia lata. Although the risk of foreign body reaction and degeneration is low for these materials, they are also associated with increased morbidity at the harvest site and longer operating time (Bang & Belal, 2016). Ease of harvest of rectus fascia compared with fascia lata makes it the preferred autograft material, despite equivalent effectiveness in managing SUI (Wein et al., 2011). Allografts are cadaveric or nonhuman in source and are subject to more extensive preimplantation processing to remove any epitopes that may sensitize the host immune system. Cadaveric human dermis, porcine or bovine dermis, small intestinal submucosa (SIS), and urinary bladder matrix (UBM) have been used as uniform acellular bioscaffolds, cell-seeded composites, and grafts functionalized with growth factors and antibodies. Acellular grafts that have been used in urogynecologic surgeries include Pelvicol (porcine dermis, CR Bard, Murray Hill, NJ), Biodesign (porcine SIS, Cook Medical, Bloomington, IN), MatriStem/Gentrix (porcine UBM, ACell, Columbia, MD), and Axis (cadaveric dermis, Coloplast, Minneapolis, MN). Many of these materials were initially intended for hernia repair before being adapted for urogynecologic procedures. Synthetic materials that are biologically augmented, through the addition of either human cells or platelet-rich plasma, have also been considered for use in POP and SUI repair (D'Angelo et al., 2019; Whooley et al., 2020).

Concepts from the field of tissue engineering are being examined for their applicability in manufacturing a more biocompatible mesh. Of note are electrospun materials, three-dimensional (3D) printed cell–extracellular matrix (ECM) bioinks, nanofibers incorporated into scaffolds, and novel crosslinking methods (Dutta, 2017; Taylor et al., 2018; Yao et al., 2019). Like grafts currently in use, mesh fabricated via these processes would be intended to provide adequate mechanical support to local tissue architecture while maintaining a local inflammatory response adequate for tissue integration into the graft and removal of any debris incurred during implantation. These methods of biofabrication favor the use of endogenous ECM proteins and growth factors, with the goal of recruiting the appropriate host cell types to the supporting matrix. Current research is directed toward refining the manufacturing process to maximize cellular integration and recreate host tissue mechanical properties.

In addition to composition, the physical dimensions, anchoring method, and mechanical phenotype of biologic grafts can vary. It is reasonable to assume that the maximum amount of force a graft can handle, as well as where that force is distributed, is influenced by both its micro- and macrostructure. *Ex vivo* biomechanical analysis suggests that the tensile strength of autologous and cadaver tissues processed into full strip slings is greater than these same tissues processed into patch suture slings (PSSs), and that the risk of suspension suture pull-through for the PSS is increased. Furthermore, the use of suspension sutures with PSSs makes sling failure most likely to occur at the insertion point by way of suture pull-through (Choe et al., 2001). Animal studies have shown that select synthetic-biologic composite grafts exhibit greater mechanical durability than pure synthetic mesh, such as increased graft elongation to failure over 84 days in primates undergoing

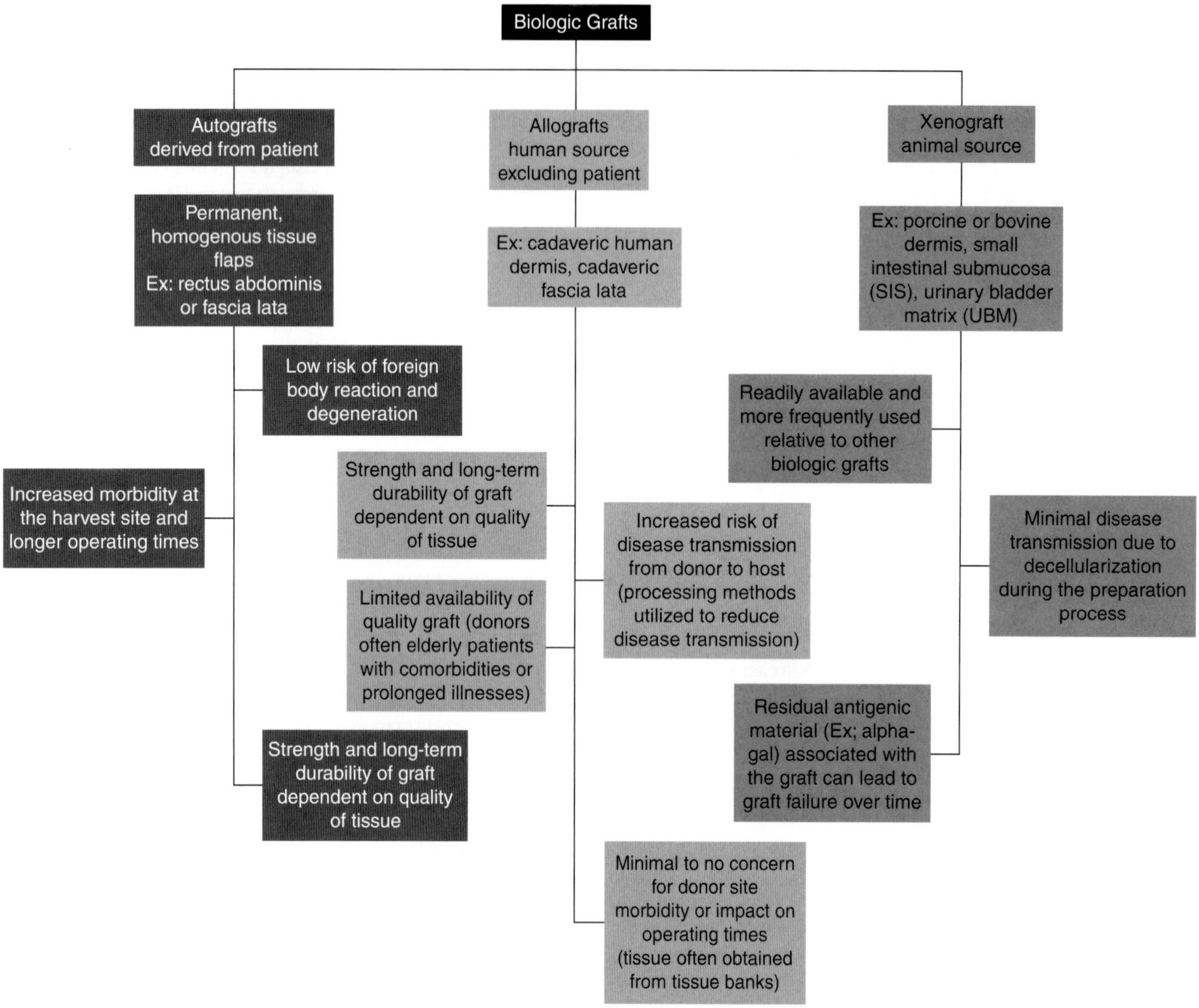

Fig. 7.11 Overview of the types of biologic grafts.

sacrocolpopexy (Liang et al., 2016) or gradually increased tensile strength over 90 days in rats undergoing abdominal fascial reconstruction (Konstantinovic et al., 2010).

Graft Processing

The ultimate goal of xenogenic graft processing is generation of a sterile, nonimmunogenic scaffold that can facilitate tissue repair and angiogenesis without provoking a harmful inflammatory response. In practice, this is difficult to achieve. Xenogenic and cadaveric grafts are subject to a variety of decellularization and crosslinking procedures that inevitably alter their mechanical and biochemical properties, as well as the host immune response. After isolation from the donor, they are exposed to mechanical, chemical, enzymatic, and/or irradiative treatments in an effort to remove any residual immunogenic components such as cell membranes, DNA, or mitochondria. Grafts intended to provide additional structural support, as is the case with POP/SUI mesh, require additional crosslinking steps to restore some lost tensile strength. The decellularization and crosslinking processes do not follow a one-size-fits-all procedure; rather, the procedure must be fine-tuned based on cell-ECM stoichiometry and the ultimate purpose of the generated acellular graft. Although many tissue-specific techniques have been developed, no "perfect" process currently exists. Presently, most xenograft processing workflows are syntheses of independently developed procedures and are highly proprietary. Awareness of the advantages and drawbacks of each procedure is important, as graft degradation, inflammation, and integration into the surrounding tissue are driven by exposed cell attachment motifs, release of matrikines, and leftover reagents and intermediates from decellularization and crosslinking processes (Wells, 2015; Dutta, 2017; Taylor et al., 2018). The current lack of standardization between research and commercial product testing procedures may be a primary contributor to the heterogeneous foreign body response associated with biologic pelvic grafts.

Current decellularization procedures combine physical, chemical, and more recently biological methods to eliminate cell remnants from ECM. In addition to freeze-thaw cycles, physical techniques involving oscillation and ultrahigh hydrostatic pressure can be used to delaminate xenografts. Chemical methods rely on detergents such as Triton X-100, sodium deoxycholate (SDC), and sodium dodecyl sulfate (SDS) to disrupt cell membranes. Grafts can be immersed in baths of these reagents for minutes to days, depending on their concentrations and the size of the graft. Differing reagent combinations, and even different solvents, can influence retention of bioactive peptides such as vascular endothelial growth factor and bone morphogenetic protein 2, as found by Ventura et al. (2019) in their experiments decellularizing porcine dermal ECM. Large, highly vascular tissues such as heart, liver, and lung can be decellularized via perfusion of chemical and enzymatic agents to lyse cells and clear out debris, thereby reducing physical stress and preserving more ECM architecture (Taylor et al., 2018; Yao et al., 2019). Biologic agents such as nucleases and proteases are used in conjunction with Triton X-100, SDC, and SDS for eradication of remaining immunogenic materials. Exposure to proteases must be controlled, however, as overexposure can result in biomechanical compromise and cleavage of cell anchoring and homing motifs.

The utilization of liquid nitrogen, detergents, and enzymes designed to degrade cell–ECM attachments in part contributes to decreasing the mechanical integrity of isolated matrix. To mitigate this, physical, chemical, and biologic crosslinking methods are being explored in both research and clinical settings. However, if a material intended to recapitulate normal tissue architecture through rebuilding absent or diseased structures is excessively crosslinked, it may lose the capacity to integrate into tissues. This problem is especially pertinent for urogynecologic grafts, given that release of growth factors and other regulatory peptides may be entirely dependent on ECM degradation (Lopresti & Brown, 2015). Therefore, choosing the correct crosslinker at the correct concentration is necessary. Physical crosslinking methods, such as photooxidation and thermal dehydrogenation, are typically not used as the primary crosslinking method in most current protocols because of their harsh reaction conditions and the disruption of ECM mechanical properties (Taylor et al., 2018; Yao et al., 2019). As with physical methods, chemical crosslinkers are not ideal, because of their biologic incompatibility. Unreacted compounds that may remain in ECM after processing have high immunogenic and/or cytotoxic potential. Glutaraldehyde is a chemical agent intended to resist degradation and promote strength by reacting with amino groups in proteins. Unintended effects of glutaraldehyde include cytotoxicity and tissue calcification. Epoxy compounds, carbodiimide (CDI), and hexamethylenediamine carbamate (HMDC) have different methods of action and adverse effects on surrounding cells. Generally, epoxy compounds confer mild crosslinking strength at the expense of toxicity, CDI crosslinks collagen with less toxicity but is prone to calcification, and HMDC crosslinks lysine residues and has increased cytotoxic activity (Yao et al., 2019).

McPherson et al. (1986) characterized an ideal concentration window of glutaraldehyde that maximized fibroblast infiltration and vascularization of crosslinked collagen while retaining resistance to degradation in animal models. However, the variable clinical performance of Pelvicol (CR Bard, Murray Hill, NJ), a glutaraldehyde-crosslinked mesh, highlights the need for more research into alternate mesh crosslinking methods. Briefly, drastic variation in the *in vivo* response to Pelvicol (e.g., encapsulation, no cell infiltration, complete degeneration, no reaction) has been proposed to be linked to crosslinking, patient age, graft size, and differing mechanical properties (Guerrero et al., 2010; Whooley et al., 2020). Recent research has delved into the usage of biologic agents as crosslinkers, with genipin as a notable example. Genipin reacts with the free amino groups of select residues in structural proteins such as collagen with little cellular toxicity. Collagen mesh crosslinked with genipin has been shown to be competitive with other suburethral sling materials in rats, although more work must be done to further characterize host response over time (Chapin et al., 2018; Yao et al., 2019). Tannic acid, proanthocyanidins (PCs), and nordihydroguaiaretic acid (NDGA) confer similar advantages. Tannic acid is a low-cost crosslinker that reacts with elastin and collagen but has some carcinogenic potential. PC crosslinks through hydrogen bonding with the same ECM proteins and may confer some antioxidant and antiinflammatory effects. NGDA covalently crosslinks amino groups in proteins with similar antioxidant effects, but it is cytotoxic at higher concentrations (Yao et al., 2019). Riboflavin is a candidate biologic crosslinker that is activated after exposure to ultraviolet A light; however, research involving this compound is mostly limited to crosslinking of decellularized ECM bioinks for 3D printing (Jang et al., 2016; Taylor et al., 2018; Dzobo et al., 2019).

Like other processing steps, sterilization of biologic grafts can compromise their structural integrity and performance *in vivo* and do not always result in complete eradication of DNA and other immunogenic compounds (Whooley et al., 2020). Common procedures include immersion in peracetic acid (PAA), gamma radiation, and exposure to ethylene oxide (EO). EO and harsh radiation do not preserve ECM structure mechanical properties as well as supercritical carbon dioxide or PAA. Early *in vitro* research has demonstrated that PAA may be preferable to other sterilization agents for promoting cell adhesion to the prepared matrix (Matuska & McFetridge, 2015). Tissue preservation after sterilization is another opportunity for a graft to undergo structural damage and loss of bioactive compounds. Depending on purpose and time to use, preservation typically means either short-term incubation in 4° C phosphate-buffered saline with antibiotics or freezing at −20° C for long-term preservation (Yao et al., 2019). Although freshly prepared grafts would be ideal for POP/SUI repair applications, preservation steps seem unavoidable to adequately supply all surgeons and researchers who use these grafts.

In Vivo Studies

Despite some amount of anatomic and cellular homology between humans, primates, and other mammals, variable experimental and clinical findings post–biologic graft implantation have complicated analysis of the host response. The structural and ECM composition of autografts, cadaveric tissues, and xenografts most certainly differs between species. Even within the same species the composition can vary based on the source organ. For example, porcine SIS and UBM differ in collagen type composition. The ratio of different collagen subtypes and any retention of foreign DNA can influence the extent of the inflammatory response and subsequent graft remodeling. The immune systems of rabbits, primates, and humans may react to grafts differently, and grafts that may have been beneficial for abdominal hernia repair may not see the same success in POP/SUI surgeries. Rabbits, for example, have higher collagenolytic activity against collagen constructs that incorporate multiple collagen fiber subtypes (Claerhout et al., 2008). Therefore, generalizing animal studies to humans and vice versa must be done with caution.

Dora (2004) analyzed the behavior of cadaveric fascia, porcine dermis, porcine SIS, polypropylene mesh, and autologous fascial grafts in 15 rabbits. Each rabbit had a section of mesh implanted on the anterior rectus fascia that was harvested at either 2, 6, or 12 weeks. The human cadaveric and porcine tissue slings exhibited a decrease in tensile strength and stiffness 12 weeks after implantation. The autologous fascial grafts did exhibit decreased tensile strength, but along with porcine SIS showed decrease in surface area at the 12-week time point. The authors described these findings as additional support for the use of synthetics in anti-incontinence procedures. Claerhout et al. (2008) investigated the efficacy of polypropylene, Pelvicol, and SIS grafts in repairing full-thickness abdominal wall defects in rabbits. Gross and histologic analysis showed integration of polypropylene into a fibrotic scar within 1 month and complete remodeling of SIS into native tissue within 2 months. Pelvicol, however, remained structurally unchanged for up to 6 months beneath a thick fibrous capsule, after which it was partially degraded. Furthermore, after 720 days of implantation, all Pelvicol implants felt stiff when palpated, likely related to encapsulation secondary to a persistent heightened foreign body response. Indeed, a persistent chronic inflammatory response was observed after implantation with Pelvicol, whereas the inflammation related to SIS tapered off by 3 months. The difference in the responses to the two biologic grafts is consistent with animal studies demonstrating a heightened and prolonged foreign-body response to crosslinked biologic grafts, whereas the host response to uncrosslinked materials is limited and consistent with a constructive remodeling response (see Graft Processing). For this reason, biologic scaffolds should be used as intended; that is, degradation by the host followed by constructive remodeling of functional tissue (Brown & Badylak, 2014).

Connor et al. (2009) used decellularized, galactose-α(1,3)-galactose terminal carbohydrate epitope (α-gal)–cleaved porcine dermal tissue to repair full-thickness abdominal wall defects in a Caribbean vervet model. α-gal is present in all mammalian tissues except for old world primates, a family group known taxonomically as Cercopitheciae to which humans belong. Humans become sensitized to this antigen by consuming meat, leading to the development of anti–α-gal antibodies. Implantation of a material that retains this antigen risks eliciting a hyperacute rejection response mediated via circulating anti–α-gal antibodies. The authors used enzymatic cleavage to remove α-gal and subsequently found that the grafts were well tolerated up to the final time point of 6 months. Gross pathology and histologic analysis revealed no herniation or scar formation and evidence of angiogenesis and fibroblast proliferation on the cellular level. Based on histology, a mixed cellular inflammatory infiltrate was present at the 2-week time point. Graft dimensions were also unchanged upon explantation. Liang et al. (2016) implanted MatriStem (a multilayered scaffold derived from UBM) and composite polypropylene-MatriStem grafts via abdominal sacrocolpopexy (ASC) in a rhesus macaque model. Gross and histologic analysis showed less apoptosis in vaginal tissue implanted with composite grafts, as well as a reduced inflammatory response (compared with previous data on polypropylene mesh). Composite mesh samples exhibited worse performance than sham in passive mechanical testing but demonstrated preserved contractility and smooth muscle thickness at sham values. This is in contrast to polypropylene mesh implants in this model, which demonstrate reduced smooth muscle contractility and thickness. ECM biomolecule composition of composite graft vaginal tissue was similar to the sham animals, with one exception being lower total collagen content. Histologic, mechanical, and collagen properties of the ECM graft resembled those of sham. From these findings, the authors concluded that augmenting synthetic mesh with ECM components could reduce negative effects associated with synthetic grafts. Following up on these findings, Liang et al. (2017) used a rhesus macaque with resected uterosacral ligament (level I) and paravaginal (level II) support (Fig. 7.12C and D) as a vaginal prolapse model to assess the regenerative ability of MatriStem to restore support to the vagina. Grafts were shaped to mimic the lost anatomy and support from both anterior and posterior aspects. Both transvaginal and transabdominal insertions of these grafts were performed. Animals were analyzed 3 months postoperatively to assess the degree of graft remodeling and incorporation into existing anatomy. Animals requiring vaginal incisions for transvaginal placement experienced decreases in vaginal stiffness and collagen content, with an increase in collagen III/I subtypes. These findings were not observed in the transabdominal group, which had values similar to the sham group. MMP-2 content was increased in both mesh implantation groups compared with sham, indicating the presence of graft remodeling activity. Most notably, regeneration of level I and II support was evidenced (Fig. 7.12E and F).

A robust library of animal and clinical studies has contributed significantly to our understanding of the *in vivo* behavior of biologic grafts of multiple origins. Autologous materials undergo limited remodeling and induce a low inflammatory response and moderate collagen production. The mechanical properties of these grafts are reported to undergo no significant changes in mechanical properties during the first 3 to 4 months postimplantation. Cadaveric allografts have shown more variable *in vivo* performance, with evidence of degradation, encapsulation, acute inflammation, cell infiltration, and vascularization all observed in various studies (Moalli, 2006). Mechanical analysis also varies from significant increase or decrease to no change in tensile strength. Host response to xenografts appears to be linked to crosslinking and degradation rate. Crosslinked collagenous materials do not facilitate cell infiltration or remodeling and degradation, whereas the opposite is true for non—crosslinked grafts. It is to be expected that crosslinking increases the mechanical integrity of grafts by boosting their resistance to degradation; however,

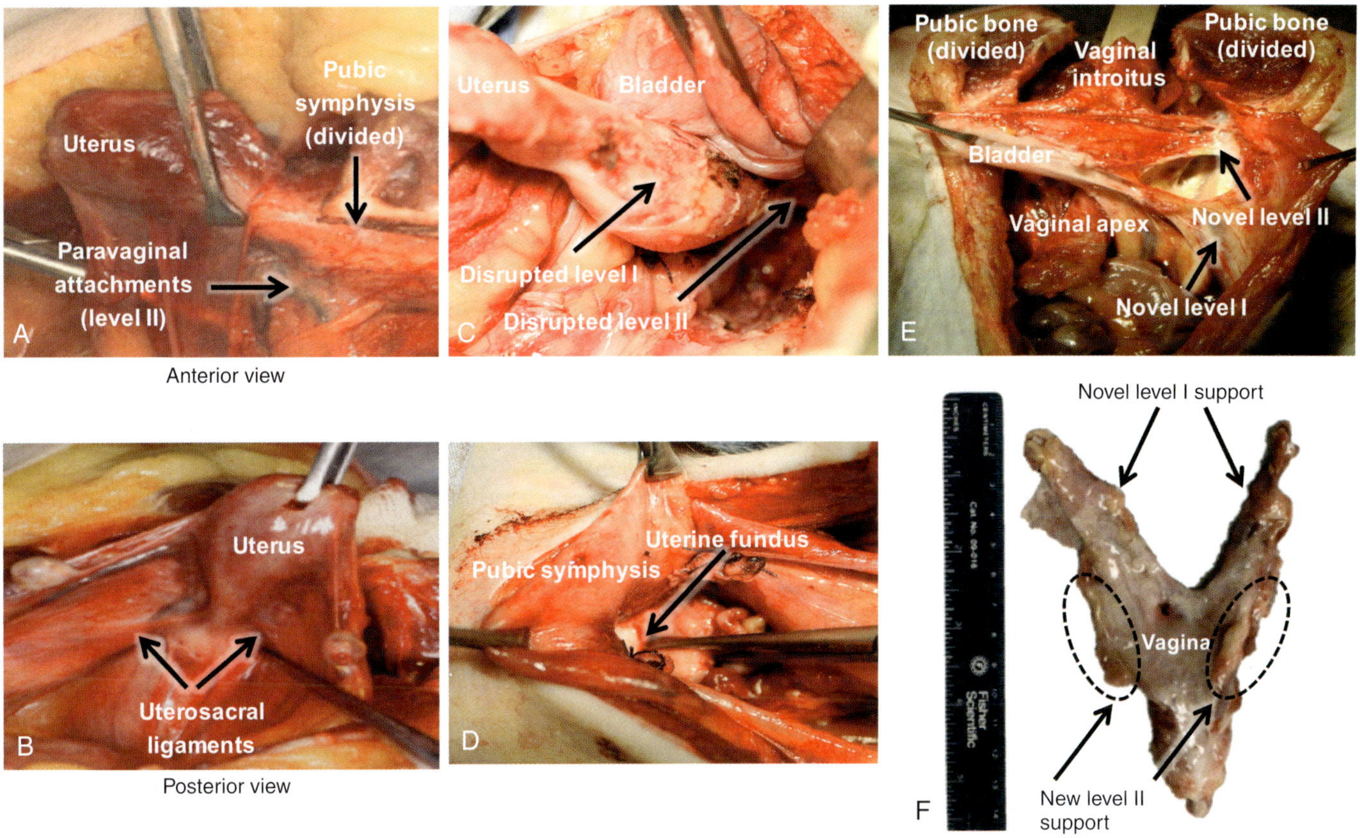

Fig. 7.12 In the normally supported vagina of the rhesus macaque, the paravaginal attachments to the pelvic sidewall (level II support) provide lateral support to the vagina (**A**), whereas the uterosacral ligaments (level I support) provide apical support to the vagina (**B**). **C**, Surgical disruption of level I and II support before implanting an extracellular matrix onto the anterior and posterior vagina. **D**, Image demonstrating free movement of the uterus and vagina below the pubic symphysis, mimicking pelvic organ prolapse. **E**, *In vivo* anatomy and **F**, morphology after dissection. Images depicting newly formed tissue that is providing novel level I and II support to the vagina following the implantation of an extracellular matrix bioscaffold after 3 months of implantation.

as stated above, the chemical toxicity associated with some of these products has limited their use. Generally, it has been observed in applications utilizing non—crosslinked bioscaffolds that porcine dermal collagen maintains mechanical stability for 3 months, whereas SIS may increase in strength up to 2 years postimplantation (Gigliobianco et al., 2015).

Gigliobianco et al. (2015) outlined five tenets for the ideal graft: ability to degrade, capacity to provoke acute inflammation, amenability to remodeling, cell permeability, and durability during the implantation procedure. On the patient level, these tenets translate to a procedure and material that should do the least harm, as complications like chronic pain and reoperation are impossible to completely eradicate. Key to clinical studies is assessment of patient quality of life over a long period of time, ideally years. As with animal studies, results can be difficult to generalize. Graft type, placement, patient sample size demographics, follow-up time, surgeon experience with the material, and concomitant procedures all influence the data collected and their significance.

Histopathologic analysis of biologic suburethral slings shows widely variable host response regarding predisposition to encapsulation, vascularization, and immunologic response. Gandhi et al. (2005) described histopathologic changes in slings fashioned from hexamethylene diisocyanate crosslinked porcine dermis grafts. The patient population of interest was a small cohort (n = 12) who reported recurrent SUI or urinary retention 6 to 67 weeks post transvaginal sling surgery. The specimens available for evaluation showed diverse inflammatory and remodeling responses. Patients with urinary retention generally had preserved grafts with only peripheral collagen deposition, whereas in patients with recurrent incontinence the graft had mostly degraded and was replaced by neovascularization and fibrosis. Some samples contained lymphocytes, whereas others implicated a more vigorous foreign body response as evidenced by the presence of histocytes and multinucleated giant cells. Woodruff et al. (2008) characterized the histopathology of pubovaginal sling grafts of varying origin, observing high variability in host response. The 24 patients in this study who had a section of transvaginally placed graft removed for biopsy 2 to 34 months after surgery had undergone surgical revision for decreased sling efficacy, urinary retention, or sling obstruction. Of this group, 14 received biologic grafts (two cadaveric fascia, three cadaveric dermis, four porcine dermis, five autologous fascia). Cadaveric graft histology showed no neovascularization, few peripheral fibroblasts, and mild to moderate graft degradation. Porcine dermis grafts showed no evidence of degradation, and instead were entirely encapsulated. Autologous fascial grafts showed moderate amounts of degradation, with moderate vascularization and peripheral fibroblast infiltration. The 10 patients who were treated with polypropylene mesh had biopsies that demonstrated little graft degradation and encapsulation, as well as moderate vascularization and uniform fibroblast penetration. Although histological studies such as these use small sample sizes and are thus hard to generalize, they outline the idea of graft failure as a multifactorial process with varied clinical presentation.

Cohort studies, randomized controlled trials, and meta-analyses of literature covering POP/SUI repair have helped shed more light on clinical outcomes for this heterogeneous group of materials and aided in comparing outcomes with synthetic grafts. Flynn et al. (2002) retrospectively observed a significant decrease in postoperative pain and disability with pubovaginal slings manufactured from allograft fascia lata relative to autograft fascia for all types of SUI (Flynn & Yap, 2002). Giri et al. (2006) prospectively compared the long-term efficacy of Pelvicol versus rectus fascia in SUI repair. Data from 101 consecutive, nonrandomized patients undergoing SUI surgery between 2000 and 2001 were analyzed. Some 36 months after surgery, low patient-perceived success rates (assessed via questionnaire and telephone interview) indicated an inferior long-term cure rate for Pelvicol. The authors reported a 46% recurrent incontinence rate and a 37.5% reoperation rate for patients treated with Pelvicol. These results led the authors to conclude that Pelvicol should not be used as a rectus fascia substitute for SUI repair, despite early reductions in morbidity. Guerrero et al. (2010) conducted a randomized controlled trial of 201 women with SUI analyzing the effectivity of Pelvicol, TVT, and fascial slings for treatment. Four assessments were conducted: baseline, 6 weeks, 6 months, and 1 year, with patient quality of life as the primary outcome. Operative complications and time, reoperation rates, and self-catheterization were analyzed as secondary outcomes. The Pelvicol arm of the trial was suspended after 1 year owing to poor outcomes, and data analysis indicated no significant difference between use of TVT and fascial slings for SUI repair. Also of note were the observation of longer operating times and more frequent self-catheterization for fascial slings, as well as shorter hospital stay for TVT. Overall, this study discouraged use of Pelvicol based on patient-reported outcomes. More recently, Peng et al. (2020) performed a retrospective review of 105 women who were treated with autologous fascia lata or rectus fascia as pubovaginal slings for SUI repair. Comparing the two, fascia lata pubovaginal slings were associated with lower blood loss and similar operative time, similar rate of complications, and similar functional outcomes (i.e., patients without SUI symptoms at 1 month, 1 year, and >1 year postimplantation) as compared with rectus fascia pubovaginal slings.

Schimpf et al. (2016) performed a meta-analysis of literature on ASC and transvaginal mesh or graft use published through 2015. All studies analyzed also included anatomic and symptomatic outcomes at a minimum of 1 year. The meta-analysis conclusions indicated that synthetic mesh was superior to native tissue repair in anterior wall POP repair regarding reported anatomic and bulge outcomes. Additionally, data collected indicated that neither biologic nor synthetic grafts inserted transvaginally led to outcome improvement in any vaginal compartments. The authors highlighted the difficulty of interpreting subjective symptom outcomes in the current literature because of the heterogeneity of reporting measures used. Hijazi et al. (2017) described a small cohort study assessing the effectiveness of transabdominal ASC and accompanying Burch colposuspension using Pelvicol. Of the 27 women included in this study, 24 were postoperatively assessed (mean follow-up time: 21 months) for changes in quality-of-life factors such as pad usage, pelvic pain, and incontinence status. Follow-up assessment indicated quality of life improvement through decreased voiding frequency, pad usage, residual urine, dysuria, and nocturia. The authors did not report any graft removal based on graft complications or rejection. However, the failure rate of the Pelvicol graft was high, at 8.3% (two patients at 3 and 11 months after surgery, respectively). Sohlberg et al. (2020) performed a population-based cohort analysis comparing outcomes of POP repair with synthetic and biologic (both autologous and xenogenic) grafts. Over a 4-year period (2005–2011), patient data from 14,192 women were collected. Synthetic grafts predominated (86%) within the cohort. Biologic grafts were associated with increased rates of surgery for recurrent POP whereas synthetic grafts were associated with increased rates of surgery for graft complications. Data analysis indicated no overall difference in repeat surgery rate despite differing predominant cause per graft type. Variation in trial design is a major contributory factor to discrepancies in reported outcomes and their significance, a problem that becomes more apparent as sample size decreases. Larger, more robust trials are required to better incorporate biologic grafts into clinical practice.

Limitations

Additional research on biologic outcomes is needed to better characterize the mechanisms for anatomic failure and complications to isolate susceptible individuals preoperatively. Unfortunately, there is still a low quantity of adequately powered randomized controlled trials, because of issues with recruitment and blinding of patients and clinical providers. Heterogeneity between POP procedures, surgeon experience, follow-up period, and materials used provides a significant challenge in generalizing trial results to a large and diverse patient population (Costantini et al., 2016). Even the largest cohort study performed to this date did not survey patient quality-of-life outcomes or differentiate between the different types of biologic or synthetic grafts used (Sohlberg et al., 2020). Although certainly not the only cause, issues with patient recruitment can possibly be attributed to public opinion of mesh and related procedures (Nager et al., 2016).

FUTURE OUTLOOK FOR SYNTHETIC MESHES AND BIOLOGIC GRAFTS

Since the initial use of synthetic and biologic grafts for POP and SUI repairs, *ex vivo* mechanical testing, computational modeling, *in vivo* animal studies, and clinical trials have all served as invaluable tools that have aided our understanding of the host response to and pathogenesis of complications associated with mesh and biologic grafts. Over the next 10 years, it is anticipated that our ability to design/develop synthetic meshes and biologic grafts that are specifically tailored for POP and SUI will only improve as our knowledge of the pathophysiology of these disorders increases. Furthermore, given that the etiology of prolapse and the anatomical defects vary from patient to patient, a movement away from the "one-size-fits-all mentality" and the development of patient-specific approaches to biomaterials are highly warranted.

Synthetic meshes have evolved over the past 3 decades from heavyweight, small-pore, high-stiffness devices to lightweight, large-pore, low-stiffness fabrics as a way to improve patient outcomes by mitigating the foreign body response via decreasing the amount of material in contact with the host. Alternative approaches include coating meshes with various biologic and chemical agents (e.g., collagen, extracellular matrix, IL-4) to modify the host response. The recent discovery of the importance of preserving geometry with tensioning and loading has increased the use of square-pored meshes (along the direction of loading) over those with hexagon or diamond pores. The limitation of current products is that most are manufactured from polymers that are substantially stiffer than the vagina—a phenomenon that is known to increase complications. Improved biologically active materials designed to rebuild or biofabricate damaged tissues are currently under development. Future studies will focus on manufacturing meshes made from softer materials, including biologics, synthetics, and composite biologic-synthetics with stiffness values that more closely mimic that of the vagina, thereby preserving both structure and function.

BIBLIOGRAPHY

Aldridge AH.Transplantation of fascia for relief of urinary stress incontinence." *Am J Obstet Gynecol.* 1942;44:398.

Amid PK. Classification of biomaterials and their related complications in abdominal wall hernia surgery. *Hernia.* 1997;1:15.

Anderson JM. Biological responses to materials. *Annu Rev Mater Sci.* 2001;31:81.

Anderson JM, Rodriguez A, Chang DT. Foreign body reaction to biomaterials. *Semin Immunol.* 2008;20:86.

Artsen AM, Liang R, Meyn L, et al. T regulatory cells and TGF-ß1: predictors of the host response in mesh complications. *Acta Biomater.* (In press).

Artsen AM, Rytel M, Liang R, et al. Mesh induced fibrosis: the protective role of T regulatory cells. *Acta Biomater.* 2019;96:203.

Bang SL, Belal M. Autologous pubovaginal slings: back to the future or a lost art? *Res Rep Urol.* 2016;8:11.

Barber MD, Brubaker L, Burgio KL, et al. Comparison of 2 transvaginal surgical approaches and perioperative behavioral therapy for apical vaginal prolapse: The OPTIMAL randomized trial. *J Am Med Assoc.* 2014;311:1023.

Barone W R, Amini R, Maiti S, et al. The impact of boundary conditions on surface curvature of polypropylene mesh in response to uniaxial loading. *J Biomech.* 2015;48:1566.

Barone WR, Knight KM, Moalli PA, Abramowitch SD. Deformation of transvaginal mesh in response to multiaxial loading. *J Biomech Eng.* 2019;141:0210011.

Barone WR, Moalli PA, Abramowitch SD. Textile properties of synthetic prolapse mesh in response to uniaxial loading. *Am J Obstet Gynecol.* 2016;215:326.e321.

Boreham MK, Wai CY, Miller RT, et al. Morphometric analysis of smooth muscle in the anterior vaginal wall of women with pelvic organ prolapse. *Am J Obstet Gynecol.* 2002;187:56.

Boreham MK, Wai CY, Miller RT, et al. Morphometric properties of the posterior vaginal wall in women with pelvic organ prolapse. *Am J Obstet Gynecol.* 2002;187:1501.

Brown BN, Badylak SF. Expanded applications, shifting paradigms and an improved understanding of host-biomaterial interactions. *Acta Biomater.* 2013;9:4948.

Brown BN, Badylak SF. Extracellular matrix as an inductive scaffold for functional tissue reconstruction. *Transl Res.* 2014;163:268.

Brown BN, Londono R, Tottey S, et al. Macrophage phenotype as a predictor of constructive remodeling following the implantation of biologically derived surgical mesh materials. *Acta Biomater.* 2012;8:978.

Brown BN, Mani D, Nolfi AL, et al. Characterization of the host inflammatory response following implantation of prolapse mesh in rhesus macaque. *Am J Obstet Gynecol.* 2015;213:668e661.

Brown BN, Ratner BD, Goodman SB, et al. Macrophage polarization: an opportunity for improved outcomes in biomaterials and regenerative medicine. *Biomaterials.* 2012;33:3792.

Chapin K, Khalifa A, Mbimba T, et al. In vivo biocompatibility and time-dependent changes in mechanical properties of woven collagen meshes: a comparison to xenograft and synthetic mid-urethral sling materials. *J Biomed Mater Res B Appl Biomater.* 2018;107:479.

Chen CC, Ridgeway B, Paraiso MF. Biologic grafts and synthetic meshes in pelvic reconstructive surgery. *Clin Obstet Gynecol.* 2007;50:383.

Choe JM, Kothandapani R, James L, Bowling D. Autologous, cadaveric, and synthetic materials used in sling surgery: comparative biomechanical analysis. *Urology.* 2001;58:482.

Claerhout F, Verbist G, Verbeken E, et al. Fate of collagen-based implants used in pelvic floor surgery: a 2-year follow-up study in a rabbit model. *Am J Obstet Gynecol.* 2008;198:94.e91.

Clemons JL, Weinstein M, Guess MK, et al. Impact of the 2011 FDA transvaginal mesh safety update on AUGS members' use of synthetic mesh and biologic grafts in pelvic reconstructive surgery. *Female Pelvic Med Reconstr Surg.* 2013;19:191.

Cobb WS, Peindl RM, Zerey M, et al. Mesh terminology 101. *Hernia.* 2009;13:1.

Connor J, McQuillan D, Sandor M, et al. Retention of structural and biochemical integrity in a biological mesh supports tissue remodeling in a primate abdominal wall model. *Regen Med.* 2009;4:185.

Conze J, Junge K, Weiss C, et al. New polymer for intra-abdominal meshes - PVDF copolymer. *J Biomed Mater Res B Appl Biomater.* 2008;87:321.

Conze J, Rosch R, Klinge U, et al. Polypropylene in the intra-abdominal position: Influence of pore size and surface area. *Hernia.* 2004;8:365.

Cosson M, Debodinance P, Boukerrou M, et al. Mechanical properties of synthetic implants used in the repair of prolapse and urinary incontinence in women: which is the ideal material? *Int Urogynecol J Pelvic Floor Dysfunct.* 2003;14:169.

Costantini E, Brubaker L, Cervigni M, et al. Sacrocolpopexy for pelvic organ prolapse: evidence-based review and recommendations. *Eur J Obstet Gynecol Reprod Biol.* 2016;205:60.

Costello CR, Bachman SL, Grant SA, et al. Characterization of heavyweight and lightweight polypropylene prosthetic mesh explants from a single patient. *Surg Innov.* 2007;14:168.

D'Angelo W, Dziki J, Badylak SF. The challenge of stress incontinence and pelvic organ prolapse. *Curr Opin Urol.* 2019;29:437.
Davis NF, McGuire BB, Callanan A, et al. Xenogenic extracellular matrices as potential biomaterials for interposition grafting in urological surgery. *J Urol.* 2010;184:2246.
Delgado LM, Bayon Y, Pandit A, Zeugolis DI. To cross-link or not to cross-link? cross-linking associated foreign body response of collagen-based devices. *Tissue Eng Part B Rev.* 2015;21:298.
Desmouliere A, Chaponnier C, Gabbiani G. Tissue repair, contraction, and the myofibroblast. *Wound Repair Regen.* 2005;13:7.
Dora CD. Time dependent variations in biomechanical properties of cadaveric fascia, porcine dermis, porcine small intestine submucosa, polypropylene mesh and autologous fascia in the rabbit model: implications for sling surgery. *J Urol.* 2004;171:1970.
Duffield JS, Lupher M, Thannickal VJ, Wynn TA. Host responses in tissue repair and fibrosis. *Annu Rev Pathol.* 2013;8:241.
Dutta RC. Competent processing techniques for scaffolds in tissue engineering. *Biotechnol Adv.* 2017;35:240.
Dzobo K, Motaung KSCM, Adesida A. Recent trends in decellularized extracellular matrix bioinks for 3D printing: an updated review. *Int J Mol Sci.* 2019;20:4628.
Engelsman AF, Van Dam GM, Van Der Mei HC, et al. In vivo evaluation of bacterial infection involving morphologically different surgical meshes. *Ann Surg.* 2010;251:133.
Feiner B, Maher C. Vaginal mesh contraction: Definition, clinical presentation, and management. *Obstet Gynecol.* 2010;115:325.
Feola A, Abramowitch S, Jallah Z, et al. Deterioration in biomechanical properties of the vagina following implantation of a high-stiffness prolapse mesh. *BJOG.* 2013;120:224.
Feola A, Barone W, Moalli P, Abramowitch S. Characterizing the ex vivo textile and structural properties of synthetic prolapse mesh products. *Int Urogynecol J Pelvic Floor Dysfunct.* 2013;24:559.
Feola A, Duerr R, Moalli P, Abramowitch S. Changes in the rheological behavior of the vagina in women with pelvic organ prolapse. *Int Urogynecol J Pelvic Floor Dysfunct.* 2013;24:1221.
Feola A, Endo M, Urbankova I, et al. Host reaction to vaginally inserted collagen containing polypropylene implants in sheep. *Am J Obstet Gynecol.* 2015;212:474.e471.
Feola A, Pal S, Moalli P, et al. Varying degrees of nonlinear mechanical behavior arising from geometric differences of urogynecological meshes. *J Biomech.* 2014;47:2584.
Flynn BJ, Yap WT. Pubovaginal sling using allograft fascia lata versus autograft fascia for all types of stress urinary incontinence: 2-year minimum followup. *J Urol.* 2002;167:608.
Gandhi S, Kubba LM, Abramov Y, et al. Histopathologic changes of porcine dermis xenografts for transvaginal suburethral slings. *Am J Obstet Gynecol.* 2005;192:1643.
Gigliobianco G, Roman Regueros S, Osman NI, et al. Biomaterials for pelvic floor reconstructive surgery: how can we do better? *Biomed Res Int.* 2015;2015:1.
Giri SK, Hickey JP, Sil D, et al. The long-term results of pubovaginal sling surgery using acellular cross-linked porcine dermis in the treatment of urodynamic stress incontinence. *J Urol.* 2006;175:1788.
Goel VK, Lim TH, Gwon J, et al. Effects of rigidity of an internal fixation device. A comprehensive biomechanical investigation. *Spine (Phila Pa 1976).* 1991;16:S155.
Goepel C, Hefler L, Methfessel HD, Koelbl H. Periurethral connective tissue status of postmenopausal women with genital prolapse with and without stress incontinence. *Acta Obstet Gynecol Scand.* 2003;82:659.
Greca FH, De Paula JB, Biondo-Simões MLP, et al. The influence of differing pore sizes on the biocompatibility of two polypropylene meshes in the repair of abdominal defects: Experimental study in dogs. *Hernia.* 2001;5:59.
Greca FH, Souza-Filho ZA, Giovanini A, et al. The influence of porosity on the integration histology of two polypropylene meshes for the treatment of abdominal wall defects in dogs. *Hernia.* 2008;12:45.
Guerrero KL, Emery SJ, Wareham K, et al. A randomised controlled trial comparing TVT, Pelvicol and autologous fascial slings for the treatment of stress urinary incontinence in women. *BJOG.* 2010;117:1493.
Gundra UM, Girgis NM, Ruckerl D, et al. Alternatively activated macrophages derived from monocytes and tissue macrophages are phenotypically and functionally distinct. *Blood.* 2014;123:e110.
Hijazi S, Echtle D, Aboumarzouk OM, Heinrich E. Abdominal sacrocolpopexy with Pelvicol xenograft and concomitant Burch colposuspension. *Int J Womens Health.* 2017;9:625.
Hinz B. Formation and function of the myofibroblast during tissue repair. *J Invest Dermatol.* 2007;127:526.
Huiskes R, Weinans H, Grootenboer HJ, et al. Adaptive bone-remodeling theory applied to prosthetic-design analysis. *J Biomech.* 1987;20:1135.
Iglesia CB, Fenner DE, Brubaker L. The use of mesh in gynecologic surgery. *Int Urogynecol J Pelvic Floor Dysfunct.* 1997;8:105.
Jackson SR, Avery NC, Tarlton JF, et al. Changes in metabolism of collagen in genitourinary prolapse. *Lancet.* 1996;347:1658.
Jallah Z, Liang R, Feola A, et al. The impact of prolapse mesh on vaginal smooth muscle structure and function. *BJOG.* 2016;123:1076.
Jang J, Kim TG, Kim BS, et al. Tailoring mechanical properties of decellularized extracellular matrix bioink by vitamin B2-induced photo-crosslinking. *Acta Biomater.* 2016;33:88.
Jelovsek JE, Barber MD, Norton P, et al. Effect of uterosacral ligament suspension vs sacrospinous ligament fixation with or without perioperative behavioral therapy for pelvic organ vaginal prolapse on surgical outcomes and prolapse symptoms at 5 years in the OPTIMAL randomized clinical trial. *J Am Med Assoc.* 2018;319:1554.
Jones HW, Rock JA. *Te Linde's Operative Gynecology.* Philadelphia: Wolters Kluwer; 2015.
Jones KA, Feola A, Meyn L, et al. Tensile properties of commonly used prolapse meshes. *Int Urogynecol J Pelvic Floor Dysfunct.* 2009;20:847.
Klinge U, Junge K, Spellerberg B, et al. Do multifilament alloplastic meshes increase the infection rate? Analysis of the polymeric surface, the bacteria adherence, and the in vivo consequences in a rat model. *J Biomed Mater Res.* 2002;63:765.
Klinge U, Junge K, Stumpf M, et al. Functional and morphological evaluation of a low-weight, monofilament polypropylene mesh for hernia repair. *J Biomed Mater Res.* 2002;63:129.
Klinge U, Klosterhalfen B. Modified classification of surgical meshes for hernia repair based on the analyses of 1,000 explanted meshes. *Hernia.* 2012;16:251.
Klinge U, Klosterhalfen B, Birkenhauer V, et al. Impact of polymer pore size on the interface scar formation in a rat model. *J Surg Res.* 2002;103:208.
Klinge U, Klosterhalfen B, Conze J, et al. Modified mesh for hernia repair that is adapted to the physiology of the abdominal wall. *Eur J Surg.* 1998;164:951.
Klinge U, Klosterhalfen B, Muller M, et al. Shrinking of polypropylene mesh in vivo: an experimental study in dogs. *Eur J Surg.* 1998;164:965.
Klinge U, Klosterhalfen B, Öttinger AP, et al. PVDF as a new polymer for the construction of surgical meshes. *Biomaterials.* 2002;23:3487.

Klosterhalfen B, Klinge U, Schemeless V. Functional and morphological evaluation of different polypropylene-mesh modifications for abdominal wall repair. *Biomaterials*. 1998;19:2235.

Knight K, Moalli PA. Mechanics of pelvic floor prosthetic devices. In: Hoyte L, Amasser M, eds. *Biomechanics of the Female Pelvic Floor*. Elsevier: 2016;149.

Konstantinovic ML, Ooze Y, Spelzini F, et al. Biomechanical findings in rats undergoing fascial reconstruction with graft materials suggested as an alternative to polypropylene. *Neurourol Urodyn*. 2010;29:488.

Kropp BP, Eppley BL, Prevel CD, et al. Experimental assessment of small intestinal submucosa as a bladder wall substitute. *Urology*. 1995;46:396.

Leveen HH, Barberio JR. Tissue reaction to plastics used in surgery with special reference to teflon. *Ann Surg*. 1949;129:74.

Liang R, Abramowitch S, Knight K, et al. Vaginal degeneration following implantation of synthetic mesh with increased stiffness. *BJOG*. 2013;120:233.

Liang R, Knight K, Barone W, et al. Extracellular matrix regenerative graft attenuates the negative impact of polypropylene prolapse mesh on vagina in rhesus macaque. *Am J Obstet Gynecol*. 2016;216:153.e151.

Liang R, Knight K, Easley D, et al. Towards rebuilding vaginal support utilizing an extracellular matrix bioscaffold. *Acta Biomater*. 2017;57:324.

Liang R, Zong W, Palcsey S, et al. Impact of prolapse meshes on the metabolism of vaginal extracellular matrix in rhesus macaque. *Am J Obstet Gynecol*. 2015;212:174.e171.

Lopresti ST, Brown BN. Chapter 4: Host response to naturally derived biomaterials. In: Badylak SF, ed. *Host Response to Biomaterials*. Oxford: Academic Press; 2015;53.

Mantovani A, Sica A, Sozzani S, et al. The chemokine system in diverse forms of macrophage activation and polarization. *Trends Immunol*. 2004;25:677.

Matuska AM, McFetridge PS. The effect of terminal sterilization on structural and biophysical properties of a decellularized collagen-based scaffold; implications for stem cell adhesion. *J Biomed Mater Res B Appl Biomater*. 2015;103:397.

McGuire EJ, Lytton B. Pubovaginal sling procedure for stress incontinence. *J Urol*. 1978;119:82.

McPherson JM, Sawamura S, Armstrong R. An examination of the biologic response to injectable, glutaraldehyde cross-linked collagen implants. *J Biomed Mater Res*. 1986;20:93.

Mills CD, Kincaid K, Alt JM, et al. M-1/M-2 Macrophages and the Th1/Th2 Paradigm. *J Immunol*. 2000;164:6166.

Moalli PA. Cadaveric fascia lata. *Int Urogynecol J Pelvic Floor Dysfunct*. 2006;17:S48.

Moalli PA, Papas N, Menefee S, et al. Tensile properties of five commonly used mid-urethral slings relative to the TVT™. *Int Urogynecol J Pelvic Floor Dysfunct*. 2008;19:655.

Moalli PA, Shand SH, Zyczynski HM, et al. Remodeling of vaginal connective tissue in patients with prolapse. *Obstet Gynecol*. 2005;106:953.

Mosser DM, Edwards JP. Exploring the full spectrum of macrophage activation. *Nat Rev Immunol*. 2008;8:958.

Murray PJ, Wynn TA. Protective and pathogenic functions of macrophage subsets. *Nat Rev Immunol*. 2011;11:723.

Nager CW, Zyczynski H, Rogers RG, et al. The design of a randomized trial of vaginal surgery for uterovaginal prolapse: vaginal hysterectomy with native tissue vault suspension versus mesh hysteropexy suspension (the study of uterine prolapse procedures randomized trial). *Female Pelvic Med Reconstr Surg*. 2016;22:182.

Nolfi AL, Brown BN, Liang R, et al. Host response to synthetic mesh in women with mesh complications. *Am J Obstet Gynecol*. 2016;215:206.e201.

Novitsky YW, Cristiano JA, Harrell AG, et al. Immunohistochemical analysis of host reaction to heavyweight-, reduced-weight-, and expanded polytetrafluoroethylene (ePTFE)-based meshes after short- and long-term intraabdominal implantations. *Surg Endosc*. 2008;22:1070.

Nygaard I, Brubaker L, Zyczynski HM, et al. Long-term outcomes following abdominal sacrocolpopexy for pelvic organ prolapse. *JAMA*. 2013;309:2016.

O'Dwyer PJ, Kingsnorth AN, Molloy RG, et al. Randomized clinical trial assessing impact of a lightweight or heavyweight mesh on chronic pain after inguinal hernia repair. *Br J Surg*. 2005;92:166.

Orenstein SB, Saberski ER, Kreutzer DL, Novitsky YW. Comparative analysis of histopathologic effects of synthetic meshes based on material, weight, and pore size in mice. *J Surg Res*. 2012;176:423.

Otto J, Kaldenhoff E, Kirschner-Hermanns R, et al. Elongation of textile pelvic floor implants under load is related to complete loss of effective porosity, thereby favoring incorporation in scar plates. *J Biomed Mater Res A*. 2014;102:1079.

Patel H, Ostergard DR, Sternschuss G. Polypropylene mesh and the host response. *Int Urogynecol J*. 2012;23:669.

Peng M, Sussman RD, Escobar C, et al. Rectus fascia versus fascia lata for autologous fascial pubovaginal sling: a single-center comparison of perioperative and functional outcomes. *Female Pelvic Med Reconstr Surg*. 2020;26:493.

Pierce LM, Rao A, Baumann SS, et al. Long-term histologic response to synthetic and biologic graft materials implanted in the vagina and abdomen of a rabbit model. *Am J Obstet Gynecol*. 2009;200:546.e541.

Rac G. Stress urinary incontinence surgery trends in academic female pelvic medicine and reconstructive surgery urology practice in the setting of the food and drug administration public health notifications SUI Surgery Trends. *Neurourol Urodyn*. 2017;36:1155.

Rosch R, Junge K, Schachtrupp A, et al. Mesh implants in hernia repair: inflammatory cell response in a rat model. *Eur Surg Res*. 2003;35:161.

Rudolph R, Utley JR, Woodward M. Contractile fibroblasts (myofibroblasts) in a painful pacemaker pocket. *Ann Thorac Surg*. 1981;31:373.

Rumian AP, Draper ER, Wallace AL, Goodship AE. The influence of the mechanical environment on remodelling of the patellar tendon. *J Bone Joint Surg Br*. 2009;91:557.

Saberski ER, Orenstein SB, Novitsky YW. Anisotropic evaluation of synthetic surgical meshes. *Hernia*. 2011;15:47.

Schimpf MO, Abed H, Sanses T, et al. Society of Gynecologic Surgeons Systematic Review. Graft and mesh use in transvaginal prolapse repair: a systematic review. *Obstet Gynecol*. 2016;128:81.

Schultheiss D, Höfner K, Oelke M, Grünewald V, Jonas U. Historical aspects of the treatment of urinary incontinence. *Eur Urol*. 2000;38(3):352–362. doi:10.1159/000020306.

Shepherd JP, Feola AJ, Abramowitch SD, Moalli PA. Uniaxial biomechanical properties of seven different vaginally implanted meshes for pelvic organ prolapse. *Int Urogynecol J Pelvic Floor Dysfunct*. 2012;23:613.

Sohlberg EM, Dallas KB, Weeks BT, et al. Reoperation rates for pelvic organ prolapse repairs with biologic and synthetic grafts in a large population-based cohort. *Int Urogynecol J*. 2020;31:291.

Svabik K, Martan A, Masata J, et al. Ultrasound appearances after mesh implantation—evidence of mesh contraction or folding? *Int Urogynecol J*. 2011;22:529.

Taylor DA, Sampaio LC, Ferdous Z, et al. Decellularized matrices in regenerative medicine. *Acta Biomater*. 2018;74:74.

Tennyson L, Rytel M, Palcsey S, et al. Characterization of the T-cell response to polypropylene mesh in women with complications. *Am J Obstet Gynecol.* 2019;220:187.e181.

Tomasek JJ, Gabbiani G, Hinz B, et al. Myofibroblasts and mechano-regulation of connective tissue remodelling. *Nat Rev Mol Cell Biol.* 2002;3:349.

Ugianskiene A, Davila GW, Su TH, FIGO Urogynecology and Pelvic Floor Committee. FIGO review of statements on use of synthetic mesh for pelvic organ prolapse and stress urinary incontinence. *Int J Gynaecol Obstet.* 2019;147:147.

US Food and Drug Administration. Urogynecologic Surgical Mesh: Update on the Safety and Effectiveness of Transvaginal Placement for Pelvic Organ Prolapse. 2011. https://www.fda.gov/media/81123/download. Accessed May 5, 2021.

Ventura RD, Padalhin AR, Park CM, Lee BT. Enhanced decellularization technique of porcine dermal ECM for tissue engineering applications. *Mater Sci Eng C Mater Biol Appl.* 2019;104:109841.

Wein AJ, Kavoussi LR, Novick AC, et al. *Campbell-Walsh Urology: Expert Consult Premium Edition: Enhanced Online Features And Print, 4-Volume Set.* Philadelphia: Elsevier Health Sciences, 2011.

Wells JM. MMP generated matrikines. *Matrix Biol.* 2015;44-46:122.

Weyhe D, Schmitz I, Belyaev O, et al. Experimental comparison of monofile light and heavy polypropylene meshes: less weight does not mean less biological response. *World J Surg.* 2006;30:1586.

Whooley J, Cunnane EM, Do Amaral R, et al. Stress urinary incontinence and pelvic organ prolapse: biologic graft materials revisited. *Tissue Eng Part B Rev.* 2020;26:475.

Wohlrab KJ, Erekson EA, Myers DL. Postoperative erosions of the Mersilene® suburethral sling mesh for antiincontinence surgery. *Int Urogynecol J Pelvic Floor Dysfunct.* 2009;20:417.

Woodruff AJ, Cole EE, Dmochowski RR, et al. Histologic comparison of pubovaginal sling graft materials: a comparative study. *Urology.* 2008;72:85.

Yamamoto N, Ohno K, Hayashi K, et al. Effects of stress shielding on the mechanical properties of rabbit patellar tendon. *J Biomech Eng.* 1993;115:23.

Yao Q, Zheng YW, Lan QH, et al. Recent development and biomedical applications of decellularized extracellular matrix biomaterials. *Mater Sci Eng C Mater Biol Appl.* 2019;104:109942.

Zong W, Stein SE, Starcher B, et al. Alteration of vaginal elastin metabolism in women with pelvic organ prolapse. *Obstet Gynecol.* 2010;115:953.

8

Description and Classification of Lower Urinary Tract Dysfunction and Pelvic Organ Prolapse

Cecile A. Ferrando and Mark D. Walters

CHAPTER OUTLINE

INTRODUCTION

The purposes of any classification system are to facilitate understanding of disease etiology and pathophysiology, to help establish and standardize treatment and research guidelines, and to avoid confusion among those who are concerned with the problem. Classification systems for voiding disorders and pelvic organ prolapse have been based on various symptoms, as well as anatomic, radiographic, and urodynamic findings. This chapter reviews the classification of voiding dysfunction in women, as well as the differential diagnosis of urinary incontinence using up-to-date terminology from the International Continence Society (ICS). Pelvic organ prolapse terminology, quantitative assessment, and staging are also reviewed. Lastly, the ICS classification system of vaginal prostheses and graft complications is presented. It is hoped that the nomenclature used in these classification systems will become more widely understood and used, and that further research will be aimed at defining their clinical applicability.

CLASSIFICATION SYSTEMS OF LOWER URINARY TRACT DYSFUNCTION

International Continence Society Classification

In 1973 the ICS established a committee for the standardization of terminology of lower urinary tract function. Over the subsequent decades, reports from this committee and its subcommittees have been considered the gold standard in establishing terminology related to lower urinary tract function and dysfunction. In 2010, the ICS terminology for lower urinary tract dysfunction was updated and incorporated into a report on terminology for female pelvic floor dysfunction (published jointly by the International Urogynecological Association [IUGA] and the ICS). In 2018, more focused ICS terminology reports were published related to nocturnal lower urinary tract function and underactive bladder. Each report highlights the importance of basing diagnoses for pelvic floor disorders on the correlation between a woman's symptoms, signs, and relevant diagnostic investigations. The following sections summarize terminology and classifications for female lower urinary tract dysfunction based on the 2010 IUGA/ICS report, as well as the ICS terminology updates from 2018.

The lower urinary tract is composed of the bladder and urethra, which work together as a functional unit to store and excrete urine. Symptoms, signs, urodynamic observations, and conditions are separate categories with unique but overlapping terminologies. Although a complete urodynamic investigation is not necessary for all symptomatic patients, some clinical or urodynamic assessment of the filling and voiding phases is essential for each patient. It is useful to examine bladder and urethral activity separately in each phase. If urodynamic studies are performed, results should clearly reflect the patient's signs and symptoms.

Filling and Storage Phase. The ICS classification of abnormalities of the storage and voiding phases is outlined in Box 8.1 and diagrammed in Fig. 8.1. Cystometry measures the pressure/volume relationship of the bladder during filling and storage and assesses bladder function in terms of bladder sensation, detrusor activity, bladder capacity, and bladder compliance.

Detrusor activity may be normal or overactive. Overactive detrusor function is characterized by involuntary detrusor contractions during filling. These contractions may be spontaneous or provoked and cannot be suppressed completely. Overactive detrusor function in the absence of a known neurologic abnormality is called idiopathic detrusor overactivity, and overactivity caused by disturbance of the nervous control mechanisms is called neurogenic detrusor overactivity. These conditions are often associated with the symptom of urinary urgency. Urgency, with or without urgency incontinence, usually with frequency and nocturia in the absence of urinary tract infection or obvious pathology, is described as overactive

BOX 8.1 The International Continence Society Classification of Lower Urinary Tract Dysfunction

I. Storage Phase

A. Bladder function during storage
  1. Detrusor activity
     a. Normal
     b. Overactive
  2. Bladder sensation
     a. Normal
     b. Increased (oversensitivity)
     c. Reduced
     d. Absent
     e. Nonspecific bladder sensations
     f. Bladder pain
     g. Urgency
  3. Bladder capacity
  4. Bladder compliance

B. Urethral function during storage
  1. Normal
  2. Incompetent
  3. Urethral relaxation (instability)

II. Voiding Phase

A. Detrusor function during voiding
  1. Normal
  2. Abnormal
     a. Underactive
     b. Acontractile

B. Urethral function during voiding
  1. Normal
  2. Abnormal
     a. Bladder outlet obstruction
     b. Dysfunctional voiding
     c. Detrusor sphincter dyssynergia

bladder (urgency) syndrome. Terminology used to describe overactive bladder is provided in Box 8.2.

Urethral function during storage can be assessed clinically (direct observation of urine loss with cough or Valsalva maneuver), urodynamically (urethral closure pressure profilometry and leak point pressure measurements), or radiographically (cystourethrography with or without video). The urethral closure mechanism may be competent or incompetent. An incompetent urethral closure mechanism is one that allows leakage of urine during activities, which may raise intraabdominal pressures in the absence of a detrusor contraction. Involuntary leakage during filling cystometry may occur during increased abdominal pressure, in the absence of a detrusor contraction

Abnormalities of storage and voiding phases

	Storage phase	Voiding phase
Bladder		
Normal	Detrusor relaxation	Detrusor contraction
Abnormal	Detrusor overactivity	Detrusor underactivity or acontractility
Urethra		
Normal	Urethral sphincter contraction	Urethral sphincter relaxation
Abnormal	Sphincter incompetence (SUI or ISD)	Urethral obstruction, dysfunctional voiding, detrusor sphincter dyssynergia

Fig. 8.1 Abnormalities of storage and voiding phases. *SUI*, Stress urinary incontinence; *ISD*, intrinsic sphincter deficiency.

BOX 8.2 International Urogynecological Association/International Continence Society Terminology for Overactive Bladder

Increased Daytime Urinary Frequency

Complaint that micturition occurs more frequently during waking hours than previously deemed normal by the woman. Seven episodes of micturition per day is felt to be the upper limit of normal, although some variations between populations may exist.[a]

Complaint from a patient who considers that she/he voids too often by day.[b]

Nocturia[c]

Complaint of interruption of sleep one or more times because of the need to micturate. Each void is preceded and followed by sleep.[a]

The number of times urine is passed during the main sleep period. Having woken to pass urine for the first time, each urination must be followed by sleep or the intention to sleep.[b]

Urgency

Complaint of a sudden, compelling desire to pass urine that is difficult to defer.[a,b]

Overactive Bladder (Urgency) Syndrome

Urinary urgency, usually accompanied by frequency and nocturia, with or without urgency urinary incontinence, in the absence of urinary tract infection (or other obvious pathology).[a,b]

Urgency (Urinary) Incontinence

Complaint of involuntary loss of urine associated with urgency. "Urgency" replaces "urge" as accepted terminology per the International Continence Society.[a]

Detrusor Overactivity

The occurrence of involuntary detrusor contractions during filling cystometry. The contractions may be spontaneous or provoked and produce a wave form on cystometrogram of variable amplitude and duration. No minimum requirement is known for the amplitude of an involuntary detrusor contraction. Detrusor overactivity, with or without urgency and/or urgency incontinence, may be phasic or terminal. Detrusor overactivity may be further qualified if the cause is known: neurogenic, when there is a relevant neurologic condition; and idiopathic, when the cause is unknown.[a]

(Modified from [a]Haylen BT, de Ridder D, Freeman RM, et al. An International Urogynecological Association (IUGA)/International Continence Society (ICS) joint report on the terminology for female pelvic floor dysfunction. *Neurourol Urodyn.* 2010;29:4. [b]Chapple CR, Osman NI, Birder L, et al. Terminology report from the International Continence Society (ICS) Working Group on Underactive Bladder (UAB). *Neurourol Urodyn.* 2018;37:2928. [c]Hashim H, Blanker MH, Drake MJ, et al. International Continence Society (ICS) report on the terminology for nocturia and nocturnal lower urinary tract function. *Neurourol Urodyn.* 2019;38:499.)

(urodynamic stress incontinence), or because of urethral relaxation in the absence of raised abdominal pressure or detrusor overactivity (urethral relaxation incompetence). The definition and significance of the latter condition await additional data.

Urinary incontinence is the complaint of any involuntary (urethral or extraurethral) leakage of urine. Urinary incontinence is a symptom, a sign, and a condition. Urinary incontinence as a symptom means that the patient states that she has involuntary urine loss. Types of incontinence symptoms include stress incontinence, urgency incontinence, mixed incontinence, nocturnal enuresis, situational incontinence, and continuous incontinence. In each specific circumstance, urinary incontinence should be further described by specifying relevant factors such as type, frequency, severity, precipitating factors, social impact, effect on hygiene and quality of life, the measures used to contain leakage, and whether or not the individual seeks or desires help because of urinary incontinence. The sign of stress incontinence denotes the observation of urine loss from the external urethral meatus synchronously with physical exertion such as a cough or Valsalva maneuver. Because symptoms and signs of urinary incontinence are sometimes misleading, accurate diagnosis often requires urodynamic investigation in addition to careful history and physical examination.

Voiding Phase. During the voiding phase, the detrusor muscle may be normal, underactive, or acontractile. Normal voiding usually is achieved by an initial voluntary reduction in intraurethral pressure (urethral relaxation) followed by a continuous detrusor contraction that leads to complete bladder emptying within a normal time span, and in the absence of obstruction. Detrusor underactivity during micturition is defined as a contraction of reduced strength and/or duration, resulting in prolonged bladder emptying and/or a failure to achieve complete bladder emptying within a normal time span. An acontractile detrusor is one that cannot be demonstrated to contract during urodynamic studies, resulting in incomplete bladder emptying.

During voiding, urethral function may be normal or abnormal. Abnormal urethral function may be caused by uncoordinated or involuntary urethral contractions, urethral stricture, or obstruction from an anatomic abnormality such as severe pelvic organ prolapse or changes after a stress incontinence procedure.

Simultaneous measurement of intravesical or detrusor pressure and urine flow is necessary to determine whether the patient's voiding is obstructive. In general, high detrusor pressures with low flow rates suggest an obstructive problem, whereas low detrusor pressures with low flow rates imply that the problem is one of detrusor underactivity or acontractility. Simultaneous external urethral sphincter electromyography is necessary to determine whether an obstructive voiding pattern is secondary to urethral overactivity or mechanical obstruction.

DIFFERENTIAL DIAGNOSIS OF URINARY INCONTINENCE

Among women complaining of urinary incontinence, the differential diagnosis includes genitourinary and nongenitourinary conditions (Box 8.3). As previously mentioned, genitourinary disorders include problems of bladder filling and storage, as well as extraurethral disorders such as fistula and congenital abnormalities. Nongenitourinary conditions that cause urinary incontinence generally are functional conditions that occur simultaneously with normal or abnormal urethral and bladder function. These conditions are most common in elderly women.

BOX 8.3 Differential Diagnosis of Urinary Incontinence in Women

Genitourinary Etiology

Filling/Storage Disorders

Urodynamic stress incontinence
Detrusor overactivity (idiopathic)
Detrusor overactivity (neurogenic)
Mixed types

Fistula

Vesical
Ureteral
Urethral

Congenital

Ectopic ureter
Epispadias

Nongenitourinary Etiology

Functional
Neurologic
Cognitive
Psychologic
Physical impairment
Environmental
Pharmacologic
Metabolic

The most common urine storage disorder in women is urodynamic stress incontinence. Bladder filling disorders caused by overactive detrusor function resulting in urgency urinary incontinence are the second most common cause of urinary incontinence. The relative likelihood of each condition causing incontinence varies with the age and health of the individual (Fig. 8.2). Underactive or acontractile detrusor function may result in voiding dysfunction or urinary incontinence. The ICS

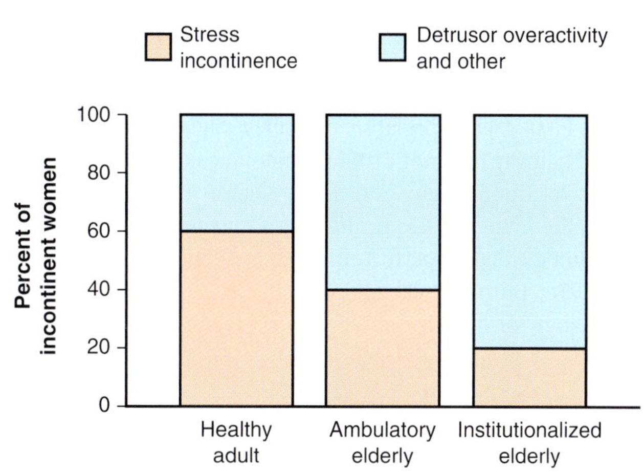

Fig. 8.2 Estimated likelihood of conditions causing incontinence in women in various age categories.

no longer recommends the term "overflow incontinence," but, if it is used, a precise definition and any associated pathophysiology, such as reduced urethral function, or detrusor overactivity/low bladder compliance, should be stated. Voiding disorders with incontinence in women usually are associated with diabetes, neurologic diseases, severe genital prolapse, or postsurgical obstruction.

Functional incontinence is associated with cognitive, psychologic, or physical impairments that make it difficult to reach the toilet or interfere with appropriate toileting. With these conditions, continent women may not have enough time to avoid an accident. Functional causes also may act synergistically with other urinary problems. For example, women with manageable detrusor overactivity may become incontinent if another disease or physical problem keeps them from reaching the toilet. Physical conditions that may cause functional incontinence include joint abnormalities, arthritic pain, or muscular weakness. An unfamiliar setting, lack of convenient toilet facilities, or other environmental factors can aggravate this condition. Dementia, psychological difficulties, and repressed or hostile behavior may be related to incontinence, especially in the institutionalized elderly. Finally, iatrogenic factors, such as pharmacotherapy, can cause or aggravate incontinence.

DESCRIPTION AND STAGING OF PELVIC ORGAN PROLAPSE

Pelvic organ prolapse refers to descent of one or more of the anterior vaginal wall, posterior vaginal wall, the uterus (cervix), or the apex of the vagina (cuff scar after hysterectomy). As with voiding dysfunction, systematic description and classification of pelvic organ prolapse are useful to help document and communicate the severity of the problem, establish treatment guidelines, and improve the quality of research by standardizing definitions. Two general classification systems are in use, although it is recommended that the ICS terminology be used routinely by clinicians and researchers.

For many years, the severity of pelvic organ prolapse has been described using criteria modified from Beecham (1980) and Baden et al. (1968). This grading system is simple to use; it is widely understood among gynecologic surgeons and has been found to have reasonable interobserver variability for all segments of the vagina and for uterine support. The most dependent position of the pelvic organs during maximum straining or standing is used and graded as normal or as first, second, or third degree. First-degree prolapse describes vaginal segments that descend halfway (but not to) the hymen; second degree describes descent to the hymen; and third degree describes prolapse beyond the hymen. Classification of posterior vaginal wall prolapse can be aided by performing a rectovaginal examination.

In 1996, Bump et al. described the ICS standardization of terminology of female pelvic organ prolapse, with the most recent ICS revision published in 2016. This most recent report focused on updating the terminology and description of symptoms, signs, investigations, and diagnoses of pelvic organ prolapse, and only added a validated simplified version to the classification system itself. The Pelvic Organ Prolapse Quantitation (POPQ) system is applied during physical examination of the external genitalia and vaginal canal and describes the topographic positions of six vaginal sites. This system is now used among clinicians and researchers as a standard method of describing degree of prolapse severity. Segments of the lower reproductive tract are intended to replace the terms cystocele, enterocele, rectocele, and urethrovesical junction, because these terms imply an unrealistic certainty as to the structures on the other side of the vaginal bulge, particularly in women who have had previous prolapse surgery.

With the bladder empty, the examiner sees and describes the maximum protrusion noted by the patient during her daily activities. The details of the examination, including criteria for the endpoint of the examination and full development of the prolapse, should be specified. Suggested criteria for demonstration of maximum prolapse include one or all of the following: protrusion of the vaginal wall becomes tight during straining by the patient; traction on the prolapse causes no further descent; the subject confirms that the size of the prolapse and the extent of the protrusion seen by the examiner are as extensive as the most severe protrusion she has had (a small handheld mirror to visualize the protrusion may be helpful); and a standing/straining examination confirms that the full extent of the prolapse was observed in the other positions used. Details about the patient position, the types of vaginal specula or retractors, the type and intensity of straining used to develop the prolapse maximally, and the fullness of the bladder should be reported.

The POPQ system is a series of site-specific measurements of the woman's pelvic organ support. It can be easily learned and taught by means of a video tutorial. Prolapse in each segment is evaluated and measured relative to the hymen (not introitus), which is a fixed anatomic landmark that can be identified consistently and precisely. The anatomic position of the six defined points for measurement should be centimeters above or proximal to the hymen (negative number) or centimeters below or distal to the hymen (positive number), with the plane of the hymen being defined as zero. For example, a cervix that protrudes 3 cm distal to the hymen should be described as +3 cm.

Six points (two on the anterior vaginal wall, two in the superior vagina, and two on the posterior vaginal wall) are located with reference to the plane of the hymen (Fig. 8.3). Descent of the anterior vaginal wall is most commonly a result of bladder prolapse (cystocele), whereas higher-stage anterior wall prolapse may be a result of uterine or vaginal vault descent or an anterior enterocele in patients with prior prolapse surgery. Although the terms cystocele and enterocele continue to be used by most gynecologists, anterior vaginal wall prolapse remains the preferred terminology. There are two anterior sites:

Point Aa: A point located in the midline of the anterior vaginal wall 3 cm proximal to the external urethral meatus, corresponding to the proximal location of the urethrovesical crease. By definition, the range of position of point Aa relative to the hymen is –3 to +3 cm.

Point Ba: A point that represents the most distal (i.e., most dependent) position of any part of the upper anterior vaginal wall from the vaginal cuff or anterior vaginal fornix to point Aa.

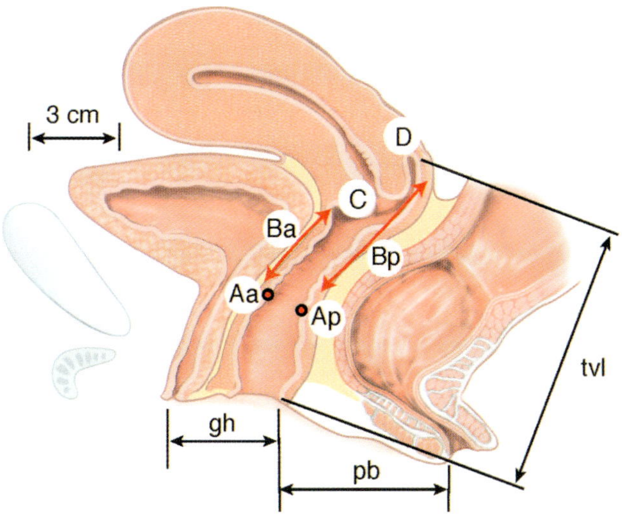

Fig. 8.3 Six sites (points *Aa, Ba, C, D, Bp,* and *Ap*), genital hiatus (*gh*), perineal body (*pb*), and total vaginal length (*tvl*) used for pelvic organ support quantitation. (From Bump RC, Mattiasson A, Bø K, et al. The standardization of terminology of female pelvic organ prolapse and pelvic floor dysfunction. *Am J Obstet Gynecol.* 1996;75:10.)

By definition, point Ba is at –3 cm in the absence of prolapse and would have a positive value equal to the position of the cuff in women with total posthysterectomy vaginal eversion.

Two points are on the superior vagina. These points represent the most proximal locations of the normally positioned lower reproductive tract and describe uterine/cervical and vaginal vault (cuff scar) prolapse.

Point C: A point that represents either the most distal (i.e., most dependent) edge of the cervix or the leading edge of the vaginal cuff (hysterectomy scar) after total hysterectomy.

Point D: A point that represents a location of the posterior fornix in a woman who still has a cervix. It represents a level of uterosacral ligament attachment to the proximal posterior cervix. It is included as a point of measurement to differentiate suspensory failure of the uterosacral cardinal ligament complex from cervical elongation. Point D is omitted in the absence of the cervix.

Two points are located on the posterior vaginal wall. Posterior vaginal wall descent is often because of rectal protrusion into the vagina (rectocele), with higher-stage prolapse usually involving prolapse of the vaginal vault and/or an enterocele. Analogous to anterior prolapse, posterior prolapse should be discussed in terms of segments of the vaginal wall rather than the organs that lie behind it. Thus, the term posterior vaginal wall prolapse is preferable to rectocele or enterocele unless the organs involved are identified by ancillary tests. If small bowel appears to be present in the rectovaginal space, the examiner should comment on this fact and clearly describe the basis for this clinical impression (e.g., by observation of peristaltic activity in the distended posterior vagina or palpation of loops of small bowel between an examining finger in the rectum and one in the vagina).

Point Ap: A point located in the midline of the posterior vaginal wall 3 cm proximal to the hymen. By definition, the range of position point Ap relative to the hymen is –3 to +3 cm.

Point Bp: A point that represents the most distal (i.e., most dependent) position of any part of the upper posterior vaginal wall from the vaginal cuff of posterior vaginal fornix to point Ap. By definition, point Bp is at –3 cm in the absence of prolapse and would have a positive value equal to the position of the cuff in a woman with total posthysterectomy vaginal eversion.

Other landmarks include the genital hiatus (gh), which is measured from the middle of the external urethral meatus to the posterior midline hymen; the perineal body (pb), which is measured from the posterior margin of the genital hiatus to the midanal opening; and the total vaginal length (tvl), which is the greatest depth of the vagina in centimeters when point C or D is reduced to its full normal position. The points and measurements are presented in Fig. 8.3. All points are measured during maximal Valsalva except tvl, which is measured at rest.

The positions of points Aa, Ba, Ap, Bp, C, and (if applicable) D with reference to the hymen are measured and recorded. Measurements may be recorded as a simple line of numbers (e.g., –3, –3, –7, –9, –3, –3, 9, 2, 2 for points Aa, Ba, C, D, Bp, Ap, tvl, gh, and pb, respectively). Alternatively, a three-by-three grid can be used to concisely organize the measurements, as shown in Fig. 8.4, or a line diagram of a configuration can be drawn, as shown in Fig. 8.5 and Fig. 8.6. Fig. 8.5 is a grid and line diagram contrasting measurements indicating normal support to those of posthysterectomy vaginal eversion. Fig. 8.6 is a grid and line diagram representing predominant anterior and posterior vaginal wall prolapse with partial vault descent.

The profile for quantifying prolapse provides a precise description of anatomy for individual patients. An ordinal staging system of pelvic organ prolapse is suggested using these measurements and can be useful for the description of populations and for research comparisons. Stages are assigned according to the most severe portion of the prolapse when the full extent of the protrusion has been demonstrated. For a stage to be assigned to an individual subject, it is essential that her quantitative description be completed first. The five stages of pelvic organ support (0–IV) are described in Box 8.4.

Anterior wall **Aa**	**Anterior wall** **Ba**	**Cervix or cuff** **C**
Genital hiatus **gh**	**Perineal body** **pb**	**Total vaginal length** **tvl**
Posterior wall **Ap**	**Posterior wall** **Bp**	**Posterior fornix** **D**

Fig. 8.4 Three-by-three grid for recording quantitative description of pelvic organ support. (From Bump RC, Mattiasson A, Bø K, et al. The standardization of terminology of female pelvic organ prolapse and pelvic floor dysfunction. *Am J Obstet Gynecol.* 1996;75:10.)

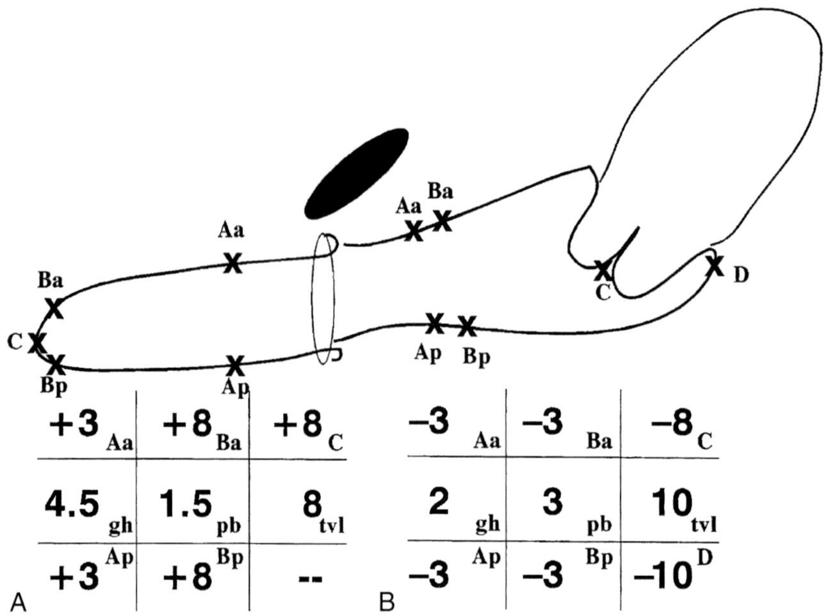

Fig. 8.5 **A**, Grid and line diagram of complete eversion of vagina. Most distal point of anterior wall (point *Ba*), vaginal cuff scar (point *C*), and most distal point of the posterior wall (point *Bp*) are all at same position (+8), and points *Aa* and *Ap* are maximally distal (both at +3). Because total vaginal length equals maximum protrusion, this is stage IV prolapse. **B**, Normal support. Points *Aa* and *Ba* and points *Ap* and *Bp* are all –3 because there is no anterior or posterior wall descent. Lowest point of the cervix is 8 cm above hymen (–8), and posterior fornix is 2 cm above this (–10). Vaginal length is 10 cm, and genital hiatus and perineal body measure 2 and 3 cm, respectively. This represents stage 0 support. (From Bump RC, Mattiasson A, Bø K, et al. The standardization of terminology of female pelvic organ prolapse and pelvic floor dysfunction. *Am J Obstet Gynecol.* 1996;75:10.)

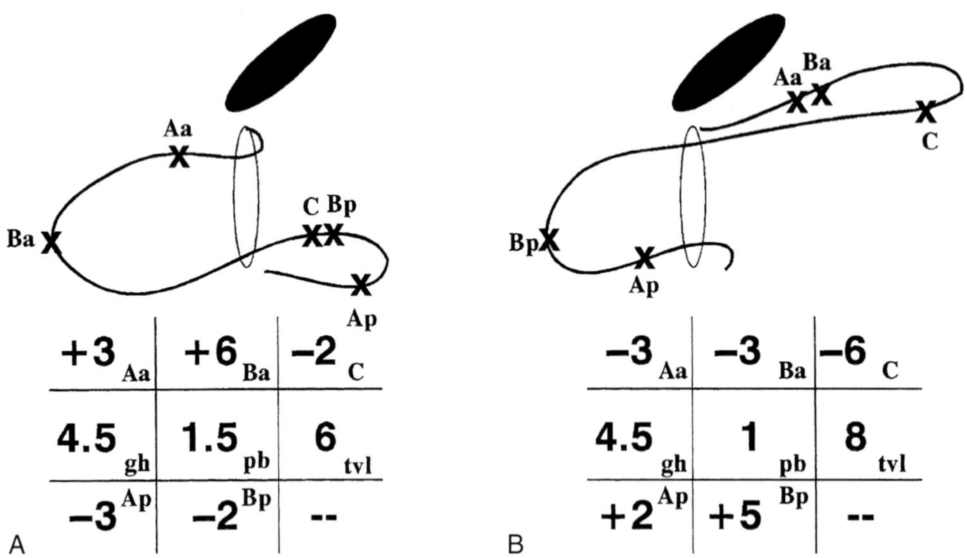

Fig. 8.6 **A**, Grid and line diagram of predominant anterior support defect. Leading point of prolapse is upper anterior vaginal wall, point *Ba* (+6). There is significant elongation of bulging anterior wall. Point *Aa* is maximally distal (+3), and vaginal cuff scar is 2 cm above hymen (C = –2). Cuff scar has undergone 4 cm of descent, because it would be at –6 (total vaginal length) if it were perfectly supported. In this example total vaginal length is not maximum depth of vagina with elongated anterior vaginal wall maximally reduced, but rather depth of vagina at cuff with point *C* reduced to its normal full extent, as specified in the text. This represents stage III Ba prolapse. **B**, Predominant posterior support defect. Leading point of prolapse is upper posterior vaginal wall, point *Bp* (+5). Point *Ap* is 2 cm distal to hymen (+2), and vaginal cuff scar is 6 cm above hymen (–6). Cuff has undergone only 2 cm of descent, because it would be at –8 (total vaginal length) if it were perfectly supported. This represents stage III Bp prolapse. (From Bump RC, Mattiasson A, Bø K, et al. The standardization of terminology of female pelvic organ prolapse and pelvic floor dysfunction. *Am J Obstet Gynecol.* 1996;75:10.)

BOX 8.4 Stages of Pelvic Organ Prolapse

Stage 0	No prolapse is demonstrated. Points Aa, Ap, Ba, and Bp are all at –3 cm, and either point C or D is between –total vaginal length (TVL) cm and –(TVL-2) cm (i.e., the quantitation value for point C or D is ≤–[TVL-2] cm). Fig. 8.5B shows stage 0.
Stage I	The criteria for stage 0 are not met, but the most distal portion of the prolapse is >1 cm above the level of the hymen (i.e., its quantitation value is <–1 cm).
Stage II	The most distal portion of the prolapse is ≤1 cm proximal to or distal to the plane of the hymen (i.e., its quantitation value is ≥–1 cm but ≤+1 cm).
Stage III	The most distal portion of the prolapse is >1 cm below the plane of the hymen but protrudes no further than 2 cm less than the TVL in centimeters (i.e., its quantitation value is >+1 cm but <+[TVL-2] cm). Fig. 8.6A shows stage III Ba prolapse, and Fig. 8.5B shows stage III Bp prolapse.
Stage IV	Essentially, complete eversion of the total length of the lower genital tract is demonstrated. The distal portion of the prolapse protrudes to at least (TVL-2) cm (i.e., its quantitation value is ≥+(TVL-2) cm). In most instances, the leading edge of stage IV prolapse is the cervix or vaginal cuff scar. Fig. 8.5A shows stage IV C prolapse.

(From Bump RC, Mattiasson A, Bø K, et al. The standardization of terminology of female pelvic organ prolapse and pelvic floor dysfunction. *Am J Obstet Gynecol.* 1996;75:10.)

Ancillary techniques for describing pelvic organ prolapse include performance of a digital rectal examination while the patient is straining; digital assessment of the contents of the rectovaginal septum during examination to differentiate between a "traction" enterocele (the posterior cul-de-sac is pulled down by the prolapsing cervix or vaginal cuff but is not distended by intestines) and a "pulsion" enterocele (the intestinal contents of the enterocele distend the rectal-vaginal septum and produce a protruding mass); cotton swab testing for the measurement of urethral axis mobility (Q-tip test); measurement of perineal descent; measurement of the transverse diameter of the genital hiatus or of the protruding prolapse; measurement of vaginal volume; description and measurement of rectal prolapse; and examination techniques differentiating between various types of defects (e.g., central vs. paravaginal defects of the anterior vaginal wall). Cystoscopy and imaging can be useful in describing pelvic organ prolapse. Imaging procedures include ultrasonography, contrast radiography, computed tomography, and magnetic resonance imaging.

Precise characterization of pelvic floor muscle strength and the description of functional symptoms are important. The reader is referred to the ICS committee document for further details (Haylen et al., 2010).

CLASSIFICATION SYSTEM OF VAGINAL PROSTHESES AND GRAFT COMPLICATIONS

With the increased use of mesh in pelvic reconstructive surgery beginning in the early 2000s, an increase in the number of patients seeking care for mesh-related complications was seen, including mesh exposure and erosion, chronic pelvic pain, dyspareunia, infection, intraoperative bladder perforations, infection, and fistula formation. In response to this, an IUGA/ICS joint report on the terminology and classification of complications arising from the insertion of prostheses and grafts in female pelvic floor surgery was published in 2011.

The IUGA/ICS classification system includes three components: category (C), time (T), and site (S). Each complication is reported using these three identifiers and then further classified (and subclassified), resulting in a numerical "CTS" code. For example, the categories of complications range from vaginal complication without epithelial separation (1) to patient compromise (7). Further divisions for each category describe the presence of symptoms including pain and/or infection as a result of the complication. Time "T" describes when the complication is clinically diagnosed (e.g., ranging from intraoperative [1] to over 12 months after surgery [4]). Site "S" describes where the prostheses or graft complication is noted, ranging from the vaginal suture line (1) to intraabdominal (5). Multiple, as well as early and late, complications are reported separately.

The ICS/IUGA classification system for vaginal prostheses and graft complications is much more comprehensive and specific than other surgical complication classification systems currently in use. However, it has been criticized for being too complex, with categories that are too broad and not clearly defined, leading to poor interrater reliability among providers. Additionally, the classification system does not lend to gradation of severity of a complication, which some critics assert is important when choosing a management plan for treatment and when relaying information about a disease process. Potentially because of these concerns, this classification system is not currently used as frequently as those for pelvic organ prolapse and urinary incontinence.

BIBLIOGRAPHY

Classification of Urinary Incontinence

Abrams P, Blaivas JG, Stanton SL, et al. Sixth report on the standardization of terminology of lower urinary tract function. Procedures related to neurophysiological investigations: electromyography, nerve conduction studies, reflex latencies, evoked potentials and sensory testing. *World J Urol.* 1986;4:2; *Scand J Urol Nephrol.* 1986;20:161; *Br J Urol* 1987;59:300.

Abrams P, Blaivas JG, Stanton SL, Andersen JT. The standardization of terminology of lower tract function. *Scand J Urol Nephrol.* 1988;114:5.

Abrams P, Cardozo L, Fall M, et al. The standardization of terminology of lower urinary tract function: report from the Standardization Sub-committee of the International Continence Society. *Am J Obstet Gynecol.* 2002;187:116.

Bates P, Bradley WE, Glen E, et al. First report on the standardization of terminology of lower urinary tract function. Urinary incontinence. Procedures related to the evaluation of urine storage: cystometry, urethral closure pressure profile, units of measurement. *Br J Urol.* 1976;48:39; *Eur Urol.* 1976;2:274; *Scand J Urol Nephrol.* 1976;11:193; *Urol Int.* 1976;32:81.

Bates P, Bradley WE, Glen E, et al. Second report on the standardization of terminology of lower urinary tract function. Procedures related to the evaluation of micturition: flow rate, pressure measurement, symbols. *Acta Urol Jpn.* 1977;27:1563; *Br J Urol.* 1977;49:207; *Scand J Urol Nephrol.* 1977;11:197.

Bates P, Bradley WE, Glen E, et al. Third report on the standardization of terminology of lower urinary tract function. Procedures related to the evaluation of micturition: pressure flow relationships, residual urine. *Br J Urol.* 1980;52:348; *Eur Urol.* 1980;6:170; *Acta Urol Jpn.* 1980;27:1566; *Scand J Urol Nephrol.* 1980;12:191.

Bates P, Bradley WE, Glen E, et al. Fourth report on the standardization of terminology of lower urinary tract function. Terminology related to neuromuscular dysfunction of lower urinary tract. *Br J Urol.* 1981;52:333; *Urology.* 1981;17:618; *Scand J Urol Nephrol.* 1981;15:169; *Acta Urol Jpn.* 1981;27:1568.

Blaivas JG. Classification of stress urinary incontinence. *Neurourol Urodyn.* 1983;2:103.

Blaivas JG, Olsson CA. Stress incontinence: classification and surgical approach. *J Urol.* 1988;139:727.

Chapple CR, Osman NI, Birder L, et al. Terminology report from the International Continence Society (ICS) Working Group on Underactive Bladder (UAB). *Neurourol Urodyn.* 2018;37:2928.

Enhorning G. Simultaneous recording of intravesical and intraurethral pressure. *Acta Chir Scand.* 1961;276:1.

Hashim H, Blanker MH, Drake MJ, et al. International Continence Society (ICS) report on the terminology for nocturia and nocturnal lower urinary tract function. *Neurourol Urodyn.* 2019;38:499.

Haylen BT, de Ridder D, Freeman RM, et al. An International Urogynecological Association (IUGA)/International Continence Society (ICS) joint report on the terminology for female pelvic floor dysfunction. *Neurourol Urodyn.* 2010;29:4.

McGuire EJ, Lytton B, Pepe V, et al. Stress urinary incontinence. *Am J Obstet Gynecol.* 1976;47:255.

Ouslander J, Staskin D, Raz S, et al. Clinical versus urodynamic diagnosis in an incontinent female geriatric population. *J Urol.* 1987;37:68.

Quigley GJ, Harper AC. The epidemiology of urethral-vesical dysfunction in the female patient. *Am J Obstet Gynecol.* 1985;151:220.

Resnick NM, Yalla SV, Laurino E. The pathophysiology of urinary incontinence among institutionalized elderly persons. *N Engl J Med.* 1989;320:1.

Wein AJ. Pathophysiology and categorization of voiding dysfunction. In: Walsh PC, Retik AB, Vaughan ED, et al, eds. *Campbell's Urology.* 7th ed. Philadelphia: WB Saunders; 1998.

Wein AJ, Barrett DM. *Voiding Function and Dysfunction.* Chicago: Mosby; 1988.

Classification of Pelvic Organ Prolapse

Baden WF, Walker T. Fundamental, symptoms, and classification. In: Baden WF, Walker T, eds. *Surgical Repair of Vaginal Defects.* Philadelphia: JB Lippincott; 1992.

Baden WF, Walker T, Lindsey JH. The vaginal profile. *Tex Med.* 1968;64:56.

Beecham CT. Classification of vaginal relaxation. *Am J Obstet Gynecol.* 1980;136:957.

Bump RC, Mattiasson A, Bø K, et al. The standardization of terminology of female pelvic organ prolapse and pelvic floor dysfunction. *Am J Obstet Gynecol.* 1996;75:10.

Hall AF, Theofrastous JP, Cundiff GW, et al. Interobserver and intraobserver reliability of the proposed International Continence Society, Society of Gynecologic Surgeons, and American Urogynecology Society pelvic organ prolapse classification system. *Am J Obstet Gynecol.* 1996;175:467.

Haylen BT, Maher CF, Barber MD, et al. An International Urogynecological Association (IUGA)/International Continence Society (ICS) joint report on the terminology for female pelvic organ prolapse (POP). *Int Urogynecol J.* 2016;27:655.

Kobak WH, Rosenberger K, Walters MD. Interobserver variation in the assessment of pelvic organ prolapse. *Int Urogynecol J.* 1996;7:121.

Steele A, Mallipeddi P, Welgoss J, et al. Teaching the pelvic organ prolapse quantitation system. *Am J Obstet Gynecol.* 1998;179:1458.

Classification of Complications Related to Vaginal Prostheses and Grafts

Gowda M, Kit LC, Reynolds WS, et al. Interobserver variability when employing the IUGA/ICS classification system for complications related to prostheses and grafts in female pelvic floor surgery. *Int Urogynecol.* 2013;24:1671.

Haylen BT, Freeman RM, Swift SE, et al. An International Urogynecological Association (IUGA)/International Continence Society (ICS) joint terminology and classification of the complications related directly to the insertion of prostheses (meshes, implants, tapes) and grafts in female pelvic floor surgery. *Neurourol Urodyn.* 2011;30:2.

Ridgeway B, Walters MD, Paraiso M, et al. Early experience with mesh excision for adverse outcomes after transvaginal mesh placement using prolapse kits. *Am J Obstet Gynecol.* 2008;199:703.e1-703.e7.

Tunitsky E, Abbott S, Barber MD. Interrater reliability of the international continence society and international urogynecological association (ICS/IUGA) classification system for mesh-related complications. *Am J Obstet Gynecol.* 2012;206:422.e1.

PART 2

Evaluation

9

Evaluation of Pelvic Floor Disorders: History, Physical Examination, and Diagnostic Testing

Lisa C. Hickman and Mark D. Walters

CHAPTER OUTLINE

INTRODUCTION

The term pelvic floor disorders includes urinary and fecal incontinence, pelvic organ prolapse, and sensory and emptying abnormalities of the lower urinary and gastrointestinal tracts. Pelvic floor disorders are common in women and often coexist, so it is important for providers to inquire about each of these conditions.

Urinary incontinence can be a symptom of which patients complain, a sign demonstrated on examination, or a condition (i.e., diagnosis) that can be confirmed by definitive studies. When a woman complains of urinary incontinence, appropriate evaluation includes exploring the nature of her symptoms and looking for physical findings. The history and physical examination are the first and most important steps in the evaluation. A preliminary diagnosis can be made with simple office and laboratory tests, with initial therapy based on these findings. If complex conditions are present, if the patient does not improve after initial therapy, or if surgery is being considered, definitive, specialized studies are usually necessary.

Sensory and emptying abnormalities of the lower urinary tract, or lower urinary tract symptoms (LUTS), refer to abnormal sensation or function associated with or following micturition. A spectrum of abnormalities have been defined and can be categorized into storage symptoms (including frequency, urgency, incontinence, and nocturia), voiding symptoms (such as difficulty with or abnormalities experienced during micturition), and postmicturition symptoms (feeling of incomplete emptying or postvoid dribbling). These may be signs of other pelvic floor disorders, such as incomplete emptying with an anterior vaginal wall prolapse, or represent their own condition, such as nocturia. Understanding the constellation of LUTS experienced by a patient through a detailed history can help direct one toward the anticipated findings on examination, as well as the indicated office, laboratory, and diagnostic tests.

Pelvic organ prolapse (POP) is a heterogeneous condition in which weaknesses of the pelvic floor musculature and connective tissue result in descent or bulging of pelvic organs into the vaginal canal. In more severe cases, prolapse can protrude beyond the hymenal ring. In anterior vaginal wall prolapse, the bladder and urethra may protrude into the vaginal canal (cystocele). Patients may have uterine prolapse or, after hysterectomy, the vaginal cuff may herniate, resulting in apical vaginal prolapse. The rectum, small bowel, and sigmoid colon also may herniate in posterior vaginal wall prolapse, resulting in rectoceles, enteroceles, and sigmoidoceles, respectively. That said, terms such as "cystocele" and "rectocele," although commonly used in clinical practice, are perhaps less precise, because they imply an unrealistic certainty as to the specific organs behind the vaginal wall at the time of physical examination.

Definitions of prolapse as a clinical condition or disease are based on measured severity or staging by Pelvic Organ Prolapse Quantification (POPQ; see Chapter 8) on examination and by assessment of relevant symptoms. Although most clinicians can recognize the extremes of normal support versus severe prolapse, most cannot objectively state at what point vaginal laxity becomes pathologic and requires intervention. There are limited data concerning the normal distribution of POP in the population and the correlations between symptoms and physical findings. In a study of 497 women, Swift (2000) demonstrated that the distribution of prolapse in a population exhibited a bell-shaped curve, with the majority of women having stage I or II prolapse by the POPQ classification system, and only 3% having stage III prolapse. This signifies that, at baseline, a majority of women, especially those who have borne children, have some degree of pelvic relaxation. However, these women are generally asymptomatic and will only develop symptoms if their prolapse increases in severity, especially if it protrudes to the hymen and beyond. Therefore, even if prolapse is found on physical examination and the patient is asymptomatic, it may not be clinically relevant or require intervention.

Swift and Barber (2010) proposed that POP, the disease, be defined as the descent of one or more of the anterior vaginal wall, posterior vaginal wall, the uterus (cervix), or the apex of the vagina beyond the hymen on straining examination (the sign of POP) associated with feeling or seeing a bulge from the vagina during daily activities (the symptom of POP). Patients with descent beyond the hymen who do not have bulge symptoms would be classified as having asymptomatic POP, and those with bulge symptoms should be classified as having symptomatic POP.

Fecal incontinence is defined as involuntary loss of mucus, liquid stool, or solid stool, whereas anal incontinence also includes the involuntary loss of flatus or mucus with or without the concurrent loss of stool. Similar to urinary incontinence, it can be a condition, a symptom, or a sign on examination. It is important to evaluate the incontinence with a thorough history, including assessment of symptom bother and physical examination of the vulva, vagina, and rectum. Appropriate management can be initiated after office assessment, reserving laboratory evaluation and ancillary diagnostic tests for individuals with concerns for infectious etiology, malignancy, or inconclusive evaluation, or when anatomic dysfunction is suspected.

Defecatory dysfunction, including obstructed defecation and constipation, is commonly found in women with pelvic floor disorders. Obstructed defecation results from incomplete evacuation of the rectum as a result of inadequate forces and/or increased resistance. Constipation, which is often defined by the Rome classification system (Drossman & Hasler, 2016), is considered chronic in nature when persisting for 6 months or more. Chronic constipation can be further classified into disordered or "slow" colonic transit, or normal transit with pelvic or anorectal dysfunction. A history should explore the specific bothersome symptoms during defecation, manipulation used to assist with defecation, and any significant changes in bowel habits that could be concerning for colorectal cancer. Similar to fecal incontinence, a physical examination involves inspection of the vulvovaginal and anorectal regions and a digital rectal exam. Although no specific symptoms or findings are sensitive and specific for defecatory dysfunction, the provider may obtain enough information to diagnose and initiate treatment. When this is not possible, or when the patient is refractory to the initial interventions, a number of sophisticated anorectal tests and imaging studies may help the provider obtain a diagnosis.

HISTORY FOR PELVIC FLOOR DISORDERS

Urinary Incontinence and Lower Urinary Tract Symptoms

Early in a patient interview, one should elicit a description of the patient's main complaint, including duration and frequency, with specific questions to differentiate amongst the known genitourinary and nongenitourinary etiologies and specific types of urinary incontinence (see Chapter 8). The initial goal should be to diligently seek out and treat all reversible causes of urinary incontinence and voiding difficulty (Box 9.1). The mnemonic DIAPPERS has long been used to remember this list (Delirium, Infections, Atrophic vaginitis, Psychological causes, Pharmacological, Endocrine, Restricted mobility, Stool impaction). A clear understanding of the severity of the problem or disability and its effect on quality of life should be sought. Assessment of physical mobility and living environment is especially important in certain patients. Questions should be asked about access to toilets or toilet substitutes and about social factors such as living arrangements, social contacts, and caregiver involvement.

Box 9.2 lists questions that are helpful in evaluating urinary incontinence in women. The first question is designed to elicit the symptom of stress urinary incontinence (i.e., urine loss with events that increase intraabdominal pressure). The symptom of stress urinary incontinence is usually (but not always) associated with the diagnosis of urodynamic stress incontinence. Questions 2 through 9 help elicit the symptoms associated with overactive bladder and urgency urinary incontinence. The symptom of urgency incontinence is present if the patient answers question 3 affirmatively. Frequency (questions 4 and 5), bedwetting (question 6), leaking with intercourse (question 8), and a sense of urgency (questions 2 and 7) are all associated with detrusor overactivity. Questions 9 and 10 help to define the severity of the problem. Questions 11 through 13 screen for urinary tract infection and neoplasia, and questions 14 through 16 are designed to elicit symptoms of voiding dysfunction.

BOX 9.1 Reversible Conditions that Cause or Contribute to Urinary Incontinence

- Urinary tract infection
- Urethritis
- Atrophic vaginitis/urethritis
- Pregnancy
- Drug side effects (see Table 9.1)
- Increased urine production
- Metabolic (hyperglycemia, hypercalcemia)
- Excess fluid intake
- Volume overload
- Stool impaction
- Impaired ability or willingness to reach toilet
- Restricted mobility
- Delirium, dementia
- Chronic illness, injury, or restraint that interferes with mobility
- Psychological causes (depression, hopelessness)

BOX 9.2 Helpful Questions in the Evaluation of Female Urinary Incontinence

1. Do you leak urine when you cough, sneeze, or laugh?
2. Do you ever have such an uncomfortably strong need to urinate that if you don't reach the toilet you will leak?
3. If "yes" to question 2, do you ever leak before you reach the toilet?
4. How many times during the day do you urinate?
5. How many times do you void during the night after going to bed?
6. Have you wet the bed in the past year?
7. Do you develop an urgent need to urinate when you are nervous, under stress, or in a hurry?
8. Do you ever leak during or after sexual intercourse?
9. How often do you leak?
10. Do you find it necessary to wear a pad because of your leaking?
11. Have you had bladder, urine, or kidney infections?
12. Are you troubled by pain or discomfort when you urinate?
13. Have you had blood in your urine?
14. Do you find it hard to begin urinating?
15. Do you have a slow urinary stream or have to strain to pass your urine?
16. After you urinate, do you have dribbling or a feeling that your bladder is still full?

Stress urinary incontinence and voiding difficulties can also coexist with anterior and apical vaginal prolapse. However, overt symptoms of stress urinary incontinence may not be present in women with advanced degrees of prolapse, owing to mechanical obstruction of the urethra that prevents urinary leakage. Instead, these women may require manual replacement of the prolapse, also known as splinting, to accomplish voiding. The prolapse increases the risk for incomplete bladder emptying and recurrent or persistent urinary tract infections and for the development of *de novo* stress incontinence after the prolapse is repaired. In addition to difficulty voiding, other urinary symptoms such as urgency, frequency, and urgency incontinence can be found in women with prolapse. However, it is not clear whether the severity of prolapse is directly associated with more irritative voiding symptoms or bladder pain.

After the urologic history, thorough medical, surgical, gynecologic, neurologic, and obstetric histories should be obtained. Certain medical and neurologic conditions, such as diabetes, stroke, and lumbar disc disease, may cause or contribute to urinary incontinence. Furthermore, strong coughing associated with chronic pulmonary disease can markedly worsen symptoms of stress incontinence. A bowel history should be noted, because chronic severe constipation has been associated with voiding difficulties, urgency, stress urinary incontinence, increased bladder capacity, and POP. A history of hysterectomy, vaginal repair with or without mesh, pelvic cancer and/or radiotherapy, or surgery for incontinence should alert the physician to the possibility of prior surgical trauma to the lower urinary tract.

A complete list of the patient's medications (including nonprescription medications) should be sought to determine whether individual drugs might influence the function of the bladder or urethra, leading to urinary incontinence or voiding difficulties. A list of drugs that commonly affect lower urinary tract function is shown in Table 9.1. In these cases, altering drug dosage or changing to a drug with similar therapeutic effectiveness but with fewer lower urinary tract side effects will often improve or "cure" the offending urinary tract symptom.

Patient histories regarding frequency and severity of urinary symptoms are often inaccurate and misleading. Urinary diaries are more reliable and require the patient to record volume and frequency of fluid intake and of voiding, usually for a 1- to 7-day period. A 3-day diary seems to be as accurate as a 7-day diary to document symptoms, and compliance is improved. Episodes of urinary incontinence and associated events or symptoms such as coughing, urgency, and pad use are noted. The number of times voided each night and any episodes of

TABLE 9.1 Medications that Can Affect Lower Urinary Tract Functions

Drug Class	Type of Medication	Lower Urinary Tract Effects
Allergy	Antihistamines	Anticholinergic actions, sedation
	Decongestants	Urinary retention, voiding difficulty
Analgesics, sedatives, and hypnotics	Benzodiazepines	Urinary retention, voiding difficulty
	Narcotics	Urinary retention, fecal impaction, sedation, delirium
Anticholinergics	Spasmolytic	Urinary retention, voiding difficulty
	Anti-Parkinson medications	Urinary retention, voiding difficulty
	Antimuscarinic	Urinary retention, voiding difficulty
Cardiac agents	Angiotensin converting enzyme inhibitors	Chronic cough, stress incontinence
	α-adrenergic agonists	Urinary retention, voiding difficulty
	α1-adrenergic blockers	Stress incontinence
	Antiarrhythmic	Decreased contractility, anticholinergic actions
	Calcium channel blockers	Urinary retention, voiding difficulty
	Diuretics	Polyuria, frequency, urgency
Dietary agents	Alcohol	Sedation, impaired mobility, diuresis
	Caffeine	Frequency, urgency
Psychotropic agents	Antidepressants	Anticholinergic actions, sedation
	Antipsychotics	Anticholinergic actions, sedation
	Sedatives/hypnotics	Sedation, muscle relaxation, confusion

bedwetting are recorded the next morning. The maximum voided volume also provides a relatively accurate estimate of bladder capacity. The physician should review the frequency/volume charts with the patient and corroborate or modify the initial diagnostic impression. If excessive frequency and volume of fluid intake are noted, restriction of excessive oral fluid intake (combined with scheduled voiding) may improve symptoms of stress and urge incontinence by keeping the bladder volume below the threshold at which urinary leaking results. Electronic bladder diaries have become widely available in recent years. These application-based diaries are easy to use and correlate well with paper diary results across age, gender, and education level. Urinary diaries are also a useful and accepted research method to measure the severity of incontinence and as an outcome measure after interventions. This is reviewed in Chapter 41.

After the history, patients can often be categorized as having probable urodynamic stress incontinence and/or probable detrusor overactivity (with or without coexistent stress incontinence, i.e., mixed urinary incontinence). Women who have the symptom of stress urinary incontinence as their only complaint have a 64% to 90% chance of having urodynamic stress incontinence confirmed on diagnostic urodynamic testing. Of these patients, 10% to 30% are found to have detrusor overactivity (alone or coexistent with urodynamic stress incontinence). Other rare conditions that can cause the symptom of stress incontinence are urethral diverticulum, genitourinary fistula, ectopic ureter, and urethral instability. Inquiry directed at differentiating amongst these conditions should be considered when an atypical history is provided by the patient or when initial therapy is not effective.

Sensory urgency, urgency incontinence, diurnal and nocturnal frequency, and bedwetting all are associated with overactive bladder. The more of these abnormal urinary symptoms the patient has, the greater the chance that she has detrusor overactivity. Cantor and Bates (1980) observed that 81% of patients with three or more of these symptoms had detrusor overactivity on cystometry.

For either diagnosis, appropriate behavioral or medical therapy can be given, and a substantial percentage of patients are expected to respond. Even patients with mixed disorders (coexistent stress and urgency urinary incontinence) respond to various forms of conservative therapy in about 60% of cases. Alternatively, the initial therapy selected for mixed incontinence should be directed toward the first occurring and most bothersome symptom, as this relates most closely to the urodynamic diagnosis. Complex causes of incontinence should be triaged for urodynamic testing or for consultation (see Box 9.3).

Pelvic Organ Prolapse

Patients with POP may present with symptoms directly related to the prolapse, such as vaginal bulge, pressure, and discomfort, and with a plethora of associated symptoms relating to voiding, defecation, and sexual dysfunction. The severity of the prolapse is not necessarily associated with increased visceral symptomatology.

BOX 9.3 Situations that Warrant Consultation for the Evaluation and Treatment of Lower Urinary Tract Dysfunction

Uncertain diagnosis and inability to develop a reasonable treatment plan based on the basic diagnostic evaluation. Uncertainty in diagnosis may occur when there is lack of correlation between symptoms and clinical findings.
Failure to respond to the patient's satisfaction to an adequate therapeutic trial, and the patient is interested in pursuing further therapy.
Consideration of surgical intervention, particularly if previous surgery failed or the patient has a high surgical risk.
The presence of other comorbid conditions:
Incontinence associated with recurrent symptomatic urinary tract infection
Persistent symptoms of difficult bladder emptying
History of previous antiincontinence surgery, radical pelvic surgery, or pelvic radiation therapy
Symptomatic pelvic prolapse, especially if beyond hymen
Abnormal postvoid residual urine
Neurologic condition such as multiple sclerosis or spinal cord lesions or injury
Fistula or suburethral diverticulum
Hematuria without infection

Vaginal prolapse in any compartment—anterior, apical, or posterior—can manifest as vaginal fullness, feeling or seeing a protruding mass or, more rarely, pain. In a study by Tan et al. (2005), the feeling of "a bulge or that something is falling outside the vagina" had a positive predictive value of 81% for POP; the lack of this symptom had a negative predictive value of 76% for predicting prolapse at or past the hymen. Not surprisingly, increased degree of prolapse, especially beyond the hymen, is associated with increased pelvic discomfort and visualization of a protrusion. The presence of vaginal bulge symptoms is a highly specific (but not sensitive) symptom for predicting the presence of prolapse beyond the hymen on a straining examination (specificity 99%–100%). A variety of questions should be asked to understand the POP impact on bladder, bowel, and sexual function (see associated sections), especially as urinary splinting and digital assistance with defecation are also common in women with advanced prolapse.

Elucidating the symptom severity is the most important component of POP evaluation. This should include how the symptoms have changed over time, whether or not the symptoms impact physical activities, and the overall effect on the patient's quality of life. This information will ultimately direct the provider to the most appropriate treatment options available to the patient.

Fecal Incontinence and Defecatory Dysfunction

Obtaining a thorough bowel history is an important component of the pelvic floor disorder evaluation. The basic inquiry should include the frequency of bowel movements, typical consistency, presence of incontinence, and any difficulty with defecation.

When patients report anal incontinence, the provider first determines whether it is incontinence of flatus, liquid stool, solid stool, mucus, or a combination. Further characterization of the incontinence should include frequency/timing of occurrence, provoking factors, pad/diaper use, stool consistency, medication history, and severity. The provider should elucidate whether the soiling is associated with urgency or is passive. A detailed inquiry of the patient's medical, surgical, obstetric, medication, and dietary histories is performed.

Similarly, if the patient reports defecatory dysfunction, a history should be obtained to determine the specific bothersome symptoms and their frequency. This may include anorectal pain with defecation, a sensation of incomplete emptying, straining to defecate, the need for manual assistance with defecation such as perineal or vaginal splinting, digital evacuation of stools, or other maneuvers to aid in defecation. A medical history may reveal conditions associated with chronic constipation, whereas inquiry of medication use may identify agents known to cause (such as opioids) or treat (stool softeners, laxatives) constipation.

POP, especially in the apical and posterior compartments, can be (but is not always) associated with defecatory dysfunction, such as pain with defecation, the need for manual assistance with defecation, and anal incontinence. These patients often have outlet-type constipation secondary to the trapping of stool within the rectal hernia, necessitating the need for splinting to reduce the prolapse and aid in defecation. Interestingly, splinting is the only symptom specifically associated with posterior compartment POP (Erekson et al., 2010). Although defecatory dysfunction remains an area that is least understood in patients with POP, clinical and radiographic studies have shown that the severity of prolapse is not strongly correlated with increased symptomatology. Further review of this topic can be found in Chapters 27 and 28.

Sexual Dysfunction

Questions regarding sexual dysfunction must be included in the evaluation of patients with pelvic floor disorders. Patients may report symptoms of dyspareunia, decreased libido and orgasm, and increased embarrassment with altered anatomy that affects body image. Urinary or fecal incontinence may also have a significant negative impact on sexual activity. Some studies, but not all, have reported that POP adversely affects sexual functioning, with subsequent improvement in sexual function after repair of prolapse. Evaluating sexual dysfunction may be especially difficult in this patient population, as factors other than pelvic floor disorders, such as menopausal symptoms, partner limitations, and functional deficits, may contribute. See Chapter 10 for further discussion of female sexual dysfunction.

Adjuncts for Obtaining Pelvic Floor Disorder History

Symptoms of pelvic floor disorders and their impact on the woman can be measured or quantified using a number of easy-to-use and validated questionnaires measuring symptom severity, quality of life, and sexual function. New tools have been reported recently, including the Comprehensive Assessment of Self-Reported Urinary Symptoms (Weinfurt et al., 2019). These outcome measures can be useful in clinical practice and in research; they are reviewed in detail in Chapter 41.

PHYSICAL EXAMINATION

General, gynecologic, rectal, and lower neurologic examinations should be performed on every woman with pelvic floor disorder. The pelvic examination is of primary importance. A bimanual examination is performed to rule out coexistent gynecologic pathology, which can occur in up to two-thirds of patients. The rectal examination further evaluates for pelvic pathology, anorectal pathology, and fecal impaction, the latter of which may be associated with voiding difficulties and incontinence in elderly women.

Gynecologic Examination

The physical examination for pelvic floor disorders should be conducted with the patient in dorsal lithotomy position, as for a routine pelvic examination. If physical findings do not correspond to symptoms, or if the maximum extent of the prolapse cannot be confirmed, the woman can be reexamined in the standing position.

Initially, the external genitalia are inspected. One should note any vulvar abnormalities, including skin irritation secondary to pad use and/or incontinence. Incontinence-associated dermatitis can be present in up to 46% of older patients with urinary incontinence (Du Moulin et al., 2008). If no displacement of the labia owing to prolapse is apparent, the labia are gently spread to expose the vestibule and hymen. Vaginal discharge can mimic incontinence, so evidence of this problem should be sought and, if present, treated. Palpation of the anterior vaginal wall and urethra may elicit urethral discharge or tenderness that suggests a urethral diverticulum, carcinoma, or inflammatory condition of the urethra. The integrity of the perineal body is evaluated, and the extent of all prolapsed parts are assessed. A retractor, a vaginal speculum, or the posterior blade of a bivalve speculum can be used to depress the posterior vagina to aid in visualizing the anterior vagina, and vice versa for the posterior vagina. Because most patients with prolapse are postmenopausal, the vaginal epithelium should be examined for atrophy and thinning because this may affect management. Healthy, estrogenized tissue, without significant evidence of POP, will be well perfused and have rugation and physiologic moisture. Atrophic vaginal tissue consistent with hypoestrogenemia appears pale, thin, and without rugation, and can be friable; this finding suggests that the urethral mucosa is also atrophic.

After the resting vaginal examination, the patient is instructed to perform the Valsalva maneuver or to cough vigorously. During this maneuver, one should note the presence and severity of stress urinary incontinence, while also observing the order of descent of the pelvic organs, as this corresponds to the relationship of the pelvic organs at the peak of increased intraabdominal pressure. The presence and severity of anterior vaginal relaxation, including cystocele and proximal urethral detachment and mobility, or anterior vaginal scarring, are estimated. Associated pelvic support abnormalities, such as rectocele, enterocele, and uterovaginal prolapse, are noted. The amount or severity of prolapse in each vaginal segment should be measured, staged, and recorded according to POPQ classification (further discussed in Chapter 8). This descriptive system contains a series of site-specific measurements of the woman's pelvic organ support. The measurements can be obtained quickly in both experienced and nonexperienced hands. It can be easily learned and taught by means of a brief video tutorial. Prolapse in each vaginal segment is evaluated and measured relative to the hymen (not introitus), which is a fixed anatomic landmark that can be identified consistently and precisely. The anatomic position of the six defined points for measurement should be centimeters above or proximal to the hymen (negative number) or centimeters below or distal to the hymen (positive number), with the plane of the hymen being defined as zero. For example, a cervix that protrudes 3 cm distal to (beyond) the hymen should be described as +3 cm. Studies have demonstrated excellent inter- and intraexaminer reliability when using the POPQ system to quantify prolapse. The POPQ system does not take into account lateral defects and perineal body prolapse, but these can be added in descriptive terms. POPQ measurements can also help predict or aid in the diagnosis of voiding dysfunction (Chae et al., 2014) and levator hiatus ballooning (Gerges et al., 2013). Despite its limitations, the POPQ system is currently the classification system used in most academic centers, research studies, and National Institutes of Health trials.

Other clinical observations and tests to help delineate prolapse include examination techniques differentiating between various types of defects (e.g., central versus paravaginal defects of the anterior vaginal wall), description and measurement of posterior prolapse, measurement of perineal descent, and measurement of the transverse diameter of the genital hiatus or of the protruding prolapse.

Regarding urinary incontinence, physical findings associated with urodynamic stress incontinence are anterior vaginal relaxation and observed transurethral urine loss with coughing or Valsalva maneuver (i.e., positive bladder stress test). Anterior vaginal wall descent usually represents bladder descent with or without concomitant urethral hypermobility. However, in about 1% of women with anterior vaginal prolapse, an anterior enterocele can mimic a cystocele on physical examination. Cotton swab testing to measure urethral axis mobility (Q-tip test) as part of the incontinence evaluation is of questionable utility. The angle of urethral inclination does not differ between continent and incontinent women with pelvic relaxation. Noblett et al. (2005) showed that essentially all women with stage II to IV prolapse by POPQ had Q-tip angle greater than 30 degrees. Furthermore, adding serial measurement of urethral inclination with a Q-tip to the history and pelvic examination does not appreciably change the sensitivity or specificity for diagnosing urodynamic stress incontinence. However, because most women with primary urodynamic stress incontinence have urethral hypermobility, a nonmobile urethra should cause one to question that diagnosis, perhaps indicating the need to perform urodynamic testing. Several other tests are available for estimating the amount of urethral mobility in women, including the measurement of Aa in the POPQ system, visualization, palpation, and ultrasonography. Determination of urethral mobility in urinary incontinence also may add value in determining which surgical therapy is most appropriate. For example, patients without hypermobility may not benefit from a retropubic suspension or midurethral sling and may be better candidates for urethral bulking.

Lateral paravaginal defects, identified as detachment of the lateral vaginal sulci, may be distinguished from central defects, seen as a midline protrusion with preservation of the lateral sulci, by using a curved forceps placed in the anterolateral vaginal sulci directed toward the ischial spine. Bulging of the anterior vaginal wall in the midline between the forceps blades implies a midline defect; blunting or descent of the vaginal fornices on either side with straining suggest lateral paravaginal defects. However, researchers have shown that the physical examination technique to detect paravaginal defects is not particularly reliable or accurate. In a study by Barber et al. (1999) of 117 women with prolapse, the sensitivity of clinical examination to detect paravaginal defects was good (92%), yet the specificity was poor (52%). Despite a high prevalence of paravaginal defects, the positive predictive value was only 61%. Less than two-thirds of women believed to have a paravaginal defect on physical examination were confirmed to possess the same at surgery. Thus, the clinical value of determining the location of midline, apical, and lateral paravaginal defects remains unknown, but may be valuable for surgical planning when identified.

For posterior vaginal prolapse, clinical examination does not always accurately differentiate between rectoceles and enteroceles. Some investigators have advocated performing imaging studies to further delineate the exact nature of the posterior wall prolapse. Traditionally, most clinicians believe they are able to detect the presence or absence of these defects without anatomically localizing them. However, little is known regarding the accuracy or utility of clinical examinations in evaluating the anatomic locations of prolapsed small or large bowel or of specific defects in the rectovaginal space. Burrows et al. (2003) found that clinical examinations often did not accurately predict the specific location of defects in the rectovaginal septum that were subsequently found intraoperatively. Clinical findings corresponded with intraoperative observations in 59% of patients and differed in 41%; sensitivities and positive predicative values of clinical examinations were less than 40% for all posterior defects. However, what remains unclear is the clinical consequence of not detecting these defects preoperatively.

Rectal Examination

Rectal and rectovaginal examinations are recommended to evaluate both bowel continence and defecatory issues, as well as to fully characterize posterior vaginal wall prolapse and perineal body descent. Inspection of the perianal region is performed with the buttocks separated. The resting anal tone should be noted, as well as any fecal soiling, scarring, hemorrhoids, anal fissures, and asymmetry or gaping of the anal opening, which can be associated with neurologic disorders. Women with disruption of the external anal sphincter may have gross abnormalities of the perineal body, with a "dove tail" sign in the area of the disrupted sphincter.

Perineal descent can be assessed by having the patient perform a Valsalva maneuver. During voluntary contraction of the anal sphincter, the perineal body should elevate. Next, a digital rectal examination is performed, noting the resistance to entry of the examining finger. Some 50% to 85% of overall resting anal tone is generated by the internal anal sphincter. Loss of resting tone suggests disruption of the internal anal sphincter and/or an injury to its sympathetic innervation (i.e., pelvic plexus injury). Anoperineal or recovaginal pocketing can be assessed by palpating anteriorly to identify weakness in the rectovaginal septum and/or perineal body. The patient then should be asked to maximally squeeze her anal sphincter. The presence of a strong voluntary anal sphincter contraction indicates intact pudendal innervation and external anal sphincter. The Digital Rectal Examination Scoring System is one scoring system that is available to evaluate sphincter tone (Table 9.2). This system correlates well with resting and squeeze pressures on manometry, and is scored from 0 to 5, with 3 representing normal anal tone. Absence or decrease of both anal sphincter tone and voluntary contraction suggests a possible sacral or peripheral nerve lesion. Preservation of resting tone in the absence of a voluntary contraction suggests a suprasacral lesion. Anal sphincter defects can also be evaluated during anal squeeze, with the examiner noting a weakness or absence of contraction in the anterior or anterolateral regions; however, agreement between digital rectal examination and ultrasonographic findings for sphincter defects is poor, calling into question the specificity of this technique. Lastly, the patient should be instructed to bear down. Digital assessment of bowel contents in the rectovaginal septum during straining examination can help to diagnose an enterocele. At this time, the examiner can also assess for POP.

In patients with pelvic floor dyssynergia, a hypercontracted and tender puborectalis muscle may not relax on command. Patients may also have paradoxical anal sphincter contraction during straining. These patients often complain of difficult or incomplete bowel emptying.

Neurologic Examination

Urinary or fecal incontinence may be the presenting symptom(s) of neurologic disease. The screening neurologic examination should evaluate mental status and sensory and motor function of both lower extremities and include a screening lumbosacral neurologic examination. The screening lumbosacral examination includes assessments of: (1) pelvic floor muscle strength, (2) anal sphincter resting tone, (3) voluntary anal contraction, and (4) perineal sensation. This simple screening examination can be performed quickly and easily as part of the gynecologic examination. When abnormalities are noted, or when an individual is suspected of having neurologic dysfunction, a comprehensive neurologic examination with particular emphasis on the lumbosacral nerve roots should be performed. This comprehensive evaluation is performed before any neurophysiologic testing, because any such testing should only be interpreted in the context of the patient's history and physical examination findings.

Mental status is determined by noting the patient's level of consciousness, orientation, memory, speech, and comprehension. The Mini-Cog screening tool, which consists of three easily administered components (three-word registration, clock drawing, and three-word recall), and other formal mental status assessments can be helpful, particularly for elderly patients. Disorders associated with mental status aberrations that may result in changes in bowel or bladder function include senile and presenile dementia, brain tumor, stroke, Parkinson disease, and normal pressure hydrocephalus.

Evaluation of the sensory and motor systems may identify an occult neurologic lesion or can help determine the level of a known lesion. Common diseases associated with sensory and motor abnormalities that can produce urologic disturbances include Parkinson disease, multiple sclerosis, cerebrovascular disease, infections, and tumors. Sacral segments 2 through 4, which contain the important neurons controlling micturition, are particularly important. Sensory function is evaluated by testing the lumbosacral dermatomes for the ability to sense light touch, pinprick, and temperature. The sensory dermatomes of interest include the perineum and perianal skin (pudendal nerve, S2–4), mons pubis and upper aspect of labia majora (ilioinguinal nerve, L1–2), front of the knees (L3–4), and sole of the foot (S1). Dermatome maps are useful for characterizing sensory deficits, although it is important to remember that there can be considerable overlap between dermatomes. To test motor function, the patient extends and flexes the hip, knee, and ankle and inverts and everts the foot. The strength and tone of the levator ani muscles and external anal sphincter are estimated digitally. The strength of the pelvic floor musculature is assessed by palpating the levator ani muscle complex bilaterally in the posterior vaginal wall approximately 2 to 4 cm cephalad to the hymen. The patient is then asked to squeeze around the examiner's fingers. Validated scales include the Brink and Oxford scales (Table 9.3). Weakness in this muscle complex can be a result of neurologic deficits or direct trauma during childbirth. Position sense and vibration should

TABLE 9.2 Digital Rectal Examination Scoring System

RESTING SCORE		SQUEEZE SCORE	
0	No discernable tone at rest, an open or patulous anal canal	0	No discernable increase in tone with squeezing effort
1	Very low tone	1	Slight increase
2	Mildly decreased tone	2	Fair increase but below normal
3	Normal	3	Normal
4	Elevated tone, snug	4	Strong squeeze
5	Very high tone, a tight anal canal, difficult to insert a finger	5	Very strong squeeze, to the point of being painful to the examiner

(From Orkin BA, Sinykin SB, Lloyd PC. The digital rectal examination scoring system (DRESS). *Dis Colon Rectum.* 2010;53:1656.)

TABLE 9.3 Grading Scales for Pelvic Muscle Strength

BRINK SCALE		MODIFIED OXFORD SCALE	
Level 0	No objective perineal function, not even to palpation	0	Lack of muscle response
Level 1	Absent objective perineal function, contraction recognized as palpation	1	Flicker or nonsustained contraction
Level 2	Weak objective perineal function, contraction recognized to palpation	2	Presence of low-intensity, but sustained, contraction
Level 3	Present objective perineal function and opposing resistance not kept for >5 seconds to palpation	3	Moderate contraction, feels like an increase in intravaginal pressure that compresses the fingers of the examiner, with small cranial elevation of the vaginal wall
Level 4	Present objective perineal function and opposing resistance kept for >5 seconds to palpation	4	Satisfactory contraction, compressing the fingers of the examiner with elevation of the vaginal wall toward the pubic symphysis
		5	Strong contraction, firm compression of the examiner's fingers with positive movement toward the pubic symphysis

(From Brink CA, Sampselle CM, Wells TJ, et al. A digital test for pelvic muscle strength in older women with urinary incontinence. *Nurs Res.* 1989;38:196; Laycock J. Clinical evaluation of pelvic floor. In: Baessler K, Schüssler B, Burgio KL, Moore K, Stanton SL, eds. *Pelvic Floor Re-Education.* London: Springer-Verlag; 1994.)

be assessed but need only be evaluated in the distal extremities. The patellar, ankle, and plantar reflex responses are tested.

Visceral sensation of the bladder and rectum can be assessed with cystometry and anal manometry, respectively. Loss of perineal sensation in a patient with bowel or bladder dysfunction, particularly if acute, should always alert the examiner to a potentially serious neurologic problem. Neurophysiologic testing and/or radiologic evaluation would be performed to assess for conus medullaris or cauda equina syndrome.

Two reflexes may help in the examination of sacral reflex activity. In the anal reflex, stroking the skin adjacent to the anus causes reflex contraction of the external anal sphincter muscle. The bulbocavernosus reflex involves contraction of the bulbocavernosus and ischiocavernosus muscles in response to tapping or squeezing of the clitoris or stroking the labia majora. Unfortunately, these reflexes can be difficult to evaluate clinically and are not always present, even in neurologically intact women.

DIAGNOSTIC TESTING

Urinary Incontinence and Lower Urinary Tract Symptoms

Perineal Pad Test. Perineal pad weighing may be used when one wants to objectively document the presence and amount of urine loss. The test should approximate activities in daily life. The total amount of urine lost during the test period is determined by weighing a collecting device such as an absorbent pad of adequate capacity that is resistant to leaking. Immediately before the test begins, the collecting device is weighed to the nearest gram. A typical test schedule is started without the patient voiding and with drinking approximately 500 mL of fluid. The patient is then asked to walk, cough, exercise, and wash her hands over the course of an hour. At the end of the 1-hour test period, or if the device becomes saturated during the test, the collecting device is removed, weighed, and replaced if indicated. If the test is regarded as representative, the patient voids, and the volume is recorded; if not, the test is repeated for an additional hour. Alternatively, the test can be performed after filling the bladder to a defined volume or at home over a 24-hour period (see Chapter 41 for more details).

The total weight of urine lost during the test period is taken to be equal to the gain in weight of the collecting device(s). In interpreting the test results, it should be remembered that a weight gain of up to 1 g may be because of weighing errors, sweating, or vaginal discharge.

Phenazopyridine hydrochloride (Pyridium) is sometimes used to aid clinicians in differentiating urinary continence from incontinence in women with disturbing vaginal wetness ("Pyridium pad test"). Patients are given Pyridium tablets and instructed to wear a sanitary pad for a given time. The pad is then removed and examined. Red-orange staining is taken as evidence that urine loss has occurred. Although this test may occasionally be useful, Wall et al. (1990) demonstrated that, although all incontinent women had pad staining, 52% of healthy, continent women also had staining, reflecting a high false-positive rate.

Pad weighing has acceptable test-retest reliability and is easy to perform in a clinical setting. It has a strong correlation with findings on a standing cough stress test (Yi et al., 2020), but a low sensitivity and poor correlation between pad gain and videographic assessment of incontinence severity. Although pad testing can confirm the presence of incontinence, it cannot determine the specific type. These shortcomings have limited acceptance of pad weighing as a routine part of the evaluation of incontinence.

Evaluation of Bladder Filling, Voiding, and Emptying. The office evaluation of incontinence should involve some assessment of voiding, detrusor function during filling, and competency of the urethral sphincteric mechanism. During the assessment, one should try to determine the specific circumstances leading to the involuntary loss of urine. If possible, such circumstances should be reproduced and directly observed during clinical evaluation. The examination is most easily initiated with the patient's bladder comfortably full. The patient is allowed to void as normally as possible in private. The time to void and the amount of urine voided are recorded. In the absence of symptoms of voiding difficulty, patients usually have normal voiding function. The incidence of asymptomatic voiding dysfunction among women with other urologic complaints is only about 3%. The patient then returns to the examination room, and the volume of residual urine is noted by transurethral catheterization or ultrasound. If a sterile urine sample has not yet been obtained for analysis, it can be obtained at this time.

Normal values for postvoid residual urine measurements have not been established; however, a study of over 1200 individuals with and without LUTS found median residual volumes of 26 mL or less (Peterson et al., 2019). Residual volumes less than 50 mL indicate adequate bladder emptying, and volumes greater than 200 mL can be considered inadequate emptying. Clinical judgment must be exercised in interpreting the significance of postvoid residual urine volumes, especially in the intermediate range of 50 to 200 mL. Because isolated instances of elevated residual urine volume may not be significant, the test should be repeated when abnormally high values are obtained. Among women with symptoms of voiding difficulty and those who appear to void abnormally or have retention, more sophisticated testing is required to determine the causes and the mechanism of the voiding dysfunction.

Retrograde bladder filling can then be performed to assess bladder sensation and an estimate of bladder capacity. This test is performed using a 50-mL syringe, without its piston or bulb, attached to the catheter and held above the bladder. The patient is then asked to sit or stand, and the bladder is filled by gravity by pouring 50-mL aliquots of sterile water into the syringe (Fig. 9.1). The patient's first bladder sensation and maximum bladder capacity are noted. The water level in the syringe should be closely observed during filling, as any rise in the water column can be secondary to a detrusor contraction. Unintended increases in intraabdominal pressure by the patient should be avoided.

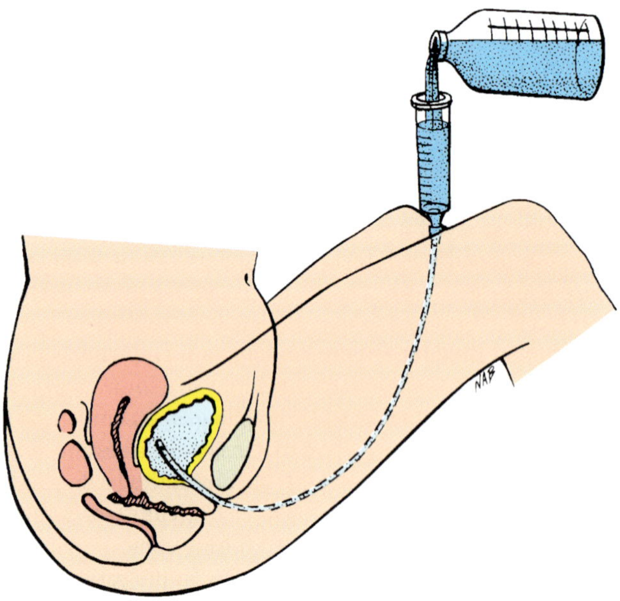

Fig. 9.1 Office evaluation of bladder filling function. In sitting or standing position with a catheter in the bladder, the bladder is filled by gravity by pouring sterile water into the syringe.

Patients without urgency and frequency who note a sensation of bladder fullness and have an estimated bladder capacity that is within normal range probably have normal bladder filling function. There seems to be no clear consensus about the definition of normal bladder capacity: values range from 300 to 750 mL. However, large bladder capacities are not always pathologic, as one-third of women with bladder capacities greater than 800 mL were urodynamically normal, and only a minority had true bladder atony.

The catheter is then removed, and the patient is asked to cough in a standing position. Loss of small amounts of urine in spurts simultaneous with the coughs strongly suggests a diagnosis of urodynamic stress incontinence. Prolonged loss of urine, leaking 5 to 10 seconds after coughing, or no urine loss with provocation indicates that other causes of incontinence, especially detrusor overactivity, may be present. Interpretation of these office tests can be difficult because of artifact introduced by rises in intraabdominal pressure caused by straining or patient movement. Borderline or negative tests should be repeated to maximize their diagnostic accuracy.

Because patients with anterior, apical, or posterior prolapse may have voiding dysfunction resulting from obstruction of the urethra, the completeness of bladder emptying should be assessed with the prolapse reduced. Kinking of the urethra may obscure any indication that urinary incontinence may be present. Therefore, it is important to assess for evidence of incontinence after reduction of the prolapse. This can be done manually or with a pessary, vaginal packing, or ring forceps at the time of the office bladder filling or urodynamic testing. If urinary leakage occurs with coughing or Valsalva maneuver after reduction of the prolapse, the urethral sphincter is probably incompetent, even if the patient is normally continent. This can occur in up to half of women with stage III or IV prolapse. In this situation, the surgeon probably should choose a midurethral sling procedure in conjunction with the prolapse repair, although this is controversial. If stress incontinence is not present even after reduction of the prolapse, an anti-incontinence procedure may not be indicated, although future studies will further help define the role of "prophylactic" bladder neck suspension or sling procedures in this setting. A clinical decision tool to help predict the risk of postoperative *de novo* stress incontinence was published by Jelovsek et al. (2014).

Indications for Urodynamics. It is recognized that, even in the most typical clinical situations, the diagnosis of incontinence based only on clinical evaluation may be uncertain. This diagnostic uncertainty may be acceptable if medical or behavioral treatment (as opposed to surgery) is planned, because of the low morbidity and cost of these treatments, and because the ramifications of noncure (continued incontinence) are not severe. Further, routine urodynamic testing may not improve outcomes when nonsurgical management or surgical management of pure stress urinary incontinence is planned. In situations where greater diagnostic certainty is needed, urodynamic testing is performed to objectively assess urine storage and evacuation. It can be performed with or without fluoroscopy and generally involves cystometry, uroflowmetry/pressure-flow studies, measures of urethral function, and electromyography. Further discussion of urodynamic testing can be found in Chapter 11.

Limited data support the need for urodynamic testing in the routine or basic evaluation of urinary incontinence. It is indicated as part of the evaluation of more complex disorders of bladder filling and voiding, such as the presence of neurologic disease and other comorbid conditions. When surgical treatment of stress incontinence is planned, urodynamic testing is usually recommended, unless the patient has an uncomplicated history and compatible physical findings of stress incontinence (positive cough stress test), has a low postvoid residual volume, and has not had previous surgery for incontinence (Nager et al., 2012). Urodynamic testing is also indicated whenever objective clinical findings do not correlate with or reproduce the patient's symptoms, or in the situation of complex cases, as it can aid in diagnosis and treatment planning. Finally, when trials of therapy are used, patients must be followed up periodically to evaluate response. If the patient fails to improve to her satisfaction, appropriate further testing is required.

Laboratory Testing. Few laboratory tests are necessary for the evaluation of incontinence. A clean midstream or catheterized urine sample should be obtained for dipstick urinalysis. Urine culture and sensitivity could be obtained when the dipstick test indicates infection. Acute cystitis can present with multiple irritative symptoms, such as dysuria, frequency, urgency, incontinence, and voiding difficulty. In these cases, treatment of the infection usually eradicates the symptoms. However, bacteriuria is often asymptomatic, especially in the elderly. Boscia et al. (1986) demonstrated that no differences in urinary symptoms were found when elderly bacteriuric subjects were compared with themselves when they were nonbacteriuric. In view of these conflicting data, it seems reasonable to examine the urine for infection in all incontinent patients and, if bacteriuria is found, to prescribe appropriate antibiotics and reevaluate the patient in several weeks.

Blood testing (blood urea nitrogen, creatinine, glucose, and calcium) is recommended if compromised renal function is suspected or if polyuria (in the absence of diuretics) is present. Urine cytology is not recommended in the routine evaluation of the incontinent patient or in the initial evaluation of microscopic hematuria in women, because of its diminished diagnostic accuracy and risk of missed cases (Shen Tan et al., 2019). Because of the low risk of urothelial cancer (≤0.5%) in asymptomatic women younger than 50 years old, with no smoking history and without gross hematuria (less than 25 red blood cells per high-powered field), further workup for malignancy is not required in this group. See Chapter 40 for further information on the evaluation of asymptomatic microscopic hematuria.

Imaging. Lateral cystourethrography in the resting and straining view can identify mobility or fixation of the bladder neck, funneling of the bladder neck and proximal urethra, and degree of cystocele. The voiding component can identify a urethral diverticulum, fistula, mass, obstruction, or vesicoureteral reflux, although in modern practice this test is usually replaced by magnetic resonance imaging (MRI). Videocystourethrography allows a dynamic assessment of the anatomy and function of the bladder base and urethra during retrograde filling with contrast material and during voiding. It is most helpful in sorting out causes of complex incontinence and voiding problems.

Ultrasonography is an alternative method of evaluating urethrovesical anatomy and is described in detail in Chapter 13. Vaginal ultrasonography accurately displays descent of the urethrovesical junction, opening of the bladder neck, and detrusor contractions. This technique is a noninvasive and accurate method of evaluating the position and mobility of the urethrovesical junction and proximal urethra in incontinent women.

Cystoscopy. Cystoscopy is indicated for the evaluation of patients with incontinence who have sterile hematuria or pyuria; irritative voiding symptoms, such as frequency, urgency, and urge incontinence, in the absence of any reversible causes; suspicion of fistula; bladder pain; recurrent cystitis; suburethral mass; suspected foreign body or mesh in the bladder or urethra; and when urodynamic testing fails to duplicate symptoms of urinary incontinence. Bladder lesions are found in less than 2% of patients with incontinence; therefore cystoscopy should not be performed routinely in patients with incontinence. See Chapter 12 for further discussion.

Pelvic Organ Prolapse

Laboratory Testing. Typically, no additional testing is required beyond a thorough history and physical examination. If patients have advanced prolapse and symptoms associated with voiding dysfunction, obtaining a postvoid residual by either bladder scan or straight catheterization may be useful. If other LUTS are present, one should obtain a urinalysis with culture if indicated. Assessment of kidney function may be important in patients with advanced prolapse, as ureteral kinking can lead to hydroureter and hydronephrosis; however, serum creatinine may not consistently predict the severity of imaging findings.

Imaging. In women with advanced prolapse, imaging of the upper tracts should be considered, as hydroureter and hydronephrosis was found in nearly one-third of women with stage 3 and two-thirds of women with stage 4 prolapse (Siddique et al., 2020). This may be especially important when expectant management is selected, as pessary use and surgical prolapse repair often result in resolution of the obstructive findings.

Pelvic ultrasonography may also be indicated for women who have postmenopausal bleeding. This may be related to abrasions from advanced prolapse, but an intrauterine etiology should be excluded. If examination findings do not correlate with symptoms, or if there is a history of previous vaginal mesh placement, an ultrasound may help with further characterization of the problem and surgical planning.

Patients with prolapse who are without symptoms of defecatory dysfunction generally do not warrant ancillary bowel testing. For example, although defecating proctography can provide additional information regarding rectal emptying, Siproudhis et al. (1993) demonstrated that it is no more sensitive at detecting rectoceles than physical examination alone. However, patients with concomitant constipation or motility disorders do merit further evaluation.

Fecal Incontinence and Defecatory Dysfunction

In patients with fecal incontinence or defecatory dysfunction, diagnostic testing can be helpful in defining the underlying etiology and inform management planning. In patients with defecatory dysfunction, it is necessary to differentiate between those with colonic motility disorders versus those with pelvic outlet symptoms. A more comprehensive discussion can be found in Chapters 27 and 28.

Laboratory Testing. Laboratory testing for fecal incontinence is reserved for individuals with suspected infectious etiologies. No laboratory tests are generally indicated for defecatory dysfunction.

Anoscopy, Proctosigmoidoscopy, and Colonoscopy. Anoscopy and proctosigmoidoscopy can be used to evaluate for prolapsing hemorrhoids and intrarectal prolapse. Colonoscopy should be considered for those who have not had age-appropriate routine screening colonoscopy or for patients who report "red flag" symptoms for colorectal cancer, such as a recent change in bowel habits, difficulty with stool evacuation, abdominal pain, unintentional weight loss, or rectal bleeding (Bharucha et al., 2013). Colitis can also be evaluated with these tests.

Ultrasonography. Endoanal ultrasound is an excellent modality for evaluating fecal incontinence when there is concern for an anatomic sphincter defect, such as in patients with a history of prior obstetric anal sphincter injury. A 360-degree probe is inserted in the anal canal to evaluate the levator, internal anal sphincter, and external anal sphincter anatomy. Three-dimensional technology can create a rendering of the anatomy and any associated defects and is considered the reference standard, with high sensitivity. Although ultrasound can be helpful for surgical planning for individuals undergoing anal sphincteroplasty, imaging is not necessary before initiating treatments such as physical therapy with biofeedback or medical management. Additionally, observed sphincter defects and symptoms do not correlate well.

Transperineal or translabial three-dimensional ultrasound has also been proposed as a modality to functionally assess pelvic floor defects. With urine in the bladder and radiopaque gel in the rectum (if desired), anatomic images can be obtained at rest, with levator contraction, and at maximum straining. Dynamic images can then be rendered to visualize the interactions between the different compartments. Although this is a relatively easy and noninvasive test to perform and has been demonstrated to have high concordance with defocography results, ultrasound, like defocography, does not correlate well with POPQ examination findings in the posterior compartment. When used for the evaluation of anal sphincter defects, transperineal and endovaginal ultrasound were associated with high specificity (85% for both) but poorer sensitivity (64% and 48%, respectively) (Roos et al., 2011).

Defecography. Defecating proctography, which involves dynamic and still fluoroscopic images of patients at rest, during defecation, and while contracting the anal sphincter, can also be used for diagnosis when rectal prolapse or intussusception is suspected. Defecography has the added advantage of providing radiographic evidence of the specific organ that is herniating into the posterior vaginal wall and is the gold standard for measuring perineal descent.

Dynamic MRI defecography provides information regarding defecation and anatomic soft-tissue defects. It has multiple advantages: it is noninvasive, does not require ionizing radiation, and is unrivaled in its depictions of pelvic soft tissue. It has shown benefit in enterocele detection in the apical and posterior compartments and correlated well with anterior and posterior compartment prolapse identified on physical examination (Lin et al., 2018). Some surgeons use this modality to help decide whether an abdominal or vaginal prolapse repair is most appropriate. However, given the costliness of this imaging modality, the clinical utility in routine practice is debatable.

Anorectal Manometry. Anorectal manometry is a useful test for patients with constipation suspected to be nonmechanical in etiology. These conditions include pelvic floor dyssynergia, rectal sensory disorders, and Hirschprung disease, and are typically managed nonsurgically. This test employs a pressure catheter with attached balloon to evaluate rectal sensation, compliance, internal anal sphincter reflexive relaxation, and manometric function. The small balloon attached to the catheter is slowly inflated in the rectum, and the patient is asked to squeeze, relax, and push during the test. This provides an assessment of reflex pathways via changes in anal sphincter muscle pressures. Next, a balloon is inflated with water, and the patient attempts to expel the balloon to simulate defecation. This should normally take less than 60 seconds. Patients with pelvic floor dyssynergia often contract the external anal sphincter inappropriately during attempts to defecate. With decreased rectal sensation, abnormally high volumes in the rectal balloon (>90 mL) are tolerated. In Hirschprung disease, there is nonrelaxation of the internal anal sphincter during distention, because of the pathologic absence of intramural ganglion cells.

Colon Transit Studies. Motility disorders can be assessed with colonic transit studies. These patients typically describe infrequent bowel movements that are not improved by a bowel regimen or conservative measures. The most commonly used test is the Sitzmark transit study, which employs a gelatin capsule taken by the patient on day 0 with 24 radiopaque markers and an abdominal x-ray that is performed on day 5 to determine how many markers are expelled. If six or more markers remain, the test is considered positive for a colon transit abnormality. A diagnosis of slow-transit constipation is made if the markers are scattered throughout the colon, whereas outlet obstruction is more likely when markers are located primarily in the rectosigmoid.

SUMMARY

Because many patients experience more than pelvic floor disorder, the evaluation starts with a thorough and comprehensive history, with importance placed on determining the impact of the condition on the patient's quality of life. Physical examination includes gynecologic, rectal, and lower neurologic examinations in addition to the general components. A variety of simple office tests can be used to evaluate prolapse, bladder function, and bowel function, with additional adjunctive diagnostic tests used for complex cases, those refractory to conservative measures, or when surgical intervention is desired.

BIBLIOGRAPHY

Introduction

Abrams P, Cardozo L, Fall M, et al. The standardization of terminology of lower urinary tract function: report from the Standardisation Sub-committee of the International Continence Society. *Neurourol Urodyn.* 2002;21:167.

Drossman DA, Hasler WL. Rome IV-functional GI disorders: disorders of gut-brain interaction. *Gastroenterology.* 2016;150:1257.

Swift SE. The distribution of pelvic organ support in a population of women presenting for routine gynecologic healthcare. *Am J Obstet Gynecol.* 2000;183:277.

Swift SE, Barber MD. Pelvic organ prolapse: defining the disease. *Female Pelvic Med Reconstr Surg.* 2010;16:201.

Swift SE, Woodman P, O'Boyle A, et al. Pelvic organ support study (POSST): the distribution, clinical definition, and epidemiologic condition of pelvic organ support defects. *Am J Obstet Gynecol.* 2005;192:795.

History of Pelvic Floor Disorders

Abrams P, Blaivas JG, Stanton SL, et al. The standardization of terminology of lower urinary tract function recommended by the International Continence Society. *Int Urogynecol J.* 1990;1:45.

ACOG Committee on Practice Bulletins – Gynecology. ACOG Practice Bulletin No. 214: Pelvic organ prolapse. *Obstet Gynecol.* 2019; 134(5):e125-142.

Barber MD. Symptoms and outcome measures of pelvic organ prolapse. *Clin Obstet Gynecol.* 2005;48:724.

Barber MD, Neubauer NL, Klein-Olarte V. Can we screen for pelvic organ prolapse without a physical examination in epidemiologic studies? *Am J Obstet Gynecol.* 2006;195:942.

Barber MD, Visco AG, Wyman JF, et al. Sexual function in women with urinary incontinence and pelvic organ prolapse. Continence Program for Women Research Group. *Obstet Gynecol.* 2002;99:281.

Bradley CS, Nygaard IE. Vaginal wall descensus and pelvic floor symptoms in older women. *Obstet Gynecol.* 2005;106:759.

Bump RC, Mattiasson A, Bø K, et al. The standardization of terminology of female pelvic organ prolapse and pelvic floor dysfunction. *Am J Obstet Gynecol.* 1996;175:10.

Burrows LJ, Meyn LA, Walters MD, Weber AM. Pelvic symptoms in women with pelvic organ prolapse. *Am J Obstet Gynecol.* 2004;104:982.

Cantor TJ, Bates CP. Comparative study of symptoms and objective urodynamic findings in 214 incontinent women. *Br J Obstet Gynaecol.* 1980;87:889.

Cundiff GW, Fenner D. Evaluation and treatment of women with rectocele: focus on associated defecatory and sexual dysfunction. *Obstet Gynecol.* 2004;104:1403.

Digesu GA, Derpapas A, Hewett S, et al. Does the onset or bother of mixed urinary incontinence symptoms help in the urodynamic diagnosis? *Eur J Obstet Gynecol Reprod Biol.* 2013;171:381.

Diokno AC, Wells TJ, Brink CA. Comparison of self-reported voided volume with cystometric bladder capacity. *J Urol.* 1987;137:698.

Ellerkmann RM, Cundiff GW, Melick CF, et al. Correlation of symptoms with location and severity of pelvic organ prolapse. *Am J Obstet Gynecol.* 2001;185:1332.

Erekson EA, Kassis NC, Washington BB, Myers DL. The association between stage II or greater posterior prolapse and bothersome obstructive bowel symptoms. *Female Pelvic Med Reconstr Surg.* 2010;16:59.

Fantl JA, Wyman JF, Wilson MS, et al. Diuretics and urinary incontinence in community-dwelling women. *Neurourol Urodyn.* 1990;9:25.

Ghetti C, Gregory WT, Edwards SR, et al. Pelvic organ descent and symptoms of pelvic floor disorders. *Am J Obstet Gynecol.* 2005;193:53.

Gormley EA, Griffiths DJ, McCracken PN, Harrison GM. Polypharmacy and its effect on urinary incontinence in a geriatric population. *Br J Urol.* 1993;71:265.

Haylen BT, de Ridder D, Freeman RM, et al. An International Urogynecological Association (IUGA)/International Continence Society (ICS) joint report on the terminology for female pelvic floor dysfunction. *Int Urogynecol J.* 2010;21:5.

Jensen JK, Nielsen FR, Ostergard DR. The role of patient history in the diagnosis of urinary incontinence. *Obstet Gynecol.* 1994;83:904.

Korda A, Krieger M, Hunter P, Parkin G. The value of clinical symptoms in the diagnosis of urinary incontinence in the female. *Aust NZ J Obstet Gynecol.* 1987;27:149.

Mateu Arrom L, Peri Cusi L, Lopez-Fando L, et al. Validation of a 3 day electronic bladder diary as an app for smart-phone. *Neurourol Urodyn.* 2019;38:764.

Melville JL, Miller EA, Fialkow MF, et al. Relationship between patient report and physician assessment of urinary incontinence severity. *Am J Obstet Gynecol.* 2003;189:76.

Nygaard I, Holcomb R. Reproducibility of the seven-day voiding diary in women with stress urinary incontinence. *Int Urogynecol J.* 2000;11:15.

Palmer C, Farhan B, Nguyen N, et al. Are electronic and paper questionnaires equivalent to assess patients with overactive bladder? *J Urol.* 2018;200:369.

Rogers RG, Villarreal A, Kammerer-Doak D, Qualls C. Sexual function in women with and without urinary incontinence and/or pelvic organ prolapse. *Int Urogynecol J Pelvic Floor Dysfunc.* 2001;12:361.

Romanzi LJ, Chaiken DC, Blaivis JG. The effect of genital prolapse on voiding. *J Urol.* 1999;161:581.

Sand PK, Hill RC, Ostergard DR. Incontinence history as a predictor of detrusor stability. *Obstet Gynecol.* 1988;71:257.

Tan JS, Lukacz ES, Menefee SA, et al. Predictive value of prolapse symptoms: a large database study. *Int Urogynecol J.* 2005;16:203.

Urinary incontinence in women. ACOG Practice Bulletin No. 155. American College of Obstetricians and Gynecolgists. *Obstet Gynecol.* 2015;126:e66.

Walters MD, Realini JP. The evaluation and treatment of urinary incontinence in women: a primary care approach. *J Am Board Fam Pract.* 1992;5:289.

Weber AM, Walters MD, Piedmonte MR. Sexual function and vaginal anatomy in women before and after surgery for pelvic organ prolapse and urinary incontinence. *Am J Obstet Gynecol.* 2000;182:1610.

Weinfurt KP, Griffith JW, Flynn KE, et al. The comprehensive assessment of self-reported urinary symptoms: a new tool for research on subtypes of patients with lower urinary tract symptoms. *J Urol.* 2019;201:1177.

Williams ME, Gaylord SA. Role of functional assessment in the evaluation of urinary incontinence, National Institutes of Health Consensus Development Conference on Urinary Incontinence in Adults, Bethesda, MD, October 3–5, 1988. *J Am Geriatr Soc.* 1990;38:296.

Wyman JF, Choi SC, Harkins SW, et al. The urinary diary in evaluation of incontinent women: a test-retest analysis. *Obstet Gynecol.* 1988;71:812.

Physical Examination

Barber MD, Cundiff GW, Weidner AC, et al. Accuracy of clinical assessment of paravaginal defects in women with anterior vaginal wall prolapse. *Am J Obstet Gyneol.* 1999;181:87.

Blaivas JG, Zayed AAH, Kamal BL. The bulbocavernosus reflex in urology: a prospective study of 299 patients. *J Urol.* 1981;126:197.

Brink CA, Sampselle CM, Wells TJ, et al. A digital test for pelvic muscle strength in older women with urinary incontinence. *Nurs Res.* 1989;38:196.

Brink CA, Wells TJ, Sampsell CM, et al. A digital test for pelvic muscle strength in women with urinary incontinence. *Nurs Res.* 1994; 43:352.

Burrows LJ, Sewell C, Leffler KS, Cundiff GW. The accuracy of clinical evaluation of posterior vaginal wall defects. *Int Urogynecol J.* 2003;14:160.

Chae JY, Park GY, Kim JH, et al. Points Aa and Ba are factors associated with preoperative voiding dysfunction in patients with cystocele. *Eur J Obstet Gynecol Reprod Biol.* 2014;174:146.

Dalpiaz O, Curti P. Role of perineal ultrasound in the evaluation of urinary stress incontinence and pelvic organ prolapse: a systematic review. *Neurourol Urodyn.* 2006;25:301.

Du Moulin MF, Hammers JP, Ambergen AW, et al. Prevalence of urinary incontinence among community-dwelling adults receiving home care. *Res Nurs Health.* 2008;31:604.

Gerges B, Kamisan Atan I, Shek KL, Dietz HP. How to determine "ballooning" of the levator hiatus on clinical examination: a retrospective observational study. *Int Urogynecol J.* 2013;24:1933.

Jeppson PC, Paraiso MF, Jelovsek JE, Barber MD. Accuracy of digital anal examination in women with fecal incontinence. *Int Urogynecol J.* 2012;23:765.

Kaushal JN, Goldner F. Validation of the digital rectal examination as an estimate of anal sphincter squeeze pressure. *Am J Gastroenterol.* 1991;86:886.

Kenton K, Shott S, Brubaker L. Vaginal topography does not correlate well with visceral position in women with pelvic organ prolapse. *Int Urogynecol J.* 1997;8:336.

Laycock J. Clinical evaluation of pelvic floor. In: Baessler K, Schüssler B, Burgio KL, Moore K, Stanton SL, eds. *Pelvic Floor Re-Education.* London: Springer-Verlag; 1994.

Mattison ME, Simsiman AJ, Menefee SA. Can urethral mobility be assessed using the pelvic organ prolapse quantification system? An analysis of the correlation between point Aa and Q-tip angle in varying stages of prolapse. *Urology.* 2006;68:1005.

Noblett K, Lane FL, Driskill CS. Does pelvic organ prolapse quantification exam predict urethral mobility in stages 0 and I prolapse? *Int Urogynecol J.* 2005;16:268.

Orkin BA, Sinykin SB, Lloyd PC. The digital rectal examination scoring system (DRESS). *Dis Colon Rectum.* 2010;53:1656.

Pirpiris A, Shek KL, Dietz HP. Urethral mobility and urinary incontinence. *Ultrasound Obstet Gynecol.* 2011;36:507.

Romanzi LJ, Polaneczky M, Glazer HI. Simple test of pelvic muscle contraction during pelvic examination: correlation to surface electromyography. *Neurourol Urodynam.* 1999;18:603.

Sampselle CM, Brink CA, Wells TJ. Digital measurement of pelvic muscle strength in childbearing women. *Nurs Res.* 1989;38:134.

Shek KL, Atan IK, Dietz HP. Can anal sphincter defects be identified by palpation? *Female Pelvic Med Reconstr Surg.* 2015;22:472.

Tulikangas PK, Lukban JC, Walters MD. Anterior enterocele: a report of three cases. *Int Urogynecol J.* 2004;15:350, 2004.

Walters MD, Shields LE. The diagnostic value of history, physical examination, and the Q-tip cotton swab test in women with urinary incontinence. *Am J Obstet Gynecol.* 1988;159:145.

Whiteside JL, Barber MD, Paraiso MF, et al. Clinical evaluation of anterior vaginal wall support defects: interexaminer and intraexaminer reliability. *Am J Obstet Gynecol.* 2004;191:100.

Diagnostic Testing

Abrams P, Klevmark B. Frequency-volume charts: an indispensable part of lower urinary tract assessment. *Scand J Urol Nephrol.* 1996;179:47.

Arnold EP, Webster JR, Loose H, et al. Urodynamics of female incontinence: factors influencing the results of surgery. *Am J Obstet Gynecol.* 1973;117:805.

Bharucha AE, Pemberton JH, Locke III GR. American Gastroenterological Association technical review on constipation. *Gastroenterology.* 2013;144:218.

Boscia JA, Kobasa WD, Abrutyn E, et al. Lack of association between bacteriuria and symptoms in the elderly. *Am J Med.* 1986;81:979.

Brocklehurst JC, Dillane JB, Griffiths L, Fry J. The prevalence and symptomatology of urinary infection in an aged population. *Gerontol Clin.* 1968;10:242.

Broekhuis SR, Kluivers KB, Hendriks JC, et al. POP-Q, dynamic MR imaging, and perineal ultrasonography: Do they agree in the quantification of female pelvic organ prolapse? *Int Urogynecol J Pelvic Floor Dysfunct.* 2009;20:541.

Brown ET, Krlin RM, Winters JC. Urodynamics: examining the current role of UDS testing. What is the role of urodynamic testing in light of recent AUA urodynamics and overactive bladder guidelines and the VALUE study? *Curr Urol Rep.* 2013;14:403.

Byrne DJ, Hamilton Stewart PA, Gray BK. The role of urodynamics in female urinary stress incontinence. *Br J Urol.* 1987;59:228.

Cameron AP, Jimbo M, Heidelbaugh JJ. Diagnosis and office-based treatment of urinary incontinence in adults. Part two: treatment. *Ther Adv Urol.* 2013;5:189.

Chahal R, Gogi NK, Sundaram SK. It is necessary to perform urine cytology in screening patients with haematuria? *Eur Urol.* 2001;39:283.

Chiarioni G, Kim SM, Vantini I, et al. Validation of the balloon evacuation test: reproducibility and agreement with findings from anorectal manometry and electromyography. *Clin Gastroenterol Hepatol.* 2014;12:2049.

Committee Opinion No. 703: Asymptomatic Microscopic Hematuria in Women. *Obstet Gynecol.* 2017;129:e168.

Croghan SM, Costigan G, O'Dwyer N, et al. Efficacy of urodynamic studies in predicting long-term outcomes of the transobturator tape: do they augment clinical assessment? *Cent European J Urol.* 2019;72:384.

Davis R, Jones JS, Barocas DA, et al. Diagnosis, evaluation and follow-up of asymptomatic microhematuria (AMH) in adults: AUA guideline. *J Urol.* 2012;188(suppl 6):2473.

Fantl JA, Bump RC, Robinson D, et al. Efficacy of estrogen supplementation in the treatment of urinary incontinence. The Continence Program for Women Research Group. *Obstet Gynecol.* 1996;88:401.

Fantl JA, Harkins SW, Wyman JF, et al. Fluid loss quantitation test in women with urinary incontinence: a test-retest analysis. *Obstet Gynecol.* 1987;70:739.

Fischer-Rasmussen W, Hansen RI, Stage P. Predictive values of diagnostic tests in the evaluation of female urinary stress incontinence. *Acta Obstet Gynecol Scand.* 1986;65:291.

Groutz A, Blaivas J, Chaikin D, et al. Noninvasive outcome measures of urinary incontinence and lower urinary tract symptoms: a multicenter study of micturition diary and pad test. *J Urol.* 2000;164:698.

Haylen BT, Frazer MI, Sutherst JR. Diuretic response to fluid load in women with urinary incontinence: optimum duration of pad test. *Br J Urol.* 1988;62:331.

Jakobsen H, Vedel P, Andersen JT. Which pad-weighing test to choose: ICS one hour test, the 48 hour home test or a 40 min test with known bladder volume? *Neurourol Urodyn.* 1987;4:23.

Jelovsek JE, Chagin K, Brubaker L, et al. A model for predicting the risk of de novo stress urinary incontinence in women undergoing pelvic organ prolapse surgery. *Obstet Gynecol.* 2014;123:279.

Kadar N. The value of bladder filling in the clinical detection of urine loss and selection of patients for urodynamic testing. *Br J Obstet Gynaecol.* 1988;95:698.

Kelvin FM, Maglinte DD. Dynamic evaluation of female pelvic organ prolapse by extended proctography. *Radiol Clin North Am.* 2003;41:395.

Kelvin FM, Maglinte DDT, Hornback JA. Dynamic cystoproctography of female pelvic floor defects and their interrelationships. *Am J Radiol.* 1997;169:769.

Kelvin FM, Hale DS, Maglinte DD, et al. Female pelvic organ prolapse: diagnostic contribution of dynamic cystoproctography and comparison with physical examination. *Am J Roentgenol.* 1999;173:31.

Kinn A-C, Larsson B. Pad test with fixed bladder volume in urinary stress incontinence. *Acta Obstet Gynecol Scand.* 1987;55:369.

Larson G, Victor A. The frequency-volume chart in genuine stress incontinent women, *Neurourol Urodyn.* 1992;1:23.

Lestar B, Penninckx F, Kerremans R. The composition of anal basal pressure. An in vivo and in vitro study in man. *Int J Colorectal Dis.* 1989;4:118.

Lin FC, Funk JT, Tiwari HA, et al. Dynamic pelvic magnetic resonance imaging evaluation of pelvic organ prolapse compared to physical examination findings. *Urology.* 2018;119:49.

Lor KY, Soupashi M, Abdel-Fattah, Mostafa A. Does pre-operative urodynamics lead to better outcomes in management of urinary incontinence in women? A linked systematic review and meta-analysis. *Eur J Obstet Gynecol Reprod Biol.* 2020;244:141.

Lose G, Gammelgaard J, Jorgenson TJ. The one-hour pad-weighing test: reproducibility and the correlation between the test result, the start volume in the bladder, and the diuresis. *Neurourol Urodyn.* 1986;5:17.

Martellucci J, Naldini G. Clinical relevance of transperineal ultrasound compared with evacuation proctography for the evaluation of patients with obstructed defecation. *Colorectal Dis.* 2011;13:1167.

Martin JL, Williams KS, Sutton AJ, et al. Systematic review and meta-analysis of methods of diagnostic assessment. *Neurourol Urodyn.* 2006;25:674.

Matsuoka H, Wexner SD, Desai MB. A comparison between dynamic pelvic magnetic resonance imaging and videoproctography in patients with constipation. *Dis Colon Rectum.* 2001;30:199.

Mohr DN, Offord KP, Owen RA, Melton III LJ. Asymptomatic microhematuria and urologic disease. A population-based study. *JAMA.* 1986;256:224.

Nager CW, Brubaker L, Litman HJ, et al. A randomized trial of urodynamic testing before stress-incontinence surgery. *N Engl J Med.* 2012;366:1987.

Nygaard I, Zmolek G. Exercise pad testing in continent exercisers: reproducibility and correlation with voided volume, pyridium staining, and type of exercise. *Neurourol Urodyn.* 1995;14:125.

Ouslander JG. Diagnostic evaluation of geriatric urinary incontinence. *Clin Geriatr Med.* 1986;2:715.

Ouslander J, Staskin D, Raz S, et al. Clinical versus urodynamic diagnosis in an incontinent female geriatric population. *J Urol.* 1987;37:68.

Perniola G, Shek C, Chong CC, et al. Defecation proctography and translabial ultrasound in the investigation of defecatory disorders. *Ultrasound Obstet Gynecol.* 2008;31:567.

Peterson AC, Smith AR, Fraser MO, et al. The distribution of post-void residual volumes in people seeking care in the symptoms of lower urinary tract dysfunction network observational cohort study with a comparison to asymptomatic populations. *Urology.* 2019;130:22.

Poston G, Joseph A, Riddle P. The accuracy of ultrasound and the measurement of changes in bladder volume. *Br J Urol.* 1983;55:361.

Quigley GJ, Harper AC. The epidemiology of urethral-vesical dysfunction in the female patient, *Am J Obstet Gynecol.* 1985;151:220.

Rimstad L, Larsen ES, Schiøtz HA, Kulseng-Hanssen S. Pad stress tests with increasing load for the diagnosis of stress urinary incontinence. *Neurourol Urodyn.* 2014;33:1135.

Richmond DH, Sutherst JR, Brown MC. Quantification of urine loss by weighing perineal pads. Observation on the exercise regimen. *Br J Urol.* 1987;59:224.

Roos AM, Abdool Z, Sultan AH, Thakar R. The predictive accuracy of endovaginal and transperineal ultrasound for detecting anal sphincter defects: The PREDICT study. *Clin Radiol.* 2011;66:597.

Ryhammer AM, Djurhuus JC, Laurberg S. Pad testing in incontinent women: a review. *Int Urogynecol J.* 1999;10:111.

Schaer GN, Koechli OR, Schuessler B, Haller U. Perineal ultrasound for evaluating the bladder neck in urinary stress incontinence. *Obstet Gynecol.* 1995;85:220.

Shen Tan W, Sarpong R, Khetrapal P, et al. Does urinary cytology have a role in haematuria investigations? *BJU Int.* 2019;123:74.

Siddique M, Ingraham C, Kudish B, et al. Hydronephrosis associated with pelvic organ prolapse: a systematic review. *Female Pelvic Med Reconstr Surg.* 2020;26:212.

Siproudhis L, Robert A, Vilotte J, et al. How accurate is clinical examination in diagnosing and quantifying pelvirectal disorders? A prospective study in a group of 50 patients complaining of defecatory difficulties. *Dis Colon Rectum.* 1993;36:430.

Swift SE, Ostergard DR. Evaluation of current urodynamic testing methods in the diagnosis of genuine stress incontinence. *Obstet Gynecol.* 1995;86:85.

Sutherst JR, Brown MC, Richmond D. Analysis of the pattern of urine loss in women with incontinence as measured by weighing perineal pads. *Br J Urol.* 1986;58:273.

Versi E, Orrego G, Hardy E, et al. Evaluation of the home pad test in the investigation of female urinary incontinence. *Br J Obstet Gynaecol.* 1996;103:162.

Wall LL, Want K, Robson I, Stanton SL. The pyridium pad test for diagnosing urinary incontinence. *J Reprod Med.* 1990;35:682.

Walters MD, Dombroski RA, Prihoda TJ. Perineal pad testing in the quantitation of urinary incontinence. *Int Urogynecol J.* 1990;1:3.

Webster GD, Sihelnik SA, Stone AR. Female urinary incontinence: the incidence, identification, and characteristics of detrusor instability. *Neurourol Urodyn.* 1984;3:235.

Weidner AC, Barber MD, Visco AC, et al. Pelvic muscle electromyography of levator ani and external anal sphincter in nulliparous women and women with pelvic floor dysfunction. *Am J Obstet Gynecol.* 2000;183:1390.

Winters JC, Dmochowski RR, Goldman HB, et al. Urodynamic studies in adults: AUA/SUFU guideline. *J Urol.* 2012;188:2464.

Yi YA, Keith CG, Graziano CE, et al. Strong correlation between standing cough test and 24-hour pad weights in the evaluation of male stress urinary incontinence. *Neurourol Urodyn.* 2020;39:319.

10

Female Sexual Function and Dysfunction: Assessment and Treatment

Erika L. Kelley, Roya L. Rezaee, and Sheryl A. Kingsberg

CHAPTER OUTLINE

INTRODUCTION

Sexual health is an important component of a woman's well-being. Evidence suggests that healthy sexual functioning is a fundamental component of a woman's sense of self and quality of life. Diminished sexual function has been found to correlate with advancing age, menopause, and economic and health problems (Cabral et al., 2013; Ornat et al., 2013). Sexual dysfunction is associated with poorer mental health and reduced vitality and social function, as well as relationship problems and undiagnosed medical conditions (Biddle et al., 2009). Sexual problems are highly prevalent in women in the United States: about 40% have sexual concerns, and nearly 12% report sexual distress (Shifren et al., 2008). Sexual functioning is best approached from a biopsychosocial perspective. There are different types of sexual dysfunction, and treatment typically is individualized and tailored to the diagnosis and to the psychological, physical, and medical etiological factors.

The World Health Organization (WHO) stipulated that the maintenance of sexual health is the physician's responsibility (WHO, 2000). In 2001, the US Surgeon General, in his Call to Action to promote sexual health as one of the goals of Healthy People 2010, described the role of health care professionals and the need for better education and preparation (Office of the Surgeon General, 2001). For these concerns to be addressed, health care professionals must understand what constitutes functional sexuality. Unfortunately, there is a culturally-driven difficulty in determining normal sexual functioning (Parish et al., 2019b). Moreover, sexual medicine is not given a high priority in medical education, which leaves many providers uncomfortable. This discomfort, ultimately, is an obstacle to competency. Additionally, many patients are unaware of, or have misconceptions about, sexual dysfunction and treatment and are hesitant to discuss these problems with their providers. This also contributes to the underdiagnosis and undertreatment of female sexual dysfunction. However, patients prefer for their health care providers to initiate conversations about their sexual health (Kingsberg et al., 2019).

This chapter will offer the provider a working knowledge of the evolving theoretical models to describe a healthy sexual response, as well as an understanding of the neurobiology of sexual function. Additionally, a framework for assessment, diagnosis, and management of sexual dysfunction in women will be outlined and will include surgical and medical conditions that can contribute to the development of sexual dysfunction.

MODELS OF FEMALE SEXUAL RESPONSE

Several models have been put forth to demonstrate the female sexual response. The female sexual response was first described by Masters and Johnson (1966) as a linear model of discrete events in which excitement always precedes arousal and then is followed by orgasm and resolution (Fig. 10.1). This model then was modified by Kaplan (1979) and Leif (1977) independently to a triphasic model that emphasized desire (and neurobiology) as a critical stage of the sexual response, in contrast to physiologic genital arousal.

In the late 1990s, Basson added her intimacy-based, nonlinear model to help explain the multifactorial character of the

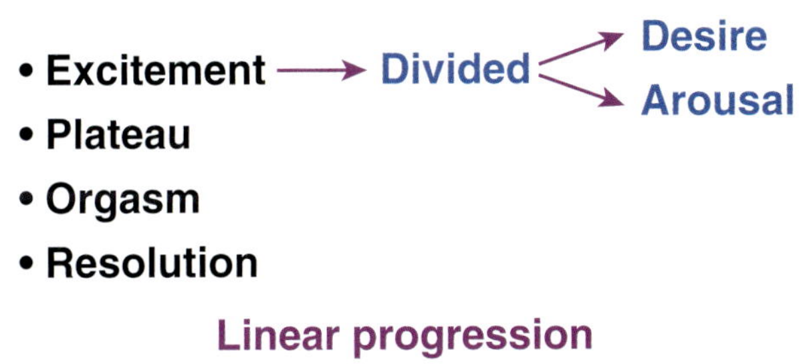

Fig. 10.1 Human sexual response: classic models. (From Masters WH, Johnson VE. *Human Sexual Response*. Boston, MA: Little Brown; 1966; Kaplan HS. Disorders of Sexual Desire and Other New Concepts and Techniques in Sex Therapy. *The New Sex Therapy*. Vol 2. New York: Bruner/Meisel U; 1979; Leif H. Inhibited sexual desire. *Med Aspects Hum Sex*. 1977;7:94.)

female sexual response. This model includes the interplay of emotional intimacy, sexual stimuli, psychological factors, and relationship satisfaction. This model also introduces the concept of receptive (or responsive) desire, the idea that arousal often precedes desire, and that women often begin a sexual encounter from a position of sexual neutrality (Basson, 2001). It encompasses the impact of biologic and nonbiologic factors on a woman's sexual response like motivation, interpersonal issues, cultural and religious beliefs, partner health, relationship quality, past sexual abuse, and distractions. These theoretical models of sexual response may reflect the variation that women experience in sexuality. This was demonstrated by The Nurses' Sexuality Study, in which nurses were asked to endorse the model that best fit their response (Sands & Fisher, 2007). Approximately 33% endorsed the Masters and Johnson model, 33% endorsed Kaplan's models, and 33% endorsed Basson's model. Of note, the women who had sexual concerns were more likely to endorse Basson's model of sexual response.

Sexual function is best considered through the lens of a biopsychosocial model (Fig. 10.2). This is an integrative, evolving model that reflects fluctuations in a woman's physical health, mental health, neurochemical balance, sociocultural factors, and interpersonal issues. It highlights that sexual function is multifactorial, and that a multidisciplinary treatment approach to sexual dysfunction is often indicated. Biological (e.g., use of medications, physical health, neurobiological factors, and endocrine functioning), psychological (e.g., depression, sexual performance anxiety, and body image), interpersonal (e.g., relationship functioning, communication skills, and history of sexual abuse), and sociocultural (e.g., religious beliefs about sex and reproduction, and gender norms) all may affect sexual function and should be assessed (Althof et al., 2005; Rosen & Barsky, 2006).

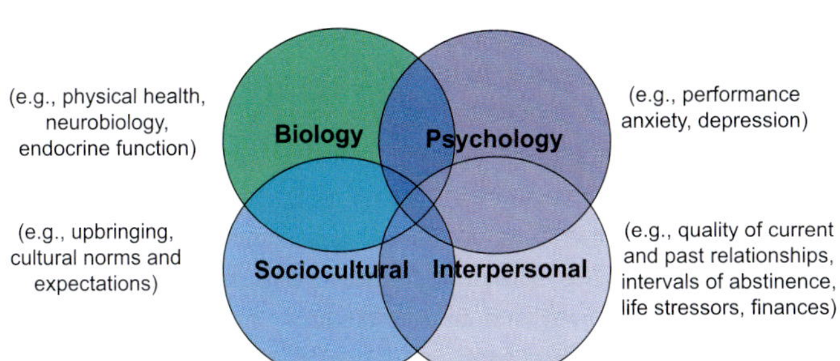

Fig. 10.2 Biopsychosocial model of female sexual response. (Modified from Kingsberg SA, Rezaee RL. Hypoactive sexual desire in women. *Menopause*. 2013;20:1284.)

PHYSIOLOGY

Female sexual response is partly determined by neurobiological factors, including hormonal and neurochemical influences in the brain and signaling between the central nervous system (CNS) and erogenous zones (e.g., genitalia). Sexual response is thought to be influenced by excitatory and inhibitory pathways in the brain, involving the hypothalamus and limbic system affecting both excitatory and inhibitory mechanisms, and the cortex and midbrain affecting inhibitory mechanisms. Excitatory factors include dopamine and melanocortins (believed to influence attention to sexual stimuli and desire), as well as norepinephrine and oxytocin (believed to influence sexual arousal). Inhibitory factors include serotonin (thought to control satiety), opioids (believed to manage sexual rewards), and endocannabinoids (thought to promote sedation) (Kingsberg et al., 2015; Pfaus, 2009). Research, largely based on animal models, indicates that the balance or summation of inhibitory and excitatory signals determines an individual's sexual response. This has been referenced as the "sexual tipping point" (Perleman, 2009). It is believed that hypoactive sexual desire disorder (HSDD) may result from hypofunctional excitatory factors, hyperfunctional inhibitory factors, or both. Imaging research showed that women with HSDD had higher activation in the medial frontal gyrus and right inferior gyrus (areas involved in attentional control of stimuli and response inhibition) than those without sexual dysfunction, providing support for hyperfunctional inhibition in women with HSDD (Arnow et al., 2009).

Furthermore, it is believed that the reward circuitry of the brain, involving the hypothalamus and basal ganglia that influence goal-directed and stimulus-directed behaviors, is a major determinant of sexual response. The prefrontal cortex exerts cognitive influence on sexual response by evaluating the reward value of a stimulus to encourage or discourage a behavior. Multiple other neurobiologic factors determine sexual response, such as attentional processes.

Sexual arousal is a normal physiologic response occurring in anticipation of, and during, sexual activity. Genital arousal occurs because of increased activity in the central and peripheral nervous system in response to physical (genital and nongenital) and nonphysical stimuli. The physiologic pathway of arousal in women is an intricate neurobiologic process that is not fully understood. The female sexual anatomy includes the mons pubis; the vulva, including the labia majora, labia minora, interlabial space, and clitoris; and the inner genitalia, including the vestibule, periurethral glans and vagina, uterus, fallopian tubes, and ovaries (Salonia et al., 2010). The cycle of arousal is initiated by genital vasocongestion driven by increased sympathetic nervous system activity. The vulva swell, exposing the introitus; the vagina lengthens and dilates; the outer third of the vagina tightens; the clitoris increases in length and diameter; and the uterus rises above the levator plate. Stimulation of the pelvic nerves induces smooth muscle relaxation and decreases the resistance within the arteries, leading to increased blood flow to the clitoris. This blood flow results from active neurogenic dilation of the sinusoidal blood spaces, which causes the corpora cavernosa of the clitoris to become engorged, and the clitoris becomes progressively more prominent. It has been noted that the vulvar structures become engorged, but they do not become erect, because the thinner tunica in women does not trap venous blood, and it therefore pools with persistent inflow and outflow (Basson, 2003). In addition, vaginal lubrication occurs as a result of increased pressure in the capillaries of the genital vasculature and transudation of fluid through the subepithelium of the vaginal walls. Secretions are a combination of androgen-dependent glands of the vulva releasing mucin and aquaporin channels in the vaginal mucosa releasing a transudate of blood serum. Extragenital changes associated with arousal include nipple erection, skin flushing, and increases in heart rate, blood pressure, and respiration rate (Parish et al., 2016).

It is likely that nitric oxide (NO), vasoactive intestinal peptide (VIP), and acetylcholine (ACh) play significant roles in sexual arousal (Meston & Frolich, 2000). Most of what we understand about their roles in female sexual excitement and response comes from studies of penile erection and sexual biology in animal models. Sexual stimulation releases NO from the vascular endothelium, which stimulates the release of guanylate cyclase, which in turn converts guanosine triphosphate into cyclic guanosine monophosphate (Salonia et al., 2010). This stimulates smooth muscle relaxation in the penile arteries and corpora cavernosum, causing blood flow to the penis. VIP and ACh also have been shown to relax smooth muscle and increase blood flow in the penis in animal models.

Before orgasm, physical changes occur, including tumescence, color change in the labia minora, lubrication, and relaxation of smooth muscles in the vaginal wall. Orgasm occurs with the release of contraction-producing agents (e.g., serotonin and oxytocin), leading to rhythmic contractions of the levator plate, uterus, and vagina, and multiple orgasms may occur if stimulation continues. The pelvic muscles repetitively contract in varying degrees of intensity and duration across women; for some women, contractions are not perceived. There is no current consensus regarding the brain regions activated during orgasm. Following orgasm, heart rate, respiration, and blood pressure immediately decrease, and detumescence, decongestion, and discontinuation and reabsorption of excess lubrication occurs (Parish et al., 2016). The time required for resolution to take place varies among women.

FEMALE SEXUAL DISORDERS

The International Society for the Study of Women's Sexual Health (ISSWSH) has published a process of care (POC) document outlining recommendations for the identification and management of sexual problems in women and describing nomenclature for female sexual dysfunction, including dysfunction in the domains of sexual desire, arousal, orgasm, and sexual pain (Parish et al., 2019a). The sexual dysfunction subtypes characterized in the POC include HSDD, female sexual arousal disorders (FSADs), persistent genital arousal disorder, female orgasmic illness syndrome, and genitopelvic pain penetration dysfunction. The POC nomenclature departs from the American Psychiatric Association's Diagnostic and Statistical Manual of Mental Disorders, Fifth Edition (DSM-5; APA, 2013), which combines desire and arousal problems into one condition (female sexual interest/arousal disorder). ISSWSH retained the separation of desire and arousal disorders in part because of research supporting the distinction between HSDD and FSAD (McCabe et al., 2016; Parish et al., 2016). In addition, whereas desire and arousal dysfunction can be comorbid, treatment of sexual dysfunction is often targeted toward the primary sexual problem. The ISSWSH POC nomenclature also differs from the DSM-5 definition of genitopelvic pain/penetration disorder (a classification combining vaginismus and dyspareunia) by including, in their classification of genitopelvic pain penetration dysfunction, difficulties associated with genital contact beyond intercourse, and hypertonicity or overactivity of the pelvic floor muscles with or without genital contact. The ISSWSH and International Consultation for Sexual Medicine nomenclature and definitions are presented in Box 10.1.

Sexual dysfunction is characterized by persistent difficulties in a domain of sexual function (desire, arousal, or orgasm) or by sexual pain that is persistent (i.e., at least 3 months' duration and occurring with ≥75% of sexual experiences) and accompanied by personal or interpersonal distress (e.g., bother, concern, unhappiness). The dysfunction must not be better accounted for by another psychiatric disorder or due exclusively to the direct physiologic effects of a substance or gynecologic or general medical condition (Table 10.1). Each disorder is further subtyped into lifelong versus acquired and generalized versus situational. Sexual problems may co-occur (McCabe et al., 2016), and the best approach for clinical practice is to identify the most problematic or primary issue and focus initial treatment there.

Hypoactive Sexual Desire Disorder

ISSWSH has also published a POC document for the identification and management of HSDD (Clayton et al., 2018). HSDD is defined as any of the following symptoms experienced for 6 or more months in duration: lack of motivation for sexual activity manifested by either (1) reduced or absent spontaneous desire (e.g., sexual thoughts, fantasies) or (2) reduced or absent responsive desire to erotic cues and stimulation or inability to maintain desire; and/or loss of desire to initiate or participate in sexual activity, including behavioral responses such as avoidance, not secondary to a sexual pain disorder. The loss of desire must include clinically significant personal distress that includes frustration, grief, incompetence, loss, sorrow, or worry (Parish et al., 2019). Decreased sexual desire is associated with negative effects, such as poor self-image, mood instability, depression, and strained relationships with partners (Biddle et al., 2009; Kingsberg, 2014).

The prevalence of HSDD is difficult to determine because it varies depending on the population surveyed and methodology used. Segraves and Woodard (2006) suggested that, if the

BOX 10.1 Classifications of Female Sexual Disorders

Hypoactive Sexual Desire Disorder

Presence of any of the following for a minimum of 6 months:

1. Lack of motivation for sexual activity as manifested by either
   a. Reduced or absent spontaneous desire (sexual thoughts or fantasies)
   b. Reduced or absent responsive desire to erotic cues and stimulation or inability to maintain desire or interest through sexual activity
2. Loss of desire to initiate or participate in sexual activity, including behavioral responses such as avoidance of situations that could lead to sexual activity, that is not secondary to sexual pain disorders

And is combined with clinically significant personal distress that includes frustration, grief, incompetence, loss, sadness, sorrow, or worry.

Female Sexual Arousal Disorder

Female cognitive arousal disorder: Characterized by the distressing difficulty or inability to attain or maintain adequate mental excitement associated with sexual activity as manifested by problems with feeling engaged or mentally turned on or sexually aroused, for a minimum of 6 months.

Female genital arousal disorder:

1. Characterized by the distressing difficulty or inability to attain or maintain adequate genital response, including vulvovaginal lubrication, engorgement of the genitalia, and sensitivity of the genitalia associated with sexual activity, for a minimum of 6 months
2. Disorders related to either/or:
   a. Vascular injury or dysfunction
   b. Neurologic injury or dysfunction

Persistent Genital Arousal Disorder

Characterized by the persistent or recurrent, unwanted or intrusive, distressing feelings of genital arousal or being on the verge of orgasm (genital dysesthesia), not associated with concomitant sexual interest, thoughts, or fantasies, for a minimum of 6 months.

May be associated with:

1. Limited resolution, no resolution, or aggravation of symptoms by sexual activity with or without aversive or compromised orgasm
2. Aggravation of genital symptoms by certain circumstances
3. Despair, emotional lability, catastrophization, or suicidality

Inconsistent evidence of genital arousal during symptoms

Female Orgasm Disorders

Characterized by the persistent or recurrent, distressing compromise of orgasm frequency, intensity, timing, or pleasure associated with sexual activity for a minimum of 6 months:

1. Frequency: orgasm occurs with reduced frequency (diminished frequency of orgasm) or is absent (anorgasmia)
2. Intensity: orgasm occurs with reduced intensity (muted orgasm)
3. Timing: orgasm occurs either later (delayed orgasm) or earlier (spontaneous or premature orgasm) than desired by the woman
4. Pleasure: orgasm occurs with absent or reduced pleasure (anhedonic orgasm, pleasure dissociative orgasm disorder)

Female Orgasmic Illness Syndrome

Characterized by the peripheral or central aversive symptoms that occur before, during, or after orgasm not related, *per se*, to a compromise of orgasm quality.

Genitopelvic Pain Penetration Dysfunction

Persistent or recurrent difficulties with one or more of the following:

1. Vaginal penetration during intercourse
2. Marked vulvovaginal or pelvic pain during genital contact
3. Marked fear or anxiety about vulvovaginal or pelvic pain in anticipation of, during, or as a result of genital contact
4. Marked hypertonicity or overactivity of pelvic floor muscles with or without genital contact

(Modified from Parish SJ, Hahn SR, Goldstein SW, et al. The International Society for the Study of Women's Sexual Health Process of Care for the identification of sexual concerns and problems in women. *Mayo Clin Proc.* 2019;94:842.)

TABLE 10.1 Examples of Psychiatric and General Health Problems that May Affect Sexual Function

General Health	Examples
Urogynecologic problems	Urinary tract infections, pelvic organ prolapse, urinary and fecal incontinence
Gynecologic problems	Pelvic pain, fibroids, unpredictable bleeding, oral contraceptive pills, vulvovaginal atrophy, postpartum period, breastfeeding, sexually transmitted infections, endometriosis, vulvar dermatoses, vulvodynia/vestibulodynia
Endocrine problems	Diabetes mellitus, thyroid disorders, hyperprolactinemia
Chronic illness	Cancer, psoriasis, rheumatoid arthritis, degenerative arthritis, hypertension, coronary artery disease, neurologic conditions, chronic pain
Malignancy/treatment	Mastectomy, gynecologic/colorectal surgery, pelvic radiation
Psychiatric problems	
Mood disorders	Major depression, bipolar depression
Anxiety disorders	
Psychotic illness	

(Modified from Parish SJ, Hahn SR, Goldstein SW, et al. The International Society for the Study of Women's Sexual Health Process of Care for the identification of sexual concerns and problems in women. *Mayo Clin Proc.* 2019;94:842.)

population studied were restricted to those reporting frequent problems with desire, then the prevalence of HSDD would be between 5.4% and 13.6%. The Prevalence of Female Sexual Problems Associated with Distress and Determinants of Treatment Seeking survey included a validated measure to evaluate more than 31,000 women over the age of 18 (Shifren et al., 2008). In this study, 8.9% of women 18 to 44 years of age, 12.3% of women 45 to 64 years of age, and 7.4% of women 65 years of age or older had low desire and distress. The Women's International Study of Health and Sexuality included women 20 to 70 years of age from the United States and Europe. It indicated that the prevalence of HSDD in the United States was 14% for premenopausal women,

9% in naturally menopausal women, 26% in surgically menopausal women 20 to 49 years of age, and 14% in surgically menopausal women 50 to 70 years of age (Leiblum et al., 2006).

Identifying the etiology of diminished desire can be challenging for both the patient and the clinician. Desire is a compilation of drive, expectations, beliefs, and motivation and is affected by the interactions of sex steroids and neurotransmitters. Laboratory testing is not typically indicated for identification of HSDD. Declining levels of androgens parallel increasing age and contribute to the decline in sexual desire, arousal, and orgasm. Women achieve peak androgen production in their mid-20s and gradually lose circulating testosterone and the adrenal preandrogens in an age-dependent fashion. By the time women reach their 60s, testosterone levels are half of what they were before age 40 years. Menopause has long been assumed to result in a decreased libido because of the decline in ovarian testosterone production. This is particularly true for women who experience a sudden loss of testosterone accompanying a surgical or chemical menopause (Kingsberg et al., 2020). Longitudinal studies suggest that relationship factors and other nonbiological changes have a stronger impact on overall desire than menopause alone (Hayes & Dennerstein, 2005). Many medications can cause sexual side effects (Table 10.2). It is critical to distinguish between various components of desire because treatments can vary based on which components have been impaired.

Although testosterone plays a role in drive, motivation, and sexual sensation, it is important to understand that there is little correlation between HSDD and serum androgen levels, and so they should not be used as a diagnostic measure of sexual dysfunction (Clayton et al., 2018; Davis et al., 2005). A global consensus position statement on the use of testosterone therapy for women describes recommendations regarding assessment of, and treatment using, testosterone based on empirical evidence and expert opinion (Davis et al., 2019). According to the statement, there is no cutoff blood level for measuring circulating androgen to diagnose sexual dysfunction. However, use of direct assays to measure testosterone in clinical practice is considered appropriate to exclude high baseline concentrations and supraphysiologic concentrations during treatment. Direct assays to measure total and free testosterone are unreliable in the female range, but liquid/gas chromatography and tandem mass spectrometry can be used to measure total testosterone with high accuracy and reproducibility (Davis et al., 2019).

Female Sexual Arousal Disorders

ISSWSH defines two subtypes of FSAD. Female cognitive arousal disorder is characterized by persistent or recurrent impairment or absence of mental excitement associated with sexual activity (i.e., feeling engaged, mentally turned on, or sexually aroused). Female genital arousal disorder is characterized by persistent or recurrent impairment or absence of physiologic responsiveness (i.e., vulvovaginal lubrication, and engorgement and sensitivity of the genitalia including the clitoris) to sexual stimulation. The inability to attain or maintain this cognitive or genital sexual responsiveness and the resulting marked personal or interpersonal distress is central to the diagnosis. Symptoms last for 6 months or more in duration. Difficulty with arousal may be associated with pain and avoidance of sexual contact. FSAD should not be diagnosed in cases where difficulties with arousal are attributed to insufficient stimulation. Conditions of vulvovaginal atrophy, infection, or inflammation, or vulvar or vaginal inflammatory disorders, vestibulodynia, and clitorodynia should be ruled out (see Parish et al., 2019).

Estimates of the prevalence of FSAD are difficult to determine, especially given changes in nomenclature over time and the common lack of assessment of associated distress or impairment. Prevalence estimates from studies on female arousal and lubrication problems ranged from 6% to 28% (Lewis et al., 2010; Parish et al., 2016). The rate of lubrication difficulties is 50% or greater, although the role of genitourinary syndrome of menopause is not commonly accounted for in prevalence studies (McCabe et al., 2016; Parish et al., 2019b).

Conditions and risk factors associated with FSAD include hormonal (e.g., decreased estrogens, diabetes, menopause), neurologic (e.g., central or peripheral nervous system disorders such

TABLE 10.2 Medications Associated with Sexual Dysfunction

Psychoactive medications	SSRIs, SNRIs, antipsychotics, barbiturates, benzodiazepines, tricyclic antidepressants, lithium, MAOIs, antiepileptics
Antihypertensive and cardiovascular medications	Lipid-lowering agents, digoxin, β blockers, α blockers, diuretis, calcium channel blockers, clonidine, hydrochlorothiazide, statins, methyldopa
Hormones	Antiandrogens (flutamide, spironolactone), progestins, oral contraceptives, GnRH agonists, estrogens, combined hormonal contraceptives, tamoxifen, aromatase inhibitors
Anticonvulsants	Carbamazepine, phenytoin, primidone
Pain medication	Nonsteroidal antiinflammatory drugs, opioids
Antihistamines and H2 receptor blockers	
Narcotics	
Amphetamines, weight loss agents	
Steroids	
Chemotherapeutic agents	
Immunosuppressants	

SSRIs, Selective serotonin reuptake inhibitors; *SNRIs*, serotonin-norepinephrine reuptake inhibitors; *MAOIs*, monoamine oxidase inhibitors; *GnRH*, gonadotropic-releasing hormone.

(Modified from Kingsberg S, Althof SE. Evaluation and treatment of female sexual disorders. *Int Urogynecol J.* 2009;20:S33.)

as multiple sclerosis), vascular (e.g., metabolic conditions including diabetes, obesity, hypertension, coronary artery disease), infectious (e.g., urinary tract, vulvar, vaginal), inflammatory (e.g., lichen planus or sclerosus, contact dermatitis), iatrogenic (e.g., pelvic irradiation and surgery), psychiatric (e.g., anxiety, depression), and psychological (e.g., negative cognitive pattern, relationship conflict) factors (Parish et al., 2019b).

Persistent genital arousal disorder, a rarer condition with no known prevalence estimates, is characterized by persistent or recurrent distressing and unwanted or intrusive feelings of genital arousal or being on the verge of orgasm that is not associated with concomitant sexual desire. Diagnosis is currently based on expert opinion, and further research is warranted on this condition and its treatment (Parish et al., 2016; Parish et al., 2019b).

Female Orgasm Disorders

Orgasm is defined as a "variable transient peak sensation of intense pleasure creating an altered state of consciousness, usually accompanied by involuntary, rhythmic contractions of the pelvic striated circumvaginal musculature, often with concomitant [vaginal], uterine and anal contractions, and myotonia that resolves the sexually induced vasocongestion [sometimes only partially], usually with an induction of well-being and contentment" (Meston et al., 2004). The ISSWSH POC defines female orgasm disorders as persistent or recurrent distressing compromise in orgasm frequency, intensity, timing (delayed or premature), and/or pleasure. Two rarer conditions, pleasure dissociative orgasm disorder and female orgasmic illness syndrome (central or peripheral aversive symptoms occurring before, during, or after orgasm that are not related to orgasm quality compromise), are currently based on expert opinion and require further research.

The cause of orgasmic dysfunction is likely multifactorial, making the prevalence difficult to evaluate, but the prevalence has been reported as 3.4% to 5.8% using the DSM-based classification of female orgasm disorder (Shifren et al., 2008). Etiologic and risk factors contributing to orgasm disorders include excitatory and inhibitory imbalances (described previously), psychosocial issues, organic factors (e.g., genital mutilation, medication, complications from genital surgery), or partner sexual dysfunction (Parish et al., 2016). Women demonstrate variability in the intensity and type of stimulation required for orgasm. Many women can attain orgasm with a specific form of sexual stimulation (e.g., manual or oral) or with a specific partner. Penetrative intercourse is not a reliable way for many women to achieve orgasm because many women require clitoral stimulation to reach orgasm.

Sexual Pain Disorders

The ISSWSH POC describes genitopelvic pain penetration dysfunction as persistent or recurrent difficulties with vaginal penetration during intercourse, and/or marked pelvic or vulvovaginal pain during genital contact, fear or anxiety about vulvovaginal/pelvic pain, and/or hypertonicity or overactivity of pelvic floor muscles with or without genital contact. Pain can occur with initial penetration, deep penetration or thrusting, or noncoital genital contact. Rates of genitopelvic pain penetration dysfunction vary across studies, in part because of varying definitions used, with a meta-analysis indicating that the incidence of painful intercourse ranges between 8% and 22% (Latthe et al., 2006).

Sexual pain likely has multiple etiologies with interdependent psychological and biological contributors. Even when an anatomic or organic cause is found, there is typically considerable stress and anxiety that maintain the pain and promote a continued avoidance of intercourse and negative sexual expectations. This cycle of pain results in a loss of desire and arousal, which perpetuate the problem. Sexual pain is considered to be a common problem over the life span of women, largely because of the multiple potential causes (Table 10.3). The International Society for the Study of Vulvovaginal Disease (ISSVD), ISSWSH, and the International Pelvic Pain Society (IPPS) published a 2015 consensus document describing nomenclature and classification of persistent vulvodynia (idiopathic chronic vulvar pain) and vulvar pain conditions, and such pain conditions are described elsewhere (Bornstein et al., 2016; Pukall et al., 2016). Factors potentially associated with these pain conditions include genetics, hormonal factors, comorbidities and other pain syndromes (e.g., irritable bowel syndrome), inflammation, and musculoskeletal factors, as well as neurological (e.g., neuroproliferation), psychosocial (e.g., depression), and structural factors (e.g., perineal descent).

TABLE 10.3 Causes of Sexual Pain

Condition	Examples
Superficial	
Anatomic variations	Congenital anomalies, labial hypertrophy, urethral diverticulum
Vulvovaginal atrophy	Estrogen deficiency, radiation
Injury or trauma	Childbirth-related, surgery, female circumcision
Inflammation or infection	Vulvar, vaginal, cervical, lower urinary tract
Generalized vulvodynia	
Vestibulodynia/vulvar vestibulitis syndrome	
Vulvar dystrophies	Lichen sclerosus, lichen planus
Inadequate lubrication/dryness	
Deep	
Endometriosis	
Myofascial pelvic pain	Hypertonus of levator muscles
Interstitial cystitis	
Infection	Cervical, uterine, lower urinary tract
Uterine fibroids	
Adhesions	Prior surgery, prior infection
Prolapse disorders	Uterine, vaginal apex, vaginal wall/bladder/rectum
Uterine position variations	Retroflexed, retroverted
Adnexal pathology	Ovarian/tubal cyst or neoplasm
Intestinal and/or rectal pathology	Irritable bowel, inflammatory bowel, dermatitis, fissure, prolapse
Other	
Psychological problems	Depression, anxiety, body image issues, stress
History of sexual abuse or negative experiences	

VARIABLES THAT CAN AFFECT SEXUAL FUNCTION

Pregnancy and the Postpartum Period

Pregnancy and childbirth are central periods in many women's lives. Although sexuality during pregnancy and the postpartum period has been insufficiently researched using validated sexual function questionnaires, data show that sexual function is altered, and that many factors may contribute to this. At 12 weeks postpartum some common issues include marital dissatisfaction, sexual pain, fatigue, and depression (De Judicibus & McCabe, 2002). Just as during other periods in a woman's life, during pregnancy and the postpartum period, women who were more satisfied with their relationships reported higher sexual function and satisfaction and greater frequency of activity than women who were less satisfied (Wittig et al., 2008).

Low desire during pregnancy and the postpartum period is not unusual, and it is well-known that desire fluctuates during pregnancy, typically decreasing in the third trimester (Lowenstein et al., 2013; Wallwiener et al., 2017). Women report worsened sexual function, including diminished sexual satisfaction, during pregnancy, which often persists for 6 to 12 months postpartum. Sexual desire during the first trimester may be lowered because of nausea, vomiting, and breast tenderness. During the third trimester, sexual activity may be less comfortable owing to the physical changes associated with pregnancy. Furthermore, although 80% to 93% of women have resumed intercourse at 12 weeks postpartum, a longitudinal study found that 34.8% of women were at risk for sexual dysfunction at 4 months postpartum (Wallwiener et al., 2017). At 6 months, 18% to 30% of women still may be experiencing sexual problems, including sexual pain (Rogers et al., 2009). Fatigue commonly is reported to contribute to loss of desire, infrequent activity, and lack of enjoyment, and fatigue and its impact continues well past 6 months.

Obstetrical events such as massive hemorrhage, preeclampsia, sepsis, and uterine rupture lead to significant changes in sexual health and well-being in women who experience these morbidities. For some, it is the physical complications of such events, whereas for others, it is a loss of interest and a fear of conceiving (Watersone et al., 2003). Body image has a variable impact on sexual function. It has been correlated positively with the highest sexual function prepregnancy, but it also has been shown to decline between the first and third trimesters, is the lowest postpartum, and remains low until 6 months postpartum (Pauls et al., 2008).

Childbirth negatively affects a woman's sexual function through physical trauma, such as perineal laceration and pudendal neuropathy. These effects can be temporary or enduring. Pain caused by perineal trauma can lead to problems with intercourse. Women who have an episiotomy complain of increased pain and delayed sexual relations compared with women who deliver over an intact perineum. Overall, sexual pain with intercourse is reported in about 41% to 67% of women 2 to 3 months after birth (Handa, 2006). Persistent sexual pain is associated strongly with operative vaginal delivery and severity of the perineal trauma. Women who experience high-order perineal lacerations demonstrate less desire to engage in sexual activities, such as touching and stroking, and are more likely to experience a delay in return to sexual activity at 6 months postpartum (Brubaker et al., 2008). Women who have fourth-degree perineal tears are much more likely to report pain with intercourse than women who did not experience lacerations at birth (Signorello et al., 2001).

The impact of the route of delivery and the resulting effects on long-term pelvic floor health continue to be investigated. In addition to the potential of causing perineal lacerations, vaginal birth has been implicated in damage to the innervation of the pelvic floor. Compression or stretch injury that occurs during delivery leads to neuropathy of the pudendal nerve, which can lead to urinary and anorectal incontinence and pelvic organ prolapse (POP). Birth may cause or worsen previously existing hypertonicity of the pelvic floor or trigger points. Spasm induced by contraction of the muscles can cause referred pain or irritative symptoms throughout the path of the pudendal nerve and adjacent structures. Because the pudendal nerve mediates some of the reflex pathways of the inherent female sexual response, the damage can result in physiologic causes of female sexual dysfunction.

This neuropathic injury may be less likely to occur when cesarean section is performed before the onset of labor, by avoiding direct perineal trauma and pudendal neuropathy. Evidence regarding the supposed protective benefits of scheduled cesarean section, however, remains inconsistent (Leeman & Rogers, 2012). The National Institutes of Health State-of-the Science Conference on Cesarean Delivery on Maternal Request indicated that, by 6 months postpartum, there is no difference in overall sexual function based on route of delivery alone, although they recognized that anal sphincter tears may be a risk factor for fecal incontinence, and that vaginal delivery is a risk factor for severe perineal lacerations (NIH Consensus SC Statement, 2006). Data using validated sexual health questionnaires suggest that women who undergo cesarean delivery have an elevated risk of sexual dysfunction that is not related to sexual pain. Any protective effect of caesarean delivery on sexual function appears to be limited to the early postnatal period and is related to the absence of perineal injury (Leeman & Rogers, 2012).

There is evidence that breastfeeding reduces a woman's sexual desire and frequency of intercourse. This may result from several factors, including decreased vaginal lubrication from high levels of prolactin (interfering with hypothalamic feedback to the ovary and decreased estrogen, which can contribute to vaginal dryness and atrophy); leaking milk; nipple sensitivity and discomfort with the potential erotic feelings from breastfeeding as a result of oxytocin production leading to a sense of sexual arousal and orgasm; and sleep disturbances that contribute to fatigue, exhaustion, and partner isolation. Finally, postnatal depression and emotional lability are related inversely to sexual enjoyment, interest, and activity. The use of selective serotonin reuptake inhibitor (SSRI) medications can compound this problem because they are commonly associated with female sexual dysfunction (Leeman & Rogers, 2012).

Genitourinary Syndrome of Menopause

Genitourinary syndrome of menopause (GSM) includes physical changes and symptoms associated with estrogen deficiency from the menopausal transition and affects more than 50% of postmenopausal women. GSM consists of vulvovaginal dryness, irritation, or burning; sexual pain; and urinary symptoms (urgency, dysuria, or recurrent urinary tract infection). GSM is associated with impaired sexual function; dyspareunia, or sexual pain, is considered the most bothersome symptom. Treatment of GSM may resolve sexual problems in postmenopausal women. Current pharmacologic treatments for GSM include vaginal hormone therapy as creams, inserts, or rings; selective estrogen-receptor modulators; and vaginal laser therapy, which is a potential option that needs more long-term safety and efficacy data (Faubion et al., 2017; NAMS 2017 Hormone Therapy Positive Statement Advisory Panel, 2017).

ISSWSH published an expert consensus panel review of the role of androgens in the treatment of GSM, summarizing evidence for efficacy of hormonal treatment (e.g., vaginal dehydroepiandrosterone [DHEA], ospemiphene, local vaginal estrogens for sexual pain because of GSM) (Simon et al., 2018). The North American Menopause Society and ISSWSH published a document with recommendations for GSM management in women with or at high risk for breast cancer (Faubion et al., 2018). These documents should be reviewed by providers to appropriately counsel patients regarding local hormone therapy, particularly as patients may have concerns about cancer risk with hormone therapy because of early public misconceptions (Kingsberg et al., 2019).

Pelvic Floor Disorders

Myofascial Pelvic Pain. The International Urogynecological Association and International Continence Society published a joint report on terminology for sexual health associated with pelvic floor dysfunction in women, which can be a useful tool in standardizing assessment in this field (Rogers et al., 2018). Various terms have been used to describe hypertonus disorders of the pelvic floor, including pelvic floor dysfunction, levator ani syndrome, pelvic floor tension myalgia, pelvic floor myofascial pain, pelvic floor spasm, and shortened pelvic floor (Fitzgerald & Kotarinos, 2003a). Although the mechanism of pelvic floor dysfunction is incompletely understood, one description of myofascial pain or pelvic floor hypertonicity is a disorder in which pain is attributed to short, tight, tender pelvic floor muscles in which trigger points are present. The pain or irritative symptoms are typically localized and may occur in the pelvis, vulva, bladder, and rectum. As the trigger points persist, the muscles weaken and over time, the surrounding muscle groups become affected, and more distant areas, such as the buttocks, thighs, and abdomen, become involved (Fitzgerald & Kotarinos, 2003b). It has also been argued that pelvic floor muscles can stretch and weaken from factors such as childbirth, aging, and increased stress leading to hypertonicity, ultimately contributing to strain on pelvic connective tissues and pelvic floor dysfunction (Wallace et al., 2019). Pelvic floor muscle hypertonus has been associated with interstitial cystitis, provoked vestibulodynia, and generalized vulvodynia and sexual pain.

The hypertonus can be a result of pain or injury, but also can be the origin of pain. Childbirth, surgery, chronic low back or hip pain, pelvic pain, recurrent vaginitis, bladder infections, dysmenorrhea, constipation or irritable bowel, neuromuscular and inflammatory disorders, chronic pain syndromes, and anxiety can all be underlying etiologies. Many women without obvious organic disease such as positive urine cultures, vaginitis, or adnexal pathology may find that their clinicians are unable to find the cause of their symptoms. This may be attributed to a lack of recognition or a lack of understanding that this diagnosis can be a cause of sexual pain or sexual dysfunction. A thorough history and directed physical examination will uncover myofascial pelvic pain as a possible cause of sexual pain. Treatment involves validating the presence of pain even in the absence of clear pathology and using a multidisciplinary approach to resolve the identified aspects of the sexual dysfunction. Pelvic floor physical therapy involving pelvic floor surface electromyography biofeedback is used to treat hypertonus of the pelvic floor that is related to vulvar pain syndromes and can be effective when accompanied by a home exercise plan. A variety of manual therapy techniques such as myofascial release, myofascial trigger point release, visceral manipulation, and neural mobilizations, as well as therapeutic exercises such as pelvic floor retraining with dilators, core stabilization, and behavioral therapies are used to benefit women with sexual pain problems. The use of botulinum toxin injected into the levator muscles is demonstrating an additive effect to pain treatment.

Overactive Bladder. Overactive bladder is characterized by urinary urgency, with or without urinary incontinence; urinary frequency; and nocturia. It often is associated with detrusor overactivity. These symptoms can be quite bothersome and have a negative effect on the overall quality of life and daily functioning. The fear of leakage during sexual stimulation and intercourse, as well as the urgency and frequency felt afterward interfere with a woman's enjoyment of sexual relations (Coyne et al., 2007). Treatment with antimuscarinic drugs and neuromodulation significantly improved sexual frequency, desire, lubrication, orgasm, satisfaction, pain, and total Female Sexual Function Index (FSFI) 6-item scoring when study populations were compared at baseline and then 3 to 12 months posttreatment (Pauls et al., 2007a; Rogers et al., 2008).

Incontinence and Prolapse. Stress urinary incontinence (SUI), anal incontinence (AI), and POP have been shown to have deleterious effects on the overall health of women because they affect their social, occupational, physiologic, physical, domestic, and sexual well-being. Studying the effects of pelvic floor disorders on sexual function has been challenging because of the inherent differences between the populations studied, the characterization of sexual dysfunction, and the use of condition nonspecific questionnaires or unvalidated measures. These issues likely do not allow for the full capture of the effects of these disorders on sexual satisfaction and function and so have resulted in conflicting data when evaluating women with pelvic floor disorders. Add to this uncertainty the fact that sexual function is multidimensional, and it is easy to understand why there is confusion. Overall, however, the effects of urinary incontinence and POP do appear to adversely affect sexual relationships and seem to depend on the severity of the symptoms, because the more significant the disorder, the greater the decrease in sexual activity and satisfaction (Tannenbaum et al., 2006). Pelvic floor symptoms are associated with poorer genital body image and reduced arousal, infrequent orgasm, and sexual pain (Handa et al., 2008; Zielinski et al., 2012). Women's self-reported body image and degree of bother from POP are associated with sexual function (Lowenstein et al., 2009). Urinary incontinence has been associated with low libido, vaginal dryness, and sexual pain, whereas low-stage or asymptomatic POP has not been associated with sexual complaints (Handa et al., 2004). Coital incontinence can occur with vaginal penetration in women with stress incontinence, and with orgasm in women with overactive bladder, and can be problematic for some women.

AI commonly occurs in combination with POP and SUI and is associated with high-order perineal lacerations, median episiotomy, and operative vaginal delivery. Posterior compartment POP can lead to defecatory dysfunction and sexual dysfunction. Detachments of the rectovaginal fascia from the perineal body can result in perineal descent, which has been associated with a variety of defecatory disorders, including constipation, rectal pain, and fecal incontinence (Bartolo et al., 1983). Pudendal neuropathy also can be a result of perineal descent separate from rectocele or laceration findings and has been identified as a mechanism for fecal incontinence. Fecal incontinence of solid stool is recognized as the most severe form of AI, and this type of AI, as well as the presence of symptoms of depression related to fecal incontinence, appears most likely to be correlated with poor sexual function (Pauls et al., 2007b). Other studies similarly indicate that women with AI, compared with those without, experience similar rates of sexual activity but poorer sexual function (Cichowski et al., 2013; Zielinski, et al., 2012). Furthermore, although many women who have had anal sphincter repair for AI still report some incontinence, repair does not correlate well with improved sexual function (Trowbridge et al., 2006). Clinicians who care for women with anal sphincter disruption and AI know how devastating these injuries can be. More studies are needed to demonstrate the sexual dysfunction and relationship interference that is associated with AI.

Surgery and Sexual Dysfunction. Few studies are designed specifically to address the role of pelvic surgery on benign gynecologic issues and female sexual dysfunction. Surgery to resolve gynecologic indications may improve, worsen, or have no effect on sexual function. Pelvic and sexual pain caused by endometriosis or adhesions may be improved after surgery or hormonal therapies (Ferrero et al., 2005). Touching the vaginal apex with the penis, digit, or cotton swab may be painful posthysterectomy owing to focal pain even after the vaginal cuff has healed. Treatment depends on the location and suspected origin of the pain. Lidocaine, antidepressants, and even surgical resection for focal areas of neuropathic pain and recurrent disease may be helpful. Physical therapy can be particularly effective for pain because of levator spasm (Lamvu et al., 2004).

Meta-analyses indicate that, after surgery for SUI, 55.5% of women experienced no change in sexual function, 31.9% experienced improved sexual function, and 13.1% experienced lowered sexual function (Jha et al., 2012), and that surgery for POP was not associated with changes in sexual function (Jha & Gray, 2015). However, most studies evaluating sexual function after surgery for SUI are small, retrospective, do not use validated questionnaires, and do not include women who were not sexually active. Often there is no assessment of baseline preoperative sexual function, and ultimately a variety of anti-incontinence and reconstructive surgeries are included. Assessment of sexual activity and function (including pain), as well as partner status and function, before and following surgical treatment is important to evaluate surgical outcomes (Rogers et al., 2018). Traditionally, maintenance of sexual function was mostly directed at the question of preserving vaginal length and caliber to allow for adequate mechanics of sexual intercourse. Vaginal anatomy assessed in this fashion previously had been found to not correlate well with sexual function, and still appears to be unrelated to sexual satisfaction (Weber et al., 1995; Weber et al. 2000). Multiple studies employing condition-specific questionnaires such as the Pelvic Organ Prolapse/Urinary Incontinence Sexual Function Questionnaire (PISQ) have demonstrated that surgical treatment for POP and SUI improves sexual function in both physical and partner domains, with coital incontinence and subsequent embarrassment resolving in the majority of women (Jha et al., 2007; Rogers et al., 2006; Roos et al., 2014). Most prospective studies demonstrate that a woman's overall sexual function improves after prolapse surgery because of a resolution of the preexisting sexual pain and the interference of the bulge (Handa et al., 2007).

Evidence indicates that surgery for POP also can lead to deterioration of sexual function. Reasons for this are sexual pain, fear of causing damage to the surgical result, new symptoms, and a disappointing result of surgery (Roos et al., 2014). The complaint of pain postoperatively is not uncommon, and typically a period of 6 months is considered to be an adequate time for symptom resolution, given that surgery often requires vaginal dissection. Prediction of who may develop postsurgery pain disorders is difficult (Rogers et al., 2018). *De novo* sexual pain can occur in up to 26% of women, particularly after posterior colporrhaphy and levator plication (Cundiff & Fenner, 2004). However, another study of sexual function following vaginal surgery found that *de novo* sexual pain rates were low (5% at 12 months and 10% at 24 months) (Lukacz et al., 2016). Prolapse repair that does not include plication of the levator musculature may have a lower rate of new-onset sexual pain. The new-onset pain also may be a result of a tight vaginal introitus. The general guidelines for tightness of "two to three fingerbreadths" may not be ideal when partner anatomy and vulvovaginal atrophy are taken into consideration. Finally, synthetic graft material may have an impact on sexual pain by affecting the pliability and movement of the vagina. Controversy now surrounds some of these grafts because they have been implicated in vaginal exposure and scarring that contributes to pain.

Few published studies have evaluated the effect on sexual function of anal sphincteroplasty for AI, and even fewer in which validated scales measuring function and fecal incontinence were used. Additionally, it is difficult to assess sexual function in this population of women, because their surgeries often are performed as a combination of procedures for SUI and POP. Some studies demonstrate that, postsurgery, women report improvement in sexual sensation and satisfaction and that they are more able emotionally to engage in sexual activity (Lewicky et al., 2004). Other authors report no difference in sexual functioning in the anal repair group compared with controls. Finally, there are insufficient data on the impact of female genital cosmetic surgery (e.g., vaginoplasty) on sexual function and on the efficacy or safety of these procedures (Rogers et al., 2018).

SCREENING AND EVALUATION FOR SEXUAL DYSFUNCTION

Identification and Assessment of a Sexual Problem

Numerous barriers interfere with communication of sexual function concerns during the typical patient–provider interaction. This lack of discussion regarding sexual concerns may be the result of incomplete or insufficient knowledge on the part of the provider, poor training in the taking of an effective sexual history, a perceived lack of office time, a limited number of approved pharmacologic options for treatment, and an uneasiness on both the part of the patient and the provider about discussing such issues. Societal stigma surrounding sexual health and misconceptions about conditions and available treatment options are also patient barriers to sexual health care (Kingsberg et al., 2019).

The ISSWSH POC outlines an algorithm for identification and assessment of HSDD (Clayton et al., 2018) and other sexual problems (Parish et al., 2019). Sexual problem identification should be a routine part of primary care, and the review of systems can be an ideal time to elicit such concerns. Postpartum and postsurgical periods and visits related to menopause must include such a discussion and assessment as well. The first step to identification is to "just ask" with direct questioning, which is critical to uncovering a patient's sexual concerns and also signals that the provider is comfortable with discussing sexual health (Kingsberg, 2006; Parish et al., 2019). Studies have shown that patients are reluctant to initiate discussions about sexual concerns but very much want their provider to set up the environment and open dialogue for this to take place (Berman et al., 2003b). Use of a ubiquity statement can be useful in normalizing the topic. A basic three-question screening algorithm can be efficient, starting by asking "are you currently involved in a sexual relationship?" If the patient answers "yes," the provider can ask "with men, women, or both?" and "do you have any sexual concerns or pain with sex?" If the patient answers "no," then the provider can ask "do you have any sexual concerns you would like to discuss or that have contributed to lack of sexual behavior?" (Kingsberg, 2006). The PEARLS mnemonic can also be a useful model to guide clinician's screening and assessment of sexual function in an empathic manner (Box 10.2). When conducting the interview, the four-step model outlined in the ISSWSH POC can provide a useful structure for eliciting the patient's story, for naming and reframing the sexual problem, and for empathic witnessing. It is important to ask about the gender of partners and also not to assume that the woman's sexual behavior is limited to one partner, or even to an identified partner or spouse.

BOX 10.2 PEARLS Mnemonic

P	The clinician should acknowledge that this is a Partnership and that they are in it together
E	The clinician should express understanding and Empathy
A	The clinician should address any unmet expectation with an Apology
R	The clinician should acknowledge any patient suffering or dissatisfaction with Respect/Reflection/Reinforcement
L	The clinician should Legitimize the patient's concerns and feelings
S	The clinician should Support the patient and emphasize that he or she will continue to work with the patient

This is a useful structure for the health professional to use to demonstrate empathy and therefore open communication, which ultimately will allow for a productive interview with the patient.
(From Cohen-Cole S. The Medical Interview: The Three Function Approach. St. Louis: Mosby-Yearbook, 1991.)

Evaluation of an Identified Problem

Many evaluation tools for sexual dysfunction are complicated and more useful in the research setting than in clinical practice. The sexual assessment questions listed in Box 10.3 can be used for an initial evaluation of sexual problems. The Brief Sexual Symptoms Checklist (Box 10.4) also may prove to be helpful. These questions help to identify the specific components of the sexual problem and address the patient's perceptions of the problem and the time line, context, and other health problems that might contribute to a sexual complaint. When choosing a questionnaire, clinicians must consider what they are hoping to accomplish and whether they are looking for generic or condition-specific information. A validated scale developed for use by clinicians not specifically trained in sexual medicine is the Decreased Sexual Desire Screener (Clayton et al., 2009). It is a five-question self-administered survey designed to help identify generalized acquired HSDD in pre- and postmenopausal women in a time-efficient manner. Another validated tool for office-based use is the Brief Profile of Female Sexual Function (Rust et al., 2007). This seven-question self-administered

BOX 10.3 Suggested Sexual Assessment Questions

How does the patient describe the problem?
How long has the problem been present?
Was the onset sudden or gradual?
Is the problem specific to a situation or partner or is it generalized?
Were there any precipitating events?
Are there problems in the women's primary sexual relationship or any sexual relationship?
Are there current life stressors that might be contributing to sexual problems?
Is there guilt, depression, or anger that is not being directly acknowledged?
Are there physical problems such as pain?
Are there problems in desire, arousal, or orgasm?
Is there a history of physical, emotional, or sexual abuse?
Does the partner have any sexual problems?

(Modified from Basson R. Taking the sexual history, part 1: eliciting the sexual concerns of your patient in primary care. *Med Aspects Human Sex.* 2000;1:13.)

BOX 10.4 Brief Sexual Symptoms Checklist for Women

Please answer the following questions about your overall sexual function

1. Are you satisfied with your sexual function?
   ___ Yes
   ___ No
   If no, then please continue.
2. How long have you been dissatisfied with your sexual function?

3a. The problem(s) with your sexual function is (mark one or more):
   ___ 1 little or no interest in sex
   ___ 2 decreased genital sensation (feeling)
   ___ 3 decreased vaginal lubrication (dryness)
   ___ 4 reaching orgasm
   ___ 5 pain during sex
   ___ 6 other

3b. Which problem is the most bothersome (circle)? 1 2 3 4 5 6

4. Would you like to talk about it with your doctor?
   ___ Yes
   ___ No

(Reprinted from Hatzichristou D, Rosen RC, Derogatis LR, et al. Recommendations for the clinical evaluation of men and women with sexual dysfunction. *J Sex Med*. 2010;7:337.)

survey measures the loss of sexual desire and function in postmenopausal women with HSDD. The PISQ is a short-form 12-question, self-administered test that measures sexual function in women with POP or urinary incontinence (Rogers et al., 2003). The FSFI six-item questionnaire is a brief self-reporting instrument to assess the areas of desire, arousal, orgasm, and pain (Isidori et al., 2010). The original 19-item version often is used in clinical trials. The Female Sexual Distress Scale is a 13-item scale assessing sexually related personal distress (DeRogatis et al., 2008).

Once a problem is identified, it is important to specify the components of the sexual response that are compromised (see Box 10.3). Answers to these sexual assessment questions not only assist in isolating the key issues and etiologies, but also serve as a basis for treatment considerations. A thorough sexual history should focus on identifying modifiable factors. Medical issues that commonly affect sexual function and are potentially modifiable include: use of oral contraceptives, presence of depression, use of medications including antidepressants, GSM, and partner sexual problems.

Physical examination may be pursued to uncover the physiologic and anatomic factors involved with the sexual complaint (Table 10.4). This is especially important for vulvar and vaginal pain to identify contributing factors such as inflammatory, hormonal, and neurologic factors. Pelvic, including vulvovaginal, examination is warranted for women with pelvic pain to help locate the source of the pain (e.g., GSM). It is imperative that the clinician pay special attention to the physical features relevant to sexual function. Each step of the examination should be explained to and agreed on by the patient, particularly in the woman with a history of abuse or pain. The provider should attempt to increase the patient's sense of control and establish a foundation of trust. The examination also is an opportunity to provide education about anatomy and female sexual function, especially if a partner is with her. No standard laboratory tests or imaging studies are required for the initial evaluation of a patient with a normal exam. For sexual pain, testing for sexually transmitted infections or other vaginal pathogens may be useful, and other tests (e.g., of thyroid function and prolactin levels) may be indicated.

Advanced-level practitioners' assessment of sexual dysfunction should aim to clarify specifiers of the condition (e.g., generalized versus situational), identify potential other biopsychosocial factors contributing to the dysfunction, and assess for less common female sexual dysfunction. Comorbid behavioral health factors should also be assessed, including history of sexual abuse and other trauma, body image concerns, relationship conflict, and

TABLE 10.4 Components and Related Conditions of a Thorough Physical Examination in Sexual Function Assessment

Component	Related Conditions
Inspection of the External Genitalia	
Vulvar skin turgor, thickness, color, integrity	Lichen sclerosus/planus, atrophy, dermatologic conditions
Pubic hair amount and distribution	Androgen level
Labial abnormalities	Previous circumcision, congenital variations, clitoromegaly
Cotton swab test	Pain mapping of the vulva and vestibule
Hymenal and urethral abnormalities	Urethral diverticulum
Vestibular, skene, and bartholin glands	Cyst, abscess
Speculum exam	Vaginal pH, genital cultures, examination for atrophy, assessment for prolapse
Digital/Bimanual Examination	
Introital assessment	Contraction, relaxation ability, tenderness, scarring
Bladder, urethra, levator muscles, pelvic floor assessment	Assess for muscle tension, tenderness, and trigger points
Uterus and adnexa, rectovaginal exam	Palpate for mobility, fixed cul-de-sac, uterosacral ligaments, vaginal length, prolapse
General Examination	
Evaluation of signs of anemia, endocrine disorders	Pallor, hair loss, thyromegaly, striae
Evaluate for signs of connective tissue disease	Dryness consistent with Sjogren syndrome, scleroderma, other
Evaluation for disabilities of movement or sensation	Neurologic disease, arthritis, chronic pain, fibromyalgia

(Modified from Phillips NA. The clinical evaluation of dyspareunia. *Int J Impot Res*. 1998;10:S177.)

psychiatric conditions (particularly depression, anxiety, and substance use disorders) (Bancroft et al., 2003). At any stage of the assessment, referral for specialized assessment and/or treatment should be considered and necessitates a practitioner's awareness of the availability of such resources.

TREATMENT OF FEMALE SEXUAL DISORDERS

Treatment of sexual concerns demands an individualized approach. Core-level treatment includes education about patient factors affecting sexual function (e.g., side effects of medication, aging) and about communication skills and the importance of foreplay and vibrators, and instruction on use of personal lubricants, moisturizers, and local hormone therapy for GSM-associated sexual pain. Referral to a specialist may be indicated. The patient is much more likely to comply with referral if the clinician verbalizes both the nature of the problem and the use of a specialist or multidisciplinary approach.

Hypoactive Sexual Desire Disorder

Treatment of lifelong HSDD or situational low desire includes education and counseling (e.g., around normative sexual function) and referral to a specialist if indicated (Clayton et al., 2018). For generalized, acquired HSDD, education (i.e., on normative sexual functioning, personal sexual and medical history variables that may impact desire, and available treatment options in the context of patient's motivation for treatment) and management of potential modifying biopsychosocial factors (see Tables 10.1 and 10.2) are considered first- and second-line treatment strategies. Third-line treatment options depend on the menopausal status of the patient. For both pre- and postmenopausal women, sex therapy (including behavior therapy, cognitive behavioral therapy [CBT], and/or mindfulness) in individual, couples, or group format with a specialist may be indicated (Clayton et al., 2018; Kingsberg et al., 2017). Behavior therapy includes sensate focus exercises (a graded series of nondemand sensual touching exercises), communication skills training, and education. CBT can assist in educating patients about normal sexual function, anatomy, and physiology. CBT helps an individual navigate areas of poor communication skills and imbalanced expectations. It allows for more productive interactions and role playing that ultimately can lead to resolution of resentment, avoidant behavior, and conflict, resulting in better intimacy. Mindfulness CBT (MCBT) focuses on increasing nonjudgmental awareness of sensation and sexual response and awareness of the present moment during sexual activity.

For premenopausal women, two medications have been approved by the US Food and Drug Administration (FDA) to treat acquired, generalized HSDD. The first, flibanserin, is a multifunctional 5-HT_{2a}-receptor antagonist and $5HT_{1a}$-recepter agonist that is taken orally, daily, at bedtime (Katz et al., 2013). There is a risk evaluation and mitigation strategy associated with the risk of syncope and hypotension. Patients should be advised to discontinue alcohol use at least 2 hours before taking flibanserin, to avoid alcohol consumption until the day after administration, and to skip the daily dose if consuming three or more standard alcoholic drinks. Severe hypotension and syncope can occur when flibanserin is used in patients with hepatic impairment or when used with moderate or strong CYP3A4 inhibitors (Sprout Pharmaceuticals, 2019). The second, bremelanotide, is a cyclic 7-amino acid melanocortin receptor agonist and is self-administered on demand, via subcutaneous injection in the thigh or abdomen 45 minutes before intended sexual activity. Bremelanotide is a synthetic analog of α-melanocyte–stimulating hormone and is an agonist that activates the melanocortin receptors MC3-R and MC4-R in the CNS. The maximum recommended doses are one dose per 24 hours and up to eight doses per month (Simon et al., 2019).

Additional CNS agents have been used in the off-label treatment of HSDD in premenopausal women, including bupropion, buspirone, and combination therapies (e.g., testosterone with sildenafil, testosterone with buspirone, and bupropion with trazadone) (Clayton et al., 2018). Bupropion is an antidepressant that has been shown to have a moderate prosexual effect and is used to treat the sexual side effects of SSRIs. It has both dopamine and norepinephrine reuptake inhibition. There is also evidence for prosexual effects of buspirone, an anxiolytic that reduces serotonin inhibition and has been used to treat sexual side effects of SSRIs. Combination therapies are hypothesized to address different subgroups of HSDD (owing to diminished excitatory response to sexual cues versus owing to enhanced sexual inhibitory mechanisms).

For postmenopausal women, there are currently no FDA-approved medications to treat HSDD. However, research on flibanserin provides support for improvement in sexual desire when it is used in postmenopausal women (Simon et al., 2014). A global consensus position statement summarizes the efficacy of, safety evidence for, and guidance for the use of off-label testosterone therapy in women to treat HSDD (Davis et al. 2019). In doses that approximate physiological testosterone concentrations for premenopausal women, research shows that testosterone therapy is effective in the treatment of HSDD in both naturally and surgically postmenopausal women (Buster et al., 2005; Braunstein et al., 2005; Davis et al., 2019; Shifren et al., 2006). Presently, no testosterone product is approved by the FDA for the treatment of HSDD. Long-term safety concerns have stalled the FDA approval of topical testosterone therapy for postmenopausal women. According to the consensus position statement (Davis et al., 2019), off-label prescribing of an approved male formulation is reasonable when hormone concentrations are maintained in the physiologic female range, where an appropriate approved female preparation is not available. Compounded "bioidentical" testosterone therapy or any preparation that results in supraphysiological concentrations of testosterone (e.g., pellets) is not recommended. Transdermal testosterone gels are FDA-approved for men and are used sometimes for women in an off-label fashion by reducing the amount applied to estimate what has been shown to be the effective dose in women (300 mcg/day). Baseline total testosterone concentration should be measured before initiation of testosterone treatment, with a repeat level evaluated 3 to 6 weeks after treatment initiation. Monitoring of response to treatment and for androgen excess via serum total testosterone levels should occur every 6 months, and testosterone treatment should be discontinued if no benefit is experienced by 6 months (Davis et al., 2019). Systematic reviews and meta-analyses have not shown benefit of systemic DHEA, a prohormone of testosterone, on female sexual dysfunction (Davis et al., 2019; Elraiyah et al., 2014).

Female Sexual Arousal Disorders

First, the clinician should identify which subtypes of FSAD may be present or overlapping (cognitive and/or genital). Current educational and psychological treatment options include learning to adequately attend to sexual sensations using masturbation and self-stimulation training alone or with one's partner and improving communication with one's partner to include frank discussions of what promotes romance and intimacy and what interferes. The use of erotica, fantasy, and sexual accessories such as adjunctive aids can be encouraged. Additional psychosocial contributing factors that should be addressed include cultural or religious factors affecting sexual guilt, stress, negative affect, and cognitive or attentional distractions during sexual activity (Kingsberg et al., 2017). MCBT and sensate focus approaches may improve sexual arousal, and MCBT can be particularly helpful for women who experience disconnection between their genital and subjective arousal levels (Brotto & Goldmeier, 2015).

Autogenic training is a psychophysiological relaxation technique with evidence for improvement in subjective and objective arousal (Stanton et al., 2018). Physiologic strategies employing phosphodiesterase inhibitors (sildenafil) have been studied in hopes of overcoming the problems of poor vasocongestion and blood flow, but engorgement did not conclusively result in subjective arousal (Berman et al., 2003a). However, there is evidence for improvements in sexual arousal in response to treatment with sildenafil citrate among women with medical conditions that are known to interfere with genital neurovascular substrates (e.g., diabetes, multiple sclerosis, or antidepressant use) (Leddy et al., 2012; Schoen & Bachmann, 2009).

Transdermal testosterone patch therapy is used off-label for treatment of low sexual arousal, with demonstrated effects on arousal from clinical trials (Davis et al., 2019). Systemic and locally administered estrogen therapy often helps postmenopausal women with FSAD resulting from GSM. GSM does not improve over time, as do the vasomotor symptoms of low estrogen states and the menopausal transition. Because of the complexity and the possible side effects and risk factors associated with systemic estrogen usage, many patients and clinicians have opted for vaginally administered minimally absorbed estrogen, which has been shown to be effective and is FDA-approved for the treatment of sexual pain caused by vulvovaginal atrophy (see GSM section earlier).

The EROS Clitoral Therapy System is the only FDA-approved device currently available to treat female sexual dysfunction. It produces clitoral vascular congestion through a vacuum apparatus and is designed to help with arousal problems. It is prescription only but can be used in conjunction with manual vibrators and handheld massagers. Femprox is an alprostadil-based cream intended for the treatment of FSAD. Alprostadil (PGE1) is a naturally occurring potent vasodilator that has an important role in the regulation of blood flow to the female reproductive tract. In Femprox, it is combined with the skin penetration enhancer dodecyl 2-(NN-dimethylamino)propionate, which is an ester of *N,N*-dimethylalanine and dodecanol. Apomorphine is a dopamine agonist that has been used as a subcutaneous injection for the treatment of Parkinson disease and has been researched as an oral treatment for arousal disorder. Bupropion also has been found to improve sexual arousal in premenopausal women with HSDD (Segraves et al., 2004). Bremelanotide (FDA-approved for HSDD in premenopausal women) has demonstrated efficacy in treating FSAD but is not FDA-approved for this indication.

Female Orgasm Disorders

There is evidence that psychotherapy and education can improve orgasm dysfunction. Many women with orgasm disorder need to learn to become comfortable with their bodies and their sexual response, and this is achieved by altering negative perspectives and decreasing anxiety. Therapy techniques include directed masturbation (or masturbation training), sensate focus exercises, and systematic desensitization. Some of the most important things that a clinician can do are to educate women about the female sexual response, to give the woman permission to explore and understand her body, and to debunk the myths that contribute to the negativity directed at self-stimulation (Kingsberg et al., 2017). Women with acquired orgasm dysfunction need to undergo assessment for the possible contributions of health conditions and medications to their sexual concerns, and need to understand that orgasmic function can change with age. Treatment of orgasm disorder is partly determined by whether or not the orgasm dysfunction exists in the context of desire and/or arousal dysfunction. Many nonpharmacological techniques employed to treat sexual arousal disorders (sensate focus, MCBT, and training in use of vibrators, erotica, and other sexual enhancement products) can be used for orgasmic disorders as well.

Few pharmacologic options have been researched for the treatment of orgasm disorders. Studies of pharmacologic treatments have focused mainly on desire and arousal dysfunction, but many of these treatments (systemic estrogen and testosterone therapy, PDE5 inhibitors) have demonstrated improvements in orgasm as well (Kingsberg et al., 2017). A clinical trial also provided some evidence that oxytocin can improve orgasm (Magon & Kalra, 2011).

Sexual Pain Disorders

Treatment for sexual pain or genitopelvic pain penetration dysfunction likely warrants a sexual medicine specialist, often in conjunction with a pelvic floor physical therapist (Faubion & Rullo, 2015). In determining a treatment strategy, it is imperative that the clinician identify a broad differential diagnosis so that treatment can be directed appropriately at the underlying physiologic, anatomic, or psychological source of the pain. A careful and in-depth evaluation must take place. The pain must be identified by its character, initial onset, initiating and alleviating factors, duration, severity, impact on self and partner, and previous treatments. The examination contains a thorough inspection of the anatomy of the vulva and may or may not include a speculum if the patient can tolerate it. A cotton swab test of the vulvar vestibule and palpation of the pelvic floor musculature must be included. Collection of vaginal discharge for testing can take place if appropriate. It often helps to separate the location of sexual pain into categories: superficial (introital), pelvic (deep), and emotional. The ISSVD, ISSWSH, and IPPS 2015 consensus document describes terminology and classification of persistent vulvar pain and vulvodynia and outlines potential contributing and modifiable factors affecting such pain (Bornstein et al., 2016). Treatment is often individualized to the specific origin of the pain and to any related behavioral causes or repercussions. Patient counseling, education, and referral to a qualified therapist should be provided, as needed.

Nonpharmacologic approaches to addressing sexual pain include CBT, MCBT, pelvic floor physical therapy, and therapist-aided exposure psychotherapy. Pelvic floor physical therapy consists of manual therapy, psychoeducation, relaxation and breathing (re)training, local tissue sensitization, electromyographic biofeedback, and instructed, progressive use of vaginal dilators (Bergeron et al., 2010; Bergeron et al., 2015). Trigger point injections may be used (often as an adjunctive therapy to pelvic floor physical therapy) to address pain associated with pelvic floor hypertonicity and pelvic pain conditions (Bartley et al., 2019). Therapist-aided exposure therapy is particularly helpful for fear or anxiety-based genitopelvic pain/penetration difficulties, and consists of psychoeducation and a systematic, graded approach to genital contact and penetration using a dilator/dilator kit (van Lankveld et al., 2006).

CONCLUSION

It is well understood that providers of health care to women have a duty to promote patient well-being. Providing education about sexual health and function, addressing changes in sexual function, and evaluating and addressing sexual complaints must be part of the standard care that is given. The task of screening for sexual dysfunction requires knowledge of the complexity of the female sexual response and the factors that affect it. Viewing this process from a biopsychosocial perspective and treating patients in an individualized fashion via a multidisciplinary approach is likely to lead to more successful outcomes.

BIBLIOGRAPHY

Althof SE, Leiblum SR, Chevret-Measson M, et al. Psychological and interpersonal dimensions of sexual function and dysfunction. *J Sex Med.* 2005;2:793.

American Psychiatric Association. *Diagnostic and Statistical Manual of Mental Disorders: DSM-5.* 5th ed. Washington, DC: American Psychiatric Publishing; 2013.

Arnow BA, Millheiser L, Garrett A, et al. Women with hypoactive sexual desire disorder compared to normal females: a functional magnetic resonance imaging study. *Neuroscience.* 2009;158:484.

Bancroft J, Loftus J, Long JS. Distress about sex: a national survey of women in heterosexual relationships. *Arch Sex Behav.* 2003;32:193.

Bartley J, Han E, Gupta P, et al. Transvaginal trigger point injections improve pain scores in women with pelvic floor hypertonicity and pelvic pain conditions. *Female Pelvic Med Reconstr Surg.* 2019;25:392.

Bartolo DC, Read NW, Jarratt JA, et al. Differences in anal sphincter function and clinical presentation in patients with pelvic floor descent. *Gastroenterology.* 1983;85:68.

Basson R. Human sex-response cycles. *J Sex Marital Ther.* 2001;27:33.

Basson R. Taking the sexual history, part 1: eliciting the sexual concerns of your patient in primary care. *Med Aspects Human Sex.* 2000;1:13.

Basson R. Sexuality and sexual disorders. *Clin Updates Women's Healthcare.* 2003; 1:1.

Bergeron S, Corsini-Munt S, Aerts L, et al. Female sexual pain disorders: a review of the literature on etiology and treatment. *Curr Sex Health Rep.* 2015;7:159.

Bergeron S, Morin M, Lord MJ. Integrating pelvic floor rehabilitation and cognitive-behavioral therapy for sexual pain: what have we learned and where do we go from here? *Sex Relat Ther.* 2010;25:304.

Berman JR, Berman LA, Toler SM, et al. Safety and efficacy of sildenafil citrate for the treatment of female sexual arousal disorder: a double-blinded, placebo controlled study. *J Urol.* 2003;170:2333.

Berman L, Berman J, Felder S, et al. Seeking help for sexual function complaints: what gynecologists need to know about the female patient's experience. *Fertil Steril.* 2003;79:572.

Biddle AK, West SL, D'Alosio AA, et al. Hypoactive sexual desire disorder in postmenopausal women: quality of life and health burden. *Value Health.* 2009;12:763.

Bornstein J, Goldstein AT, Stockdale CK, et al. 2015 ISSVD, ISSWSH, and IPPS consensus terminology and classification of persistent vulvar pain and vulvodynia. *J Sex Med.* 2016;13:607.

Braunstein GD, Sundwall DA, Katz M, et al. Safety and efficacy of a testosterone patch for the treatment of hypoactive sexual desire disorder in surgically menopausal women: a placebo-controlled trial. *Arch Intern Med.* 2005;165:1571.

Brotto LA, Goldmeier D. Mindfulness interventions for treating sexual dysfunctions: the gentle science of finding focus in a multitask world. *J Sex Med.* 2015;12:1687.

Brubaker L, Handa VL, Bradley CS, et al. Sexual function 6 months after first delivery. *Obstet Gynecol.* 2008;111:1040.

Buster JE, Kingsberg SA, Aguirre O, et al. Testosterone patch for low sexual desire in surgically menopausal women: a randomized trial. *Obstet Gynecol.* 2005;105:944.

Cabral PU, Canário AC, Spyrides MH, et al. Determinants of sexual dysfunction among middle-aged women. *Int J Gynaecol Obstet.* 2013;120:271.

Cichowski SB, Komesu YM, Dunivan GC, Rogers RG. The association between fecal incontinence and sexual activity and function in women attending a tertiary referral center. *Int Urogynecol J.* 2013;24:1489.

Clayton AH, Goldfischer ER, Goldstein I, et al. Validation of the decreased sexual desire screener (DSDS): a brief diagnostic instrument for generalized acquired female hypoactive sexual desire disorder (HSDD). *J Sex Med.* 2009;6:730.

Clayton AH, Goldstein I, Kim NN, et al. The International Society for the Study of Women's Sexual Health process of care for management of hypoactive sexual desire disorder in women. *Mayo Clin Proc.* 2018;93:467.

Cohen-Cole S. *The Medical Interview: The Three Function Approach.* St. Louis: Mosby Yearbook; 1991.

Coyne KS, Margolis MK, Brewster-Jordan J, et al. Evaluating the impact of overactive bladder on sexual health in women: what is relevant? *J Sex Med.* 2007;4:124.

Cundiff GW, Fenner D. Evaluation and treatment of women with rectocele: focus on associated defecatory and sexual dysfunction. *Obstet Gynecol.* 2004;104:1403.

Davis SR, Baber R, Panay N, et al. Global consensus position statement on the use of testosterone therapy for women. *J Clin Endocrinol Metab.* 2019;104:4660.

Davis SR, Davison SL, Donath S, Bell RJ. Circulating androgen levels and self-reported sexual function in women. *JAMA.* 2005;294:91.

De Judicibus MA, McCabe MP. Psychological factors and sexuality of pregnant and postpartum women. *J Sex Res.* 2002;39:94.

DeRogatis L, Clayton A, Lewis-D'Agostino D, et al. Validation of the female sexual distress scale-revised for assessing distress in women with hypoactive sexual desire disorder. *J Sex Med.* 2008;5:357.

Elraiyah T, Sonbol MB, Wang Z, et al. The benefits and harms of systemic dehydroepiandrosterone (DHEA) in postmenopausal women with normal adrenal function: a systematic review and meta-analysis. *J Clin Endocrinol Metab.* 2014;99:3536.

Faubion SS, Larkin LC, Stuenkel CA, et al. Management of genitourinary syndrome of menopause in women with or at high risk for breast cancer: consensus recommendations from The North American Menopause Society and The International Society for the Study of Women's Sexual Health. *Menopause.* 2018;25:1.

Faubion SS, Rullo JE. Sexual dysfunction in women: a practical approach. *Am Fam Physician.* 2015;92:281.

Faubion SS, Sood R, Kapoor E. Genitourinary syndrome of menopause: Management strategies for the clinician. *Mayo Clin Proc.* 2017;92:1842.

Ferrero S, Esposito F, Abbamonte LH, et al. Quality of sex life in women with endometriosis and deep dyspareunia. *Fertil Steril.* 2005;83:573.

Fischman SH, Rankin EA, Soeken KL, Lenz ER. Changes in sexual relationships in postpartum couples. *JOGNN.* 1986;15:58.

Fitzgerald MP, Kotarinos R. Rehabilitation of the short pelvic floor. I: background and patient evaluation. *Int Urogynecol J Pelvic Floor Dysfunct.* 2003a;14:261.

Fitzgerald MP, Kotarinos R. Rehabilitation of the short pelvic floor. II: treatment of the patient with the short pelvic floor. *Int Urogynecol J Pelvic Floor Dysfunct.* 2003b;14:269.

Handa VL. Sexual function and childbirth. *Semin Perinatol.* 2006;30:253.

Handa VL, Cundiff GW, Change HH, Helzlsouer KJ. Female sexual function and pelvic floor disorders. *Obstet Gynecol.* 2008;111:1045.

Handa VL, Harvery L, Cundiff GW, et al. Sexual function among women with urinary incontinence and pelvic organ prolapse. *Am J Obstet Gynecol.* 2004;191:751.

Handa VL, Zyczynski HM, Brubaker L, et al. Sexual function before and after sacrocolpopexy for pelvic organ prolapse. *Am J Obstet Gynecol.* 2007;197:629.

Hatzichristou D, Rosen RC, Derogatis LR, et al. Recommendations for the clinical evaluation of men and women with sexual dysfunction. *J Sex Med.* 2010;7:337.

Hayes R, Dennerstein L. The impact of aging on sexual function and sexual dysfunction in women: a review of population based studies. *J Sex Med.* 2005;2:317.

Isidori AM, Pozza C, Esposito K, et al. The Female Sexual Function Index (FSFI): Development and validation of a 6-item version of the female sexual function index (FSFI) as a diagnostic tool for female sexual dysfunction. *J Sex Med.* 2010;7:1139.

Jha S, Ammenbal M, Metwally M. Impact of incontinence surgery on sexual function: a systematic review and meta-analysis. *J Sex Med.* 2012;9:34.

Jha S, Gray T. A systematic review and meta-analysis of the impact of native tissue repair for pelvic organ prolapse on sexual function. *Int Urogynecol J.* 2015;26:321.

Jha S, Moran P, Greenham H, Ford C. Sexual function following surgery for urodynamic stress incontinence. *Int Urogynecol J Pelvic Floor Dysfunct.* 2007;18:845.

Kaplan HS. Disorders of Sexual Desire and Other New Concepts and Techniques in Sex Therapy. *The New Sex Therapy*. Vol 2. New York: Bruner/Meisel U; 1979.

Katz M, DeRogatis LR, Ackerman R, et al. Efficacy of flibanserin in women with hypoactive sexual desire disorder: results from the BEGONIA trial. *J Sex Med.* 2013;10:1807.

Kingsberg SA. Taking a sexual history. *Obstet Gynecol Clin N Am.* 2006;33:535.

Kingsberg SA. Attitudinal survey of women living with low sexual desire. *J Women's Health (Larchmt).* 2014;23:817.

Kingsberg SA, Althof SE. Evaluation and treatment of female sexual disorders. *Int Urogynecol J.* 2009;20:S33.

Kingsberg SA, Althof S, Simon JA, et al. Female sexual dysfunction—medical and psychological Treatments, Committee 14. *J Sex Med.* 2017;14:1463.

Kingsberg SA, Clayton AH, Pfaus JG. The female sexual response: current models, neurobiological underpinnings and agents currently approved or under investigation for the treatment of hypoactive sexual desire disorder. *CNS Drugs.* 2015;29:915.

Kingsberg SA, Larkin LC, Liu JH. Clinical effects of early or surgical menopause. *Obstet Gynecol.* 2020;135:1.

Kingsberg SA, Schaffir J, Faught BM, et al. Female sexual health: Barriers to optimal outcomes and a roadmap for improved patient-clinician communications. *J Women's Health (Larchmt).* 2019;28:432.

Lamvu G, Robinson B, Zolnoun D, Steege JF. Vaginal apex resection: a treatment option for vaginal apex pain. *Obstet Gynecol.* 2004;104:1340.

Latthe P, Latthe M, Say L, et al. WHO systematic review of prevalence of chronic pain: a neglected reproductive health morbidity. *BMC Public Health.* 2006;6:177.

Leddy LS, Yang CC, Stuckey BG, et al. Influence of sildenafil on genital engorgement in women with female sexual arousal disorder. *J Sex Med.* 2012;9:2693.

Leeman LM, Rogers RG. Sex after childbirth: postpartum sexual function. *Obstet Gynecol.* 2012;119:657.

Leiblum SR, Koochaki PE, Rodenberg CA, et al. Hypoactive sexual desire disorder in postmenopausal women: US results from the Women's International Study of Health and Sexuality (WISHeS). *Menopause.* 2006;13:46.

Leif H. Inhibited sexual desire. *Med Aspects Hum Sex.* 1977;7:94.

Lewicky CE, Valentin C, Saclarides TJ. Sexual function following sphincteroplasty for women with third- and fourth-degree perineal tears. *Dis Colon Rectum.* 2004;47:1650.

Lewis RW, Fugl-Meyer KS, Corona G, et al. Definitions/epidemiology/risk factors for sexual dysfunction. *J Sex Med.* 2010;7:1598.

Lowenstein L, Gamble T, Sanses TV, et al. Sexual function is related to body image perception in women with pelvic organ prolapse. *J Sex Med.* 2009;6:2286.

Lowenstein L, Mustafa S, Burke Y. Pregnancy and normal sexual function. Are they compatible? *J Sex Med.* 2013;10:621.

Lukacz ES, Warren LK, Richter HE, et al. Quality of life and sexual function 2 years after vaginal surgery for prolapse. *Obstet Gynecol.* 2016;127:1071.

Magon N, Kalra S. The orgasmic history of oxytocin: love, lust, and labor. *Indian J Endocrinol Metab.* 2011;15:S156.

Masters WH, Johnson VE. *Human Sexual Response*. Boston, MA: Little Brown; 1966.

McCabe M, Sharlip ID, Atalla E, et al. Definitions of sexual dysfunctions in women and men: a consensus statement from the Fourth International Consultation on Sexual Medicine. *J Sex Med.* 2016;13:135.

McCabe M, Sharlip IR, Lewis R, et al. Incidence and prevalence of sexual dysfunction in women and men: A consensus statement from the Fourth International Consultation on Sexual Medicine 2015. *J Sex Med.* 2016;13:144.

McCoy NL. The McCoy Female Sexuality Questionnaire. *Qual Life Res.* 2000;9:739.

Meston CM, Frolich PE. The neurobiology of sexual function. *Arch Gen Psychiatry.* 2000;57:1012.

Meston CM, Levin RJ, Sipski ML, et al. Woman's orgasm. *Ann Rev Sex Res.* 2004;15:173.

NAMS 2017 Hormone Therapy Position Statement Advisory Panel. The 2017 hormone therapy position statement of The North American Menopause Society. *Menopause.* 2017;24:728.

NIH State-of-the Science Conference Statement on Cesarean Delivery on Maternal Request. *NIH Consensus SC Statements.* 2006;23:1.

Office of the Surgeon General (US); Office of Population Affairs (US). *The Surgeon General's Call to Action to Promote Sexual Health and Responsible Sexual Behavior.* Rockville, Maryland: Office of the Surgeon General (US); 2001. Available at: http://www.ncbi.nlm.nih.gov/books/NBK44216/. Accessed 12/12/12.

Ornat L, Martínez-Dearth R, Muñoz A, et al. Sexual function, satisfaction with life and menopausal symptoms in middle-aged women. *Maturitas.* 2013;75:261.

Parish SJ, Goldstein AT, Goldstein SW, et al. Toward a more evidence-based nosology and nomenclature for female sexual dysfunctions-Part II. *J Sex Med.* 2016;13:1888.

Parish SJ, Hahn SR, Goldstein SW, et al. The International Society for the Study of Women's Sexual Health Process of Care for the identification of sexual concerns and problems in women. *Mayo Clin Proc.* 2019;94:842.

Parish SJ, Meston CM, Althof SE, et al. Toward a more evidence-based nosology and nomenclature for female sexual dysfunctions-part III. *J Sex Med.* 2019;16:452.

Pauls RN, Marinkovic SP, Silva WA, et al. Effects of sacral neuromodulation on female sexual function. *Int Urogynecol J Pelvic Floor Dysfunct.* 2007;18:391.

Pauls RN, Occhino JA, Dryfhout VL. Effects of pregnancy on female sexual function and body image: a prospective study. *J Sex Med.* 2008;5:1915.

Pauls RN, Silva WA, Rooney CM, et al. Sexual function after vaginal surgery for pelvic organ prolapse and urinary incontinence. *Am J Obstet Gynecol.* 2007a;197:622.

Pauls RN, Silva WA, Rooney CM, et al. Sexual function following anal sphincteroplasty for fecal incontinence. *Am J Obstet Gynecol.* 2007b;197:618.

Perelman MA. The sexual tipping point: a mind/body model for sexual medicine. *J Sex Med.* 2009;6:629.

Pfaus JG. Pathways of sexual desire. *J Sex Med.* 2009;6:1506.

Phillips NA. The clinical evaluation of dyspareunia. *Int J Impot Res.* 1998;10:S117.

Pukall CF, Goldstein AT, Bergeron S. Vulvodynia: definition, prevalence, impact and pathophysiological factors. *J Sex Med.* 2016;13:291.

Rogers RG, Bachmann G, Jumadilova Z, et al. Efficacy of tolterodine on overactive bladder symptoms and sexual and emotional quality of life in sexually active women. *Int Urogynecol J Pelvic Floor Dysfunct.* 2008;19:1551.

Rogers RG, Borders N, Leeman L, Albers L. Does spontaneous genital tract trauma impact postpartum sexual function? *J Midwifery Women's Health.* 2009;54:98.

Rogers RG, Coates KW, Kammerer-Doak D, et al. A short form of the Pelvic Organ Prolapse/Urinary Incontinence Sexual Questionnaire (PISQ-12). *Int Urogynecol J.* 2003;14:164.

Rogers RG, Kammerer-Doak DN, Darrow A, et al. Does sexual function change after surgery for stress urinary incontinence and/or pelvic organ prolapse? A multicenter prospective study. *Am J Obstet Gynecol.* 2006;195:e1.

Rogers RG, Pauls RN, Thaker R., et al. An International Urogynecological Association (IUGA)/International Continence Society (ICS) joint report on the terminology for the assessment of sexual health of women with pelvic floor dysfunction. *Neurourol Urodyn* 2018;8:1.

Roos AM, Thakar R, Sultan AH, et al. The impact of pelvic floor surgery on female sexual function: a mixed quantitative and qualitative study. *BJOG.* 2014;121:92.

Rosen RC, Barsky JL. Normal sexual response in women. *Obstet Gynecol Clin North Am.* 2006;33:515.

Rosen R, Brown C, Heiman J, et al. The Female Sexual Function Index (FSFI): a multidimensional self-report instrument for the assessment of female sexual function. *J Sex Marital Ther.* 2000;26:191.

Rust J, DeRogatis L, Rodenberg C, et al. Development and validation of a new screening tool for hypoactive sexual desire disorder: The Brief Profile of Female Sexual Function (B-PSFS). *Gynecol Endocrinol.* 2007;23:638.

Rust J, Golombok S. The Golombok-Rust Inventory of Sexual Satisfaction (GRISS). *Br J Clin Psychol.* 1985;24:63.

Salonia A, Giraldi A, Chivers ML, et al. Physiology of women's sexual function: basic knowledge and new findings. *J Sex Med.* 2010;7:2637.

Sands M, Fisher MA. Women's endorsement of models of female sexual response; the nurses' sexuality study. *J Sex Med.* 2007;4:708.

Schoen C, Bachmann G. Sildenafil citrate for female sexual arousal disorder: a future possibility? *Nat Rev Urol.* 2009;6:216.

Segraves RT, Clayton A, Croft H. Bupropion sustained release (SR) for the treatment of hypoactive sexual desire disorder (HSDD) in nondepressed women. *J Sex Marital Ther.* 2004;27:303.

Segraves R, Woodard T. Female hypoactive sexual desire disorder. History and current status. *J Sex Med.* 2006;3:408.

Shifren JL, Davis SP, Moreau M, et al. Testosterone patch for the treatment of hypoactive sexual desire disorder in naturally menopausal women: results from the INTIMATE NM1 Study. *Menopause.* 2006;13:770.

Shifren JL, Monz BU, Russo PA, et al. Sexual problems and distress in United States women: prevalence and correlates. *Obstet Gynecol.* 2008;12:970.

Signorello LB, Harlow BL, Chekos AK, Repke JT. Postpartum sexual function and its relationship to perineal trauma: a retrospective study of primiparous women. *Am J Obstet Gynecol.* 2001;184:881.

Simon JA, Goldstein I, Kim NN. The role of androgens in the treatment of genitourinary syndrome of menopause (GSM): International Society for the Study of Women's Sexual Health (ISSWSH) expert consensus panel review. *Menopause.* 2018;25:837.

Simon JA, Kingsberg SA, Portman D, et al. Long-term safety and efficacy of bremelanotide for hypoactive sexual desire disorder. *Obstet Gynecol.* 2019;134:909.

Simon JA, Kingsberg SA, Shumel B, et al. Efficacy and safety of flibanserin in postmenopausal women with hypoactive sexual desire disorder: results of the SNOWDROP trial. *Menopause.* 2014;21:633.

Sprout Pharmaceuticals. *Addyi (flibanserin) Tablets, for Oral Use* [package insert]. Bridgewater, NJ: Sprout Pharmaceuticals, Inc.; 2019.

Stanton AM, Hizon G, Nichols LM, Meston CM. One session of autogenic training increases acute subjective sexual arousal in premenopausal women reporting sexual arousal problems. *J Sex Med.* 2018;15:64.

Symonds T, Boolell M, Quirk F. Development of a questionnaire on sexual quality of life in women. *J Sex Marital Ther.* 2005;31:385.

Tannenbaum C, Corcos J, Assalian P. The relationship between sexual activity and urinary incontinence in older women. *J Am Geriatr Soc.* 2006;54:1220.

Trowbridge ER, Morgan D, Trowbridge MJ, et al. Sexual function, quality of life and severity of anal incontinence after sphinctero-plasty. *Am J Obstet Gynecol.* 2006;195:1753.

van Lankveld JJ, ter Kuile MM, de Groot HE, et al. Cognitive-behavioral therapy for women with lifelong vaginismus: a randomized waiting-list controlled trial of efficacy. *J Consult Clin Psychol.* 2006;75:168.

Wallace SL, Miller LD, Mishra K. Pelvic floor physical therapy in the treatment of pelvic floor dysfunction in women. *Curr Opin Obstet Gynecol.* 2019;31:485.

Wallwiener S., Müller M, Doster A, et al. Sexual activity and sexual dysfunction of women in the perinatal period: a longitudinal study. *Arch Gynecol Obstet.* 2017;295:873.

Watersone M, Wolfe C, Hooper R, Bewley S. Postnatal morbidity after childbirth and severe obstetric morbidity. *BJOG.* 2003;110:128.

Weber AM, Walters MD, Piedmont MR. Sexual function and vaginal anatomy in women before and after surgery for pelvic organ prolapse and urinary incontinence. *Am J Obstet Gynecol.* 2000; 182:1610.

Weber AM, Walters MD, Schover LR, Mitchinson A. Vaginal anatomy and sexual function. *Obstet Gynecol.* 1995;86:946.

Wittig K, Santitila P, Alanko K, et al. Female sexual function and its associations with number of children, pregnancy and relationship satisfaction. *J Sex Marital Ther.* 2008;34:89.

World Health Organization. *Education and Treatment in Human Sexuality: The Training of Health Professionals. Report of a WHO meeting.* Albany, NY: Q Corporation; 2000.

Zielinski R, Miller J, Low LK, et al. The relationship between pelvic organ prolapse, genital body image, and sexual health. *Neurourol Urodyn.* 2012;31:1145.

11

Urodynamics: Indications, Techniques, Interpretation, and Clinical Utility

Mickey M. Karram and Ayman Mahdy

CHAPTER OUTLINE

INTRODUCTION TO URODYNAMICS

The term *urodynamics* means observation of the changing function of the lower urinary tract (LUT) over time. Specifically, urodynamic studies are a number of interactive diagnostic tests that can be used to obtain functional information about bladder filling, urine storage, and voiding.

To understand the fundamental value of urodynamics, one should realize that the female bladder responds similarly to a variety of pathologies. Symptoms do not always accurately reflect the physiologic state of the bladder. For example, a patient may feel that her bladder is full when it is nearly empty, or that her bladder is contracting when it is not. The validity of any urodynamic diagnosis is linked to the patient's symptoms and the reproduction of these symptoms during the testing session. To obtain the most accurate, clinically relevant interpretation of urodynamic studies, the urodynamicist should clearly understand LUT function and should correlate urodynamic data with other clinical information. Ideally, the urodynamicist should be the physician who takes the history, reviews the voiding diary, performs the physical examination, interprets other tests, explains the diagnosis, and develops a reasonable management plan.

Results of urodynamic investigations should be recorded in a way that can be communicated among physicians and other health care personnel. For this reason, the recommendations detailed in the standardization reports of the International Continence Society (ICS) should be followed (Schäfer et al., 2002).

Normal Bladder Physiology

A prerequisite to performing and interpreting a urodynamic study is having a full understanding of normal LUT function (see Chapter 3). During filling, a normal adult bladder should act as a low-pressure reservoir. It has the inherent ability of responding to filling (when done at a physiologic rate) with an almost imperceptible change in intravesical and detrusor pressure (P_{det}). This high compliance of the bladder is due primarily to its elastic and viscoelastic properties. During filling, the bladder outlet should be closed and remain closed even during increases in intraabdominal pressure. There is a gradual increase in urethral pressure during bladder filling contributed to in part by the striated sphincter of the urethra and perhaps also by smooth sphincteric elements as well. This can be detected by measuring urethral pressure but also can be seen on electromyography (EMG). The normal opening vesical pressure in an adult female bladder should be in the range of 2 to 6 cm H_2O, with it only increasing to approximately 10 cm H_2O at maximum capacity.

Bladder filling should be associated with appropriate sensation. Most women will feel a first sensation of bladder filling between 75 and 150 mL, feel an urge to void between 300 and 400 mL, and have a maximum capacity or strong desire to void between 400 and 700 mL. Although many factors are involved in the initiation of micturition in adults, it is intravesical pressure that creates the sensation of distention that is primarily responsible for the initiation of a normal voluntarily induced emptying of the bladder. This also involves inhibition of the striated sphincter of the urethra and an inhibition of all aspects of any spinal sympathetic reflexes evoked during filling. A decrease in outlet resistance occurs with adaptive shaping and funneling of the relaxed bladder outlet, leading to efficient voiding. Fig. 11.1 demonstrates a storage and micturition reflex in a neurologically intact female.

Functional Classification of Lower Urinary Tract Dysfunction

To be able to formulate the appropriate questions to be answered by a urodynamic study, the clinician must have a clear understanding of the possible or potential causes of symptoms. The functional classification of LUT dysfunction as proposed and popularized by Wein (1981) is a simple, clinically relevant way of classifying LUT dysfunction. Wein proposed that functional abnormalities of the LUT can be broadly divided into failure of the bladder to adequately store urine or failure of the bladder to adequately empty. Failure of the bladder to store urine results from bladder overactivity (involuntary contractions or decreased compliance), decreased outlet resistance (sphincter deficiency), heightened or altered sensation, or a combination of these various abnormalities. Failure of the bladder to empty results from decreased bladder contractility, increased outlet resistance, or a combination of both. Finally, a combined dysfunction of failure to store and empty is also potentially feasible.

To use a functional classification appropriately, there must be an understanding of the physiology of urine storage and voiding, as well as knowledge regarding the various disease states that can cause LUT dysfunction. The advantage of a simple classification such as this is that it helps to clarify treatment options for a given patient. Simply determining whether there is a problem with storage, emptying, or both, as well as assessing bladder and urethral (outlet) function, can commonly lead to a correct urodynamic diagnosis with institution of appropriate therapy. The clinician should always focus on the urodynamic finding that is most likely to explain a particular symptom, and, more importantly, how a particular finding may

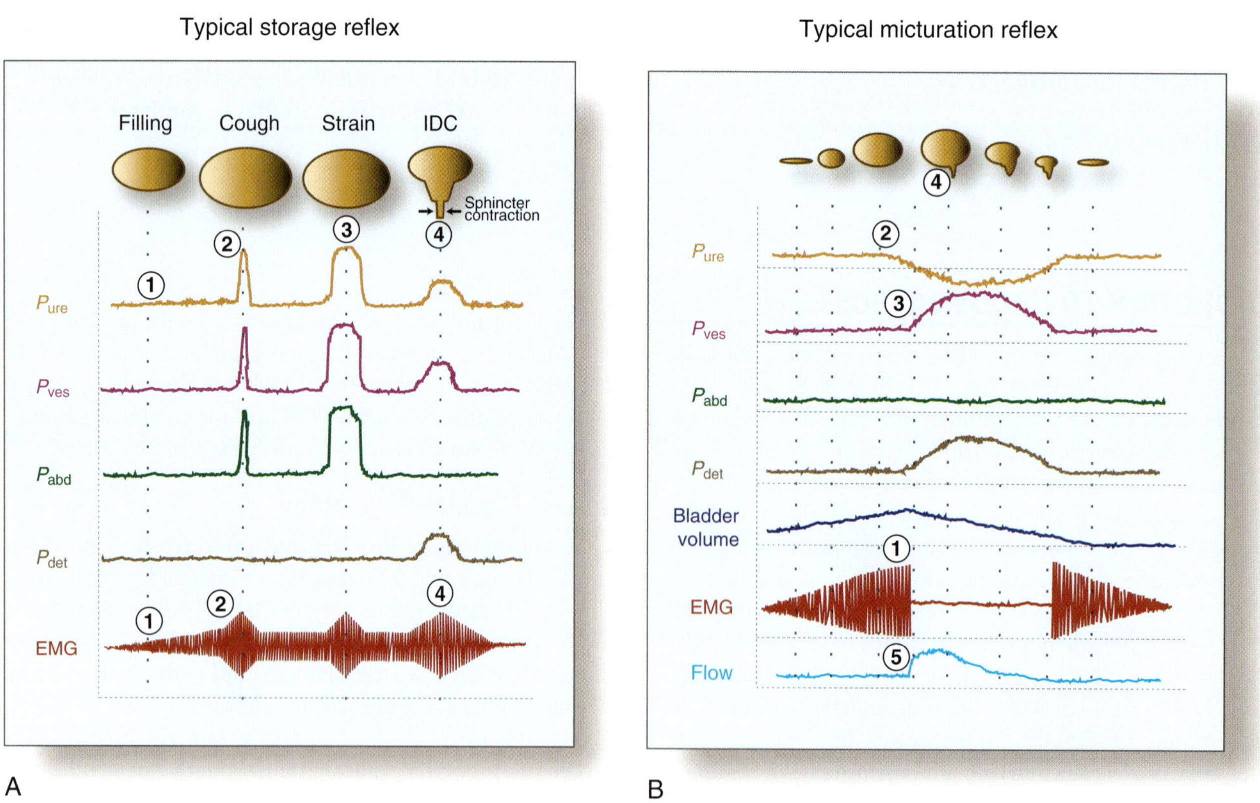

Fig. 11.1 **A**, Typical storage reflex in a neurologically intact woman; note increased electromyographic (*EMG*) activity during filling, coughing, straining, and an uninhibited detrusor contraction. This indicates an intact synergistic pelvic floor response. **B**, Typical micturition reflex in a neurologically intact woman. Note complete loss of EMG activity simultaneous with an increase in detrusor pressure at initiation of voiding. *IDC*, Involuntary detrusor contraction; P_{abd}, intraabdominal pressure; P_{det}, detrusor pressure; P_{ure}, urethral pressure; P_{ves}, intravesical pressure.

ultimately affect the patient and her subsequent treatment. See Box 11.1 for a variety of disease states categorized using this classification.

Role of Urodynamics in Clinical Practice

Although urodynamic testing has been frequently used in the evaluation of women with LUT dysfunction, level 1 evidence–based "indications" for its use are surprisingly few. The clinical question that must always be asked is whether the results of a urodynamic evaluation will either alter the outcome of the proposed management plan or be able to identify a potentially life-threatening situation (e.g., neurogenic voiding dysfunction). Urodynamic studies should be considered in clinical situations in which the testing is felt to be needed to make an accurate diagnosis, to assist in making an appropriate treatment plan, or to determine the impact of a disease state that has the potential to cause irreversible damage to the urinary tract, such as spinal cord injury. Hosker et al. (2009) summarized the role of urodynamics in clinical practice by listing the following situations in which urodynamic studies should be considered:

1. To identify or rule out factors contributing to LUT dysfunction and assess their relative importance.
2. To obtain information about other aspects of LUT dysfunction.
3. To predict the consequences of LUT dysfunction on the upper urinary tract.
4. To predict the outcome, including undesirable side effects, of a contemplated treatment.
5. To confirm the effects of an intervention or understand the mode of action of a particular type of treatment (especially a new one).
6. To understand the reasons for failure of previous treatments for symptoms or for LUT function in general.

URODYNAMIC EQUIPMENT

The ICS has developed recommendations for the minimum requirements for the equipment used to conduct urodynamic studies. These include three measurement channels (two for pressure and one for flow), a display on either a printer or a monitor, and a method of secure storage of the recorded pressures (Schäfer et al., 2002). The infused volume and voided volume may be recorded graphically or numerically. There also must be a method of event recording to mark information about sensation, leakage, and additional comments during the study. Cystometry transducers are devices that convert an applied pressure into an electrical signal. Pressure to be measured may be transmitted indirectly to the transducer using an open-ended or sealed catheter filled with liquid or gas or directly when the transducer is small and mounted on the tip of the catheter (microtip transducer). The transducer is normally calibrated against atmospheric pressure, with a zero reference level being the superior edge of the symphysis pubis. The customary unit of measurement for pressure during urodynamics is cm H_2O. The standard catheter for routine urodynamics is a transurethral double-lumen catheter (Schäfer et al., 2002). The urethral catheters should be as small as possible, but not so small as to dampen pressure transmission or limit the desired filling rate. The smallest available is a 6-French double-lumen catheter; this allows the fill and void sequence to be repeated without recategorization.

More recently, air-charged catheters have become popular for pressure measurement. These catheters have miniature air-filled balloons placed circumferentially around a polyethylene catheter. The catheters are disposable and single-use. Practical advantages over fluid-filled pressure lines revolve around

BOX 11.1 Modified Functional Classification of Voiding Dysfunction

I. Failure to Store
1. Bladder abnormality
   - A. Detrusor overactivity
     - i. Involuntary contractions
       - a. Idiopathic
       - b. Inflammatory
       - c. Outlet obstruction
       - d. Neurogenic
     - ii. Impaired compliance
       - a. Neurogenic
       - b. Fibrosis
       - c. Idiopathic
     - iii. Combination
   - B. Bladder hypersensitivity
     - i. Infection/inflammation
     - ii. Idiopathic
     - iii. Psychologic
     - iv. Neurogenic
     - v. Combination
2. Incompetent outlet
   - A. Urodynamic SUI
     - i. Anatomic (hypermobility)
     - ii. ISD
     - iii. Combination
   - B. Neurologic disease
     - i. ISD

II. Failure to Empty
1. Bladder abnormality
   - A. Neurogenic
   - B. Idiopathic
   - C. Myogenic
   - D. Psychogenic
2. Outlet abnormality
   - A. Anatomic
     - i. Obstruction—post–incontinence surgery
     - ii. Distortion—(e.g., pelvic organ prolapse)
     - iii. External compression
   - B. Functional
     - i. Smooth sphincter dyssynergia
     - ii. Striated sphincter dyssynergia
     - iii. Dysfunctional voiding
   - C. Combination

ISD, Intrinsic sphincter deficiency; *SUI*, stress urinary incontinence.

the fact that there is no hydrostatic pressure effect to account for, so there is no need to position anything at the level of the symphysis pubis or to flush the system through to exclude air, which is essential when using a fluid-filled system. With that said, many urodynamic "standard measurements" have been determined using fluid-filled systems. There are few studies directly comparing air-charged catheters with standard fluid-filled catheters; however, current evidence suggests the two are not interchangeable. One comparative study found that air-charged catheters consistently produce higher mean pressures than water-filled catheters and suggested that caution must be used when comparing urodynamic parameters using air-charged and water-filled catheters (Digesu et al., 2014). Another study found that pressure recordings from air-charged catheters and fluid-filled systems appear to be interchangeable for some urodynamic parameters, such as intravesical pressure (P_{ves}) at Valsalva maneuver, if the baseline pressure is compensated, but not for fast-changing pressure signals such as coughs (Sheng & Kirschner-Hermanns, 2019).

Although it is beyond the scope of this chapter to discuss the various commercially available urodynamic systems, most are computer-based digital systems that allow for easy data storage and post-processing. Available systems can range in price from several thousand dollars to more than $100,000 for a video urodynamic system. Despite constant nuanced improvements in systems and software, the clinician performing the study remains the most important constant in data collection and interpretation. In certain clinical settings, a simple three-channel system (Fig. 11.2) may be adequate, whereas large referral centers that evaluate complex cases or have a high percentage of patients with neurogenic bladder may require a more sophisticated system with the potential for video assessment (Fig. 11.3). Several modern urodynamic systems that are wireless and use Bluetooth technology have become available. These systems have the advantage of allowing more patient flexibility and privacy, as the catheters are not tethered to the urodynamic machine, because the signal can be sent wirelessly (up to 30 m) from the transducer to the urodynamic machine.

PERFORMING A URODYNAMIC EVALUATION

Urodynamic procedures should be performed with a clear indication and with a specific question or questions that hopefully can be answered by the study. The procedure must be performed interactively with the patient and should include continuous and careful observation of the collected data. Artifacts are best corrected as they occur, because they are often difficult to correct after the study is completed. It is valuable for the urodynamicist to have a clear understanding of the patient's symptoms and pertinent physical examination findings, practical experience with the equipment being used, and an understanding of quality control, with the ultimate goal of determining whether the questions that the procedure attempted to answer have been appropriately addressed. Obviously, a prerequisite to this is a good understanding of pertinent anatomy and physiology of the LUT, as well as the biomechanics and physics of the urodynamic study. The test should be explained to the patient in advance. Although complications are rare, certain morbidities such as urinary retention, hematuria, urinary tract infection, and pain can occur.

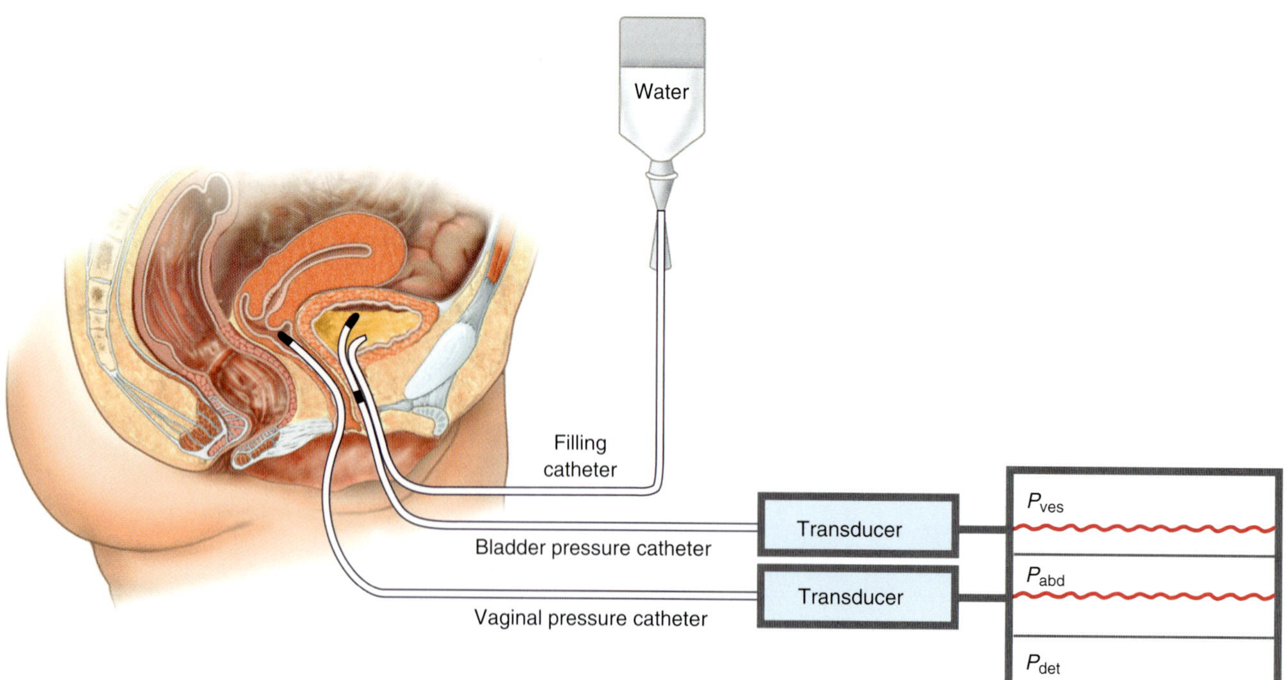

Fig. 11.2 Subtracted cystometry. Intravesical and intraabdominal pressures are measured, and true detrusor pressure is electronically derived ($P_{ves} - P_{abd}$). P_{ves}, Bladder pressure; P_{abd}, abdominal pressure; P_{det}, detrusor pressure.

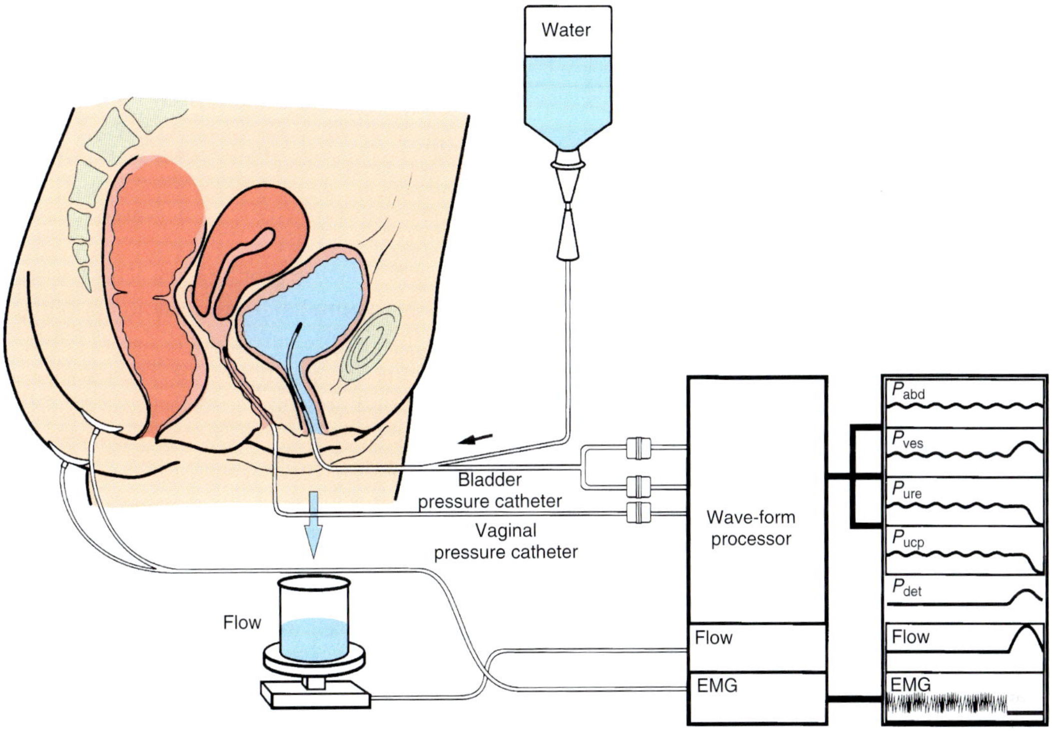

Fig. 11.3 Multichannel urodynamics. Intravesical, intraabdominal, and intraurethral pressures are measured. True detrusor pressure (P_{det}) and urethral closure pressure (P_{ucp}) are electronically derived. Electromyography (*EMG*) and flow studies are also performed. P_{ves}, Bladder pressure; P_{abd}, abdominal pressure; P_{det}, detrusor pressure; P_{ure}, urethral pressure; P_{ucp}, urethral closure pressure.

Based on the American Urological Association (AUA) "Best Practice Policy Statement," assuming the preprocedure urine is negative for a urinary tract infection, preprocedure antibiotic prophylaxis is not indicated except in high-risk patients (Box 11.2). The antimicrobial agents of choice are fluoroquinolones or trimethoprim/sulfamethoxazole. In patients who are allergic to both medications, the alternatives include a combination of aminoglycosides and ampicillin, first- or second-generation cephalosporin, or amoxicillin/clavulanate (Foon et al., 2012). If a preprocedure urinary tract infection is diagnosed, the condition should be treated before the procedure. The American Heart Association no longer recommends the use of antibiotic prophylaxis before genitourinary procedures solely to prevent infective endocarditis. For patients who have had previous orthopedic surgery, there is no indication for antibiotic prophylaxis if the urine culture is negative and patients are not high risk.

BOX 11.2 Risk Factors for Infection

Advanced age
Anatomic anomalies of the urinary tract
Poor nutritional status
Smoking
Chronic corticosteroid use
Immunodeficiency
Externalized catheters
Colonized endogenous/exogenous material
Distant coexistent infection
Prolonged hospitalization

Because micturition is normally a private act, the study setting should be quiet, to provide as little distraction as possible. The number of observers should be limited to as few as possible to minimize patient embarrassment.

A list of problems or questions that should be solved or answered by the urodynamic studies should be made before any testing is performed. A good practice is to decide on the questions before starting the study and then potentially design the study to answer those questions with the idea of customizing every study to a specific patient and her issues. It is also important to explain to the patient exactly why the tests are being performed and how the results may affect the treatment plan that will be proposed. The following is a brief description of the various tests that can be performed during a urodynamic evaluation.

1. Postvoid residual (PVR) urine volume: This is an objective assessment of how well a woman empties her bladder. It can be performed by ultrasound, bladder scan, or direct catheterization. An elevated PVR indicates a problem with emptying but does not really provide any information regarding the etiology of the dysfunction. A persistently elevated PVR may prompt further testing. Although no specific number has been agreed on to define what a normal PVR is, most would agree that a PVR less than 50 mL or a PVR less than 80% of the total bladder volume would be considered normal.
2. Uroflowmetry is a measurement of the rate of urine flow over time (Fig. 11.4). It is also an assessment of bladder emptying. A normal uroflow is a bell-shaped curve (Fig. 11.5).

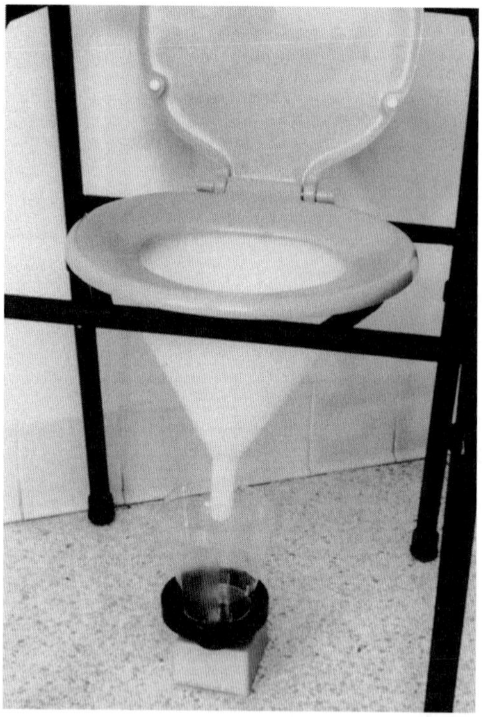

Fig. 11.4 Special commode and flowmeter used for spontaneous uroflowmetry.

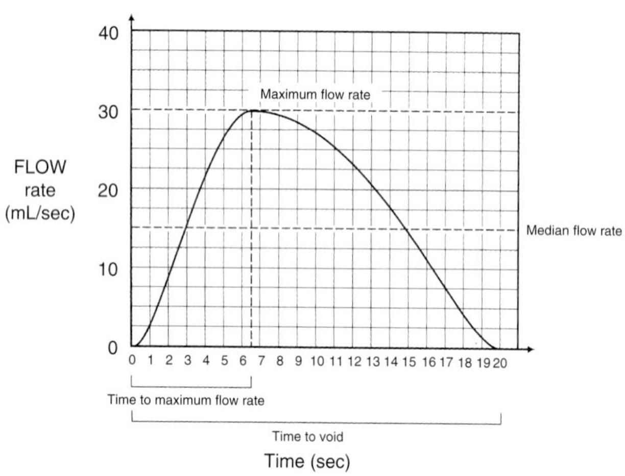

Fig. 11.5 Graphic representation of normal uroflow curve.

When the flow rate is reduced, or the pattern is altered, this may indicate bladder underactivity or bladder outlet obstruction (BOO).

3. Cystometrogram (CMG): Filling cystometry is the method by which the pressure/volume relationship of the bladder is measured during bladder filling. The test starts when filling commences and ends when the patient and urodynamicist decide that permission to void has been given. Although single-channel cystometry has been described, it is recommended that subtracted CMG be performed using the total vesical pressure and abdominal pressure by catheter placements in the bladder and rectum or vagina to calculate the true P_{det}, which is the vesical pressure minus the abdominal pressure. Also, leak point pressure measurements are obtained during filling cystometry.
4. EMG is the study of electronic potentials produced by the depolarization of muscle membranes. In the case of urodynamics, EMG measurement is usually performed with patch electrodes placed in close proximity to the striated sphincter muscles of the perineum. The test is mostly used to assure appropriate coordination between the pelvic floor muscles and LUT. EMG activity is measured during both filling and voiding.
5. Urethral pressure profilometry (UPP): This is measurement of the intraluminal pressure along the length of the urethra. The urethral pressure is defined as the fluid pressure needed to just open a closed urethra. The UPP is obtained by withdrawal of a pressure sensor catheter along the length of the urethra.
6. Pressure-flow studies of voiding are the method by which the relationship between pressure in the bladder and urine flow rate is measured during bladder emptying. P_{det} is measured with a simultaneous measurement of flow. The voiding phase starts when permission to void is given or when uncontrollable voiding begins and ends when the patient considers that voiding has finished.

Fig. 11.6 demonstrates a typical setup for a multichannel urodynamic assessment. The technique of performing a full urodynamic assessment in our laboratory is as follows:

1. The patient presents with a symptomatically full bladder. She voids spontaneously in a uroflow chair. A PVR urine volume is obtained via a transurethral catheter.
2. With the patient in the supine position on a urodynamic chair, the abdominal catheter is placed into the vagina and taped to the inside of the leg. If the patient has severe vaginal prolapse or has undergone previous vaginal surgery resulting in a narrowed vagina, the catheter is placed into the rectum. A dual microtransducer catheter with a filling port is then placed into the bladder. The patient is moved to a sitting position, and the catheter is secured to a mechanical puller (if urethral pressure studies are anticipated) or to the inside of the leg, so that the proximal transducer is near the midurethra (area of maximum urethral closure pressure).
3. After the catheters are appropriately placed, the subtraction is checked by asking the patient to cough. Cough-induced pressure spikes should be seen on the P_{ves}, intraabdominal pressure, and urethral pressure channels, but not on the true P_{det} channel. If there is an inappropriate deflection on the P_{det} channel, it is usually secondary to inaccurate placement of the vaginal (or rectal) catheter. If repositioning the catheter does not correct the problem, all connections and calibration techniques should be rechecked. Video 11.1 demonstrates appropriate calibration and subtraction during cough spikes and Valsalva.
4. Bladder filling is begun. First sensation, first desire to void, and strong desire to void are recorded. Throughout the filling portion of the examination, the patient is asked to perform provocative activities, such as coughing and straining. The external urethral meatus is constantly observed for any involuntary urine loss. The first set of provocative maneuvers should be performed at a volume between 150 and 250 mL. If the patient has urodynamic stress incontinence, leak point pressures can

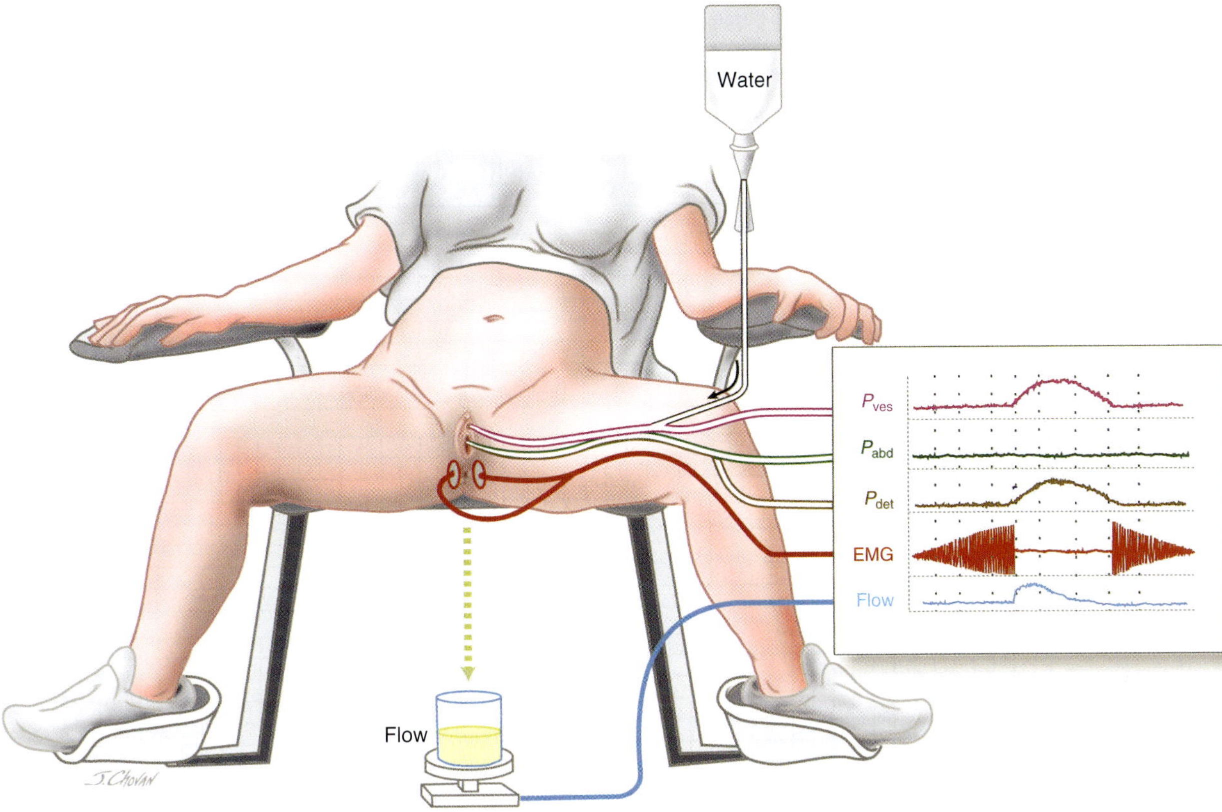

Fig. 11.6 Setup for urodynamic testing. The patient is typically seated on the urodynamic chair after the catheters have been placed. Abdominal and vesical pressures are measured by catheters in the bladder and vagina or rectum. The machine automatically calculates true detrusor pressure (P_{det}) by subtracting intraabdominal pressure (P_{abd}) from intravesical pressure (P_{ves}). Electromyography (*EMG*) activity using surface electrodes and urinary flow is also measured.

be obtained. Any abnormal rise in true P_{det} is noted. If the patient's symptoms are reproduced during filling, then the test can be completed in the sitting position. If they are not, the patient should be asked to stand and repeat provocative maneuvers in an attempt to reproduce her symptoms.

5. At the completion of filling, urethral pressure and flow studies can be performed, if indicated.

Fig. 11.7 illustrates an example of filling and voiding urethrocystometry. No urodynamic abnormalities are noted in this study.

INTERPRETATION OF SPECIFIC TESTS

Uroflowmetry

Uroflowmetry is noninvasive and inexpensive and is best used as a screening test for patients who may have voiding dysfunction. Many clinicians feel that uroflowmetry should routinely precede all other urodynamic studies. It is easy to perform and quickly provides data on both storage and emptying symptoms. The study should be conducted with as much privacy as possible, with patients being asked to void when they feel they have a normal desire. The addition of a PVR measurement, usually by ultrasound, adds value to this study. Normal voiding includes detrusor muscle contraction, coordinated bladder outlet relaxation, low voiding pressure, and a smooth arc-shaped flow curve (Schäfer et al., 2002). It should be noted that uroflowmetry alone is insufficient to diagnose BOO, because it cannot distinguish true obstruction from poor detrusor contractility. Because small, voided volumes affect the curved shape, only voided volumes of at least 150 mL are interpretable (Fig. 11.8). Because women have very short urethras with minimal outlet resistance, generally speaking the only factors influencing female outflow are the strength of the detrusor muscle, the urethral resistance, and the degree of relaxation of the sphincter mechanism. The most common conditions associated with increase in outlet resistance are previous antiincontinence surgery or significant anatomic distortion, usually from pelvic organ prolapse.

Urine flow may be described in terms of flow rate and flow pattern and may be continuous or intermittent. Flow rate (Q) is defined as the volume of fluid expelled via the urethra per unit time and is expressed in milliliters per second (mL/s). Certain information is necessary in interpreting the tracing, including the volume voided, the environment and position in which the patient passed urine, whether the bladder filled naturally or by a catheter, and whether diuresis was stimulated by fluid or diuretics. If filling was by catheter, the type of fluid used should be stated; it should also be stated whether the flow study was part of another investigation. Maximum flow rate (Q_{max}) is the maximum measured value of the flow rate after correction for

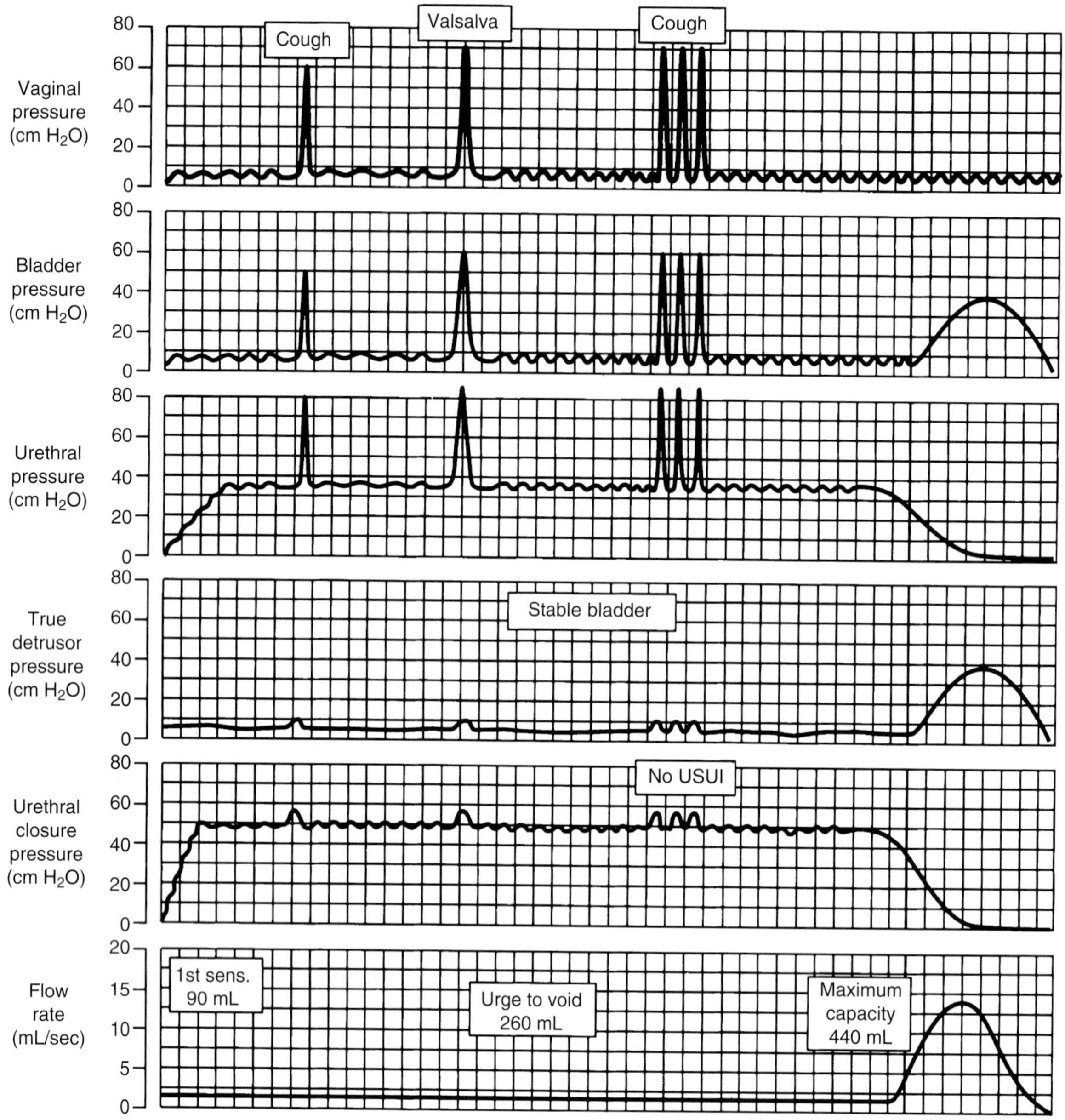

Fig. 11.7 Normal filling and voiding subtracted cystometry. Note that provocation in the form of coughing and straining does not provoke any abnormal rise in true detrusor pressure. At maximum capacity on command, a detrusor contraction is generated, and voiding is initiated. *USUI*, Urodynamic stress urinary incontinence.

artifacts. Voided volume is the total volume expelled via the urethra.

Flow time is the time over which measurable flow occurs. Average flow rate is voided volume divided by flow time. The average flow should be interpreted with caution if flow is interrupted or if there is a terminal dribble. Time to maximum flow is the elapsed time from onset of flow to maximum flow.

Most experts agree that a study can be considered normal if the patient voids at least 200 mL over 15 to 20 seconds and if it is recorded as a smooth single curve with a Q_{max} greater than 20 mL/s (Fig. 11.5). Q_{max} values of less than 15 mL/s with a voided volume greater than 200 mL are generally considered abnormal. However, because flow rate is determined by the relationship between detrusor force and urethral resistance, and because these factors may vary considerably and still produce adequate bladder emptying, a precise definition of a normal or a low flow rate cannot be made. The maximum urinary flow rate (MUFR) and average urinary flow rate are the two most important uroflowmetry parameters.

The clinical usefulness of uroflowmetry has been hampered by the lack of absolute values defining normal limits. These normal limits would need to be over a wide range of voided volumes, ideally in the form of nomograms. Haylen et al. (1989) performed uroflowmetry on 249 female volunteers between ages 16 and 63 years. Uroflowmetry was performed on each woman in a completely private environment, and a second uroflow study was obtained in 46 of those women. The MUFR and the average urinary flow rate of the first voids were

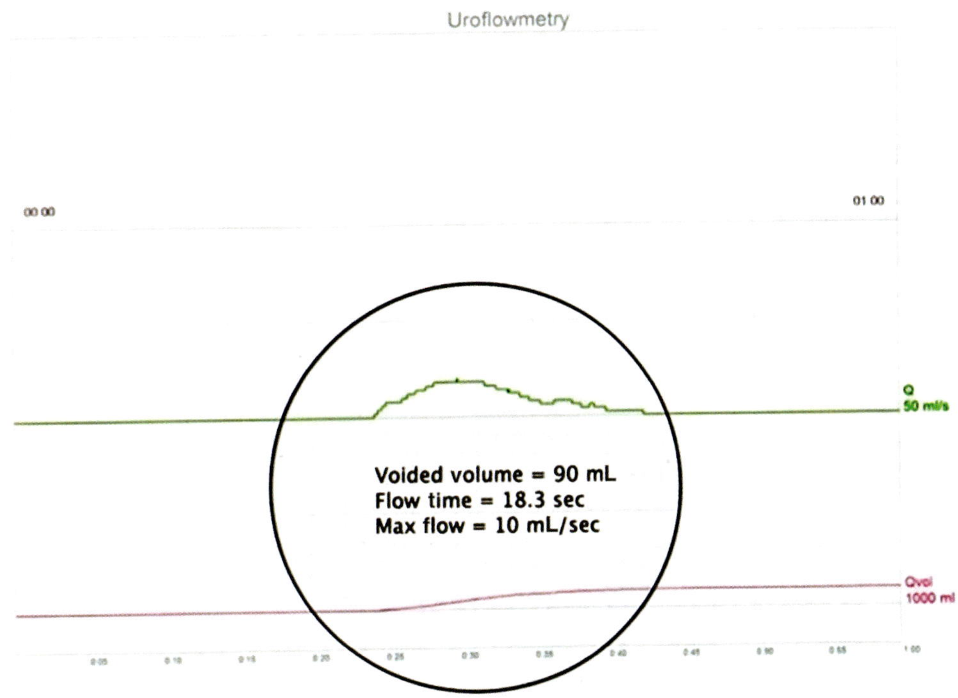

Fig. 11.8 Uroflow curve from a void of only 90 mL. Data obtained are not useful, because the voided volume was less than 150 mL.

compared with respective voided volumes. By using statistical formulations of both voided volumes and urine flow rates, relationships between the two variables were obtained. This allowed the construction of nomograms, which are shown in Fig. 11.9. The previously described nomograms refer to free flowmetry voids and are not applicable to flow rates obtained during a pressure-flow study, because all urethral catheters can be expected to have the effect of decreasing urine flow rates for the equivalent voided volume. In 1999, Haylen et al. completed a further study of 250 symptomatic women who were consecutively referred for urogynecologic assessment, which included urodynamics. Flow data for these women were converted to centiles from the Liverpool nomograms. The authors noted a decreased flow rate in symptomatic women in general, and specifically in women with genital prolapse. In contrast to asymptomatic women, there is a decline in flow rates with age, and final urodynamic diagnosis shows that women with various combinations of stress incontinence, overactive bladder (OAB),

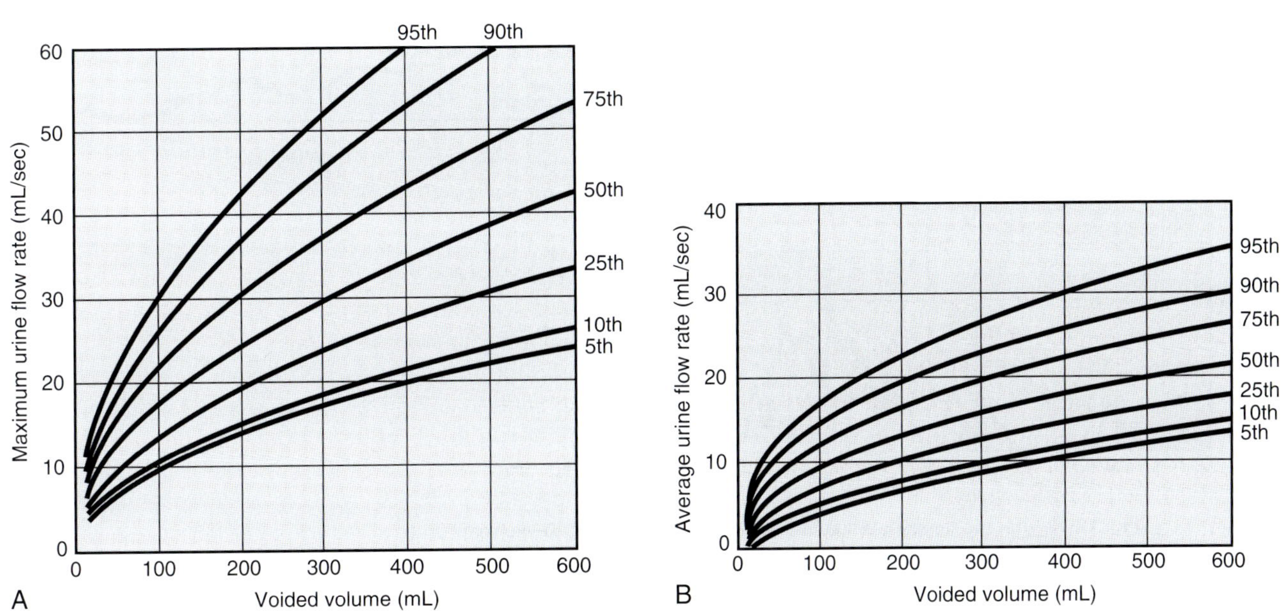

Fig. 11.9 A, Liverpool maximum flow rate nomogram for women; curves are centiles. **B**, Liverpool average flow rate nomogram for women; curves are centiles.

or voiding dysfunction have flow rates that are significantly different than those of asymptomatic women.

Curve patterns refer to the configuration of the uroflowmetric curve. Continuous flow that shows a rapidly increasing flow rate that reaches the maximum within one-third of the total voiding time is usually considered normal (Fig. 11.10A). Fig. 11.10B demonstrates what has been termed a superflow pattern, in which there is a very rapid acceleration to a high MUFR.

Flow is considered intermittent when the flow rate drops and subsequently increases. Intermittent flow rates are described as multiple-peak patterns when there is a downward deflection of the flow rate that does not reach 2 mL/s (Fig. 11.10C). When the downward deflection of the flow rate reaches 2 mL/s or less (Fig. 11.10D), an interrupted pattern occurs. Obstructed voiding patterns are much less common in women than in men, and usually produce a low, flat tracing (Fig. 11.10E).

Abnormal uroflowmetric parameters can occur secondarily to factors that affect detrusor contractility, urethral resistance, or both. Also, inappropriate contraction of pelvic floor muscles can affect flow rates. Detrusor contractility can be affected by neuropathic lesions, pharmacologic manipulation, intrinsic detrusor muscle or bladder wall dysfunction, or psychogenic inhibition. Urethral resistance can be altered by tissue trophic changes producing atrophy or fibrosis, drug effects such as

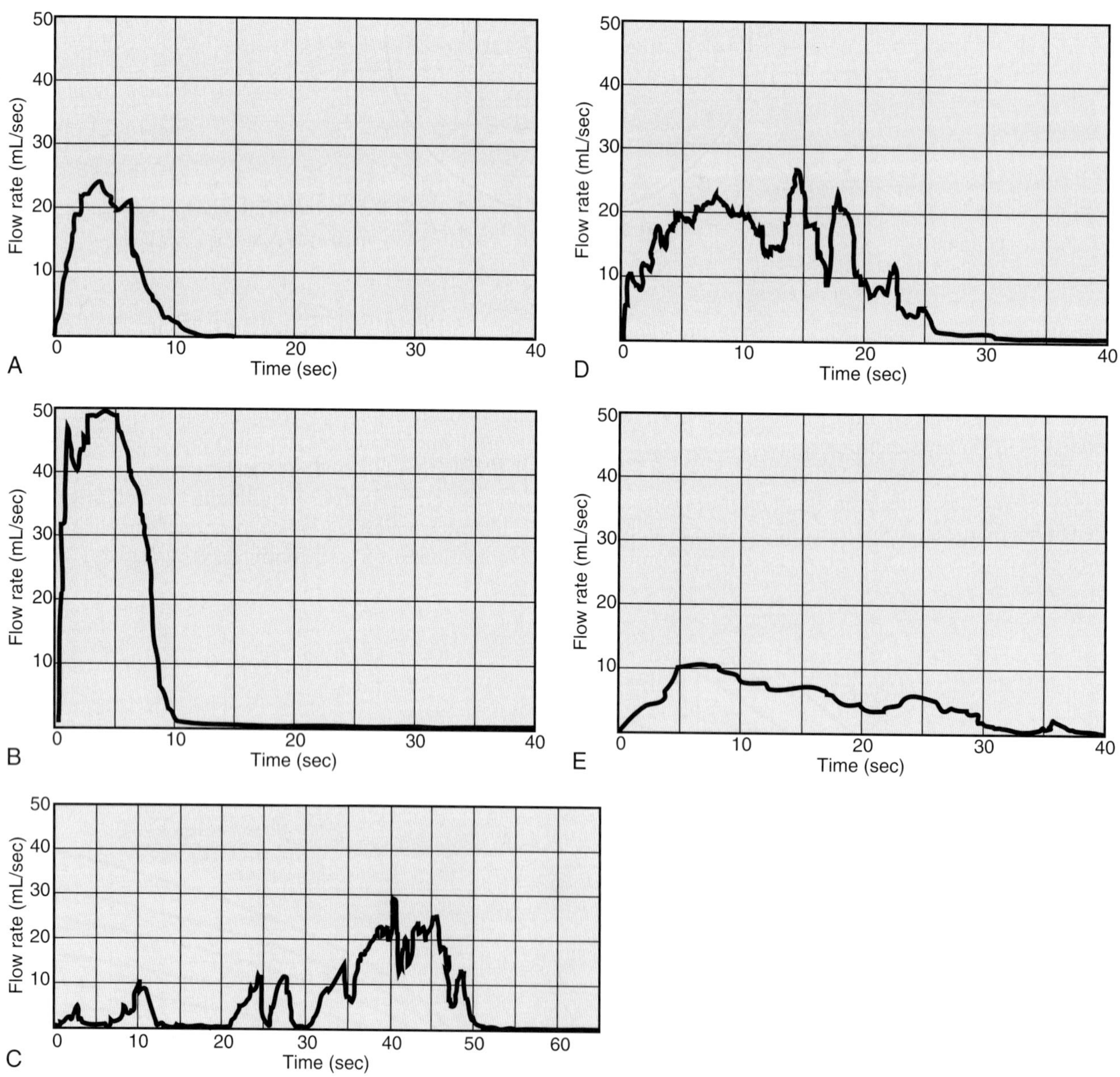

Fig. 11.10 Graphic representation of various uroflow patterns. **A**, Normal curve; voided volume of 145 mL; maximum urinary flow rate (MUFR) 23 mL/s. **B**, Superflow pattern; voided volume of 330 mL; MUFR 49 mL/s. **C**, Intermittent flow rate with multiple peak pattern. This tracing is characteristic of voluntary urethral sphincter activity. **D**, Intermittent flow rate with interrupted pattern. This is a characteristic pattern seen when abdominal pressure is used to expel urine. **E**, Reduced urine flow rate secondary to detrusor outflow obstruction.

alpha-adrenergic stimulators or blockers, neuropathic striated muscle contraction, pain or fear, and urethral axis distortion secondary to severe pelvic organ prolapse. Outlet obstruction secondary to an intraurethral lesion or stricture is exceedingly rare in women. Extraurethral lesions, such as vaginal masses or cysts, or a large enterocele or rectocele may externally compress the urethra, resulting in obstructed voiding. Inability to relax pelvic floor muscles appropriately can cause prolonged flow times. This may occur after a traumatic delivery or pelvic floor reconstructive surgery, or as part of any disease state that causes vaginal pain. Detrusor-external (or striated) sphincter dyssynergia is a condition in which there is lack of coordination between the detrusor muscle and the external striated urethral sphincter. This leads to obstructed voiding and is always secondary to a neurologic lesion, most classically high spinal cord trauma. In the nervous and anxious but neurologically intact patient, the urethra may be closed by pelvic floor contracture. Urethral closure may be attributed to contraction of the intraurethral striated muscle or contraction of the pelvic floor musculature. This condition has been termed dysfunctional voiding.

If uroflow measures are normal in patients complaining of symptoms of voiding difficulty, further investigation is unnecessary, but abnormal flow rates may require further urodynamic testing. Uroflowmetry is a simple urodynamic investigation that is useful as a preliminary screening test to distinguish patients who need more extensive studies from those who do not. Uroflowmetry is also an integral part of a full urodynamic study performed for more complex problems.

Filling Cystometry

Cystometry is the urodynamic study used to describe the pressure/volume relationship of the bladder. One should also collect information on bladder sensation during filling. Normal bladder sensation is usually judged at three defined points: a first sensation of bladder filling, a first desire to void, and a strong desire to void (Fig. 11.11). Although specific parameters are not given for these various changes in sensation, increased bladder sensation is defined as an early first sensation of bladder filling or an early strong desire to void that occurs at what is felt to be a low bladder volume and ultimately persists, whereas reduced bladder sensation is a diminished sensation through bladder filling. P_{det} during filling should be very low, with no involuntary contractions. Detrusor overactivity (DO) is defined as involuntary detrusor contractions during filling that may be spontaneous or provoked (Fig. 11.12 and Video 11.2). DO is classified as either neurogenic (when there is a relevant neurologic condition) or idiopathic (when there is no identifiable cause). Bladder compliance describes the relationship between the change in bladder volume and change in P_{det}. Compliance is calculated by dividing the volume change by the change in P_{det} during that change in bladder volume. It is expressed in mL/cm H_2O. Although it is difficult to define what normal compliance

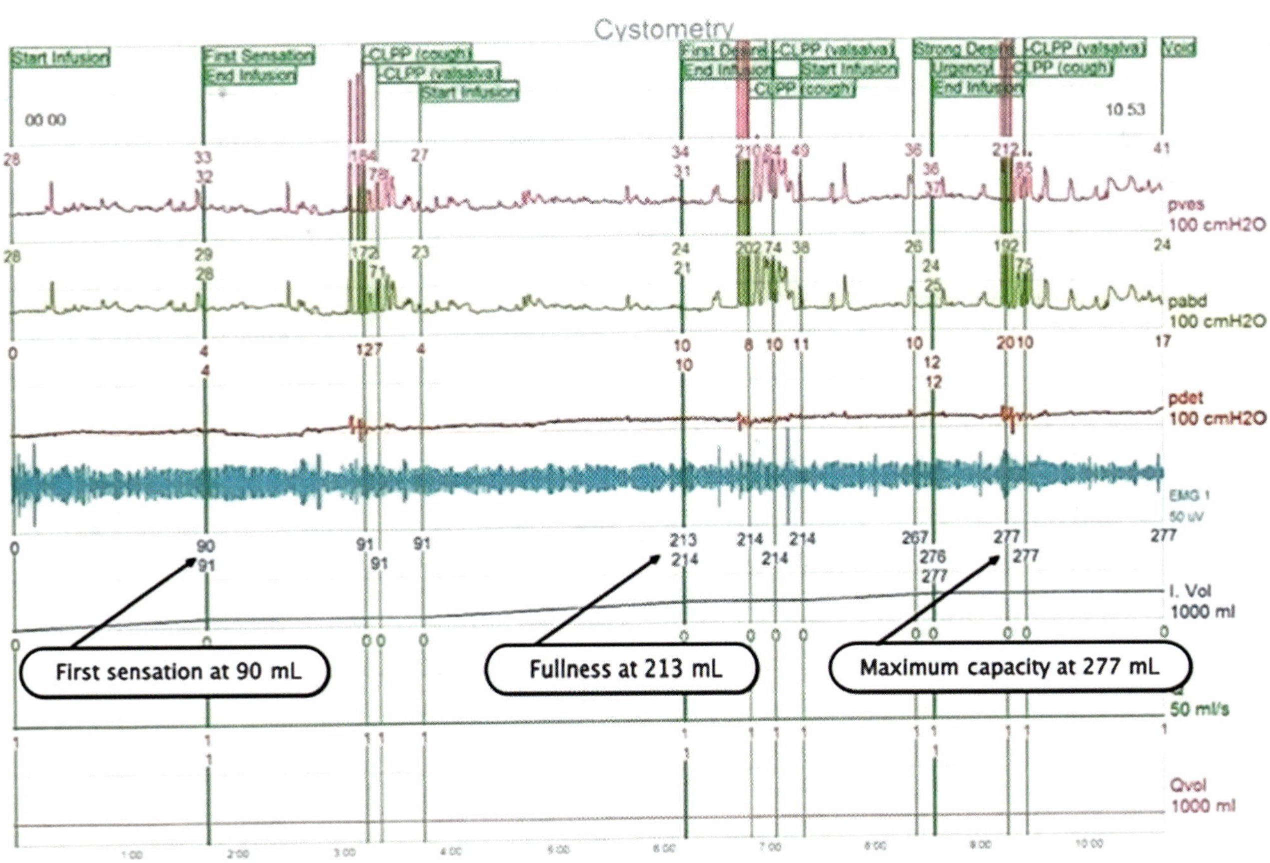

Fig. 11.11 Filling cystometry; first sensation, fullness, and maximum capacity are noted. Detrusor remained stable during filling, and no stress incontinence was demonstrated.

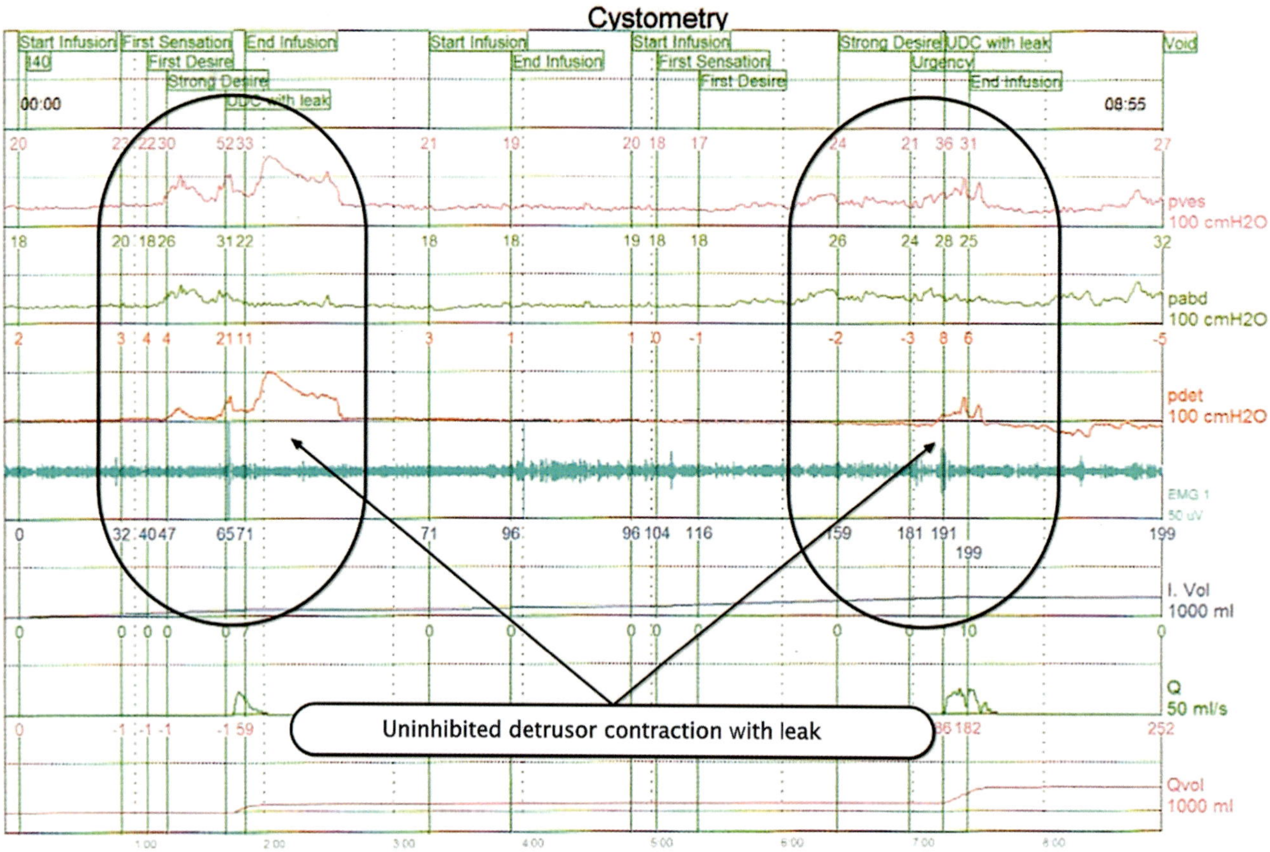

Fig. 11.12 Filling cystometry in a patient with detrusor overactivity; note that two uninhibited bladder contractions occurred during the filling portion of the test.

is in terms of mL/cm H_2O, several authors have shown that the mean values for compliance in healthy subjects range from 46 to 124 mL/cm H_2O (Hosker, 2009; Sørensen et al., 1989; Van Waalwijk Van Doorn et al., 1992). Because of these wide-ranging values, it is more practical from a clinical standpoint to use absolute pressure instead of a compliance number. For example, it has been shown that urine storage pressure greater than 40 cm H_2O can be associated with harmful effects to the upper tract (McGuire et al., 1981). In general, prolonged storage at high pressures can lead to upper tract deterioration.

When there appears to be an abnormal rise in true P_{det}, the urodynamicist must determine if this rise is caused by poor bladder compliance (Fig. 11.13) or best classified as DO (Fig. 11.14). Abnormal bladder compliance is going to be more common in certain subsets of patients, including women with neurogenic disease, a history of radiation or multiple bladder surgeries, multiple bladder tumor resections, a defunctionalized bladder after long-term anuria, long-term indwelling catheterization, recurrent bladder infections, or long-standing BOO. In patients with abnormal bladder compliance during filling cystometry, there will be a steep rise in P_{det} that is usually parallel to bladder filling. Abnormal compliance is related to filling; DO is not. Most of the time, if you stop infusing fluid, the P_{det} will plateau in cases of low compliance but continue to rise toward the peak with DO (Fig. 11.11 and 11.12). With continuation of filling, assuming there is no "pop-off" effect, as noted by leakage from the urethra or vesicoureteral reflux, the P_{det} will continue to rise in low compliance, but a detrusor contraction will usually end, resulting in a significant drop in P_{det} ultimately returning to the baseline pressure before the DO (Videos 11.2 and 11.3).

The condition of urodynamic stress incontinence is defined as involuntary loss of urine simultaneous with a rise in abdominal pressure in the absence of any rise in true P_{det} (Fig. 11.15; Video 11.4). This diagnosis is made during filling cystometry. Provocation in the form of coughing, straining, and heel bouncing in the sitting (and, if necessary, standing) position should be performed at different volumes throughout the testing session. Once the diagnosis is made, Valsalva and cough leak point pressure measurements can be obtained if felt to be clinically indicated.

Leak Point Pressures

There are two distinct types of leak point pressures that can be measured in an incontinent patient. The first is an abdominal leak point pressure sometimes termed either a Valsalva leak point pressure (VLPP) or cough leak point pressure; the second is a detrusor leak point pressure (DLPP). These pressures are independent of each other and conceptually measure completely different things. An abdominal leak point pressure, whether measured during cough or Valsalva, is a measure of the intrinsic sphincter strength of the urethra or its ability to resist leakage with increases in abdominal pressure. It is specifically

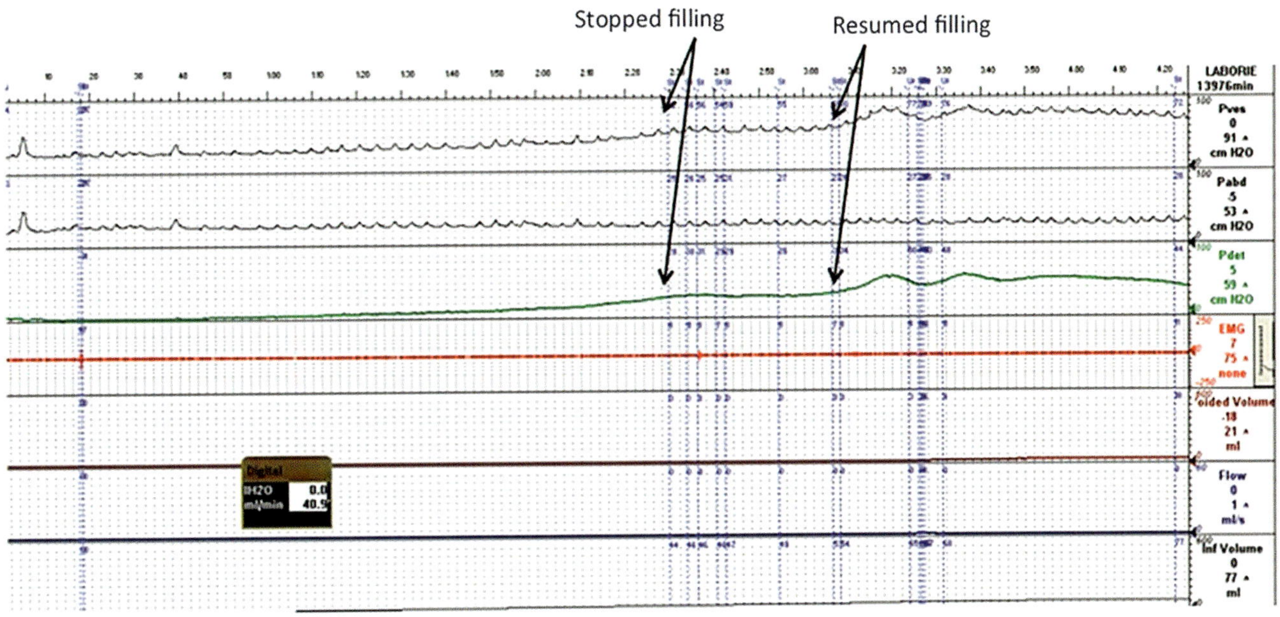

Fig. 11.13 Multichannel filling cystometry in a patient with poor bladder compliance. Note steady rise in true detrusor pressure with plateaus when filling stops and increases when filling is resumed.

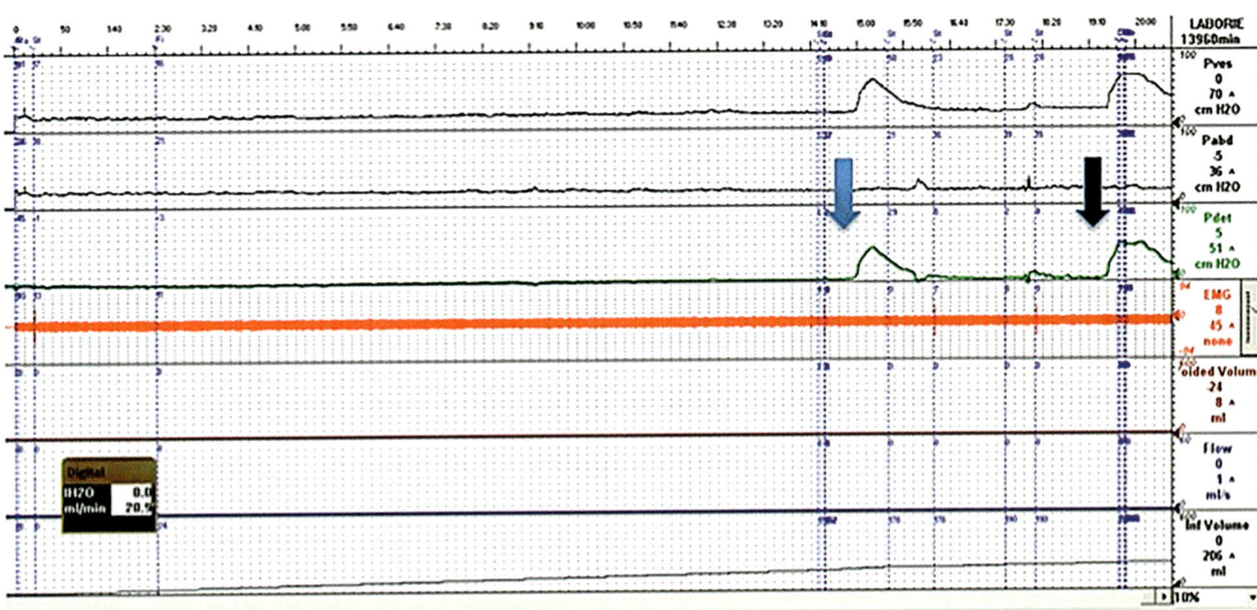

Fig. 11.14 Multichannel filling cystometry in a patient with detrusor overactivity. Note that detrusor pressure returns to baseline after completion of contraction.

defined as the intravesical pressure at which urine leakage occurs because of an increased abdominal pressure in the absence of a detrusor contraction. Thus, it is an objective assessment of the amount of abdominal pressure required to overcome outlet resistance and create leakage. This test is applicable to patients with urodynamic stress incontinence. Theoretically, the lower the abdominal leak point pressure, the weaker the sphincter. There is no normal abdominal leak point pressure, because patients without stress incontinence will not leak at any volume or physiologic abdominal pressure. The pressure should be a measure of the total (absolute) abdominal pressure required to cause leakage, not the change in pressure. The reading is taken from the vesicle channels, because it is usually a cleaner channel to obtain the pressure, assuming there are no involuntary contractions of the detrusor. A Valsalva effort is the most reliable method of provocation; however, if the patient cannot Valsalva on command, coughing can be used (Figs. 11.16 and 11.17; Video 11.5).

The second type of leak point pressure is the DLPP, which is a measure of P_{det} in patients with decreased bladder compliance. It is defined as the lowest P_{det} at which urine leakage occurs in the absence of either a detrusor contraction or an increase in abdominal pressure (Video 11.6). From a clinical perspective, a DLPP is most useful in patients with lower motor

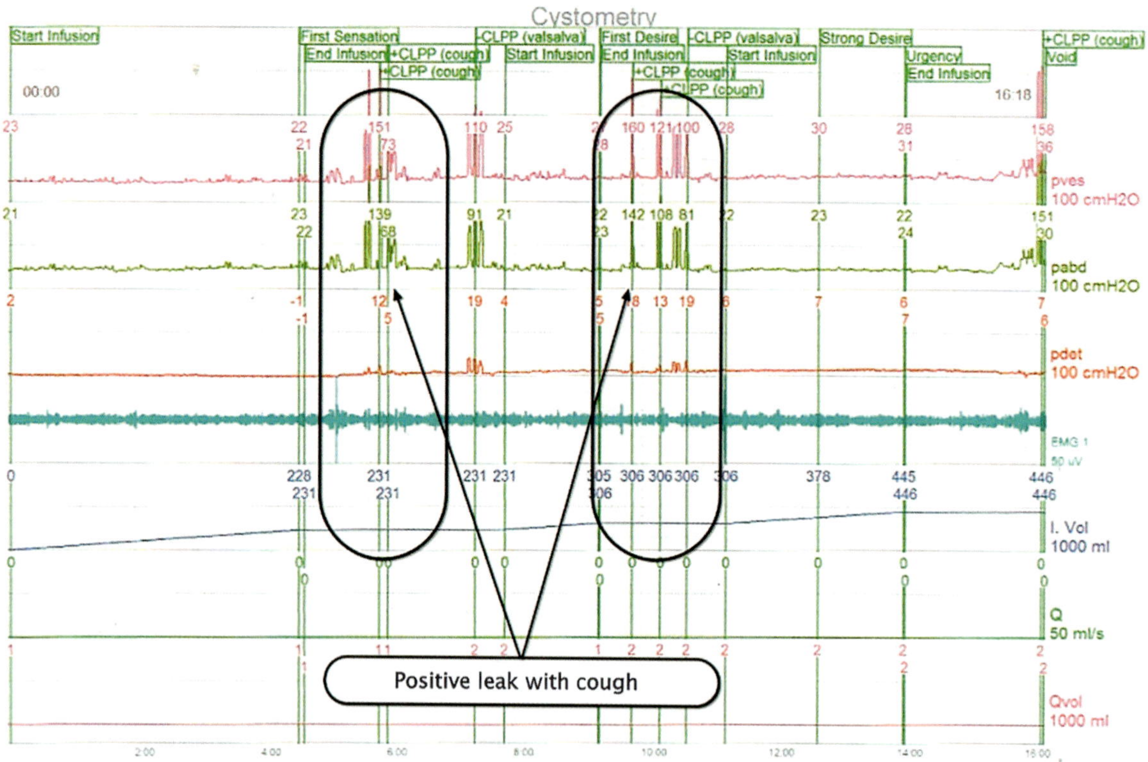

Fig. 11.15 Filling cystometry demonstrating the condition of urodynamic stress incontinence. Urine leakage occurred simultaneous with a cough (rise in intraabdominal pressure) in the absence of any rise in true detrusor pressure.

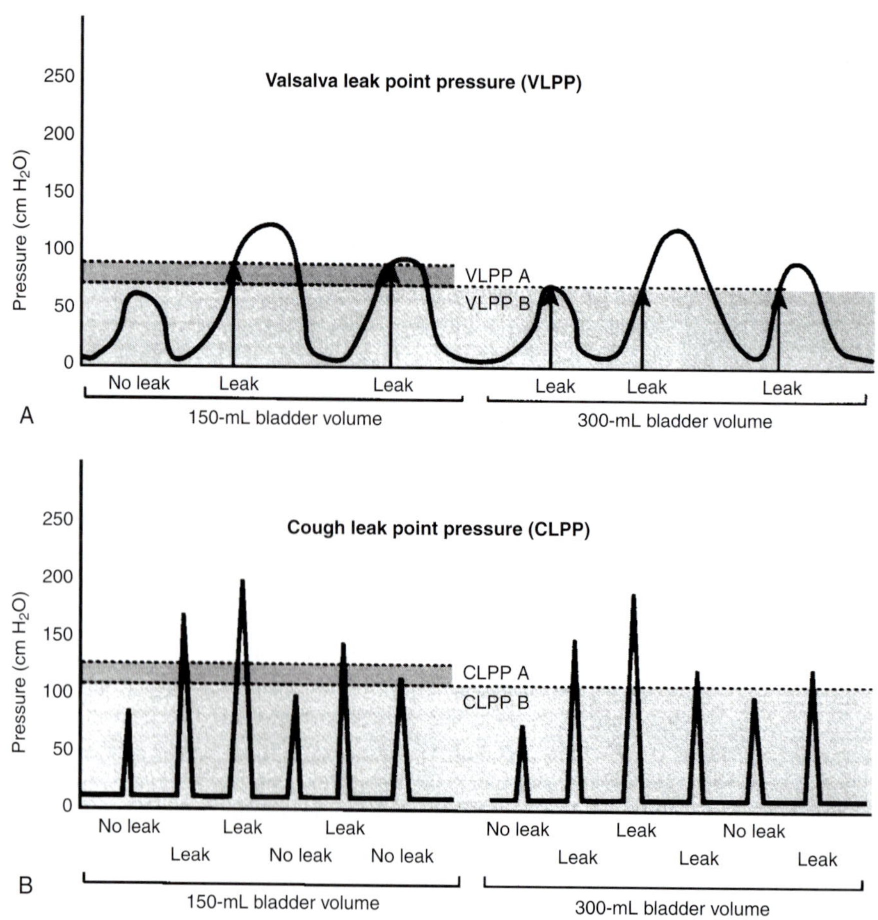

Fig. 11.16 A, Graphic representation of Valsalva leak point pressure measurement at bladder volumes of 150 and 300 mL. Leak point pressures tend to decrease with increased bladder volume. **B**, Graphic representation of cough leak point pressure at bladder volumes of 150 and 300 mL. Note the difficulty involved in isolating the cough that generates the minimal amount of abdominal pressure required to produce leakage.

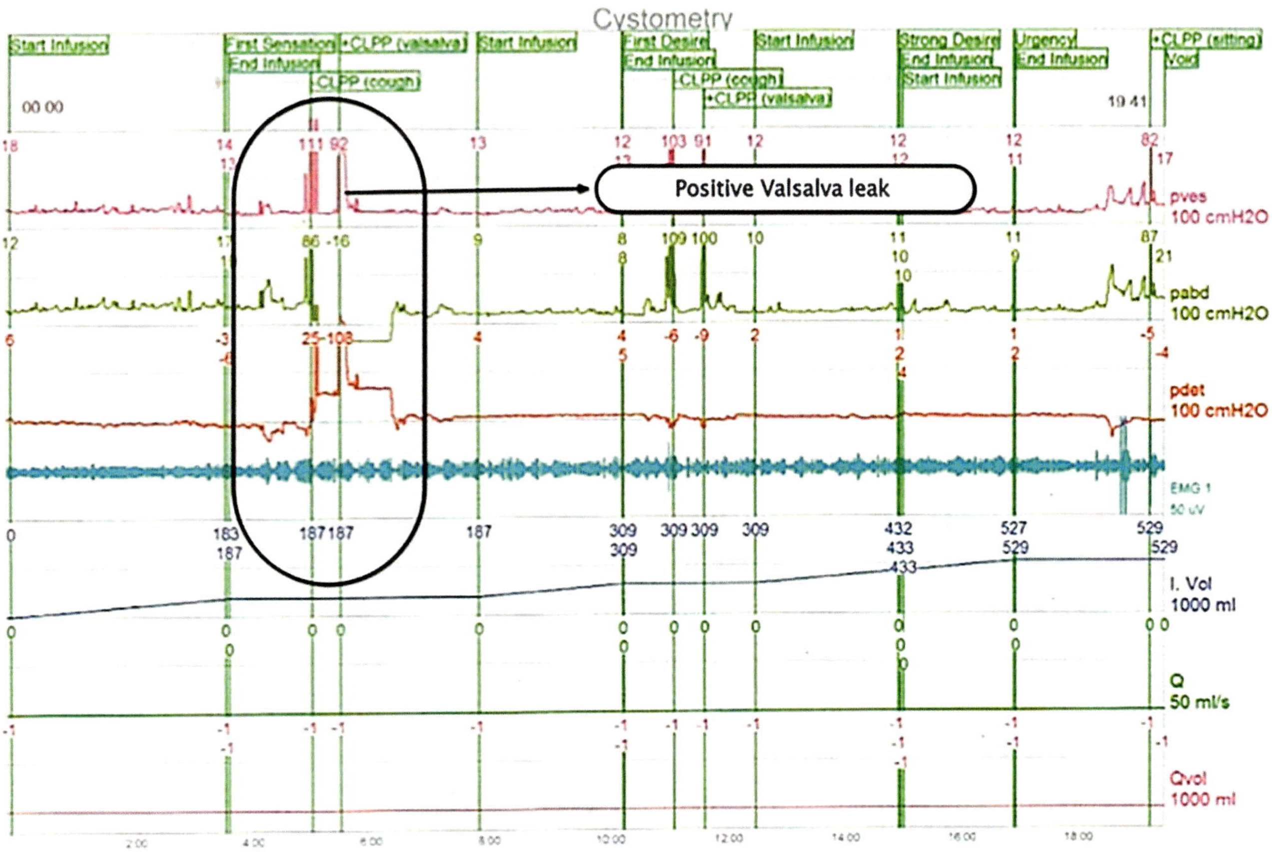

Fig. 11.17 Filling cystometry. Valsalva leak point pressure of 92 cm H_2O is noted in sitting position at a volume of 187 mL.

neuron disease causing decentralization, and rarely in nonneurogenic patients with abnormal bladder compliance, which can occur after multiple bladder surgeries, radiation therapy, tuberculosis cystitis, and other rare situations or conditions. In general, the higher the DLPP, the more likely the upper urinary tract could be damaged because of intravesical pressure being transferred to the ureters and the kidneys. McGuire (1981) showed that DLPPs greater than 40 cm H_2O would result in hydronephrosis or vesicoureteral reflux in 85% of myelodysplastic patients.

Urethral Pressure Profilometry

Urethral pressure profilometry (UPP) indicates the intraluminal pressure along the length of the urethra with the bladder at rest. The maximum urethral pressure is the maximum pressure of the measured profile. The maximum urethral closure pressure is the difference between the maximum urethral pressure and the intravesical pressure (Fig. 11.18). The functional urethral length (FUL) is the length of the urethra along which the urethral pressure exceeds the intravesical pressure, and the anatomic urethral length is the total length of the urethra. The pressure transmission ratio is the increment in urethral pressure on stress as a percentage of the simultaneously reported increment in vesical pressure.

UPP involves the withdrawal of a catheter through the urethra at a constant rate of speed. Pressure is measured along the entire urethral length, as well as in the bladder. UPP can be performed using open or balloon catheters perfused with liquid or gas, catheter-mounted (microtip) transducers, or fiberoptic catheters, as well as air-charged catheters (Fig. 11.18).

Normal values for maximal urethral closure pressure (MUCP) and FUL vary widely among women; however, most continent women will have an FUL of approximately 3 cm and an MUCP between 40 and 60 cm H_2O. Although many authors have used an MUCP of less than 20 cm H_2O to define intrinsic sphincter deficiency (ISD) in women with urodynamic stress urinary incontinence (SUI), this definition has many of the same problems that hamper the definition and diagnosis of ISD.

In 2002, the ICS standardization subcommittee concluded that the clinical utility of UPP is unclear (Lose & Brostrøm, 2002), stating that there are no urethral pressure measurements that:

1. Discriminate urethral incompetence from other disorders.
2. Provide a measure of the severity of the condition.
3. Provide a reliable indicator to surgical success.

Electromyography

EMG studies have become popular components of a urodynamic assessment. Muscle depolarization is detected by an electrode placed in or near a muscle. The test can be done with needle or surface electrodes; however, surface electrodes with self-adhesive skin patches that are applied over the skin of the anal sphincter are the most commonly used during a urodynamic assessment. The surface electrodes have a significant advantage over needle electrodes regarding patient convenience and comfort, as well as ease of doing the test. Although using a

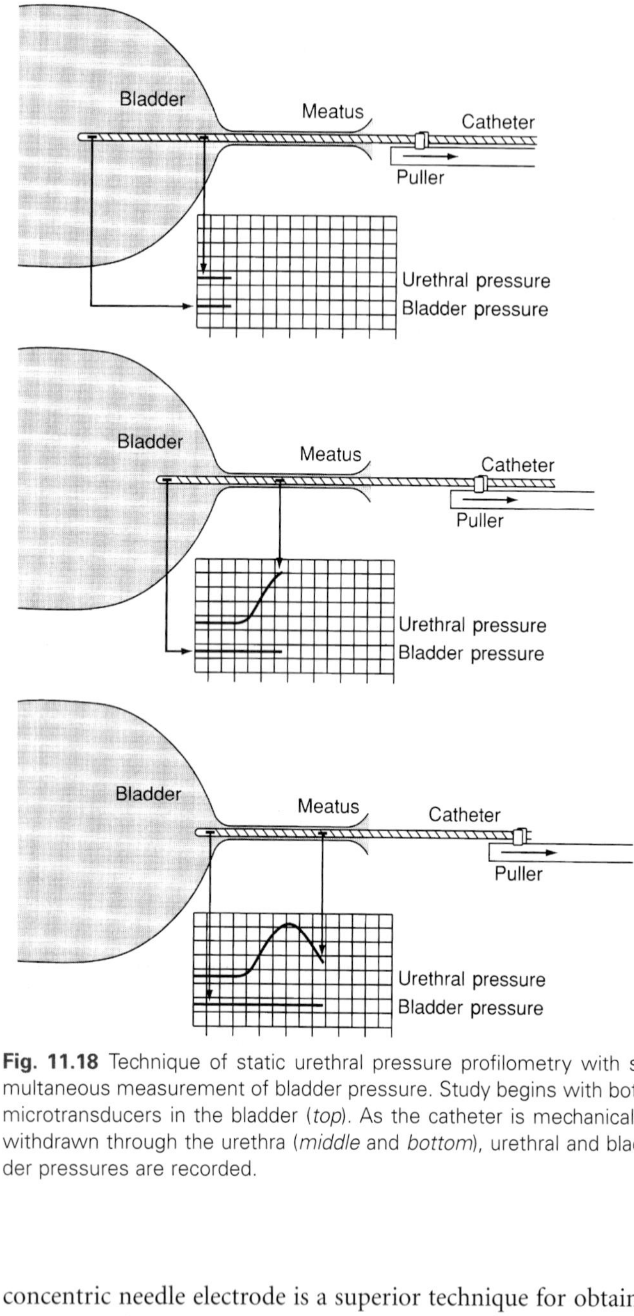

Fig. 11.18 Technique of static urethral pressure profilometry with simultaneous measurement of bladder pressure. Study begins with both microtransducers in the bladder (*top*). As the catheter is mechanically withdrawn through the urethra (*middle* and *bottom*), urethral and bladder pressures are recorded.

concentric needle electrode is a superior technique for obtaining a signal source of EMG activity of the striated external urethral sphincter muscle, the information obtained by the perianal surface electrodes will suffice in the evaluation of most women with LUT dysfunction. In a neurologically intact individual, EMG activity should increase during filling and provocation to prevent any leakage. Normal voiding requires external sphincter relaxation followed by contraction of the detrusor. Failure of the sphincter to relax or stay completely relaxed during micturition is abnormal. Thus, normally, EMG activity decreases before a voluntary bladder contraction; however, it is not abnormal for EMG activity to increase with an involuntary contraction as part of a guarding reflex to inhibit the detrusor contraction. Some question the clinical utility of routine EMG during urodynamic performance, and others argue that it remains a good objective method to assure appropriate synergistic responses during filling, voiding, and provocation.

Pressure-Flow Studies

Because uroflowmetry can provide only limited information, pressure-flow studies represent a natural progression. However, if uroflowmetry is normal, the information obtained in a pressure-flow study is largely unnecessary. In contrast, in those with voiding symptoms and an abnormal MUFR and/or peak flow velocity, pressure-flow studies are necessary to determine the cause. Flow rate depends on both the outlet resistance and the contractile properties of the detrusor, as well as the volume of fluid in the bladder. A low flow rate may be associated with a high voiding pressure or a below-normal voiding pressure. Similarly, the finding of a normal flow rate does not exclude BOO, because normal flow may be maintained by a high voiding pressure.

Some women have normal flow rates in the absence of a detrusor contraction. This may be because sphincteric relaxation, either alone or assisted by increased intraabdominal pressure from straining, is sufficient to produce a normal flow rate. Pressure-flow studies are essential for a complete functional classification of LUT disorders and an objective assessment of the basis of a patient's voiding dysfunction.

These studies are usually performed after a cystometric evaluation. In most patients, it is clear when bladder filling should be stopped. However, if the patient has little sensation, it is important to use the functional bladder capacity from the frequency–volume chart as a guide to cystometric capacity. At this point, if a separate filling catheter is being used, it is removed; the intravesical catheter is left in place. An intravaginal or intrarectal catheter records intraabdominal pressure to assess whether the patient uses a Valsalva maneuver to void and to electronically derive true P_{det}. Thus, these studies involve the monitoring of abdominal, intravesical, and true P_{det} synchronously with flow (Fig. 11.19 and 11.20). External sphincter EMG activity and urethral pressure also may be measured. To ensure that proper pressure transmission is occurring, the patient should be asked to cough before being allowed to void. With the patient in a sitting position, she is then instructed to void to completion if possible. It is important during the voiding phase to respect the patient's privacy. Few women are able to void in the presence of others, so it may be necessary for the practitioner to leave the room for her to initiate voiding. Video 11.7 demonstrates a voiding mechanism with an appropriate detrusor contraction, and Video 11.8 demonstrates a voiding mechanism with significant Valsalva effort.

Pressure-flow studies are invasive because the patient is asked to void around catheters. It is important to appreciate the limitations of pressure-flow studies, as well as the differences between the patient's performance during urodynamic testing and her normal voiding. This is best judged by asking the patient and by comparing the noninstrumented urine flow rate with the flow rate obtained from the pressure-flow study.

Voiding in a urodynamic laboratory can be affected by a variety of factors. It is estimated that approximately 30% of women who void without problems at home are unable to void on command in the urodynamic laboratory. This is hardly surprising, because they are surrounded by complex equipment, have catheters in their bladder and vagina or rectum, and are usually being observed by strangers.

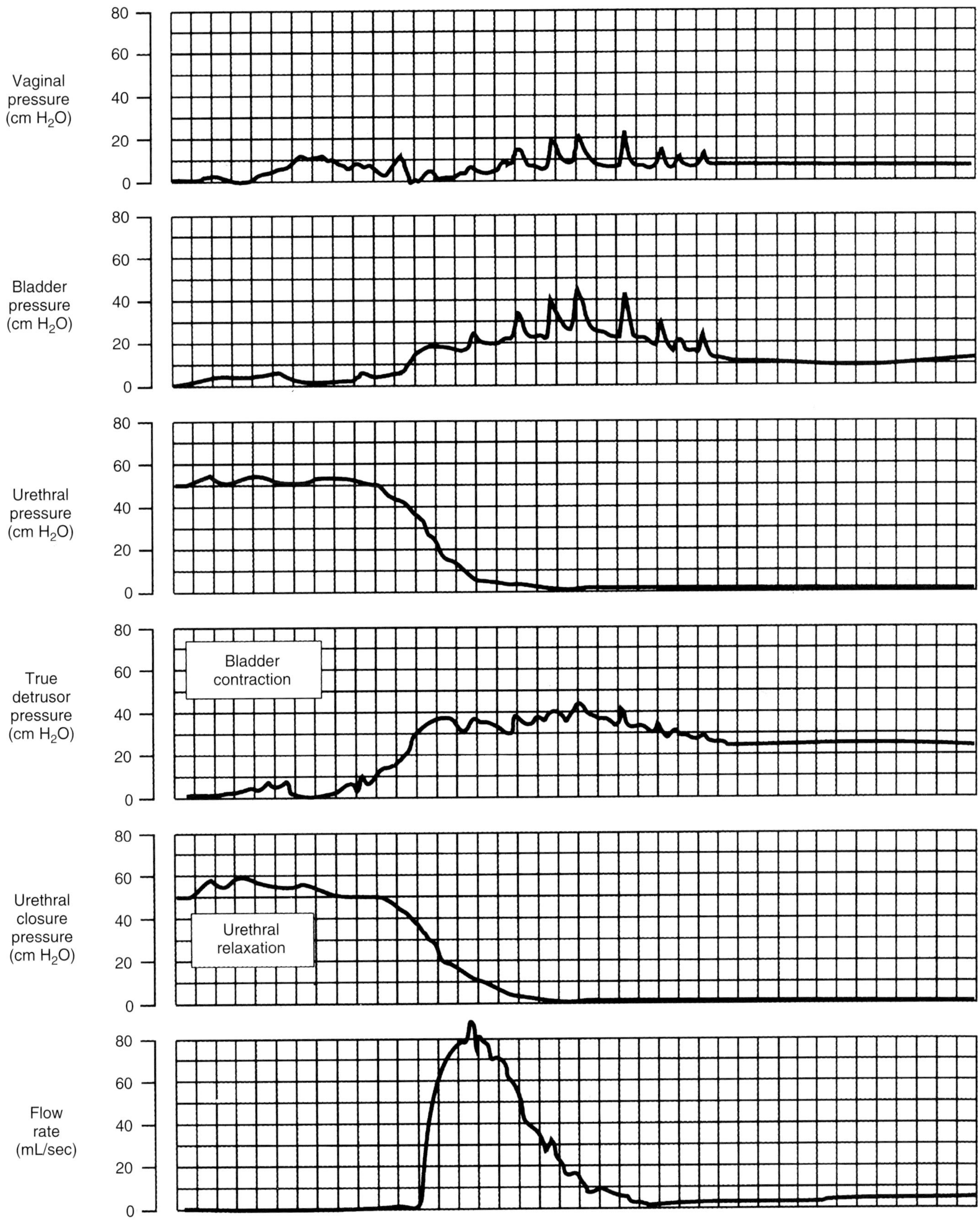

Fig. 11.19 Pressure-flow study in a patient who voids with urethral relaxation and bladder contraction. Note minimal Valsalva effort.

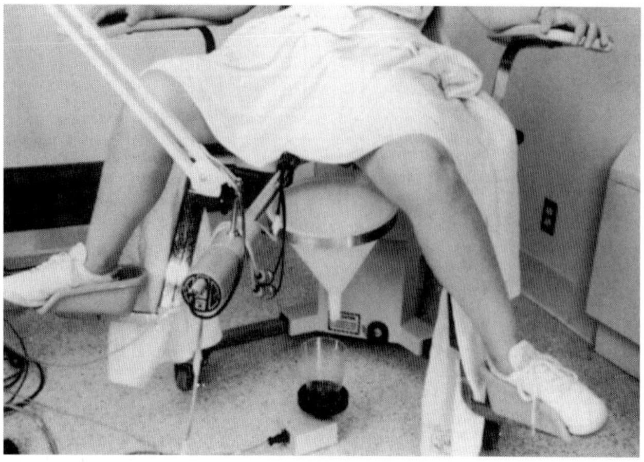

Fig. 11.20 Pressure-flow study in a patient who has voiding dysfunction after suburethral sling procedure. The study is consistent with outlet obstruction in that the flow is reduced and detrusor pressure is elevated.

Fast filling or overfilling of the bladder may make normal voiding difficult. Studies that compared ambulatory urodynamics (natural bladder filling) with conventional urodynamics show that voiding pressures are higher with natural filling. This implies that the detrusor may be incompletely stimulated, partially inhibited, or mechanically less efficient if it is overfilled or filled too fast.

During the voiding phase, the detrusor muscle may be normal, acontractile, or underactive. Normal voiding is usually achieved by a voluntarily initiated continuous detrusor contraction that is sustained and can be suppressed. An underactive detrusor during micturition implies that the detrusor contraction is of inadequate magnitude or duration (or both) to effect bladder emptying within a normal time span.

During voiding, urethral function may be normal or abnormal. A normal urethra opens during voiding and is continuously relaxed to allow the bladder to be emptied at a normal pressure. Abnormal urethral function may be secondary to urethral overactivity or a mechanical obstruction, such as a urethral stricture or tumor. BOO, regardless of the cause, is characterized by increased P_{det} and reduced urine flow rate, seen by observing the synchronous values of flow rate and P_{det} during voiding (Video 11.9). In mechanical obstruction, which is rare in females, the voiding pressures are constantly elevated. If the obstruction is caused by urethral overactivity, the voiding pressures may fluctuate. Urethral overactivity is characterized by the urethra contracting during voiding or the urethra failing to relax. In detrusor external sphincter dyssynergia (DESD), the patient's phasic contractions of the intrinsic urethral striated muscle are simultaneous with the detrusor contraction. This produces a very high voiding pressure and an interrupted flow. The urodynamic characteristic of this type of urethral overactivity is a fall in flow rate accompanied by a rising P_{det} that then falls when the urethra relaxes, leading to a resumption of urine flow. Another form of urethral overactivity is called dysfunctional voiding. This is most commonly seen in children who are neurologically normal but complain of urinary incontinence or recurrent infections. The interrupted flow in these children is caused by pelvic floor overactivity rather than contractions of the intrinsic striated muscle.

Depending on age, menopausal status, total voided volume, and the presence or absence of LUT dysfunction, women void by any combination of a detrusor contraction, abdominal straining, and urethral relaxation.

It is difficult to ascertain whether abdominal straining that occurs during a pressure-flow study is real or artifactually induced by the surroundings and presence of indwelling catheters. The patient should always be asked to void normally and in as relaxed a way as possible. If the patient has an acontractile detrusor, voiding can be achieved only by straining. If the detrusor contracts during voiding, but the patient also strains, then the tracing is more difficult to interpret. It is also difficult to understand precisely what effect straining has on urine flow. In patients without obstruction, straining increases flow, but it does not produce the same increase in flow as that achieved by a P_{det} rise of the same magnitude (Video 11.8).

Although pressure-flow studies are an established and accepted urodynamic modality, what constitutes a normal voiding mechanism is poorly understood, as is the normal range for P_{det} during voiding in women. Most of the previously published literature has been derived from male subjects in whom pressures are abnormally high secondary to outflow obstruction.

Because there is no highly prevalent condition such as benign prostatic hypertrophy in women that causes female obstruction, it has been very difficult to establish nomograms. Because voiding dynamics differ in women, nomograms derived for men cannot be used in women. As mentioned, anatomic differences allow women to void by simply relaxing their pelvic floor, or by increasing abdominal pressure by straining. Small elevations in P_{det} or decreases in flow rates, which might be considered insignificant in a male, may be consistent with BOO in a female. Thus, clinicians should always have a high index of suspicion for BOO in women with a prior history of an antiincontinence procedure, chronic cystitis, pelvic organ prolapse, or incomplete bladder emptying.

Numerous investigators have attempted to establish cutoff values for pressure and flow to diagnose outlet obstruction in women (Chassagne et al., 1998; Lemack & Zimmern, 2000). These studies, however, have some limitations in that obstruction was predefined clinically, and only patients with anatomic obstruction were included. A study by Defreitas et al. (2004) used normal asymptomatic women as the control group and found the highest sensitivity and specificity for predicting obstruction was obtained with Q_{max} less than 12 mL/s and P_{det} Q_{max} greater than 25 cm H_2O. Blaivas and Groutz (2000) created a nomogram defining voiding obstruction in women using Q_{max} from a noninstrumented uroflow and a maximum P_{det} from the pressure-flow study. More recently, an analysis of the urodynamic data from the Trial of Mid-Urethral Slings (TOMUS) study noted that the difference between these two values increases as voided volumes increase (Mueller et al., 2015), concluding that values from a pressure-flow study and noninstrumented uroflow cannot be used interchangeably, as has been suggested by the Blaivas–Groutz nomogram for obstruction in women.

The main clinical use of pressure-flow studies is to document the mechanism of abnormal voiding. If a patient has symptoms and signs of abnormal voiding, has low flow rates, and voids with a high P_{det}, she is probably voiding against an obstruction. On the other hand, if a patient has low flow rates and voids with minimal or no rise in P_{det}, then her voiding dysfunction is probably secondary to an acontractile or underactive detrusor. As previously mentioned, the limiting factor is that there is no clear cutoff between normal and abnormally high P_{det} during voiding.

The clinical setting in which pressure-flow studies are most useful in women is in the patient who has undergone pelvic surgery and has developed postoperative voiding dysfunction. The dysfunction may be secondary to denervation, resulting in an underactive or acontractile detrusor, but more commonly the dysfunction is secondary to increased outlet resistance produced from the surgery. Voiding dysfunction or retention occurs in 3% to 20% of patients after various operations to correct stress incontinence. It is always a clinical dilemma whether urethrolysis or a takedown of the repair will restore normal voiding. Filling cystometry and pressure-flow studies may be helpful in this setting. If the patient is able to void around a catheter and is noted to have a high P_{det} with a low flow rate (Fig. 11.21), then she is obstructed, and relieving the obstruction should improve voiding (Nitti & Raz, 1994).

Although some previous studies have shown that a preoperative pressure flow study may be predictive of postoperative voiding dysfunction after an antiincontinence procedure (Bhatia & Bergman, 1984), others have shown that the only true predictor is a preoperative elevated PVR volume (Kobak et al., 2001). Thus, at the present time it remains controversial whether there is a role for preoperative pressure-flow studies in women with SUI and/or pelvic organ prolapse as a predictor of postoperative voiding dysfunction.

URODYNAMICS AND SPECIFIC CONDITIONS

Stress Urinary Incontinence

The role of urodynamics in SUI in women has been recently debated. Urodynamic studies have been cited historically as being potentially beneficial for diagnosing the condition of urodynamic stress incontinence, assessing urethral function with either VLPPs or maximum urethral closure pressures, and also potentially predicting postoperative voiding dysfunction based on preoperative pressure-flow studies.

Recently, many data have questioned whether there is any beneficial role for urodynamics in women with straightforward symptoms of stress incontinence in which the sign of stress incontinence is demonstrable in an office setting. Nager et al. (2012) published the results of the Value of Urodynamic Evaluation (VALUE) trial, a randomized trial focused on the role of urodynamics in women with SUI. Six hundred thirty women meeting criteria for an antiincontinence procedure were randomized to

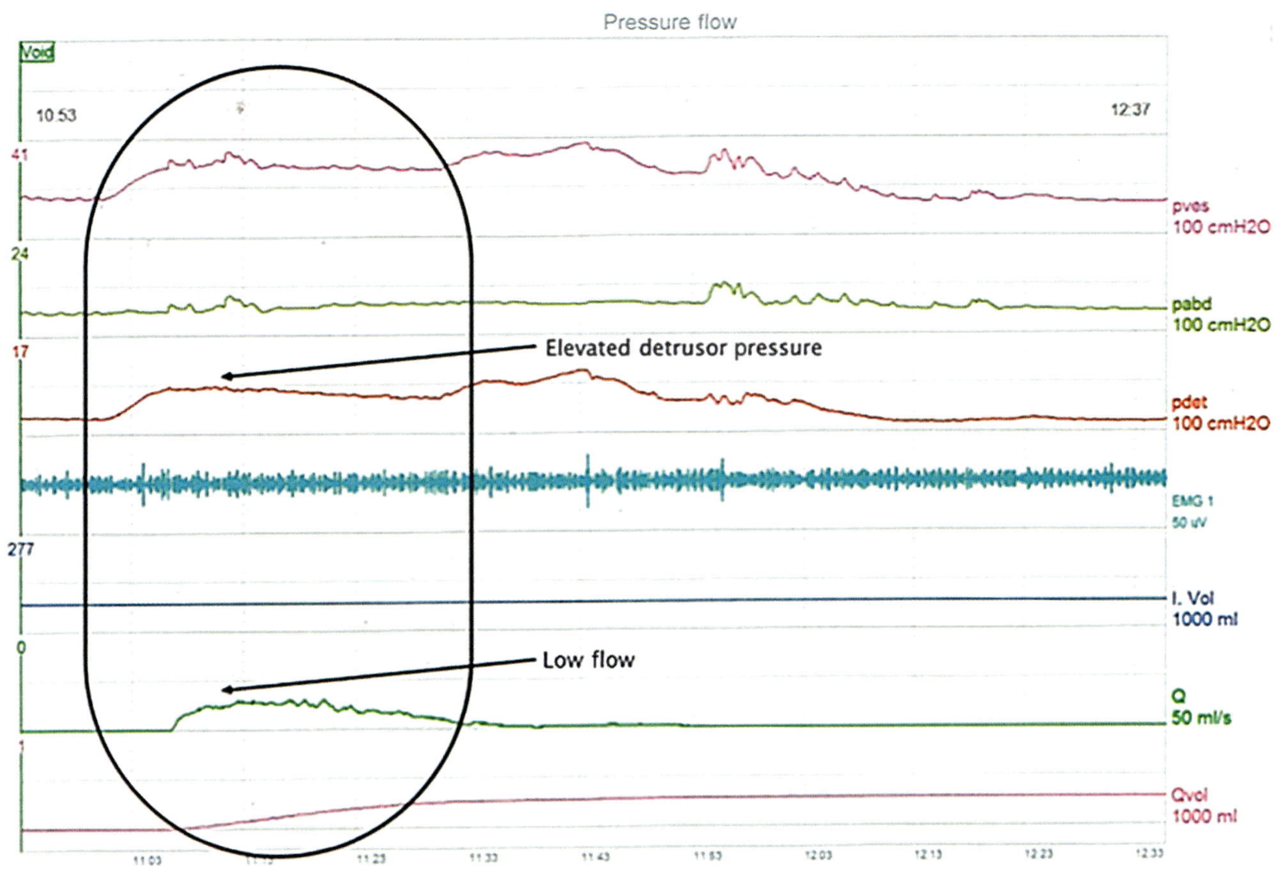

Fig. 11.21 Technique for performing pressure-flow studies. The patient must be able to void around the catheters.

preoperative urodynamics or a simple office-based evaluation. The primary outcome of the study was treatment success, defined as a 70% reduction or more from baseline to 12 months in the urogenital distress inventory and a patient global impression of improvement response of "very much better" or "much better" at 12 months. Secondary outcomes sought to determine if preoperative urodynamic findings in women with stress-predominant incontinence would affect surgical outcome, with the secondary outcomes being cost and utility of performing urodynamics. At 12 months, no significant difference was seen between the urodynamic testing group and the office evaluation–only group with respect to treatment success (76.9% and 77.2%, respectively). When secondary outcomes were examined, there was no difference between the two groups for changes in incontinence severity index or patient global impression of improvement. The study concluded that, in a woman with straightforward symptoms of SUI, urodynamics did not improve the rate of treatment success, and thus showed no benefit over a simple office evaluation in which the sign of stress incontinence was objectively demonstrated.

Based on the VALUE trial, women with symptoms of stress incontinence who meet the following criteria gain no benefit from a urodynamic evaluation before SUI surgery:

1. Stress-predominant urinary incontinence symptoms.
2. Positive urine stress test.
3. PVR less than 150 mL.
4. A mobile urethra.
5. Stage 0 to 2 pelvic organ prolapse.
6. No prior incontinence surgery or pelvic radiation.

A more recent follow-up study looking at the cost of preoperative urodynamics in a secondary analysis of the VALUE trial noted that $13 million to $33 million could be saved annually by not performing preoperative urodynamics studies (Norton et al., 2016). Incorporating these data into diagnostic and treatment algorithms will significantly reduce the number of women undergoing preoperative urodynamics prior to placement of a midurethral sling (Lloyd et al., 2018).

In their October 2006 document, the UK National Institute of Health and Clinical Excellence stated that urodynamics in women with pure SUI is no longer recommended. Urodynamics was indicated only in women with urinary incontinence where there was a clinical suspicion of either mixed incontinence (coexistent DO), in women who have previously undergone surgery for SUI and developed recurrent incontinence, in women who have had previous anterior compartment prolapse surgery, and in women with symptoms suggestive of significant voiding dysfunction.

In the Netherlands, the Value of Urodynamics Before Stress Incontinence Surgery study (van Leijsen et al., 2009) was performed to further assess this question. This multicenter randomized controlled trial examined the role of urodynamics in women with symptoms of SUI who had urodynamic findings that were discordant with history and physical findings and were then randomized to receive either a midurethral sling or individual treatment. Individual treatment included pessary, medical treatment, physiotherapy, or surgery at the discretion of the provider. The primary outcome was clinical improvement in incontinence as measured by the validated Dutch version of the long form of the Urogenital Distress Inventory, with a secondary outcome being cost. The study concluded that, in women with uncomplicated SUI, an immediate midurethral sling operation is not inferior to individually tailored treatment based on urodynamics.

Urethral function or lack thereof has been traditionally assessed with UPP and/or VLPPs. Data from the Stress Incontinence Surgical Treatment Efficacy (SISTEr) trial (Albo et al., 2007) indicated that VLPP did not correlate with several other indices of SUI severity or with urodynamic parameters such as volume of first leakage, volume of first sensation, and presence of DO. In the TOMUS study (Richter et al., 2010), preoperative urodynamics was performed before randomization to a retropubic midurethral sling or a transobturator midurethral sling procedure and repeated at 12 months after surgery. Patients and surgeons were blinded to the findings of the preoperative urodynamics so that they would not be influenced in their treatment decision. The study showed that VLPP did not impact surgical outcome. The supine empty bladder stress test, which indicates a low threshold for leakage in a supine position with an empty bladder, was thought to correlate with more severe forms of incontinence and lower VLPPs; however, in a study by Nager et al. (2010), VLPP and urethral closure pressure showed a moderate correlation to each other but little to no correlation to the empty supine stress test. Measurement of maximum urethral closure pressure is a technically demanding test with low reproducibility. This variability in findings is evident in the numerous definitions of ISD as determined by the maximum urethral closure pressure. Urodynamics studies from the TOMUS trial would suggest a limited future for the utilization of UPPs in clinical practice.

A great deal of information is available on the potential use of urodynamics as a predictor of the development of LUT symptoms following antiincontinence procedures. As previously mentioned, based on the results of the SISTEr trial, the predictive value of a urethral function test, specifically a VLPP, was not confirmed. A similar study by Nager et al. (2008) also noted that there were no urodynamic predictors that could be identified as useful for predicting the development of *de novo* postoperative DO after an antiincontinence procedure. Lemack et al. (2008) published their findings on the relationship between VLPP and urodynamic study findings. Voiding dysfunction was defined as the need for surgical revision to improve voiding at any point 6 weeks postoperatively. In an analysis of the 579 participants from the SISTEr trial, there were no urodynamic parameters that predicted which patients would develop voiding dysfunction following a pubovaginal sling or Burch colposuspension. Miller and colleagues (2003) attempted to predict who would develop urinary retention following a pubovaginal sling in a study of 98 women who had a cadaveric fascia lata sling procedure for SUI. In the final analysis of the 73 women who voided preoperatively without evidence of a detrusor contraction, 19% developed urinary retention postoperatively compared with 0% in those who voided with the detrusor contraction. The authors concluded that women who void with a weak or absent detrusor contraction are more likely to have postoperative urinary retention. Alperin et al. (2008) studied clinical and urodynamic parameters in 200 women who underwent a retropubic synthetic midurethral sling procedure for SUI. In the final analysis, which included 92 patients who were directly questioned preoperatively about their incontinence, none of the questions except increased daytime frequency were predictive of the development of *de novo* DO postoperatively. In addition, 56% of patients with a P_{det} greater than 15 cm H_2O during filling cystometry developed *de novo* urge incontinence, compared with 21% of patients whose pressure during filling cystometry was less than 15 cm H_2O.

In a study of 79 women undergoing tension-free vaginal tape surgery for SUI, Wang and Chen (2003) concluded that women with normal pressure-flow studies were more likely to have a better quality of life and pad test results as compared with patients with abnormal pressure-flow studies, as determined by a Q_{max} of less than 12 mL/s and a P_{det} Q_{max} of greater than 20 cm H_2O. Although these preliminary data may suggest a role for urodynamics before an antiincontinence procedure to predict postoperative voiding dysfunction and *de novo* urge incontinence, more conclusive data are required to determine whether this information would truly impact the management of women with stress incontinence. Currently, a clear role for urodynamics in patients with SUI appears to be limited to those with complex symptoms, concurrent voiding dysfunction/elevated PVR, concurrent neurologic disease, and prior incontinence surgery or pelvic radiation.

Pelvic Organ Prolapse

The role of urodynamic testing in predicting incontinence in women undergoing surgery for pelvic organ prolapse has been debated for many years. At the present time, there is no question that symptomatic pelvic organ prolapse that causes anatomic distortion to the urethra and LUT can mask the presence of urinary incontinence and will, in a certain percentage of women, become unmasked after surgical correction of the prolapse. In 2008, the Colpopexy and Urinary Reduction Efforts (CARE) trial (Visco et al., 2008) was published by the Pelvic Floor Disorders Network (PFDN). One goal of the CARE trial was to assess the importance of prolapse reduction in predicting SUI after sacral colpopexy. Preoperative urodynamics were performed, and clinicians were blinded to the results. At the time of sacral colpopexy, patients were randomized to receive either a Burch urethropexy or no antiincontinence procedure. The study ended early, because the Burch colposuspension group had a significantly lower rate of SUI than the no antiincontinence procedure group. In the trial, five different methods of reduction were used (pessary, manual reduction, swabs, forceps, and a half a speculum). SUI without prolapse reduction was uncommon, seen in only 3.7% of women, all of whom had advanced prolapse. Overall, there was a 19% incidence of urodynamic SUI with prolapse reduction, with speculum reduction having the highest incidence of SUI at 30% and pessary the lowest at 6%. Furthermore, women who developed SUI on prolapse reduction were more likely to report postoperative SUI at 3 months. Similarly, the PFDN's Outcomes Following Vaginal Prolapse Repair and Midurethral Sling trial found that women with advanced prolapse without incontinence symptoms who received a prophylactic midurethral sling had significantly less *de novo* SUI after surgery than those who did not, and that a preoperative stress test provided little differentiation between those who would benefit from a prophylactic sling and those who would not (Wei et al., 2012). The debate continues between those in favor of a prophylactic SUI treatment at the time of prolapse repair and others who worry about the potential risks of performing a surgical procedure that may never have been needed. Online clinical risk prediction models exist that provide a more accurate prediction of who will develop *de novo* stress incontinence for an individual than do complex urodynamics or a simple bladder stress test (Jelovsek et al., 2014). Although the incorporation of a bladder stress test result into this prediction model improves its accuracy, there is no evidence that a full urodynamic evaluation is beneficial in these patients (Jelovsek et al., 2019). Given the current data, a reasonable approach to these patients would be to perform a basic reduction maneuver as part of an office bladder stress test to help guide counseling around prophylactic antiincontinence surgery at the time of prolapse repair. Electronic multichannel urodynamic testing is not necessarily required. This is assuming that the patients with symptomatic prolapse have no LUT symptoms. In patients who do have LUT symptoms in conjunction with their prolapse, or who have evidence of voiding difficulty or outlet obstruction as denoted by high PVR, a more precise evaluation that could include a formal urodynamic assessment should be considered.

Overactive Bladder

In women with OAB, it is common practice to initiate nonsurgical management in the form of behavioral therapy, timed voiding, and pharmacologic therapy without a urodynamic diagnosis. Before considering a urodynamic evaluation for failure of drug therapy, the reason for failure should be explored, because many times better patient compliance or increasing drug dosage may be warranted. Urodynamic evaluation should be considered when conservative and drug therapy fail to adequately improve symptoms in a patient who is considering more invasive therapeutic interventions. Whether to discontinue antimuscarinic therapy before a urodynamic assessment is controversial. Stopping the drugs increases the likelihood of observing DO if present, whereas continuing them allows evaluation of the mechanism underlying residual refractory symptoms.

The two main urodynamic diagnoses associated with OAB are DO and increased sensation during filling. It must be emphasized that many women with OAB and urge incontinence may not have demonstrable DO on filling cystometry (Hashim & Abrams, 2006). In some patients with OAB symptoms, the ultimate urodynamic diagnosis turns out to be stress incontinence. Additional diagnoses that can be relevant to managing OAB include BOO and inefficient bladder emptying.

During filling cystometry, ideally the patient should be seated or standing, because OAB symptoms are more commonly experienced in an upright position. However, if there is severe DO at low volumes, it may be difficult to ascertain if urinary stress incontinence is also present. Sometimes a second filling in the supine position will make the DO less overt (Al-Hayek et al., 2008), allowing an increase in bladder capacity to sufficiently test for the possibility of coexistent stress incontinence. The urodynamic report should clearly state whether the OAB symptoms were reproduced during the testing session.

Mixed Urinary Incontinence

When symptoms of stress incontinence coexist with OAB symptoms, urodynamic assessment can help provide useful information regarding which condition is more severe, as well as specifically document the urodynamic stress incontinence. In a patient who complains of mixed incontinence symptoms, the probability of reproducing the stress incontinence is much higher than the probability of demonstrating DO as the cause of the patient's urge incontinence. This is why the results of the study must be closely correlated with the patient's symptoms before determining an appropriate management plan. Fig. 11.22 demonstrates a filling cystometric study demonstrating urodynamic SUI and consistent DO.

Voiding Symptoms and Outlet Obstruction

Voiding symptoms are symptoms that deviate from the norm during or after micturition. These symptoms can be experienced at the beginning of the urination (hesitancy), during urination (slow stream, intermittency, straining to void, spraying [splitting] of urinary stream, and position-dependent micturition), or at the end of the urination (feeling of incomplete bladder emptying, need to immediately revoid, and postmicturition leakage). The most extreme voiding symptom is complete urinary retention. As previously mentioned, voiding symptoms can be bladder-related (detrusor underactivity or acontractile detrusor) and/or BOO-related. They may also be related to a lack of synergy between the bladder and the outlet. Urodynamics can provide valuable information in the evaluation of female voiding symptoms. Uroflowmetry provides an initial evaluation of the patient's voiding status, with the least chance for circumstantial voiding abnormalities. This is because the test is done before urodynamic catheter insertion and in a test environment that is as close as possible to the patient's real life. Specific attention should be paid to the voided volume, the Q_{max}, and the flow curve. Although abnormal uroflowmetry can diagnose voiding abnormalities, it cannot differentiate between detrusor and BOO-related voiding symptoms. A normal uroflow in a patient with voiding symptoms most likely represents a situation where the patient perceives her voiding is abnormal, when in reality it is not.

The next important piece of information is the PVR volume. It should be kept in mind that a normal PVR does not rule out BOO. Consistently high PVR, on the other hand, usually indicates a voiding abnormality.

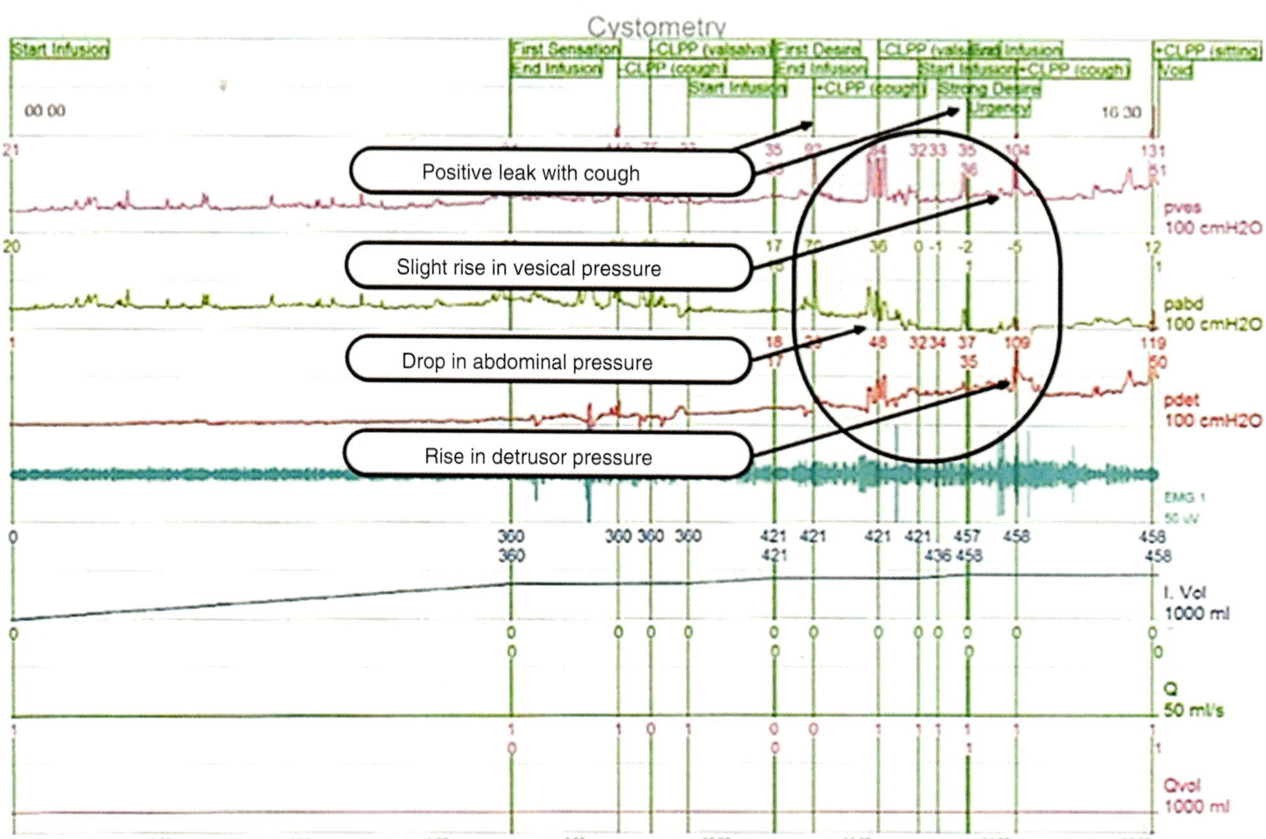

Fig. 11.22 Filling cystometry in a patient with coexistent stress incontinence and detrusor overactivity. At a volume of 421 mL, coughing produces urodynamic stress incontinence, then at a volume of 457 mL there is a rise in vesical and true detrusor pressure that is associated with significant urgency. Note that a portion of the rise in true detrusor pressure is artifactual secondary to a drop in abdominal pressure.

Filling cystometry in the setting of voiding symptoms may provide some additional information. Patients who have BOO may also have DO. Reduced or absent bladder sensation (usually with increased cystometric capacity) is a common finding in patients with abnormal detrusor contraction strength during voiding. The latter combination is more commonly seen in the setting of neuropathic diseases that affect both bladder sensation and contractility. This pattern can also be seen in patients who have encountered detrusor damage secondary to chronic bladder distention.

Pressure-flow studies correlate the flow rate to P_{det} during voiding. In general, women are low-pressure voiders. Therefore, it is not uncommon to see normal urine flow with a low or even absent detrusor contraction. High P_{det}, on the other hand, with low urine flow rate usually represents a form of BOO (Video 11.9).

Neurogenic Bladder

Certain neurologic diseases are associated with bladder and urethral dysfunction. Although at times generalizations can be made about the type of dysfunction based on the disease and level of the lesion, these inferences are not reliable. Patients with neurogenic bladder will present with storage symptoms, emptying symptoms, or both. The goals of treating patients with neurogenic bladder is to treat their urinary incontinence, assure efficient bladder emptying, avoid neurogenic bladder-related complications, and avoid any upper urinary tract deterioration. Urodynamic studies are very commonly indicated in these patients, because valuable information can be retrieved. Filling cystometry can assess for abnormal bladder compliance and DO; pressure-flow studies can differentiate BOO from impaired detrusor contractility as a cause of impaired bladder emptying; and EMG studies can assist in diagnosing DESD, which carries a risk for vesicoureteral reflux and renal failure. The use of video urodynamics in the setting of neurogenic bladder can add some anatomic details and will be discussed later in this chapter. Video 11.10 demonstrates poor detrusor compliance and ISD in a patient with spina bifida, and Video 11.11 demonstrates detrusor external sphincter dysnergia in a patient with multiple sclerosis (MS).

An important consideration when contemplating a urodynamic study on a neurogenic bladder patient is to weigh the risks of the study against the potential benefit of the information that will be obtained. Urodynamic studies may increase the risk of urinary tract infections, which is already high in this population. Also, some neurogenic bladder patients are at increased risk for autonomic dysreflexia, a condition that is life threatening and can be induced by bladder filling. These patients should be monitored for symptoms and signs of autonomic dysreflexia. If the condition is diagnosed, prompt bladder emptying should be performed, which will usually resolve the symptoms.

VIDEO URODYNAMICS

Video urodynamic (VUD) testing consists of simultaneous measurement of the typical urodynamic parameters in conjunction with imaging of the LUT (Fig. 11.23). It is thought by most to provide the most precise evaluation of LUT dysfunction (McGuire et al., 1996). VUDs are similar to conventional

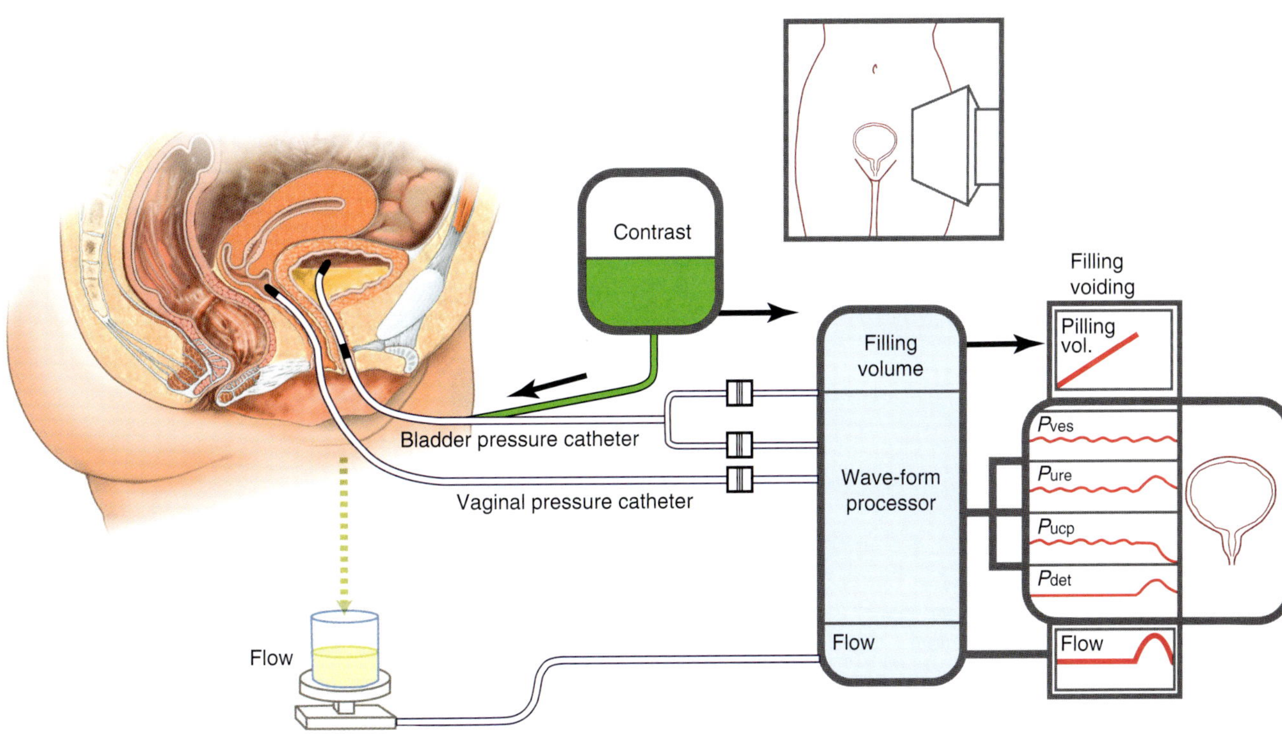

Fig. 11.23 Video urodynamic testing. Multichannel urodynamic tests are performed with the addition of fluoroscopy, allowing simultaneous visualization of the lower urinary tract during recording of pressures. Contrast is used as the filling media. P_{ves}, Intravesical pressure; P_{det}, detrusor pressure; P_{ucp}, urethral closure pressure.

urodynamics, with the addition of contrast media as the filling solution and the use of fluoroscopy. This allows for simultaneous anatomic and functional evaluation of the LUT.

Indications

Although the indications for VUD testing are controversial, most would agree they are most useful in women with a known neurologic condition that is felt to affect LUT function. In 2009, the Fourth Consultation on Incontinence Committee on dynamic testing made the following grade B/C recommendation on the basis of the available evidence-based literature (Hosker et al., 2009): patients with suspected neurogenic dysfunction of the LUT should receive comprehensive urodynamic evaluation including VUDs, if possible, to establish the state and function of the lower tract. VUDs can identify certain pathologies and are important when trying to answer a specific clinical question. The AUA Urodynamics Guidelines state: "VUDS can be performed in properly selected patients to localize the level of obstruction, particularly for diagnosing primary bladder neck obstruction" (Brown et al., 2013; Winters et al., 2012). In younger patients with voiding dysfunction, VUDs can differentiate between functional obstruction and dysfunctional voiding (Brown et al., 2013).

A VUD study can provide objective documentation of the effect of the neurologic lesion on vesicourethral function, as well as assess for the presence of certain risk factors that could decompensate the upper urinary tract. These risk factors include DESD, low bladder compliance, and sustained high-magnitude detrusor contractions. Without effective therapy, patients with these risk factors have up to an 85% chance of developing hydronephrosis, vesicoureteral reflux, and/or urosepsis within 5 years (McGuire et al., 1981). In cases of impaired compliance in which there is compensation by a pop-off mechanism of vesicoureteral reflux, the impaired compliance may not be identified unless the reflux is also recognized by fluoroscopy. Also, an accurate DLPP can be obtained in cases where it would otherwise be impossible to observe any leakage.

In women with BOO, VUD testing is the only way to localize the exact level of obstruction. If there is no obvious anatomic cause of obstruction, VUDs can differentiate between functional causes of obstruction, such as primary bladder neck obstruction and dysfunctional voiding. Other indications may include any patient who is at high risk for complicated voiding dysfunction for whom an accurate diagnosis cannot otherwise be obtained. This could include unexplained urinary retention in women, prior radical pelvic surgery, urinary diversion, prerenal or postrenal transplant, or prior pelvic radiation. Finally, VUDs may be helpful in some women with severe recurrent SUI and ISD, as visualizing the urethra during provocation may be clinically useful. Table 11.1 reviews possible indications for VUDs and lists additional information that can be obtained by this technique compared with conventional urodynamics.

Technique

The Video Urodynamic Lab. The urodynamic room should be set up in a way that minimizes patient discomfort and anxiety. The room should be large enough to fit all the equipment necessary for the procedure, including the fluoroscopy machine and the fluorocompatible chair (Fig. 11.24). The disposables required for the procedure should be kept and organized in cabinets within the room to avoid running in and out of the room during the procedure. A C-arm is preferable over fixed fluoroscopy machines, because it allows different angles of view and flexibility during patient positioning.

TABLE 11.1 Possible Indications for Video Urodynamics With Potential Findings that Could Not be Obtained With Conventional Urodynamics

Possible Indication for Video Urodynamics	Potential Findings
Neurogenic bladder	• Vesicoureteral reflux • DESD • DSSD • The cause of neurogenic bladder (e.g., sacral agenesis, spina bifida, spine deformities or fractures)
Unexplained urinary retention	• In cases of bladder outlet obstruction, exact location is identified • Functional obstruction • Dysfunctional voiding
Cases at risk for poor bladder compliance: • Previous radical pelvic surgery • Pelvic irradiation • Chronic cystitis • Long-term indwelling catheter • History of long-term anuria (e.g., patient who was on hemodialysis then received renal transplant)	• Vesicoureteral reflux • Bladder diverticula • Bladder trabeculations
Cases of recurrent incontinence after one or more previous surgeries	• Open bladder neck at rest • Intrinsic urethral sphincter deficiency • Bladder and/or urethral diverticulum • Urogenital fistula • Filling defects in the bladder (radiolucent stones, foreign bodies, bladder tumors, etc.)

DESD, Detrusor external sphincter dyssynergia; *DSSD*, Detrusor smooth sphincter dyssynergia.

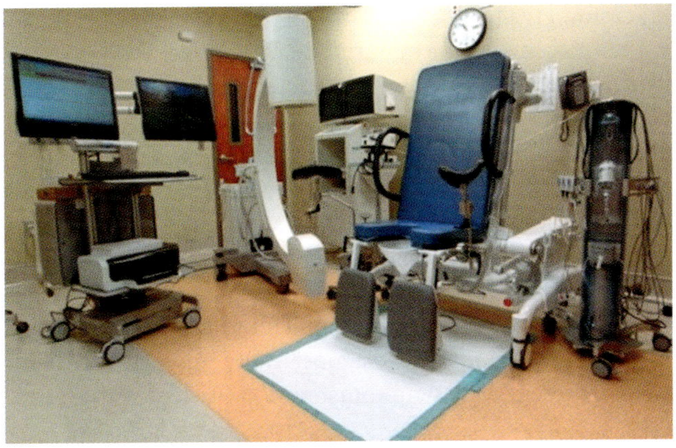

Fig. 11.24 Video urodynamic laboratory.

Patient Positioning. VUD testing can be done in the supine, sitting, or standing positions. The test is usually begun in the sitting position, with the understanding that changing patient position may become necessary at certain points of the test. For example, changing from the sitting to the standing positions may be necessary to demonstrate SUI. Likewise, a change from a supine to a lateral position may be needed to further localize certain anatomic findings such as bladder or urethral diverticula.

Radiation Exposure. VUD testing comes with the cost of risking radiation exposure to both the staff and patient. In a study of radiation exposure during VUDs in the pediatric population, Ngo et al. (2011) reported a mean radiation exposure of 10 mGy per study. Radiation exposure has many known biological effects, including the risk for secondary cancer (Brenner & Hall, 2007). This makes it crucial to take all possible precautions to minimize radiation exposure for both the staff and patients. The staff should wear lead protection shields and use radiation exposure monitors to track their cumulative exposure time. The number of images should be kept to a minimum and only taken for the high-yield parts of the study. Intermittent (as opposed to continuous) fluoroscopy should be used. Modern fluoroscopy machines are equipped with the "last image hold" feature that can keep the last image frozen so the physician can use that image as a reference for next steps without the need to repeat that image. Other important features of modern fluoroscopy machines include "pulsed fluoroscopy," in which the radiation beams are emitted in intermittent pulses, and a "dose-spreading" technique. During VUDs, most of the images are focused on the pelvic area, which may predispose certain areas of the patient's skin to radiation. One way to avoid this is to rotate the fluoroscope around a central area within the anatomy of interest. Furthermore, it is advisable to keep the image source away from the patient, while keeping the image receptor close to her (Mahesh, 2001).

Performing the Video Study. The actual technique of VUD testing is very similar to the technique used for conventional urodynamics, except that contrast is the filling media, and fluoroscopic images are obtained during filling and voiding. The study usually begins with a noninstrumented uroflow, as previously described. The authors generally obtain five basic images during VUDs. The first is a scout film to visualize any significant radiopaque shadows or bony abnormalities within the pelvic region. After filling is started, a second image assures appropriate positioning of the urodynamic catheter in the bladder. The next image is usually taken as continuous fluoroscopy during Valsalva and cough stress tests. This is done at an initial bladder volume of 150 mL. If the patient does not leak at the initial filling volumes, we repeat this step after every 100 mL of infused contrast until the patient reaches her maximum cystometric capacity, or until an obvious abnormality such as SUI, impaired compliance, or DO is demonstrated. A voiding film is obtained during the emptying phase of the study. This image is particularly important to assess the bladder outlet in patients with obstructive voiding symptoms. The last image is taken after the patient voids to completion to assess for any PVR contrast. Additional images are taken during the test as needed, such as during rises in true P_{det} or when low bladder compliance is noticed to identify any vesicoureteral reflux and/or urinary incontinence.

Interpretation

The scout film should be free of abnormal radiopaque shadows in the pelvic region. This film should be examined for bony lesions such as spine fracture, plates and screws, spina bifida, sacral agenesis, and so on. These lesions may predispose to neuropathic disease and development of neurogenic bladder. Bony anatomic abnormalities also may contraindicate certain treatments, such as sacral nerve stimulation. In patients who were previously treated for urinary incontinence, the initial fluoroscopy image may show a migrated or malpositioned sacral neuromodulator lead or a radiopaque bulking agent at the bladder neck area.

Patients with neuropathy and LUT dysfunction can present clinically with incontinence, which may be of bladder origin (DO or impaired compliance) or sphincter origin. They also may present with difficulty emptying, which can be of bladder origin (impaired detrusor contractility) or sphincter origin (dyssynergia). Finally, some neuropathic patients may present with upper urinary tract decompression with hydroureter, hydronephrosis, and even renal insufficiency without any bothersome LUT symptoms.

During bladder filling, the cystogram should be free of filling defects, and the bladder outline should be smooth without sacculae or diverticula. The ureters should not be seen during the filling cystogram or during the voiding cystourethrogram. The bladder neck should be closed during the filling phase of the study, regardless of patient position or activity (resting, Valsalva, or cough). The lower border of the bladder should be at the level of the symphysis pubis. Deviation from these normal findings during filling cystometry may suggest bladder and/or bladder outlet pathology. Examples include ISD, bladder diverticula, vesicoureteral reflux, cystocele, bladder tumors, bladder stones or foreign bodies, and previously injected urethral bulking agents.

During filling the P_{det} should be closely observed. Any rise in P_{det} needs to be looked at closely to determine if it is simple accommodation or a true decrease in compliance. Also, DO, particularly if the contraction is sustained and of low amplitude, can be confused with impaired compliance. If filling is stopped and the pressure returns to baseline, then the compliance is not impaired. A number of pop-off mechanisms can make bladder compliance appear better than it actually is. Examples of this would be vesicoureteral reflux, which basically means that bladder pressure is being transferred to the reflexing renal unit, which, over time, will be harmful to the upper tract. Fig. 11.25 demonstrates vesicoureteral reflux into a transplanted kidney. Another example is a large bladder diverticulum that may protect the upper tract. Finally, an incompetent outlet may be a pop-off mechanism. It may only become apparent when outlet resistance is increased, which can be demonstrated during filling cystometry by occluding the urethra. It can occur surgically after placement of a suburethral sling.

During the voiding phase, the bladder neck should be open, and the urethra should be relaxed and free of strictures, diverticula, or filling defects. This part of the study is aimed at diagnosing BOO. The diagnosis of BOO in women is more difficult than in men, because there is a lack of standardized nomograms available to help establish the diagnosis. Furthermore, it is well-known that many women can void to completion without a significant rise in P_{det}. This makes it difficult to use P_{det} parameters as they are used in men to diagnose BOO. Also, women with BOO may present with symptoms more consistent with storage

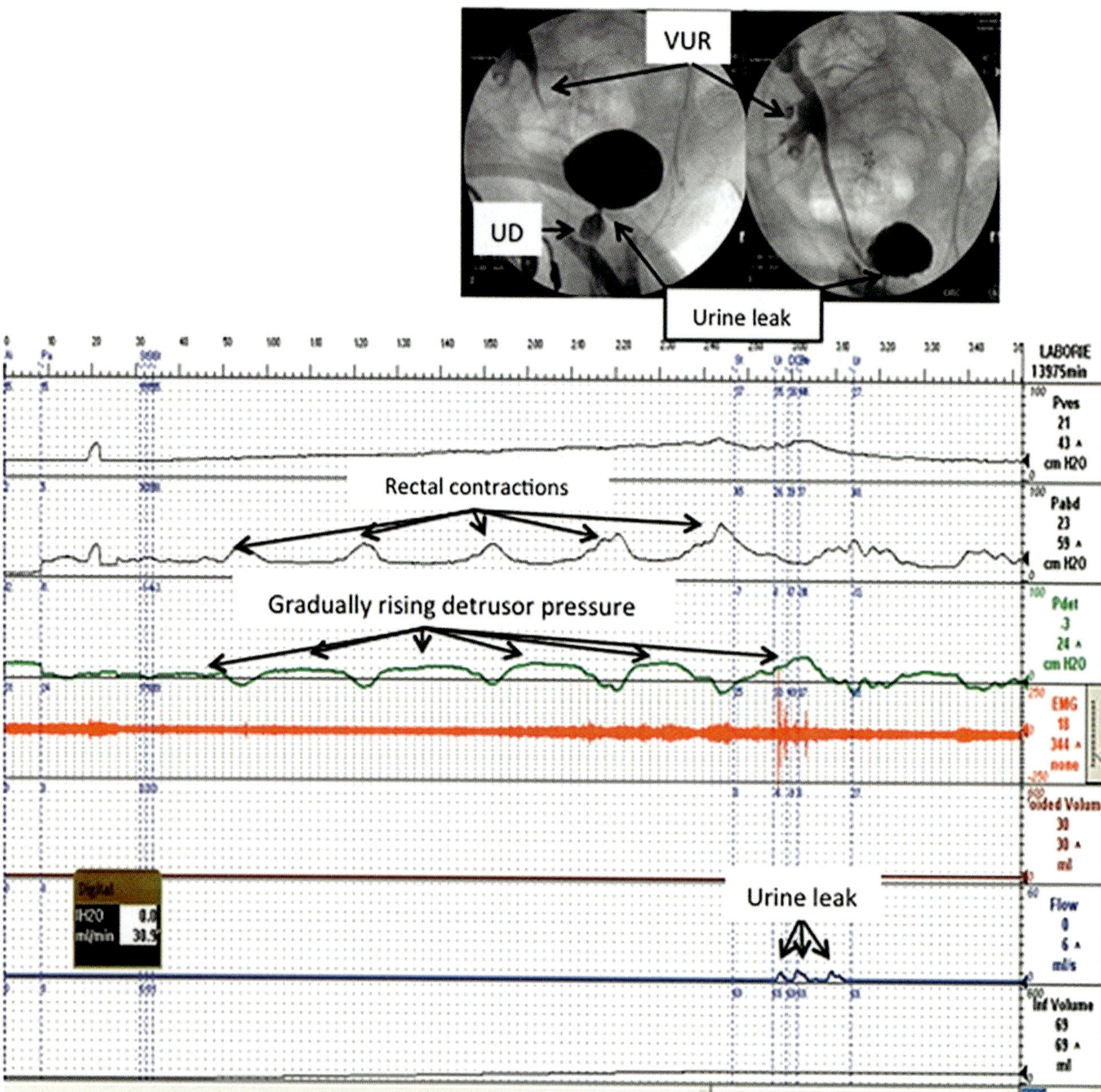

Fig. 11.25 Video urodynamic tests on a 44-year-old woman with urinary incontinence 4 months after a renal transplant. Before renal transplant, the patient was anuric for 7 years. Video urodynamic studies demonstrate a low bladder capacity, low bladder compliance (notice gradual rise in detrusor pressure that is partially masked by rectal contractions), vesicoureteral reflux into the transplanted kidney, and leak per urethra, as well as a possible urethral diverticulum.

abnormalities, such as urgency and frequency, in contrast to the typical symptoms consistent with difficult voiding.

BOO in women can be either anatomic or functional (Fig. 11.26). Anatomic causes are primarily iatrogenic. In a retrospective study of 86 women with anatomic BOO, Brucker et al. (2013) found antiincontinence surgery to be the most common cause. Other causes included pelvic organ prolapse, external compression, urethral diverticulum, and urethral stricture. Functional BOO, on the other hand, refers to failure of relaxation of the bladder neck and/or the urethral sphincter in coordination with detrusor muscle contraction during urination. VUDs have the unique advantage of differentiating different forms of female BOO. This is because of their ability not only to capture the P_{det} uroflow parameters, but also to localize the level of obstruction. Diagnosis of anatomic BOO is largely based on the history and physical examination, which are usually able to detect the cause. In the patient with functional BOO with a history of neurogenic bladder (typically suprasacral lesions), failure of sphincter relaxation is termed *DESD* (Fig. 11.27). If the patient has no history suggestive of neurogenic bladder, the condition is termed

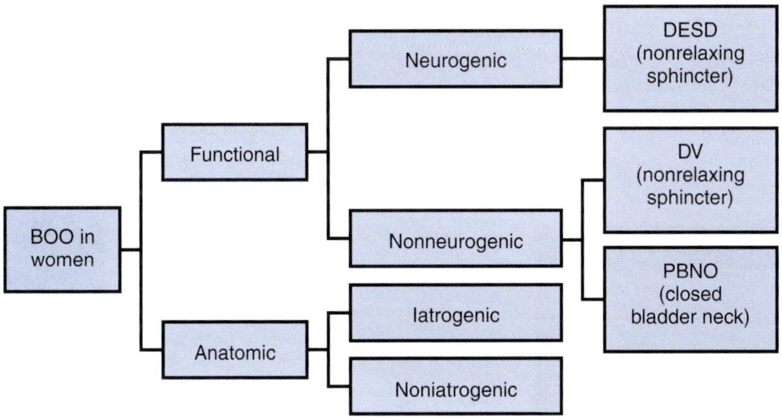

Fig. 11.26 Classification of bladder outlet obstruction in women. *BOO*, Bladder outlet obstruction; *DV*, dysfunctional voiding; *DESD*, detrusor external sphincter dyssynergia; *PBNO*, primary bladder neck obstruction.

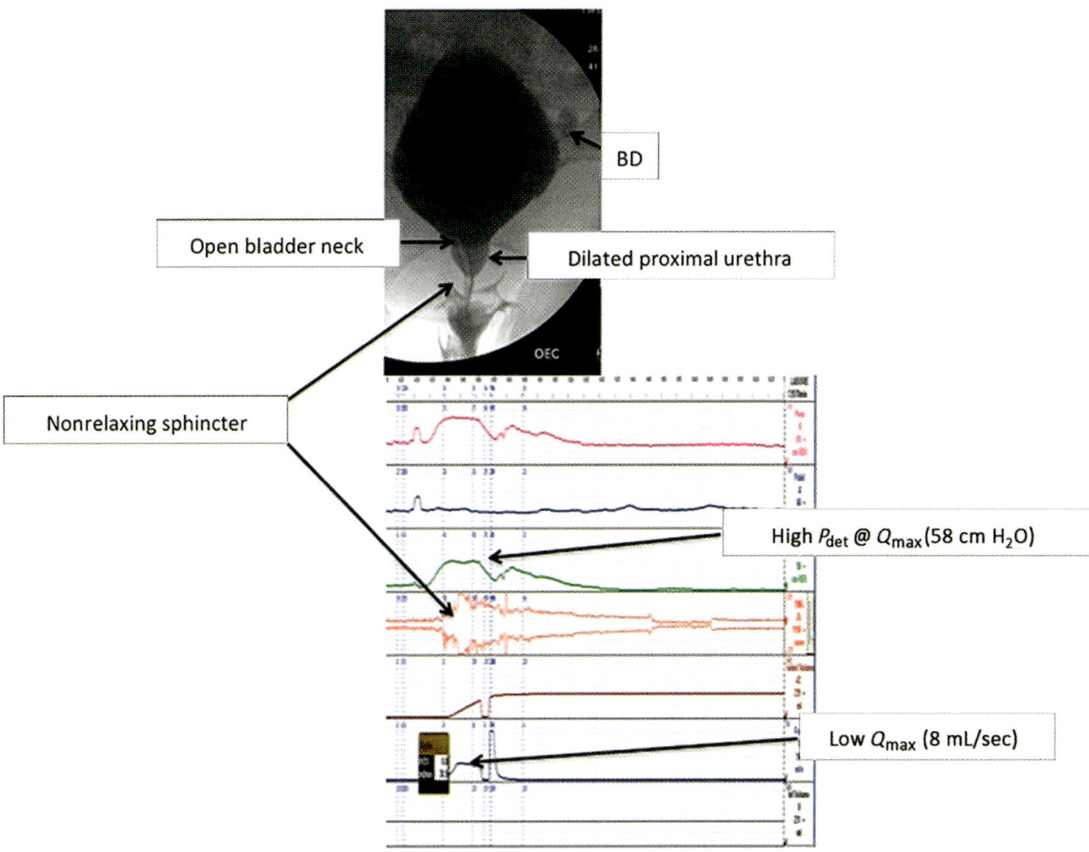

Fig. 11.27 Video urodynamic tests showing detrusor external sphincter dyssynergia (DESD) in a patient with T6 spinal cord injury. The classic findings of DESD as shown in the study include high detrusor pressure, low urine flow, open bladder neck, dilated proximal urethra, and nonrelaxing sphincter. Note also the small bladder diverticulum.

dysfunctional voiding. Primary bladder neck obstruction is the term used to describe the rare patient who is neurologically intact and shown on VUDs to have a closed bladder neck during attempts at voiding.

CASE DISCUSSIONS

Case 1: A 49-Year-Old Female with Recurrent Stress Urinary Incontinence and History of a Pelvic Fracture (Figs. 11.28 A & B)

MM is a 49-year-old female who presented with recurrent SUI. Pertinent in her medical history is a motor vehicle accident with subsequent pelvic fracture that was fixed with a plate and screws. After the accident, she developed severe SUI, which was initially treated with a transobturator sling. On presentation, she was soaking through 12 protective pads per day. General and focused neurological examinations were unremarkable. Vaginal examination revealed urethral hypermobility, an exposed piece of the polypropylene mesh in the left vaginal sulcus, no pelvic organ prolapse, negative empty supine stress test, and no vaginal atrophy. Because the patient has recurrent incontinence with a history of pelvic fracture, VUDs were obtained.

Urodynamic Findings

Uroflowmetry. Patient voided 118 mL in 22 seconds with a PVR of 40 mL. The flow curve showed a normal bell-shaped pattern. Although the voided volume was less than 150 mL, the uroflow parameters were all within the normal range.

Filling Cystometry (Fig. 11.28A). The filling cystometry was performed using Omnipaque with a filling rate of 50 mL/min. The first sensation of bladder filling occurred at a volume of

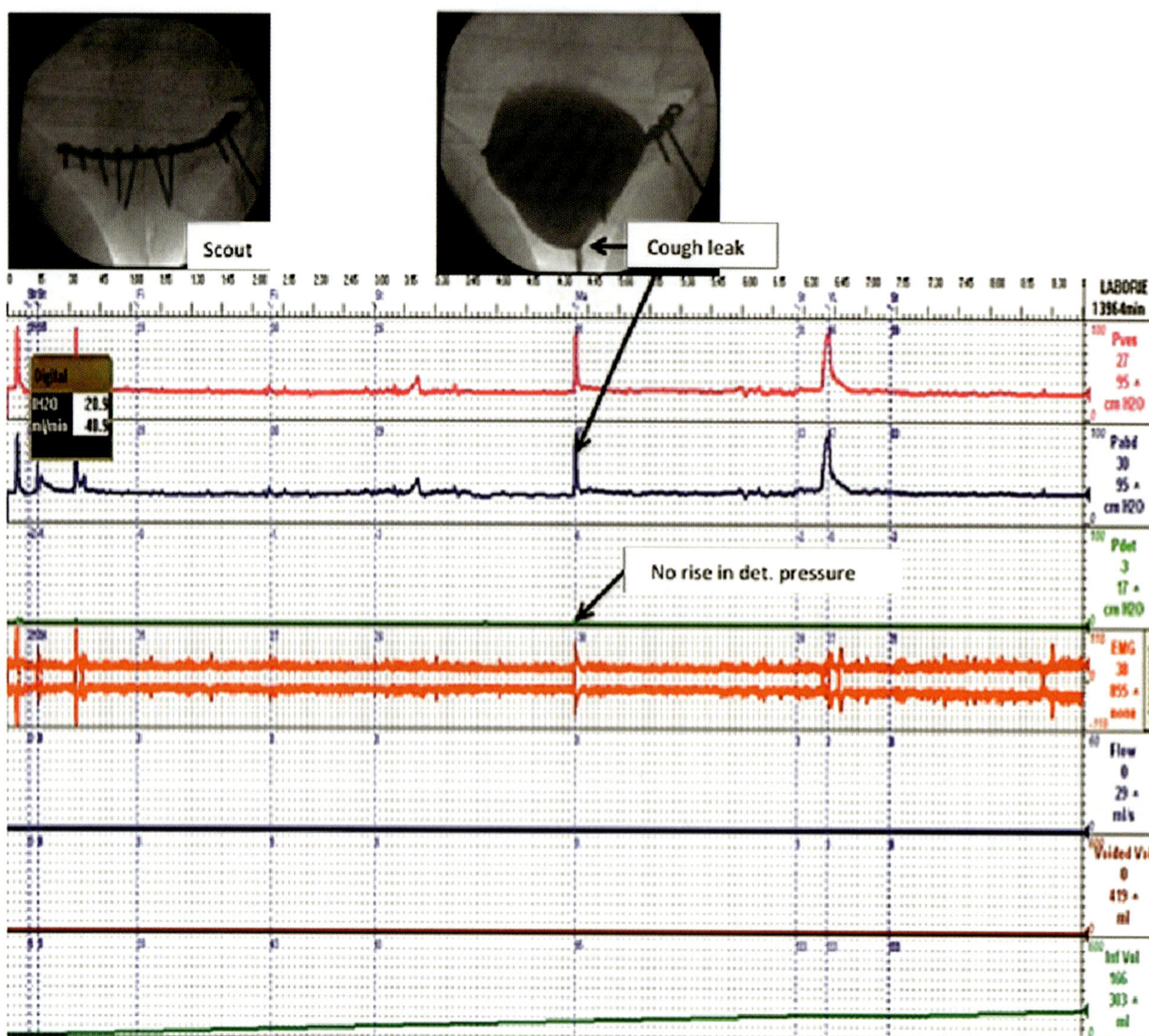

A

Fig. 11.28 Case 1. A, Filling cystometry in a patient with history of pelvic fracture and recurrent stress urinary incontinence (SUI). Note stable detrusor with normal compliance. Urodynamic SUI is demonstrated at a volume of 150 mL with a cough leak point pressure of 96 cm H_2O.

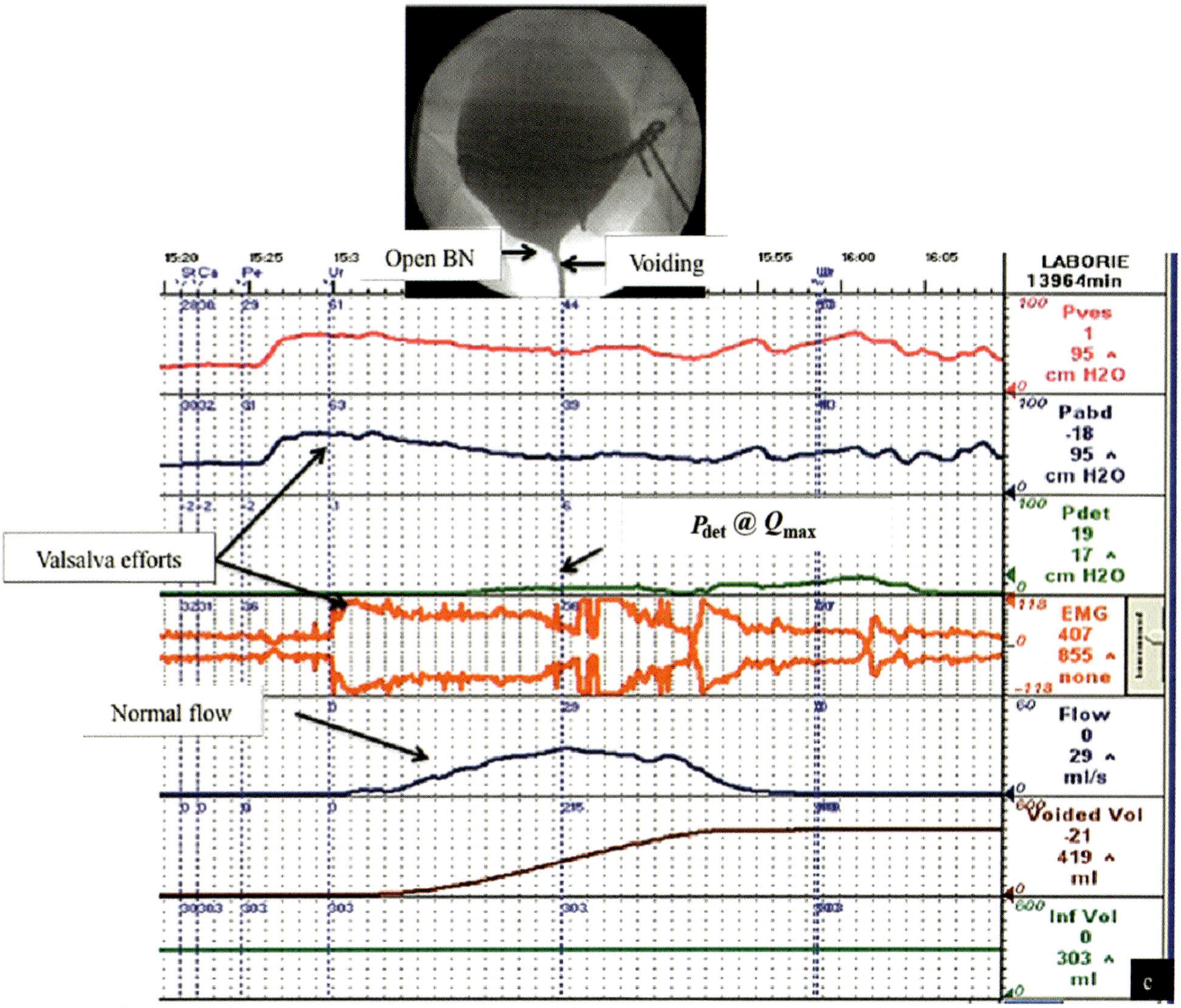

B

Fig. 11.28 Cont'd B, Pressure-flow study in a patient with a history of pelvic fracture and recurrent SUI. Note good flow with minimal rise in detrusor pressure and significant Valsalva effort.

20 mL, desire to void at 61 mL, and strong desire to void at 303 mL. Because the first sensation occurred at a very low volume, impaired bladder sensation was excluded. Urodynamic stress incontinence was demonstrated at a volume of 150 mL, with a cough leak point pressure of 96 cm H_2O. The filling phase of the study demonstrated a stable detrusor with normal bladder compliance.

Pressure-Flow Study (Fig. 11.28B). The patient voided 315 mL with a Q_{max} of 29 mL/s and a P_{det} at Q_{max} of 6 cm H_2O. This finding, in conjunction with the initial uroflow and low PVR, rules out BOO in this patient. There is an increase in the intraabdominal pressure, which reflects an additional Valsalva effort during voiding.

Electromyography. EMG activity responds appropriately to cough, which reflects an intact guarding reflex even though this guarding reflex failed to prevent stress leakage. During voiding, the pelvic floor muscles and the external sphincter should be completely relaxed; thus EMG activity should be silent. In this case, the increased EMG activity during voiding was likely related to the possibility that she may have a discoordinated pelvic floor response, which is not clinically significant because she emptied well with an adequate flow.

Fluoroscopic Findings. The scout film (Fig. 11.28A) shows the plate and screws in the pubic region. The cystogram (see Fig. 11.28A) showed the bladder neck to be wide open during cough, with visible urethral leakage.

During voiding (Fig. 11.28B), the bladder neck is open, with no evidence of urethral obstruction. The urethra is a little distorted, probably related to the previous pelvic fracture and/or previous sling procedure. Note the minimal rise in P_{det}, with a good urine flow secondary to a significant Valsalva effort. A postvoid film confirmed complete bladder emptying.

Discussion. This patient has recurrent SUI, which initially developed after a motor vehicle accident resulting in a pelvic fracture. The pathogenesis of her SUI is probably a disruption of the periurethral attachments with subsequent urethral hypermobility. Another possible mechanism is neuropathic ISD secondary to a significant pelvic fracture. The VUDs confirmed SUI and ruled out BOO. Also noted were bony changes related to the previous pelvic fracture. The patient ultimately underwent excision of the exposed sling and insertion of a synthetic retropubic sling. Her SUI improved, but she ultimately needed an additional urethral bulking agent injection to make her completely dry.

In summary, VUD in this patient allowed a complete assessment of the condition of her pelvic bones and the position of the metal plates, which may have influenced any future surgical procedure. In addition, neurogenic bladder, which could have resulted from pelvic nerve damage, was ruled out.

Case 2: A 56-Year-Old Female With Multiple Sclerosis and Urinary Incontinence (Fig. 11.29)

AK is a 56-year-old female who was diagnosed with MS 15 years before presentation. During the course of her disease, she had developed urge urinary incontinence that was complicated by paraplegia and limited mobility. Initially her incontinence was managed with an indwelling Foley catheter. On examination, the patient was wheelchair-bound with an otherwise normal body habitus. Pelvic examination was unremarkable; the urethra was normal, and the Foley catheter was noted to be draining clear urine. Focused neurologic examination was positive for paraplegia, with what appeared to be a normal pudendal nerve sensory distribution.

Urodynamic Findings

Uroflowmetry. The patient had a Foley catheter inserted so no uroflow study could be obtained.

Filling Cystometry (Fig. 11.29). The patient did not experience any sensation during filling cystometry. She started to leak secondary to poor bladder compliance and ISD at a volume of 68 mL. The lowest value of the P_{det} at which the patient started to leak without a detrusor contraction or increased intraabdominal pressure was 14 cm H_2O (DLPP). VLPP and cough leak point pressure could not be assessed because of the small bladder volume. Bladder compliance improved toward the end of the study after the bladder had emptied.

Electromyography. The EMG shows a synergistic response of increased muscle activity during high P_{det} in an attempt to prevent leakage. No pressure-flow study could be performed because the patient had involuntarily emptied her bladder during filling.

Fluoroscopy. Cystogram showed a small bladder volume, open bladder neck during filling, and leakage of contrast through the urethra. There is also right vesicoureteral reflux. The urodynamic diagnosis for this patient is a low cystometric capacity, with impaired bladder compliance, ISD, and right vesicoureteral reflux.

Discussion. MS is a disease of neural demyelination that affects women twice as often as men. The disease affects mostly the cervical spinal cord but can also affect the brain and other spinal cord segments. Voiding dysfunction occurs in up to 90% of MS patients, with urinary incontinence occurring in 37% to 72% of those affected. The goals of treating patients with suspected neurogenic bladder are to keep the patient dry, maintain

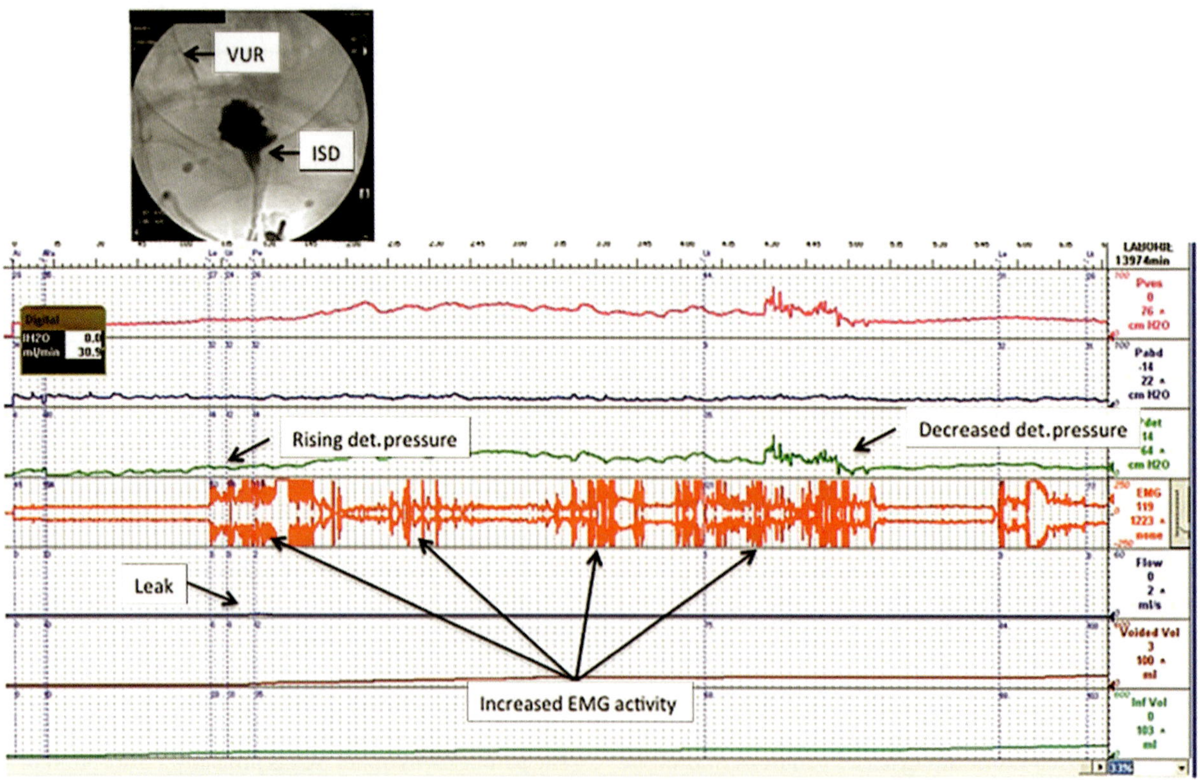

Fig. 11.29 Case 2. Video urodynamics in a patient with multiple sclerosis. Notice the rise in detrusor pressure during filling with no concomitant rise in the abdominal pressure. Also noted is the right vesicoureteral reflux and the leak per urethra occurring at low pressures.

sufficient bladder emptying, and avoid neurogenic bladder–related complications. The main complaint of this patient was urinary incontinence; VUDs showed low cystometric capacity and impaired bladder compliance with leakage. Because she could not ambulate, she would not benefit from any therapy that would only improve her micturition warning time; thus, there is no role for medical or minimally invasive treatment options for urge urinary incontinence in this case.

The patient has an indwelling Foley catheter that, when used for long periods, has known associated risks of infection, encrustation, and potential for development of bladder cancer. The indwelling urethral catheter also carries risk for urethral erosion, fistula, and worsening of leakage. A suprapubic tube could be considered as an alternative, with the advantage of avoiding the urethra, but the patient may still continue to leak through the urethra. Furthermore, the suprapubic tube carries similar risks for recurrent urinary tract infection, encrustation, and bladder mucosal changes. Based on this complicated situation, different forms of urinary diversion (continent and incontinent) were discussed with the patient, because this approach would assure tubeless drainage, and hence avoid the indwelling catheter–related complications. Because she had reasonable manual dexterity, the patient elected to proceed with a continent urinary diversion. Given the small bladder capacity and right vesicoureteral reflux, bladder augmentation was concomitantly performed. Because there were also concerns about constant urethral leakage postoperatively, an obstructive rectus fascia sling was also placed. In the setting of continent urinary diversion, the authors prefer an obstructive biologic sling over bladder neck closure for treatment of ISD, because this allows for future urinary endoscopic procedures.

VUDs detected the important finding of vesicoureteral reflux that could have been missed if conventional urodynamic studies alone had been performed.

Case 3: Urinary Incontinence After Pelvic Irradiation (Fig. 11.30)

TL is a 60-year-old female referred for severe, long-standing urinary incontinence. She has a history of cervical cancer treated with hysterectomy and pelvic irradiation 22 years ago. She had been tried on different antimuscarinic medications, without significant improvement. She also had failed Interstim therapy and intravesical Botox injection. She eventually had an indwelling Foley catheter placed in the hopes of temporarily relieving her severe leakage; however, catheter placement resulted in recurrent urinary tract infections, pain, and intermittent hematuria. On examination, the patient was moderately obese, and, although she was able to walk, she frequently used a wheelchair. Vaginal examination demonstrated severe vaginal atrophy with vaginal stenosis. The Foley catheter was noted to be draining cloudy urine.

Urodynamic Findings

Uroflow Study. This study was not done, because the patient had an indwelling Foley catheter.

Filling Cystometry (Fig. 11.30). The bladder was initially filled to capacity of 40 mL, with a first desire to void at 28 mL. She did not reach a normal desire to void secondary to terminal DO at 40 mL. Repeat bladder filling at a slower rate was done with the hope of obtaining a filling volume sufficient to evaluate for SUI. The second attempt at filling resulted in another episode of terminal DO at an infusion volume of 81 mL. There was also evidence of gradually increasing P_{det} (although of low amplitude) with filling, suggesting poor bladder compliance. This was hard to confirm because of the low filling volumes. Because the bladder was completely emptied with terminal DO, no pressure-flow studies could be obtained.

Fluoroscopy. The scout film showed the Interstim lead to be in a good position. Cystogram showed low cystometric capacity and vesicoureteral reflux, as well as urethral leakage with each bout of terminal DO. Her final urodynamic diagnosis was terminal DO, low cystometric capacity, poor bladder compliance, left vesicoureteral reflux, and normal position of the previously placed sacral neuromodulator lead.

Discussion. Urinary incontinence after pelvic irradiation can have multiple etiologies. SUI may develop secondary to a fibrotic (pipe stem) urethra and subsequent ISD. Urge incontinence and DO may occur secondary to detrusor damage, resulting in poor bladder compliance and capacity. Detrusor damage and/or urethral stricture secondary to urethral fibrosis and scarring may result in urinary retention with overflow urinary incontinence. Finally, in patients who develop extensive tissue necrosis after radiation, vesicovaginal fistula may develop, resulting in severe continuous urine leakage. The VUDs confirmed a contracted bladder with terminal DO, poor bladder compliance, and left vesicoureteral reflux. Also, the sacral neuromodulator lead was seen in a normal position, which excludes technical factors as an explanation for failure of neuromodulation. The patient was counseled about different options and ultimately underwent a transverse colon conduit. The transverse colon was used in this case to avoid the possibility of using irradiated small bowel.

Case 4: Female Urethral Stricture (Fig. 11.31)

A 49-year-old female was referred with a diagnosis of a urethral stricture with high PVR volumes and symptoms of urgency and frequency. She had received multiple urethral dilations in the past in an attempt to relieve the urethral stricture. She was eventually kept on daily urethral self-calibration, noting that she could not urinate if she missed 1 day of self-calibration. The diagnosis of urethral stricture had been made on urethroscopy, noting urethral bleeding when an attempt was made to advance the scope through the stricture. Otherwise her genitourinary examination was normal. PVR volume in the office was 200 mL. The patient was counseled about the need for suprapubic tube insertion as a temporary measure for her urine retention. This would allow healing of the urethra, and a more precise evaluation could then be performed.

Urodynamic Findings. VUDs were performed to assess her bladder and the proximal end of the stricture, and to rule out vesicoureteral reflux secondary to BOO. There was no uroflow study or PVR obtained, because the patient had a suprapubic

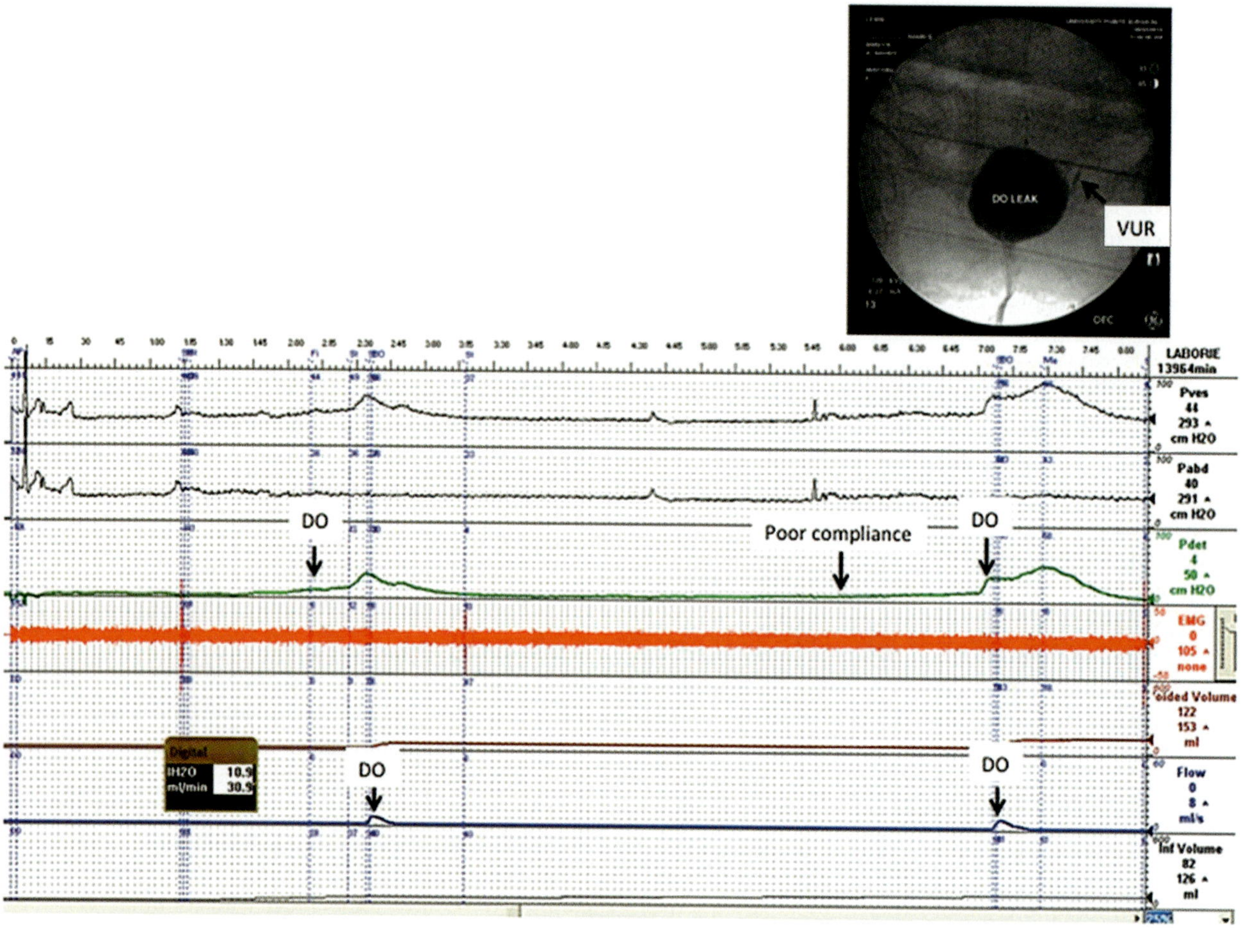

Fig. 11.30 Case 3. Video urodynamic tracing and cystogram showing two episodes of terminal detrusor overactivity with leakage, questionable bladder compliance, and left vesicoureteral reflux. Note also the position of the Interstim lead and the leakage per urethra on the cystogram.

catheter in place. The suprapubic tube was clamped to allow for bladder filling. This phase of the study was normal, with normal cystometric capacity, bladder sensation, and compliance. There was no DO or leak with cough or Valsalva. The pressure-flow study (Fig. 11.31) noted that the patient spontaneously voided a few drops of contrast, even though she had a P_{det} of 85 cm H_2O. The voiding cystogram confirmed a dilated bladder neck and proximal part of the urethra, with narrowing at the distal part. Also noted was a small bladder diverticulum.

Discussion. Urethral stricture is a rare cause of female BOO requiring a high index of suspicion for diagnosis. Possible clues are obstructive voiding symptoms in a patient who has a history of urethral trauma, urethral infections, or urethral surgery. Oftentimes, as in this case, a cystoscope cannot pass through the stricture and therefore does not provide details about the proximal extent of the stricture. A retrograde urethrogram could be attempted but is technically difficult in females and has a low clinical yield. Evaluation of the proximal part of the urethra can be obtained with a voiding cystogram or antegrade cystoscopy by passing a scope through the suprapubic tube tract. Because this patient had significant storage symptoms in conjunction with a known anatomic problem, VUDs were performed, which involved a voiding cystogram as well as filling cystometry to exclude the possibility of vesicoureteral reflux secondary to BOO. The study showed the classic picture of BOO, with high P_{det} and absence of significant urine flow. The study confirmed that the patient has good detrusor contractility and normal bladder compliance and capacity. Because she had previously undergone multiple urethral dilations that failed to correct the stricture urethral, reconstruction using a vaginal skin flap was performed.

AMERICAN UROLOGICAL ASSOCIATION/ SOCIETY OF URODYNAMICS, FEMALE PELVIC MEDICINE & UROGENITAL RECONSTRUCTION GUIDELINES ON URODYNAMIC STUDIES IN ADULTS

A review of the literature was performed that resulted in a guideline statement regarding the utilization of urodynamic tests after the evaluation and symptom characterization of a patient with LUT dysfunction (Winters et al., 2012). The goal was to identify peer-reviewed publications relevant to using urodynamic tests for making a diagnosis, determining prognosis, guiding clinical management decisions, and improving patient outcomes in patients with various LUT symptoms. The

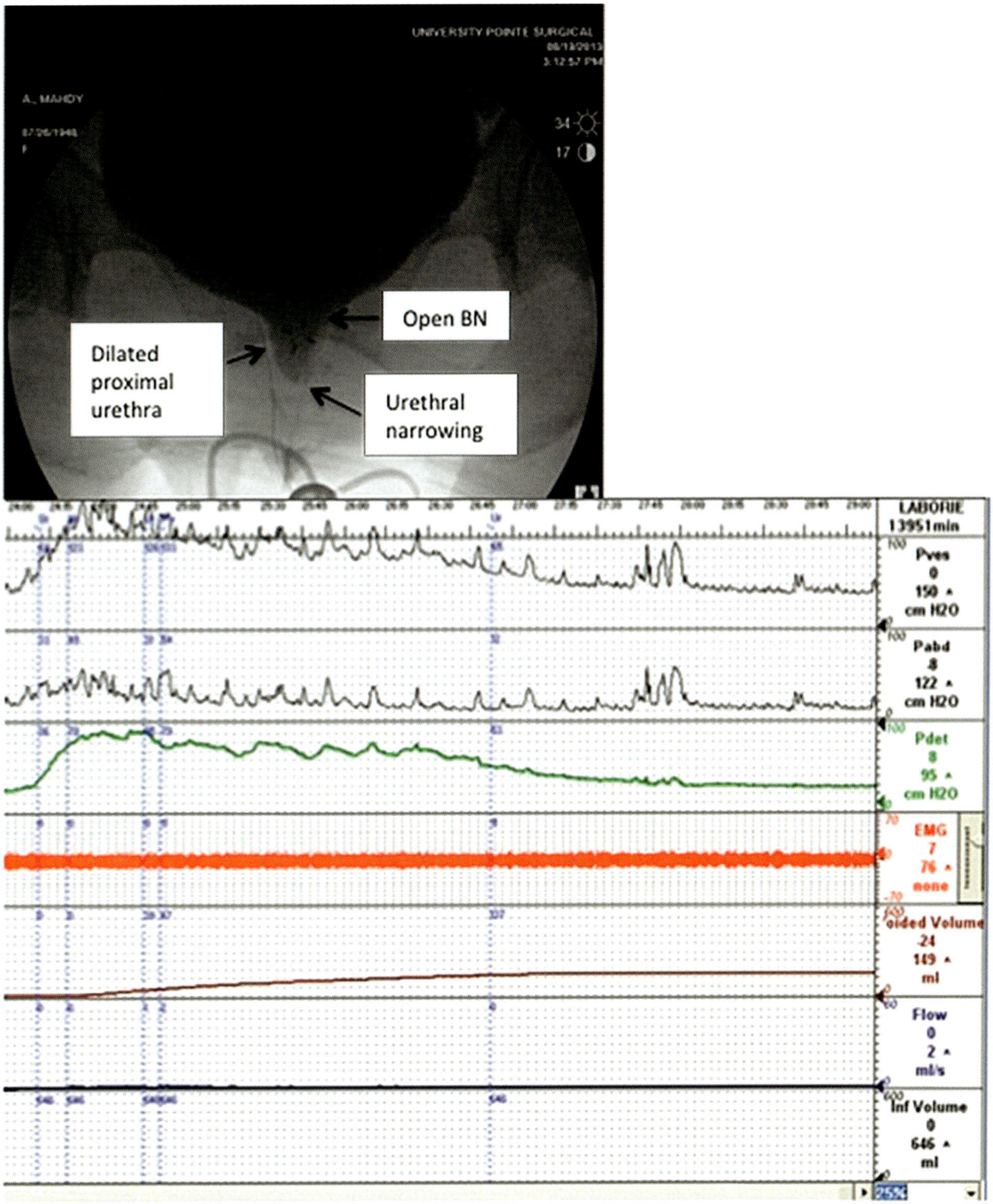

Fig. 11.31 Case 4. Pressure-flow study during video urodynamics showing the typical high detrusor pressure, and barely detectable urine flow. Voiding cystogram shows an open bladder neck, dilated proximal urethra, and narrow distal urethra. These are characteristics of bladder outlet obstruction secondary to urethral stricture.

review identified 393 studies that were used to create an evidence base for characterizing the statements presented in the guidelines as standard recommendations or options. Based on the available evidence, each guideline was assigned a strength rating of A (high), B (moderate), or C (low). In the absence of any sufficient evidence, additional information is provided as clinical principles and expert opinion. The guideline was intended to serve as a tool to facilitate the most effective utilization of urodynamic testing as part of a comprehensive evaluation of patients presenting with LUT dysfunction. The following is a review of these guidelines specific to women.

1. Clinicians who are making the diagnosis of urodynamic stress incontinence should assess urethral function. Although not a universal finding, poor urethral function suggested by a

lower cough or VLPP and/or maximum urethral closure pressure tends to predict less optimal outcomes with some types of therapy. Some clinicians may use this information about urethral function to guide appropriate surgical treatment decisions. (Evidence grade C)

2. Surgeons considering invasive therapy in patients with SUI should assess PVR urine volumes. An elevated PVR can be suggestive of detrusor underactivity, BOO, or a combination of both. Patients with an elevated preoperative PVR are at increased risk for transient or permanent postoperative voiding difficulties following urethral bulking injection or SUI surgery. (Expert opinion)
3. Clinicians may perform multichannel urodynamic studies in patients with both symptoms and physical findings of SUI who are considering invasive, potentially morbid, or irreversible treatments. Urodynamic studies are not absolutely necessary as a component of the preoperative evaluation of a patient with uncomplicated stress incontinence. These findings are comparable with the published Urinary Incontinence Treatment Network multicenter trial that concluded that urodynamic studies did not enhance the predictive value regarding treatment outcomes compared with office assessment alone. (Evidence grade C)
4. Clinicians should perform repeat stress testing with the urethral catheter removed in patients suspected of having SUI who did not demonstrate this finding with the catheter in place during urodynamic testing. More than 50% of women with SUI symptoms who do not demonstrate SUI with the urethral catheter in place will do so when it is removed. (Evidence grade C)
5. In women with high-grade pelvic organ prolapse but without the symptoms of SUI, clinicians should perform bladder stress testing with reduction of the prolapse. Multichannel urodynamics with prolapse reduction may be able to assess for occult stress incontinence and detrusor dysfunction in these women with associated LUT symptoms. If the presence of SUI would change the surgical treatment plan, stress testing with prolapse reduction should be performed to evaluate for occult SUI. This can be done independently or during urodynamic testing. Prolapse can be reduced with a number of tools including a pessary, ring forceps, or vaginal packing. The investigator should be aware that the instrument used for pelvic organ prolapse reduction may also obstruct the urethra, creating a falsely elevated VLPP or preventing the demonstration of SUI. Multichannel urodynamics can also assess the presence of detrusor dysfunction in women with high-grade pelvic organ prolapse. Urodynamics with the prolapse reduced may facilitate evaluation of detrusor function and determine if elevated PVR or urinary retention is caused by detrusor underactivity or outlet obstruction or both. This may help to predict postoperative bladder function once the prolapse has been surgically repaired. (Evidence grade C)
6. Clinicians may perform multichannel filling cystometry when it is important to determine if altered compliance, DO, or other urodynamic abnormalities are present or not in patients with urgency incontinence in whom invasive and potentially morbid or irreversible treatments are considered. Cystometry is the mainstay investigation assessing urinary storage. Urodynamics may have a role when conservative and drug therapy fail and a patient desires more invasive treatment options for OAB. A patient with refractory urgency incontinence may have concurrent diagnoses of SUI or BOO, and correction of these associated conditions may greatly improve the symptoms related to urinary urgency. In the setting of mixed urinary incontinence, urodynamics may contribute by aiding in symptom correlation; however, these tests may not precisely predict outcomes of treatment. (Evidence grade C)
7. Clinicians may perform pressure-flow studies in patients with urgency incontinence or voiding dysfunction after bladder outlet procedures to evaluate BOO. Clinicians should consider pressure-flow testing to assess BOO in patients with refractory urgency symptoms after bladder outlet procedures. However, in women with significant elevations of PVR, urinary retention or definite alterations in voiding symptoms that occurred after an antiincontinence procedure strongly implies BOO; thus, urodynamics may not be necessary before intervention. (Expert opinion)
8. Clinicians should counsel patients with urgency incontinence and mixed incontinence that the absence of DO on a single urodynamic study does not exclude it as a causative agent for their symptoms. The technical reasons for the inability to elicit the finding of DO in certain individuals, whether spontaneous or provoked, are unclear. Thus, it is very important to try to replicate symptoms precisely. Despite this, urodynamics may not diagnose DO even in the patients who are very symptomatic. Therefore, urodynamic findings should be interpreted in the context of the global assessment including examination, diaries, residual urine, and other pertinent information. (Clinical principles)

CONCLUSION

Although urodynamic studies have been available to clinicians and researchers for many years, only recently has significant effort been put toward assessing the true benefit and potential clinical utilization of these tests. As mentioned, multiple recent trials have helped establish procedural guidelines and reference points for practitioners using urodynamic studies. Multichannel urodynamic tests are useful for the assessment of bladder neuropathy and voiding dysfunction. The use of VLPP and UPP measurements to assess urethra dysfunction has produced disappointing results. The evolving consensus appears to be that urodynamics is not necessary in all cases of pure SUI and has a limited predictive role for LUT symptoms after antiincontinence procedures. Until more definitive studies are published about the use of urodynamic studies in women, these studies should be used judiciously, with both patient and practitioner having a clear understanding as to why the urodynamic study is being performed and what clinically relevant information may be obtained.

VUD testing is the most sophisticated evaluation tool for LUT symptoms. It provides the advantages of combining anatomic and functional evaluation of complex symptoms using fluoroscopy and contrast media. Although the test provides invaluable data in certain clinical situations, the benefit of the test should be balanced against the cost, invasiveness, radiation hazards, and morbidity. The most frequent indication for VUD studies is neurogenic bladder, because it can assess for vesicoureteral reflux. Also, in situations when anatomic abnormalities of the LUT are expected, and when BOO is suspected, VUD is preferable over conventional urodynamic studies.

BIBLIOGRAPHY

Abrams P. *Urodynamics*. 2nd ed. London: Springer; 1997.

Blaivas J. Multichannel urodynamic studies. *Urology.* 1984;23:421.

Brown ET, Krlin RM, Winters JC. Urodynamics: examining the current role of UDS testing. What is the role of urodynamic testing in light of recent AUA urodynamics and overactive bladder guidelines and the VALUE study? *Curr Urol Rep.* 2013;14:403.

Dass AK, Lo TS, Khanuengkitkong S, Tan YL. Bacteriuria and safety of female urodynamic studies. *Int Urogynecol J Pelvic Floor Dysfunct.* 2013;24:677.

Diokno AC, Normolle DP, Brown MB, et al. Urodynamic tests for female geriatric urinary incontinence. *Urology.* 1990;36:431.

Foon R, Toozs-Hobson P, Latthe P. Prophylactic antibiotics to reduce the risk of urinary tract infections after urodynamic studies. *Cochrane Database Syst Rev.* 2012;10:CD008224. doi:10.1002/14651858.CD008224.pub2.

Griffiths DJ. Uses and limitations of mechanical analogies in urodynamics. *Urol Clin North Am.* 1979;6:143.

Hosker G, Rosier P, Gajewski J, et al. Dynamic testing. In: Abrams P, Cardoza L, Khoury S, Wein A, eds. *Incontinence; 4th International Consultation on Incontinence.* Birmingham, United Kingdom: Health Publications; 2009.

Jelovsek JE, Chagin K, Brubaker L, et al. A model for predicting the risk of de novo stress urinary incontinence in women undergoing pelvic organ prolapse surgery. *Obstet Gynecol.* 2014;123:279.

Jelovsek JE, Ploeg JMV, Roovers JP, Barber MD. Validation of a model predicting de novo stress urinary incontinence in women undergoing pelvic organ prolapse surgery. *Obstet Gynecol.* 2019;133:683.

Kozomara M, Mehnert U, Seifert B, Kessler TM. Is detrusor contraction during rapid bladder filling caused by cold or warm water? A Randomized, Controlled, Double-Blind Trial. *J Urol.* 2018;199:223.

Lenherr SM, Clemens JQ. Urodynamics: with a focus on appropriate indications. *Urol Clin North Am.* 2013;40:545.

Lloyd JC, Dielubanza E, Goldman HB. Trends in urodynamic testing prior to midurethral sling placement—What was the value of the VALUE trial? *Neurourol Urodyn.* 2018;37:1046.

Massey A, Abrams P. Urodynamics of the female lower urinary tract. *Urol Clin North Am.* 1985;12:231.

Norton PA, Nager CW, Brubaker L, et al. The cost of preoperative urodynamics: a secondary analysis of the VALUE trial. *Neurourol Urodyn.* 2016;35:81.

Öztürk E, Hamidi N, Yikilmaz TN, et al. Effect of listening to music on patient anxiety and pain perception during urodynamic study: randomized controlled trial. *Low Urin Tract Symptoms.* 2019;11:39.

Rowan D, James ED, Kramer AE, et al. Urodynamic equipment: technical aspects. Produced by the International Continence Society Working Party on Urodynamic Equipment. *J Med Eng Technol.* 1987;1:57.

Schäfer W, Abrams P, Liao L, et al. International Continence Society. Good urodynamic practices: uroflowmetry, filling cystometry, and pressure-flow studies. *Neurourol Urodyn.* 2002;21:261.

Solomon ER, Ridgeway B. Interventions to decrease pain and anxiety in patients undergoing urodynamic testing: a randomized controlled trial. *Neurourol Urodyn.* 2016;35:975.

Sørensen S. Urethral pressures during bladder filling. *Scand J Urol Nephrol Suppl.* 1989;125:45.

VanLeijsen SA, Kluivers KB, Mol BW, et al. Value of urodynamics before stress urinary incontinence surgery: a randomized controlled trail. *Obstet Gynecol.* 2013;121:999.

Wei JT, Nygaard I, Richter HE, et al. A midurethral sling to reduce incontinence after vaginal prolapse repair. *N Engl J Med.* 2012;366:2358.

Wein AJ, Barrett DM. *Voiding Function and Dysfunction.* Chicago: Mosby; 1988.

Wein AJ. Classification of neurogenic voiding dysfunction. *J Urol.* 1981;125:605.

Winters JC, Dmochowski RR, Goldman HB, et al. Urodynamic studies in adults: AUA/SUFU guideline. *J Urol.* 2012;188:2464.

Cystometry

Al-Hayek S, Belal M, Abrams P. Does the patient's position influence the detection of detrusor overactivity? *Neurourol Urodyn.* 2008;27:279.

Alperin M, Abrahams-Gessel S, Wakamatsu MM. Development of de novo urge incontinence in women post sling: the role of preoperative urodynamics in assessing the risk. *Neurourol Urodyn.* 2008;27:407.

Arnold EP. Proceedings: cystometry–postural effects in incontinent women. *Urol Int.* 1974;29:185.

Bates CP, Whiteside CG, Turner-Warwick R. Synchronous cine/pressure/flow cystourethrography with special reference to stress and urge incontinence. *Br J Urol.* 1970;42:714.

Bates P, Bradley WE, Glen E, et al. First report on the standardization of terminology of the lower urinary tract function. Urinary incontinence. Procedures related to the evaluation of urine storage: cystometry, urethral closure pressure profile, units of measurement. *Br J Urol.* 1976;48:39; *Eur Urol.* 1976;2:274; *Scand J Urol Nephrol.* 1976;11:193; *Urol Int.* 1976;32:81.

Bradley WE, Timm GW, Scott FB. Cystometry: III. Cystometers. *Urology.* 1975;5:843.

Bradley WE, Timm GW, Scott FB. Cystometry: V. Bladder sensation. *Urology.* 1975;6:654.

Cass AS, Ward BD, Markland C. Comparison of slow and rapid fill cystometry using liquid and air. *J Urol.* 1970;104:104.

Colstrup H, Andersen JT, Walter S. Detrusor reflex instability in male intravesical obstruction. Fact or artifact? *Neurourol Urodyn.* 1982;1:183.

Coolsaet BL, Blok C, Van Venrooij GE, et al. Subthreshold detrusor instability. *Neurourol Urodyn.* 1985;4:309.

Digesu GA, Derpapas A, Robshaw P, et al. Are the measurements of water-filled and air-charged catheters the same in urodynamics? *Int Urogynecol J.* 2014;25:123.

Enhorning G. Simultaneous recording of intravesical and intraurethral pressure. *Acta Chir Scand Suppl.* 1961;suppl 276:1.

Fossberg E, Beisland HO, Sauder S. Sensory urgency in females. Treatment with phenylpropanolamine. *Eur Urol.* 1981;7:157.

Gleason DM, Bottaccini MR, Reilly RJ. Comparison of cystometrograms and urethral profiles with gas and water media. *Urology.* 1977;9:155.

Hashim H, Abrams P. Is the bladder a reliable witness for predicting detrusor overactivity? *J Urol.* 2006;175:191.

Hashim H, Abrams P. Pharmacological management of women with mixed urinary incontinence. *Drugs.* 2006;66:591.

Jorgensen L, Lose G, Andersen JT. Cystometry: H_2O or CO_2 as filling medium? A literature survey of the influence of the filling medium on the qualitative and the quantitative cystometric parameters. *Neurourol Urodyn.* 1988;7:343.

Lapides J, Friend CR, Ajemian EP. Denervation supersensitivity as a test for neurogenic bladder. *Surg Gynecol Obstet.* 1962;114:141.

Lemack GE, Krauss S, Litman H, et al. Normal preoperative urodynamic testing does not predict voiding dysfunction after Burch colposuspension versus pubovaginal sling. *J Urol.* 2008;180:2076.

McCarthy TA. Validity of rectal pressure measurements as indication of intraabdominal pressure changes during urodynamic evaluation. *Urology.* 1982;20:657.

McGuire EJ, Savastano JA. Stress incontinence and detrusor instability/urge incontinence. *Neurourol Urodyn.* 1985;4:313.

McGuire EJ, Woodside JR, Norden TA, et al. Prognostic value of urodynamic testing in myelodysplastic patients. *J Urol.* 1981;126:205.

Miller EA, Amundsen CL, Toh KL, Flynn BJ, Webster GD. Preoperative urodynamic evaluation may predict voiding dysfunction in women undergoing pubovaginal sling. *J Urol.* 2003;169:2234.

Nager CW, Brubaker L, Litman HJ, et al. A randomized trial of urodynamic testing before stress-incontinence surgery. *N Engl J Med.* 2012;366:1987.

Nager CW, FitzGerald M, Kraus SR, et al. Urodynamic measures do not predict stress continence outcomes after surgery for stress urinary incontinence in selected women. *J Urol.* 2008;179:1470.

Nager CW. The urethra is a reliable witness: simplifying the diagnosis of stress urinary incontinence. *Int Urogynecol J.* 2012;23:1649.

Nager CW. Urinary Incontinence Treatment Network. Re: Comments on "A randomized trial of urodynamic testing before stress-incontinence surgery" (*N Engl J Med* 2012;366:1987) From the Italian Society of Urodynamics. *Neurourol Urodyn.* 2013;32:303.

Ouslander JG, Staskin D, Raz S, et al. Clinical versus urodynamic diagnosis in an incontinent geriatric female population. *J Urol.* 1987;137:68.

Penders L, De Leval J. Simultaneous urethrocystometry and hyperactive bladders: a manometric differential diagnosis. *Neurourol Urodyn.* 1985;4:89.

Sand PK, Bowen LW, Ostergard DR. Uninhibited urethral relaxation: an unusual cause of incontinence. *Obstet Gynecol.* 1986;l68:645.

Sheng W, Kirschner-Hermanns R. Comparison of air-filled and water-filled catheters for use in cystometric assessment. *Int Urogynecol J.* 2019;30:2061.

Sutherst JR, Brown MC. Comparison of single and multichannel cystometry in diagnosing bladder instability. *BMJ.* 1984;288:1720.

van Waalwijk van Doorn ESC, Gommer E. Ambulatory urodynamics. *Curr Opin Obstet Gynecol.* 1995;7:378.

van Waalwijk van Doorn ESC, Remmers A, Janknegt RA. Conventional and extramural ambulatory urodynamic testing of the lower urinary tract in female volunteers. *J Urol.* 1992;147:1319.

Visco AG, Brubaker L, Nygaard J, et al. The role of preoperative urodynamic testing in stress-continent women undergoing sacrocolpopexy: the Colpopexy and Urinary Reduction Efforts (CARE) randomized surgical trial. *Int Urogynecol J Pelvic Floor Dysfunct.* 2008;19:607.

Wang AC, Chen MC. The correlation between preoperative voiding mechanism and surgical outcome of the tension-free vaginal tape procedure, with reference to quality of life. *BJU Int.* 2003;91:502.

Weir J, Jacques PF. Large-capacity bladder: a urodynamic survey. *Urology.* 1974;4:544.

Zimmern P, Litman H, Nager C, et al. Pre-operative urodynamics in women with stress urinary incontinence increases physician confidence, but does not improve outcomes. *Neurourol Urodyn.* 2014;33:302.

Leak Point Pressures

Albo ME, Richter HE, Brubaker L, et al. Burch colposuspension versus fascial sling to reduce urinary stress incontinence. *N Engl J Med.* 2007;356:2143.

Bump RC, Elser DM, Theofrastous JP, et al. Valsalva leak point pressures in women with genuine stress incontinence: reproducibility, effect of catheter caliber, and correlations with other measures of urethral resistance. *Am J Obstet Gynecol.* 1995;173:551.

Cummings JM, Boulier JA, Parra RO, Wozniak-Petrofsky J. Leak point pressures in women with urinary stress incontinence: correlation with patient history. *J Urol.* 1997;157:818.

Decter RM, Harpster L. Pitfalls in determination of leak point pressure. *J Urol.* 1992;148:588.

Gray M, King CJ. Urodynamic evaluation of the intrinsically incompetent sphincter. *J Urol Nurs.* 1993;13:67.

Hosker G. Is it possible to diagnose intrinsic sphincter deficiency in women? *Curr Opin Urol.* 2009;19:342.

Howard D, Miller JM, DeLancey JO, Ashton-Miller JA. Differential effects of cough, Valsalva, and continence status on vesical neck movement. *Obstet Gynecol.* 2000;95:535.

Hsu TH, Rackley RR, Appell RA. The supine stress test: a simple method to detect intrinsic urethral sphincter dysfunction. *J Urol.* 1999;162:460.

McCormack M, Pike J, Kiruluta G. Leak point of incontinence: a measure of the interaction between outlet resistance and bladder capacity. *J Urol.* 1993;150:1452.

McGuire EJ, Fitzpatrick CC, Wan J, et al. Clinical assessment of urethral sphincter function. *J Urol.* 1993;150:1452.

McGuire EJ, Woodside JR, Bordern TA, et al. Prognostic value of urodynamic testing in myelodysplastic patients. *J Urol.* 1981;126:205.

McLennan MT, Bent AE. Supine empty stress test as a predictor of low Valsalva leak point pressure. *Neurourol Urodyn.* 1998;17:121.

McLennan MT, Melick CE, Bent AE. Leak-point pressure clinical application of values at two different volumes. *Int Urogynecol J.* 2000;11:136.

Miklos JR, Sze EHM, Karram MM. A critical appraisal of the methods of measuring leak-point pressures in women with stress incontinence. *Obstet Gynecol.* 1995;86:349.

Nager CW, Kraus SR, Kenton K, et al. Urodynamics, the supine empty bladder stress test, and incontinence severity. *Neurourol Urodyn.* 2010;29:1306.

Nitti VW, Combs AJ. Correlation of Valsalva leak point pressure with subjective degree of stress urinary incontinence in women. *J Urol.* 1996;155:281.

Noblett KL, Jensen JK, Ostergard DR. The relationship of body mass index to intra-abdominal pressure as measured by multichannel cystometry. *Int Urogynecol J Pelvic Floor Dysfunct.* 1997;8:323.

O'Connell HE, McGuire EJ. Leak point pressure. In: O'Donnell PD, ed. *Urinary Incontinence.* St. Louis: Mosby; 1997.

Richter HE, Albo ME, Zyczynski HM, et al. Retropubic versus transobturator midurethral slings for stress incontinence. *N Engl J Med.* 2010;362:2066.

Siltberg H, Larsson G, Victor A. Cough-induced leak-point pressure – a valid measure for assessing treatment in women with stress incontinence. *Acta Obstet Gynecol Scand.* 1998;77:1000.

Sultana CJ. Urethral closure pressure and leak-point pressure in incontinent women, *Obstet Gynecol.* 1995;86:839.

Swift SE, Ostergard DR. A comparison of stress-leak-point pressure in incontinent women. *Obstet Gynecol.* 1995;85:704.

Swift SE, Ostergard DR. Evaluation of current urodynamic test methods in the diagnosis of genuine stress urine incontinence. *Obstet Gynecol.* 1995;86:85.

Swift SE, Utrie JW. The need for standardization of the Valsalva leak-point pressure. *Int Urogynecol J.* 1996;7:227.

Theofrastous JP, Bump RC, Elser DM, et al. Correlation of urodynamic measures of urethral resistance with clinical measures of incontinence severity in women with pure genuine stress incontinence. *Am J Obstet Gynecol.* 1995;173:407.

Theofrastous JP, Cundiff GW, Harris RI, Bump RC. The effect of vesical volume on Valsalva leak-point pressures in women with genuine stress urinary incontinence. *Obstet Gynecol.* 1996;7:13.

van Leijsen SA, Kluivers KB, Mol BW, et al. Protocol for the value of urodynamics prior to stress incontinence surgery (VUSIS) study: a multicenter randomized controlled trial to assess the cost effectiveness of urodynamics in women with symptoms of stress urinary incontinence in whom surgical treatment is considered. *BMC Womens Health.* 2009;9:22.

Wan J, McGuire EJ, Bloom DA, et al. Stress leak point pressure: a diagnostic tool for incontinent children. *J Urol.* 1993;150:700.

Weber AM. Leak point pressure measurement and stress urinary incontinence: a review. *Curr Womens Health Rep.* 2001;1:45.

Urethral Pressure Profilometry

Asmussen M, Ulmsten U. Simultaneous urethrocystometry and urethral pressure profile measurement with a new technique. *Acta Obstet Gynecol Scand.* 1975;54:385.

Asmussen M, Ulmsten U. The role of urethral pressure profile measurement in female patients with urethral carcinoma. *Ann Chir Gynaecol.* 1982;71:122.

Baker KR, Drutz HP. Retropubic colpourethropexy: clinical and urodynamic evaluation in 289 cases. *Int Urogynecol J.* 1991;2:196.

Bhatia NN, McCarthy TA, Ostergard DR. Urethral pressure profiles of women with diverticula. *Obstet Gynecol.* 1981;58:375.

Blaivas JG, Olsson CA. Stress incontinence: classification and surgical approach. *J Urol.* 1988;139:727.

Bowen LW, Sand PK, Ostergard DR. Unsuccessful Burch retropubic urethropexy: a case controlled urodynamic study. *Am J Obstet Gynecol.* 1989;160:452.

Brown M, Wickham JEA. The urethral pressure profile. *Br J Urol.* 1969;41:211.

Bump RC, Copeland WE, Hurt WG, et al. Dynamic urethral pressure profilometry pressure transmission ratio determinations in stress-incontinent and stress-continent subjects. *Am J Obstet Gynecol.* 1988;159:749.

Bump RC, Fantl JA, Hurt WG. Dynamic urethral pressure profilometry pressure transmission ratio determinations after continence surgery: understanding the mechanism of success, failure, and complications. *Obstet Gynecol.* 1988;72:870.

Bump RC, Hurt WG, Addison WA, et al. Reliability and correlation of measurements during and after bladder neck surgery. *Br J Urol.* 1998;82:628.

Edwards L, Malvern J. The urethral pressure profile: theoretical considerations and clinical applications. *Br J Urol.* 1974;46:325.

Enhorning G, Miller ER, Hinman F. Urethral closure studies with cine roentgenography and bladder urethral recording. *Surg Gynecol Obstet.* 1964;118:507.

Farghaly SA, Shah J, Worth P. The value of transmission–pressure ratio in the assessment of female stress incontinence. *Arch Gynecol.* 1985;237:366.

Haeusler G, Tempfer C, Heinzi H, et al. Value of urethral pressure profilometry in the female incontinent patient: a prospective trial with an 8-channel urethral catheter. *Urology.* 1998;52:1113.

Hilton P, Stanton SL. A clinical and urodynamic evaluation of the Burch colposuspension for genuine stress incontinence. *Br J Obstet Gynaecol.* 1983;l90:934.

Hilton P. Unstable urethral pressure: toward a more relevant definition. *Neurourol Urodyn.* 1988;6:411.

Horbach NS, Blanco JS, Ostergard DR, et al. A suburethral sling procedure with polytetrafluorethylene for the treatment of genuine stress incontinence in patients with low urethral closure pressure. *Obstet Gynecol.* 1988;71:648.

Kauppila A, Penttinen J, Häggman VM. Six-microtransducer catheter connected to computer in evaluation of urethral closure function of women. *Urology.* 1989;33:159.

Koonings PP, Bergman A, Ballard CA. Low urethral pressure and stress urinary incontinence in women: risk factor for failed retropubic surgical procedure. *Urology.* 1990;36:245.

Lose G, Brostrøm S. Low-pressure urethra in women: what does it mean and what can it be used for? *Int Urogynecol J Pelvic Floor Dysfunct.* 2002;13:215.

McGuire EJ, Lytton B, Pepe V, et al. Stress urinary incontinence. *Obstet Gynecol.* 1976;47:255.

McGuire EJ. Urodynamics findings in patients after failure of stress incontinence operations. *Prog Clin Biol Res.* 1981;78:351.

Messelink EJ, Dabholwala NF, Vrij V, et al. Multichannel urethral pressure profiles: reproducibility and three-dimensional representation. *J Endourol.* 1997;11:211.

Millar HD, Baker LE. Stable ultraminiature catheter-tip pressure transducer. *Med Biol Eng.* 1973;11:86.

Myers DL, Lasala CA, Hogan JW, et al. The effect of posterior wall support defects on urodynamic indices in stress urinary incontinence. *Obstet Gynecol.* 1998;91:710.

Quadri G, Magatti F, Belloni C, et al. Marshall-Marchetti-Krantz urethropexy and Burch colposuspension for stress urinary incontinence in women with low pressure and hypermobility of the urethra: Early results of a prospective randomized clinical trial. *Am J Obstet Gynecol.* 1999;181:12.

Richardson DA, Ramahi A, Chaiss E. Surgical management of stress incontinence in patients with low urethral pressure. *Gynecol Obstet Invest.* 1991;31:106.

Richardson DA. Value of the cough pressure profile in the evaluation of patients with stress incontinence. *Am J Obstet Gynecol.* 1986;155:808.

Rosenzweig BA, Bhatia NN, Nelson AL. Dynamic urethral pressure profilometry pressure transmission ratio: what do the numbers really mean? *Obstet Gynecol.* 1991;77:586.

Rud T. Urethral pressure profile in continent women from childhood to old age. *Acta Obstet Gynecol Scand.* 1980;59:331.

Sand PK, Bowen LW, Ostergard DR. Uninhibited urethral relaxation: an unusual cause of incontinence. *Obstet Gynecol.* 1986;68:645.

Sand PK, Bowen LW, Panganiban R, et al. The low pressure urethra as a factor in failed retropubic urethropexy. *Obstet Gynecol.* 1987;69:399.

Sand PK, Winkler H, Blackhurst DW, et al. A prospective randomized study comparing modified Burch retropubic urethropexy and suburethral sling for treatment of genuine stress incontinence with low-pressure urethra. *Am J Obstet Gynecol.* 2000;182:30.

Swift SE, Rust PF, Ostergard DR. Intrasubject variability of the pressure-transmission ratio in patients with genuine stress incontinence. *Int Urogynecol J Pelvic Floor Dysfunct.* 1996;7:312.

Tapp AJS, Cardozo L, Versi E, et al. The prevalence of variation of resting urethral pressure in women and its association with lower urinary tract function. *Br J Urol.* 1988;61:314.

Ulmsten U, Hendriksson L, Iosif S. The unstable female urethra. *Am J Obstet Gynecol.* 1982;144:93.

Versi E, Cardozo L, Studd J. Distal urethral compensatory mechanisms in women with an incompetent bladder neck who remain continent, and the effect of the menopause. *Neurourol Urodyn.* 1990;9:579.

Versi E, Cardozo L. Urethral instability: diagnosis based on variations of the maximum urethral pressure in normal climacteric women. *Neurourol Urodyn.* 1986;5:535.
Versi E. Discriminant analysis of urethral pressure profilometry data for the diagnosis of genuine stress incontinence. *Br J Obstet Gynaecol.* 1990;97:251.
Ward GH, Hosker GL. The anisotropic nature of urethral occlusive forces. *Br J Obstet Gynaecol.* 1985;92:1279.
Weber AM. Is urethral pressure profilometry a useful diagnostic test for stress urinary incontinence? *Obstet Gynecol Surv.* 2001;58:720.
Weil A, Reyes H, Bischoff P, et al. Modification of urethral rest and stress profiles after different types of surgery for urinary stress incontinence. *Br J Obstet Gynaecol.* 1984;91:46.

Flow Studies

Abrams P, Torrens M. Urine flow studies. *Urol Clin North Am.* 1979;6:71.
Akikwala TV, Fleischman N, Nitti VW. Comparison of diagnostic criteria for female bladder outlet obstruction. *J Urol.* 2006;176:2093.
Backman KA. Urinary flow during micturition in normal women. *Acta Chir Scand.* 1965;130:357.
Barnick CG, Cardozo LD, Benness C. Use of routine videocystourethrography in the evaluation of female lower urinary tract dysfunction. *Neurourol Urodyn.* 1989;8:447.
Bergman A, Bhatia NN. Uroflowmetry: spontaneous versus instrumented. *Am J Obstet Gynecol.* 1984;150:788.
Bergman A, Karram M, Bhatia N. Urethral syndrome: a comparison of different treatment modalities. *J Reprod Med.* 1989;34:157.
Bhatia NN, Bergman A, Karram MM. Changes in urethral resistance following incontinence surgery. *Urology.* 1989;34:200.
Bhatia NN, Bergman A. Urodynamic predictability of voiding following incontinence surgery. *Obstet Gynecol.* 1984;63:85.
Bhatia NN, Bergman A. Use of preoperative uroflowmetry and simultaneous urethrocystometry for predicting risk of prolonged postoperative bladder drainage. *Urology.* 1986;28:440.
Blaivas JG, Groutz A. Bladder outlet obstruction nomogram for women with lower urinary tract symptomatology. *Neurourol Urodyn.* 2000;19:553.
Chassagne S, Bernier PA, Haab F, et al. Proposed cutoff values to define bladder outlet obstruction in women. *Urology.* 1998;51:408.
Cucchi A. Acceleration of flow rate as a screening test for detrusor instability in women with stress incontinence. *Br J Urol.* 1990; 65:17.
Defreitas GA, Zimmern PE, Lemack GE, Shariat SF. Refining diagnosis of anatomic female bladder outlet obstruction: comparison of pressure-flow study parameters in clinically obstructed women with those of normal controls. *Urology.* 2004;64:675.
Drach GW, Ignatoff J, Layton T. Peak urinary flow rate: observations in female subjects and comparison to male subjects. *J Urol.* 1979;122:215.
Drake WM. The uroflowmeter: an aid to the study of lower urinary tract. *J Urol.* 1948;59:650.
Fantl AJ, Smith PJ, Schneider V, et al. Fluid weight uroflowmetry in women. *Am J Obstet Gynecol.* 1983;145:1017.
Griffiths DJ. Basics of pressure-flow studies. *World J Urol.* 1995;13:30.
Groutz A, Blaivas JG, Sassone AM. Detrusor pressure uroflowmetry studies in women: effect of a 7Fr transurethral catheter. *J Urol.* 2000;164:109.
Groutz A, Blaivas JG. Non-neurogenic female voiding dysfunction. *Curr Opin Urol.* 2002;12:311.
Hashim H, Abrams P. Flow meter urine testing: a practical proposition in patients attending for urodynamics? *BJU Int.* 2006;97:1027.
Haylen BT, Ashby D, Sutherst JR, et al. Maximum and average flow rates in normal male and female populations: the Liverpool nomograms. *Br J Urol.* 1989;64:30.
Haylen BT, Parys BT, Anyaegbunam WI, et al. Urine flow rates in male and female urodynamic patients compared with Liverpool nomograms. *Br J Urol.* 1990;65:483.
Karl C, Gerlach R, Hannappel J, et al. Uroflow measurements: their information yield in a long-term investigation of pre- and postoperative measurements. *Urol Int.* 1986;41:270.
Kobak WH, Walters MD, Piedmonte MR. Determinants of voiding after three types of incontinence surgery: a multivariable analysis. *Obstet Gynecol.* 2001;97:86.
Lemack GE, Baseman AG, Zimmern PE. Voiding dynamics in women: a comparison of pressure-flow studies between asymptomatic and incontinent women. *Urology.* 59:42, 2002.
Lemack GE, Zimmern PE. Pressure flow analysis may aid in identifying women with outflow obstruction. *J Urol.* 2000;163:1823.
Massey A, Abrams P. Urodynamics of the female lower urinary tract. *Urol Clin North Am.* 1985;12:231.
Meunier P. Study of micturition parameters in healthy young adults using a uroflowmetric method. *Eur J Clin Invest.* 1983;13:25.
Mueller ER, Litman H, Rickey LR, et al. Comparison of flowrates and voided volumes during non-instrumented uroflowmetry and pressure-flow studies in women with stress incontinence. *Neurourol Urodyn.* 2015;34:549.
Nitti VW, Raz S. Obstruction following anti-incontinence procedures: diagnosis and treatment with transvaginal urethrolysis. *J Urol.* 1994;152:93.
Nitti VW, Tu LM, Gitlin J. Diagnosing bladder outlet obstruction in women. *J Urol.* 1999;161:1535.
Nitti VW. Evaluation of the female with neurogenic voiding dysfunction. *Int Urogynecol J Pelvic Floor Dysfunct.* 1999;10:119.
Saxton HM. Urodynamics: the appropriate modality for the investigation of frequency, urgency, incontinence, and voiding difficulties. *Radiology.* 1990;175:307.
Solomon E, Yasmin H, Duffy M, et al. Developing and validating a new nomogram for diagnosing bladder outlet obstruction in women. *Neurourol Urodyn.* 2018;37:368.
Stanton SL, Ozsoy C, Hilton P. Voiding difficulties in the female: prevalence, clinical and urodynamic review. *Obstet Gynecol.* 1983;61:144.
Susset JG, Brissot RB, Regnier CH. The stop-flow technique: a way to measure detrusor strength. *J Urol.* 1982;127:489.
Susset JG, Picker P, Kretz M, et al. Critical evaluation of uroflometers and analysis of normal curves. *J Urol.* 1983;109:874.
Tanagho EA, McCurrey E. Pressure and flow rate as related to lumen caliber and entrance configuration. *J Urol.* 1971;105:583.
Tanagho EA, Miller ER. Initiation of voiding. *Br J Urol.* 1970;42:175.
van Garrelts B, Strandell P. Continuous recording of urinary flow-rate. *Scand J Urol Nephrol.* 1972;6:224.
van Garrelts B. Analysis of micturition: a new method of recording the voiding of the bladder. *Acta Chir Scand.* 1956;112:326.
Walter S, Olesen KP, Nordling J, et al. Bladder function in urologically normal middle aged females. *Scand J Urol Nephrol.* 1979;13:249.
Walters MD. Mechanism of continence and voiding, with International Continence Society classification of dysfunction. *Obstet Gynecol Clin North Am.* 1989;16:773.
Yalla SV, Blunt KJ, Fam BA, et al. Detrusor–urethral sphincter dyssynergia. *J Urol.* 1977;118:1026.

Video Urodynamics

Abrams P, Cardozo L, Fall M, et al. The standardisation of terminology of lower urinary tract function: report from the Standardisation

Sub-committee of the International Continence Society. *Neurourol Urodyn.* 2002;21:167.
Aron BS, Schlesinger A. Complications of radiation therapy: the genitourinary tract. *Semin Roentgenol.* 1974; 9:65.
Barrett DM. Disposable (infant) surface electrocardiogram electrodes in urodynamics: a simultaneous comparative study of electrodes. *J Urol.* 1980;124:663.
Brenner DJ, Hall EJ. Computed tomography – an increasing source of radiation exposure. *N Engl J Med.* 2007;357:2277.
Brown ET, Krlin RM, Winters JC. Urodynamics: examining the current role of UDS testing. What is the role of urodynamic testing in light of recent AUA urodynamics and overactive bladder guidelines and the VALUE study? *Curr Urol Rep.* 2013;14:403.
Brucker BM, Fong E, Shah S, et al. Urodynamic differences between dysfunctional voiding and primary bladder neck obstruction in women. *Urology.* 2012;80:55.
Brucker BM, Shah S, Mitchell S, et al. Comparison of urodynamic findings in women with anatomical versus functional bladder outlet obstruction. *Female Pelvic Med Reconstr Surg.* 2013;19:46.
Caruso DJ, Kanagarajah P, Cohen BL, et al. What is the predictive value of urodynamics to reproduce clinical findings of urinary frequency, urge urinary incontinence, and/or stress urinary incontinence? *Int Urogynecol J.* 2010;21:1205.
Chancellor MB, Blaivas JG, Kaplan SA, Axelrod S. Bladder outlet obstruction versus impaired detrusor contractility: the role of outflow. *J Urol.* 1991;145:810.
Ciancio SJ, Mutchnik SE, Rivera VM, Boone TB. Urodynamic pattern changes in multiple sclerosis. *Urology.* 2001;57:239.
Costantini E, Mearini E, Pajoncini C, et al. Uroflowmetry in female voiding disturbances. *Neurourol Urodyn.* 2003;22:569.
Hosker G, Rosier P, Gajewski J, et al. Dynamic testing. In: Abrams P, Cardoza L, Khoury S, Wein A, eds. *Incontinence; 4th International Consultation on Incontinence.* Birmingham, United Kingdom: Health Publications; 2009:413.
Kuo HC. Videourodynamic characteristics and lower urinary tract symptoms of female bladder outlet obstruction. *Urology.* 2005;66:1005.
Mahesh M. Fluoroscopy: patient radiation exposure issues. *Radiographics.* 2001;21:1033.
McGuire EJ, Cespedes RD, Cross CA, O'Connell HE. Videourodynamic studies. *Urol Clin North Am.* 1996;23:309.
McGuire EJ, Woodside JR, Borden TA, Weiss RM. Prognostic value of urodynamic testing in myelodysplastic patients. *J Urol.* 1981;126:205.
Ngo TC, Clark CJ, Wynne C, Kennedy II WA. Radiation exposure during pediatric videourodynamics. *J Urol.* 2011;186:1672.
Patel R, Nitti V. Bladder outlet obstruction in women: prevalence, recognition, and management. *Curr Urol Rep.* 2001;2:379.
Scarpero HM, Padmanabhan P, Xue X, Nitti VW. Patient perception of videourodynamic testing: a questionnaire based study. *J Urol.* 2005;173:555.
Schaeffer AJ, Schaeffer EM. Infections of the urinary tract. In Wein AJ, Kavoussi LR, Novick AC, Partin AW, Peters CA, eds. *Campbell-Walsh Urology.* 9th ed. Philadelphia: Saunders-Elsevier; 2007.

12

Endoscopic Assessment of the Lower Urinary Tract

Geoffrey W. Cundiff

CHAPTER OUTLINE

HISTORICAL PERSPECTIVE

The first endoscopic technique for evaluating the female urethra and bladder was described by Bozzini in 1805 and used candlelight reflected through a funnel in the urethra. Nineteenth-century refinements to this crude instrument included a surrounding cannula and, later, a lens system to provide magnification of the field of view. Despite efforts to improve illumination using reflective mirrors, an alcohol lamp, a platinum wire loop, and, finally, an incandescent light source, visualization remained poor without bladder distention. Consequently, by the end of the nineteenth century, cystoscopy was merely an adjunct to the established practice of urethral dilation and bimanual palpation of the bladder.

Kelly (1894) changed the role of cystoscopy by developing an innovative technique that provided adequate bladder distention. The cystoscope, essentially a hollow tube without a lens, was introduced, using an obturator with the patient in the knee-chest position. The negative intraabdominal pressure created in this position allowed air to distend the bladder when the cystoscope was introduced. A head mirror was used to reflect an electric light into the bladder for illumination. This simple technique dramatically enhanced the accessibility of cystoscopy to all physicians.

The twentieth century saw many innovations in cystoscopy. Hopkins and Kopany (1954) introduced a fiberoptic telescope and, later, a rod lens system, which dramatically improved light transmission and resolution. Their rod lens design is the system used in today's rigid cystoscopes. Replacement of the air chamber with a series of glass rods with optically finished ends, separated by intervening air spaces, provides a wider viewing field and permits a change in the viewing angle. The innovation of angled telescopes improved the extent of visualization and facilitated more invasive and operative procedures, largely used during this time in the new subspecialty of urology.

Robertson (1973), known as the American "father of urogynecology," reintroduced cystoscopy to the field of gynecology with his Robertson urethroscope. This instrument addressed the deficiencies of the cystoscope for viewing the urethra by applying the rod lens technology of the Hopkins cystoscope to a shorter straight-on telescope with a nonfenestrated sheath designed specifically for viewing the urethra. He also outlined a technique, dynamic urethroscopy, for evaluating incontinent women. Dynamic urethroscopy offered a simple office procedure that considerably improved the clinical evaluation of the lower urinary tract of the time.

The most recent development in cystoscopy is the flexible cystoscope. A flexible cystoscope takes advantage of the flexibility of the fiberoptic lens system to create a cystoscope that bends, thereby increasing the range of the field of view. Some authors report an improved view of the bladder neck using a flexible fiber cystoscope, whereas others advocate flexible cystoscopy to limit the necessary instrumentation and improve patient tolerance.

INDICATIONS

Cystourethroscopy is an indispensable procedure for today's urogynecologist, with both diagnostic and operative indications. Diagnostic indications include hematuria, lower urinary tract symptoms, urinary incontinence, urethral diverticula, and urogenital fistulas.

The differential diagnosis of hematuria is extensive but includes conditions that are primarily renal or postrenal in origin. Endoscopy is useful in the diagnosis of postrenal conditions, including neoplasms of the bladder and urethra, urethral polyps, chronic cystitis, recurrent cystitis, interstitial cystitis, urolithiasis, and foreign bodies.

The differential diagnosis for lower urinary tract symptoms is extensive, including many nebulous conditions. Possible causes include acute cystitis, chronic cystitis, radiation cystitis, urethral pain syndrome, urethral diverticula, urethritis, and interstitial cystitis. Other conditions that may cause similar symptoms include detrusor overactivity, urolithiasis, suture or mesh in the bladder or urethra, partial urinary retention, and moderate to severe pelvic organ prolapse. Cystourethroscopy is indicated when the presenting symptoms strongly suggest a diagnosis of urethral diverticulum, interstitial cystitis, urolithiasis, foreign body, or tumor, as well as for patients who do not respond to initial therapy. Endoscopy should be avoided in the presence of an active urinary tract infection.

There is general agreement that cystoscopy is indicated for patients complaining of persistent incontinence or voiding symptoms following incontinence surgery, but there is less agreement about the role of cystoscopy in the baseline evaluation of patients with urinary incontinence. The refinement of urodynamic evaluation since the 1980s has demonstrated its superiority for diagnosing the common causes of urinary incontinence such as urodynamic stress incontinence and detrusor overactivity. However, urodynamic testing provides little information about lower urinary tract anatomy, which can be achieved with urethrocystoscopy. Anatomic abnormalities, such as urethral diverticula, urogenital fistulas, and intravesical foreign bodies causing detrusor overactivity, might be suspected based on history or urodynamic tests but require an anatomic assessment for confirmation. Cystourethroscopy also can reveal unsuspected neoplasia in the incontinent patient.

Cystourethroscopy also has value in the diagnosis of intrinsic sphincter deficiency, which has no standardized diagnostic criteria. Some advocate a single urodynamic parameter to make the diagnosis, such as leak point pressure or urethral pressure profilometry. In the absence of validated standard criteria for diagnosing intrinsic sphincter deficiency, we advocate combining clinical measures of severity, urodynamic evidence of poor urethral resistance, and an anatomic evaluation of urethral coaptation. Cystourethroscopy is perhaps the simplest way to achieve such an anatomic evaluation of the urethrovesical junction (UVJ).

The last decade has seen an increase in patients suffering from complications related to midurethral slings and prolapse procedures that include transvaginal placement of mesh. Endoscopic evaluation of the lower urinary tract is an essential component of the evaluation of lower urinary tract symptoms associated with prior surgical implantation of mesh and is listed in recent diagnostic algorithms. Endoscopy also has a major role in treating some of these mesh complications (Video 12.1).

Operative cystourethroscopy in the female lower urinary tract includes minor procedures that can be performed in an ambulatory setting through an operative cystoscope, as well as the use of a cystoscope to facilitate other operations. In the former category, cystourethroscopy is commonly used to perform urethral bulking injections and intravesical botulinum toxin type A injections. In the latter category, intraoperative cystoscopy is an important adjuvant to midurethral sling procedures and facilitates the surgical repair of urinary tract fistula and urethral diverticula. It is also invaluable to evaluate the ureters and bladder mucosa for inadvertent damage at the time of surgery and to ensure the safe placement of ureteral catheters and suprapubic catheters.

INSTRUMENTATION

Rigid Cystoscope

There are three components to the rigid cystoscope: the telescope, the bridge, and the sheath (Fig. 12.1). Each is available with various options to facilitate its role under different circumstances. The telescope transmits light to the bladder cavity and an image to the viewer. Telescopes designed for cystoscopy are available with several viewing angles, including 0 degrees (straight), 30 degrees (forward-oblique), 70 degrees (lateral), and 120 degrees (retroview), to facilitate inspection of the entire bladder wall (Videos 12.2 and 12.3). Although the 0-degree lens is ideal for urethroscopy, it is insufficient for cystoscopy. The 30-degree lens provides the best view of the bladder base and posterior wall, and the 70-degree lens permits inspection of the anterior and lateral walls. The retroview of the 120-degree lens is not usually necessary for cystoscopy of the female bladder but can be useful for evaluating the urethral opening into the bladder. Angled telescopes have a field marker to help facilitate orientation, visible as a blackened notch at the outside of the visual field opposite the angle of deflection.

The cystoscope sheath provides a vehicle for introducing the telescope and distending medium into the vesical cavity. Sheaths are available in various calibers, ranging from 17 to 28 French for adults and smaller calibers for pediatric patients. Cystoscopic sets include obturators that fit the sheath and smooth the end to minimize trauma during introduction to the urethra. When the telescope, which measures 15 French, is placed within the sheath, it only partially fills the lumen, leaving an irrigation-working channel. The smaller sheath is better tolerated for diagnostic procedures, whereas the larger-caliber sheaths provide space to accommodate instruments in the irrigation-working channel. The proximal end of the sheath has two irrigating ports: one for introduction of the distending medium and another for removal of the medium. The distal end of the cystoscope sheath is fenestrated to permit use of instrumentation in the angled field of view. It is also beveled, opposite the fenestrae. Many urogynecologists forego the sheath obturator in introducing the cystoscope to the relatively short and straight female urethra, instead using the bevel to depress the posterior urethral wall, increasing the comfort of introduction of the cystoscope. Bevels increase with the diameter of the cystoscope, and larger sheaths may require an obturator for atraumatic placement.

The bridge serves as a connector between the telescope and sheath and forms a watertight seal with both. It may also have

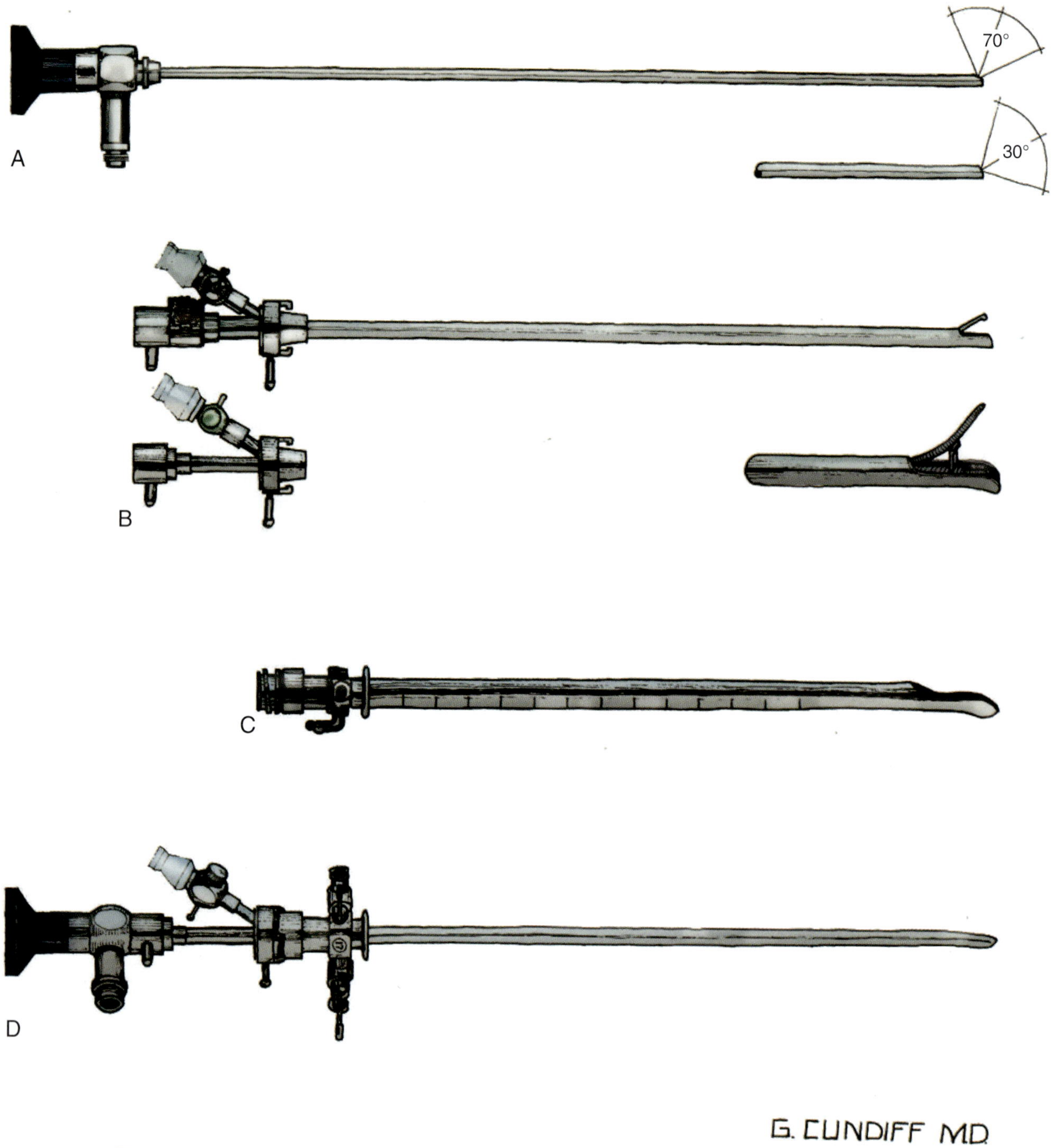

Fig. 12.1 Rigid cystoscopes used in urology and urogynecology. **A**, Telescopes (*top to bottom*): 70-degree and 30-degree lens. **B**, Bridges (*top to bottom*): catheter-deflecting bridge and diagnostic bridge. **C**, Sheath. **D**, Assembled rigid cystoscope.

one or two ports for the introduction of instruments into the irrigation-working channel. The Albarran bridge is a variation that has a deflector mechanism at the end of an inner sheath (see Fig. 12.1). When placed in the cystoscope sheath, the deflector mechanism is located at the distal end of the inner sheath within the fenestra of the outer sheath. In this location, elevation of the deflector mechanism assists the manipulation of instruments and ureteral catheters within the field of view.

Rigid Urethroscope

The rigid urethroscope is a modification of the cystoscope designed exclusively for evaluation of the urethra (Fig. 12.2). Because it is primarily a diagnostic instrument, it does not have a bridge. The telescope is shorter and has a 0-degree viewing angle, which provides an optimal circumferential view of the urethral lumen, because the mucosa in front of the urethroscope is distended by the distention medium.

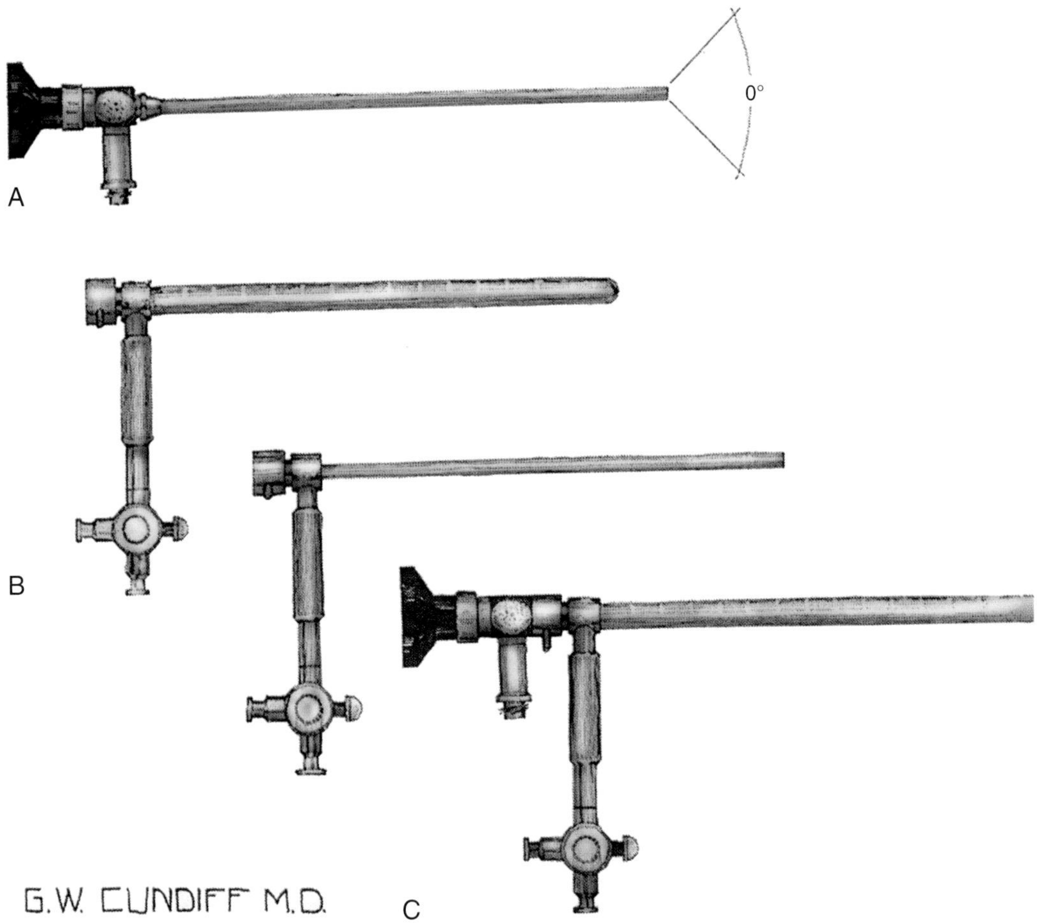

Fig. 12.2 Rigid urethroscope. **A**, Telescope, 0 degrees. **B**, Sheaths (*top to bottom*): 24 and 15 French. **C**, Urethroscope.

The urethroscope sheath is designed to maximize distention of the urethral lumen. The proximal end of the sheath has a single irrigating port, and the telescope only partially fills the sheath, leaving space for the irrigant to flow around it. Sheaths are available in 15- and 24-French calibers. If tolerated, the larger sheath is useful, because it provides the best view of the urethral lumen by providing more rapid fluid flow for maximal distention.

Flexible Cystoscope

Unlike the rigid cystoscope, the flexible cystoscope combines the optical systems and irrigation-working channel in a single unit. The coated tip is 15 to 18 French in diameter and 6 to 7 cm in length; the working unit makes up half the length. The optical system consists of a single image-bearing fiberoptic bundle and two light-bearing fiberoptic bundles. The fibers of these bundles are coated, parallel coherent optical fibers that transmit light even when bent. The fiber coating results in a somewhat granular image, and the delicate 5- to 10-μm diameter makes them susceptible to damage. Gentle handling is essential to good visualization and instrument longevity. The flexibility of the fibers permits a distal tip-deflecting mechanism, controlled by a lever at the eyepiece that will deflect the tip 290 degrees in a single plane. The optical fibers are fitted to a lens system that magnifies and focuses the image. The irrigation-working port enters the instrument at the eyepiece opposite the deflecting mechanism (see Video 12.2).

Many urologists prefer the flexible cystoscope because of improved patient comfort. However, the short length of the female urethra means that rigid cystoscopy is well tolerated by most women. Moreover, there are several disadvantages to the flexible cystoscope. The flow rate of the irrigation-working channel is approximately one-fourth that of a similar-size rigid cystoscope and is further curtailed by the passage of instruments down this channel. Some tip deflection is also lost with use of the instrument channel. In addition, because the view afforded by the flexible cystoscope is not as clear as that of a rigid cystoscope, greater operator skill is required to completely visualize the vesical cavity. There is no difference in the postprocedural morbidity compared with rigid cystourethroscopy.

Light Sources and Video Monitors

Although any light source that provides adequate illumination via a fiberoptic cable is sufficient, a high-intensity (xenon) light source is recommended for the use of video monitoring or photography. The cable attaches to the telescope at the eyepiece. Light cables are usually fiberoptic, although fluid-filled cables are also available; they tend to be more expensive and more durable.

Fiberoptic cables use flexible optic fibers that are comparable to those of the flexible cystoscope and are similarly prone to damage.

Although all cystoscopic procedures can be performed with direct visualization through the eyepiece, video monitoring eliminates awkward positioning required for direct visualization. It permits video documentation, which facilitates teaching. The video camera attaches directly to the eyepiece and should be maintained in an upright orientation. Changing the direction of view is accomplished by rotating the cystoscope without moving the camera.

Distending Media

The three types of distention media are nonconductive fluids, conductive fluids, and gases. Cystourethroscopy is feasible with carbon dioxide, but most practitioners prefer to use water or saline to distend the bladder and urethra. A liquid medium prevents the carbon dioxide from bubbling and washes away blood or debris that can limit visualization. Moreover, the bladder volumes achieved using liquid medium more accurately approximate physiologic volumes.

The choice of liquid medium depends on the planned procedure. For diagnostic cystourethroscopy, sterile water is an ideal medium that is readily available and inexpensive. If absorption of a large volume of fluid into the vascular space is anticipated, an osmotic solution such as normal saline should be used. Similarly, if electrocautery is to be used, a nonconducting solution, such as glycine, should be used. A liquid medium is instilled via gravity through a standard intravenous infusion set. The bag should be at a height of approximately 100 cm above the patient's pubic symphysis to provide adequate flow.

Operative Instrumentation

A wide range of instrumentation is available for use through a cystoscope. Those most pertinent to urogynecology are grasping forceps with a rat tooth or alligator jaws, biopsy forceps, and scissors. These instruments can be obtained in semirigid or flexible varieties and come in various diameters. A flexible monopolar ball electrode is useful for electrocautery during operative cystoscopy. A specialized sheath with a mechanism to advance and retract a long needle is useful for urethral injections and intravesical bladder injections.

Instrument Care

Blood and debris should be removed from the equipment promptly to avoid accumulation in crevices and pitting of metal surfaces. The most common method of sterilization is immersion in a 2% activated glutaraldehyde solution (Cidex; Surgikos, Inc., Arlington, TX). Cystourethroscopic equipment should be soaked for 20 minutes and then transferred to a basin of sterile water until ready for use. Longer soaks shorten the life of the telescope by deteriorating the lens system and seals. If more permanent storage is desired, the scopes are cleaned with detergent and water, rinsed, and stored. Once a week, the inside and outside of the scopes should be cleaned with alcohol. The irrigating ports and locking mechanisms should be lubricated regularly with super oil.

CYSTOURETHROSCOPIC TECHNIQUE

A complete evaluation of the lower urinary tract includes both urethroscopy and cystoscopy. A convenient approach involves beginning with urethroscopy and then performing cystoscopy. Diagnostic urethroscopy provides an evaluation of the urethral mucosa and UVJ. Diagnostic cystoscopy permits evaluation of the vesical cavity and ureteral function. In addition to the description below, videos are available that review and demonstrate cystourethroscopic technique (see Videos 12.2 and 12.3).

Diagnostic Urethroscopy

The urethral meatus is cleansed with disinfectant, and, with distention medium flowing, the urethroscope is advanced into the external urethral meatus. The scope is advanced while the center of the urethra lumen is maintained in the center of the operator's visual field, and the urethra lumen, distended by the infusing medium, is visualized to the UVJ. Dynamic urethroscopy is performed after the bladder has a volume of 300 mL. The urethroscope is withdrawn until the UVJ closes one-third of the way, and the response of the urethra to the requested patient instruction to "hold your urine" and "squeeze your rectum" commands are evaluated. The urethroscope is then withdrawn until the UVJ is two-thirds closed, and its response to a Valsalva maneuver and cough is observed (Fig. 12.3). The normal response is UVJ closure with all of these commands.

The urethroscope is then positioned so that the UVJ is one-third closed, and its response to bladder filling is observed. Bladder volumes are noted for the patient's sensations of feeling fullness and maximum capacity. The maneuvers at the UVJ are repeated, and the patient attempts to void. If voiding occurs, the urethra opens, and water escapes around the sheath. The normal UVJ should close over the urethoscope in response to the command "hold your urine." The urethroscope is next withdrawn, while a vaginal finger massages the urethra against the scope. Exudate or diverticular openings may be seen.

Diagnostic Cystoscopy

Cystoscopy is performed using a 30- or 70-degree rigid telescope with a 17-French sheath. Topical anesthetics are typically avoided during urethroscopy because they can affect the color of the urethral mucosa and function of the continence mechanism. After urethroscopy, however, 2% lidocaine jelly may be used on the cystoscope sheath as a lubricant and a topical anesthetic.

The cystoscope is placed into the urethral meatus with the bevel directed posteriorly and advanced to the bladder under direct vision. An obturator is not necessary when using a diagnostic 17-French sheath, because downward pressure on the posterior lumen of the urethra with the blunt bevel is well tolerated by a majority of women. The infusion of water is maintained at a slow rate until the patient reports fullness, or until a volume of approximately 300 to 400 mL is reached.

Orientation is easily established by identifying an air bubble anteriorly at the dome of the bladder. This serves as a landmark during the remainder of the examination. Beginning at the dome superior to the UVJ, the survey progresses in

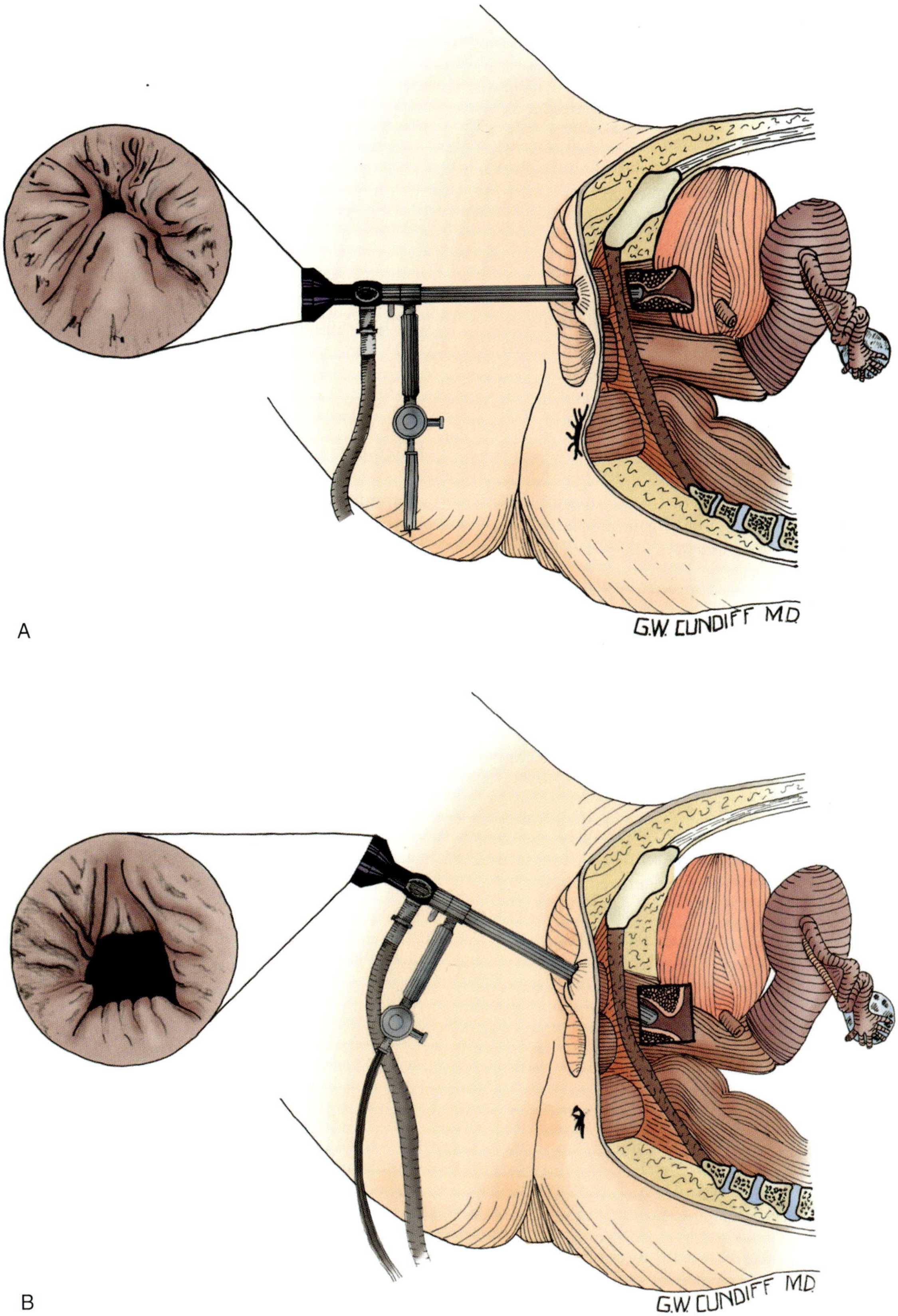

Fig. 12.3 Evaluating urethral hypermobility using dynamic urethroscopy. **A**, Urethroscope is positioned to view the urethrovesical junction (UVJ; window cut away to visualize the UVJ). **B**, As the patient coughs, the UVJ opens (the urethroscope is elevated to follow the UVJ, visualized through cutaway).

12 sweeps, corresponding to the points on a clock (Fig. 12.4). Orientation is maintained by placing the field marker directly opposite the portion of the bladder to be inspected. The trigone and ureteral orifices are viewed by angling the scope downward at a 30-degree angle and laterally. Visualization of the bladder base can be difficult in patients with a large cystocele unless the prolapse is reduced with a finger in the vagina. The mucosa is examined for color, vascularity, trabeculation, and abnormal lesions such as plaques or masses. Once the survey is complete, the telescope is removed while the sheath is left in place. This allows the bladder to drain and permits measurement of the volume of drained fluid. The approach to diagnostic cystoscopy using a flexible cystoscope follows an approach similar to that described for rigid cystoscopy.

Infection of the urinary tract is one potential cause of morbidity associated with cystourethroscopy, yet the actual rate of procedure-related bacteriuria is not well defined. In the literature, the rate of bacteriuria after cystoscopy ranges from 2.9% to 6% (Clenon et al., 2019; Cundiff et al., 1999). Many clinicians use prophylactic antibiotics, including antibiotic bladder irrigation in lieu of oral antibiotics. The most common prophylactic regimen used for cystoscopy is oral nitrofurantoin. Although antibiotic prophylaxis is commonly used, the evidence suggests that there is no need for antibiotic prophylaxis after cystoscopy and urodynamic investigation (Clenon et al., 2019; Cundiff et al., 1999).

Intraoperative Assessment of Lower Urinary Tract Integrity. The majority of ureteral injuries occur during gynecologic operations, and lower urinary tract injury is one of the most common reasons for medical litigation against gynecologists. Estimates of the incidence of injury to the ureters during major gynecologic surgery range from 0.4% to 2.5%. The incidence of lower urinary tract injury is higher for some urogynecologic operations, and most authorities recommend perioperative cystourethroscopy after all urogynecology procedures. Decision analyses and cost-effectiveness studies show value to using perioperative cystourethroscopy after benign gynecologic surgeries,

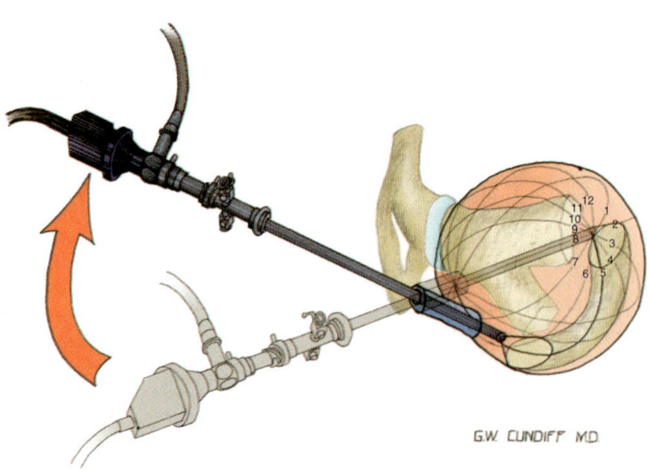

Fig. 12.4 Diagnostic cystoscopy. A survey of vesical cavity is made by making 12 sweeps from the superior bladder to the urethrovesical junction. The 5 o'clock sweep is demonstrated.

which have an incidence of lower urinary tract injury of 1.5% to 2.0% (Visco et al., 2001).

The approach to assessment of the integrity of the bladder mucosa after pelvic surgery is similar to the approach described for diagnostic cystoscopy. A thorough survey of the bladder is made, with special attention paid to the portions of the bladder potentially jeopardized by the procedure. Inspection of the anterior and lateral aspects of the mucosa is important after a mid-urethral sling or retropubic urethropexy, whereas inspection of the trigone is warranted after a difficult vaginal hysterectomy or dissection of an enterocele from the base of the bladder. Assessment of ureteral integrity should be considered after any retropubic dissection, total laparoscopic or robotic hysterectomy, apical support procedures, culdoplasty, or colpocleisis, and in other complex situations whenever there is a suspicion of ureteral injury. Intravenous administration of indigo carmine or sodium fluorescein approximately 5 minutes before initiating cystoscopy stains the urine and facilitates visualization of the ureteral orifices during efflux.

Suprapubic Teloscopy. Suprapubic teloscopy is an alternative to transurethral cystoscopy for evaluating the lower urinary tract during pelvic surgery. Transurethral cystoscopy is well suited to pelvic surgery performed via a vaginal approach but is challenging during a laparotomy in the supine position, whereas suprapubic teloscopy allows endoscopy via an abdominal approach. Because of the simplicity of the technique, suprapubic teloscopy compares favorably with the alternatives of open cystotomy or dissection of ureters in terms of required operating time and morbidity.

Suprapubic teloscopy is an extraperitoneal technique that begins with closure of the anterior peritoneum to prevent contamination of the peritoneal cavity with spilled urine. The bladder cavity is filled through a triple-lumen transurethral Foley catheter to at least 400 mL. A 1- to 2-cm purse-string suture is placed into the muscularis layer of the dome of the bladder, using a No. 2.0 absorbable suture. Two absorbable stay sutures can be placed within the purse string, but with a full-thickness purchase to facilitate introduction of the telescope. A stab incision made between the stay sutures provides an opening for insertion of the telescope. Because distention of the bladder is achieved through the transurethral catheter, use of the sheath and bridge are unnecessary. The purse string is tightened sufficiently to prevent leakage without limiting the movement of the telescope (Fig. 12.5). A 30-degree telescope provides the best view of the trigone and ureteral orifices while also permitting a thorough bladder survey. Identifying the transurethral Foley catheter bulb and the trigone beneath the bulb is useful to provide orientation. If suprapubic catheterization is planned, the catheter can be placed through the same stab incision when teloscopy is completed.

Cystoscopic Passage of Ureteral Catheters. The absence of efflux of urine from the ureteral orifices during pelvic surgery is an indication for the passage of ureteral catheters to evaluate for potential obstruction. Ureteral catheters are available in various sizes and with a number of specialized tips. The most useful

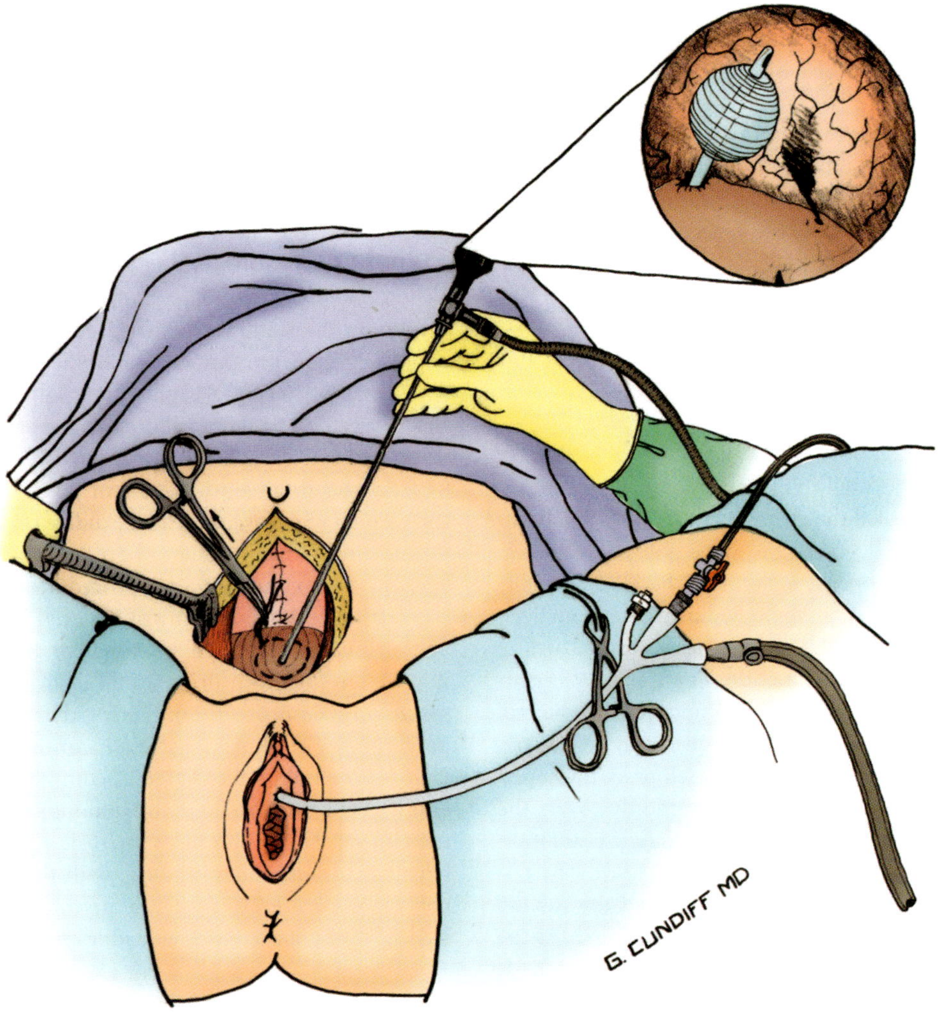

Fig. 12.5 Intraoperative teloscopy.

catheters for assessing ureteral patency are the general-purpose catheter and the whistle-tip catheter. Although available in sizes from 3 to 12 French, the most useful catheter calibers are in the 4- to 7-French range. They have graduated centimeter markings for judging the length of insertion.

Once the ureteral orifice is located, the ureteral catheter is advanced into the field of view. Although the deflecting mechanism of the Albarran bridge facilitates ureteral catheterization, it is usually not essential to its completion. The catheter is placed just outside the fenestrated end of the cystoscope, with the catheter tip oriented in the axis of the ureteral lumen. The tip is threaded into the ureteral orifice by advancing the entire cystoscope. Once the tip enters the ureteral orifice, the catheter is gently advanced until it meets resistance as it passes into the renal pelvis, which is generally 25 to 30 cm. If the catheter is to be left in place, it should be secured to a transurethral catheter and connected to a drainage device. Gentle technique is essential to preventing hematuria and resulting colic. The use of a glide wire or fluoroscopy with retrograde passage of contrast medium also facilitates safe catheter passage. Other potential complications include perforation and ureteral spasm, but with proper methods the risk of complication is small.

Operative Cystoscopy

Several minor operative cystoscopy procedures are easily performed in the office, including biopsy of mucosal lesions, removal of small foreign bodies or intravesical sutures, and intravesical botulinum toxin type A injection. Several useful considerations simplify the technique. Because the focal length of the optics provides the best view immediately in front of the telescope, this is where operative procedures should take place. After introduction of the cystoscope into the bladder and instillation of a sufficient volume of fluid to view the entire bladder wall, the instrument is introduced into the operative port and advanced until it is visible just at the end of the cystoscope. Gross movements are made by moving the cystoscope, and minor adjustments are made by moving the instrument itself. This approach keeps the operation in the optimal field of view. Irrigation at a brisk rate helps to keep the field from being obscured by blood. The bleeding that occurs with biopsy is usually minor, but if excessive hemorrhage occurs, this can be controlled with electrocautery.

Because these procedures require a larger cystoscope sheath (>22 French) and may cause some patient discomfort, local anesthesia is recommended. Intravesical instillation of anesthetic is often sufficient but can be augmented by a bladder pillar block. For bladder instillation, the bladder is catheterized and drained; 50 mL of a 4% lidocaine solution is instilled and left in place for 5 minutes. The bladder pillar block can be placed before the lidocaine is drained from the bladder. The block is performed by injecting 5 mL of 1% lidocaine 5 mm submucosally at the bladder pillars. After placement of a bivalve speculum, the bladder pillars are located in the lateral fornices at 2 and 10 o'clock with respect to the cervix.

CYSTOURETHROSCOPIC FINDINGS

Normal and abnormal findings seen during cystourethroscopy are described here and reviewed in Videos 12.2 and 12.4.

Normal Findings

The urethral mucosa is normally pink and smooth, with a posterior longitudinal ridge called the urethral crest. The UVJ is typically round or an inverted horseshoe shape and is completely coapted until the irrigant opens the lumen. The UVJ normally closes briskly and has minimal mobility with Valsalva maneuver.

In its normal state, the bladder mucosa has a smooth surface with a pale pink to glistening white hue. The translucent mucosa affords easy visualization of the branched submucosal vasculature. As the mucosa of the dome gives way to the trigone, it thickens, and a granular texture develops. A thickened white membrane with a villous contour commonly covers the reddened granular surface of the trigone. Histologic evaluation of this layer reveals squamous metaplasia (Fig. 12.6). The trigone is triangular, with the inferior apex directed toward the UVJ and the ureteral orifices forming the superior apices. As the cystoscope is advanced past the UVJ, the trigone is apparent at the bottom of the field. The interureteric ridge is a visible elevation that forms the superior boundary of the trigone and runs between the ureteral orifices. The intramural portions of the ureters can often be seen as they course from the lateral aspect of the bladder toward the trigone and ureteral orifices. There is marked variation in the ureteral orifices, but they are generally circular or slit-like openings at the apex of a small mound. With efflux of urine, the slit opens, and the mound retracts in the direction of the intramural ureter.

When distended, the bladder is roughly spherical, but numerous folds of mucosa are evident in the empty or partially filled bladder. The uterus and cervix can usually be seen indenting the posterior wall of the bladder, which creates posterolateral pouches where the bladder drapes over the uterus into the paravaginal spaces. At times, visualization of the bowel peristalsis is possible through the bladder wall.

Pathologic Findings

Urethroscopic Pathologic Examination. In the urethral pain syndrome, the urethra is reddened, and exudate sometimes can be expressed from the posterior urethral glands. Fronds (feathery structures with a central capillary) or polyps (bulbous structures) may be seen in the proximal urethra or at the UVJ and have been associated with chronic inflammation. Urethral diverticula appear as ostia, usually along the lateral or posterior surface of the urethra, which may have expressed exudate on palpation (Fig. 12.7). Rarely, foreign material, such as exposed polypropylene mesh, can be seen after midurethral sling procedures.

A stricture is a narrowing of the urethra that typically occurs at the meatus, although proximal or midurethral narrowing may also result from prior urethral surgery. Hypoestrogenism results in pale urothelium. During dynamic urethroscopy, the patient with urodynamic stress incontinence cannot close the UVJ to the "hold" and "squeeze" commands, and the UVJ generally opens and descends in response to cough and Valsalva maneuvers. The patient with intrinsic sphincter deficiency may have a rigid, immobile urethra, with the UVJ unresponsive to commands. In severe cases, the urethral lumen may be visualized from the meatus to the bladder neck.

Cystoscopic Pathologic Examination. Pathologic conditions affecting the bladder can be categorized as mucosal lesions or structural variations. Mucosal lesions are either inflammatory or neoplastic, although their coexistence is common.

Despite its common use to describe infection of the bladder, cystitis in its broadest definition refers to inflammation of the bladder mucosa, of which there are several varieties. Cystoscopy should be avoided in the presence of active infectious cystitis,

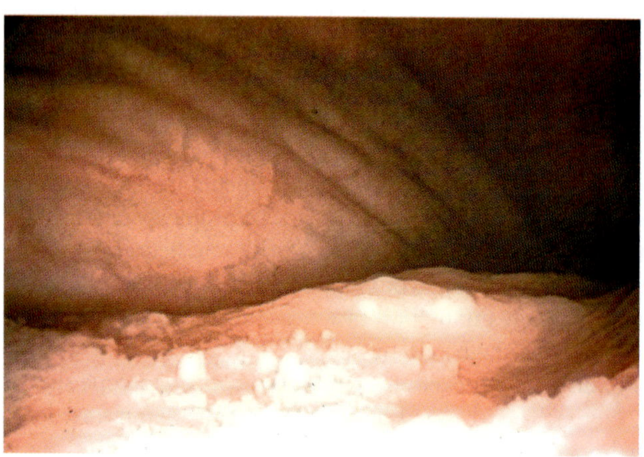

Fig. 12.6 Trigone demonstrating squamous metaplasia.

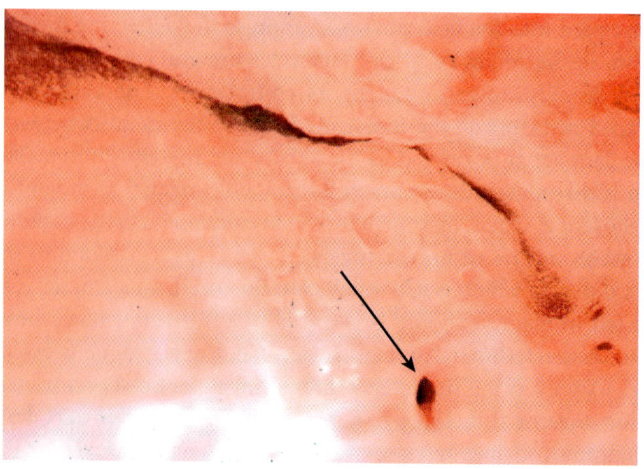

Fig. 12.7 Urethroscopic view of the orifice of a suburethral diverticulum (*arrow*). The proximal urethral orifice is at the upper right side.

but, if performed inadvertently, it may provide varying findings. In its mildest form, bacterial cystitis can be rather inconspicuous, with little more than pink- or peach-colored macules or papules. With increasing severity, mucosal edema and hypervascularity are evident, with loss of the submucosal vascular pattern and marked vascular dilation. In hemorrhagic cystitis, this can progress to individual or confluent mucosal hemorrhages and may be associated with hematuria in addition to irritative voiding symptoms.

The symptoms of hematuria and irritative voiding are typical of several other, less common inflammatory conditions that can often be distinguished on cystoscopy. The hemorrhagic cystitis that follows bladder infusion with toxins such as cyclophosphamide is characterized by diffuse mucosal hemorrhage. In radiation cystitis, areas of hemorrhage are surrounded by pale mucosa, which may be fibrotic and hypovascular. A chronic indwelling urethral or suprapubic catheter produces an inflammatory reaction of the mucosa directly in contact with the catheter. Mucosal changes range from pseudopapillary edema and submucosal hemorrhage to vesical fibrosis.

Interstitial cystitis, another form of chronic inflammation, is often associated with hematuria and fibrosis. The pathognomonic lesions appear on refilling the bladder, after initially filling to maximum cystometric capacity. General anesthesia is usually required to fill to maximum cystometric capacity, because the fibrosis and associated pain often make filling intolerable. Glomerulations are the primary finding in very mild cases. These petechial hemorrhages are small, red dots that may coalesce to form larger hemorrhagic areas. Rare petechiae are seen in normal patients, especially on the posterior wall and trigone, caused by cystoscope trauma. In contrast, interstitial cystitis patients have at least 10 to 20 glomerulations per field of vision. The classic Hunner ulcer is seen in more severe cases of interstitial cystitis. These ulcers appear as velvety red patches or linear cracks with a granulating base and surrounding vascular congestion.

Recurrent or chronic inflammation can produce characteristic lesions as well. Inflammatory polyps are often identified at the UVJ if the cystoscope is retracted into the proximal urethra and the infusion is interrupted to allow them to float into the field of view. They are usually translucent with a villous appearance but can become large enough to partially fill the urethral lumen. Cystitis cystica consists of clear mucosal cysts usually found in multiple areas over the bladder base. The cysts are formed by single layers of subepithelial transitional cells, which degenerate with central liquefaction. Cystitis glandularis has a similar appearance to cystitis cystica, but the cysts are not clear, and they have a less uniform contour. As in cystitis cystica, the mechanism of formation is a glandular metaplasia. In cystitis glandularis, however, there is involvement of multiple layers, including the mucous-producing glandular epithelium. Both lesions are associated with chronic irritation of the bladder mucosa and are commonly surrounded by marked inflammation. The association of cystitis glandularis with adenovillous carcinoma of the bladder has led to the belief that cystitis glandularis may be a precursor of adenocarcinoma. A proposed metaplastic transformation from epithelial hyperplasia through cystitis glandularis and finally to adenocarcinoma is based on a case presented by Shaw et al. (1958) of a gradual transition of cystitis glandularis to adenocarcinoma over a 5-year period. There have been two subsequent reports of transformation of cystitis glandularis to adenocarcinoma.

Although bladder cancer is twice as common in men as in women, it is the most common genitourinary neoplasm in women. The vast majority of cases occur past the fifth decade. Transitional cell carcinoma is the most common histologic type, followed by adenocarcinoma and squamous cell carcinoma. Transitional cell carcinoma is usually induced by a carcinogen; tobacco, dyes, and organic chemicals are known carcinogens for the transitional epithelium. Adenocarcinoma is more common with bladder extrophy. Squamous cell carcinoma has been reported with long-term indwelling catheters. Cystoscopic appearance is variable, depending on histologic type and grade, but usually reveals a raised lesion with a villous feathery or papillary appearance. Circumferential inflammation is ubiquitous. Superficial transitional cell carcinoma may be multicentric or may have associated carcinoma *in situ*. Carcinoma *in situ* can be disturbingly inconspicuous, often mimicking the macules or plaques of infectious cystitis.

Vesical and ureteral structural variations may be anatomic or functional anomalies. Auxiliary ureteral orifices are examples of rare anatomic anomalies that are indicative of renal collecting anomalies. When present, they often enter the vesical wall slightly superior to the trigone and in near proximity to the other ureteral orifice. Ureteroceles are caused by laxity of the distal ureteral lumen, with herniation into the vesical cavity during efflux.

Trabeculations are smooth ridges that become evident with distention of the bladder to volumes approaching maximum cystometric capacity. They appear as interlaced cords of different diameters with intervening sacculations. They represent hypertrophied detrusor musculature associated with detrusor overactivity and functional or anatomic bladder obstruction. A bladder diverticulum can occur when high intravesical pressure produces an enlargement of the intervening sacculations. The thick muscular band that creates the neck varies in diameter and gives way to outpouchings of bladder mucosa. The interior of the diverticulum has been reported to be the site of neoplasm in approximately 7% of cases.

Fistulas also may be encountered at cystoscopy. Approximately 75% of vesicovaginal fistulas (Fig. 12.8) result from abdominal hysterectomies. They may also occur after vaginal hysterectomies, urologic procedures, vaginal mesh procedures, radiation, cancer, and obstetric trauma. Post hysterectomy fistulas are usually located in the bladder base superior to the interureteric ridge, corresponding to the level of the vaginal cuff. The fistulous openings range from small to several centimeters in diameter. In the immediate postoperative state, the surrounding mucosa is edematous and hyperemic; in later stages, the mucosa has a smooth appearance. In contrast, vesicoenteric fistulas uniformly have a surrounding inflammatory reaction, often with bulbous edema, and the fistulous tract is not discernible in two-thirds of cases.

Bladder calculi may result from urinary stasis or the presence of a foreign body, or an inflammatory exudate may coalesce and serve as a nidus for stone formation. They can become attached

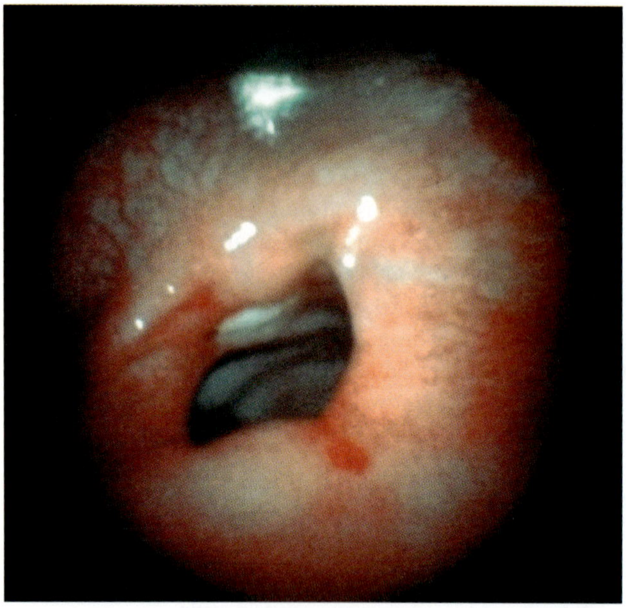

Fig. 12.8 Vesicovaginal fistula (*bottom*).

to small areas of exposed mesh, slings, or nonabsorbable sutures. Stones have extremely variable cystoscopic appearances in terms of color, size, and shape but generally have an irregular surface. Foreign bodies and stones are usually accompanied by varying degrees of general or localized inflammatory reaction.

BIBLIOGRAPHY

Historical Perspective

Gunning JE, Rosenzweig BA. Evolution of endoscopic surgery. In: White RA, Klein SR, eds. *Endoscopic Surgery*. St. Louis: Mosby; 1991.

Hopkins HH, Kopany NS. A flexible fiberscope, using static scanning. *Nature*. 1954;179:39.

Kelly HA. The direct examination of the female bladder with elevated pelvis: the catheterization of the ureters under direct inspection, with and without elevation of the pelvis. *Am J Obstet Dis Women Child*. 1894;25:1.

Ridley JH. Indirect air cystoscopy. *South Med J*. 1951;44:114.

Robertson JR. Air cystoscopy. *Obstet Gynecol*. 1968;32:328.

Robertson JR. Gynecologic urethroscopy. *Am J Obstet Gynecol*. 1973;115:986.

Robertson JR. Office cystoscopy: substituting the culdescope for the Kelly cystoscope. *Obstet Gynecol*. 1966;28:219.

Instrumentation

Aso Y, Yokoyama M, Fukutani K, et al. New trial for fiberoptic cystourethroscopy: the use of metal sheath. *J Urol*. 1976;115:99.

Bagley DH, Huffman JL, Lyon ES. *Urologic Endoscopy: A Manual and Atlas*. Boston: Little, Brown and Co.; 1985.

Clayman RV, Reddy P, Lange PH. Flexible fiber optic and rigid-rod lens endoscopy of the lower urinary tract: a prospective controlled comparison. *J Urol*. 1984;131:715.

Cundiff GW, Quinlan DJ, van Rensburg JA, Slack M. Foundation for an evidence informed algorithm for treating pelvic floor mesh complications: a review. *BJOG*. 2018;125:1026.

Figueroa TE, Thomas R, Moon TD. A comparison of rigid with flexible instruments. *J La State Med Soc*. 1987;139:26.

Fowler CG, Badenoch DF, Thakar DR. Practical experience with flexible fiberscope cystoscopy in out-patients. *Br J Urol*. 1984;56:618.

Fowler CG. Fiberscope urethrocystoscopy. *Br J Urol*. 1984;56:304.

Matthews PN, Bidgood KA, Woodhouse RJ. CO_2 cystoscopy using a flexible fiberoptic endoscopy. *Br J Urol*. 1984;56:188.

Matthews PN, Skewes DG, Kothari JJ, et al. Carbon dioxide versus water for cystoscopy: a comparative study. *Br J Urol*. 1983;55:364.

Quiroz LH, Shobeiri SA, Nihira MA, et al. Randomized trial comparing office flexible to rigid cystoscopy in women. *Int Urogynecol J*. 2012;23:1625.

Cystourethroscopic Technique

AAGL. AAGL practice report: practice guidelines for intraoperative cystoscopy in laparoscopic hysterectomy. *J Minim Invasive Gynecol*. 2012;19:407.

Aldridge CW, Beaton JH, Nanzig RP. A review of office urethroscopy and cystometry. *Am J Obstet Gynecol*. 1978;131:432.

Bootsma AM, Laguna Pes MP, Geerlings SE, Goossens A. Antibiotic prophylaxis in urologic procedures: a systematic review. *Eur Urol*. 2008;54:1270.

Clark KR, Higgs MJ. Urinary infection following out-patient flexible cystoscopy. *Br J Urol*. 1990;66:503.

Clenon EK, Acevedo AM, Sajadi K. Safety and effectiveness of zero antimicrobial prophylaxis protocol for outpatient cystourethroscopy. *BJU Int*. 2019;123:E29.

Cundiff GW, Bent AE. The contribution of urethrocystoscopy to a combined urodynamic and urethrocystoscopic evaluation of urinary incontinence in women. *Int J Urogynecol*. 1996;7:307.

Cundiff GW, McLennan MT, Bent AE. Randomized trial of antibiotic prophylaxis for combined urodynamics and cystourethroscopy. *Obstet Gynecol*. 1999;93:749.

Denholm SW, Conn IG, Newsam JE, et al. Morbidity following cystoscopy: comparison of flexible and rigid techniques. *Br J Urol*. 1990;66:503.

Fozard JB, Green DF, Harrison GS, et al. Asepsis and out-patient cystoscopy. *Br J Urol*. 1983;55:680.

Ibeanu OA, Chesson RR, Echols KT, et al. Urinary tract injury during hysterectomy based on universal cystoscopy. *Obstet Gynecol*. 2009;113:6.

Manson AL. Is antibiotic administration indicated after out-patient cystoscopy? *J Urol*. 1988;140:316.

Marier R, Valenti AJ, Madri JA. Gram-negative endocarditis following cystoscopy. *J Urol*. 1978;119:134.

Richards B, Bastable JR. Bacteriuria after outpatient cystoscopy. *Br J Urol*. 1977;49:561.

Robertson JR. Dynamic urethroscopy. In: Ostergard DR, ed. *Gynecologic Urology and Urodynamics*. 2nd ed. Baltimore: Williams & Wilkins; 1985.

Robertson JR. Gas endoscopy. In: Raz S, ed. *Female Urology*. Philadelphia: WB Saunders; 1983.

Romero RE, Hicks TH, Galindo GH, et al. Evaluation of the importance of cystoscopy in staging gynecologic carcinomas. *J Urol*. 1979;121:64.

Sand PK, Hill RC, Ostergard DR. Supine urethroscopic and standing cystometry as screening methods for the detection of detrusor instability. *Obstet Gynecol*. 1987;70:57.

Scotti RJ, Ostergard DR, Guillaume AA, et al. Predictive value of urethroscopy as compared to urodynamics in the diagnosis of genuine stress incontinence. *J Reprod Med*. 1990;35:772.

Siff LN, Hill AJ, Jallad K, Harnegie MP, Barber MD. Intraoperative evaluation of urinary tract injuries at the time of pelvic surgery: a systematic review. *Female Pelvic Med Reconstr Surg*. 2020;26:655.

Uehling DT. The normal caliber of the adult female urethra. *J Urol.* 1978;120:176.

Visco AG, Taber KH, Weidner AC, et al. Cost-effectiveness of universal cystoscopy to identify ureteral injury at hysterectomy. *Obstet Gynecol.* 2001;97:685.

Cystourethroscopic Findings

Anderson MJ. The incidence of diverticula in the female urethra. *J Urol.* 1967;98:96.

Davis BL, Robinson DG. Diverticula of the female urethra: assay of 120 cases. *J Urol.* 1970;104:850.

Edwards PD, Hurm RA, Jaesehke WH. Conversion of cystitis glandularis to adenocarcinoma. *J Urol.* 1972;108:568.

Gillenwater JY, Wein AJ. Summary of the National Institute of Arthritis, Diabetes, Digestive and Kidney Diseases workshop on interstitial cystitis, National Institutes of Health, Bethesda, Maryland, August 28-29, 1987. *J Urol.* 1988;140:203.

Hunner GL. A rare type of bladder ulcer in women: report of cases. *Trans South Surg Gynecol Assoc.* 1914;27:247.

Lee RA. Diverticulum of the urethra. Clinical presentation, diagnosis and management. *Clin Obstet Gynecol.* 1984;27:490.

Lyon RP, Smith DR. Distal urethral stenosis. *J Urol.* 1963;89:414.

MacDermott JP, Charpied GC, Tesluk H, et al. Can histological assessment predict the outcome in interstitial cystitis? *Br J Urol.* 1991;67:44.

Marshall FC, Uson AC, Melicow MM. Neoplasm and caruncles of the female urethra. *Surg Gynecol Obstet.* 1960;110:723.

Messing EM, Stamey TA. Interstitial cystitis: early diagnosis, pathology, and treatment. *Urology.* 1978;12:381.

Mufson MA, Belshe RB, Horrigan TJ, et al. Cause of acute hemorrhagic cystitis in children. *Am J Dis Child.* 1973;126:605.

Numazaki Y, Kumasaka T, Yano N, et al. Further study on acute hemorrhagic cystitis due to adenovirus type II. *N Engl J Med.* 1973;289:344.

Richardson FH. External urethroplasty in women: technique and clinical evaluation. *J Urol.* 1969;101:719.

Shaw JL, Gislason GJ, Imbriglia JE. Transition of cystitis glandularis to primary adenocarcinoma of the bladder. *J Urol.* 1958;79:815.

Susmans D, Rubenstein AB, Dakin AR, et al. Cystitis glandularis and adenocarcinoma of the bladder. *J Urol.* 1971;105:6.

13

Radiologic Studies of the Lower Urinary Tract and Pelvic Floor

Denicia S. Dwarica, Gennady Slobodov, and Lieschen H. Quiroz

CHAPTER OUTLINE

INTRODUCTION

Pelvic floor disorders (PFDs), including urinary incontinence (UI), pelvic organ prolapse (POP), and anorectal disorders, are prevalent conditions that have a significant negative impact on women's quality of life. The main approach to evaluating these conditions starts with a detailed history and physical examination, along with evaluation of pelvic muscle function, strength, and integrity. The pelvic floor anatomy may be described as comprising an anterior, a middle, and a posterior compartment. The bladder and urethra comprise the anterior compartment; the vagina and uterus comprise the middle compartment; and the rectum, anal canal, and sigmoid comprise the posterior compartment.

Because of the complexity of PFDs, physical examination can have limitations, especially when the severity of symptoms does not correlate with examination findings. Imaging diagnostic evaluations such as dynamic anorectal physiologic tests, magnetic resonance imaging (MRI), and ultrasound imaging, among others, serve as adjunct tools to physical examination. Radiographic imaging can complement the evaluation of PFDs by revealing clinically occult abnormalities in patients with a complex presentation. Although imaging plays a limited role in the evaluation of a straightforward case, it is valuable and informative in complex cases and when multiple compartments of the pelvic floor are involved. Many imaging modalities have been used to evaluate the pelvic floor, including x-ray, computed tomography (CT), MRI, barium contrast defecography, and pelvic floor ultrasound.

In this chapter we will review various imaging modalities used in clinical practice and in research to investigate PFDs.

PLAIN FILM OF THE ABDOMEN

A plain film of the abdomen is not appropriate for evaluation of pelvic floor dysfunction. It is, however, useful as a scout film with an intravenous pyelography (IVP) and may be of benefit in the evaluation of urinary calculi. With the introduction of newer, nonionizing imaging techniques, other modalities are preferred when evaluating PFDs. A plain film can help with the evaluation of upper and lower urinary tract urolithiasis. Figs. 13.1A and B show plain films of a right ureteral stone and multiple ureteral stones, respectively. Plain films are also valuable in evaluating the position of ureteral stents (Fig. 13.2).

INTRAVENOUS PYELOGRAPHY, COMPUTED TOMOGRAPHY UROGRAM, AND RETROGRADE PYELOGRAPHY

IVP is still frequently used to evaluate the urinary tract, even with the emergence of newer technologies. Advantages of this imaging modality include safety, low cost, wide availability, and its ability to provide information on the functional status of the urinary collecting system. Disadvantages to IVP include the exposure to iodine dye and radiation, and it is contraindicated

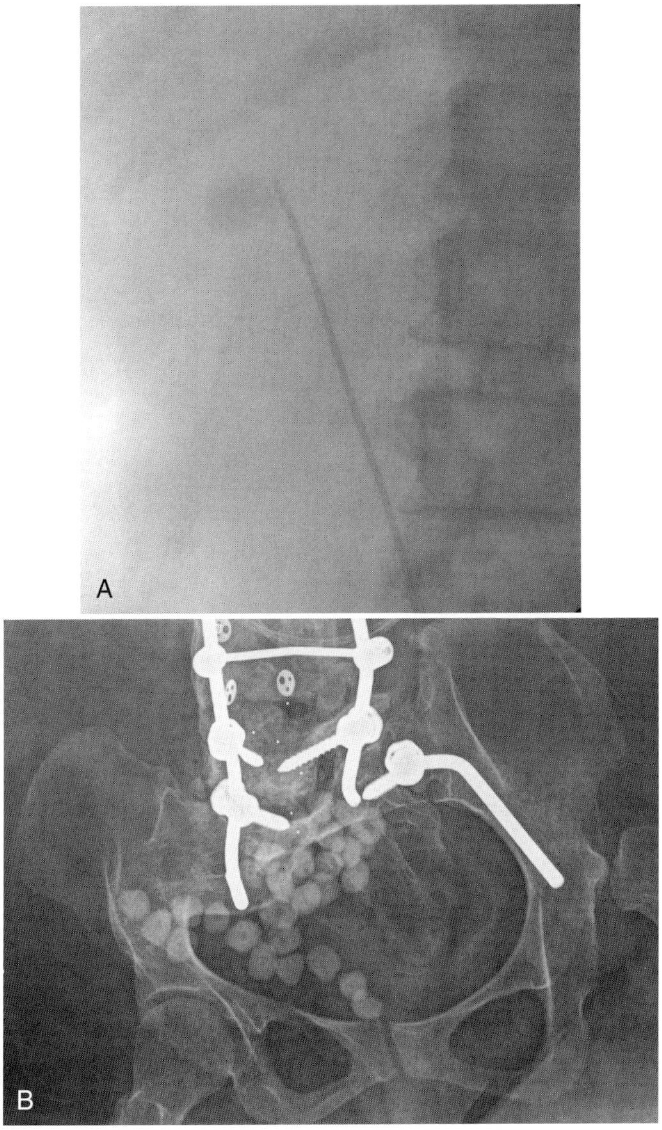

Fig. 13.1 Plain x-ray films of right kidney stones (**A**) and multiple bladder stones (**B**).

in pregnancy, in those with congestive heart failure, and in those with renal insufficiency.

IVP is a mainly historic technique that is now infrequently used in the evaluation of the urinary tract. IVP is most commonly used in the setting of an acute trauma to assess bilateral renal moieties. Computed tomography urogram (CTU) has gradually replaced IVP in the evaluation of the urinary collecting system and is currently the gold standard for evaluation of hematuria, urinary stone detection, and characterization of renal masses. Two of the most common indications for CTU are the evaluation of ureteral obstruction as a result of stones, gynecologic or genitourinary malignancy, pelvic mass, or POP and the evaluation of postoperative complications after gynecologic surgery.

Diagnosing collecting system injury is essential to identifying cases that may require surgical management. Although many collecting system injuries may spontaneously resolve, the persistence of urine extravasation may require a urinary diversion with a

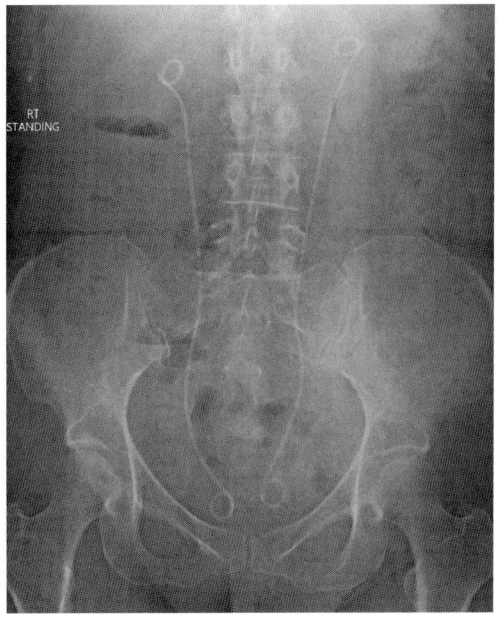

Fig. 13.2 Plain x-ray film of bilateral ureteral catheters.

percutaneous nephrostomy tube, double-J ureteral stent, or surgical treatment (see Chapter 24). Because collecting system injuries may be occult on arterial and venous phase imaging, the use of delayed contrast excretory phase imaging is vital in the setting of a suspected renal injury following trauma. The main diagnostic sign of a ureteric injury is visualization of contrast extravasation (shown as urinary ascites in Fig. 13.3), although more elusive findings may include mild ureteral dilation, deviation, or delayed function (Fig. 13.4).

If the IVP and CT results are inconclusive, retrograde pyelography is indicated. Retrograde pyelogram is the most accurate, dedicated imaging test to evaluate the location and degree of ureteric injury, especially in cases where cystoscopy is also indicated. At the time of cystoscopy, the contrast medium is injected

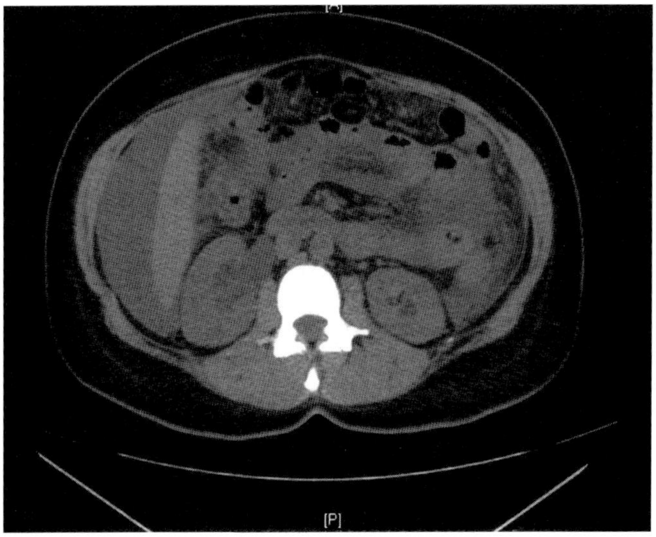

Fig. 13.3 Computed tomography urogram demonstrating urinary ascites from a ureteric injury.

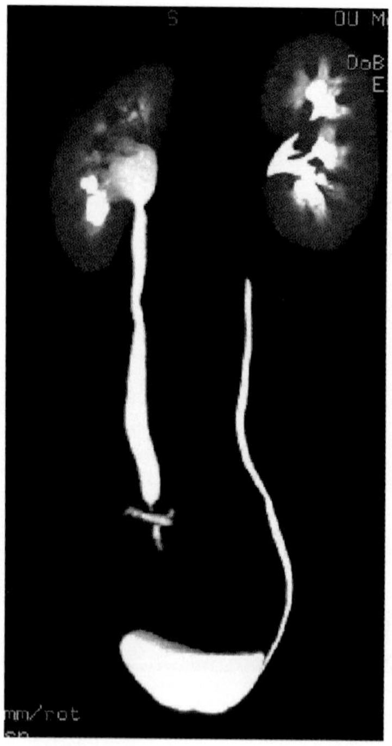

Fig. 13.4 Computed tomography urogram demonstrating right ureteral obstruction secondary to suture ligation at the time of hysterectomy.

into the upper urinary tract through a ureteral catheter under fluoroscopy (fluoroscopy is a modification of x-ray which is used to image the continuous movement of internal structures) (Fig. 13.5). Disadvantages of retrograde pyelogram include a higher rate of infection compared with the anterograde approach, and the possibility of systemic absorption of contrast extravasation. See Chapters 24 and 40 for more information on

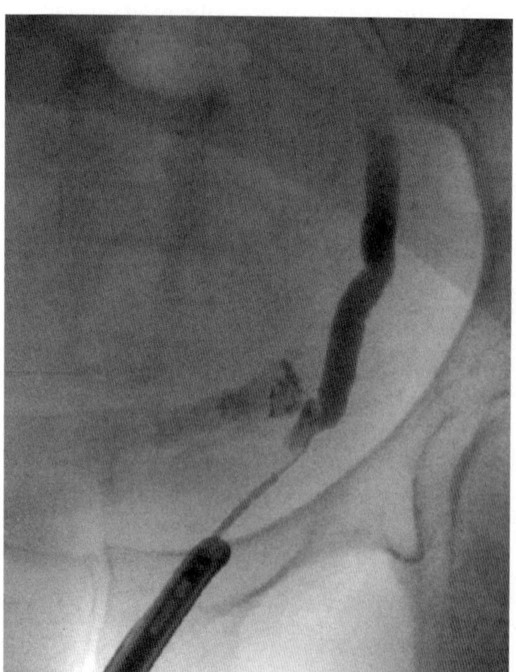

Fig. 13.5 Retrograde pyeleography demonstrating a left ureterovaginal fistula.

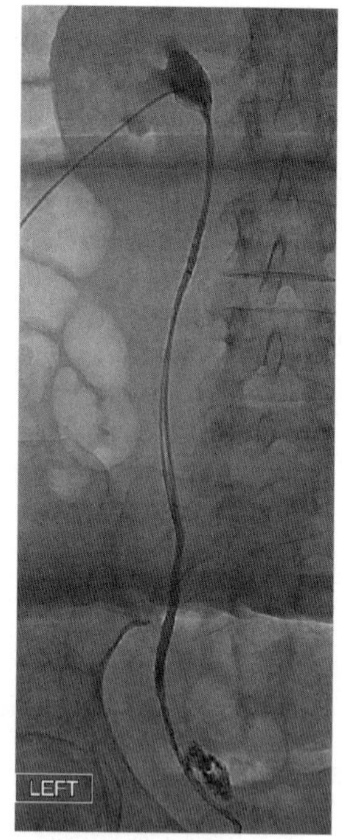

Fig. 13.6 Antegrade pyleography or nephrostogram.

the indications, technique, and interpretation of retrograde pyelography. The integrity of the renal collecting system may also be evaluated by anterograde pyelography (Fig. 13.6). However, this approach is only indicated when there is an indication for percutaneous puncture of the renal pelvis, such as at the time of percutaneous nephrostomy to relieve an obstructive or infected renal collection system.

CYSTOGRAPHY AND VOIDING CYSTOURETHROGRAPHY

Cystography may be considered in the evaluation of bladder integrity in the setting of traumatic injury to the pelvis. Historically, cystography was done with plain films, but today it is most commonly done with CT (i.e., CT cystography). Cystography is also a useful tool in the evaluation of fistulas between the bladder and adjacent organs and in the setting of assessing bladder integrity after a cystotomy repair. This method may be useful to identify vesicovaginal, vesicoenteric, or vesicouterine fistulas, although small fistula tracts may be too small to be radiologically apparent (Fig. 13.7).

A voiding cystourethrogram (VCUG) is a dynamic radiologic study used to evaluate bladder and urethral abnormalities with voiding. Currently its main clinical application is in the evaluation of vesicoureteral reflux. Historically, this test has also been used in the evaluation of bladder or urethral diverticuli. This test is no longer recommended for routine evaluation of urethral diverticula, because it incurs the risk of radiation exposure and has a limited sensitivity as low as 65%. Upright VCUG has also been used to evaluate cystoceles and urethral hypermobility in pre- and postoperative patients, although it is rarely used in clinical practice today. Current limitations of this examination in pelvic floor dysfunction include patient exposure to

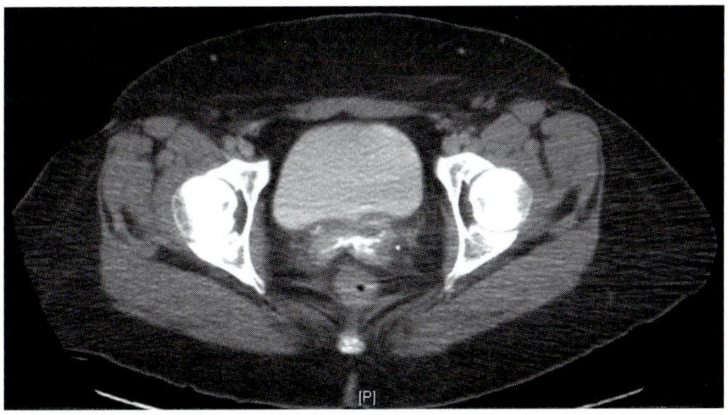

Fig. 13.7 Computed tomography cystography showing vesicovaginal fistula in a patient after hysterectomy. Extravasation of contrast into the vagina is noted.

radiation, patient discomfort, and the fact that imaging is confined to just the anterior compartment and lacks visualization of surrounding structures.

FLUOROSCOPY AND DEFECOGRAPHY

Fluoroscopy is a modification of x-ray examination that is used to visualize the continuous movement of internal structures. Many imaging modalities have previously been used to evaluate the pelvic floor, including CT, MRI, and barium defecography.

Defecography, or fluoroscopic proctography, is an established method used to dynamically evaluate the mechanics of rectal emptying. Defecography is able to image dynamic physiologic rectal emptying under radiographic guidance. However, owing to the physiologic nature of the emptying mechanism, this evaluation is dependent on the voluntary control of the pelvic floor and passive emptying of the rectum from the patient's point of view. A normal defecography study is conducted in three phases: rest, evacuation, and recovery. In the resting phase (with normal sphincter function), the anal canal should be closed. Measurements of the anorectal junction (ARJ) and the anorectal angle (ARA) are obtained during the resting phase. Evacuation is initiated by pelvic floor descent, which begins the defecation process. This is characterized by a descent of the ARJ from rest to opening of the rectal canal, normally occurring within a few seconds. When the canal is empty, it empties quickly, normally within 30 seconds. At this time, anatomy or mechanical abnormalities are evaluated following significant straining/Valsalva. The recovery phase follows evacuation and is typically shown by the return of tone to the internal sphincter and levator ani. At this time, the anal canal is closed, the ARA becomes more acute, and the ARJ and pelvic floor elevate to return to their resting positions. A notable advantage of defecography is that it enables patients to replicate their symptoms, because it requires patients to be upright, thereby replicating a more physiologic positioning for rectal emptying. In addition, organs of the anterior and posterior compartments of the pelvic floor can be examined, so that a patient can be evaluated for anterior and posterior prolapse concomitantly. See Video 13.1 for a detailed demonstration of the indications, technique, and normal and abnormal findings of defecography. Overall, defecography is useful for evaluating the interaction between rectal evacuation, the pelvic organs, and the pelvic floor musculature. The most significant disadvantage is that it requires multiple organs to be opacified, thereby exposing patients to a high level of radiation. See Chapter 28 for additional discussion on the use of defecography in the evaluation of constipation and rectal evacuation disorders.

ULTRASOUND

Techniques

The basic structures to include for the pelvic floor ultrasound examination include the pubic symphysis, the urethra, the bladder, the vagina, the uterus (if present), the endoanal canal, the levator plate, and the levator ani muscle complex. The integrity of the levator ani muscle complex is usually evaluated by documenting its insertion at the inferior portion of the pubic symphysis and measuring the dimensions of the levator hiatus. More than one modality may be required for proper identification of all relevant anatomic structures. All ultrasound modalities should include a two-dimensional (2D) assessment of the pelvic floor and a dynamic assessment with imaging at rest (static assessment) and then with squeeze and Valsalva maneuvers (dynamic assessment), followed by three-dimensional (3D) and four-dimensional (4D) assessments if available. Lastly, an evaluation of the anal sphincter may be performed. Indications for pelvic floor ultrasound are listed in Box 13.1.

Perineal Ultrasound and Introital Ultrasound

For perineal ultrasound, the patient is placed in the dorsal lithotomy position (with hips flexed and abducted). If stirrups are not available on the examination table, the patient may be placed on the lateral position. The patient is asked to empty her bladder before the examination or to have a moderate amount

BOX 13.1 Indications for Pelvic Floor Ultrasound

- Urinary incontinence
- Recurrent urinary tract infections
- Persistent dysuria
- Symptoms of voiding dysfunction
- Symptoms of pelvic organ prolapse
- Obstructed defecation
- Anal incontinence
- Vaginal discharge or bleeding after pelvic floor surgery
- Pelvic or vaginal pain after pelvic floor surgery
- Dyspareunia
- Vaginal cyst or mass
- Synthetic implants (slings, meshes, and bulking agents)
- Levator ani muscle assessment after childbirth
- Obstetric perineal injury
- Obstetric anal sphincter injury
- Perineal cyst or mass

(From AIUM/IUGA practice parameter for the performance of Urogynecological ultrasound examinations. Int Urogynecol J 30, 1389–1400 (2019). https://doi.org/10.1007/s00192-019-03954-5.)

of urine in the bladder without discomfort. Requirements for 2D perineal ultrasound include a B-mode capable 2D ultrasound system and a 3.5- to 6-MHz transducer. A curved abdominal transducer is placed on the perineum/vulva. The transducer may be covered with a non—powdered glove or transducer cover. Ultrasound gel is applied to the transducer, and it is then placed firmly on the perineum. The examination is started with midsagittal images of the pelvis, which are obtained at rest, during squeeze, and with the Valsalva maneuver. Midsagittal images of the pelvic organs are demonstrated (bladder, vagina, uterus, and rectum) with relation to the pelvic floor at the level of the pubic symphysis (Fig. 13.8). From the midsagittal view, the following structures should be identified from ventral to dorsal: symphysis pubis (SP), urethra, bladder neck, vaginal canal, uterus, cervix, anorectal canal, and the central portion of the puborectalis muscle. The examiner can visualize in real-time and measure the degree of pelvic prolapse at rest and with Valsalva maneuvers. The bladder neck undergoes subjective and objective evaluation for hypermobility. Findings of pelvic floor dyssynergia may be noted as a paradoxical movement of the pelvic floor during these maneuvers; similarly, an atonic pelvic floor is characterized by a lack of levator plate movement with prompted squeeze. Observation of coordinated pelvic floor lift by ultrasound may be indicative of pelvic floor dysfunction. Parting the labia and varying the degree of pressure of the transducer may improve image quality. By rotating the transducer 90 degrees, one can obtain a coronal view, and by placing a dorsal inclination on the transducer, the anal canal and sphincter complex can be visualized and examined. Once adequate images are obtained, the transducer is removed from the perineum and cleaned.

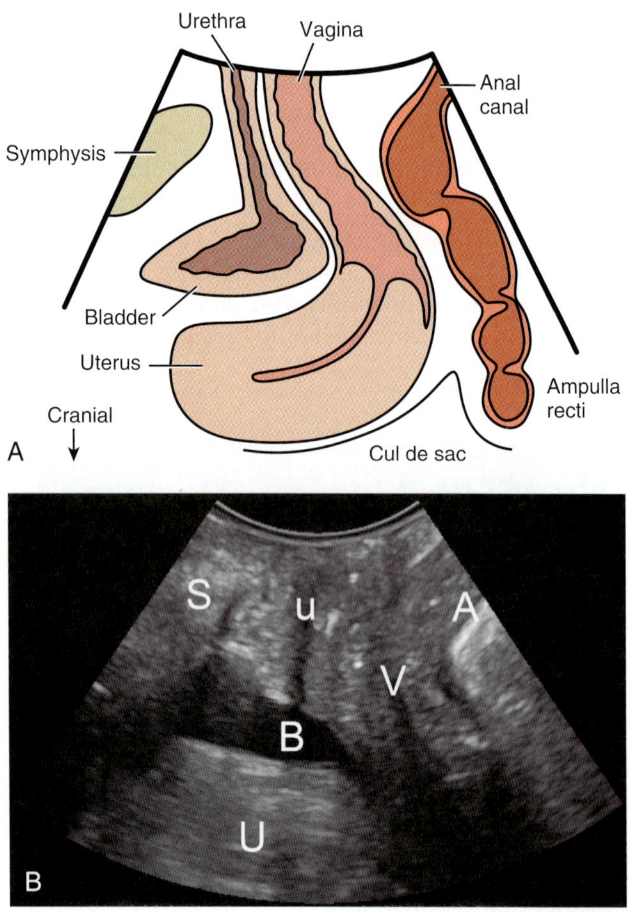

Fig. 13.8 **A**, A schematic diagram and **(B)**, the ultrasound image showing a midsagittal view on two-dimensional transperineal ultrasound (Voluson E6 with RAB 4-8 MHz transducer [GE Healthcare, Wauwatosa, WI]). *A*, Anal canal; *V*, vagina; *u*, urethra; *U*, uterus; *B*, bladder; *S*, symphysis pubis. (**A** from Dietz HP. Pelvic floor ultrasound: a review. *Am J Obstet Gynecol.* 2010;202:321. With permission.)

The 2D images can be integrated into 3D volume data either by freehand acquisition of images or by using a transducer equipped with a motor to allow for automatic acquisition of images. To perform the examination, the patient is placed in the same position as described for 2D ultrasound. The 3D-capable transducer is placed firmly on the perineum, maintaining a midsagittal orientation. The transducer is then held in place while the images are obtained at rest, during squeeze, and with the Valsalva maneuver. The 3D postprocessing of the images can be performed with the appropriate software. The 4D imaging entails the real-time acquisition of data to produce and save image cineloops. To perform 4D ultrasound, images are recorded during a prompted maneuver such as a squeeze or maximal Valsalva maneuver. This allows for instant acquisition of ultrasound volumes, optimized versions of which may then be viewed in orthogonal planes or rendered views (Fig. 13.9A and B).

Introital pelvic floor ultrasound requires an endocavitary front fire transducer. Similar steps are performed by obtaining images of the pubic symphysis, urethra, vagina, and anal canal with an initial midsagittal view. This will allow for an initial static image of the urethrovesical junction and ARA. A dynamic assessment of the pelvic floor is obtained by having the patient perform squeeze and Valsalva maneuvers, followed by a 3D assessment of the levator ani complex, if the 3D modality is available. Lastly, the anal sphincter complex may be imaged in the axial plane, specifically noting the integrity of the external anal sphincter (EAS) and internal anal sphincter (IAS) (Fig. 13.10).

Endovaginal Ultrasonography. Endovaginal ultrasound (EVUS) of the pelvic floor also begins with a 2D static and dynamic assessment of the pelvic floor. An endocavitary transducer such as a high-resolution, multifrequency, 9- to 16-MHz transducer is used (linear array 360-degree 3D transducer or radial array 360-degree 3D transducer). EVUS is routinely performed with the patient in the dorsal lithotomy position with a comfortable amount of urine in the bladder (Fig. 13.11A and B). To perform the exam, the transducer is inserted into the vagina in a neutral position, avoiding excessive pressure on the surrounding structures. Typically it is performed at rest, with a Valsalva maneuver, and during pelvic floor muscle contraction.

During the 2D assessment, the transducer is introduced into the vagina until the urethrovaginal junction is visualized. At this time, any anterior compartment, including the urethra or bladder neck, can be visualized, and any dynamic maneuvers, such as squeeze or Valsalva, can also be performed. Note that these movements can be impeded by the presence of the transducer in the vaginal canal. The transducer may then be

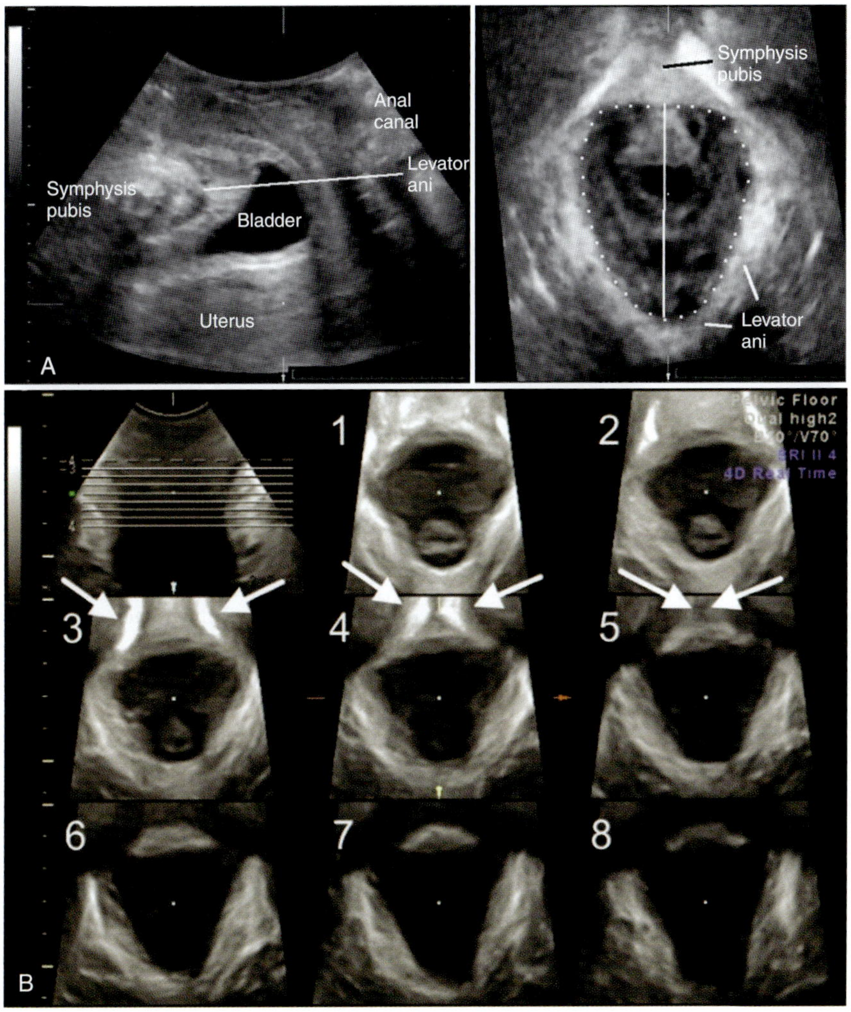

Fig. 13.9 **A**, Translabial three-dimensional ultrasound images in the midsagittal plane (*left*) and oblique axial plane (*right*) showing identification of the plane of minimal hiatal dimensions on Valsalva maneuver. The horizontal line in the image on the *left* illustrates the identification of the plane of minimal hiatal dimensions in the midsagittal plane and is equivalent to the vertical line in the image on the *right*. The *dotted line* in the image on the *right* illustrates the minimal hiatal area on Valsalva, which was measured at 19 cm^2, indicating normal distensibility of the hiatus. (From Dietz HP, Shek C, De Leon J, Steensma AB. Ballooning of the levator hiatus. *Ultrasound Obstet Gynecol.* 2008;31:676.) **B**, Tomographic ultrasound imaging in the C (axial) plane for assessment of levator integrity. Slice 1 is the caudal slice; slice 8 is the most cranial slice. The *arrows* indicate the symphysis pubis. (From AIUM/IUGA practice parameter for the performance of urogynecological ultrasound examinations: developed in collaboration with the ACR, the AUGS, the AUA, and the SRU. *Int Urogynecol J.* 2019;30:1389.)

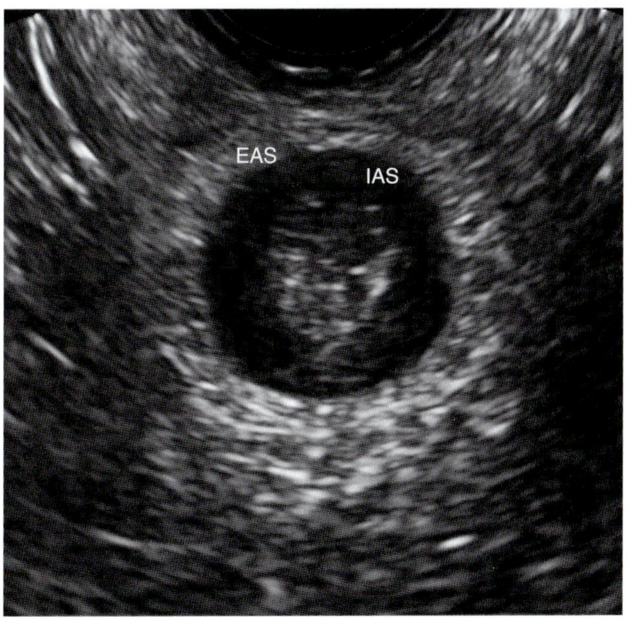

Fig. 13.10 Transperineal view showing an intact anal sphincter complex. *EAS*, External anal sphincter; *IAS*, internal anal sphincter.

advanced to visualize the urethrovesical junction, and it is at this time that the 3D volume acquisition, if available, can be started. The scan starts at the urethrovesical junction and continues until 6 cm caudally to include the perineal body as an anatomic landmark. Postprocessing may be performed on the scanner, but is easier to carry out using the free software, which can be installed on any computer. Video 13.2 shows an example of 3D postprocessing of a 3D volume from an EVUS and includes measurements of minimal levator hiatus, the ARA, and levator ani integrity. This allows for the volume to be exported to an external drive and viewed and analyzed at any time. The software allows manipulation of the 3D cube in the x, y, and z planes, as well as linear, angle, area, and volume measurements (Fig. 13.12). As with other ultrasound modalities, the 3D volume obtained is useful in visualizing levator ani muscle integrity or defects, for describing and measuring vaginal masses, and for localizing and characterizing slings, mesh, and other foreign bodies (Fig. 13.13).

Transrectal Ultrasonography. Endoanal ultrasound is useful for the evaluation of anal sphincter defect or pathology and is

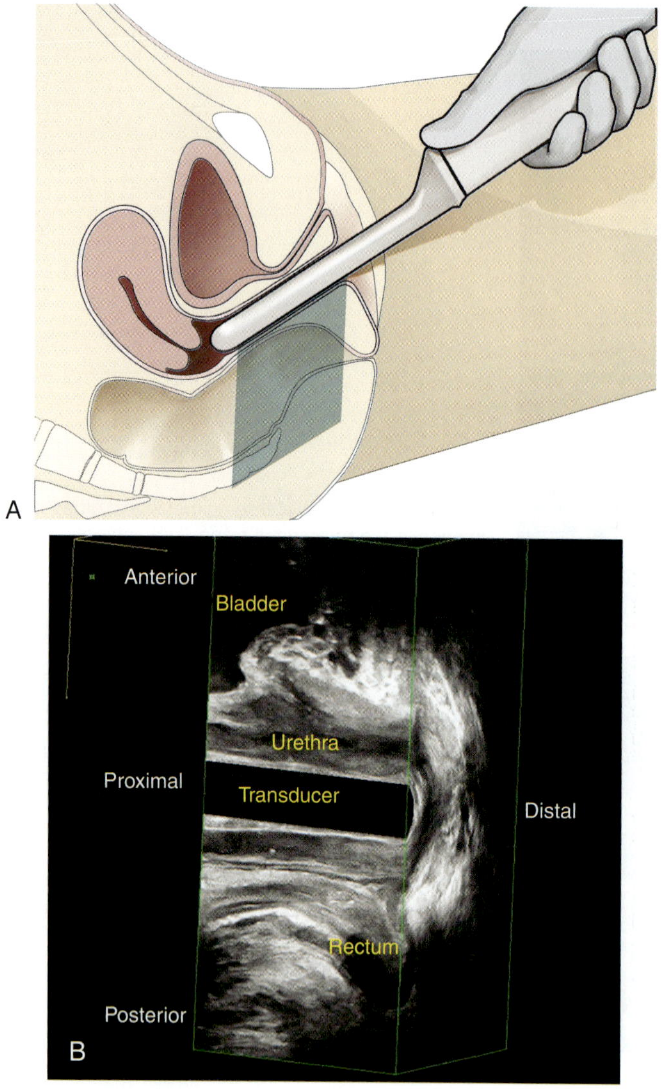

Fig. 13.11 **A**, Schematic of placement of three-dimensional (3D) endovaginal transducer. **B**, 3D endovaginal ultrasound volume.

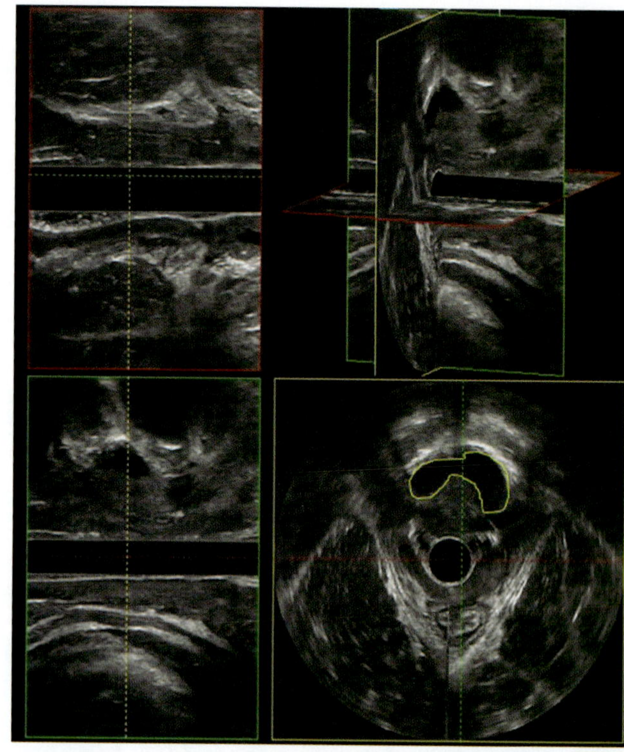

Fig. 13.12 Three views of urethra diverticulum on the x, y, and z planes using three-dimensional endovaginal sonography.

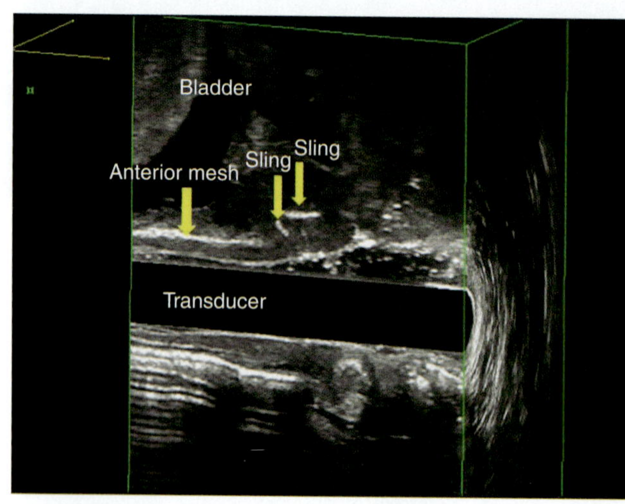

Fig. 13.13 Three-dimensional ultrasound showing anterior mesh and two midurethral slings.

performed with a high-resolution, multifrequency, mechanical 360-degree rotational transducer. This method has been regarded as the "gold standard" in the evaluation of the anal sphincter complex. The patient is placed in the lithotomy, lateral, or prone position. Some clinicians prefer the left lateral position when performing this ultrasound. If in lithotomy position, the transducer is inserted gently at a 45-degree angle until the levator plate is visualized posteriorly. Irrespective of patient positioning, the transducer should be positioned so that the anterior aspect of the anal canal is superior on the screen, at the 12 o'clock position. The distal end of the transducer should be at the level of the puborectalis muscle or 6 cm into the anal canal. The mechanical rotational transducer, once activated, automatically obtains 3D images. In addition to obtaining detailed views of the anal sphincter complex, this method may be useful in imaging the pelvic anatomy of individuals with a short or absent vagina. The IAS is a continuous smooth muscle hypoechoic ring, the EAS is a striated muscle hyperechoic ring, and the conjoint longitudinal muscle consists of a mixed echogenicity layer between the two sphincters (Fig. 13.14).

APPLICATIONS OF ULTRASOUND IN EVALUATING DISORDERS OF THE LOWER URINARY TRACT AND PELVIC FLOOR

Anterior Compartment

The anterior compartment of the pelvis is often assessed with transperineal ultrasounds and EVUSs. Considering the inherent displacement of adjacent tissue with EVUS, transperineal

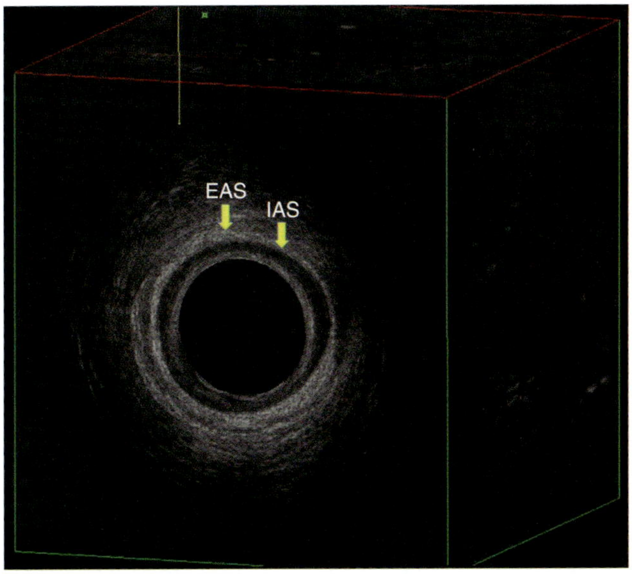

Fig. 13.14 Example of a normal three-dimensional endoanal ultrasound. *EAS*, External anal sphincter; *IAS*, internal anal sphincter.

ultrasound may be preferred for visualizing bladder neck descent, urethral hypermobility, cystocele, and cystourethrocele. On transperineal and introital ultrasound, the position of the urethrovesical junction at rest and at maximal Valsalva may be measured relative to the central line of the SP or its inferoposterior margin. It is recommended to use the posterior inferoposterior margin of the SP as a reference. On Valsalva, the bladder neck and proximal urethra are noted to rotate in the inferior and posterior directions. The distal urethra remains stable because of its tethering to the SP and pelvic side walls. There is no standard measurement to define hypermobility of the urethra, but movement cutoffs of 20, 25, or 30 mm have been proposed. However, there is no current standard definition for urethral hypermobility on ultrasound, and similar measurements have been found in asymptomatic nulliparous women. Perhaps an observation of greater importance is hypomobility of the urethra. A fixed or hypomobile urethra considerably increases the risk of failure after placement of a midurethral sling. In a study by Lo et al. (2016), repeat sling surgery for UI in patients with limited urethral mobility diagnosed by either Q-tip test or ultrasound was associated with a four times greater risk of sling failure. Similarly, Viereck et al. (2015) also noted that patients treated with tension-free vaginal tape who had decreased bladder neck mobility of 10 mm or less on ultrasound had a two-fold higher risk of failure from the procedure. Clinically, the finding of urethral hypomobility increases the risk of sling failure and may prompt consideration of other treatment options.

A 3D EVUS can be used to provide a detailed anatomic depiction of anterior compartment structures, including the trigone, the compressor urethra, and the urogenital sphincter. The examiner is also able to measure the components of the urethral complex, including urethral width, length, and volume. Ultrasound is also an excellent tool for visualizing vaginal cysts and masses, including Skene's gland cysts, urethral diverticula, and Garner's duct cysts.

The female urethra is a complex organ that plays a central role in UI, and thus normal anatomy, innervation, position, and proper relation to the surrounding pelvic floor structures ensure its normal function. Signs and symptoms of pelvic floor dysfunction often overlap with signs and symptoms of urethral diverticula, ectopic ureters, urethral tumors, and periurethral cystic lesions. Ectopic ureters and ureteroceles are usually diagnosed in childhood and rarely present in adults. Nevertheless, these conditions should be considered in patients with urinary tract infections or UI, as surgery can correct these disorders. EVUS has been used in the diagnosis of ectopic and dystopic ureters. Moreover, on rare occasions ultrasound is helpful in distinguishing pathology mimicking anterior vaginal wall prolapse, such as a vaginal cyst, vaginal myoma, Skene's gland cyst, or urethral diverticulum.

Urinary Incontinence

Various ultrasound techniques and findings have been taken into account in the evaluation of UI. One of the initial steps in the evaluation of UI involves the measurement of a postvoid residual, which may be accomplished with ultrasound, allowing for the estimation of bladder volume in millimeters. Evaluation of the bladder neck in the context of UI was one the first procedures to be performed by perineal ultrasound. Findings such as urethral hypermobility and bladder funneling have been noted in association with UI but may also be observed in asymptomatic women with normal urethral sphincters and in women with urge incontinence. Currently there is insufficient evidence that ultrasound evaluation is of significant clinical benefit in the standard evaluation of UI.

Urethral and Periurethral Abnormalities

A urethral diverticulum is a localized outpouching of the urethral mucosa into the surrounding nonurothelial tissues. This is an uncommon condition that is found mainly in adult women, and it is a diagnosis that is often overlooked in patients presenting with elusive lower urinary tract symptoms (e.g., UI, dysuria, dyspareunia, vaginal mass). The delay in diagnosis of this condition can lead to chronic morbidity, including urethral calculus formation, chronic or recurrent urinary tract infections, or, rarely, malignant transformation. Previously, contrast-enhanced radiography (e.g., voiding cystourethrography, retrograde double-balloon positive pressure urethrography) was used to evaluate women for urethral diverticulum. However, these procedures are invasive and technically difficult, and the contrast-dependent studies are only able to visualize diverticula that are patent enough to allow filling with contrast material. Therefore the preferred imaging techniques are MRI or ultrasound (Fig. 13.15).

Ultrasound can help differentiate a diverticulum from other periurethral cystic lesions such as ectopic ureters, calcifications, and injected material, and can be very useful in surgical planning. It can offer invaluable information such as shape, size, and location in relation to the urethra and bladder. It is also a useful tool in the diagnosis and monitoring of urethral tumors. Ultrasound provides a noninvasive tool to evaluate and monitor vaginal masses. A rare clinical example is that of urethral leiomyoma (a rare benign smooth muscle tumor that may grow in

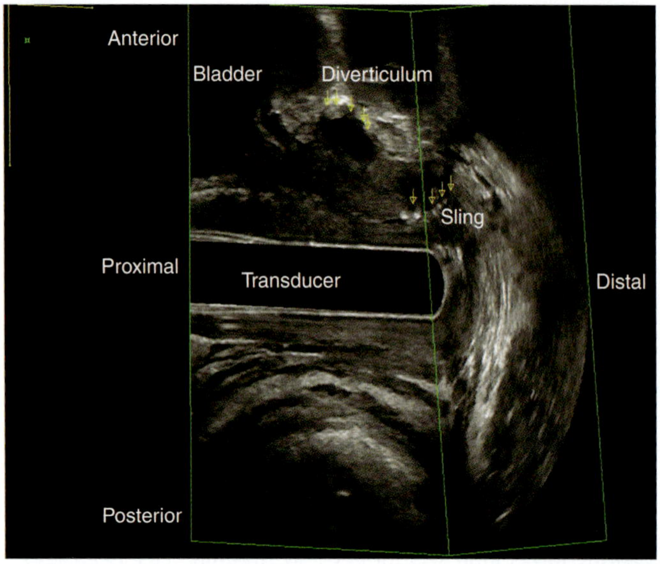

Fig. 13.15 Three-dimensional ultrasound volume showing the location of a urethral diverticulum and a midurethral sling (*yellow arrows*).

pregnancy and may be associated with lower urinary tract symptoms), which may be monitored with ultrasound during the course of the pregnancy or until surgery is indicated. There are conflicting reports of the clinical significance of measurements of bladder wall thickness and the association with detrusor instability. Detrusor hypertrophy may appear asymmetric on ultrasound, and the reduced repeatability of these sonographic measurements limits their clinical utility.

Posterior Compartment

POP of the posterior and apical compartment, particularly sigmoidoceles and enteroceles, can be difficult to diagnose by physical examination alone. In the posterior compartment, ultrasound provides visualization of defects of the rectovaginal septum (rectocele) and measurements of the ARA. The anatomical abnormalities associated with defecatory dysfunction are easily visualized on dynamic ultrasound scans. Many clinicians use the term "rectocele" to refer to any prolapse of the posterior vaginal wall; a true rectocele is defined as the herniation of the anterior rectal wall into the vagina. Although there is no standardization, a proposed measurement involves measuring the depth of the rectocele perpendicular to the expected line of contour of the rectal wall. Some studies describe a rectocele based on definitions used in defecography, with first-degree less than 1 cm in depth, second-degree 2 to 4 cm in depth, and third-degree greater than 4 cm in depth. During Valsalva, several other important aspects can be visualized, including descent of an enterocele, movement of the puborectalis, and ARA to evaluate for pelvic floor dyssynergy, as well as visualization of intussusception. Assessment of the anal canal is typically performed with endoanal ultrasound, which will be discussed later.

An enterocele is a hernia of the most inferior point of the abdominal cavity into the vagina or pouch of Douglas. On ultrasound, it is visualized as the downward movement of abdominal contents into the vagina, ventral to the rectal ampulla and anal canal, whereas a sigmoidocele is seen by differentiating hyperechoic stool movement from the surrounding tissue. It is important to differentiate a sigmoidocele from an enterocele in planning a surgical procedure. Intussusception, on the other hand, occurs when the rectal wall telescopes into the rectal lumen, and may involve the rectal mucosa or the full thickness of the rectal wall. Pelvic floor dyssynergy is typically described as a lack of normal relaxation of the puborectalis muscle during defecation. This can be a difficult condition to verify through clinical examination. On ultrasound, dyssynergy is visualized as narrowing of the ARA, shortening of the levator hiatus, and thickening of the puborectalis muscle.

Postoperative Findings and Synthetic Mesh Materials

Ultrasound is the best imaging modality for visualizing synthetic vaginal mesh implants used in pelvic floor surgeries, such as those used for POP and UI. Polypropylene is one of the most commonly used mesh products in vaginal surgery and is highly echogenic on ultrasound. Ultrasound can determine the size, shape, position, distortion, and mobility of the implants. The position of the mesh is typically along the posterior vaginal wall (sometimes extending to the perineal body), along the anterior wall, or near the midurethra in the case of midurethral slings. When palpating the vaginal wall, it may be difficult to discern implanted mesh (which may be shrunken, contracted, or folded) from the surrounding scar tissue. Fig. 13.16 shows an example of vaginal mesh and a sling in the anterior compartment. In the case of midurethral slings, ultrasound can help distinguish transobturator versus retropubic slings. A 3D ultrasound is helpful in locating and "mapping" the location of the synthetic material on axial, sagittal, and coronal images relative to the bladder neck. Fig. 13.17 shows an example of a folded transobturator sling visualized on ultrasound. Figs. 13.18A and B show the cystoscopic finding of a calcified left anterior vaginal mesh erosion in

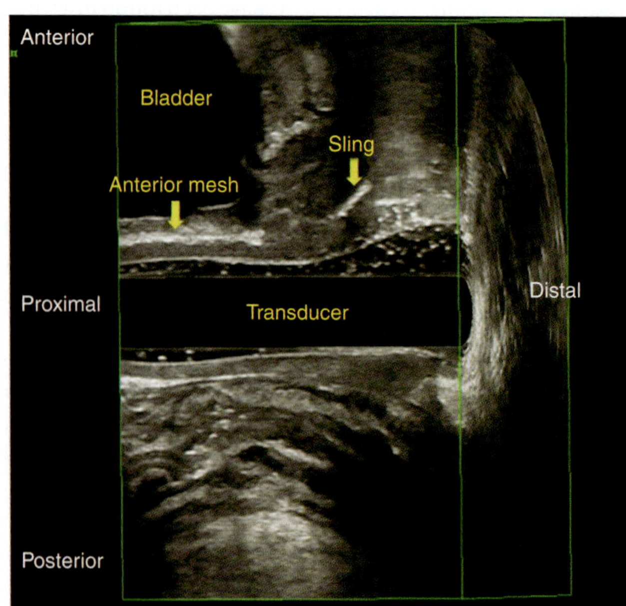

Fig. 13.16 Three-dimensional ultrasound volume. Anterior vaginal mesh and slings are labeled.

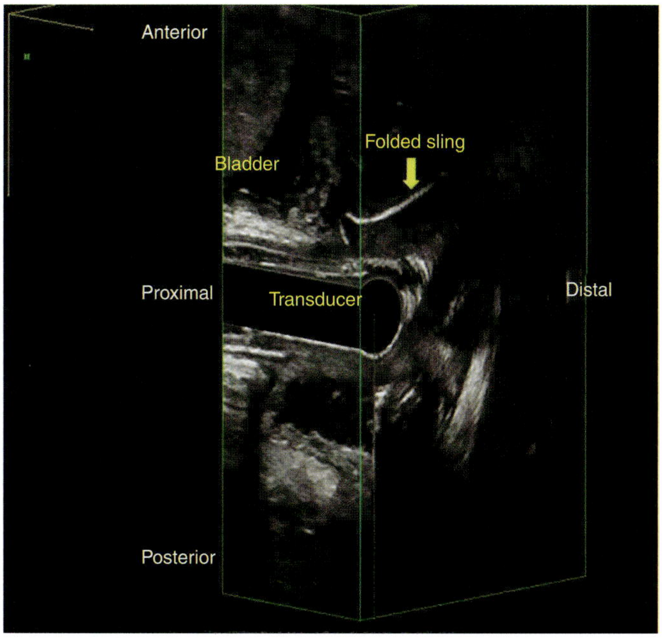

Fig. 13.17 A folded midurethral sling is noted on three-dimensional ultrasound in a patient complaining of voiding dysfunction with an elevated postvoid residual.

the bladder and the corresponding image on ultrasound. This can be helpful in planning a procedure to remove permanent synthetic materials in the absence of an operative report, or as adjunctive imaging in cases where the synthetic materials appear to be displaced. It is also a useful tool in the evaluation of patients who have persistent symptoms after mesh resection because it allows for the visualization of mesh remnants. Other foreign bodies such as urethral bulking agents can also easily be seen on ultrasound (Fig. 13.19). Video 13.3 shows a 3D EVUS illustrating the details of vaginal mesh and a sling. In this case, the patient was diagnosed with mesh erosion on cystoscopy after gross hematuria. She had a prior anterior vaginal mesh and sling, and the 3D ultrasound identified the left arm of the vaginal mesh in the bladder.

Fecal Incontinence

Endoanal ultrasound is traditionally known as the gold standard for morphological assessment of the anal canal. When performing endoanal ultrasound, the anal canal is divided into three levels in the axial plane: upper, middle, and lower. The uppermost level is marked proximally by the puborectalis muscle and distally by the ring of the IAS. The middle level is marked by the complete ring of the IAS and EAS and by visualization of the transverse perinei muscles. The lower level is marked by the subcutaneous part of the EAS. Fig. 13.14 shows an example of normal IAS and EAS anatomy on 3D endoanal ultrasound. Video 13.4 shows an example of 3D endoanal ultrasound with an intact IAS and an EAS defect from about 10 to 2 o'clock.

Endoanal ultrasound is often the diagnostic test of choice in patients presenting with fecal incontinence and a history of a traumatic childbirth. Fig. 13.20 shows an example of an EAS defect with an intact IAS. By defining the margins of disruption, ultrasound provides invaluable information for the surgeon if surgical repair is considered. Several studies have compared transperineal with endoanal imaging, showing moderate to good interrater agreement. Fig. 13.21, from Dietz (2018), shows transperineal imaging of the anal sphincter. The advantage of an exoanal approach is that it reduces patient discomfort while minimizing distortion of the anal sphincter canal. Future research comparing imaging methods as they correlate with patient symptoms is needed in this field.

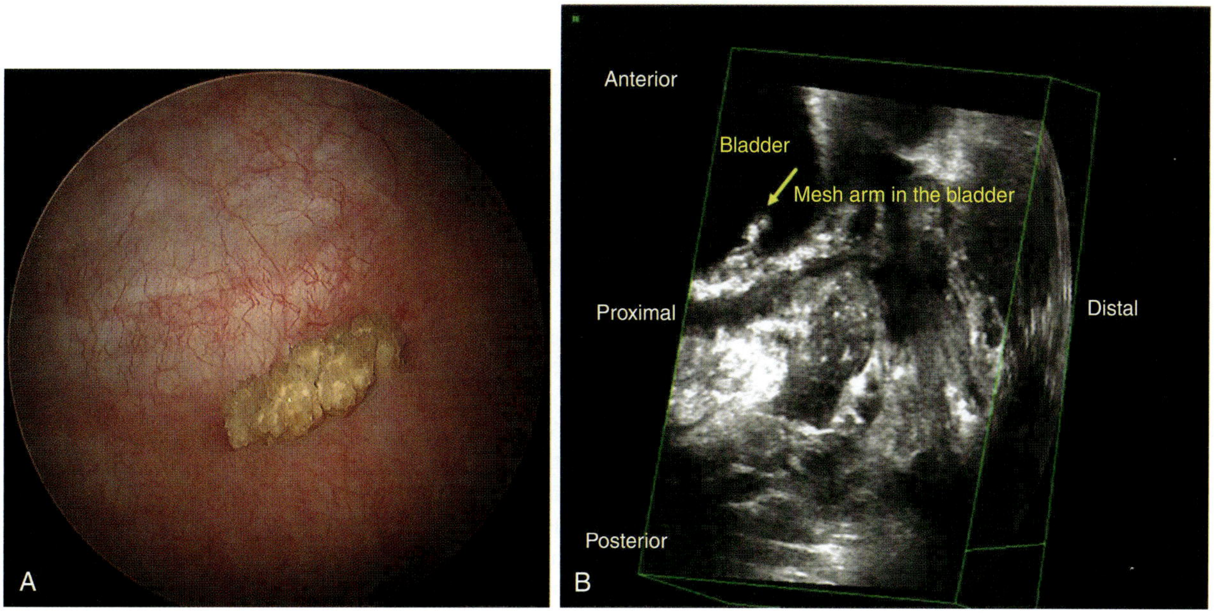

Fig. 13.18 **A**, Mesh erosion in the bladder noted at the time of cystoscopy in a patient at the time of gross hematuria workup. This same patient had a history of anterior vaginal mesh and sling placement. **B**, Three-dimensional ultrasound of this same patient allowed for visualization of the anterior vaginal mesh, confirmed as the area of mesh noted in the bladder.

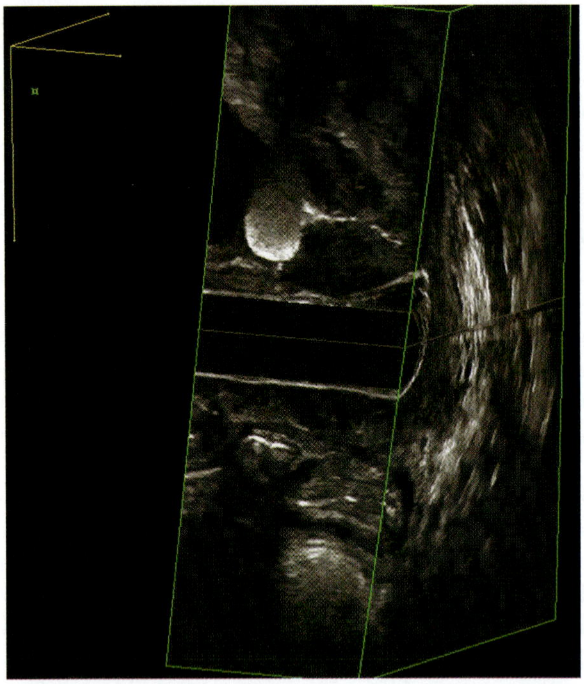

Fig. 13.19 Three- dimensional ultrasound. Sagittal view of urethral bulking agent noted as a hyperechoic sphere.

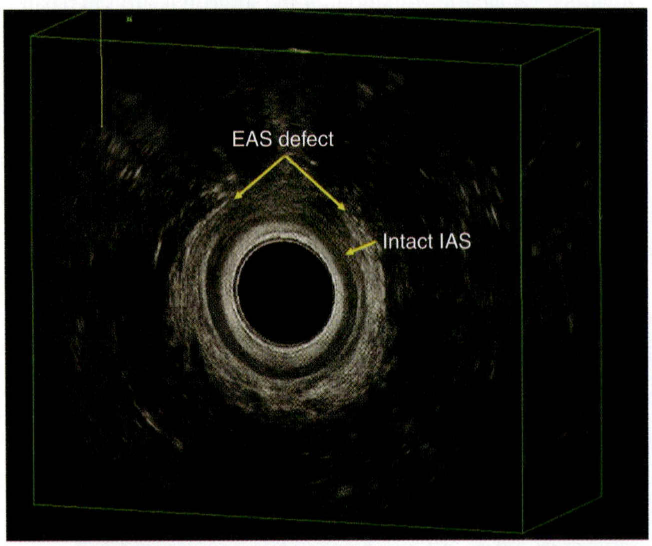

Fig. 13.20 Three- dimensional endoanal ultrasound showing an intact internal anal sphincter (hypoechoic ring) and a defect of the external anal sphincter (hyperechoic) from the 10 to the 2 o'clock positions. *IAS,* Internal anal sphincter; *EAS,* external anal sphincter.

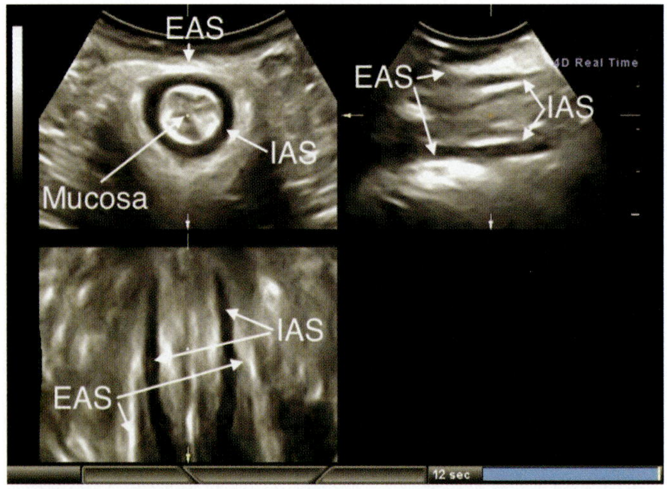

Fig. 13.21 Orthogonal views of external anal sphincter and internal anal sphincter and anal mucosa on three-dimensional/four-dimensional translabial sphincter imaging. The *top left image* is the coronal plane; *top right* is midsagittal; and *bottom left* is an axial view of the anal canal. *IAS,* Internal anal sphincter; *EAS,* external anal sphincter. (From Dietz HP. Exoanal imaging of the anal sphincters. *J Ultrasound Med.* 2018;37:263.)

MAGNETIC RESONANCE IMAGING

MRI is an important diagnostic and research tool in the evaluation of pelvic floor anatomy. It allows for multiplanar imaging and soft-tissue differentiation because of its high spatial resolution. It provides a global view of the surrounding pelvic viscera, has no known adverse biologic effects, and is not operator-dependent. MRI combines high-resolution images with soft-tissue contrast, and provides a noninvasive and objective approach to the evaluation of PFDs (Boyadzhyan et al. 2008; Comiter et al. 1999; Hoyet et al. 2001; Maglinte et al. 1999). MRI encompasses dynamic and static images. Dynamic images are captured at maximum stress to the pelvic floor, including defecography, to visualize pelvic organ mobility, pelvic floor weakness, POP, and associated compartment defects (Comiter et al. 1999; Grassi et al. 2007; Cufler et al. 2002). Static images visualize pelvic floor anatomy and defects in supportive structures (El Sayed et al. 2017). The disadvantages of MRI are that it is the most expensive modality, it is time-consuming, and it is not always readily available.

Yang et al. (1991) first described the use of MRI for the evaluation of pelvic floor descent at maximal strain. Since that time, MRI has been used for the evaluation UI, POP, defecatory dysfunction, pelvic pain, and descending perineal syndrome, among other indications. MRI also provides detailed information regarding the anatomy of the levator ani muscles (Strohbehn et al. 1996).

Patient Preparation

The patient is examined in a 1.5-T MRI unit with a phased array coil at minimum. The patient can be examined in supine position with the knee elevated on a high pillow to facilitate straining and evacuation, with the coil centered low on the pelvis to ensure complete visualization of prolapsed organs. The bladder should be moderately filled (El Sayed et al 2017). MRI can also be performed in an upright low–field strength open magnet with the patient sitting on a modified MRI-safe commode (Fielding et al. 1996; Boyadzhyan et al. 2008; El Sayed et al. 2008). Although the sitting position is more physiologic, upright magnets are not readily available at most centers. Iacobellis et al. (2020) compared MRI defecography in both upright and supine positions in the same set of patients and showed significantly lower position of the bladder and vagina, but not of the ARJ, at defecation during the upright MRI. Before imaging, the patient is instructed on the dynamic and evacuation phase of the examination. The patient is instructed to squeeze as if trying to prevent the escape of urine or feces and to hold this position for the duration of the sequence. For maximal straining, the patient is instructed to bear down as much as possible, as though constipated and trying to defecate. For evacuation, the patient is instructed to repeat evacuation until the rectum is emptied. Provision of a diaper for protection ensures patient compliance (El Sayed et al. 2017).

Ultrasound gel is usually recommended to distend the rectum. The rectum is distended to visualize the ARJ, rectoceles, and intussusceptions, and to evaluate the efficacy of rectal evacuation (El Sayed et al. 2017).

Magnetic Resonance Imaging Protocol

Static MRI sequences are obtained at rest, whereas dynamic MRI sequences are obtained during straining, squeezing, and evacuation (defecation). High-resolution T2-weighted images in three planes are recommended for static images, whereas steady-state (or balanced-state free precession sequence) in the sagittal plane is recommended for dynamic sequences. Each dynamic sequence should not exceed 20 seconds, to allow for breath holding. Optional MRI sequences can be added for further assessment of pelvic floor relaxation, including axial and coronal dynamic sequences during maximum straining. A dynamic MRI study for PFD is considered diagnostic if a clear movement of the abdominal wall is seen during squeezing and straining. If no evacuation of rectal content is observed, or if it takes more than 30 seconds to evacuate two-thirds of the rectal content, anismus is considered (El Sayed et al. 2017).

Pelvic Floor Measurements

The pubococcygeal line (PCL), drawn on the sagittal plane from the inferior aspect of the pubic symphysis to the last coccygeal joint, is the recommended reference line to measure POP (Betschart et al 2013). The midpubic line (MPL) is the line extending caudally along the long axis of the pubic symphysis. Both these lines serve as landmarks for clinical staging, with the PCL corresponding to the levator plate and the MPL corresponding to the level of the hymen. In the anterior compartment, the organ-specific reference point is the most inferior aspect of the bladder base (B); in the middle compartment, the organ-specific reference point is the anterior cervical lip (most distal edge of the cervix) (C), or the vaginal vault in the case of previous hysterectomy (V); and in the posterior compartment, the organ-specific reference point is the ARJ (El Sayed et al. 2008; Maccioni et al. 2013; Elshazly et al. 2010; Singh et al. 2003; Halligan et al. 1995; Yang et at 1991). The distance from each reference point is measured perpendicularly to the PCL at rest and at maximum strain on sagittal images (Mortele et al. 2007; Halligan et al. 1995). Staging systems to describe prolapse exist with both the MPL and the PCL. These reference lines have shown only moderate correlation with clinical staging, which may partially be caused by a difference in anatomical landmarks between studies.

The "HMO" system is used to grade POP, as well as pelvic floor laxity, and includes evaluation of the "H-line", "M-line," and organ-specific prolapse (Comiter et al. 1999). The H-line measures the width of the pelvic floor hiatus in the anteroposterior dimension and is measured from the inferior tip of the pubic symphysis to the posterior circular fibers of the ARJ. A normal H-line at rest is 6 cm or less. The M-line is drawn perpendicularly from the PCL to the posterior extent of the H-line at the posterior aspect of the ARJ. The M-line represents the degree of pelvic floor descent, and at rest is typically 2 cm or less (Reiner et al. 2013). The H-line, the M-line, and the levator plate angles are evaluated in the sagittal plane. The transverse width of the levator hiatus and the iliococcygeus angle are assessed in the axial and coronal plane during maximum straining (El Sayed et al 2008). Fig. 13.22 shows dynamic MRI images using MPL as a reference point in a patient with descending perineum syndrome and the landmarks of the HMO system used in grading prolapse.

The urethral angle is measured to assess for urethral hypermobility in the anterior compartment. The ARA and levator plate angle are measures of pelvic floor relaxation in the posterior compartment (Khatri et al 2017). The ARA is defined as the line drawn from the posterior border of the rectum and a line along the central axis of the anal canal on sagittal plane at rest, while squeezing, and at maximum strain (Elshazly et al. 2010; Shorvon et al. 1989). A normal ARA at rest ranges from 93 to 127 degrees (Schreyer et al. 2012; Mortele et al. 2007; Bartram et al. 1988; Shorvon et al. 1989; Khatri et al. 2017). The ARA should widen during defecation and narrow during Kegel by 15 to 20 degrees (Khatri et al. 2017; Mortele et al. 2007). The levator plate angle is measured between the levator plate and the PCL in the posterior compartment. The levator plate angle has been shown to be significantly higher during strain in patients with POP (Hoyte et al. 2001). Widening of the levator plate angle during strain or defecation by more than 10 degrees compared with baseline angle at rest indicates loss of pelvic support (Fielding et al. 2003; Khatri et al. 2017).

Functional Abnormalities on Dynamic Magnetic Resonance Imaging

Functional evaluation of the pelvic floor is described with respect to the anterior, middle, and posterior compartments. These can also be defined, respectively, as the urethral support system, which maintains urinary continence; the vaginal support system, which prevents prolapse; and the anal sphincter complex, which maintains anal continence. Functional evaluation is performed with reference to the PCL. UI on MRI imaging is defined by the visualized loss of urine through the urethra during maximal straining (El Sayed et al. 2008). Urethral hypermobility is reported if present (Halligan et al. 1995). The end of the evacuation phase is necessary to identify rectal intussusception (Broekhuis et al. 2009). The change in the ARA during the dynamic and evacuation sequences compared with at rest demonstrates puborectalis muscle function. The ARA should sharpen during squeezing and become more obtuse during straining and evacuation (El Sayed et al. 2017; Maccioni et al. 2013; Shorvon et al. 1989; Yang et al. 1991).

Anterior Compartment. Assessment of the anterior compartment includes evaluation of the bladder and the urethra. Anterior wall prolapse is defined on MRI imaging by descent greater than 1 cm below the PCL (Yang et al. 1991). Dynamic MRI in the supine position is highly sensitive (100%) for anterior vaginal prolapse (Gousse et al. 2008). The urethral angle (measured between the urethral axis and a vertical line drawn at the external meatus) is easily identified on midline sagittal T2-weighted images at rest. Change in urethral angle is used to access urethral mobility before and after surgery in patients with stress UI. Bladder outlet obstruction can be assessed when a voiding phase has been captured during image acquisition (Khatri et al. 2017; Showalter et al. 2001).

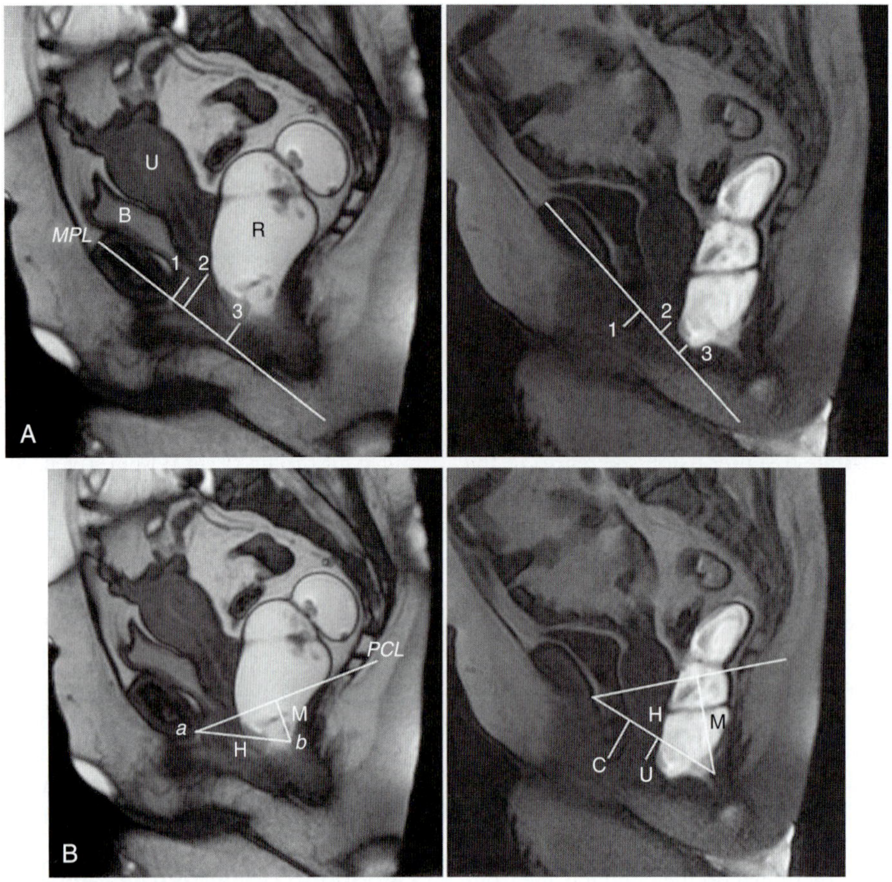

Fig. 13.22 **A**, Midsagittal T2-weighted steady-state free precession image obtained at rest (*left*) and T1-weighted gradient-recalled echo image at maximal pelvic floor descent during evacuation (*right*) show measurements of the three pelvic floor compartments (*1*, anterior; *2*, middle; *3*, posterior) with the midpubic line (*MPL*) used as a reference line. **B**, Midsagittal T2-weighted image obtained at rest shows landmarks used in the "HMO" system. (*left*) The landmarks are the inferior aspect of the symphysis pubis *(a)* and the posterior wall of the rectum at the level of the anorectal junction *(b)*. The H-line *(H)* represents the anteroposterior hiatal width and extends from *a* to *b*. The M-line *(M)* represents hiatal descent and extends perpendicularly from the pubococcygeal line (*PCL*) to the posterior end of the H-line. (*right*) Midsagittal T1-weighted multiphase gradient-recalled echo image during evacuation shows measurements of organ prolapse according to the HMO system. *C*, cystocele; *U*, uterus; *B*, bladder; *R*, rectum. (From Reiner CS, Weishaupt D. Dynamic pelvic floor imaging: MRI techniques and imaging parameters. *Abdom Imaging*. 2013;38:903.)

Middle Compartment. The middle compartment comprises the uterus, cervix, and vagina. MRI has high sensitivity for apical prolapse (Gousse et al. 2000). Paravaginal support defects may result in a more horizontal orientation of the vagina on sagittal images, and the normal "H" shape of the vagina may be disrupted on axial images. Severe uterine prolapse or the presence of uterine masses may obscure prolapse of the anterior or posterior compartments (Khatri et al. 2017).

Posterior Compartment. Compared with clinical examination, MRI offers a more comprehensive evaluation the posterior compartment (Maubon et al. 2003; Fletcher et al. 2003). MRI is best able to identify pelvic visceral and levator descent in women with obstructed defecation (Healy et al. 1997). MRI also aids in the evaluation of an enterocele, posterior vaginal wall prolapse, rectal intussusception, anal incontinence, pelvic floor dyssynergia, and descending perineal syndrome (Khatri et al. 2017).

Dynamic MRI is advantageous for the diagnosis of enterocele from a posterior vaginal wall prolapse. It also allows for characterization of contents within the enterocele sac (Tunn et al. 2000; Lienemann et al. 2000; Gupta et al. 2012). MRI allows for the diagnosis of clinically occult enteroceles by comprehensively evaluating the interaction between the pelvic floor and viscera. In one study by Attenberger et al. (2015), MRI changed the management of 59% patients relative to clinical diagnosis.

MRI defecography provides a global assessment of pelvic floor function and anatomical abnormality. It is better tolerated by patients, but it is not as sensitive as defecography in detecting trapping rectoceles and rectal intussusception (Zafar et al. 2017). Patient positioning may also make a difference in MRI defecography. In a study by Schawkat et al. (2018), more patients were able to evacuate in lateral position when compared with supine position, with similar grades of pelvic floor descent Fig. 13.23.

MRI defecography has about a 70% sensitivity for the diagnosis of rectal intussusception (Dvorkin et al. 2004). MRI is also

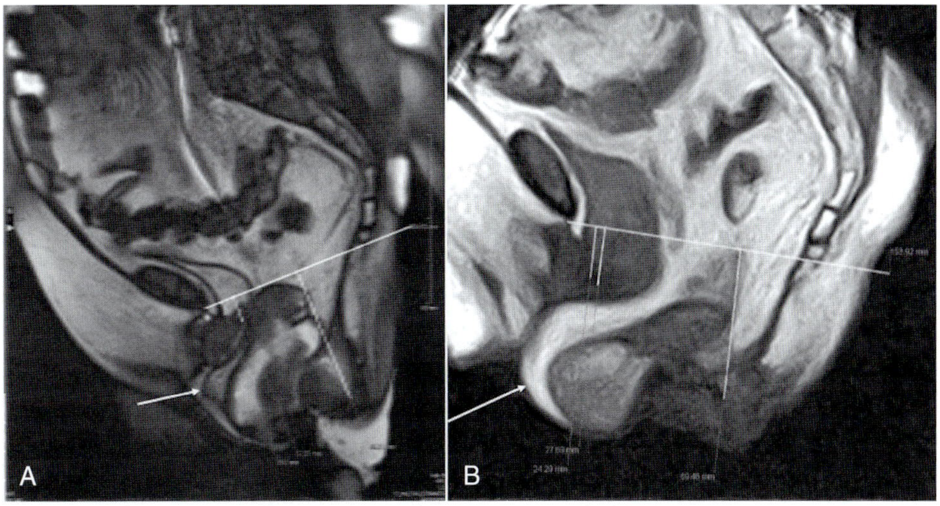

Fig. 13.23 Magnetic resonance imaging defecography. T2-weighted dynamic sequences in the sagittal plane acquired in the supine position (**A**) and in the sitting position on a dedicated magnet (**B**), during evacuation. Note the pathological perineal descent with the presence of median pelvic floor hernia (omentocele, *white arrow*) in Douglas' space causing an eversion of the vaginal wall, better seen in the sitting position (*arrow* in **B**). (From Iacobellis F, Reginelli A, Berritto D, et al. Pelvic floor dysfunctions: how to image patients? *Jpn J Radiol.* 2020;38:47.)

able to assess for atrophy or defects in the anal sphincter complex and can concomitantly be used to diagnose rectal prolapse or posterior compartment prolapse (Terra et al. 2006; Hetzer et al. 2006).

Structural Anatomy and Defects on Static Magnetic Resonance Imaging

MRI allows for direct visualization of multiple pelvic structures (including the levator muscles) without having to opacify the small bowel, bladder, or vagina with contrast. The levator muscles can be assessed for areas of asymmetric thickening or atrophy, focal defects, scarring, ballooning, or focal eventration. Anatomic evaluation should also report the presence or absence of the uterus and cervix.

A 3D model of the pelvic floor can be generated from MRI. In a study by Li et al. (2015) designed to assess the morphological features of the levator ani and bony pelvis in women with prolapse, four patterns of levator ani morphology were demonstrated among women with and without prolapse. There were significant differences in the width and length of the levator hiatus and in the levator symphysis gap between women with prolapse and healthy controls. A 3D stress-MRI allows for localization of pelvic organs during maximal Valsalva (Luo et al. 2012; Larson et al. 2010). The 3D MRI models used to characterize posterior vaginal wall prolapse have demonstrated increased folding of the vagina and an overall downward displacement in the upper two-thirds of the vagina. Forward protrusion, perineal descent, and distal widening are sometimes seen as well (Luo et al. 2012).

Stress Urinary Incontinence. SUI is associated with atrophy, laxity, and thinning of the levator ani muscles on MRI. Stress-incontinent women were found to have an oblique urethropelvic ligament, an inverted U-shaped vaginal lumen, and an increase in the distance between the SP and the bladder neck. In contrast, continent controls have more horizontal urethropelvic ligaments, closer proximity of the bladder neck to the SP, and an H-shaped vagina, with the anterior vaginal wall conforming well to the urethra. Morgan et al. (2009) evaluated urethral sphincter anatomy, urethral function, and pelvic floor function using MRI, and found that a smaller striated urogenital sphincter is associated with stress urinary incontinence and worse pelvic floor function.

Kirschner-Hermanns et al. (1993) identified degeneration of the levator ani muscles in 45% of stress incontinent women. Li et al. (2018) used MRI to show that de novo SUI was associated with levator ani muscle injury, vesical neck downward movement, and urethral sphincter dysfunction. Additionally, vesical neck funneling on sagittal images were found to be a predictor for SUI. MRI accurately showed the presence of urethral diverticulum with up to 100% sensitivity (Blander et al., 2001; Ockrim et al., 2009). Therefore MRI is considered a reference standard technology for diagnosing and characterizing urethral diverticulum (see Chapter 37). The ability of MRI to differentiate between solid and cystic masses also makes this imaging modality instrumental in distinguishing urethral diverticulum from other periurethral masses and differentiating between benign and malignant processes. Foster et al. (2007) showed that the use of preoperative MRI altered the management of urethral diverticulum in 15% of patients.

Pelvic Organ Prolapse. Pelvic organ support is currently understood on three levels, based on the work of Delancey et al. (1992). MRI measurements of pelvic landmark angles reliably differentiate between women with and without uterine prolapse and correlate best with point C on the POP Quantification system (Ginath et al. 2011). Women with prolapse more often have defects in the levator ani and generate less vaginal closure force during maximal contraction than controls

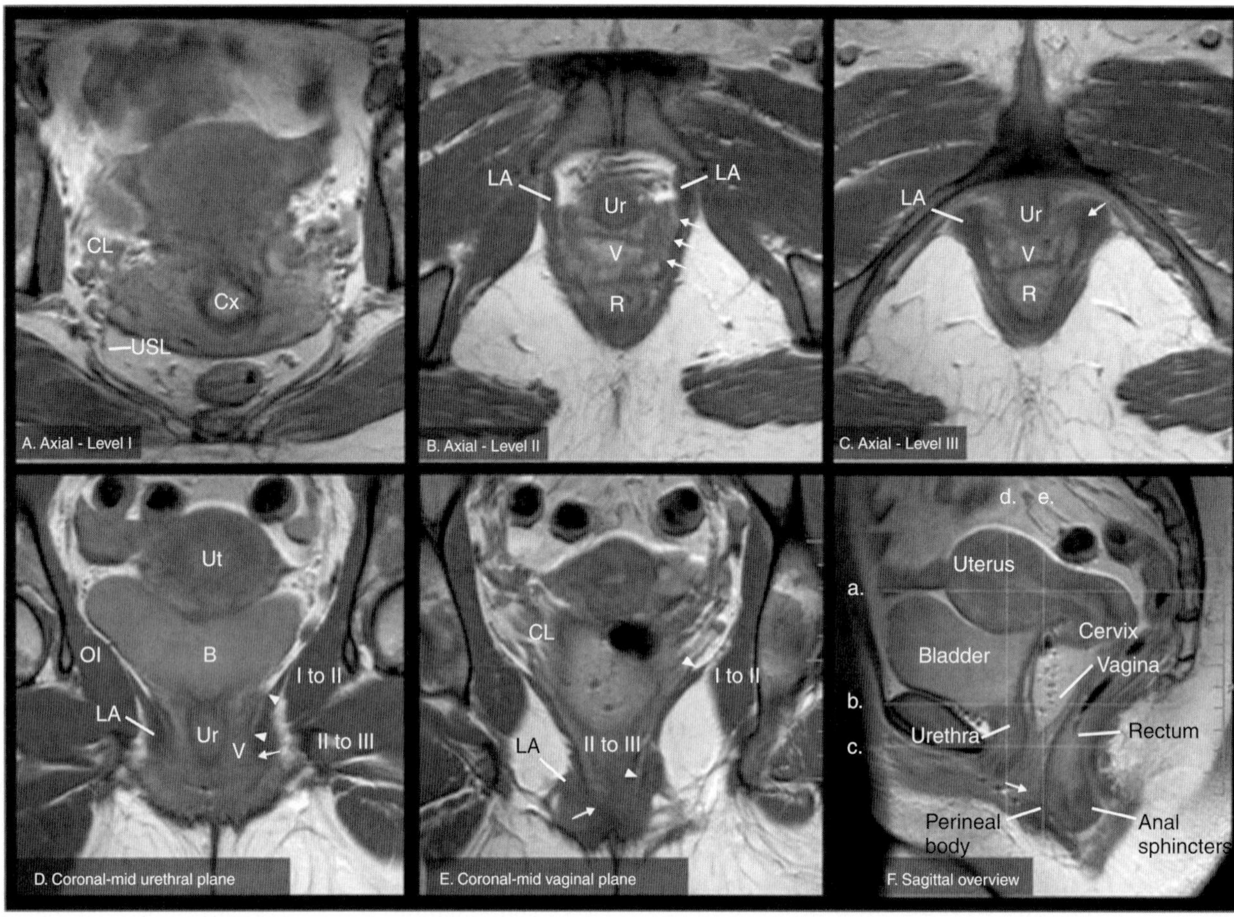

Fig. 13.24 Magnetic resonance imaging characteristics of levels of support. T2-weighted proton-density images at rest; orthogonal planes. Bilateral features have been indicated on one side so the other side can be viewed without marking. The first row contains axial scans at levels I, II, and III. **A**, Level I: apical support structures known as cardinal and uterosacral ligaments are visible. **B**, Level II: the vagina can be identified adjacent to the levator ani muscle, but with a distinct border between these two structures (*white arrows*). **C**, Level III: loss of separation between vagina and levator ani muscles where they are fused to the vagina (*white arrow*). The second row displays two coronal scan planes (**D** and **E**), as well as a sagittal scan plane (**F**) for orientation. **D**, Midurethral coronal scan: *white arrowheads* show the transition between levels I and II where the vagina contacts the pelvic wall and levels II and III where the vagina becomes fused with the levator. *White arrow* shows the loss of separation. **E**, Midvaginal coronal scan: the cardinal ligaments are visible, and the transition between levels I and II, as well as between levels II and III, can be identified; fusion of the levator and vagina is shown. *White arrowheads* show the transition between levels I and II where the vagina contacts the pelvic wall and levels II to III where the vagina becomes fused with the levator. *White arrow* shows the loss of separation. Sagittal scan: the perineal body can be seen where it is fused with the distal vagina (*arrow*). The locations of the other planes are indicated by *dashed lines*. *Ut*, Uterus; *B*, bladder; *LA*, levator ani muscle; *Ur*, urethra; *V*, vagina; *CL*, cardinal ligament; *USL*, uterosacral ligament; *Cx*, cervix; *R*, rectum; *OI*, obturator internus muscle. (From Huebner M, DeLancey JOL. Levels of pelvic floor support: what do they look like on magnetic resonance imaging? *Int Urogynecol J.* 2019;30:1593. With permission.)

(Delancey et al. 2007). The interobserver agreement of POP staging using MRI is excellent (Lakeman et al. 2012). Fig. 13.24 shows MRI illustrations of the characteristics of the Delancey levels of support.

MRI for the evaluation of POP is typically performed in the supine or seated position. However, one recent study by Grob et al. (2019) reported that upright MRI scanning of patients with advanced POP both at rest and during straining shows a significantly larger extent of the prolapse than that observed during supine straining. MRI demonstrates the interactions among pelvic organ protrusion, levator ani descent, and hiatal enlargement. In prolapse, the levator area increases more than the protrusion area, and both the urogenital hiatus and levator hiatus are larger. The odds of prolapse for an increase in the urogenital hiatus are three times larger than for the levator hiatus (Sammarco et al. 2017). At maximal Valsalva on MRI, structures are more caudal in women with posterior prolapse. The posterior vaginal wall is longer; this length strongly correlates with prolapse size (Lewicky-Gaupp et al. 2010).

MRI may also be used to evaluate the therapeutic outcomes after reconstructive surgery. Dynamic MRI diagnosed substantially more patients with recurrent or *de novo* POP in the posterior compartment compared with clinical examination (Alt et al. 2018).

Conclusion

MRI can rapidly image the entire pelvic floor and is highly reproducible between examiners. However, the limitations of MRI include variability in technique and interpretation methods, nonphysiologic positioning when performed supine, relative high cost, and the need for the opacification of the bladder for posterior compartment imaging (Ahmad et al. 2015). Studies that use MRI include a small number of subjects and comparisons of isolated defects. Furthermore, findings from 2D and 3D MRI studies are still considered investigational and have not yet been fully validated clinically or surgically. Nevertheless, the direct visualization of pelvic contents and musculature, high inherent soft tissue and contrast resolution, lack of exposure to ionizing radiation, and its relatively noninvasive nature strengthen the utilization of this important diagnostic and research tool for assessment of pelvic floor dysfunction.

BIBLIOGRAPHY

AIUM/IUGA practice parameter for the performance of urogynecological ultrasound examinations: developed in collaboration with the ACR, the AUGS, the AUA, and the SRU. *Int Urogynecol J.* 2019;30:1389.

AIUM/IUGA practice parameter for the performance of urogynecological ultrasound examinations: developed in collaboration with the ACR, the AUGS, the AUA, and the SRU. *J Ultrasound Med.* 2019;38:851.

Abdool Z, Sultan AH, Thakar R. Ultrasound imaging of the anal sphincter complex: a review. *Br J Radiol.* 2012;85:865.

Ahmad AN, Hainsworth A, Williams AB, Schizas AM. A review of functional pelvic floor imaging modalities and their effectiveness. *Clin Imaging.* 2015;39:559.

Alt CD, Benner L, Mokry T, et al. Five-year outcome after pelvic floor reconstructive surgery: evaluation using dynamic magnetic resonance imaging compared to clinical examination and quality-of-life questionnaire. *Acta Radiol.* 2018;59:1264.

Arqués JL, Rodríguez E, Nuñez M, Medina M. Antimicrobial activity of nisin, reuterin, and the lactoperoxidase system on Listeria monocytogenes and Staphylococcus aureus in cuajada, a semisolid dairy product manufactured in Spain. *J Dairy Sci.* 2008;91:70.

Attenberger UI, Morelli JN, Budjan J, et al. The value of dynamic magnetic resonance imaging in interdisciplinary treatment of pelvic floor dysfunction. *Abdom Imaging.* 2015;40:2242.

Bartram CI, Turnbull GK, Lennard-Jones JE. Evacuation proctography: an investigation of rectal expulsion in 20 subjects without defecatory disturbance. *Gastrointest Radiol.* 1988;13:72.

Beer-Gabel M, Teshler M, Schechtman E, Zbar AP. Dynamic transperineal ultrasound vs. defecography in patients with evacuatory difficulty: a pilot study. *Int J Colorectal Dis.* 2004;19:60.

Betschart C, Chen L, Ashton-Miller JA, Delancey JO. On pelvic reference lines and the MR evaluation of genital prolapse: a proposal for standardization using the Pelvic Inclination Correction System. *Int Urogynecol J.* 2013;24:1421.

Bharucha AE. Pelvic floor: anatomy and function. *Neurogastroenterol Motil.* 2006;18:507.

Blander DS, Rovner ES, Schnall MD, et al. Endoluminal magnetic resonance imaging in the evaluation of urethral diverticula in women. *Urology.* 2001;57:660.

Boyadzhyan L, Raman SS, Raz S. Role of static and dynamic MR imaging in surgical pelvic floor dysfunction. *Radiographics.* 2008;28s:949.

Brandes S, Coburn M, Armenakas N, McAninch J. Diagnosis and management of ureteric injury: an evidence-based analysis. *BJU Int.* 2004;94:277.

Broekhuis SR, Fütterer JJ, Barentsz JO, et al. A systematic review of clinical studies on dynamic magnetic resonance imaging of pelvic organ prolapse: the use of reference lines and anatomical landmarks. *Int Urogynecol J Pelvic Floor Dysfunct.* 2009;20:721.

Chou CP, Levenson RB, Elsayes KM, et al. Imaging of female urethral diverticulum: an update. *Radiographics.* 2008;28:1917.

Comiter CV, Vasavada SP, Barbaric ZL, et al. Grading pelvic prolapse and pelvic floor relaxation using dynamic magnetic resonance imaging. *Urology.* 1999;54:454.

Dane B, Baxter AB, Bernstein MP. Imaging genitourinary trauma. *Radiol Clin North Am.* 2017;55:321.

DeLancey JO. Anatomic aspects of vaginal eversion after hysterectomy. *Am J Obstet Gynecol.* 1992;166:1717, discussion 24.

DeLancey JO. The hidden epidemic of pelvic floor dysfunction: achievable goals for improved prevention and treatment. *Am J Obstet Gynecol.* 2005;192:1488.

DeLancey JO, Morgan DM, Fenner DE, et al. Comparison of levator ani muscle defects and function in women with and without pelvic organ prolapse. *Obstet Gynecol.* 2007;109:295.

Denson L, Shobeiri SA. Three-dimensional endovaginal sonography of synthetic implanted materials in the female pelvic floor. *J Ultrasound Med.* 2014;33:521.

Dietz HP. Ultrasound imaging of the pelvic floor. Part II: three-dimensional or volume imaging. *Ultrasound Obstet Gynecol.* 2004;23:615.

Dietz HP. Ultrasound imaging of the pelvic floor. Part I: two-dimensional aspects. *Ultrasound Obstet Gynecol.* 2004;23:80.

Dietz HP. The evolution of ultrasound in urogynecology. *Ultrasound Obstet Gynecol.* 2010;36:655.

Dietz HP. Pelvic floor ultrasound: a review. *Am J Obstet Gynecol.* 2010;202:321.

Dietz HP. Pelvic floor ultrasound: a review. *Clin Obstet Gynecol.* 2017;60:58.

Dietz HP. Exoanal imaging of the anal sphincters. *J Ultrasound Med.* 2018;37:263.

Dietz HP, Haylen BT, Vancaillie TG. Female pelvic organ prolapse and voiding function. *Int Urogynecol J Pelvic Floor Dysfunct.* 2002;13:284.

Dietz HP, Moegni F, Shek KL. Diagnosis of levator avulsion injury: a comparison of three methods. *Ultrasound Obstet Gynecol.* 2012;40:693.

Dietz HP, Barry C, Lim YN, Rane A. Two-dimensional and three-dimensional ultrasound imaging of suburethral slings. *Ultrasound Obstet Gynecol.* 2005;26:175.

Dietz HP, Shek C, De Leon J, Steensma AB. Ballooning of the levator hiatus. *Ultrasound Obstet Gynecol.* 2008;31:676.

Digesu GA, Khullar V, Cardozo L, Salvatore S. The open bladder neck: a significant finding? *Int Urogynecol J Pelvic Floor Dysfunct.* 2004;15:336.

Dvorkin LS, Hetzer F, Scott SM, et al. Open-magnet MR defaecography compared with evacuation proctography in the diagnosis and management of patients with rectal intussusception. *Colorectal Dis.* 2004;6:45.

El Sayed RF, El Mashed S, Farag A, et al. Pelvic floor dysfunction: assessment with combined analysis of static and dynamic MR imaging findings. *Radiology.* 2008;248:518.

El Sayed RF, Alt CD, Maccioni F, et al. Magnetic resonance imaging of pelvic floor dysfunction - joint recommendations of the ESUR and ESGAR Pelvic Floor Working Group. *Eur Radiol.* 2017;27:2067.

Elshazly WG, El Nekady Ael A, Hassan H. Role of dynamic magnetic resonance imaging in management of obstructed defecation case series. *Int J Surg.* 2010;8:274.

Fabrizio AC, Alimi Y, Kumar AS. Methods of evaluation of anorectal causes of obstructed defecation. *Clin Colon Rectal Surg.* 2017;30:46.

Fielding JR. MR imaging of pelvic floor relaxation. *Radiol Clin North Am.* 2003;41:747.

Fielding JR, Versi E, Mulkern RV, et al. MR imaging of the female pelvic floor in the supine and upright positions. *J Magn Reson Imaging.* 1996;6:961.

Fielding JR, Griffiths DJ, Versi E, et al. MR imaging of pelvic floor continence mechanisms in the supine and sitting positions. *AJR Am J Roentgenol.* 1998;171:1607.

Fletcher JG, Busse RF, Riederer SJ, et al. Magnetic resonance imaging of anatomic and dynamic defects of the pelvic floor in defecatory disorders. *Am J Gastroenterol.* 2003;98:399.

Foley CL, Greenwell TJ, Gardiner RA. Urethral diverticula in females. *BJU Int.* 2011;108:20.

Foster RT, Amundsen CL, Webster GD. The utility of magnetic resonance imaging for diagnosis and surgical planning before transvaginal periurethral diverticulectomy in women. *Int Urogynecol J Pelvic Floor Dysfunct.* 2007;18:315.

Ginath S, Garely A, Luchs JS, et al. MRI pelvic landmark angles in the assessment of apical pelvic organ prolapse. *Arch Gynecol Obstet.* 2011;284:365.

Goei R, Kemerink G. Radiation dose in defecography. *Radiology.* 1990;176:137.

Gousse AE, Barbaric ZL, Safir MH, et al. Dynamic half Fourier acquisition, single shot turbo spin-echo magnetic resonance imaging for evaluating the female pelvis. *J Urol.* 2000;164:1606.

Grassi R, Lombardi G, Reginelli A, et al. Coccygeal movement: assessment with dynamic MRI. *Eur J Radiol.* 2007;61:473.

Grob ATM, Olde Heuvel J, Futterer JJ, et al. Underestimation of pelvic organ prolapse in the supine straining position, based on magnetic resonance imaging findings. *Int Urogynecol J.* 2019;30:1939.

Gufler H, DeGregorio G, Dohnicht S, et al. Dynamic MRI after surgical repair for pelvic organ prolapse. *J Comput Assist Tomogr.* 2002;26:734.

Gupta S, Sharma JB, Hari S, et al. Study of dynamic magnetic resonance imaging in diagnosis of pelvic organ prolapse. *Arch Gynecol Obstet.* 2012;286:953.

Halligan S, Bartram CI, Park HJ, Kamm MA. Proctographic features of anismus. *Radiology.* 1995;197:679.

Healy JC, Halligan S, Reznek RH, et al. Patterns of prolapse in women with symptoms of pelvic floor weakness: assessment with MR imaging. *Radiology.* 1997;203:77.

Hetzer FH, Andreisek G, Tsagari C, et al. MR defecography in patients with fecal incontinence: imaging findings and their effect on surgical management. *Radiology.* 2006;240:449.

Hoyte L, Schierlitz L, Zou K, et al. Two- and 3-dimensional MRI comparison of levator ani structure, volume, and integrity in women with stress incontinence and prolapse. *Am J Obstet Gynecol.* 2001;185:11.

Huang WC, Yang JM. Bladder neck funneling on ultrasound cystourethrography in primary stress urinary incontinence: a sign associated with urethral hypermobility and intrinsic sphincter deficiency. *Urology.* 2003;61:936.

Huebner M, DeLancey JOL. Levels of pelvic floor support: what do they look like on magnetic resonance imaging? *Int Urogynecol J.* 2019;30:1593.

Iacobellis F, Brillantino A, Renzi A, et al. MR imaging in diagnosis of pelvic floor descent: supine versus sitting position. *Gastroenterol Res Pract.* 2016;2016:6594152.

Iacobellis F, Reginelli A, Berritto D, et al. Pelvic floor dysfunctions: how to image patients? *Jpn J Radiol.* 2020;38:47.

Javadian P, Quiroz LH, Shobeiri SA. In vivo ultrasound characteristics of vaginal mesh kit complications. *Female Pelvic Med Reconstr Surg.* 2017;23:162.

Johnsen NV, Dmochowski RR, Guillamondegui OD. Clinical utility of routine follow-up cystography in the management of traumatic bladder ruptures. *Urology.* 2018;113:230.

Joshi G, Kim EY, Hanna TN, et al. CT cystography for suspicion of traumatic urinary bladder injury: indications, technique, findings, and pitfalls in diagnosis: RadioGraphics Fundamentals Online Presentation. *Radiographics.* 2018;38:92.

Kapoor DS, Thakar R, Sultan AH. Obstetric anal sphincter injuries: review of anatomical factors and modifiable second stage interventions. *Int Urogynecol J.* 2015;26:1725.

Kelvin FM, Maglinte DD. Dynamic evaluation of female pelvic organ prolapse by extended proctography. *Radiol Clin North Am.* 2003;41:395.

Khatri G, de Leon AD, Lockhart ME. MR imaging of the pelvic floor. *Magn Reson Imaging Clin N Am.* 2017;25:457.

Khullar V, Salvatore S, Cardozo L, et al. A novel technique for measuring bladder wall thickness in women using transvaginal ultrasound. *Ultrasound Obstet Gynecol.* 1994;4:220.

Kirschner-Hermanns R, Wein B, Niehaus S, et al. The contribution of magnetic resonance imaging of the pelvic floor to the understanding of urinary incontinence. *Br J Urol.* 1993;72:715.

Kong JP, Bultitude MF, Royce P, et al. Lower urinary tract injuries following blunt trauma: a review of contemporary management. *Rev Urol.* 2011;13:119.

Lakeman MM, Zijta FM, Peringa J, et al. Dynamic magnetic resonance imaging to quantify pelvic organ prolapse: reliability of assessment and correlation with clinical findings and pelvic floor symptoms. *Int Urogynecol J.* 2012;23:1547.

Larson KA, Yousuf A, Lewicky-Gaupp C, et al. Perineal body anatomy in living women: 3-dimensional analysis using thin-slice magnetic resonance imaging. *Am J Obstet Gynecol.* 2010;203:494.e15.

Lekskulchai O, Dietz HP. Detrusor wall thickness as a test for detrusor overactivity in women. *Ultrasound Obstet Gynecol.* 2008;32:535.

Lewicky-Gaupp C, Yousuf A, Larson KA, et al. Structural position of the posterior vagina and pelvic floor in women with and without posterior vaginal prolapse. *Am J Obstet Gynecol.* 2010;202:497.e1.

Li N, Cui C, Cheng Y, et al. Association between magnetic resonance imaging findings of the pelvic floor and de novo stress urinary incontinence after vaginal delivery. *Korean J Radiol.* 2018;19:715.

Li R, Song Y, Ma M. Relationship between levator ani and bony pelvis morphology and clinical grade of prolapse in women. *Clin Anat.* 2015;28:813.

Lienemann A, Anthuber C, Baron A, Reiser M. Diagnosing enteroceles using dynamic magnetic resonance imaging. *Dis Colon Rectum.* 2000;43:205, discussion 12.

Lo TS, Pue LB, Tan YL, Wu PY. Risk factors for failure of repeat midurethral sling surgery for recurrent or persistent stress urinary incontinence. *Int Urogynecol J.* 2016;27:923.

Luo J, Larson KA, Fenner DE, et al. Posterior vaginal prolapse shape and position changes at maximal Valsalva seen in 3-D MRI-based models. *Int Urogynecol J.* 2012;23:1301.

Maccioni F. Functional disorders of the ano-rectal compartment of the pelvic floor: clinical and diagnostic value of dynamic MRI. *Abdom Imaging.* 2013;38:930.

Maglinte DD, Bartram C. Dynamic imaging of posterior compartment pelvic floor dysfunction by evacuation proctography: techniques, indications, results and limitations. *Eur J Radiol.* 2007;61:454.

Maglinte DD, Kelvin FM, Fitzgerald K, et al. Association of compartment defects in pelvic floor dysfunction. *AJR Am J Roentgenol.* 1999;172:439.

Maubon A, Aubard Y, Berkane V, et al. Magnetic resonance imaging of the pelvic floor. *Abdom Imaging.* 2003;28:217.

Morgan DM, Umek W, Guire K, et al. Urethral sphincter morphology and function with and without stress incontinence. *J Urol.* 2009;182:203.

Mortele KJ, Fairhurst J. Dynamic MR defecography of the posterior compartment: Indications, techniques and MRI features. *Eur J Radiol.* 2007;61:462.

Newhouse JH, Amis Jr ES, Bigongiari LR, et al. Radiologic investigation of patients with hematuria. American College of Radiology. ACR Appropriateness Criteria. *Radiology.* 2000;215:687.

Nygaard I, Barber MD, Burgio KL, et al. Prevalence of symptomatic pelvic floor disorders in US women. *JAMA.* 2008;300:1311.

Ockrim JL, Allen DJ, Shah PJ, Greenwell TJ. A tertiary experience of urethral diverticulectomy: diagnosis, imaging and surgical outcomes. *BJU Int.* 2009;103:1550.

Oom DM, West RL, Schouten WR, Steensma AB. Detection of anal sphincter defects in female patients with fecal incontinence: a comparison of 3-dimensional transperineal ultrasound and 2-dimensional endoanal ultrasound. *Dis Colon Rectum.* 2012;55:646.

Pannu HK, Javitt MC, Glanc P, et al. ACR Appropriateness Criteria pelvic floor dysfunction. *J Am Coll Radiol.* 2015;12:134.

Perniola G, Shek C, Chong CC, et al. Defecation proctography and translabial ultrasound in the investigation of defecatory disorders. *Ultrasound Obstet Gynecol.* 2008;31:567.

Petros PE, Ulmsten UI. An integral theory of female urinary incontinence. Experimental and clinical considerations. *Acta Obstet Gynecol Scand Suppl.* 1990;153:7.

Petros PE, Ulmsten UI. An integral theory and its method for the diagnosis and management of female urinary incontinence. *Scand J Urol Nephrol Suppl.* 1993;153:1.

Petros PE, Woodman PJ. The integral theory of continence. *Int Urogynecol J Pelvic Floor Dysfunct.* 2008;19:35.

Reiner CS, Weishaupt D. Dynamic pelvic floor imaging: MRI techniques and imaging parameters. *Abdom Imaging.* 2013;38:903.

Romanzi LJ, Groutz A, Blaivas JG. Urethral diverticulum in women: diverse presentations resulting in diagnostic delay and mismanagement. *J Urol.* 2000;164:428.

Ros C, Martinez-Franco E, Wozniak MM, et al. Postpartum two- and three-dimensional ultrasound evaluation of anal sphincter complex in women with obstetric anal sphincter injury. *Ultrasound Obstet Gynecol.* 2017;49:508.

Rostaminia G, White DE, Quiroz LH, Shobeiri SA. Visualization of periurethral structures by 3D endovaginal ultrasonography in midsagittal plane is not associated with stress urinary incontinence status. *Int Urogynecol J.* 2012;24:1145.

Rostaminia G, Peck J, Quiroz L, Shobeiri SA. Levator Plate Upward Lift on Dynamic Sonography and Levator Muscle Strength. *J Ultrasound Med.* 2015;34:1787.

Rostaminia G, White D, Hegde A, et al. Levator ani deficiency and pelvic organ prolapse severity. *Obstet Gynecol.* 2013;121:1017.

Royal SA, Slovis TL, Kushner DC, et al. Hematuria. American College of Radiology. ACR Appropriateness Criteria. *Radiology.* 2000;215:841.

Sammarco AG, Nandikanti L, Kobernik EK, et al. Interactions among pelvic organ protrusion, levator ani descent, and hiatal enlargement in women with and without prolapse. *Am J Obstet Gynecol.* 2017;217:614.e1.

Santiago AC, O'Leary DE, Quiroz LH, et al. An ultrasound approach to the posterior compartment and anorectal dysfunction. *Int Urogynecol J.* 2015;26:1393.

Santoro GA, Fortling B. The advantages of volume rendering in three-dimensional endosonography of the anorectum. *Dis Colon Rectum.* 2007;50:359.

Santoro GA, Shobeiri SA, Petros PP, et al. Perineal body anatomy seen by three-dimensional endovaginal ultrasound of asymptomatic nulliparae. *Colorectal Dis.* 2016;18:400.

Santoro GA, Wieczorek AP, Stankiewicz A, et al. High-resolution three-dimensional endovaginal ultrasonography in the assessment of pelvic floor anatomy: a preliminary study. *Int Urogynecol J Pelvic Floor Dysfunct.* 2009;20:1213.

Santoro GA, Wieczorek AP, Shobeiri SA, et al. Interobserver and interdisciplinary reproducibility of 3D endovaginal ultrasound assessment of pelvic floor anatomy. *Int Urogynecol J.* 2011;22:53.

Santoro GA, Wieczorek AP, Dietz HP, et al. State of the art: an integrated approach to pelvic floor ultrasonography. *Ultrasound Obstet Gynecol.* 2011;37:381.

Schaer GN, Perucchini D, Munz E, et al. Sonographic evaluation of the bladder neck in continent and stress-incontinent women. *Obstet Gynecol.* 1999;93:412.

Schawkat K, Pfister B, Parker H, et al. Dynamic MRI of the pelvic floor: comparison of performance in supine vs left lateral body position. *Br J Radiol.* 2018;91:20180393.

Schreyer AG, Paetzel C, Fürst A, et al. Dynamic magnetic resonance defecography in 10 asymptomatic volunteers. *World J Gastroenterol.* 2012;18:6836.

Serati M, Salvatore S, Cattoni E, et al. Ultrasound measurement of bladder wall thickness in different forms of detrusor overactivity. *Int Urogynecol J.* 2010;21:1405.

Shobeiri SA, Rostaminia G, White D, Quiroz LH. The determinants of minimal levator hiatus and their relationship to the puborectalis muscle and the levator plate. *BJOG.* 2013;120:205.

Shobeiri SA, Rostaminia G, White D, et al. Evaluation of vaginal cysts and masses by 3-dimensional endovaginal and endoanal sonography. *J Ultrasound Med.* 2013;32:1499.

Shorvon PJ, McHugh S, Diamant NE, et al. Defecography in normal volunteers: results and implications. *Gut.* 1989;30:1737.

Showalter PR, Zimmern PE, Roehrborn CG, Lemack GE. Standing cystourethrogram: an outcome measure after anti-incontinence procedures and cystocele repair in women. *Urology.* 2001;58:33.

Singh K, Jakab M, Reid WM, et al. Three-dimensional magnetic resonance imaging assessment of levator ani morphologic features in different grades of prolapse. *Am J Obstet Gynecol.* 2003;188:910.

Sioutis D, Thakar R, Sultan AH. Overdiagnosis and rising rate of obstetric anal sphincter injuries (OASIS): time for reappraisal. *Ultrasound Obstet Gynecol.* 2017;50:642.

Steensma AB, Oom DM, Burger CW, Schouten WR. Assessment of posterior compartment prolapse: a comparison of evacuation proctography and 3D transperineal ultrasound. *Colorectal Dis.* 2010;12:533.

Strohbehn K, Ellis JH, Strohbehn JA, DeLancey JO. Magnetic resonance imaging of the levator ani with anatomic correlation. *Obstet Gynecol.* 1996;87:277.

Sultan AH. The role of anal endosonography in obstetrics. *Ultrasound Obstet Gynecol.* 2003;22:559.

Sultan AH, Kamm MA, Talbot IC, et al. Anal endosonography for identifying external sphincter defects confirmed histologically. *Br J Surg.* 1994;81:463.

Terra MP, Stoker J. The current role of imaging techniques in faecal incontinence. *Eur Radiol.* 2006;16:1727.

Tunn R, Picot A, Marschke J, Gauruder-Burmester A. Sonomorphological evaluation of polypropylene mesh implants after vaginal mesh repair in women with cystocele or rectocele. *Ultrasound Obstet Gynecol*. 2007;29:449.

Tunn R, Paris S, Taupitz M, et al. MR imaging in posthysterectomy vaginal prolapse. *Int Urogynecol J Pelvic Floor Dysfunct*. 2000;11:87.

Tunn R, Schaer G, Peschers U, et al. Updated recommendations on ultrasonography in urogynecology. *Int Urogynecol J Pelvic Floor Dysfunct*. 2005;16:236.

van Gruting IMA, Stankiewicz A, Kluivers K, et al. Accuracy of four imaging techniques for diagnosis of posterior pelvic floor disorders. *Obstet Gynecol*. 2017;130:1017.

Viereck V, Kuszka A, Rautenberg O, et al. Do different vaginal tapes need different suburethral incisions? The one-half rule. *Neurourol Urodyn*. 2015;34:741.

Wang S, Lang JH, Zhou HM. Symptomatic urinary problems in female genital tract anomalies. *Int Urogynecol J Pelvic Floor Dysfunct*. 2009;20:401.

Weidner AC, Low VH. Imaging studies of the pelvic floor. *Obstet Gynecol Clin North Am*. 1998;25:825, vii.

Wu JM, Vaughan CP, Goode PS, et al. Prevalence and trends of symptomatic pelvic floor disorders in U.S. women. *Obstet Gynecol*. 2014;123:141.

Yang A, Mostwin JL, Rosenshein NB, Zerhouni EA. Pelvic floor descent in women: dynamic evaluation with fast MR imaging and cinematic display. *Radiology*. 1991;179:25.

Yang JM, Huang WC, Yang SH. Transvaginal sonography in the diagnosis, management and follow-up of complex paraurethral abnormalities. *Ultrasound Obstet Gynecol*. 2005;25:302.

Yang JM, Yang SH, Huang WC. Two- and three-dimensional sonographic findings in a case of distal urethral obstruction due to a paraurethral tumor. *Ultrasound Obstet Gynecol*. 2005;25:519.

Yune JJ, Quiroz L, Nihira MA, et al. The location and distribution of transurethral bulking agent: 3-dimensional ultrasound Study. *Female Pelvic Med Reconstr Surg*. 2016;22:98.

Zafar A, Seretis C, Feretis M, et al. Comparative study of magnetic resonance defaecography and evacuation proctography in the evaluation of obstructed defaecation. *Colorectal Dis*. 2017;19:O204.

PART 3

Management of Stress Urinary Incontinence and Pelvic Organ Prolapse

14

Stress Urinary Incontinence and Pelvic Organ Prolapse: Nonsurgical Management

Diane K. Newman and Holly E. Richter

CHAPTER OUTLINE

INTRODUCTION

Stress urinary incontinence (SUI) is an involuntary loss of urine on effort, physical exertion, or with an increase in the intraabdominal pressure upon sneezing or coughing (Haylen et al., 2010). Pelvic organ prolapse (POP) is clinically defined as "the descent of one or more of the anterior vaginal wall, posterior vaginal wall, the uterus (cervix) or the apex of the vagina (vaginal vault or cuff scar after hysterectomy)" (Haylen et al., 2016). Nonsurgical management of SUI and POP should be offered to all patients. Most women are not aware of the existence of nonsurgical treatments for incontinence and prolapse, and they are often relieved that treatment options other than surgery are available. Behavioral treatment, the current "gold standard" conservative approach for SUI, improves bladder control by changing the incontinent patient's behavior, including learning skills for preventing urine loss. Multicomponent behavioral interventions include pelvic floor muscle training (PFMT) and exercise, stress and urgency suppression strategies, and biofeedback. As part of the first-line treatment, estrogen optimizes urogenital tissue health and relieves some lower urinary tract symptoms, a common genitourinary syndrome of menopause (Portman et al., 2014; Rahn et al., 2014). Although no US Food and Drug Administration (FDA)-approved medications exist for the treatment of SUI, certain medications, including duloxetine, may offer effective treatment for mild to moderate stress incontinence. Pessaries stabilize the proximal urethra, and urethral inserts (no longer available) acted by increasing urethral pressure. Pessaries also provide support for symptomatic POP. Such devices provide valuable alternatives to surgery.

This chapter describes the full range of nonsurgical options for the treatment of SUI and POP, allowing us to offer a broad spectrum of less invasive treatment options in an individualized manner. Optimal behavioral therapy for urinary incontinence depends on several factors, including the type and severity of incontinence; the presence of associated conditions, such as prolapse or other pelvic pathology; prior surgical or nonsurgical therapy; the patient's medical status; and the patient's ability and willingness to actively participate in and adhere to treatment. Similarly, nonsurgical therapy for prolapse may be used in women with significant medical comorbidities that preclude them from having surgery, those who do not wish to undergo surgical therapy, or those who want a temporizing measure before surgical intervention. Evidence-based approaches exist for the full spectrum of conservative therapy for the management of SUI and POP.

THE BLADDER DIARY: A VALUABLE CLINICAL TOOL

Before initiating nonsurgical treatment for incontinence, it is advisable to have the patient complete a bladder diary for 3 to 7 days. At a minimum, the patient should record the time and circumstances of each incontinence episode. The bladder diary assists the clinician in determining the type and severity of urine loss and in planning appropriate intervention. If the woman has associated urgency urinary incontinence (UUI) and overactive bladder symptoms of urgency and frequency, the type and amount of fluid intake, the frequency of urination, and the urgency associated with each can also be recorded (Newman & Burgio, 2020) This information can identify women who may benefit from more frequent urination to avoid a full bladder, especially during physical activity. It may also reveal cases in which voiding frequency is excessive and may be contributing to reduced bladder capacity and urgency. Using the diary, the circumstances of incontinence can be reviewed with the patient, and instructions can be given that are specific to the patient's situation. During treatment, the number of incontinent episodes can be monitored to determine the efficacy of treatment and to guide further intervention. Although more burdensome, it is also suggested that women record voided volumes for a 24-hour period by completing a frequency-volume bladder diary (Fig. 14.1). This record can identify patients with abnormal urine production, especially those with increased nighttime urine production resulting in nocturia.

Frequency-Volume Bladder Diary

Time	Trips to bathroom	Urine Leakage	If Leaked? Reason for Urine Leakage	Drinks How much and what kind?
Note each time you urinate (pee)	*Amount of urine (in oz)?*	*Check each time you have a bladder leak*	*Activity at the time? Sneeze, lifting, exercising, etc.*	*Enter number of cups and glasses* *1 glass = 6 oz* *1 cup = 4 oz*
6:00 a.m. awake	12 oz	✓	coughing	½ glass of water
6:30 a.m.				1½ glasses of water
8:00 a.m.	10 oz			
10 a.m.	7 oz			1 cup coffee
12 p.m.	Forgot to measure			8 oz of soda, 1 glass of milk, 2 glasses of water
2:30 p.m.				½ glass of water
4:30 p.m.				8 oz can of iced tea
5 p.m.	6 oz	✓	exercising	2 glasses of water
7 p.m.				1 glass of water, 2 glasses of wine
10 p.m. – to bed	10 oz			

Circle the product you are using

Write the number of products used: 2

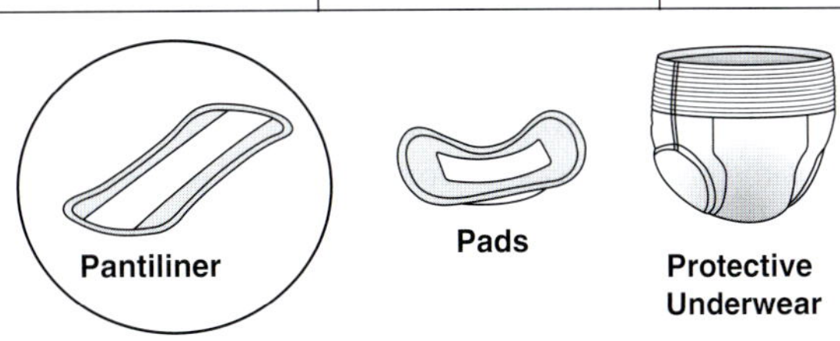

Fig. 14.1 Sample frequency-volume bladder diary. *Source:* Courtesy of Diane K. Newman, DNP.

In addition to the value of the bladder diary to the clinician, completing a daily diary appears to benefit the patient directly. As a form of self-monitoring, it enhances the patient's awareness of her voiding habits and incontinence patterns, and it facilitates her recognition of the relationship between her activities and incontinence. Specifically, understanding clearly the precipitants of urine leakage optimizes the patient's readiness to implement the continence skills she learns through behavioral treatment.

BEHAVIORAL INTERVENTION: PELVIC FLOOR MUSCLE TRAINING AND EXERCISE

PFMT and exercise are the foundation of behavioral treatment for SUI and may be beneficial for the treatment and prevention of POP (Dumoulin et al., 2017). A Cochrane review of PFMT-based treatments concluded that these treatments were effective for both SUI and mixed urinary incontinence (Dumoulin et al., 2018) and can reduce urgency, but women with pure SUI may have better outcomes (Bo & Herbert, 2013). Gynecologist Arnold Kegel first popularized PFMT in the late 1940s. He asserted that women with SUI lack awareness and coordination of the pelvic floor muscles (PFMs) and that SUI could be resolved with PFMT (Kegel, 1948; Kegel, 1956). Through the years, this intervention has evolved both as a behavioral therapy and a physical therapy, combining principles from both fields into a widely accepted conservative treatment for SUI and UUI.

Literature on outpatient behavioral treatment with PFMT and exercise has demonstrated that it is effective for reducing SUI, UUI, and mixed incontinence in most patients who cooperate with training. Behavioral treatments have been recognized for their efficacy by multiple organizations and panels, including the International Consultation on Incontinence and the American Urological Association Guideline on Overactive Bladder (Dumoulin et al, 2017; Gormley et al., 2015; Hartman et al., 2009). Although the majority of women are not cured with this approach, most can achieve significant improvement.

Teaching Pelvic Floor Muscle Control

The goal of behavioral interventions for SUI is to teach patients how to improve urethral closure by contracting PFMs during physical activities that cause urine leakage, such as coughing, sneezing, or lifting. In patients who have a combination of SUI and UUI, quick PFM contractions are performed to lessen urgency sensations before voiding. The premise is that a deliberate PFM contraction will prevent urine loss, increasing intraurethral pressure by raising the urethra and pressing it toward the symphysis pubis, preventing urethral descent, limiting its downward movement during increases in abdominal pressure, and improving structural support of the pelvic organs (Berghmans et al., 1998). PFMT may result in hypertrophy of the striated PFM, thus increasing the external mechanical pressure on the urethra. Intensive PFMT is also hypothesized to reinforce structural support of the bladder neck in women (Bo, 1995; Bo et al., 2004). Using biofeedback or other teaching methods, patients are taught to identify the PFMs and to isolate, contract, and relax them selectively (without increasing intraabdominal pressure).

Many women fail PFM exercise by religiously exercising the wrong muscles. Helping women identify and isolate the correct muscles is an essential yet often overlooked step. The most common approach to PFMT is to give women a pamphlet or brief verbal instructions to "lift the pelvic floor" or to interrupt the urinary stream during voiding. This approach is generally ineffective, most likely because most women do not properly identify the PFMs or do not persist long enough to reap the benefits of behavioral treatment. It is more effective to begin treatment by ensuring that the patient understands which muscles to use. This understanding is often accomplished by palpating the vagina during pelvic examination and guiding her with verbal feedback to find the proper muscles. The levator ani can be palpated just proximal to the hymeneal ring (Fig. 14.2), at the 4 and 8 o'clock positions, to determine strength and to determine whether palpation reproduces any discomfort or tenderness (Newman et al., 2018).

Biofeedback is not a treatment in itself but a teaching technique that helps patients learn by giving them immediate feedback on their bladder or pelvic muscle activity. Kegel (1948) introduced a biofeedback device he called the perineometer, consisting of a pneumatic chamber that was placed in the vagina and a handheld pressure gauge that registered increased vaginal pressure generated by pelvic muscle contraction (Fig. 14.3). This device provided immediate visual feedback to the woman learning to identify her PFMs and monitoring her practice.

Current biofeedback instruments are computerized. Pelvic muscle activity can be measured using vaginal or anal manometry (pressure measurement) or surface electrode electromyography (most common), with a probe or perianal surface skin electrodes. Signals are augmented through a computer, and muscle activity is displayed on a monitor where patients can receive immediate visual or auditory feedback. Patients learn better control through operant conditioning (learning by trial and error) by observing the results of their attempts to control bladder and PFM responses (Fig. 14.4). Biofeedback-assisted

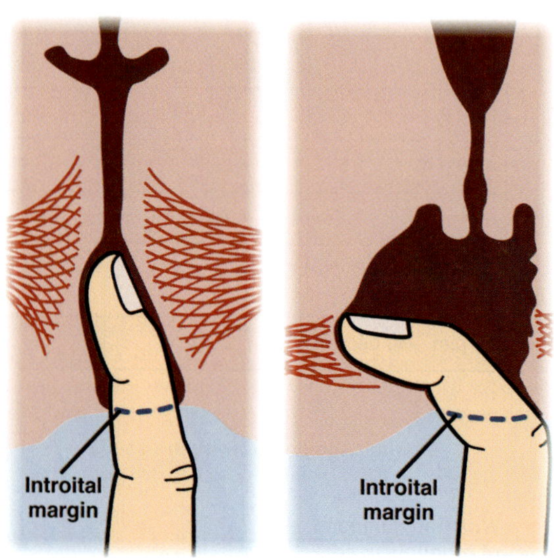

Fig. 14.2 Digital palpation of the levator ani muscle. *Source:* Courtesy of Diane K. Newman, DNP.

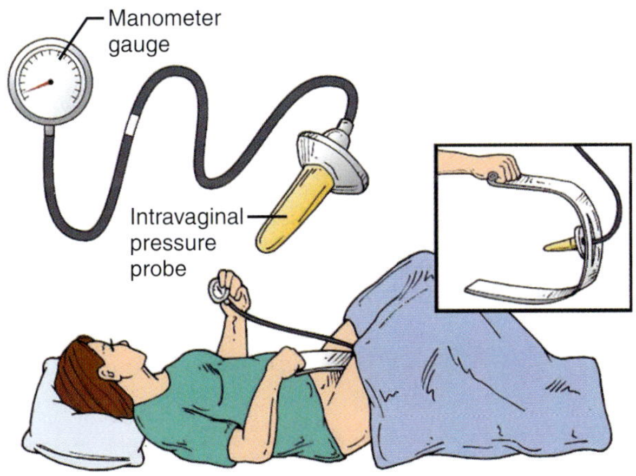

Fig. 14.3 Example of Dr. Arnold Kegel's perineometer. *Source:* Courtesy of Diane K. Newman, DNP.

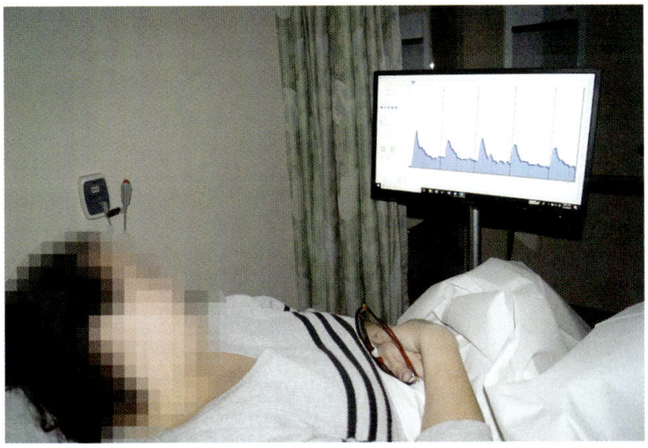

Fig. 14.4 Female patient viewing EMG-biofeedback assisted pelvic muscle contraction. *Source:* Courtesy of Diane K. Newman, DNP.

behavioral training has been tested in several studies, producing mean reductions of incontinence ranging from 60% to 85% (Dumoulin et al., 2017). Patients can usually identify their PFMs in a single session; treatment may require less repetition of biofeedback than was originally thought.

The most common problem in identifying the PFMs is that women tend to contract other muscles, typically the rectus abdominis or gluteal muscles, instead of or in conjunction with PFM. Contracting abdominal muscles is counterproductive because it increases pressure on the bladder rather than the urethra. Women commonly will perform a straining Valsalva maneuver or fail to activate all layers of the pelvic musculature. Thus, it is important to notice these incorrect responses and to teach the patient to relax other muscle groups when contracting the PFMs. To avoid bearing down, the clinician should instruct the woman to not hold her breath or to count out loud during the muscle contraction. Coordinated training of transversus abdominis muscles has also been recommended by some clinicians, because it is believed that these muscles facilitate PFM contraction. However, in a systematic review of the literature, Bo and colleagues (2009) noted an absence of evidence for this type of training, and it remains controversial.

Daily Exercise to Improve Strength and Control

Once patients learn to properly contract and relax the pelvic muscles selectively, a program of daily exercise is prescribed. The purpose of the daily regimen is not only to increase muscle strength, but also to enhance the skill of using the muscles through practice. The optimal exercise regimen has yet to be determined; however, good results are generally achieved by performing 45 to 50 exercises per day. To avoid muscle fatigue, the exercises should be spaced across the day, usually in two to three sessions (Box 14.1). Patients generally find it easiest to practice their exercises in the lying position at first. But they should be encouraged to practice in the sitting or standing positions as well, so they become comfortable using their muscles to avoid SUI, which primarily occurs in the standing position.

Programs should be individualized (Dumoulin et al., 2017; Newman et al., 2018; Newman & Burgio, 2020), but one approach is to recommend a series of "quick flicks" or 1- to 2-second contractions, followed by sustained contractions (endurance contractions) of 5 seconds, building to 10 seconds. The patient is encouraged to aim for a high level of concentrated effort with each PFM contraction, as greater contraction intensity is associated with improvement in PFM strength. Each muscle contraction is followed by a period of relaxation using a 1:1 or 1:2 ratio, allowing the muscles to recover between contractions.

Using PFMs to Prevent Stress Incontinence: Stress Strategies

Although exercise alone can improve urethral support and continence status, optimal results depend on patients learning to use their muscles actively to prevent urine loss during physical exertion. With practice and encouragement, patients can develop the habit of consciously contracting the PFMs to occlude the urethra before and during coughing, sneezing, or any other physical activities that have precipitated urine leakage. This skill has been referred to as the "stress strategy" (Burgio, 1989) and the "Knack maneuver" (Miller et al., 1998; Miller et al., 2008). Miller et al. (1998; 2008) demonstrated immediate reduction in the volume of urine leakage with a cough when anticipatory PFM contraction was used. Some women will benefit simply from learning how to control their PFMs and use them to prevent incontinence episodes (Miller et al., 1998). Others will need a more comprehensive program of PFM rehabilitation to increase strength and skill.

Using PFMs to Prevent Urgency Incontinence: Urgency Suppression Strategies

Traditionally, PFMT and exercise were used almost exclusively for SUI. However, voluntary PFM contractions can also inhibit a detrusor contraction, and this skill is a part of a behavioral treatment involving an urgency suppression strategy for patients with urgency, frequency, and/or UUI. Patients are taught a new way to respond to the sensation of urgency: instead of rushing to the toilet, which increases intraabdominal pressure and exposes patients to visual cues that can trigger incontinence, patients are encouraged to pause, sit down if possible, relax the entire body, and contract the PFM repeatedly to diminish urgency, inhibit

BOX 14.1 Instructions for Daily Pelvic Muscle Exercises

Pelvic Muscle Training for Women

What and Where Are Your Pelvic Muscles?
Your pelvic muscles support your bladder, uterus, and rectum. These muscles surround your vagina. These muscles are like a sling or hammock in the bottom of your pelvis, which is why they are called pelvic *floor* muscles. If they weaken, they cannot support these organs and may cause bladder control problems. Keeping the muscles strong by training them can help prevent urine leakage. You can make these muscles stronger by doing exercises (often called *Kegel* exercises).

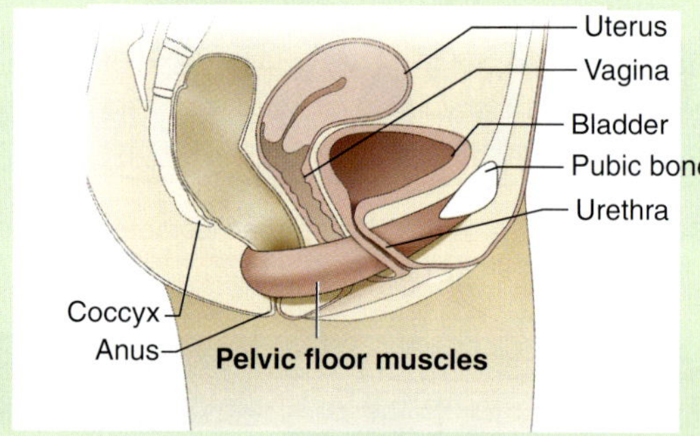

Finding the Proper Pelvic Muscles
Without tensing the muscles of your leg, buttocks or stomach, imagine that you are trying to control the passing of gas or pinching off a stool. Or imagine you are in an elevator full of people and you feel the urge to pass gas. What do you do? You squeeze or pull in the ring of muscles around your rectum— these are your pelvic muscles. You should feel a lifting sensation in the area around the vagina or a pulling in of your rectum.

Types of Exercises
There are 2 types of muscle exercises you will need to practice: <u>*quick* (2-second) or short squeezes and *slow* (10-second) or long squeezes.</u> To do the short or quick ones, squeeze your pelvic muscles quickly and hard, and then relax it. For the slow or long ones, squeeze or tighten your pelvic muscles and hold this for a count of 10 seconds, then relax the muscles for the same amount of time.

Prescription – This your Pelvic Floor Muscle Training session:

<u>Short quick squeeze –</u> **Squeeze the muscle quickly and hard for 2 seconds and then relax.** **<u>Long squeeze –</u>** **Squeeze the muscle & hold for a count of 5 seconds to start and build to a count of <u>10 seconds</u>; then relax for a count of <u>10</u>.** **When you have done both types of exercises in all 3 positions, you will have done one session.**	***TRAINING SESSION (Do 2 sessions every day)*** **Lying Down** Do <u>5</u> exercises: <u>2</u> seconds **SHORT/QUICK** Do <u>5</u> exercises: <u>5-10</u> seconds **LONG** **Sitting** Do <u>5</u> exercises: <u>2</u> seconds **SHORT/QUICK** Do <u>5</u> exercises: <u>5-10</u> seconds **LONG** **Standing** Do <u>5</u> exercises: <u>5-10</u> seconds **SHORT/QUICK** Do <u>5</u> exercises: <u>5-10</u> seconds **LONG** **Do 2 Exercise Sessions every day. One Session when you wake up and one at bedtime.**

Special Tips:

- Always empty your bladder before you exercise.
- Count out loud with the long squeezes so you keep breathing while you exercise!
- Keep your stomach, leg, and buttock muscles relaxed. Put your hand on your stomach, it should not move or tense when you squeeze you pelvic muscles.
- Be sure to rest your muscle after each squeeze.

Times to Use the Muscle
If you leak urine in one specific position only, like when standing, then follow these steps:
- Increase the number of exercises for that position only, or
- Add additional exercises each day in that position only.
- If you have overactive bladder symptoms of strong urgency to empty your bladder, squeeze your pelvic floor muscles a couple of times. Often, this will quiet the bladder down and the urge to empty your bladder will pass. Then, if you need to empty your bladder, walk calmly and slowly to the bathroom.

detrusor contraction, and prevent urine loss. When urgency subsides, they are to proceed to the toilet at a normal pace.

Behavioral training for UUI has been tested in several clinical series using pre-post designs and also in randomized trials. In controlled trials using intention-to-treat models, the mean reduction of incontinence episodes ranges from 60% to 80% (Burgio et al., 1998; Burgio et al., 2002).

Pelvic Floor Muscle Training and Exercise for Pelvic Organ Prolapse

PFMT has been used for the treatment of POP. By improving PFM strength, it is thought that training can lead to improved structural support for pelvic organs. In addition, active contraction of PFMs can be taught to brace against increases in intraabdominal pressure and thus protect the pelvic floor during coughing, sneezing, or any activity that increases pressure on the pelvic floor.

There is a small amount of literature on the effectiveness of PFMT for POP, including five randomized trials comparing training with no treatment (Braekken et al., 2010a; Braekken et al., 2010b; Ghroubi et al., 2008; Hagen et al., 2009; Piya-Anant et al., 2003). The evidence indicates that training has a beneficial effect on PFM function, prolapse symptom burden, prolapse severity, and quality of life (Dumoulin et al., 2017).

Adherence and Maintenance

PFMT and exercise require the active participation of a motivated patient (Dumoulin et al., 2015a). It is often challenging to remember to use the PFMs strategically in daily life and to persist in a regular exercise regimen to maintain strength and skill. This reliance on patient behavior change represents the major limitation of this treatment approach. In addition, improvement with behavioral treatment is gradual, usually evident by the fourth week of training and continuing for up to 6 months. Herein lies the challenge for behavioral treatment: sustaining the patient's motivation for long enough that she will experience noticeable change in her bladder control.

It is important in initiating behavioral treatment to communicate realistic expectations and make it clear to the patient that it may take weeks to months for symptom improvement, and that the improvement may be irregular, with "good" days and "bad" days. Success with symptom improvement will depend on consistent practice and use of her new skills. The patient who understands the usual course of treatment will be better prepared to persist until results are achieved. Clinicians can provide support by scheduling follow-up appointments to track and reinforce patient progress, make adjustments to the exercise regimen, and encourage persistence.

Measurement of adherence to PFM exercise and behavioral strategies is poor (Borello-France et al., 2010; Dumoulin et al., 2015b). There is very little research on methods to identify barriers and improve adherence (Alewijnse et al., 2003; Borello-France et al., 2010; Borello-France et al., 2013; Dumoulin et al., 2015b). Borello-France and colleagues (2013) reported on adherence to PFM exercise and bladder control strategies as a secondary analysis of a multisite randomized controlled trial comparing three interventions for stress-predominant UI: intravaginal continence pessary, multicomponent behavioral therapy (including PFMT and bladder control strategies), and pessary and behavioral therapy combined (Richter et al., 2010). The authors concluded that adherence to PFM exercises and bladder control strategies, when implemented by trained interventionists, can be high and sustained over time.

Electrical Stimulation

Pelvic floor electrical stimulation has been used for the treatment of urinary incontinence since 1952 (Huffman et al., 1952). In this original study, electrical stimulation was added to PFM exercises to treat SUI in women who had failed treatment with exercise alone; seven of 17 women were cured. Fifteen years later, pelvic floor electrical stimulation was reported by Moore and Schofield (1967) using a vaginal probe, and thereafter this treatment was more widely used.

Pelvic floor electrical stimulation stimulates pudendal nerve afferents, activating pudendal and hypogastric nerve efferents, causing contraction of smooth and striated periurethral and pelvic muscles. This stimulation provides a form of passive exercise, with the goal of improving the urethral closure mechanism. In addition, electrical stimulation can be useful in teaching PFM contraction to women who cannot identify or contract these muscles voluntarily. Stimulation can be applied using surface electrodes, delivering transcutaneous electrical stimulation via suprapubic, sacral, or external anal skin surface electrodes or intravaginal or intrarectal sensors for 15 minutes at a time, one to three times per day. An alternative, noninvasive approach that may be easier and less embarrassing for women is to administer electrical stimulation via surface skin electrodes on a garment that holds the electrodes around the pelvic area to ensure satisfactory recruitment of the PFM (Dmochowski et al., 2019). The literature on pelvic floor electrical stimulation in women indicates that it is effective for improving SUI (Stewart et al., 2017) and urgency and mixed urinary incontinence compared to sham or no treatment (Dumoulin et al., 2017).

Weighted Vaginal Cones

Weighted vaginal cones provide a progressive muscular load during the performance of PFMT. A systematic review was performed of 23 small trials involving 1806 women, of whom 717 received cones (Herbison & Dean, 2013). The overall quality of the trials was not optimal. Use of cones was found to be better than no active treatment, but there was inconclusive evidence for a subjective cure between cones and PFMT. It has been recommended that, for motivated women with SUI, vaginal cones with supervised training sessions can be a first-line therapy (Dumoulin et al., 2016).

WEIGHT LOSS AND URINARY INCONTINENCE

Epidemiologic research has established obesity as a strong, independent risk factor for prevalent and incident incontinence, including both SUI and UUI (Brown et al., 1996; Brown et al., 1999; Hunskaar, 2008; Nambiar et al., 2018; Phelan et al., 2012; Subak et al., 2009a). There is a clear dose-response effect: each

5-unit increase in body mass index is associated with a 20% to 70% increase in the risk of prevalent incontinence and a 30% to 60% increase in the odds of 5- to 10-year incident incontinence. Furthermore, intervention studies show that weight loss has a beneficial effect on incontinence (Hunskaar, 2008; Subak et al., 2009b). Urinary symptoms significantly improve in morbidly obese women with dramatic weight loss (45–50 kg) after bariatric surgery (Bump et al., 1992; Burgio et al., 2007; Deitel et al., 1988) and when women lose as little as 5% of their baseline weight with behavioral weight loss programs (Subak et al., 2002; Subak et al., 2005), a reasonable goal for many overweight or obese women. Pooled data from a recent meta-analysis and systematic review on the effect of bariatric surgery on urinary incontinence in obese women revealed that bariatric surgery significantly reduced the incidence of urinary incontinence at 6 and 12 months and improved pelvic floor symptoms as measured by the Pelvic Floor Distress Inventory-20 (Zhang et al., 2020).

Lifestyle interventions, specifically weight loss, have demonstrated credible efficacy in the reduction of SUI symptoms. In a randomized controlled trial (RCT) in which overweight and obese women with incontinence were given a self-administered behavioral program and randomized to a 6-month behavioral weight loss program or control intervention, the weight loss group showed a 47% reduction in frequency of incontinence, significantly greater than the 28% shown by the control group (Subak et al., 2009b). Group differences were significant for stress incontinence and total incontinence after 12 months and for urgency incontinence after 18 months (Wing et al., 2010). The weight loss group also had greater patient satisfaction ratings at 6, 12, and 18 months. Because modest weight loss is achievable for many women, it should be considered in the first-line behavioral treatment of women with stress, urgency, or mixed urinary incontinence. In general, significant weight loss (15–20 body mass index units) decreases urinary incontinence, and moderate weight loss is effective if combined with PFM exercises (Dumoulin et al., 2016).

COMPLEMENTARY AND ALTERNATIVE THERAPIES FOR URINARY INCONTINENCE

According to the viewpoint of traditional Chinese medicine, acupuncture could impact SUI symptoms by reinforcing "qi," the vital substance constituting the human body, and promote bladder function recovery, presumably via the autonomic nervous system (Knardahl et al., 1998). The only Cochrane review on this subject (Wang et al., 2013) reviewed 17 studies, but only one small trial of acupuncture versus medication met the inclusion criteria. A greater number of women in the acupuncture group improved compared with midodrine (73% vs. 33%, respectively); however, cure rates were low and did not differ between groups (13% vs. 7%). More robust research is needed in this area of treatment.

Yoga, a system of philosophy, lifestyle, and physical practice, originated in India and has been used in managing several medical conditions, including musculoskeletal disorders, cardiovascular disorders, stress, depression, and anxiety (Taneja, 2014). Only two studies of yoga for the treatment of SUI, with a total of 49 subjects, were included in a recent systematic review (Wieland et al., 2019), and the quality of the data was lacking. In general, yoga participants sustained benefit, but there is insufficient evidence to prescribe yoga as a standard-of-care nonsurgical therapy for SUI.

ESTROGEN AND STRESS URINARY INCONTINENCE

Estrogen is discussed separately from other pharmacologic therapies for SUI because it should be a generalized recommendation for many women for optimized urogenital tissue health. The prevalence of symptomatic urogenital atrophy in postreproductive women may approach 50%, and, because the lower urinary tract and vagina develop from the same embryologic origin, it is not surprising that estrogen receptors are present throughout the vagina, urethra, bladder trigone, pelvic connective tissue, and pelvic muscles. Decreased estrogen effect and the resulting urogenital atrophy, now commonly referred to as genitourinary syndrome of menopause, produce symptoms of vaginal and vulvar dryness, pruritus, dyspareunia, and vaginitis, recurrent urinary tract infections and lower urinary tract symptoms such as dysuria, urinary frequency, urinary urgency, nocturia and incontinence. Painful urination or "urethral syndrome" secondary to decreased estrogen effect responds to local estrogen therapy, as do nocturia, irritative bladder symptoms, and recurrent urinary tract infections. As the use of oral estrogen has been noted to worsen urinary incontinence symptoms (Cody et al., 2012), this current discussion will focus on the use of intravaginal estrogen.

Estrogen exerts beneficial effects in the urethra by increasing the concentration of α-adrenergic receptors in the urethra and bladder, improving vascularity and perfusion of the periurethral tissue, and increasing thickness of the urethral epithelium. These changes facilitate coaptation and increase urethral pressure (Ewies & Alfhaily, 2010). A Cochrane review assessed the effect of systemic and intravaginal estrogenin women symptomatic for or with a urodynamic diagnosis of stress, urgency, or mixed urinary incontinence (Cody et al., 2012). There was evidence that intravaginal estrogen may improve incontinence (relative risk [RR], 0.74; 95% confidence interval (CI), 0.64-0.86), but little long-term data exist. Further, there was noted improvement in voiding frequency and urinary urgency. Subsequent systematic reviews noted that, compared with placebo, vaginal estrogens improved vaginal dryness, dyspareunia, urinary urgency, frequency, SUI, and UUI. Urinary tract infection rates were also diminished (Rahn et al., 2014; Rahn et al., 2015).

Urogenital atrophy is an FDA-approved indication for estrogen therapy. Lower urinary tract symptoms associated with atrophy also significantly improve with intravaginal estrogen therapy. Therefore we strongly recommend optimizing urogenital tissue health as first-line treatment with intravaginal estrogen therapy, before or concurrently with behavioral therapy, pessary use, or any other nonsurgical treatment, and before surgical intervention for SUI. When the uterus is present, progestin treatment may be considered on an individual basis,

TABLE 14.1 Vaginal Estrogen Products

Product	Dosage	Manufacturer
Estradiol cream Estrace vaginal cream	0.1 mg/g	Allergan, Inc., Madison, NJ
Conjugated estrogens cream Premarin vaginal cream	0.625 mg/g	Pfizer Pharmaceuticals Inc., New York, NY
Estradiol vaginal ring Estring, Femring	2 mg/3 months	Pfizer Pharmaceuticals Inc., New York, NY; Millicent Pharma, Inc., Dunkalk, Ireland
Estradiol vaginal tablets Vagifem	10 μg/tablet	Novo Nordisk Health Care AG, Inc., Plainsboro, NJ

although, when used as directed, serum estrogen levels do not rise above postmenopausal levels (Rahn et al., 2014). We typically recommend approximately 0.5 g of vaginal estrogen cream nightly for 2 weeks, with maintenance doses of 0.5 g two to three times per week thereafter. Estrogen rings and tablets have standardized recommended regimens (Table 14.1).

OTHER PHARMACOLOGIC THERAPIES FOR STRESS URINARY INCONTINENCE

Numerous medications have been used to treat SUI (Andersson et al., 2009); however, none have level 1 data showing robust benefit above placebo or have FDA approval for this primary indication (Table 14.2). Pharmacotherapy for SUI takes advantage of the effects of certain medications on increasing urethral outlet resistance that is mediated by sympathetic, parasympathetic, and somatic innervation coordinated by the central nervous system. Increased outlet resistance may occur in theory with α-adrenergic agonists, β-adrenergic antagonists and agonists, tricyclic antidepressants, and serotonergic and noradrenergic reuptake inhibitors (Cannon & Chancellor, 2003; Cannon & Yoshimura, 2003).

α- and β-Adrenergic Agonists

In a Cochrane review analyzing data from 1099 women, 673 of whom received an adrenergic medication (phenylpropanolamine, 11 trials; midodrine, two trials; norepinephrine, three trials; clenbuterol, three trials, terbutaline, one trial; eskornade, one trial; and Ro 115-1240, one trial), there was limited evidence of adrenergic agonist efficacy over placebo for incontinence episodes (Alhasso et al., 2005). Potential side effects of all α-adrenergic medications include hypertension, anxiety, hemorrhagic stroke, cardiac arrhythmias, palpitations, tremor, weakness, insomnia, and headache. These results were confirmed in another systematic review (Shamliyan et al., 2008).

TABLE 14.2 Other Pharmacologic Therapies for Stress Urinary Incontinence

Drug Type	Drug Name	Dosage
Serotonin/norepinephrine reuptake inhibitor	Duloxetine	40 mg bid
α-Adrenergic agonist	Midodrine	2.5 mg tid
	Pseudoephedrine hydrochloride	15 mg bid, 30 mg bid, tid, qid
β-Agonist/antagonist	Clenbuterol	0.02 mg bid
	Propanolol	10 mg bid to 40 mg tid
Tricyclic antidepressant	Imipramine hydrochloride	10 mg qhs (older patients) 25 mg tid, 75 mg bid

β-Adrenergic Receptor Antagonists

β-adrenergic blocking agents should theoretically potentiate the activity of norepinephrine on α-receptors and increase urethral outlet resistance. Early studies demonstrated efficacy with propranolol in patients with SUI; however, subsequent RCTs have not been as successful. At this time, the role of β-adrenergic receptor antagonists in treating SUI is limited. Significant potential side effects include heart failure, lethargy, and pulmonary compromise.

Tricyclic Antidepressants

Tricyclic antidepressants, in particular doxepin and imipramine hydrochloride, improve SUI symptoms by decreasing bladder contractility and increasing urethral resistance. It is thought that they exert central and peripheral anticholinergic effects at some sites. They block the active transport system in the presynaptic nerve ending responsible for the reuptake of norepinephrine and serotonin. They act as sedatives, presumably centrally, but potentially related to antihistaminic properties. No placebo-controlled trials of the effects of tricyclic antidepressants on SUI exist (Andersson et al., 2009; Mariappan et al., 2005). A recent double-blind, randomized, placebo-controlled crossover trial in 16 healthy women showed no difference in the increase in opening urethral pressure between those receiving imipramine and those receiving placebo; there were 13 adverse events related to imipramine in seven subjects. Based on these data, the authors did not recommend off-label use of imipramine for the treatment of SUI (Kornholt et al., 2019). Side effects associated with tricyclic antidepressants include dry mouth, blurred vision, urinary retention, constipation, orthostatic hypotension, sedation, tremors, sexual side effects, fatigue, rash, jaundice, and weakness. Older patients in particular are prone to side effects such as disorientation, falls, heart rhythm abnormalities, and decreased force of cardiac contraction. Lower doses should be used in older patients; we typically start with a 5- to 10-mg nightly dose to determine tolerance and titrate up from there (Table 14.2).

Duloxetine

Serotonergic and noradrenergic reuptake inhibitors suppress parasympathetic activity and enhance sympathetic and somatic activity in the lower urinary tract, promoting urine storage. The dual serotonin-norepinephrine reuptake inhibitor duloxetine has shown clinical efficacy for SUI compared with placebo in 10 trials including 3944 subjects randomized to duloxetine or placebo, PFMT, or both (Mariappan et al., 2005). The maximum duration of treatment was 12 weeks. Efficacy of treatment was significantly better with duloxetine versus placebo with respect to quality of life and perception of improvement. Individual studies demonstrated a significant reduction of incontinence episode frequency by 50% with duloxetine (RR 1.56, 95% CI 1.46–1.66) and global improvement (RR 1.24, 95% CI 1.14–1.36) (Li et al., 2013). However, meta-analysis of the stress pad test and the 24-hour pad test showed no difference between duloxetine and placebo. Subjective cure favored duloxetine. Although duloxetine does not have FDA approval for the treatment of SUI in the United States, there has been regulatory approval for this indication in the European Union since 2004. Side effects associated with duloxetine include nausea, fatigue, dry mouth, and insomnia. Nausea was the most common reason for discontinuation in the clinical trials.

URETHRAL DEVICES

Urethral Inserts

A urethral insert acts as a mechanical barrier to prevent urinary leakage by sealing the urethral lumen. Usually these devices have a means to prevent intravesical migration (a tab at the meatus), a mechanism to maintain the device in its proper place at the bladder neck (e.g., balloon, fins), and a device or mechanism to permit removal for voiding (e.g., string, pump) (Deng, 2018). The intraurethral prosthesis with valves device is for chronic use and is not addressed here. Other inserts (e.g., FemSoft, Rochester Medical, Stewartville, MN) are no longer available. In a Cochrane systematic review addressing the use of mechanical devices for urinary incontinence in women (Lipp et al., 2014), data obtained from three small, randomized trials studying intraurethral inserts reflected insufficient evidence, both objectively and subjectively, for recommending their use.

Urethral Occlusive Devices

From a historical perspective, numerous external occlusive devices existed that essentially blocked urine loss through the external urethral meatus. Issues of cost, comfort, patient acceptability of manipulating their genitalia to apply the device, and concerns of lifelong dependence were at the forefront of deciding whether to use these products. There were several reusable external urethral occlusive devices for SUI, and none are currently on the market.

THE INS AND OUTS OF PESSARY USE

Historically, the use of pessaries has been reserved for those patients who decline surgery for SUI or POP or for those who are not surgical candidates because of significant medical comorbidities. Some practitioners extend indications for pessary use to pregnancy-related prolapse and prolapse and incontinence in older women. However, current US and Canadian practice guidelines suggest that all women interested in prolapse or SUI treatment should be offered a pessary as an alternative to surgical therapy (Robert et al., 2013; ACOG Practice Bulletin, 2019). Two studies by Clemons et al. (2004a; 2004b) showed that age greater than 65 years, severe comorbidity, and maintenance of urinary continence were significant predictors of continued pessary use after 1 year for women with POP, but high-quality evidence remains limited regarding the choice of pessary and management of pessary use. A recent survey of nurse providers (323 respondents) in the United States showed a range of responses in terms of pessary care. Physicians and advanced practice registered nurses (e.g., nurse practitioners) provided up to 80% of the care, and 86% of care occurred in the office setting. Care routines varied, most often including 3-month interval follow-up with speculum vaginal examinations, and no routine use of vaginal products. On-the-job mentoring was the primary knowledge source. This study noted a need for evidence-based guidelines for optimal care, based on patient outcomes, satisfaction, and costs of care (O'Dell et al., 2016). Even urogynecologists have not come to consensus regarding indications for pessaries and their management (Cundiff et al., 2000). Although clinicians have in the past had to rely on descriptive studies, manufacturers' recommendations, and clinical experience when managing patients who elect pessary treatment, level I evidence supporting pessary use as an alternative treatment to surgery for SUI and prolapse is slowly increasing.

Efficacy of Pessaries and Vaginal Devices for Stress Urinary Incontinence

Pessaries effectively manage SUI in some women during exercise and in daily life. Continence pessaries are placed transvaginally and are designed to prevent urine loss by stabilizing and supporting the urethra and bladder neck, increasing urethra length, and providing gentle compression of the urethra against the pubic bone during increases in intraabdominal pressure. This structural arrangement can reduce and often prevent stress-related incontinence (Newman & Burgio, 2020). Most outcomes have been short-term, and most study sizes have been small (Table 14.3). The Ambulatory Treatments for Leakage Associated with Stress trial, a robust level I study performed by the Pelvic Floor Disorders Network, consisted of three treatment arms: behavioral therapy alone (including PFMT), pessary alone, and combined behavioral therapy and pessary (Richter et al., 2010). The primary outcomes were treatment efficacy using the Urogenital Distress Inventory stress incontinence subscale of the Pelvic Floor Distress Inventory and the Patient Global Impression of Improvement. Secondary outcomes included the proportion of patients with a 75% reduction of incontinence episodes on 7-day bladder diary and patient satisfaction.

Overall, at 3 months, pessaries were not as effective as behavioral intervention in terms of patient satisfaction (75% in behavioral group vs. 63% in pessary group, $P = .02$) or proportion of patients with no bothersome urinary incontinence symptoms (49% in behavioral group vs. 33% in pessary group, $P = .006$). Both groups were similar in reported patient perception of improvement and in prolapse-specific symptom distress and bother (Kenton et al., 2012). Combining behavioral and pessary treatment was significantly better than pessary alone, but not better than behavioral therapy alone. Therefore, combined therapy was not considered superior to single-modality therapy, because to be clinically superior, combined therapy had to be better than both single-modality therapies. Group differences were not sustained to 12 months, but treatment satisfaction remained greater than 50% for all treatment groups by per-protocol analysis. Factors noted to be predictive of success and satisfaction with the use of

TABLE 14.3 Pessary Use for Urinary Incontinence

Investigators	N	Indication	Time of Follow-Up	Outcomes
Bhatia and Bergman (1985)	30	Stress incontinence	None	Cough pressure profile 24/30 patients continent
Suarez et al. (1991) (contraceptive diaphragm)	12	Stress incontinence	None	Subjective cure 9/12
Nygaard (1995) (randomized trial; pessary vs. tampon vs. no device)	18	Exercise incontinence	None	Total of 36% pessary users continent; 58% tampon users continent
Abu-Sitta et al. (1995)	11	Stress incontinence	4 days	Pad test, urine loss significantly decreased
Kondo et al. (1997) (bladder neck support prothesis)	77	Stress and mixed incontinence	12 weeks	Subjective pad test, 29% continent, 51% decreased severity by >50%, 81% combined subjective/objective some or maximum benefit
Davila et al. (1999) (Introl device,[a] UroMed, Needham, MA)	70	Stress and mixed incontinence	1 month	Total of 53/70 completed trial; significant improvement pad tests, diaries, high subjective improvement and quality of life
Robert and Mainprize (2002)	38	Stress incontinence	1 year	Total of 6/38 continued pessary use pad test, voiding diary, IIQ, UDI
Farrell et al. (2004)	100	Stress and mixed incontinence, prolapse	11 months	Total of 79% resolution symptoms 2 weeks; 55% of patients with stress, 63% of patients with mixed incontinence successfully fitted with pessary, 59% patients continued use
Donnelly et al. (2004)	119	Stress incontinence	6 months	Total of 89% successful pessary fitting, 55% continued pessary use for 6 months
Richter et al. (2010) (randomized trial)	446	Stress incontinence	Primary outcome 3, 6, and 12 months	At 3 months, no bothersome UI symptoms in the behavioral group 49% vs. 33% in the pessary group, $P = .006$; treatment satisfaction 75% of behavioral group vs. 63% pessary group, $P = .02$; no difference PGI-I, 49% behavioral group, 40% pessary group, $P = .10$. Combination behavioral and pessary treatment was significantly better than pessary by PGI-I and PFDI, but not better than behavioral therapy. Group differences not sustained to 12 months, but treatment satisfaction remained >50% for all treatment groups

[a]Device no longer available.

IIQ, Incontinence Impact Questionnaire; *UDI*, Urogenital Distress Inventory; *UI*, urinary incontinence; *PGI-I*, Patient Global Impression of Improvement; *PFDI*, Pelvic Floor Distress Inventory.

all three nonsurgical approaches included being menopausal, having a higher educational status, having no history of previous incontinence surgery, and having lower incontinence frequency (Schaffer et al., 2012).

The most recent Cochrane review on mechanical devices for the management of UI (Lipp et al., 2014) summarized the results of eight randomized trials reflecting the use of standard available intravaginal pessaries, tampons, and other intravaginal and intraurethral devices. As most trials were small, outcome measures were diverse, and few trials included control/no-treatment groups, the data regarding the use of mechanical devices for treatment of UI are still unclear.

The Impressa is an over-the-counter intravaginal device for women over the age of 21 years with SUI (Kimberly-Clark Worldwide International, Inc., Irving, TX). It is a disposable, one-time use tampon-like device that comprises a core, cover, and applicator (Fig. 14.5). The core is composed of a flexible anchor and support poles made of resin and covered with medical-grade silicone, and the cover is made of biocompatible nylon mesh that stretches between the arms of the support poles to provide support without obstructing urinary flow or

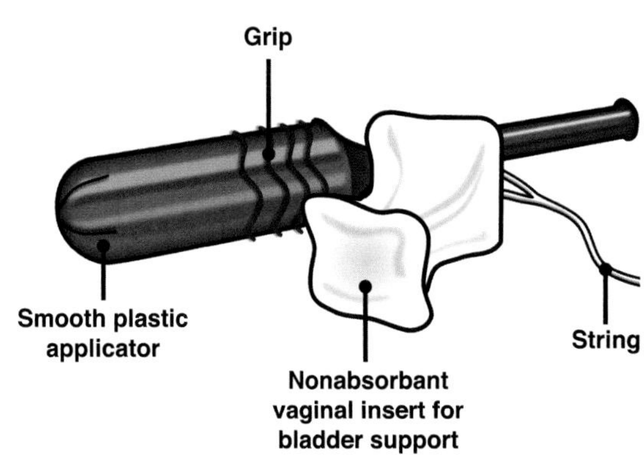

Fig. 14.5 Impressa over-the-counter intravaginal device for stress urinary incontinence (*Source:* Courtesy of Diane K. Newman, DNP.).

vaginal secretions. The device is inserted and removed similar to a vaginal tampon and comes in three sizes. It is not absorbent and should be removed during menstruation. It is not necessary to remove it before urination or defecation.

In an open-label controlled study, 60 women with severe urodynamic stress incontinence tested the device for 28 days.

Some 85% of participants achieved a greater than 70% reduction in pad weight gain, and mean pad weight gain decreased from 17g per 8 hours to 2 g per 8 hours. A high degree of satisfaction was reported, and 70% of participants reported 90% improvement (Ziv et al., 2008; Ziv et al., 2009). Adverse effects included 27 cases of vaginal discomfort, 15 cases of vaginal pain, 14 cases of vaginal spotting (mild), and one case of candidiasis. There were no vaginal excoriations, sores, ulcers, scratches, or inflammation on vaginal exam (Ziv et al., 2008).

Efficacy of Pessaries for Pelvic Organ Prolapse

Table 14.4 reports study outcomes for pessary treatment of POP, including several published randomized trials in this area. Satisfactory outcomes have been reported for stage II or greater prolapse using the Gellhorn and ring diaphragm pessaries. In one of the first prospective studies of pessaries for prolapse, after 2 to 6 months 77% to 92% of women with successful pessary fitting were satisfied; and, using intention-to-treat analysis, 44% to 67% of women who were treated initially with a pessary for prolapse were satisfied (Clemons et al., 2004b). A randomized crossover trial later confirmed that clinically meaningful improvement occurred in patient-reported pelvic floor symptom bother and functional impact with pessary treatment after 3 months for women treated with a ring versus Gellhorn pessary, with no difference in outcomes between the two pessary types (Cundiff et al., 2007). Both pessary types improved pelvic floor symptoms commonly attributed to POP, including most notably bulge and pressure symptoms, but improvement also occurred in obstructive and irritative urinary and defecatory symptoms. Two additional randomized trials compared pessary to PFMT treatment in women with symptomatic prolapse, and both reported greater prolapse-specific symptom improvement with pessary treatment (at 12–24 months) compared with PFMT (Cheung et al., 2016; Panman et al. 2016). Recent data support pessary treatment as a long-term option, with continuation rates of approximately 80% over 2- to 5-year periods (Lone et al., 2011; Mao et al., 2019; Wolff et al., 2017).

Pessary Placement and Management

More than 100 different kinds of pessaries have been described, with numerous materials used. Currently, according to Cooper Surgical, Inc. (Trumbull, CT) brochures, there are six to nine sizes of 13 Milex pessary models used for SUI, POP, or both, with the majority made of silicone or plastic (Fig. 14.6). Silicone is nonallergenic, does not absorb odors or secretions, is resistant to repeat cleansing and autoclaving, and is soft and

TABLE 14.4 Pessary Use for Pelvic Organ Prolapse

Investigators	*N*	Indication	Time of Follow-Up	Outcomes
Sulak et al. (1993)	101	Prolapse	Mean 16 months	50% continued use
Wu et al. (1997)	110	Prolapse		66% of those used at 1 month, continued for >12 months
Clemons et al. (2004a, 2004b)	73	Symptomatic prolapse, stage II or greater	2 months	92% patient satisfaction at 2 months
Cundiff et al. (2007) (randomized crossover trial; ring with support vs. Gellhorn pessary)	134	Stages II–IV prolapse	3 months	92% successful pessary fitting; 60% (1st period) and 57% (2nd period) continuation of pessary at 3 months; clinically and statistically significant improvements in POPDI scale, obstructive and irritative subscales of UDI and obstructive and irritative subscales of CRADI; no difference in improvement between pessary types; 67% (ring) and 61% (Gellhorn) of participants had high satisfaction rates
Cheung et al. (2016) (randomized trial; ring pessary with PMFT vs. PFMT alone)	276	Stages I–III prolapse	12 months	Pessary continuation rate 60% at 12 months; POPDI and POPIQ decreased in both groups, but mean score differences were higher in pessary group (POPDI: −29.7 vs.−4.7, $P < .01$; POPIQ: −29.0 vs. 3.5, $P < .01$); prolapse symptoms reported as "improved" by 60% vs. 28% in pessary vs. control group, $P < .001$
Panman et al. (2016) (randomized trial; pessary vs. PFMT)	162	Symptomatic prolapse at or beyond hymen; age 55 years and older	24 months	57% successful pessary fitting and 74% continuation of pessary at 24 months; no difference in change of PFDI-20 score between groups (primary outcome); greater improvement in POPDI-6 with pessary (mean difference −3.2 points, 95% CI −6.3 to 0.0, $P < .047$); direct medical costs over the 2-year study were $309 and $437 (mean difference $128, 95% CI $27–$236) per person for pessary and PFMT, respectively

CI, Confidence interval; *CRADI*, Colorectal-Anal Distress Inventory; *PFDI-20*, Pelvic Floor Distress Inventory-20; *PFMT*, pelvic floor muscle training; *POPDI*, Pelvic Organ Prolapse Distress Inventory; *POPDI-6*, Pelvic Organ Prolapse Distress Inventory-6; *POPIQ*, Pelvic Organ Prolapse Impact Questionnaire; *UDI*, Urinary Distress Inventory.

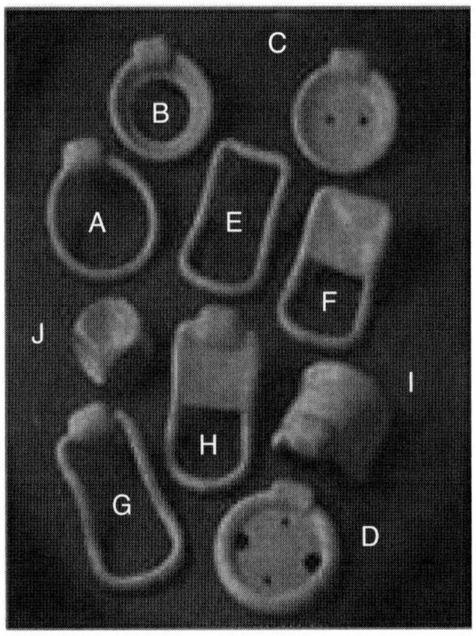

Pessary	Indication (SUI +)
A. Incontinence ring	
B. Incontinence ring with support	1st- or 2nd-degree uterine/vault prolapse and/or mild cystocele
C. Incontinence dish	Mild 1st- or 2nd-degree uterine prolapse
D. Incontinence dish w/ support	1st- or 2nd-degree uterine/vault prolapse and/or mild cystocele
E. Hodge	Narrow vaginal introitus
F. Hodge with support	Narrow vaginal introitus; mild cystocele
G. Hodge with incontinence knob	Narrow vaginal introitus + stabilization of the UVJ
H. Hodge with incontinence knob and support	Narrow vaginal introitus + stabilization of the UVJ + mild cystocele
I. Gehrung with incontinence knob	Cystocele and/or rectocele
J. Cube	SUI during strenuous exercise (insert just before exercise begins)

Fig. 14.6 Pessary types and indications. *SUI,* Stress urinary incontinence; *UVJ,* urethrovaginal junction.

pliable. If a pessary contains latex, ensure that the patient does not have a latex allergy before using it.

It is thought that the pessary restores continence by stabilizing the proximal urethra and urethrovesical junction, thereby facilitating pressure transmission to the urethra. Pessaries improve urinary incontinence in some women by increasing urethral functional length, urethral closure pressures, and cough profiles. Pessaries used for POP can also create or worsen SUI by supporting the prolapsed vagina and relieving bladder neck obstruction. This "occult" SUI occurred in 21% of the women who were successfully fitted with a pessary in a study by Clemons et al. (2004b).

Pessaries provide pelvic organ support by creating a functional obstruction within the vagina. Two categories of pessaries exist for prolapse: support and space-filling. The ring pessary (with diaphragm) is a commonly used support pessary, and the Gelhorn pessary is a commonly used space-filling pessary. Ring and other support pessaries are commonly recommended for stage I and II prolapse, whereas space-filling pessaries are for stage III and IV prolapse. Manufacturers' recommendations for pessary selection can be found in Table 14.5 (LeKan-Rutledge et al., 2003).

Pessary placement involves consideration of several issues, primarily the patient's motivation to use the pessary. Other issues include her medical and cognitive status, manual dexterity, current sexual function, type and duration of exercise, and status of the vaginal walls and cervix. We strongly recommend treatment of the vagina with estrogen if the patient is hypoestrogenic, and

TABLE 14.5 Guidelines for Pessary Selection

PROLAPSE									
1st to 2nd Degree	2nd to 3rd Degree	Sexually Active	Vaginal Wall	Urinary Stress Incontinence	Cystocele	Rectocele	Incompetent Cervix	Retro Displacement	Most Commonly Used
X		X							Ring
X		X							Ring with support
X									Shaatz
X									Incontinence dish
X									Dish with support
X									Hodge with support
	X								Donut
	X								Gellhorn (flex 95% rigid)
	X								Inflatoball
	X	X	X	X	X	Mid X			Cube, tandem cube
	X	X			X	Mid X			Gehrung
	X	X		X		Mid X			Gehrung with knob
									Incontinence ring
									Hodge w-knob
		X			Mid X		X	X	Smith, Hodge, Risser

(Modified from Milex Products, Inc., Chicago, IL.)

maintenance of estrogen treatment using any of the regimens discussed previously. We provide a consensus approach for the fitting and management of intravaginal pessaries below (Palumbo, 2000; Poma, 2000).

Steps to Fitting a Pessary

At an initial pessary fitting, it is helpful to be able to use a pessary fitting kit comprised of a variety of pessary types and sizes. These are separate from pessaries used for treatment and are reusable. The patient should be examined in lithotomy position after emptying her bladder. Estimation of pessary size can be performed digitally by placing a finger into the posterior vaginal fornix and measuring the distance to the pubis. It can also be measured with the use of ring forceps to reduce the prolapse or bladder neck. After the approximate size is determined, the appropriate type is selected (Table 14.5) based on the patient's needs and activity level. The clinician should use a dry glove to better grasp the pessary, and water-soluble lubricants as needed. On insertion, guide the pessary posteriorly to avoid the urethra. Proper size is ensured by being able to sweep the index finger between the pessary and the vaginal wall; the pessary should feel comfortable to the patient. When fitted, the patient is asked to stand, perform Valsalva, and cough to ensure that the pessary is retained. Also assess that the pessary is providing the desired urethral support and leakage control. Furthermore, ensure that the patient is able to void with the pessary in place or is able to remove the pessary to void before sending her home.

Insertion tips include the following: use of a water-soluble lubricant for insertion; folding or collapsing the pessary to reduce its size; and, when the pessary is inside the vagina, pushing it high to an area behind the symphysis pubis. When instructing the patient to insert and remove the pessary, determine whether it is done best in a standing or supine position, depending upon the patient's dexterity.

Ring pessaries with or without support are the most commonly used for SUI. They are the easiest to fold, insert, and remove. Continence pessaries (with a knob), rings, and dishes with support are also easy to fold, insert, and remove. Gellhorn and cube pessaries are typically more difficult to insert and remove. They are held in place by significant space occupation and suction, and they offer strong support. The suction of the cube pessary needs to be broken before removal. Cube pessaries should be removed daily; Gellhorns can stay in longer (up to 6–8 weeks). Donut pessaries, which are very popular, are considered a space-fitting pessary for large vaginal vault prolapse or procidentia. Donut pessaries should be removed and cleaned every 2 to 3 days if possible.

Follow-Up Recommendations

After the initial fitting, the patient should return within 7 days and then at 4 to 6 weeks, depending on her independence with the pessary, her proficiency in placement and removal, and her cognitive and motor abilities. After this initial follow-up, continued follow-up is at 6- to 12-month intervals at the discretion of the provider and depending on the patient's ability to insert and remove the pessary effectively. For patients who self-manage their pessary, it should be removed regularly (ideally at least weekly) and cleaned with soap and water (Robert et al., 2013). If the patient has to return for removal and cleaning by a provider, this is typically performed at 2- to 3-month intervals, although longer follow-up intervals may be reasonable based on new level 1 evidence. One trial randomized 60 women with a ring pessary to follow-up at 3 or 6 months. Although not statistically different, complications were more common in the 6-month follow-up group (30% vs. 10%, $P = .06$), including vaginal ulcerations, vaginitis, and pessary dislodgement (Tam et al., 2019). A larger noninferiority trial of 130 women using office-based care of prolapse or incontinence pessaries found that follow-up at 3 or 6 months was appropriate, because the between-group difference in rates of vaginal epithelial abnormalities at 48 weeks did not exceed a prespecified difference of 7.5% (vaginal epithelial abnormalities occurred in 7.4% with 3-month visits and in 1.7% with 6-month visits) (Probst et al., 2020).

On each return for follow-up, ensure that the pessary is placed properly and that it provides adequate support of the prolapse. If the patient is using the pessary for incontinence symptoms, check that her symptoms are resolved or stable. Because pessaries are fit by a process of trial and error, it is common to change the pessary size or type at least once after the initial fitting. Check the pessary's integrity, and check the patient's vaginal tissue for irritation, pressure sores, ulcerations, and estrogen status.

Complications

Although few absolute contraindications for pessary use exist (evident vaginal mesh erosion, silicone allergy), relative contraindications include placement in the setting of an active vaginal infection or significant ulceration and the potential for noncompliance with follow-up (Al-Shaikh et al., 2018).

Vaginal discharge and odor may signal an indication for removal and cleaning or a possible complication of pessary use, such as infection or erosion. An increase in bacterial vaginosis has been seen with pessary use. If the pessary does not stay in place, it is unlikely to cause erosion; conversely, the pessary may be too tight, and thus could lead to irritation or erosions. There may be *de novo* or increased SUI with reduction of vaginal prolapse. Vaginal abrasions, erosions or ulcerations, rare vesicovaginal or rectovaginal fistulas, small bowel entrapment, bilateral hydronephrosis, and urosepsis have all been described.

Another potential complication is the forgotten or incarcerated pessary. Therefore, whenever possible, the family or other health care professionals should help the debilitated or memory-impaired patient ensure adequate pessary care. Patient education is vital for successful pessary use, and a review of female anatomy may be helpful before pessary placement. We also discuss, in an individualized manner, the schedule of removal and cleaning of the pessary. It is important to counsel the patient to call for concerns or problems related to pessary use.

CONCLUSION

Credible first-line nonsurgical treatment modalities exist for the treatment of SUI and POP. These options allow providers to align patient expectations of treatment with outcomes. Nonsurgical treatment approaches should be discussed with all women seeking care for these prevalent conditions. Combinations of behavioral, medical, and other unique treatments such as pessaries should be offered and potentially implemented in most patients before offering surgical treatment of SUI and prolapse.

BIBLIOGRAPHY

Introduction

Haylen BT, deRidder D, Freeman RM, et al. An International Urogynecological Association (IUGA)/International Continence Society (ICS) joint report on the terminology for female pelvic floor dysfunction. *Int Urogynecol J.* 2010;21:5.

Haylen BT, Maher CF, Barber MD, et al. An International Urogynecological Association (IUGA)/International Continence Society (ICS) joint report on the terminology for female pelvic organ prolapse (POP). *Neurourol Urodyn.* 2016;35:137.

Portman DJ, Gass ML, Vulvovaginal Atrophy Terminology Consensus Conference Panel. Genitourinary syndrome of menopause: new terminology for vulvovaginal atrophy from the International Society for the Study of Women's Sexual Health and the North American Menopause Society. *Menopause.* 2014;21:1063.

Rahn DD, Carberry C, Sanses TV, et al. Vaginal estrogen for genitourinary syndrome of menopause: a systematic review. *Obstet Gynecol.* 2014;124:1147.

The Bladder Diary: A Valuable Clinical Tool

Newman DK, Burgio KL. Conservative management of urinary incontinence: behavioral and pelvic floor therapy and urethral and pelvic devices. In: Partin AW, Dmochowski RR, Kavoussi LR, Peters CA, eds. *Campbell-Walsh-Wein Urology.* 12th ed. Philadelphia: Elsevier; 2020:2722.

Behavioral Intervention: Pelvic Floor Muscle Training and Exercise

Alewijnse D, Mesters I, Metsemakers J, vanden Borne B. Predictors of long-term adherence to pelvic floor muscle exercise therapy among women with urinary incontinence. *Health Educ Res.* 2003;18:511.

Berghmans LC, Hendriks HJ, Bo K, et al. Conservative treatment of stress urinary incontinence in women: a systematic review of randomized clinical trials. *Br J Urol.* 1998;82:181.

Bo K, Herbert RD. There is not yet strong evidence that exercise regimens other than pelvic floor muscle training can reduce stress urinary incontinence in women: a systematic review. *J Physiother.* 2013;59:159.

Bo K, Morkved S, Frawley H, Sherburn M. Evidence for benefit of transversus abdominus training alone or in combination with pelvic floor muscle training to treat female urinary incontinence: a systematic review. *Neurourol Urodyn.* 2009;28:368.

Bo K, Talseth T. Single blind randomized controlled trial of pelvic floor exercises, electrical stimulation, vaginal cones, and no treatment in management of genuine stress incontinence in women. *BMJ.* 1999;318:487.

Bo K. Pelvic floor muscle exercise for the treatment of stress urinary incontinence: an exercise physiology perspective. *Int Urogynecol J.* 1995;6:282.

Bo K. Pelvic floor muscle training is effective in treatment of female stress urinary incontinence, but how does it work? *Int Urogynecol J Pelvic Floor Dysfunct.* 2004;15:76.

Borello-France D, Burgio KL, Goode PS, et al. Adherence to behavioral interventions for stress incontinence: rates, barriers, and predictors. *Phys Ther.* 2013;93:757.

Borello-France D, Burgio KL, Goode PS, et al. Adherence to behavioral interventions for urge incontinence when combined with drug therapy: adherence rates, barriers, and predictors. *Phys Ther.* 2010;90:1493.

Braekken IH, Majida M, Engh ME, Bo K. Can pelvic floor muscle training reverse pelvic organ prolapse and reduce prolapse symptoms? An assessor-blinded, randomized, controlled trial. *Am J Obstet Gynecol.* 2010a;203:170.

Braekken IH, Majida M, Engh ME, Bo K. Morphological changes after pelvic floor muscle training measured by 3-dimensional ultrasonography: a randomized controlled trial. *Obstet Gynecol.* 2010b;115:317.

Burgio KL, Pearce KL, Lucco AJ. *Staying Dry: A Practical Guide to Bladder Control.* Baltimore: Johns Hopkins Press; 1989:67.

Burgio KL, Goode PS, Locher JL, et al. Behavioral training with and without biofeedback in the treatment of urge incontinence in older women: a randomized controlled trial, *JAMA.* 2002;288:2293.

Burgio KL, Locher JL, Goode PS, et al. Behavioral versus drug treatment for urge incontinence in older women: a randomized clinical trial. *JAMA.* 1998;23:1995.

Deng DY. Urologic devices. In: Newman DK, Rovner ES, Wein AJ, eds. *Clinical Application of Urologic Catheters and Products.* Switzerland: Springer International Publishing; 2018:173.

Dmochowski R, Lynch CM, Efros M, Cardozo L. External electrical stimulation compared with intravaginal electrical stimulation for the treatment of stress urinary incontinence in women: a randomized controlled noninferiority trial. *Neurourol Urodyn.* 2019;38:1834.

Dumoulin C, Adewuyi T, Booth J, et al. Adult conservative management. In: Abrams P, Cardozo L, Wagg A, Wein A, eds. *Incontinence, 6th International Consultation on Incontinence.* Bristol, UK: International Continence Society; 2017:1443.

Dumoulin C, Alewijnse D, Bo K, et al. Pelvic-floor-muscle training adherence: tools, measurements and strategies-2011 ICS State-of-the-Science Seminar Research Paper II of IV. *Neurourol Urodyn.* 2015a;34:615.

Dumoulin C, Cacciari LP, Hay-Smith EJC. Pelvic floor muscle training versus no treatment, or inactive control treatments, for urinary incontinence in women. *Cochrane Database Syst Rev.* 2018;10:CD005654.

Dumoulin C, Hay-Smith J, Frawley H, et al. 2014 consensus statement on improving pelvic floor muscle training adherence: International Continence Society 2011 State-of-the-Science Seminar. *Neurourol Urodyn.* 2015b;34:600.

Dumoulin C, Hunter KF, Moore K, et al. Conservative management for female urinary incontinence and pelvic organ prolapse review 2013: Summary of the 5th International Consultation on Incontinence. *Neurourol Urodyn.* 2016;35:15.

Ghroubi S, Kharrot O, Chaari M, et al. Effect of conservative treatment in the management of low-degree urogenital prolapse. *Ann Readapt Med Phys.* 2008;51:96.

Glazener CM, Herbison GP, MacArthur C, et al. Randomized controlled trial of conservative management of postnatal urinary and faecal incontinence: six year follow-up. *BMJ.* 2005;330:337.

Goode PS, Burgio KL, Locher JL, et al. Behavioral training with and without pelvic floor electrical simulation in the behavioral treatment of stress incontinence in women: a randomized controlled trial. *JAMA.* 2003;290:345.

Gormley EA, Lightner DJ, Faraday M, Vasavada SP, American Urological Association, Society of Urodynamics Female Pelvic

Medicine. Diagnosis and treatment of overactive bladder (non-neurogenic) in adults: AUA/SUFU guideline amendment. *J Urol.* 2015;193:1572.

Hagen S, Stark D, Glazener C, et al. A randomized controlled trial of pelvic floor muscle training for stages I and II pelvic organ prolapse. *Int Urogynecol J Pelvic Floor Dysfunct.* 2009;20:45.

Hagen S, Stark D. Conservative prevention and management of pelvic organ prolapse in women. *Cochrane Database Syst Rev.* 2011; 12:CD003882.

Hahn I, Sommar S, Fall M. A comparative study of pelvic floor training and electrical stimulation for treatment of genuine female stress urinary incontinence. *Neurourol Urodyn.* 1991;10:545.

Hartmann KE, McPheeters ML, Biller DH, et al. *Treatment of Overactive Bladder in Women. Evidence Report/Technology Assessment Number 187 (Prepared by the Vanderbilt Evidence-based Practice Center under Contract No. 290-2007-10065-I).* Rockville, MD: Agency for Healthcare Research and Quality (AHRQ); 2009.

Herbison GP, Dean N. Weighted vaginal cones for urinary incontinence. *Cochrane Database Syst Rev.* 2013;(7):CD002114.

Huffman JW, Osborne SL, Sokol JK. Electrical stimulation in treatment of intractable stress incontinence. *Arch Phys Med.* 1952;33:674.

Kegel AH. Progressive resistance exercise in the functional restoration of the perineal muscles. *Am J Obstet Gynecol.* 1948;56:238.

Kegel AH. Stress incontinence of urine in women: physiologic treatment. *J Int Coll Surg.* 1956;25:487.

Miller JM, Ashton-Miller JA, DeLancey JO. A pelvic muscle precontraction can reduce cough-related urine loss in selected women with mild SUI. *J Am Geriatr Soc.* 1998;46:870.

Miller JM, Sampselle C, Ashton-Miller J, et al. Clarification and confirmation of the Knack maneuver: the effect of volitional pelvic floor muscle contraction to preempt expected stress incontinence. *Int Urogynecol J Pelvic Floor Dysfunct.* 2008;19:773.

Moore T, Schofield PF. Treatment of stress incontinence by maximum perineal electrical stimulation. *Br Med J.* 1967;3:150.

Morkved S, Bo K. Effect of postpartum pelvic floor muscle training in prevention and treatment of urinary incontinence: a one-year follow-up. *Br J Obstet Gynaecol.* 2000;107:1022.

Newman DK, Borello-France D, Sung VW. Structured behavioral treatment research protocol for women with mixed urinary incontinence and overactive bladder symptoms. *Neurourol Urodyn.* 2018;37:14.

Newman DK, Burgio KL. Conservative management of urinary incontinence: behavioral and pelvic floor therapy and urethral and pelvic devices. In: Partin AW, Dmochowski RR, Kavoussi LR, Peters CA, eds. *Campbell-Walsh-Wein Urology*, 12th ed. Philadelphia: Elsevier; 2020:2722.

NIH Consensus Conference. Urinary incontinence in adults. *JAMA.* 1989;261:2685.

Piya-Anant M, Therasakvichya S, Leelaphatanadit C, Techatrisak K. Integrated health research program for the Thai elderly: prevalence of genital prolapse and effectiveness of pelvic floor exercise to prevent worsening of genital prolapse in elderly women. *J Med Assoc Thai.* 2003;86:509.

Richter HE, Burgio KL, Brubaker L, et al. Continence pessary compared with behavioral therapy or combined therapy for stress incontinence. *Obstet Gynecol.* 2010;115:609.

Stewart F, Berghmans B, Bo K, Glazener CMA. Electrical stimulation with non-implantable devices for stress urinary incontinence in women. *Cochrane Database Syst Rev.* 2017;12:CD012390.

Sung MS, Hong JY, Choi YH, et al. FES-biofeedback versus intensive pelvic floor muscle exercise for the prevention and treatment of genuine stress incontinence. *J Korean Med Sci.* 2000;15:303.

Woodley SJ, Boyle R, Cody JD, et al. Pelvic floor muscle training for prevention and treatment of urinary and faecal incontinence in antenatal and postnatal women. *Cochrane Database Syst Rev.* 2017;12:CD007471.

Yamanishi T, Yasuda K, Sakakibara R, et al. Pelvic floor electrical stimulation in the treatment of stress incontinence: an investigational study and a placebo controlled double-blind trial. *J Urol.* 1997;158:2127.

Weight Loss and Urinary Incontinence

Brown J, Grady D, Ouslander J, et al. Prevalence of urinary incontinence and associated risk factors in postmenopausal women. Heart & Estrogen/Progestin Replacement Study (HERS) Research Group. *Obstet Gynecol.* 1999;94:66.

Brown J, Seeley D, Feng J, et al. Urinary incontinence in older women: who is at risk? Study of Osteoporotic Fractures Research Group. *Obstet Gynecol.* 1996;87:715.

Bump R, Sugerman H, Fantl J, et al. Obesity and lower urinary tract function in women: effect of surgically induced weight loss. *Am J Obstet Gynecol.* 1992;166:392.

Burgio KL, Richter HE, Clements RH, et al. Changes in urinary and fecal incontinence symptoms with weight loss surgery in morbidly obese women. *Obstet Gynecol.* 2007;110:1034.

Deitel M, Stone E, Kassam HA, et al. Gynecologic-obstetric changes after loss of massive excess weight following bariatric surgery. *J Am Coll Nutr.* 1988;7:147.

Dumoulin C, Hunter KF, Moore K, et al. Conservative management for female urinary incontinence and pelvic organ prolapse review 2013: Summary of the 5th International Consultation on Incontinence. *Neurourol Urodyn.* 2016;35:15.

Hunskaar S. A systematic review of overweight and obesity as risk factors and targets for clinical intervention for urinary incontinence in women. *Neurourol Urodyn.* 2008;27:749.

Nambiar AK, Bosch R, Cruz F, et al. EAU guidelines on assessment and nonsurgical management of urinary incontinence. *Eur Urol.* 2018;73:596.

Phelan S, Kanaya AM, Subak LL, et al. Weight loss prevents urinary incontinence in women with type 2 diabetes; results from the Look AHEAD trial. *J Urol.* 2012;187:939.

Subak LL, Johnson C, Whitcomb E, et al. Does weight loss improve incontinence in moderately obese women? *Int Urogynecol J Pelvic Floor Dysfunct.* 2002;13:40.

Subak LL, Richter HE, Hunskaar S. Obesity and urinary incontinence: epidemiology and clinical research update. *J Urol.* 2009a;182:2.

Subak LL, Whitcomb E, Shen H, et al. Weight loss: a novel and effective treatment for urinary incontinence. *J Urol.* 2005;174:190.

Subak LL, Wing R, West DS, et al. Weight loss to treat urinary incontinence in overweight and obese women. *N Engl J Med.* 2009b;360:481.

Wing RR, West DS, Grady D, et al. Effect of weight loss on urinary incontinence in overweight and obese women: results at 12 and 18 months. *J Urol.* 2010;184:1005.

Zhang J, Gao L, Liu M, Liu C. Effect of bariatric surgery on urinary incontinence in women: a meta-analysis and systematic review. *Female Pelvic Med Reconstr Surg.* 2020;26:207.

Complementary and Alternative Therapies for Urinary Incontinence

Knardahl S, Elam M, Olausson B, Wallin BG. Sympathetic nerve activity after acupuncture in humans. *Pain.* 1998;75:19.

Taneja DK. Yoga and health. *Indian J Community Med.* 2014;39:68.

Wang Y, Zhishun L, Peng W, et al. Acupuncture for stress urinary incontinence in adults. *Cochrane Database Syst Rev.* 2013;7:CD009408.

Wieland LS, Shrestha N, Lassi ZS, et al. Yoga for treating urinary incontinence in women. *Cochrane Database Syst Rev.* 2019;2:CD012668.

Estrogen and Stress Urinary Incontinence

Cody JD, Jacobs ML, Richardson K, et al. Oestrogen therapy for urinary incontinence in post-menopausal women. *Cochrane Database Syst Rev.* 2012;10:CD001405.

Ewies AA, Alfhaily F. Topical vaginal estrogen therapy in managing postmenopausal urinary symptoms: a reality or a gimmick? *Climacteric.* 2010;13:405.

Rahn DD, Carberry C, Sanses TV, et al. Vaginal estrogen for genitourinary syndrome of menopause: a systematic review. *Obstet Gynecol.* 2014;124:1147.

Rahn DD, Ward RM, Sanses TV, et al. Vaginal estrogen use in postmenopausal women with pelvic floor disorders: a systematic review and practice guidelines. *Int Urogynecol J.* 2015;26:3.

Other Pharmacologic Therapies

Alhasso A, Glazener CMA, Pickard R, et al. Adrenergic drugs for urinary incontinence in adults (Cochrane review). In: *Cochrane Library, Issue 2.* Chichester, England: John Wiley & Sons, Ltd; 2005.

Andersson KE, Chapple CR, Cardozo L, et al. Pharmacological treatment of urinary incontinence. In: Abrams P, Cardozo L, Khoury S, Wein A, eds. *Incontinence: 4th International Consultation on Incontinence.* Birmingham, UK: Health Publication Ltd; 2009.

Cannon TW, Chancellor MB. Pharmacotherapy for stress urinary incontinence. *Rev Urol.* 2003;5:135.

Cannon TW, Yoshimura N, Chancellor MB. Innovations in pharmacotherapy for stress urinary incontinence. *Int Urogynecol J.* 2003;14:367.

Kornholt J, Sonne DP, Riis T, et al. Effect of imipramine on urethral opening pressure: a randomized, double-blind, placebo-controlled crossover study in healthy women. *Neurourol Urodyn.* 2019;38:1076.

Li J, Yang L, Pu C, et al. The role of duloxetine in stress urinary incontinence: a systematic review and meta-analysis. *Int Urol Nephrol.* 2013;45:679.

Mariappan P, Alhasso AA, Grant A, N'Dow JMO. Serotonin and noradrenaline reuptake inhibitors (SNRI) for stress urinary incontinence in adults. *Cochrane Database Syst Rev.* 2005;3:CD004742.

Shamliyan TA, Kane RL, Wyman J, Wilt TJ. Systematic review: randomized, controlled trials of nonsurgical treatments for urinary incontinence in women. *Ann Intern Med.* 2008;148:459.

Urethral Devices

Cottenden A, Bliss DZ, Buckley M, et al. Management using continence products. In Abrams P, Cardozo L, Khoury S, Wein A, eds. *Incontinence: 4th International Consultation on Incontinence.* Birmingham, UK: Health Publication Ltd; 2009.

Dunn M, Brandt D, Nygaard I. Treatment of exercise incontinence with a urethral insert: a pilot study in women. *Phys Sportsmed.* 2002;30:45.

Lipp A, Shaw C, Glavind K. Mechanical devices for urinary incontinence in women. *Cochrane Database Syst Rev.* 2014;12:CD001756.

Ins and Outs of Pessary Use

Al-Shaikh G, Syed S, Osman S, et al. Pessary use in stress urinary incontinence: a review of advantages, complications, patient satisfaction, and quality of life. *Int J Womens Health.* 2018;10:195.

American College of Obstetricians and Gynecologists' Committee on Practice Bulletins—Gynecology and American Urogynecologic Society. Pelvic Organ Prolapse: ACOG Practice Bulletin, Number 214. *Obstet Gynecol.* 2019;134(5):e126.

Cheung RY, Lee JH, Lee LL, et al. Vaginal pessary in women with symptomatic pelvic organ prolapse: a randomized controlled trial. *Obstet Gynecol.* 2016;128:73.

Clemons JL, Aguilar VC, Tillinghast TA, et al. Risk factors associated with an unsuccessful pessary fitting trial in women with pelvic organ prolapse. *Am J Obstet Gynecol.* 2004a;190:345.

Clemons J, Aguilar VC, Tillinghast TA, et al. Patient satisfaction and changes in prolapse and urinary symptoms in women who were fitted successfully with a pessary for pelvic organ prolapse. *Am J Obstet Gynecol.* 2004b;190:1025.

Cundiff GW, Amundsen CL, Bent AE, et al. The PESSRI study: symptom relief outcomes of a randomized crossover trial of the ring and Gellhorn pessaries. *Am J Obstet Gynecol.* 2007;196:405.e1.

Cundiff GW, Weidner AC, Visco AG, et al. A survey of pessary use by members of the American Gynecologic Society. *Obstet Gynecol.* 2000;95:931.

Donnelly MJ, Powell-Morgan S, Olsen AL, Nygaard IE. Vaginal pessaries for the management of stress and mixed urinary incontinence. *Int Urogynecol J Pelvic Floor Dysfunct.* 2004;15:302.

Farrell SA, Singh B, Aldakhil L. Continence pessaries in the management of urinary incontinence in women. *J Obstet Gynaecol Can.* 2004;26:113.

Kenton K, Barber M, Wang L, et al. Pelvic floor symptoms improve similarly after pessary and behavioral treatment for stress incontinence. *Female Pelvic Med Reconstr Surg.* 2012;18:118.

LeKan-Rutledge D, Doughty D, Moore KN, Wooldridge L. Promoting social continence: products and devices in the management of urinary incontinence. *Urol Nurs.* 2003;23:416.

Lipp A, Shaw C, Glavind K. Mechanical devices for urinary incontinence in women. *Cochrane Database Syst Rev.* 2014;12:CD001756.

Lone F, Thakar R, Sultan AH, et al. A 5-year prospective study of vaginal pessary use for pelvic organ prolapse. *Int J Gynaecol Obstet.* 2011;114:56.

Mao M, Xu T, Kang, J, et al. Factors associated with long-term pessary use in women with symptomatic pelvic organ prolapse. *Climacteric.* 2019;22:478.

Newman DK, Burgio KL. Conservative management of urinary incontinence: behavioral and pelvic floor therapy and urethral and pelvic devices. In: Partin AW, Dmochowski RR, Kavoussi LR, Peters CA, eds. *Campbell-Walsh-Wein Urology,* 12th ed. Philadelphia: Elsevier; 2020:2722.

O'Dell K, Atnip S, Hooper G, Leung K. Pessary practices of nurse-providers in the United States. *Female Pelvic Med Reconstr Surg.* 2016;22:261.

Palumbo MV. Pessary placement and management. *Ostomy Wound Manage.* 2000;46:40.

Panman CM, Wiegersma M, Kollen BJ, et al. Effectiveness and cost-effectiveness of pessary treatment compared with pelvic floor muscle training in older women with pelvic organ prolapse: 2-year follow-up of a randomized controlled trial in primary care. *Menopause.* 2016;23:1307.

Poma PA. Nonsurgical management of genital prolapse. A review and recommendations for clinical practice. *J Reprod Med.* 2000;45:789.

Probst K, Mellen C, O'Sullivan DM, et al. Timing of office-based pessary care: a randomized controlled trial. *Obstet Gynecol.* 2020;135:100.

Richter HE, Burgio KL, Brubaker L, et al. Continence pessary compared with behavioral therapy or combined therapy for stress incontinence. *Obstet Gynecol.* 2010;115:609.

Robert M, Mainprize TC. Long-term assessment of the incontinence ring pessary for the treatment of stress incontinence. *Int Urogynecol J.* 2002;13:326.

Robert M, Schulz JA, Harvey MA, Urogynaecology Committee. Technical update on pessary use. *J Obstet Gynaecol Can.* 2013;35:664.

Schaffer J, Nager CW, Xiang F, et al. Predictors of success and satisfaction of non-surgical therapy for stress urinary incontinence. *Obstet Gynecol.* 2012;120:91.

Tam MS, Lee VYT, Yu ELM, et al. The effect of time interval of vaginal ring pessary replacement for pelvic organ prolapse on complications and patient satisfaction: a randomised controlled trial. *Maturitas.* 2019;128:29.

Wolff B, Williams K, Winkler A, et al. Pessary types and discontinuation rates in patients with advanced pelvic organ prolapse. *Int Urogynecol J.* 2017;28:993.

Ziv E, Stanton SL, Abarbanel J. Efficacy and safety of a novel disposable intravaginal device for treating stress urinary incontinence. *Am J Obstet Gynecol.* 2008;198:594.e1.

Ziv E, Stanton SL, Abarbanel J. Significant improvement in the quality of life in women treated with a novel disposable intravaginal device for stress urinary incontinence. *Int Urogynecol J.* 2009;20:651.

15

Retropubic Operations for Stress Urinary Incontinence

Mark D. Walters

CHAPTER OUTLINE

INTRODUCTION

Since 1949, when Marshall et al. first described retropubic urethrovesical suspension for the treatment of stress urinary incontinence (SUI), retropubic procedures have proved to be consistently curative. Although numerous terminologies and variations of retropubic repairs have been described, the basic goal remains the same: to suspend and stabilize the anterior vaginal wall, and thus the bladder neck and proximal urethra, in a retropubic position. This prevents their descent and allows urethral compression against a stable suburethral layer. Selection of a retropubic approach (versus a vaginal approach) depends on many factors, such as the need for laparotomy or laparoscopy for other pelvic prolapse or disease, the amount of pelvic organ prolapse, the status of the intrinsic urethral sphincter mechanism, the age and health status of the patient, any history of previous sling or mesh complications, the patient's desire for future fertility, the preference and expertise of the surgeon, and the preferences of an informed patient.

Historically, few data differentiated one retropubic procedure from another. The three most studied and popular retropubic procedures were the Burch colposuspension, the Marshall–Marchetti–Krantz (MMK) procedure, and the paravaginal defect repair. We no longer perform the MMK procedure, so this operation will not be described. We prefer the Burch colposuspension for urodynamic stress incontinence with bladder neck hypermobility and adequate resting urethral sphincter function, and sometimes combine it with a paravaginal defect repair when the patient has stage II or III anterior vaginal prolapse or when a concurrent sacrocolpopexy is to be done. The surgical techniques described here are contemporary modifications of the original operations: Tanagho (1976) described the modified Burch colposuspension; and the paravaginal defect repair was described by Richardson et al. (1981) and Shull and Baden (1989) (paravaginal repair), and by Turner-Warwick (1986) and Webster and Kreder (1990) (vaginal obturator shelf repair). Although less critically studied, the paravaginal defect repair was regionally popular and widely performed in the United States. The operations described do not represent one correct technique, but a commonly used and proven method.

This chapter describes retropubic suspension procedures that use an abdominal wall incision for direct access into the space of Retzius. The use of laparoscopy, robotic assistance, and mini-incision laparotomy to enter the retropubic space and perform these and similar procedures is usually preferred, and is based on whether other concurrent surgeries need to be done and on what is most desired by and possible for the surgeon and the informed patient. For a review of retropubic anatomy, see Video 15.1.

INDICATIONS FOR RETROPUBIC PROCEDURES

Retropubic urethrovesical suspension procedures are indicated for women with the diagnosis of urodynamic SUI and a hypermobile proximal urethra and bladder neck. It is now most frequently used for patients with SUI who have contraindications to or who do not desire a mesh sling, or for those having concomitant laparoscopic or open procedures. Although retropubic procedures can be used for intrinsic sphincter deficiency with urethral hypermobility, other, more obstructive, operations such as a retropubic bladder neck or midurethral sling probably yield better long-term results.

To diagnose urodynamic SUI, clinical and urodynamic (simple or complex) tests must be performed to evaluate bladder filling, storage, and emptying. Clinically, the urethra is shown to be incompetent by visually observing loss of urine simultaneous with increases in intraabdominal pressure (a positive cough stress test). Urodynamics may also be used for diagnosis. Abnormalities of bladder-filling function, such as detrusor overactivity, can coexist with urethral sphincter incompetence in up to 30% of patients and may be associated with a lower cure rate after retropubic surgery.

Women with SUI should generally have a trial of conservative therapy before corrective surgery is offered. Conservative treatment comes in the form of pelvic muscle exercises, bladder retraining, pharmacologic therapy, and mechanical devices such as pessaries. Eligible and willing postmenopausal patients with atrophic urogenital changes should be prescribed vaginal estrogen before surgery is considered.

SURGICAL TECHNIQUES

Operative Setup and General Entry into the Retropubic Space

The patient is supine with the legs supported in a slightly abducted position, allowing the surgeon to operate with one hand in the vagina and the other in the retropubic space. The vagina, perineum, and abdomen are sterilely prepped and draped in a fashion that permits easy access to the lower abdomen and vagina. A three-way 16- or 20-French Foley catheter with a 20- to 30-mL balloon is inserted sterilely into the bladder and kept in the sterile field. The drainage port of the catheter is left to gravity drainage, and the irrigation port is connected to sterile water, with or without blue dye, as desired. One perioperative intravenous dose of an appropriate antibiotic should be given as prophylaxis against infection within 1 hour before the incision is made. Appropriate thromboprophylaxis is given.

A small Pfannenstiel incision is made. During intraperitoneal surgery, the peritoneum is opened, the surgery is completed, and the cul-de-sac is plicated, if necessary. The retropubic space is then exposed. Staying close to the back of the pubic bone, the surgeon's hand is introduced into the retropubic space, and the bladder and urethra are gently moved downward. Sharp dissection is not usually necessary in primary cases. To aid visualization of the bladder, 100 mL sterile water with methylene blue or indigo carmine dye may be instilled into the bladder after the catheter drainage port is clamped.

If the surgery is being done with laparoscopy or with robotic assistance, the intraperitoneal ports are placed as preferred by the surgeon, and the bladder is filled with 200 to 300 mL sterile water. An incision in the anterior abdominal wall peritoneum 2 to 3 cm above the bladder is made between the umbilical ligaments and, using mostly blunt dissection, the bladder is pushed downward, exposing the retropubic space. The surgeon should mostly dissect in the midline toward the pubic symphysis, then bluntly dissect bilaterally until both Cooper's ligaments and obturator internus muscles are seen and cleared of areolar tissue. Suturing and knot-tying are done endoscopically using standard techniques noted later.

If previous retropubic sling or other bladder neck suspension procedures have been performed, dense adhesions and/or mesh fragments from the anterior vaginal and bladder wall and urethra to the symphysis pubis are often present. These adhesions and/or mesh should be dissected sharply from the pubic bone until the anterior bladder wall, urethra, and vagina are free of adhesions and are mobile. Mesh strips from prior slings can be removed if necessary. If identification of the urethra or lower border of the bladder is difficult, one may perform a small cystotomy, which, with a finger inside the bladder, helps to define the bladder's lower limits for easier dissection, mobilization, and elevation.

Burch Colposuspension

After the retropubic space is entered, the urethra and anterior vaginal wall are depressed. Minimal dissection should be performed in the midline over the urethra or at the urethrovesical junction, thus protecting the delicate musculature of the urethra from surgical trauma. Attention is directed toward the tissue on either side of the urethra. The surgeon's nondominant hand is placed in the vagina, palm facing upward, with the index and middle fingers on each side of the proximal urethra. Most of the overlying fat should be cleared away, using a swab mounted on a curved forceps. This dissection is accomplished with forceful elevation of the surgeon's vaginal finger until glistening white periurethral fascia and vaginal wall are seen (Fig. 15.1). This area is extremely vascular, with a rich, thin-walled venous plexus that should be avoided, if possible. The position of the urethra and the lower edge of the bladder is determined by palpating the Foley balloon and by partially distending the bladder to define the rounded lower margin of the bladder as it meets the anterior vaginal wall.

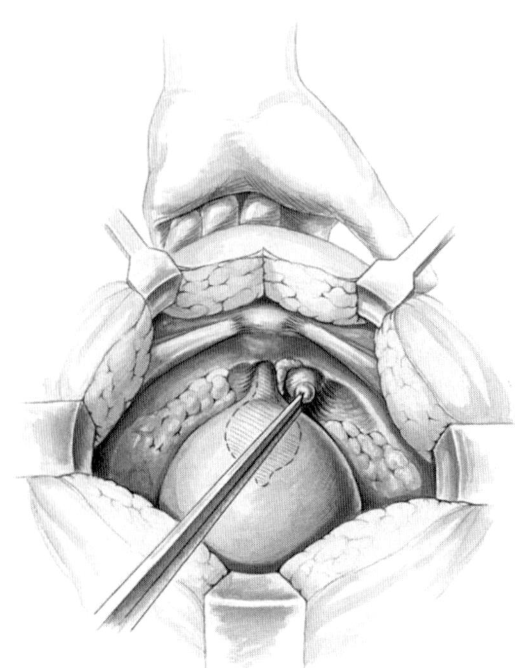

Fig. 15.1 Dissection of the lateral retropubic space. After forceful elevation of the surgeon's finger placed vaginally, the fat overlying the glistening white periurethral fascia is cleared in preparation for suture placement.

Once dissection lateral to the urethra is completed and vaginal mobility is judged to be adequate by using the vaginal fingers to lift the anterior vaginal wall upward and forward, sutures are placed. No. 0 or 1 delayed absorbable or nonabsorbable suture is placed as far laterally in the anterior vaginal wall as is technically possible. We apply two sutures of No. 0 braided polyester on an SH needle (Ethibond; Ethicon, Inc., Somerville, NJ) bilaterally, using double bites for each suture. The distal suture is placed approximately 2 cm lateral to the proximal third of the urethra. The proximal suture is placed approximately 2 cm lateral to the bladder wall at or slightly proximal to the level of the urethrovesical junction. When placing the sutures, one should take a full thickness of vaginal wall, excluding the epithelium, with the needle parallel to the urethra (Fig. 15.2, inset). This maneuver is best accomplished by suturing over the surgeon's vaginal finger at the appropriate selected sites. On each side, after the two sutures are placed, they are passed through the pectineal (Cooper's) ligament so that all four suture ends exit above the ligament (Fig. 15.2). Before the sutures are tied, a 1 × 4 cm strip of Gelfoam may be placed, if desired, between the vagina and obturator fascia below the Cooper's ligament to aid adherence and hemostasis.

As noted previously, this area is extremely vascular, and visible vessels should be avoided when possible. When excessive bleeding occurs, it can be controlled by direct pressure, sutures, application of thrombotic agents, or vascular clips. Less severe bleeding usually stops with direct pressure and after tying the suspension sutures.

After all four sutures are placed in the vagina and through the Cooper's ligaments, the assistant ties first the distal sutures and then the proximal ones, while the surgeon elevates the vagina with the vaginal hand. When tying the sutures, one does not have to be concerned about whether the vaginal wall meets the Cooper's ligament, so one should not place too much tension on the vaginal wall. A suture bridge is usually found between the two points. After the sutures are tied, one can easily insert two fingers between the pubic bone and the urethra, thus preventing compression of the urethra against the pubic bone. Vaginal fixation and urethral support depend more on fibrosis and scarring of periurethral and vaginal tissues over the obturator internus and levator fascia than on the suture material itself.

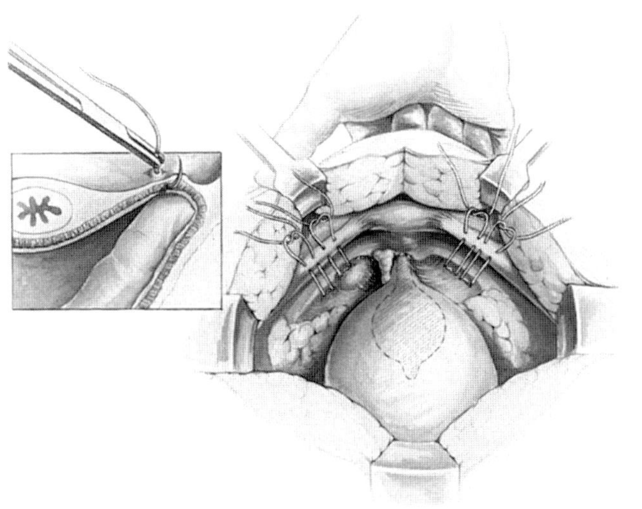

Fig. 15.2 Technique of Burch colposuspension. After the two sutures are placed on each side, they are passed through the pectineal (Cooper's) ligament, so that all four suture ends exit above the ligament to facilitate knot tying. *Inset:* When placing the sutures, one should take a full thickness of vaginal wall, excluding the epithelium, with the needle parallel to the urethra. This maneuver is best achieved by suturing over the finger placed vaginally.

Video 15.2 demonstrates our technique for laparoscopic Burch colposuspension

Paravaginal Defect Repair

The object of the paravaginal defect repair is to reattach, bilaterally, the anterolateral vaginal sulcus with its overlying endopelvic fascia to the pubococcygeus and obturator internus muscles and fascia at the level of the arcus tendineus fasciae pelvis. The retropubic space is entered, and the bladder and vagina are depressed and pulled medially to allow visualization of the lateral retropubic space, including the obturator internus and levator muscles, and the fossa containing the obturator neurovascular bundle. Blunt dissection can be carried dorsally from this point until the ischial spine is palpated. The arcus tendineus fasciae pelvis is often visualized as a white band of tissue running over the pubococcygeus and obturator internus muscles from the back of the lower edge of the symphysis pubis toward the ischial spine. A lateral paravaginal defect representing avulsion of the vagina off the arcus tendineus fasciae pelvis or of the arcus tendineus fasciae pelvis off the obturator internus muscle may be visualized (Fig. 15.3).

The surgeon's nondominant hand is inserted into the vagina. While gently retracting the vagina and bladder medially, the surgeon elevates the anterolateral vaginal sulcus. Starting near the vaginal apex, a suture is placed, first through the full thickness of the vagina (excluding the vaginal epithelium) and then deep into the obturator internus fascia or arcus tendineus fasciae pelvis, 1 to 2 cm anterior to its origin at the ischial spine. After this first stitch is tied, additional (3–5) sutures are placed through the vaginal wall and overlying fascia and then into the

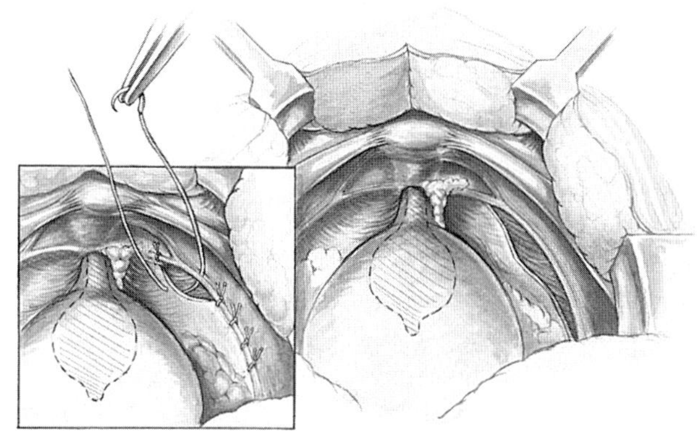

Fig. 15.3 Lateral paravaginal defect and technique of paravaginal defect repair. Five or six sutures are placed, first through the full thickness of the vagina (excluding the vaginal epithelium) and then into the obturator internus fascia or arcus tendineus fasciae pelvis, 3–4 cm below the obturator fossa.

obturator internus at about 1-cm intervals toward the pubic ramus (Fig. 15.3, inset). The most distal sutures should be placed as close as possible to the pubic ramus, into the pubo-urethral ligament; alternatively, Burch colposuspension sutures can be placed bilaterally at the level of the bladder neck and urethra if the patient has SUI. No. 2-0 or 0 delayed absorbable or nonabsorbable suture on a medium-sized, tapered needle is usually used for the paravaginal repair.

This procedure leaves free space between the symphysis pubis and the proximal urethra, but also provides secure support so that rotational descent of the proximal urethra and bladder base is prevented with sudden increases in intraabdominal pressure. According to Turner-Warwick (1986), this avoids overcorrection and fixation of the periurethral fascia, which might compromise the functional movements of the urethra and bladder base and lead to obstruction and voiding difficulty. This principle may explain why the paravaginal defect repair usually results in spontaneous voiding on the first or second postoperative day. In fact, the vaginal obturator shelf repair was used to correct dysfunctional voiding symptoms in patients after previous retropubic surgery. Video 19.5 in Chapter 19 demonstrates the technique of laparoscopic paravaginal repair.

General Intraoperative and Postoperative Procedures

To make sure that intravesical suture placement or ureteral obstruction has not occurred, cystoscopy (or a small cystotomy) should be performed to document ureteral patency and the absence of intravesical sutures after retropubic procedures. Intravenous injection of an appropriate dye before cystoscopy aids visualization of urine from the ureters.

Closed suction drains in the retropubic space are used only as necessary when hemostasis is incomplete and there is concern about postoperative hematoma. The bladder is routinely drained with a suprapubic or transurethral catheter for 1 to 2 days. After that time, the patient is allowed to begin voiding trials, and post-void residual urine volumes are checked, either with the suprapubic catheter or by intermittent self-catheterization.

CLINICAL RESULTS

Many early studies reported clinical experiences with retropubic urethral suspension procedures for SUI. Quality studies, including prospective randomized trials, have been conducted comparing Burch colposuspension to synthetic midurethral and fascial slings. Only a few studies have assessed the paravaginal defect repair for SUI. Studies using subjective outcome measures generally report that over 90% of women are continent after this procedure. However, in a prospective randomized trial, Columbo et al. (1996) found that only 61% of women were continent 3 years after a paravaginal defect repair, compared with 100% of women continent after a Burch colposuspension. We currently believe that the paravaginal defect repair should be used only selectively for anatomic correction of anterior vaginal wall prolapse, but not as primary treatment of SUI.

Multiple studies with objective measures of cure reported that the Burch colposuspension is effective for women with urodynamic SUI. At 3 to 24 months after surgery, 59% to 100% of patients became continent, for an overall average cure rate of about 85%. At 3 to 7 years, continence rates range from 63% to 89%, for an average rate of 77%. Although objectively incontinent, a small percentage of additional patients were judged to be improved and were satisfied with the surgical results. The overall reported absolute failure rate is about 14% at 5 to 7 years.

In an excellent study, Eriksen et al. (1990) reported on 91 women with urodynamic SUI, with or without detrusor overactivity, who had undergone Burch colposuspension. Urodynamic evaluation was done on 76 patients after 5 years. Stress incontinence was cured in 71% of patients with stable bladders preoperatively and in 57% of those with mixed stress incontinence and detrusor overactivity, a nonsignificant difference. After 5 years, only 52% of the study group was completely dry and free of complications; about 30% needed further incontinence therapy.

Several studies assessed women more than 10 years after undergoing a Burch procedure. Alcalay et al. (1995) followed a cohort of 109 women (out of a group of 366 eligible women) who underwent Burch colposuspension between 1974 and 1983. The mean follow-up interval was 13.8 years. Both subjective and objective outcome measures were collected during the follow-up period. The cure of incontinence was found to be time-dependent, with a decline for 10 to 12 years and then a plateau at 69%. Cure rates were significantly lower in women who had had previous bladder neck surgery. Approximately 10% of patients required at least one additional surgery to cure stress incontinence. Confirming this, Jonsson Funk et al. (2012) showed that, after 9 years, only 10.8% of women had repeat surgery for stress incontinence after a Burch procedure.

In the first prospective, multicenter, randomized trial of open Burch colposuspension and tension-free vaginal tape (TVT) for urodynamic stress incontinence, Ward and Hilton (2002) found no significant difference between surgeries in terms of objective cure rates. Bladder injury was more common during the TVT procedure; delayed voiding, operation time, and return to normal activity were all longer after colposuspension. When these authors analyzed their data at 2 years and ignored subject withdrawals, no differences were seen between procedures, with objective cure rates of 81% for TVT and 80% for colposuspension. Jelovsek et al. (2008) reported that laparoscopic Burch also had similar long-term efficacy as TVT sling after 4 to 8 years' follow-up.

In 2007, Albo et al., representing the Urinary Incontinence Treatment Network, published a definitive multicenter, randomized, clinical trial comparing Burch colposuspension with autologous rectus fascia pubovaginal sling. A total of 655 women were randomized and observed for 24 months. Cure rates of SUI (using strict definitions) were lower for women who underwent the Burch colposuspension (49% vs. 66%; $P < .001$). However, more women who underwent the sling procedure had complications, such as urinary tract infections, voiding dysfunction, and postoperative urge incontinence.

The Cochrane review from 2017 examined 55 trials involving a total of 5417 women and concluded that open Burch colposuspension is effective for SUI, especially in the long term. Continence rates at 1 year are approximately 85% to 90%, and at 5 years are about 70%. In 2010, Novara et al. published a systematic review and meta-analysis of the comparative data on colposuspensions compared with all slings. They concluded that patients treated with retropubic midurethral slings experienced slightly higher continence rates than those treated with Burch colposuspension, but that bladder perforations were more common with retropubic slings. This general finding has since been verified, although the difference in cure rates between the procedures is small, perhaps 5%. A study of the Danish National Patient Registry by Foss Hansen et al. (2016) showed the 5-year reoperation rates for pubovaginal slings, retropubic midurethral slings, and Burch procedures to be similar at 6%, with transobturator slings at 9% and urethral bulking at 44%. Another study using the Finnish national registry showed the 10-year reoperation rate to be higher for Burch than for retropubic slings (8.3/1000 woman-years vs. 4.8/1000 woman-years).

For years, Burch colposuspension was the antiincontinence procedure of choice in women who had an open abdominal sacrocolpopexy (ASC). There has been a recent reevaluation of this, both for women with clinical or occult SUI and for those who are continent. Brubaker et al. (2008) showed improved continence rates when a Burch colposuspension was done with ASC, whether or not the patient had SUI. This advantage of adding Burch to ASC has not been universally reported, so the use of this as a prophylactic antiincontinence procedure performed at the same time as ASC remains controversial. Midurethral slings are now frequently combined with ASC to treat clinical and occult SUI. Several reviews, including one from the Cochrane database, conclude that adding an antiincontinence procedure (Burch or sling) to ASC reduces the risk of postoperative SUI, but that short-term voiding difficulties and adverse events are more frequent. This should be discussed with the patient in counseling, noting that it is also reasonable to postpone the procedure for SUI and do it in a second surgery later if needed.

Clinical conditions that increase the risk of surgical failure for retropubic colposuspension are shown in Box 15.1. They include baseline urge symptoms, obesity, menopause, prior hysterectomy, prior antiincontinence procedures, and more advanced prolapse. Advanced age and concomitant hysterectomy do not appear to be associated with lower rates of cure after colposuspension. Urodynamic findings that increase the risk of surgical failure include signs of intrinsic urethral sphincter deficiency (however defined), abnormal perineal electromyography, and concurrent overactive bladder. Patients with intrinsic sphincter deficiency probably are better treated with a more obstructive operation such as a sling procedure if the urethra is hypermobile, or with urethral injections of a bulking agent if the urethra is nonmobile.

Detrusor overactivity or urge incontinence may coexist in up to 30% of patients with urodynamic SUI. The term mixed incontinence is used to describe this condition. In addition, about 15% of patients with urodynamic SUI who preoperatively had a stable cystometrogram develop *de novo* detrusor overactivity after a colposuspension procedure. The course of the overactive bladder after a retropubic repair in patients with mixed incontinence is unpredictable. Interestingly, some studies demonstrate that 50% to 60% of patients with mixed incontinence are cured of overactive bladder symptoms by surgical support of the bladder neck. A much smaller percentage (~5%–10%) have worsening of urgency, and the remainder (20%–30%) have persistence. Unfortunately, preoperative urodynamic parameters do not accurately predict the course of overactive bladder after incontinence surgery. For this reason, we believe that women with mixed incontinence should initially receive nonsurgical therapy. Karram and Bhatia (1989) found that 32% of women with mixed incontinence became dry after nonsurgical therapy. These data suggest that initial nonsurgical therapy will save up to one-third of patients the cost and morbidity of incontinence surgery.

BOX 15.1 Conditions that Decrease the Chance of Cure of Incontinence After Retropubic Colposuspension

Clinical

Greater baseline urge incontinent symptoms
Hypoestrogenic state—not receiving hormone replacement therapy
Obesity
Prior hysterectomy
Prior procedures to correct stress urinary incontinence
More advanced prolapse

Urodynamic

Detrusor overactivity (preoperative or postoperative)
Intrinsic urethral sphincter deficiency
Lower maximal urethral pressure
Lower leak point pressure
Lower functional urethral length
Open bladder neck at rest on video-urodynamics
Nonmobile bladder neck
Abnormal perineal electromyography

Surgical

Intraoperative blood loss >1000 mL
Concurrent abdominal sacrocolpopexy

MECHANISMS OF CURE

Retropubic suspension procedures elevate and stabilize the bladder neck and proximal urethra in a high retropubic position. This results, at least partially, in mechanical compression of the urethra against the stable, elevated anterior vaginal wall and/or the posterosuperior aspect of the symphysis pubis during episodes of increased abdominal pressure. The principal urodynamic change in urethrovesical function postoperatively, although no longer commonly measured, is increased pressure transmission to the urethra, relative to the bladder, during elevations in intraabdominal pressure. Resting urethral pressure and functional urethral length are unchanged, which suggests that the intrinsic function of the urethra is not altered appreciably by this type of surgery. If the retropubic procedure fails to elevate and stabilize the urethra, the patient may continue to have stress incontinence postoperatively; conversely, appropriate elevation of the bladder neck and urethra, accompanied by pressure transmission ratios near 100%, results in continence in most patients. This concept is supported by a study by Penttinen et al. (1989), who noted a significant negative correlation between postoperative bladder neck mobility and pressure transmission ratios, indicating that correction of the urethrovesical anatomic disorder eliminates the functional disorder and restores continence.

Burch procedures probably tend to overelevate and fix the urethra in a retropubic position. Patients usually experience decreased flow rates and increased detrusor pressure at maximal flow. These observations suggest that an additional mechanism results, probably partial outflow obstruction. Bump et al. (1988) determined that patients with postoperative voiding abnormalities and detrusor instability had pressure transmission ratios significantly greater than 100%, which supports the hypothesis that obstruction may have a role in postcontinence surgery voiding dysfunction and detrusor overactivity. Paravaginal defect repair procedures do not overelevate the bladder neck and proximal urethra; thus they may have somewhat lower cure rates for stress incontinence, but with fewer postoperative problems such as urgency and voiding dysfunction.

COMPLICATIONS

Short-Term Postoperative

As with most pelvic surgeries, the most common complications with Burch colposuspension are surgical site infections, excessive bleeding (with or without blood transfusion), port site complications (if laparoscopy is used), medical and anesthetic complications, and urinary tract infections. In a review, Mainprize and Drutz (1988) summarized the postoperative complications (excluding urinary retention) of open MMK procedures (Table 15.1), thus providing a comprehensive summary for all open retropubic surgeries. Wound complications and urinary infections are the most common surgical complications. Direct surgical injury to the urinary tract rarely occurs. Bladder lacerations occurred in 0.7% of patients; sutures through the bladder and urethra and catheters sewn into the urethra occurred in 0.3% of patients. Ureteral obstruction occurred in 0.1% of patients. Accidental placement of sutures into the bladder during colposuspension or paravaginal defect repair, resulting in vesical stone formation, painful voiding, recurrent cystitis, or fistula, can occur but are rare (Table 15.1).

TABLE 15.1 Postoperative Complications in 2712 Marshall–Marchetti–Krantz Procedures

Type of Complication	Percent
Wound, total	5.5
Infection or hematoma	3.4
Hernia or dehiscence	1.8
Other	0.3
Urinary tract infection	3.9
Osteitis pubis	2.5
Direct surgical injury to the urinary tract	1.6
Bladder tears	0.7
Urethral obstruction	0.5
Sutures through bladder or urethra with or without catheter sewn in	0.3
Ureteral obstruction or hydronephrosis	0.1
Fistula	0.3
Death	0.2

(Modified from Mainprize TC, Drutz HP. The Marshall–Marchetti–Krantz procedure: a critical review. *Obstet Gynecol Surv.* 1988;43:724.)

Ureteral obstruction occurs rarely after Burch colposuspension and results from ureteral stretching or kinking after elevation of the vagina and bladder base. One study reported three unilateral ureteral obstructions and three bilateral ureteral obstructions in 483 Burch colposuspensions (1.2%). All patients were treated successfully with removal of sutures and ureteral stenting. No cases of transected ureters have been reported. Eriksen et al. (1990) found that 1 of 75 patients (1.3%) observed for 5 years after Burch procedures had absent unilateral renal function caused by presumed complete ureteral obstruction. This patient had developed only transient postoperative fever.

Lower urinary tract fistulas are uncommon after retropubic procedures, with various types occurring after 0.3% of MMK procedures. Fistulas are probably less common after Burch and paravaginal defect repairs because the sutures are placed several centimeters lateral to the urethra.

Postoperative Voiding Difficulties

The incidence of voiding difficulties after colposuspension varies widely, although patients rarely have urinary retention after 30 days. In our hands, the mean number of days to complete voiding after open Burch procedure is 7 days—substantially longer than seen with midurethral slings. Eriksen et al. (1990) found that only two of 91 patients had delayed spontaneous micturition after Burch colposuspension when the catheter was removed the third day postoperatively. Some 15% of these patients had residual urine volumes of 100 to 300 mL the fifth day after surgery.

Colposuspension can change the original micturition pattern and introduce an element of obstruction that can disturb the balance between voiding forces and outflow resistance, resulting in immediate postoperative, as well as late, voiding difficulties. Urodynamic findings that may occur after colposuspension include decreased flow rate, increased detrusor pressure at maximal flow, and increased urethral resistance.

Urodynamic tests may be used to predict early postoperative voiding difficulties, although their predictive value has not been demonstrated consistently. Bhatia and Bergman (1984) found that all patients with adequate detrusor contraction and flow rates preoperatively were able to resume spontaneous voiding by the seventh postoperative day after Burch colposuspension. One-third of patients who voided without detrusor contraction required bladder drainage for 7 days or longer. No patients with decreased flow rates and absent detrusor contraction during voiding were able to void less than 7 days postoperatively. These authors believed that use of a Valsalva maneuver during voiding may further lead to postoperative voiding difficulties, perhaps by intensifying obstruction at the bladder neck. In a study by Kobak et al. (2001), risk factors for prolonged voiding after Burch colposuspension included advanced age, previous incontinence surgery, increased first sensation to void, high postvoid residual volume, and postoperative cystitis. Abdominal straining during voiding was not associated with prolonged voiding after surgery.

Overactive Bladder

Overactive bladder is a recognized postoperative complication of retropubic procedures. Detrusor overactivity as demonstrated on cystometrogram has been reported in 7% to 27% of patients with urodynamic SUI and stable bladders preoperatively, with follow-up of up to 5 years after Burch colposuspension. Postoperative overactive bladder is more common in patients with previous bladder neck surgery and in those with mixed detrusor overactivity and urodynamic SUI preoperatively. In a study of 148 patients with urodynamic SUI and stable bladders preoperatively, Steel et al. (1986) reported that 24 patients (16.2%) had postoperative detrusor overactivity on cystometrogram 6 months after surgery. A total of 10 of the 24 patients with overactive bladder were completely asymptomatic. Of the 14 symptomatic patients, four improved with drugs aimed at correcting the urgency. The remaining 10 patients (6.8%) remained symptomatic with overactive bladder 3 to 5 years after surgery.

The mechanism for this phenomenon is unknown. As noted previously, excessive urethral elevation or compression can lead to partial outflow obstruction and resulting urgency. Whatever the mechanism, postoperative overactive bladder predictably occurs in a small but significant number of patients. Patients undergoing retropubic urethropexy should understand that the operation may cause urgency and urge incontinence, even if it cures their stress incontinence.

Osteitis Pubis

Osteitis pubis is a painful inflammation of periosteum, bone, cartilage, and ligaments of structures of the anterior pelvic girdle. It is a recognized postoperative complication of urologic and radical gynecologic procedures involving the prostate gland or urinary bladder. In urogynecology, osteitis pubis occurs after 0.74% to 2.5% of MMK procedures and only rarely after Burch procedures; the incidence is partially related to the diagnostic criteria used. It also can occur rarely after placement of artificial urinary sphincters and after radical pelvic surgery for gynecologic malignancies.

The cause of osteitis pubis is unclear. It may result from infection, from trauma to the periosteum, or from impaired circulation in the vessels around the symphysis pubis. The disease typically occurs 2 to 12 weeks postoperatively. Osteitis pubis is characterized by suprapubic pain radiating to the thighs that is exacerbated by walking or abduction of the lower extremities, marked tenderness and swelling over the symphysis pubis, and radiographic evidence of bone destruction with separation of the symphysis pubis. The clinical course varies from prolonged, progressive debilitation over several months to spontaneous resolution after several weeks. Suggested conservative treatments include rest, physical therapy, steroids, and nonsteroidal antiinflammatory agents. Whatever the therapy, noninfectious osteitis pubis tends to be self-limiting.

Recalcitrant cases may result from pubic osteomyelitis. Diagnosis is made by bone biopsy and bacterial culture. Kammerer-Doak et al. (1998) found positive cultures in 71% of patients with clinical osteitis pubis who failed to respond to conservative therapy. Treatments are antibiotics, incision and drainage if abscess formation occurs, or symphyseal wedge resection or debridement.

Enterocele and Rectocele

Burch (1968) first reported that enteroceles occurred in 7.6% of cases after the Burch procedure, but only two-thirds of those patients required surgical correction. Langer et al. (1988) reported that 13.6% of patients who had undergone Burch procedures but not hysterectomy or cul-de-sac obliteration developed an enterocele 1 to 2 years postoperatively. Alcalay et al. (1995) noted that 26% of patients underwent a rectocele repair during a 10- to 20-year follow-up period after Burch colposuspension, and 5% underwent an enterocele repair. Although not all authors agree, performing a Burch colposuspension may increase the risk of developing apical or posterior vaginal prolapse in the future. This observation is consistent with other types of vaginal reconstructive surgery in which it has been observed that suspension of one vaginal segment can predispose to new prolapse in the other, unrepaired segment. Therefore, whenever possible, a cul-de-sac obliteration in the form of uterosacral plication, Moschcowitz procedure, or McCall culdoplasty should be performed at the time of retropubic colposuspension to prevent enterocele formation, although the true efficacy of this prophylactic maneuver is unknown. Rectocele repair should be done as indicated for symptomatic or large rectoceles, although care should be taken to avoid a resulting midvaginal ridge; the postoperative rate of dyspareunia may be as high as 38% when these two procedures are combined.

ROLE OF HYSTERECTOMY IN THE TREATMENT OF INCONTINENCE

Gynecologists often perform hysterectomies at the time of retropubic or vaginal surgery for SUI. Langer et al. (1988) assessed the effect of concomitant hysterectomy during Burch colposuspension on the cure rate of SUI. Some 45 patients were randomly assigned to receive colposuspension only or colposuspension plus abdominal hysterectomy and cul-de-sac obliteration. Using urodynamic investigations 6 months after surgery, the rate of cure for stress incontinence between the two groups did not differ statistically (95.5% and 95.7% for the no-hysterectomy and hysterectomy groups, respectively). This study clearly showed that hysterectomy adds little to the efficacy of Burch colposuspension in curing SUI. In general, hysterectomies should be performed only for specific uterine pathology or for the treatment of uterovaginal prolapse.

PREGNANCY AFTER RETROPUBIC SURGERY

Most physicians suggest that the patient finish childbearing before surgical correction of stress incontinence is attempted. Few data demonstrate the continence status when pregnancy or vaginal delivery occurs after a retropubic repair or sling. Thus, although surgical treatment for stress incontinence generally should be reserved for women who have finished childbearing, no data convincingly demonstrate that a pregnancy and vaginal delivery would or would not be satisfactory for women after retropubic surgery. Most surgeons prefer not to place polypropylene midurethral slings if the woman desires more pregnancies, although data on this are scarce as well. We believe that an elective caesarean delivery would be an acceptable option for patients who become pregnant after a Burch colposuspension, if desired after careful review of the pertinent risks and benefits.

BIBLIOGRAPHY

Surgical Technique

Burch JC. Urethrovaginal fixation to Cooper's ligament for correction of stress incontinence, cystocele, and prolapse. *Am J Obstet Gynecol.* 1961;81:281.

Hill AJ, Jallad K, Walters MD. Laparoscopic Burch colposuspension using a 3-trocar system: tips and tricks. *J Minim Invasive Gynecol.* 2017;24:344.

Lind LR, Gunn GC, Mattox TF, Stanford EJ. Mini-incision Burch urethropexy: a less invasive method to accomplish a time-tested procedure for treatment of genuine stress incontinence. *Int Urogynecol J.* 2004;15:20.

Marshall VF, Marchetti AA, Krantz KE. The correction of stress incontinence by simple vesicourethral suspension. *Surg Gynecol Obstet.* 1949;88:509.

Meltomaa SS, Haarala MA, Taalikka MO, et al. Outcome of Burch retropubic urethropexy and the effect of concomitant abdominal hysterectomy: a prospective long-term follow-up study. *Int Urogynecol J.* 2001;12:3.

Richardson AC, Edmonds PB, Williams NL. Treatment of stress urinary incontinence due to paravaginal fascial defect. *Obstet Gynecol.* 1981;57:357.

Shull BL. How I do the abdominal paravaginal repair. *J Pelvic Surg.* 1995;1:43.

Shull BL, Baden WF. A six-year experience with paravaginal defect repair for stress urinary incontinence. *Am J Obstet Gynecol.* 1989;160:1432.

Tanagho EA. Colpocystourethropexy: the way we do it. *J Urol.* 1976;116:751.

Turner-Warwick R. Turner-Warwick vagino-obturator shelf urethral repositioning procedure. In Debruyne FMJ, van Kerrebroeck EVA, eds. *Practical Aspects of Urinary Incontinence.* Dordrecht, The Netherlands: Martinus Nijhoff; 1986.

Webster GD, Kreder KJ. Voiding dysfunction following cystourethropexy: its evaluation and management. *J Urol.* 1990;144:670.

Results and Mechanism of Cure

Albo ME, Richter HE, Brubaker L, et al. Burch colposuspension versus fascial sling to reduce urinary stress incontinence. *N Engl J Med.* 2007;356:2143.

Alcalay M, Monga A, Stanton SL. Burch colposuspension: a 10–20 year follow up. *Br J Obstet Gynaecol.* 1995;102:740.

Baessler K, Christmann-Schmid C, Maher C, et al. Surgery for women with pelvic organ prolapse with or without stress urinary incontinence. *Cochrane Database Syst Rev* 2018;8:CD013108.

Bergman A, Elia G. Three surgical procedures for genuine stress incontinence: five-year follow-up of a prospective randomized study. *Am J Obstet Gynecol.* 1995;173:66.

Bidmead J, Cardozo L. Retropubic urethropexy (Burch colposuspension). *Int Urogynecol J.* 2001;12:262.

Black NA, Downs SH. The effectiveness of surgery for stress incontinence in women: a systematic review. *Br J Urol.* 1996;78:497.

Brubaker L, Nygaard I, Richter HE, et al. Two-year outcomes after sacrocolpopexy with and without Burch to prevent stress urinary incontinence. *Obstet Gynecol.* 2008;112:49.

Bump RC, Fantl JA, Hurt WG. Dynamic urethral pressure profilometry pressure transmission ratio determinations after continence surgery: understanding the mechanism of success, failure, and complications. *Obstet Gynecol.* 1988;72:870.

Columbo M, Milani R, Vitobello D, et al. A randomized comparison of Burch colposuspension and abdominal paravaginal defect repair for female stress urinary incontinence. *Am J Obstet Gynecol.* 1996;175:78.

Conrad DH, Pacquee S, Saar TD, et al. Long-term patient-reported outcomes after laparoscopic Burch colposuspension. *Aust N Z J Obstet Gynaecol.* 2019;59:850.

Cosson M, Boukerrou M, Narducci F, et al. Long-term results of the Burch procedure combined with abdominal sacrocolpopexy for treatment of vault prolapse. *Int Urogynecol J.* 2003;14:104.

Costantini E, Lazzeri M, Bini V, et al. Pelvic organ prolapse repair with and without concomitant Burch colposuspension in incontinent women: a randomised controlled trial with at least 5-year follow-up. *Obstet Gynecol Int.* 2012;2012:967923.

Costantini E, Lazzeri M, Bini V, et al. Burch colposuspension does not provide any additional benefit to pelvic organ prolapse repair in patients with urinary incontinence: a randomized surgical trial. *J Urol.* 2008;180:1007.

Eriksen BC, Hagen B, Eik-Nes SH, et al. Long-term effectiveness of the Burch colposuspension in female urinary stress incontinence. *Acta Obstet Gynecol Scand.* 1990;69:45.

Foss Hansen M, Lose G, Kesmodel US, Gradel KO. Reoperation for urinary incontinence: a nationwide cohort study, 1998-2007. *Am J Obstet Gynecol.* 2016;214:263.

Freites J, Stewart F, Omar MI, et al. Laparoscopic colposuspension for urinary incontinence in women. *Cochrane Database Syst Rev.* 2019;12:CD002239.

Herbertsson G, Iosif CS. Surgical results and urodynamic studies 10 years after retropubic colpourethrocystopexy. *Acta Obstet Gynecol Scand.* 1983;72:298.

Hertogs K, Stanton SL. Mechanism of urinary continence after colposuspension: barrier studies. *Br J Obstet Gynaecol.* 1985;92:1184.

Hilton P, Stanton SL. A clinical and urodynamic assessment of the Burch colposuspension for genuine stress incontinence. *Br J Obstet Gynaecol.* 1983;90:934.

Holdo B, Verelst M, Svenningsen R, et al. Long-term clinical outcomes with the retropubic tension-free vaginal tape (TVT) procedure compared to Burch colposuspension for correcting stress urinary incontinence (SUI). *Int Urogynecol J.* 2017;28:1739.

Jelovsek JE, Barber MD, Karram MM, et al. Randomised trial of laparoscopic Burch colposuspension versus tension-free vaginal tape: long-term follow up. *BJOG.* 2008;115:219.

Jonsson Funk M, Siddiqui NY, Kawasaki A, Wu JM. Long-term outcomes after stress urinary incontinence surgery. *Obstet Gynecol.* 2012;120:83.

Karram MM, Bhatia NN. Management of coexistent stress and urge urinary incontinence. *Obstet Gynecol.* 1989;73:4.

Kraus SR, Lemack GE, Richter HE, Urinary Incontinence Treatment Network, et al. Changes in urodynamic measures two years after Burch colposuspension or autologous sling surgery. *Urology.* 2011;78:1263.

Kurkijarvi K, Aaltonen R, Gissler M, Makinen J. Reoperations for female stress urinary incontinence: a Finnish national register study. *Eur Urol Focus.* 2018;4:754.

Langer R, Ron-El R, Neuman N, et al. The value of simultaneous hysterectomy during Burch colposuspension for urinary stress incontinence. *Obstet Gynecol.* 1988;72:866.

Lapitan MC, Cody JD, Mashayekhi A. Open retropubic colposuspension for urinary incontinence in women. *Cochrane Database Syst Rev.* 2017;7:CD002912.

Laursen H, Farlie R, Rasmussen KL, et al. Colposuspension Burch: an 18 year follow-up study. *Neurourol Urodyn.* 1994;13:445.

Mainprize TC, Drutz HP. The Marshall–Marchetti–Krantz procedure: a critical review. *Obstet Gynecol Surv.* 1988;43:724.

Moon YJ, Jeon MJ, Kim SK, Bai SW. Comparison of Burch colposuspension and transobturator tape when combined with abdominal sacrocolpopexy. *Int J Gynaecol Obstet.* 2011;112:122.

Novara G, Artibani W, Barber MD, et al. Updated systematic review and meta-analysis of the comparative data on colposuspensions, pubovaginal slings, and midurethral tapes in the surgical treatment of female stress urinary incontinence. *Eur Urol.* 2010;58:218.

Penttinen J, Lindholm EL, Käär K, Kauppila A. Successful colposuspension in stress urinary incontinence reduces bladder neck mobility and increases pressure transmission to the urethra. *Arch Gynecol Obstet.* 1989;244:233.

Richter HE, Brubaker L, Stoddard AM, Urinary Incontinence Treatment Network, et al. Patient related factors associated with long-term urinary continence after Burch colposuspension and pubovaginal fascial sling surgeries. *J Urol.* 2012;188:485.

Richter HE, Diokno A, Kenton K, Urinary Incontinence Treatment Network, et al. Predictors of treatment failure 24 months after surgery for stress urinary incontinence. *J Urol.* 2008;179:1024.

Sand PK, Bowen LW, Panganiban R, Ostergard DR. The low pressure urethra as a factor in failed retropubic urethropexy. *Obstet Gynecol.* 1987;69:399.

Van der Ploeg JM, van der Steen A, Zwolsman S, et al. Prolapse surgery with or without incontinence procedure: a systematic review and meta-analysis. *BJOG.* 2018;125:289.

Ward K, Hilton P. Prospective multicentre randomized trial of tension-free vaginal tape and colposuspension as primary treatment for stress incontinence. *BMJ.* 2002;325:1.

Ward K, Hilton P. A prospective multicenter randomized trial of tension-free vaginal tape and colposuspension for primary urodynamic stress incontinence: two-year follow-up. *Am J Obstet Gynecol.* 2004;190:324.

Complications

Bhatia NN, Bergman A. Urodynamic predictability of voiding following incontinence surgery. *Obstet Gynecol.* 1984;63:85.

Burch JC. Cooper's ligament urethrovesical suspension for stress incontinence. *Am J Obstet Gynecol.* 1968;100:764.

Cardozo LD, Stanton SL, Williams JE. Detrusor instability following surgery for genuine stress incontinence. *Br J Urol.* 1979;51:204.

Castellani D, Pucci M, Dellabella M. A bladder stone 28 years after Burch colposuspension. *Urology.* 2020;138:e1.

Galloway NTM, Davies N, Stephenson TP. The complications of colposuspension. *Br J Urol.* 1987;60:122.

Glass Clark SM, Huang Q, Sima AP, Siff LN. Effect of surgery for stress urinary incontinence on female sexual function. *Obstet Gynecol.* 2020;135:352.

Kammerer-Doak DN, Cornella JL, Magrina JF, et al. Osteitis pubis after Marshall–Marchetti–Krantz urethropexy: a pubic osteomyelitis. *Am J Obstet Gynecol.* 1998;179:586.

Kjohede P, Noren B, Ryden G. Prediction of genital prolapse after Burch colposuspension. *Acta Obstet Gynecol Scand.* 1996;75:849.

Kobak WH, Walters MD, Piedmonte MR. Determinants of voiding after three types of incontinence surgery. *Obstet Gynecol.* 2001;97:86.

Kwon CH, Culligan PJ, Koduri S, et al. The development of pelvic organ prolapse following isolated Burch retropubic urethropexy. *Int Urogynecol J.* 2003;14:321.

Rosenthal RE, Spickard WA, Markham RD, et al. Osteomyelitis of the symphysis pubis: a separate disease from osteitis pubis. *J Bone Joint Surg.* 1982;64:123.

Shapiro R, Hajiran A, Zaslau S. Delayed presentation of suture erosion following Burch colposuspension. *Case Rep Obstet Gynecol.* 2017;2017:8178361.

Steel SA, Cox C, Stanton SL. Long-term follow-up of detrusor instability following the colposuspension operation. *Br J Urol.* 1986;58:138.

Turner-Warwick RT. The pathogenesis and treatment of osteitis pubis. *Br J Urol.* 1960;32:464.

Wang AC, Chen M. Comparison of tension-free vaginal taping versus modified Burch colposuspension on urethral obstruction: a randomized controlled trial. *Neurourol Urodyn.* 2003;22:185.

Weber AM, Walters MD, Piedmonte MR. Sexual function and vaginal anatomy in women before and after surgery for pelvic organ prolapse and urinary incontinence. *Am J Obstet Gynecol.* 2000;182:1610.

Wiskind AK, Creighton SM, Stanton SL. The incidence of genital prolapse after the Burch colposuspension. *Am J Obstet Gynecol.* 1992;167:399.

Zyczynski HM, Albo ME, Goldman HB, et al. Change in overactive bladder symptoms after surgery for stress urinary incontinence in women. *Obstet Gynecol.* 2015;126:423.

16

Biologic Bladder Neck Slings for Stress Urinary Incontinence

Mickey M. Karram and Mallorie L. Hoover

CHAPTER OUTLINE

INTRODUCTION

The concept of using a patient's own tissue as a "sling" to provide support under the urethra to treat urinary incontinence dates to the beginning of the twentieth century; however, it was not until the last quarter of the century that the procedure gained widespread appreciation and evolved into its current identity. Initially, the procedure was described as using a strip of mobilized abdominal muscle (either rectus or pyramidalis). One end of the strip was freed from its attachment, passed under the bladder neck, and then reaffixed to the abdominal muscle wall, thus forming a "U"-shaped sling of muscle tissue around the bladder outlet. Subsequently, overlying abdominal fascia was included in the sling, and eventually replaced the muscle altogether. In 1942, Aldridge reported his fascial suburethral sling procedure, which is the forerunner of the modern pubovaginal sling. Aldridge described the procedure as a salvage-type operation for those women who had failed previous operations for stress incontinence. For the sling, he used rectus fascial strips that remained attached to the anterior abdominal wall and were passed bilaterally along the urethra and sutured together under the bladder neck. The final innovation involved using an isolated strip of fascia suspended by free sutures that were then tied to the abdominal wall directly or on top of the abdominal rectus sheath.

Despite its roots as an autologous procedure, many different types of materials have been used as sling substitutions, including various sources of autologous tissue, allografts, xenografts, and synthetic materials. Almost all these attempts at substitution have been made to help limit patient morbidity, as the procedure requires the additional morbidity of a sling tissue harvest site. Nevertheless, the most popular variety of the pubovaginal sling remains associated with the use of autologous rectus abdominis fascia.

Regardless of the material used, the pubovaginal sling is meant to be placed at the proximal urethra and bladder neck. The concept of the autologous pubovaginal sling involves supporting the proximal urethra and bladder neck with a piece of graft material, achieving continence either by providing a direct compressive force on the urethra/bladder outlet or by reestablishing a reinforcing platform or hammock against which the urethra is compressed during increased abdominal pressure. The sling is suspended with free sutures on each end that are either attached directly to the abdominal wall musculature or tied to each other on the anterior surface of the abdominal wall. The long-term success of the procedure relies not on the integrity of the suspensory sutures, but rather on the healing and fibrotic process involving the sling, which occurs primarily where the sling passes through the endopelvic fascia.

INDICATIONS

The pubovaginal sling is a surgical option for both primary and recurrent stress urinary incontinence (SUI). Although pioneered as a surgical treatment for intrinsic sphincter deficiency (ISD), its indications have been broadened to encompass all types of SUI. Because of its reliable results and durable outcomes, it is one of the main standards of treatment of SUI and has been used extensively as a primary therapy for SUI (both for ISD and urethral hypermobility), as a salvage procedure for recurrent SUI, as an adjunct for urethral and bladder reconstruction, and even as a way to functionally "close" the urethra to abandon urethral access to the bladder altogether. Another indication is in patients with SUI who decline to have a synthetic material implanted because of long-term concerns related to synthetic mesh. Also, women who have recurrent incontinence or experience a complication after implantation of a synthetic sling (such as vaginal erosion) may be good candidates for the autologous fascial sling. Finally, we prefer to use an autologous sling in patients who have been irradiated, who have had urethral injuries, and who are undergoing either simultaneous or prior urethrovaginal fistula or diverticulum repair.

SLING MATERIALS

With the increasing popularity of primary sling procedures, the escalating demand for minimally invasive techniques, and the need for nonmesh options, numerous materials have become available for use in suburethral slings. Current biologic materials can be categorized as autologous fascia, allograft fascia, or xenograft fascia. Within these categories, different variants can be subgrouped into individual materials: autologous (rectus fascia, fascia lata, vaginal wall), allograft (freeze-dried irradiated cadaveric fascia lata, solvent dehydrated cadaveric fascia lata, fresh frozen cadaveric fascia lata, cadaveric dermis), and xenograft (porcine dermis, porcine intestinal submucosa) which has been used historically but is no longer commercially available. Autologous rectus fascia and fascia lata are the most common materials in use, and the standard to which the outcome of other new materials should be compared. Both have been studied extensively and have proven to be efficacious and reliable. Of the two, most surgeons prefer rectus fascia as an autologous material because it is easier and quicker to harvest.

The application of newer tissue harvesting technologies has made multiple human- and animal-based materials available. The theoretical rationale for using allografts and xenografts for suburethral slings is reinforcement of inherently weak endopelvic fascia. Allogenic grafts harvested from cadaveric donors are widely used and do not seem to carry a significant risk of erosion or infection. Cadaveric fascia lata and cadaveric dermis provide reasonable efficacy, although durability remains an issue because higher failure rates compared with allogenic grafts have been reported in some studies. The long-term durability of allograft fascia continues to be studied, and there seems to be wide variability in the quality of tissue, depending on its source and processing. The type of sling material probably does not significantly affect cure rates, provided that the characteristics of the chosen material are considered carefully, however it may affect durability.

Synthetic graft materials of various designs and substances have been used as sling material. As with other types of synthetic graft materials, monofilament, large-pore weave grafts (type I mesh) are recommended for implantation in the vagina. Good efficacy can be achieved with synthetic mesh; although synthetic mesh also poses risks of unique complications, including infection, vaginal extrusion, and genitourinary erosion. Thus, synthetic slings are currently not usually recommended for use underneath the proximal urethra or bladder neck.

SURGICAL TECHNIQUES

Rectus Fascia Pubovaginal Sling

Preoperative Considerations. We recommend starting vaginal estrogen in postmenopausal women with vaginal atrophy at least 4 to 6 weeks before surgery. Tissue integrity improves with estrogen, and this may provide clinical benefits to the patient. No studies, however, have shown improved outcomes by using estrogen before and/or after prolapse or incontinence surgery. Informed consent should be methodical; it is a process rather than a single event. In addition to discussing the usual risks encountered in a major operation (infection, hemorrhage, injury to adjacent organs, and medical and anesthesia complications), a frank conversation should take place regarding the expected outcomes, the likelihood of SUI recurrence, the potential of voiding dysfunction, and the risk of prolonged catheterization. Additionally, because the use of a fascial (or other) graft is planned, delineating the unique set of risks related to these procedures is prudent.

Pubovaginal sling procedures are generally carried out with the patient under general anesthesia, but spinal or epidural anesthesia is also possible. Full patient paralysis is not warranted but may facilitate rectus fascia closure after fascial harvest. Perioperative antibiotics are administered with appropriate skin and vaginal floral coverage (e.g., a cephalosporin). Antibiotics should be given within 60 minutes of incision to achieve minimal inhibitory concentrations in the skin and tissues by the time the incision is made. This has now become a mandated quality-of-care measure in the United States.

In general, all patients undergoing vaginal surgery are at moderate risk for thromboembolic events and require a prevention strategy. Low-dose unfractionated heparin (5000 units every 12 hours) or low-molecular-weight heparins (e.g., 40 mg enoxaparin or 2500 units of dalteparin), an intermittent pneumatic compression device, or a combination of these are recommended. Either form of heparin should be started 2 hours before surgery, and the compression stockings placed on the patient in the operating room before incision. These treatment approaches should be continued until the patient is ambulatory.

Positioning

The patient is placed in the low lithotomy position with legs in stirrups, and the abdomen and perineum are sterilely prepared and draped to provide access to the vagina and the lower abdomen. The bladder is drained with a Foley catheter. A weighted vaginal speculum is placed, and either lateral labial retraction sutures or a self-retaining retractor system are used to facilitate vaginal exposure.

Abdominal Incision and Fascial Harvest. An 8- to 10-cm Pfannenstiel incision is made (approximately 3–5 cm above the pubic bone), and the dissection is carried down to the level of the rectus fascia with a combination of electrocautery and blunt dissection, sweeping the fat and subcutaneous tissue clear of the fascia (Fig. 16.1).

Harvest of the rectus abdominis fascia can be carried out in a transverse or vertical orientation. Typically, a fascial segment measuring at least 8 cm in length and 1.5 to 2 cm in width is harvested. The fascial segment to be resected is delineated with a surgical marking pen or electrocautery, and then incised sharply with a scalpel, scissors, or electrocautery along the drawn lines. Although virgin fascia is preferred, the presence of fibrotic rectus fascia does not prohibit its use. If resecting the

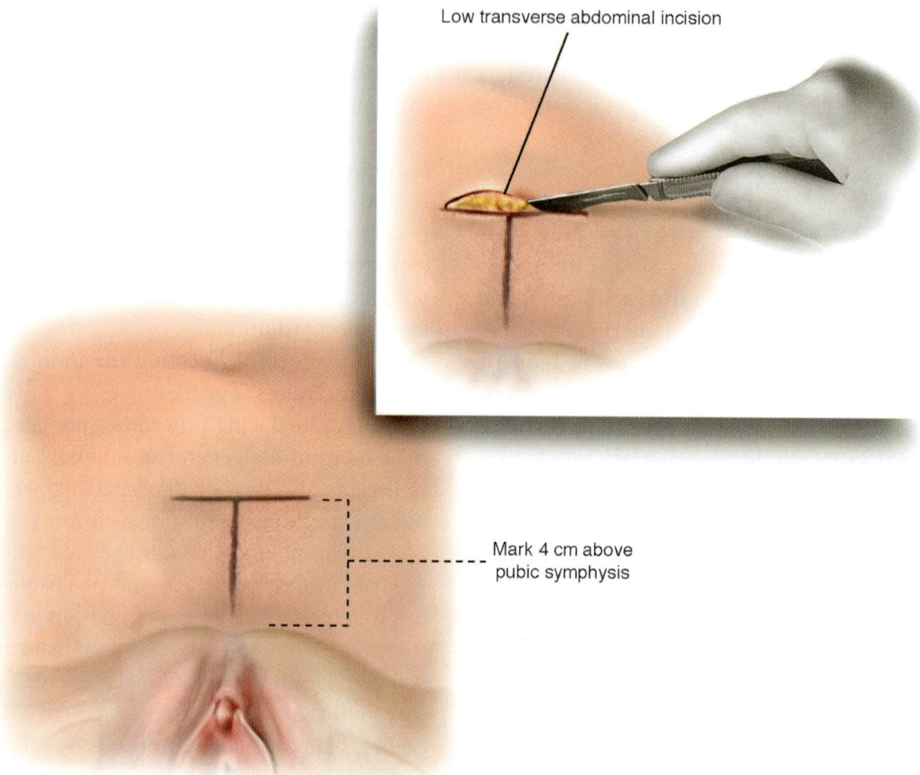

Fig. 16.1 Delineate the location of skin incision before initiating the procedure. The incision should measure 8 to 10 cm and be located about 3-5 cm above the symphysis pubis. A vertical incision is also feasible, although it is less a esthetic.

fascia close and parallel to the symphysis pubis, it is advisable to leave at least 1 cm attached, so as to facilitate closure and approximation to the superior fascial edge. Use of small Army/Navy retractors permit retraction of skin edges, thus allowing access through a smaller skin incision (Fig. 16.2).

To prepare the fascial sling for use, a No. 1 permanent (e.g., polypropylene) suture is affixed to each end using a running stitch to secure the suture to the sling. Defatting of the sling may be done if necessary (Fig. 16.3).

The fascial defect is closed using a heavy-gauge (No. 1 or 0) delayed absorbable suture in a running fashion. Mobilization of the rectus abdominis fascial edges may be required to ensure appropriate tension-free approximation. It is important to ensure that adequate anesthesia with muscular relaxation/paralysis is present when the closure is being done. Although cellulitis and hematomas are uncommon, meticulous hemostasis and copious wound irrigation are done before skin closure.

Vaginal Dissection. Vaginal dissection proceeds with a midline or inverted "U" incision. Injectable saline or local analgesic, such as 1% lidocaine, may be used to hydrodissect the subepithelial tissues. Vaginal flaps are created with sufficient mobility so as to ensure tension-free closure over the sling. Dissection is carried laterally and anteriorly until the endopelvic fascia is encountered. The endopelvic fascia is incised and dissected from the posterior surface of the pubis to enter the retropubic space. This dissection can, at times, be done bluntly, but often, especially in recurrent cases, requires sharp dissection with Mayo scissors (Fig. 16.4). To penetrate this fascia, the tips of the scissors should advance toward the ipsilateral shoulder, staying in direct contact with the posterior surface of the pubic bone.

Passing Retropubic Needles or Clamp. Stamey needles or long clamps are passed on each side through the retropubic space from the open abdominal wound immediately posterior to the pubic bone. Distal control of the needles is maintained by finger guidance through the vaginal incision, and the tip of the needle is advanced adjacent to the posterior surface of the pubic bone so as to avoid inadvertent bladder injury. Proper bladder drainage must be assured to minimize injury to the bladder, which may be closely adherent to the pubis, especially if a prior retropubic procedure has been performed (Fig. 16.5).

Cystoscopy to Rule Out Injury. Careful cystoscopic examination of the bladder after passing the needles is mandatory to rule out accidental bladder injury. As the injuries to the bladder typically occur at the 1 and 11 o'clock positions, use of the 70-degree lens is warranted, and the bladder must be completely filled to expand any mucosal redundancy. Wiggling the needles or clamps can help to localize their position relative to the bladder wall.

Deploying and Tensioning the Sling. The free ends of the sutures affixed to the sling are threaded into the ends of the

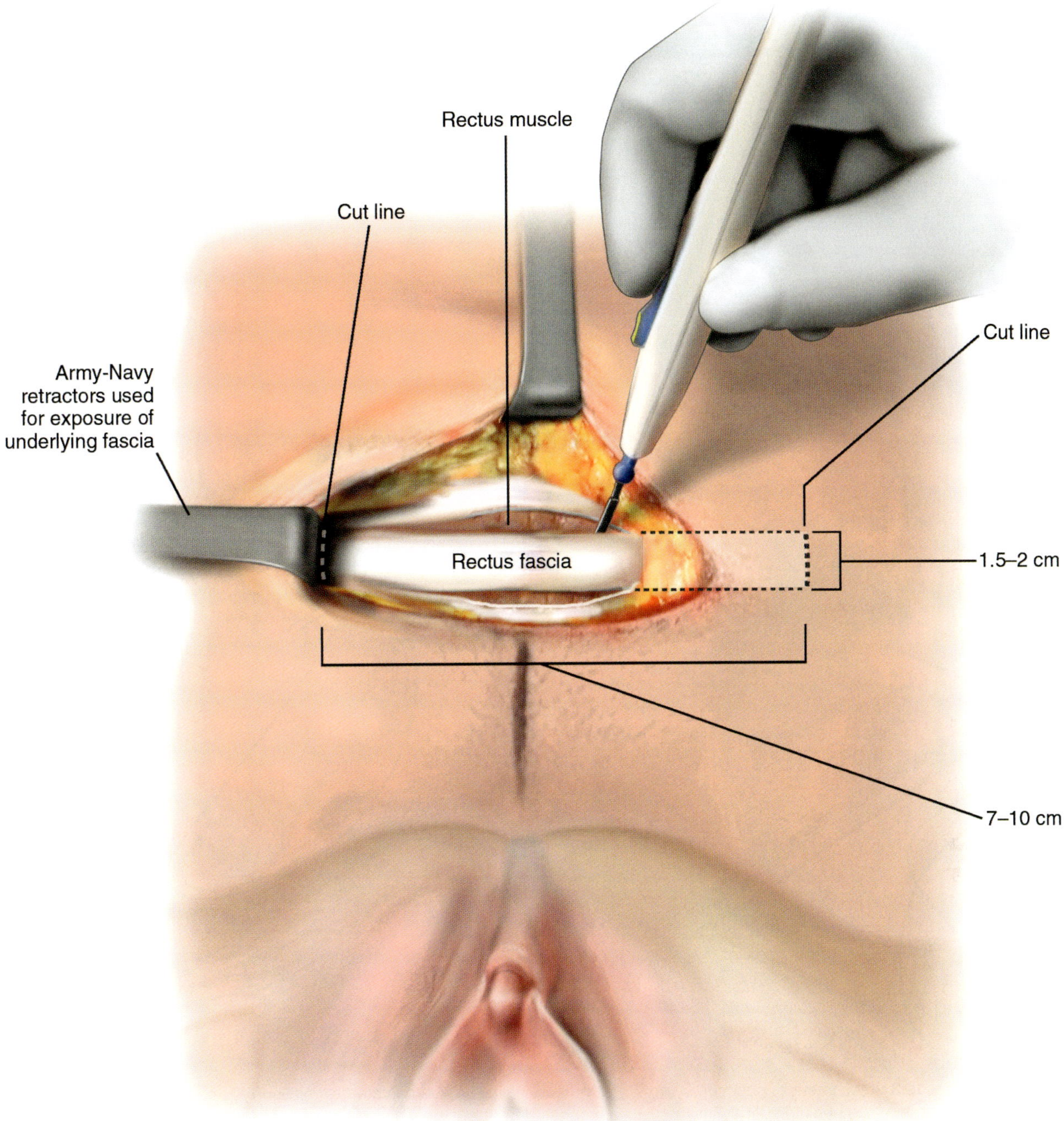

Fig. 16.2 Fascial strip resection. After deciding on the optimal location for excision, mark the area with electrocautery or a surgical marking pen. Then proceed to resecting strip using a scalpel or electrocautery. The strip should measure 8 to 10 cm and be 1.5 to 2 cm wide. If attempting to use a small skin incision, Army/Navy retractors may be helpful in enhancing exposure.

Stamey needles or similar device or grasped with the clamp, and each suture is pulled up to the anterior abdominal wall through the retropubic space. Care is taken to maintain the orientation of the sling so that it is centered and flat at the bladder neck (Fig. 16.6). Some surgeons prefer to fix the sling in the midline to the underlying periurethral tissue with several delayed absorbable sutures; alternatively, it can be left unattached and lying free under the bladder neck.

Various techniques for tensioning the sling are applicable. To ensure adequate "looseness," the author prefers to tie the sutures across the midline while holding a right-angle clamp or Mayo scissor between the sling material and the posterior urethral surface. Tensioning of the sling also may be accomplished by direct vision of proximal urethra/bladder neck coaptation with rigid cystoscopy while gently pulling up on the free ends of the sling sutures.

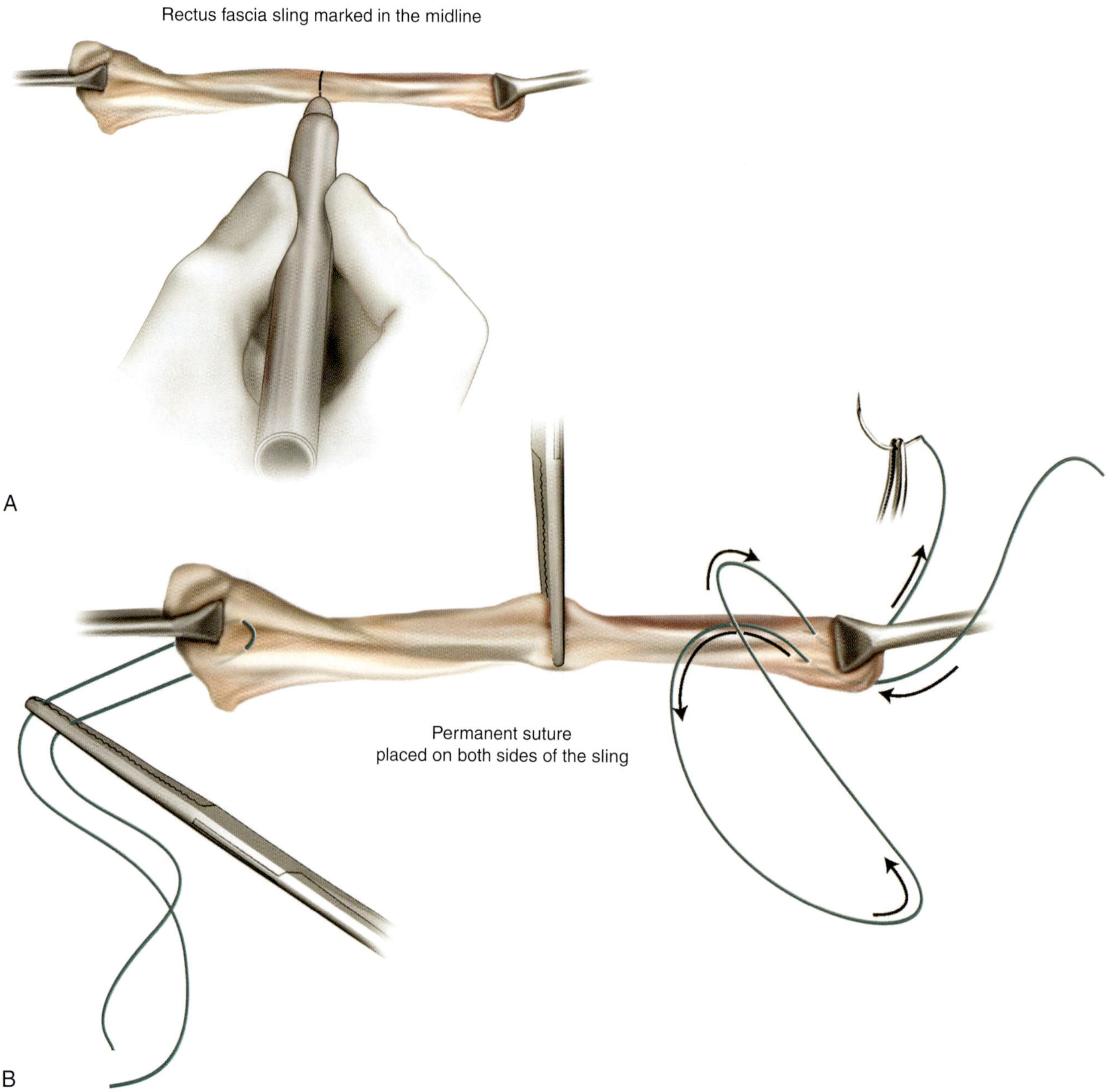

Fig. 16.3 Attachment of suspensory arms to the fascial sling. **A**, Demarcate the midline of the fascial sling with a marking pen then gently grasp it with a hemostat. **B**, Attach a polyester suture (such as Ethibond Excel) to each of the ends of the fascial sling after stripping it of any adipose tissue attached to it. Ensure that the initial entry and exit points of the polyester sutures are on the same side of the strip originally abutting the rectus muscles.

The abdominal skin incision is closed with No. 3-0 and 4-0 absorbable sutures. The vaginal mucosa is closed with No. 2-0 or 3-0 absorbable sutures. The authors prefer to close the vagina after the tensioning procedure has been completed, whereas some surgeons complete this step before the tensioning (Video 16.1; Autologous rectus fascia sling).

A bladder catheter is left indwelling, and a vaginal gauze packing is placed. The catheter and vaginal packing may be removed after 24 hours, and a trial of voiding done. If the patient is unable to void, she is taught intermittent self-catheterization, or an indwelling Foley is left in place for 1 week.

Harvest of Autologous Fascia Lata

Autologous tissue from the iliotibial fascial band of the lateral thigh (fascia lata) has been used with great success as an alternative to abdominal rectus fascia for pubovaginal sling. Although incurring the morbidity of a secondary incision at a site remote from the abdomen, harvesting fascia lata may be suitable in cases in which abdominal fascia may be of poor quality, if extensive abdominal procedures have been previously performed, or in patients with significant central obesity or large pannus.

Harvest of fascia lata may require separate positioning, skin preparation, and sterile draping in addition to those for the

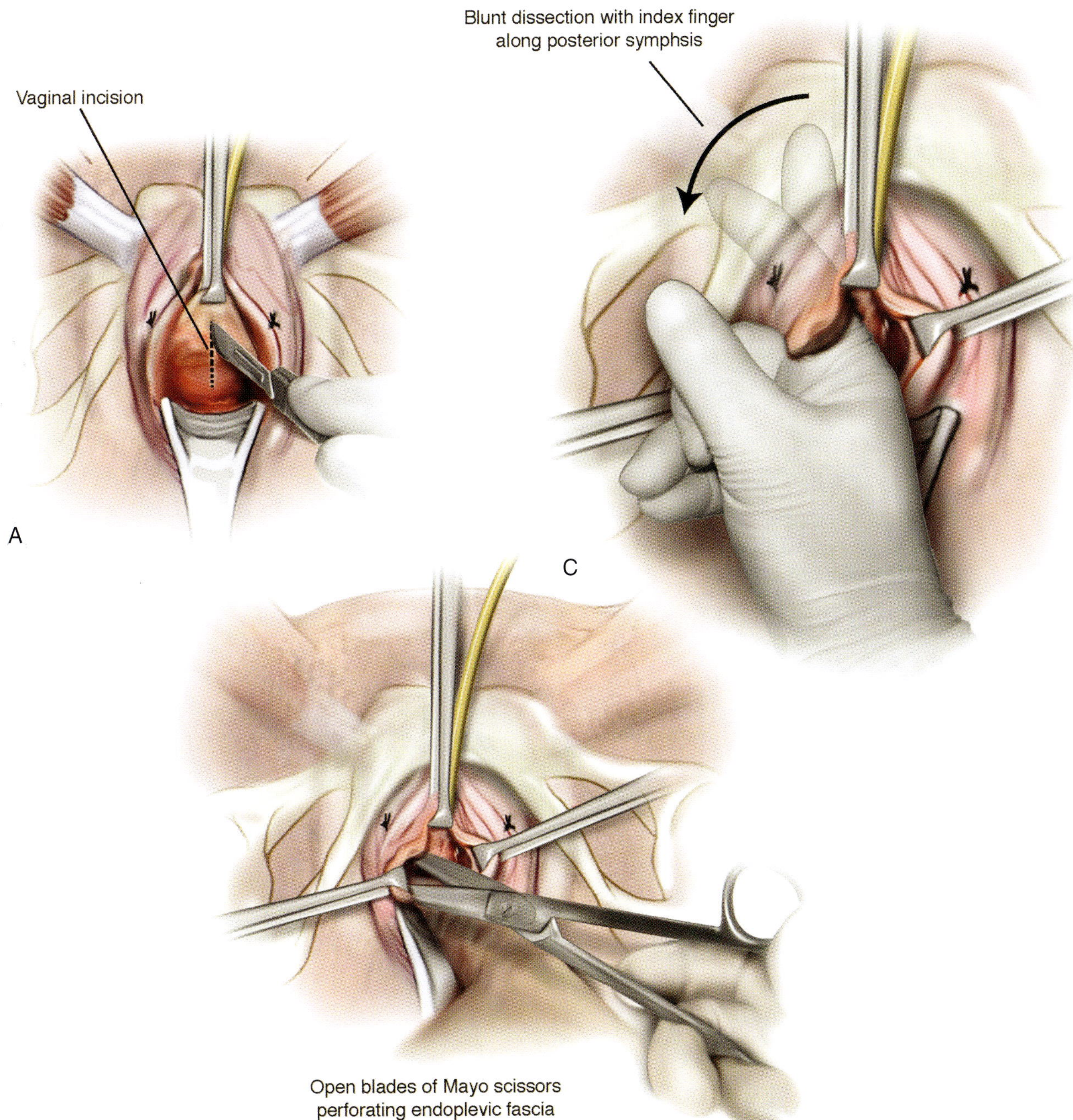

Fig. 16.4 Vaginal dissection. **A**, A vertical or inverted U-shaped incision is used on the vaginal mucosa overlying the midurethra and bladder. **B**, Careful dissection is carried out to the pubic rami bilaterally until the urogenital diaphragm is identified. Then it is sharply penetrated with the help of Mayo scissors. **C**, To develop the space, the opening created should be digitally enlarged by sweeping the index finger against the arch of the symphysis pubis. The same procedure is repeated on the opposite side.

vaginal procedure. To access the lateral aspect of the distal thigh, the leg is medially rotated and adducted. Two transverse incisions, approximately 5 to 6 cm in length, are made: the distal approximately 4 to 6 cm superior to the lateral femoral condyle, and the proximal 8 cm cranially to the first. The incision is carried down through the fatty tissue to the level of the fascia, and the fascia cleared either sharply or bluntly for an appropriate distance to attain a graft 8 × 2 cm in size. The fascial strip is harvested, using both incisions as needed for exposure. Once the graft is removed, the fascial defect is not repaired, and the subcutaneous tissue and skin are closed in multiple layers with absorbable suture. A Penrose drain can be secured in place through a separate stab incision and may be removed after 24 hours. Alternatively, a dedicated fascial stripper may be used for graft harvest when a full strip of fascia is desired. Other than tissue harvest, the remainder of the procedure is similar to that described above, except that a small suprapubic incision (5–6 cm) can be used.

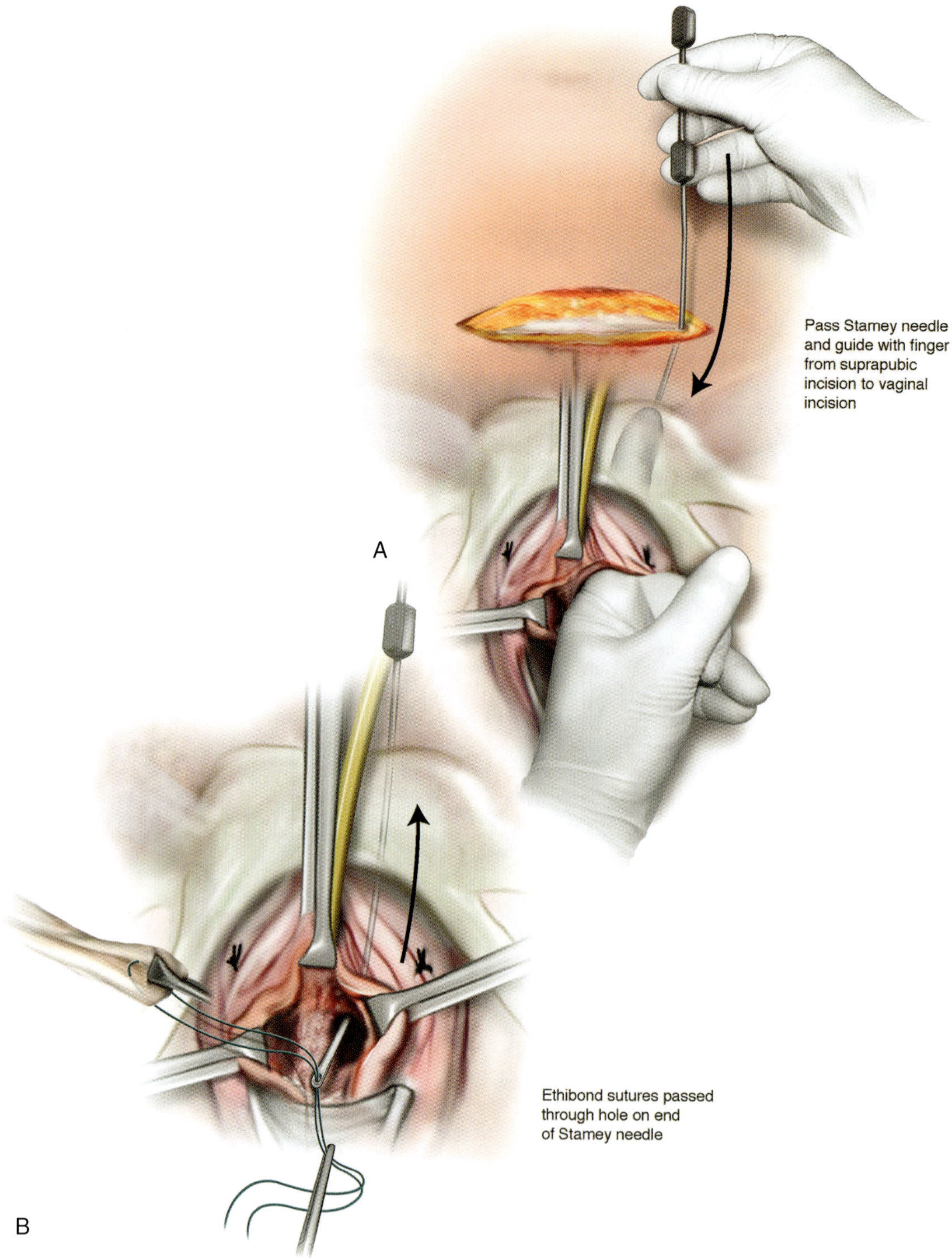

Fig. 16.5 Placement of the sling. **A**, Insert the Stamey needle through the rectus fascia and guide it into the vagina with the index finger in contact with the tip of the needle. **B**, Thread both ends of the polyester suture into the eye of the Stamey needle and then retract carefully until the suture ends are delivered abdominally at the level of the fascia.

OUTCOMES

Studies show that pubovaginal slings, in general, are highly effective, with success rates between 50% and 75% (depending on definition of cure) when followed for up to 10 years (Norton & Brubaker, 2006). In 2011, a review reported 4-year follow-up with improvement or cure in 100% of patients with uncomplicated stress incontinence and up to 93% in the more complicated cases (Blaivas & Chaikin, 2011). The same authors reported that most failures were caused by urge incontinence and happened within the first 6 months postoperatively; 3% of these patients were felt to have developed *de novo* urge incontinence.

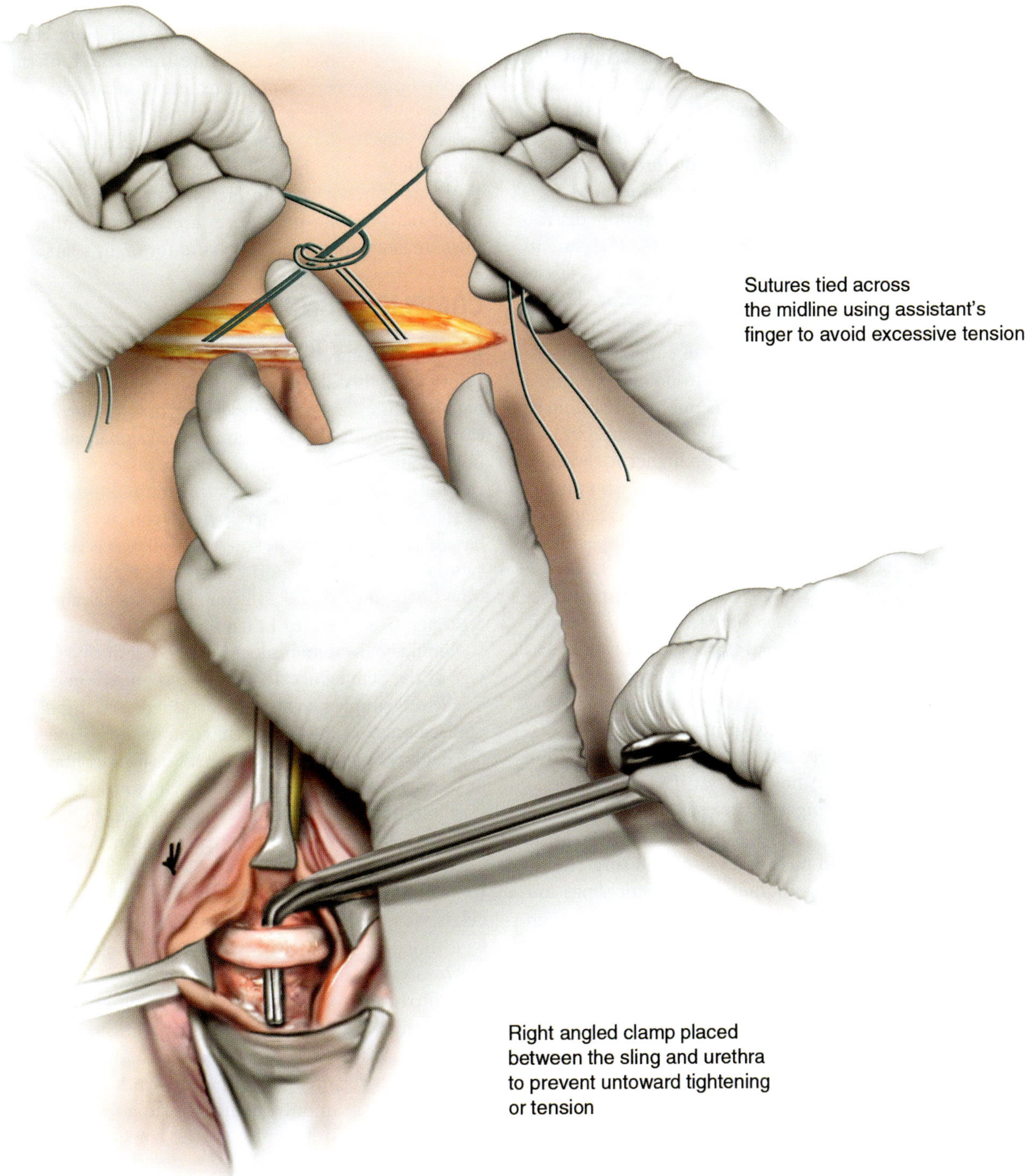

Fig. 16.6 Tensioning of the sling. Sling tensioning is done by tying the suspensory sutures abdominally above the fascial closure line. The sutures are tied across the assistant's index finger to avoid excessive tensioning. This is done concurrently with a right-angle clamp being placed between the pubovaginal sling and the vagina.

In the majority of reported cases in the literature, the suburethral sling procedure has been used predominantly as a treatment for patients with recurrent SUI after previous antiincontinence surgeries. Used for recurrent SUI, the objective cure rates recorded in the literature range between 61% and 100%, with a mean cure rate of 85%. The reported literature related to the use of pubovaginal fascial sling as a first procedure is limited, but a mean continence rate of 94% is quoted by Jarvis (1994).

Two large cohort studies have been done assessing the results of pubovaginal fascial sling for SUI. Morgan et al. (2000) reported a long-term follow-up of 247 women with types II and III incontinence after rectus fascia pubovaginal sling. These patients were followed urodynamically, as well as with quality-of-life questionnaires. At a mean follow-up of 51 months (range, 22–68 months), continence rates were 88% overall, with a 91% cure rate for type II and 84% for type III stress incontinence. Preoperative urge incontinence resolved in 81 of 109 patients (74%), whereas *de novo* urgency developed in 7% of women. Secondary procedures were required in 14 patients for management of incontinence, and five required urethrolysis. Of the 247 women, 235 (95%) completed questionnaires, and 92% reported a high degree of satisfaction with low symptom distress scores. In another study by Chaikin et al. (1998), 251 patients were followed for more than 1 year after implantation of a fascial sling; 92% of patients were objectively cured or improved. Most of the postoperative incontinence was urge incontinence. Permanent urinary retention developed in 2% of patients.

In one of the most important studies to date, 655 women with SUI were randomized to rectus fascia pubovaginal sling or Burch colposuspension in the SISTEr trial (Albo et al., 2007). At 24 months after surgery, success rates were higher for women who underwent the sling procedure than for those who underwent Burch colposuspension, for both the overall category of success (47% vs. 38%; $P = .01$) and the category specific to stress incontinence (66% vs. 49%; $P < .001$). However, women who underwent the sling procedure had more urinary tract infections, difficulty voiding, and postoperative urge incontinence. A 5-year extended follow-up of this important study was reported by Brubaker et al. (2012). Patients were evaluated yearly for a minimum of 5 years. Overall, continence at 5 years was lower in the Burch urethropexy group than in the fascial sling group ($P = .002$). Patient satisfaction declined with time in both groups ($P = .001$); however, satisfaction remained higher in the pubovaginal sling group versus the Burch group ($P = .03$).

In a systematic review and meta-analysis of SUI surgeries by Novara et al. (2010), retropubic midurethral synthetic slings and autologous pubovaginal slings were similarly effective, although patients with pubovaginal slings had more voiding problems after surgery. The Cochrane review on suburethral slings from 2020 identified 34 trials involving 3244 patients; 14 trials compared pubovaginal sling to synthetic midurethral sling. Depending on how continence and important differences in continence were defined, the review concluded that the efficacy of pubovaginal slings is not better than that of synthetic midurethral slings. Limited evidence suggested that the pubovaginal sling might result in superior continence at 10 years (51% vs. 32%: odds ratio 2.22, 95% confidence interval 1.07–4.61); however, synthetic midurethral slings have fewer perioperative complications (Saraswat et al., 2020). In a recent prospective nonrandomized study comparing synthetic midurethral sling to rectus fascia pubovaginal sling, 91 (45%) women chose a pubovaginal sling, and 110 (55%) chose a midurethral sling. Although follow-up was short (12 months), there was no statistical difference in subjective cure rate, and adverse events were comparable (Mock et al., 2015).

A study using the National Surgical Quality Improvement Program database evaluated 161 women who underwent an autologous fascial sling procedure from 2005 to 2015. A total of 126 (78.3%) had rectus fascia, and 35 (21.7%) had fascia lata harvest. The primary outcomes of the study were composite postoperative adverse events, readmission, and reoperation. There were no significant differences in operative time, length of stay, rate of reoperation, adverse events, or readmission rates between the two different harvest sites (Cardenas-Trowers et al., 2020).

The intermediate and long-term results for suburethral slings suggest that the 10-year continence rate is similar to the 1-year continence rate. In fact, Bidmead and Cardozo (2000) noted that, if sling procedures are successful after 6 months, they are likely to remain successful for many years.

COMPLICATIONS

Lower Urinary Tract Injury

Injury to the bladder or urethra can result from any of the vaginal procedures previously described for stress incontinence. This can occur during the dissection of the vaginal epithelium off the underlying fascia or during the lateral dissection below the inferior pubic ramus, when penetrating the endopelvic fascia. Injury to the urethra and bladder is more common in patients who have had previous anterior vaginal wall or bladder neck surgery. Cystotomy and urethrotomy should be repaired in layers at the time of the injury, and continuous bladder drainage instituted postoperatively for 7 to 14 days to allow adequate healing.

Should inadvertent bladder injury occur during retropubic passage of the Stamey needles and be recognized on cystoscopy, the needle can simply be withdrawn and repassed through the retropubic space, and the procedure continued as planned. Unrecognized injury or suture penetration in the bladder lumen may result in postoperative irritative bladder symptoms, persistent urinary tract infection, or formation of bladder calculi. Injury to the ureter during all sling operations for stress incontinence is rare.

Pelvic Visceral Injuries and Blood Loss

Pelvic visceral injuries and pelvic hematomas are rare and can be avoided or minimized by adequate dissection of the endopelvic fascia and retropubic space and careful needle passage in close proximity to the posterior surface of the pubic bone, with distal needle control with the surgeon's finger. If an inadvertent cystotomy or urethrotomy were to occur, the injury should be appropriately repaired. In contrast to synthetic sling placement, which would commonly require aborting the procedure, a biologic sling could still be placed after concurrent intraoperative repair of the injury.

Miscellaneous Surgical Complications

Superficial wound infection, subcutaneous seromas, and abdominal fascial hernias are uncommon. In obese patients, the use of a subcutaneous drain may be necessitated to prevent fluid loculations. Sling erosions with autologous tissue are exceedingly rare.

Voiding Dysfunction

Most of the chronic complications after biologic sling procedures relate to voiding dysfunction and urge symptoms. Modifications designed to achieve greater stabilization, such as anchorage to the pubic bone, do not seem to result in improvement over existing techniques, and carry a risk of osteomyelitis at the site of anchorage.

Studies have reported development of *de novo* urgency and storage symptoms in up to 23% of patients, with 11% of patients reporting voiding dysfunctions and up to 7.8% requiring long-term self-catheterization (Norton & Brubaker, 2006). The few randomized controlled trials (RCTs) comparing pubovaginal slings to tension-free vaginal tape (TVT) have had flawed methodology; thus, their outcomes are questionable (Novara et al., 2010). Basok et al. (2008) showed an increased rate of *de novo* urgency in the pubovaginal sling group compared with the intravaginal slingplasty group, whereas Sharifiaghdas and Mortazavi (2008) showed equal efficacy between pubovaginal and retropubic midurethral synthetic slings on follow-up. The most scientifically valid RCT was performed by Arunkalaivanan and Barrington (2003) and showed equal subjective cure rates, as well as complication rates, when a biologic pubovaginal sling was compared with TVT. In this study, the pubovaginal sling was of porcine origin. When comparing autologous versus allograft slings, Flynn and Yap (2002) showed equal effectiveness in control of stress incontinence over 2 years, with reduced postoperative discomfort in the allograft group. Recurrent SUI developed in up to 10% of patients in both groups. Autologous pubovaginal slings were compared with Burch colposuspension in a multicenter RCT (SISTEr trial) that showed superiority of fascial slings in controlling incontinence, despite an increased morbidity profile (Albo et al., 2007). A 2010 meta-analysis compared pubovaginal and midurethral synthetic slings and found that equal subjective cure rates and equal overall effectiveness were reported.

Transient urinary retention may occur in up to 20% of patients and requires intermittent self-catheterization until resolution (typically 2–4 weeks). Prolonged (persisting >4–6 weeks) postoperative voiding dysfunction, including *de novo* urgency, urgency incontinence, and/or obstructive symptoms, may occur to some degree in up to 25% of patients. Less than 3% of women require subsequent urethrolysis for treatment of prolonged retention/obstructive voiding symptoms. Some surgeons routinely teach patients intermittent self-catheterization in the preoperative period to facilitate its use, if necessary, postoperatively.

Technical Tips

Given that substantial bleeding can occur during vaginal dissection, harvesting the autologous fascia and preparing the sling by affixing sutures should be performed before vaginal dissection, such that the sling may be inserted and deployed in a timely manner, and blood loss can be minimized. Retropubic bleeding occurring during dissection will almost always resolve with sling placement, and time should not be expended with prolonged attempts at hemostasis.

When performing an autologous pubovaginal sling in the setting of urethral reconstruction (e.g., urethrovaginal fistula or diverticulum resection) or as tissue interposition, harvesting fascia and preparing and deploying the sling with passage of the retropubic sutures, but not tensioning, should all be performed before the delicate urethral reconstruction. Once the reconstruction is finished, the sling can be affixed in the appropriate location and tensioned. Damage to the reconstruction can occur through traction or direct injury if the sling is deployed after reconstruction.

Surface orientation of the autologous sling material during placement of the graft does not matter; by convention, the body "side" or underside of the graft is placed on the body "side" of the patient.

Sling tensioning, for most women, can be accomplished with the "two finger" distance over the fascia. However, in women who have had multiple procedures and who have a nonmobile urethra, the sling tension should be more significant. We prefer using a one-fingerbreadth knot with concomitant cystoscopic evidence of an impression ("lip" or "ledge") being created on the ventrum of the urethra.

BIBLIOGRAPHY

Albo ME, Richter HE, Brubaker L, et al. Burch colposuspension versus fascial sling to reduce urinary stress incontinence. *N Engl J Med.* 2007;356:2143.

Aldridge AH. Transplantation of fascia for relief of urinary stress incontinence. *Am J Obstet Gynecol.* 1942;44:398.

Anger JT, Litwin MS, Wang Q, et al. Complications of sling surgery among female Medicare beneficiaries. *Obstet Gynecol.* 2007;109:707.

Arunkalaivanan AS, Barrington JW. Randomized trial of porcine dermal sling (Pelvicol implant) vs. tension-free vaginal tape (TVT) in the surgical treatment of stress incontinence: a questionnaire-based study. *Int Urogynecol J Pelvic Floor Dysfunct.* 2003;14:17.

Basok EK, Yildirim A, Atsu N, et al. Cadaveric fascia lata versus intravaginal slingplasty for the pubovaginal sling: surgical outcome, overall success and patient satisfaction rates. *Urol Int.* 2008;80:46.

Bidmead J, Cardozo L. Sling techniques in the treatment of genuine stress incontinence. *Br J Obstet Gynaecol.* 2000;107:147.

Blaivas JG, Chaikin DC. Pubovaginal fascial sling for the treatment of all types of stress urinary incontinence: surgical technique and long-term outcome. *Urol Clin North Am.* 2011;38:7.

Blaivas JG, Jacobs BZ. Pubovaginal fascial sling for the treatment of complicated stress urinary incontinence. *J Urol.* 1991;145:1214.

Blaivas JG, Olsson CA. Stress incontinence: classification and surgical approach. *J Urol.* 1988;139:727.

Brubaker L, Richter HE, Norton PA, et al. 5-year continence rates, satisfaction and adverse events of burch urethropexy and fascial sling surgery for urinary incontinence. *J Urol.* 2012;187:1324.

Cardenas-Trowers OO, Stewart R, Meriwether KV, et al. Comparison of perioperative outcomes of autologous bladder neck fascial slings based on fascial harvest site: a secondary analysis of the national surgical quality improvement program database. *Female Pelvic Med Reconstr* Surg. 2020;26:526.

Chaikin DC, Rosenthal J, Blaivas JG. Pubovaginal fascial sling for all types of stress urinary incontinence: long-term analysis. *J Urol.* 1998;160:1312.

Dmochowski RR, Blaivas JM, Gormley EA, et al. Update of AUA guideline on the surgical management of female stress urinary incontinence. *J Urol.* 2010;183:1906.

Flynn BJ, Yap WT. Pubovaginal sling using allograft fascia lata versus autograft fascia for all types of stress urinary incontinence: 2-year minimum follow-up. *J Urol.* 2002;167:608.

Gomelsky A, Dmochowski RR. Bladder neck pubovaginal slings. *Expert Rev Med Devices.* 2005;2:327.

Groutz A, Blaivas JG, Hyman MJ, Chaikin DC. Pubovaginal sling surgery for simple stress urinary incontinence: analysis by an outcome score. *J Urol.* 2001;165:1597.

Huang YH, Lin AT, Chen KK, et al. High failure rate using allograft fascia lata in pubovaginal sling surgery for female stress urinary incontinence. *Urology.* 2001;58:943.

Jarvis GJ. Surgery for genuine stress incontinence. *Br J Obstet Gynecol.* 1994;101:371.

McGuire EJ, Lytton B. Pubovaginal sling procedure for stress incontinence. *J Urol.* 1978;167:1120.

Mock S, Angelle J, Reynolds WS, et al. Contemporary comparison between retropubic midurethral sling and autologous pubovaginal sling for stress urinary incontinence after the FDA advisory notification. *Urology.* 2015;85:321.

Morgan Jr TO, Westney OL, McGuire EJ. Pubovaginal sling: 4-year outcome analysis and quality-of-life assessment. *J Urol.* 2000;163:1845.

Norton P, Brubaker L. Urinary incontinence in women. *Lancet.* 2006;367:57.

Novara G, Artibani W, Barber MD, et al. Updated systematic review and meta-analysis of the comparative data on colposuspensions, pubovaginal slings, and midurethral tapes in the surgical treatment of female stress urinary incontinence. *Eur Urol.* 2010;58:218.

Ogah J, Cody DJ, Rogerson L. Minimally invasive synthetic suburethral sling operations for stress urinary incontinence in women: a short version Cochrane review. *Neurourol Urodyn.* 2011;30:284.

Richter HE, Varner RE, Sanders E, et al. Effects of pubovaginal sling procedure on patients with urethral hypermobility and intrinsic sphincteric deficiency: would they do it again? *Am J Obstet Gynecol.* 2001;184:14.

Saraswat L, Rehman H, Omar MI, et al. Traditional suburethral sling operations for urinary incontinence in women. *Cochrane Database Syst Rev.* 2020;1:CD001754.

Sharifiaghdas F, Mortazavi N. Tension-free vaginal tape and autologous rectus fascia pubovaginal sling for the treatment of urinary stress incontinence: a medium-term follow-up. *Med Princ Pract.* 2008;17:209.

Smith ARB, Dmochowski R, Hilton P, et al. Committee 14: Surgery for urinary incontinence in women. In: Abrams P, Cardozo L, Khoury S, Wein A, eds. *Incontinence: 4th International Consultation on Incontinence.* Paris, France: Health Publication Ltd; 2009.

Tcherniakovsky M, Fernandes CE, Bezerra CA, et al. Comparative results of two techniques to treat stress urinary incontinence: synthetic transobturator and aponeurotic slings. *Int Urogynecol J.* 2009;20:961.

Wilson WJ, Winters JC. Is there still a place for the pubovaginal sling at the bladder neck in the era of the midurethral sling? *Curr Urol Rep.* 2005;6:335.

17

Synthetic Midurethral Slings for Stress Urinary Incontinence

Matthew D. Barber, Mark D. Walters, and Mickey M. Karram

CHAPTER OUTLINE

INTRODUCTION

Synthetic midurethral slings (MUSs) have become the most popular surgical procedures performed for the treatment of stress urinary incontinence (SUI) in the twenty-first century. Few operations in gynecology or urology have been as well studied or have gained such wide acceptance. These procedures generally have been shown to be minimally invasive, and have high efficacy, low morbidity, and a relatively quick recovery. This chapter discusses synthetic retropubic, transobturator (TOT), and single-incision MUSs. Because the efficacy data are few, we do not discuss variations that use biologic materials for the slings. A complete discussion of autologous fascia bladder neck slings is found in Chapter 16.

RETROPUBIC MIDURETHRAL SLINGS

Retropubic MUSs were developed in the mid-1990s in an attempt to create a minimally invasive surgical treatment for SUI. Until this time, incontinence procedures aimed at suspending or supporting the proximal urethra and bladder neck. Ulmsten and Petros (1995) described a rationale for a more distally placed suburethral sling based on concepts they termed the "integral theory." This theory was based on the presumption that the pubourethral ligaments support the midurethra and attach to the pubic bones, acting as a backboard for the midurethra. This backboard allows for compression of the midurethra against it when intraabdominal pressure increases, thus maintaining continence. The theory states that the absence of the backboard support causes a loss of this watertight seal, and SUI develops. By passing a strip of supportive material (loosely woven polypropylene) under the midurethra in women with SUI, this "backboard" action could theoretically be replicated. The strip of polypropylene is left loose or "tensionless," and direct compression of the urethra is avoided. In its earliest configuration, placement of the MUS was achieved through an anterior vaginal wall dissection at the level of the midurethra. Placement of the sling material was accomplished by passing the arms of the tape (sling) in a retropubic fashion through the anterior abdominal wall with the aid of specially designed trocars. Available data from anatomic dissections, ultrasound, and magnetic resonance imaging do not necessarily support Ulmsten and Petros' description of the role of the pubourethral ligaments in urinary continence; nevertheless, MUSs have been shown through clinical studies to be the safest and most effective surgical treatment for SUI currently available. The primary mechanism of action for MUS is thought by most to be midurethral kinking against or around the sling with increased intraabdominal pressure.

The first commercially available retropubic MUS was tension-free vaginal tape (TVT; Ethicon, Somerville, NJ; Fig. 17.1), which

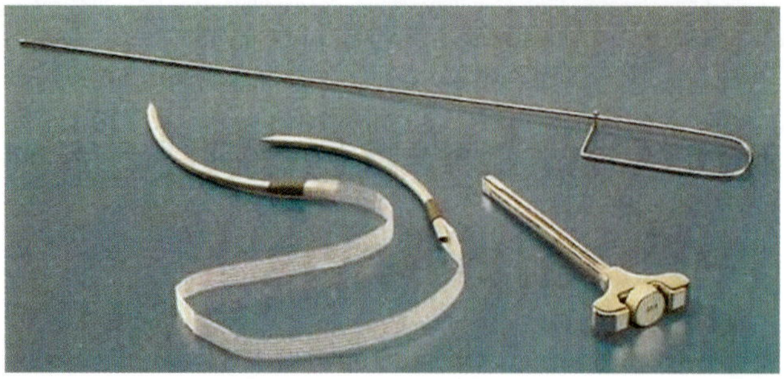

Fig. 17.1 Tension-free vaginal tape instrumentation, including (*clockwise from top*) a Foley catheter guide, needle introducer/handle, and specially designed needles attached to synthetic suburethral sling tape. (Courtesy Ethicon Inc., Somerville, NJ.)

consisted of a narrow polypropylene mesh strip with two specially designed trocars. The trocars were inserted through a small vaginal incision and passed on each side of the urethra through the retropubic space to two exit locations in the suprapubic area of the anterior abdominal wall. Passage of the trocars from the vaginal incision to the anterior abdominal wall has been described as the "bottom-up" approach. Several other retropubic sling "kits" with minor modifications also are available, including a "top-down" approach whereby the trocars are passed retropubically from the anterior abdominal wall to the vaginal incision, and the tape is attached to the vaginal end of the trocar and then pulled back up through the retropubic space to the abdominal wall.

Indications, Patient Selection, and Types of Slings

The indications for retropubic MUS placement include symptomatic SUI or occult stress incontinence significantly affecting the patient's quality of life. Patients should have failed conservative treatments for SUI. Initial studies assessing functionality of the retropubic MUS mostly included "ideal" women—those who were not obese (body mass index [BMI] >35 kg/m^2), who had stress-predominant incontinence with a mobile urethra, and who had no prolapse. In time, studies also documented excellent outcomes in women who were overweight, had recurrent or mixed urinary incontinence, had intrinsic sphincter deficiency (ISD), and in whom the procedure could be performed in conjunction with a vaginal prolapse repair. Retropubic anatomy, prior surgery, body habitus, and surgeon experience are important variables to consider in surgical planning.

Absolute contraindications to the procedure include any important structure potentially in the path of the trocars or sling, such as a pelvic kidney or vascular graft, low ventral hernias, pregnancy, and active oral anticoagulation. Relative contraindications include any previous condition that would put the patient at high risk for significant pelvic adhesions, creating the risk for small bowel to be firmly adhered to the back of the pubic bone, such as a history of a ruptured appendix with peritonitis or stage 4 endometriosis. In such circumstances, a TOT sling would be a preferred procedure, because the retropubic space would be completely avoided.

Other patients in whom a synthetic sling is probably inappropriate include those with contraindications to permanent mesh implantation, including prior mesh complications or prior pelvic irradiation. Smoking also increases the risk of mesh complications and should be considered when choosing the type of continence surgery. Additionally, MUSs should generally be avoided in those who are undergoing concurrent or have undergone prior urethral reconstruction. Examples of this clinical situation include urethral diverticulectomy, urethrovaginal fistula repair, or urethral injury secondary to prior sling placement or pelvic fracture. Although there are few reports of MUS use in this setting, experience with synthetic material in the setting of urethral reconstruction has demonstrated a high rate of erosion (Morgan et al., 1985). In contrast, excellent outcomes have been reported with the use of a biologic pubovaginal sling (see Chapter 16) in the setting of reconstruction, with an 88% cure rate after diverticulectomy in 16 patients and an 86% cure rate after genitourinary fistula repair in seven patients, with no reported erosions (Carey et al., 2002). Also, a synthetic MUS is not the preferred procedure in the case of neurogenic incontinence, such as in a patient with spina bifida. Because patients with neurogenic incontinence are already dependent on clean intermittent self-catheterization, a tension-free MUS may not provide the necessary compression to achieve continence between catheterizations. Biologic pubovaginal slings have been used successfully in patients with neurogenic causes of SUI, successfully providing occlusion at the bladder neck, with continence rates of 95% in one study (Austin et al., 2001).

Surgical Technique

Bottom-to-Top (See Video 17.1)

1. Preoperative considerations. Single-dose intravenous perioperative antibiotics are given for skin and vaginal flora coverage. The antibiotic classes commonly used include intravenous cephalosporins and fluoroquinolones. Antiembolic prophylaxis is given as indicated. Sterile urine should be confirmed before the procedure; some physicians postpone surgery if an active urinary tract infection is documented.
2. Patient positioning and preparation. The patient is positioned in the dorsal lithotomy position, with legs supported in Allen or candy cane stirrups and all pressure points padded appropriately. The perineum and vagina are prepared, and surgical draping is placed to allow access to the vagina and suprapubic area.
3. Anesthesia. We prefer to use general anesthesia; however, some surgeons prefer intravenous sedation with local anesthesia to allow the cough stress test to be performed to facilitate appropriate tensioning of the sling. Because approximately 50% of cases are done in conjunction with a prolapse repair, all surgeons need to be well versed in tensioning techniques under general anesthesia (see step 8).
4. Vaginal dissection. The anterior vaginal wall is hydrodissected with a combination of lidocaine and epinephrine, with the goal of completely blanching the anterior vaginal wall at the level of the mid- to distal urethra. A scalpel is used to make an incision from just below the external urethral meatus to the level of the midurethra. The vaginal wall is sharply dissected with Metzenbaum scissors off the posterior urethra, creating small tunnels to the inferior pubic ramus (Fig. 17.2). Sharp dissection is required, because the distal anterior vaginal wall and posterior urethra are fused at this level. Some physicians prefer to hydrodissect along the trocar trajectory bilaterally before passing the trocars.

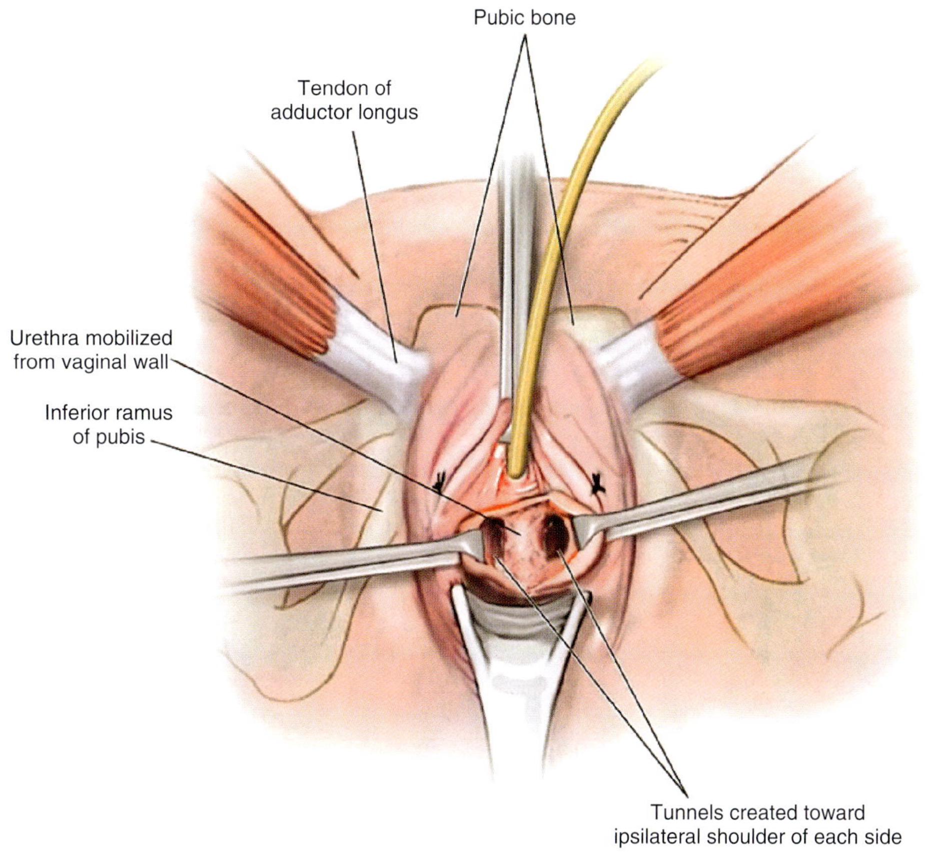

Fig. 17.2 Vaginal incision for a retropubic midurethral sling. Tunnels are created bilaterally to allow trocars to come into direct contact with the inferior pubic ramus.

5. Trocar passage. A catheter guide is placed in the indwelling Foley catheter so that the urethra and bladder neck can be displaced away from where the trocar is inserted. The trocar tip is inserted into the previously dissected tunnel on each side, lateral to the urethra, and advanced to the undersurface of the pubic bone. The tip of the trocar should be sandwiched between the index finger of the surgeon's nondominant hand placed in the anterior vaginal fornix and the undersurface of the interior pubic ramus. Care is taken not to "button-hole" into the vaginal lumen at the fornix. The tip of the needle is carefully advanced through the endopelvic fascia into the retropubic space (Fig. 17.3). When the resistance of the endopelvic fascia is overcome, and the tip of the needle is in the retropubic space, the handle of the trocar is dropped, and the needle is advanced through the retropubic space as it hugs the back of the pubic bone (Fig. 17.4). The next resistance felt is the rectus muscle and anterior abdominal fascia. The needle is advanced through these structures to exit through the previously made suprapubic stab wound (see Fig. 17.4). Fig. 17.5 illustrates the appropriate passage of the needle through the retropubic space when viewed from above, as well as examples of incorrect passage of the trocar.
6. Cystoscopy. Careful cystoscopy is performed with a 70-degree scope to evaluate the bladder for inadvertent trocar injury with the trocar in place. If such an injury were to occur, it would generally be visualized in the anterolateral aspect of the bladder (usually the area between 1 o'clock and 3 o'clock on the left side and 9 o'clock and 11 o'clock on the right side). If the trocar is seen, or if there is any creasing of the bladder mucosa that does not disappear with bladder distention, the trocar should be withdrawn and repassed. When the bladder is perforated (which occurs in approximately 3%–5% of cases), it is most often because the surgeon has allowed the trocar to migrate too medially, or away from the back of the pubic bone in a cephalad direction (see Fig. 17.5A and C). During repassage of the trocar, great care should be taken to hug the back of the pubic bone. In such cases, the patient may still proceed with the postoperative voiding trial without the need for discharge with an indwelling catheter, because the bladder perforation is very small and usually in a high, nondependent portion of the bladder. If excessive hematuria is present, or if the base or trigone of the bladder is perforated, postoperative bladder drainage should be continued for at least a few days. If bladder perforations occur on multiple attempts, the surgeon should consider another approach that avoids the retropubic space, such as TOT MUS.
7. For passage of the sling, the trocar tips are disconnected from the handle, and the mesh and its plastic sheath are pulled up through the suprapubic stab wound along the trocar trajectory.
8. Tensioning. Sling tensioning is very subjective. It may be done using a No. 8 Hegar dilator, Mayo scissor, or surgical clamp, such as a right-angled clamp, inserted between the posterior urethra and the suburethral portion of the sling if the patient is receiving general anesthesia (Fig. 17.6). Some surgeons prefer to perform the procedure using a local anesthetic and use a cough stress test. Regardless of tensioning

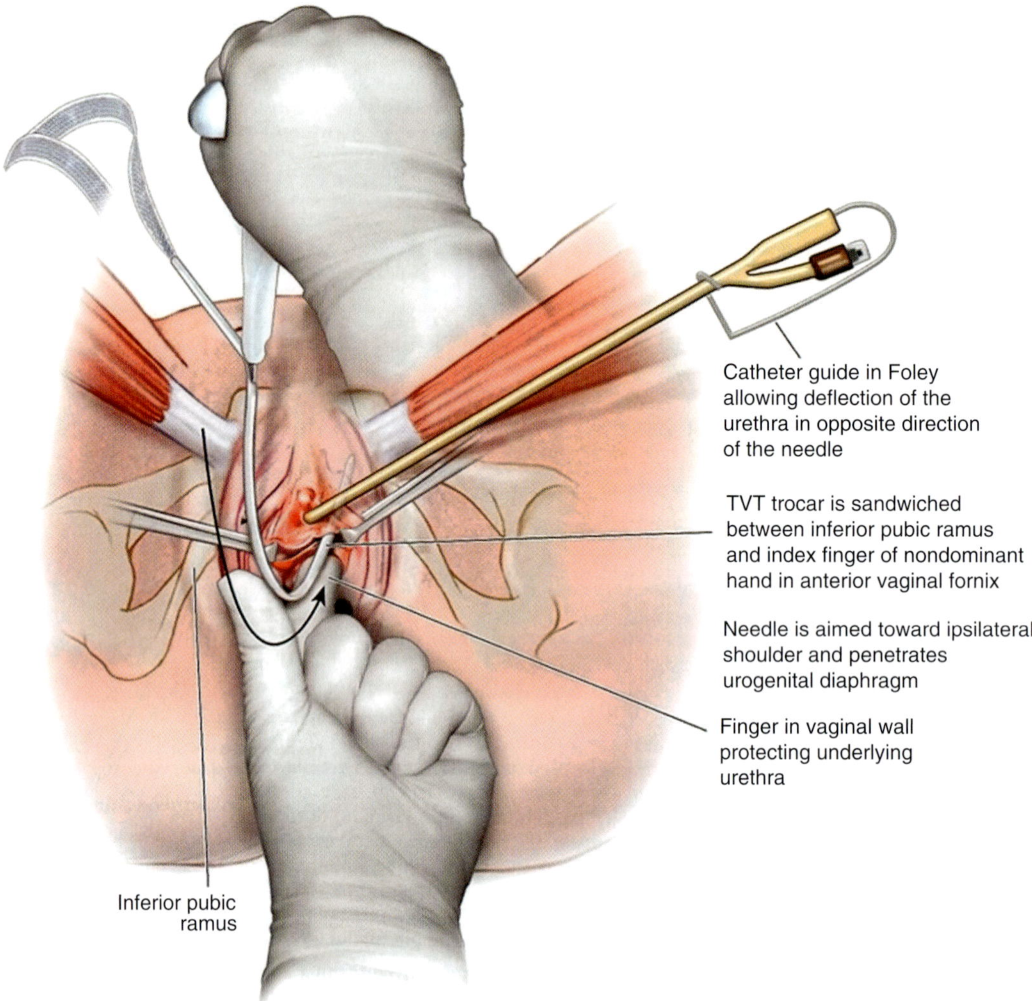

Fig. 17.3 Technique for initial passage of trocars through the vaginal incision toward the retropubic space. *TVT*, Tension-free vaginal tape.

technique, the ultimate endpoint is to create a laxity in the mesh manifested by a ricochet of the mesh back toward the urethra if it is pulled on vaginally using a right-angled clamp, as well as avoiding direct contact of the mesh with the underside of the urethra. Then the plastic sheaths covering the mesh, if present, are removed, and tension of the mesh is rechecked. The mesh is suprapubically resected flush with the skin, making sure the skin is mobilized away from the mesh ends before skin closure.

9. The vaginal wound is copiously irrigated and closed with a running 2-0 or 3-0 polyglycolic acid suture. The suprapubic stab wounds are closed with an absorbable suture or liquid tissue adhesive.
10. The catheter may be removed in the recovery room, and the patient is discharged after confirming voiding efficiency. If unable to void, the patient is taught intermittent self-catheterization, or an indwelling Foley catheter is placed.

Top-to-Bottom

1. Vaginal dissection. The vaginal incision should be larger than that described for the bottom-to-top technique, because the dissection must allow the index finger of the surgeon's nondominant hand to be placed into the incision to pick up the tip of the needle as it passes into the vaginal incision.
2. Top-to-bottom trocar passage. Before passage of the trocars, complete drainage of the bladder is ensured. At the previously marked puncture sites in the suprapubic region, a stab incision is made on each side. The incisions should be well within the pubic tubercles bilaterally. A trocar is inserted into the first of the suprapubic incisions, aligned with the sagittal axis of the body, and then carefully punctures through the anterior rectus sheath. By angling caudally and "walking off" the superior posterior edge of the pubic bone, the trocar is advanced into the retropubic space, maintaining close contact with the posterior surface of the pubic bone. Concurrently, the surgeon's finger is inserted into the previously dissected periurethral space on the ipsilateral side to control the distal tip of the trocar. In a controlled manner, the trocar is progressively advanced until the tip is visible in the vaginal incision. Cystoscopy, as previously described, is performed to confirm that the needle did not penetrate the bladder. The same maneuver is performed on the contralateral side (Fig. 17.7A and B).

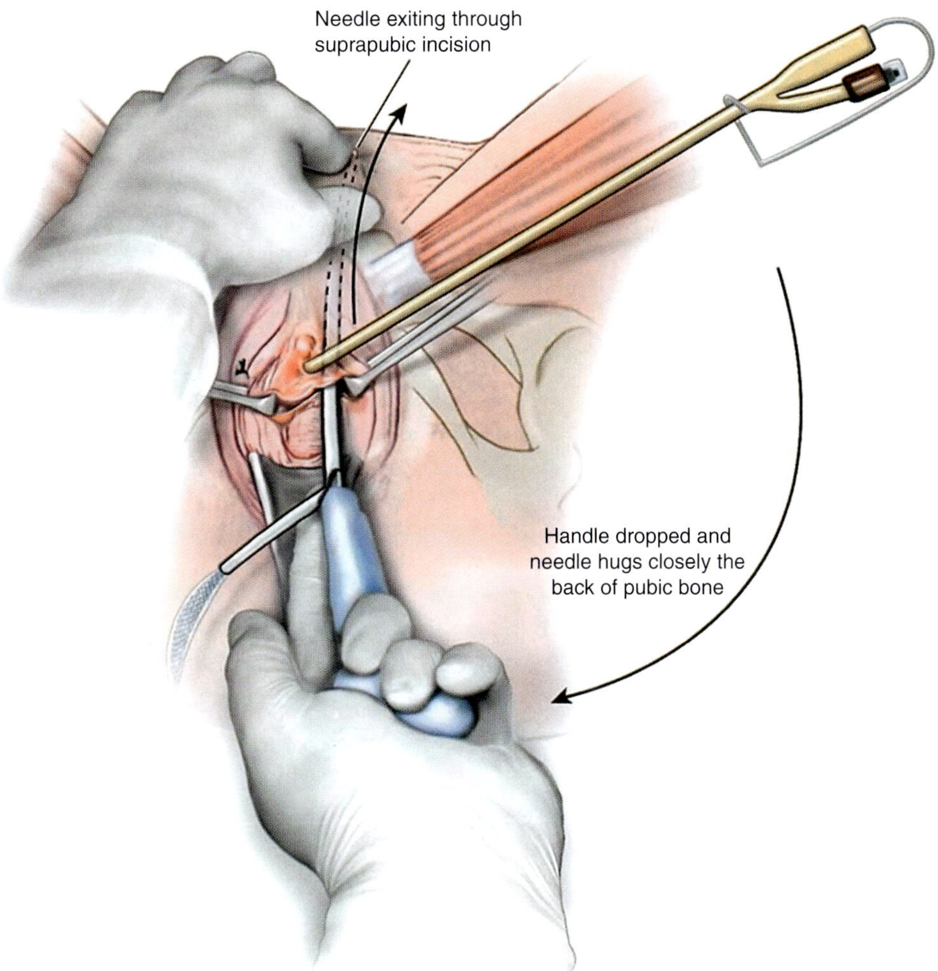

Fig. 17.4 Technique for passage of trocars through the retropubic space.

3. Loading the mesh. The mesh is attached to the trocars, and the trocars are withdrawn through the suprapubic stab wounds. The sling is tensioned as previously described for the bottom-to-top technique (Fig. 17.6).

TRANSOBTURATOR MIDURETHRAL SLINGS

Indications, Patient Selection, and Types of Slings

Because retropubic MUS require blind passage of a trocar through the retropubic space, inadvertent bladder perforation occurs in 3% to 5% of cases. Also, vascular and bowel injuries that resulted in significant morbidity and mortality have been reported, albeit very rarely. In the hope of avoiding these complications, DeLorme described the TOT technique for MUS placement in 2001; this was published by Dargent et al. (2002). The inside-out variation was described by de Leval (2003).

As with retropubic synthetic slings, this is a minimally invasive MUS using a synthetic tape; however, it is placed using a TOT approach rather than a retropubic one, almost eliminating any potential for bladder or bowel perforation and major vascular injury. Specially designed needles are passed either from the inner groin into the vaginal incision (outside-in technique) or from the vaginal incision into the inner groin (inside-out technique). When the procedure is performed in an appropriate fashion, the needle, and subsequently the sling, pass through (from the outside in) the subcutaneous fat, gracilis tendon, adductor brevis, obturator externus, obturator membrane, and obturator internus (Whiteside & Walters, 2004). TOT slings use the basic concept of midurethral support with the sling placed underneath the urethra; resistance against the urethra is generated when intraabdominal pressure increases, which increases outlet resistance and prevents SUI.

TOT slings have become a popular surgical treatment for SUI. The technique has been shown to be a low-risk procedure with effectiveness comparable to most other surgical options. TOT slings are associated with a lower risk of urethral obstruction, urinary retention, and subsequent need for sling release compared with retropubic slings. For primary cases, a TOT sling demonstrates similar rates of cure compared with retropubic synthetic slings, with fewer bladder perforations and postoperative irritative voiding symptoms (Ford et al., 2017). Also, as mentioned, rare but catastrophic bowel and major vessel injuries are almost eliminated. The tradeoff is that patients experience more complications referable to the groin, such as pain and leg weakness or numbness, with the

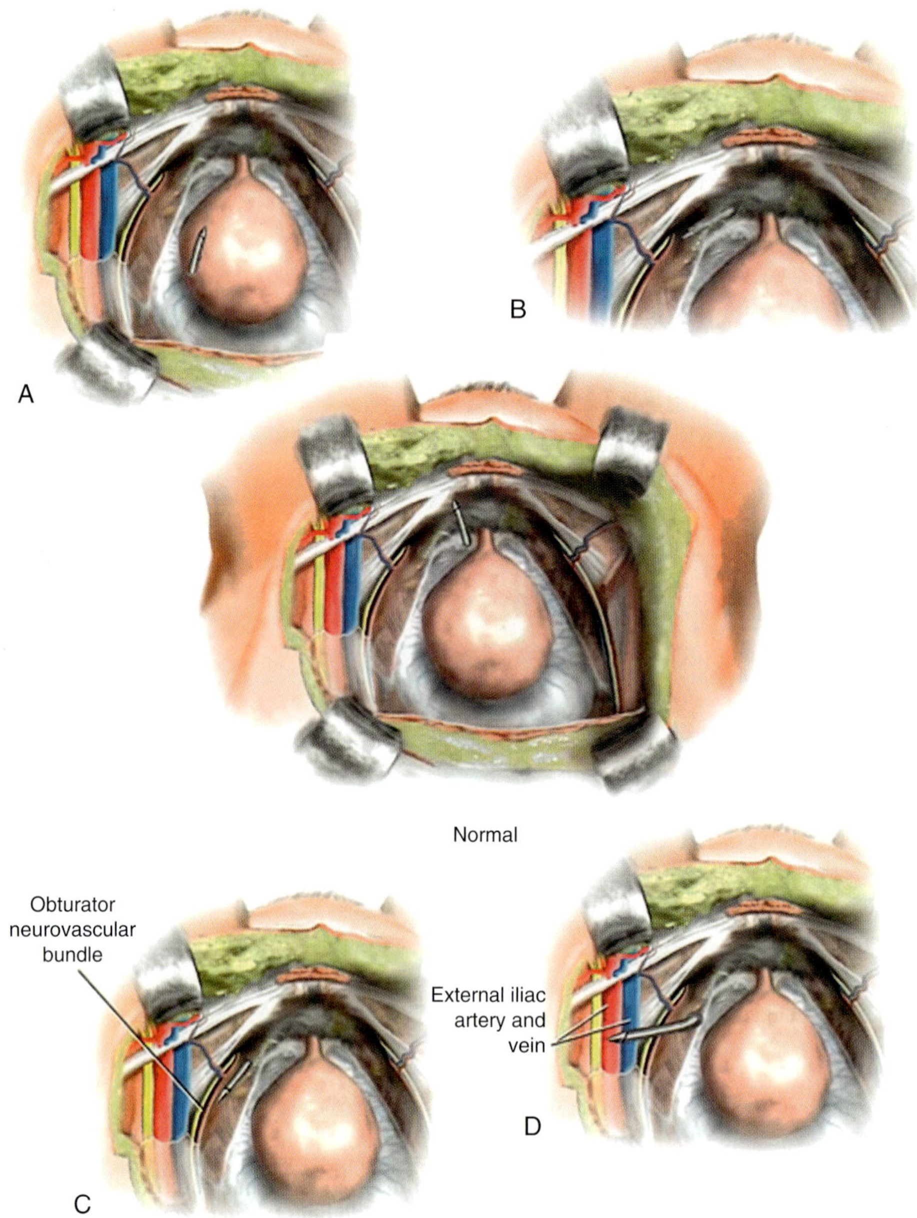

Fig. 17.5 Correct placement of the tension-free vaginal tape (TVT) trocar into the retropubic space (center). Incorrect TVT placements include: **A**, Placement of the TVT device through the bladder, typically at its lateral edge or slightly near the dome; **B**, lateral deviation of the trocar either caused by aiming it lateral to the ipsilateral shoulder or to external rotation of the device; **C**, placement of the trocar too cephalad and lateral so that it approaches the obturator neurovascular bundle; and **D**, significant lateral deviation of the trocar, risking damage to the external iliac artery or vein.

TOT approach. Retropubic slings may be more effective for recurrent incontinence and in women with ISD, although the data supporting this statement are difficult to interpret because of controversy regarding how best to define and diagnose ISD.

Indications for TOT sling placement are the same as for retropubic MUS, with the possible exception of recurrent incontinence or ISD. Contraindications include pregnancy, groin abscesses, chronic infection or pain, and active anticoagulation. TOT slings are also commonly placed in women undergoing repair of pelvic organ prolapse in the hope of preventing the *de novo* development of SUI (occult incontinence).

Surgical Technique

As previously mentioned, TOT slings can be placed inside-to-outside or outside-to-inside. The indications, effectiveness, and frequency of complications seem to be similar between the two groups (Ford et al., 2017; Madhuvrata et al., 2012; Novara et al., 2010). At the present time, the decision regarding which approach to use is based mostly on the preference and experience of the surgeon.

Inside-Out (See Video 17.2)

1. Preoperative considerations. Single-dose intravenous perioperative antibiotics are given for skin and vaginal flora

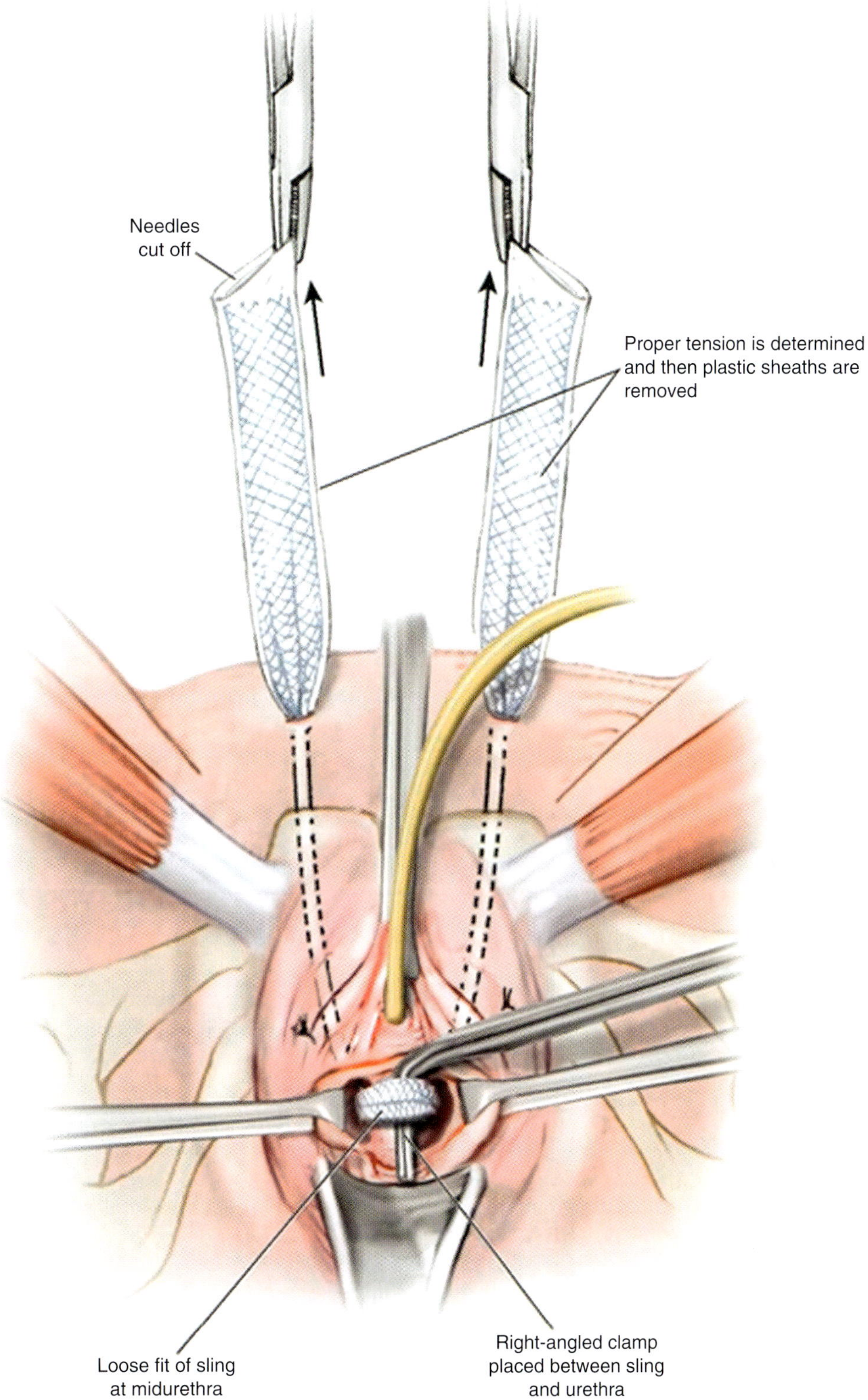

Fig. 17.6 Technique for tensioning a retropubic midurethral sling.

coverage. The antibiotic classes commonly used include intravenous cephalosporins and fluoroquinolones. Antiembolic prophylaxis is given as indicated. Sterile urine should be confirmed before the procedure; some physicians postpone the surgery if an active urinary tract infection is documented.

2. Patient positioning and preparation. The patient is positioned in the dorsal lithotomy position, with legs supported in Allen or candy cane stirrups and all pressure points padded appropriately. The perineum and vagina are prepared, and surgical draping is placed to allow access to the vagina and inner groin.

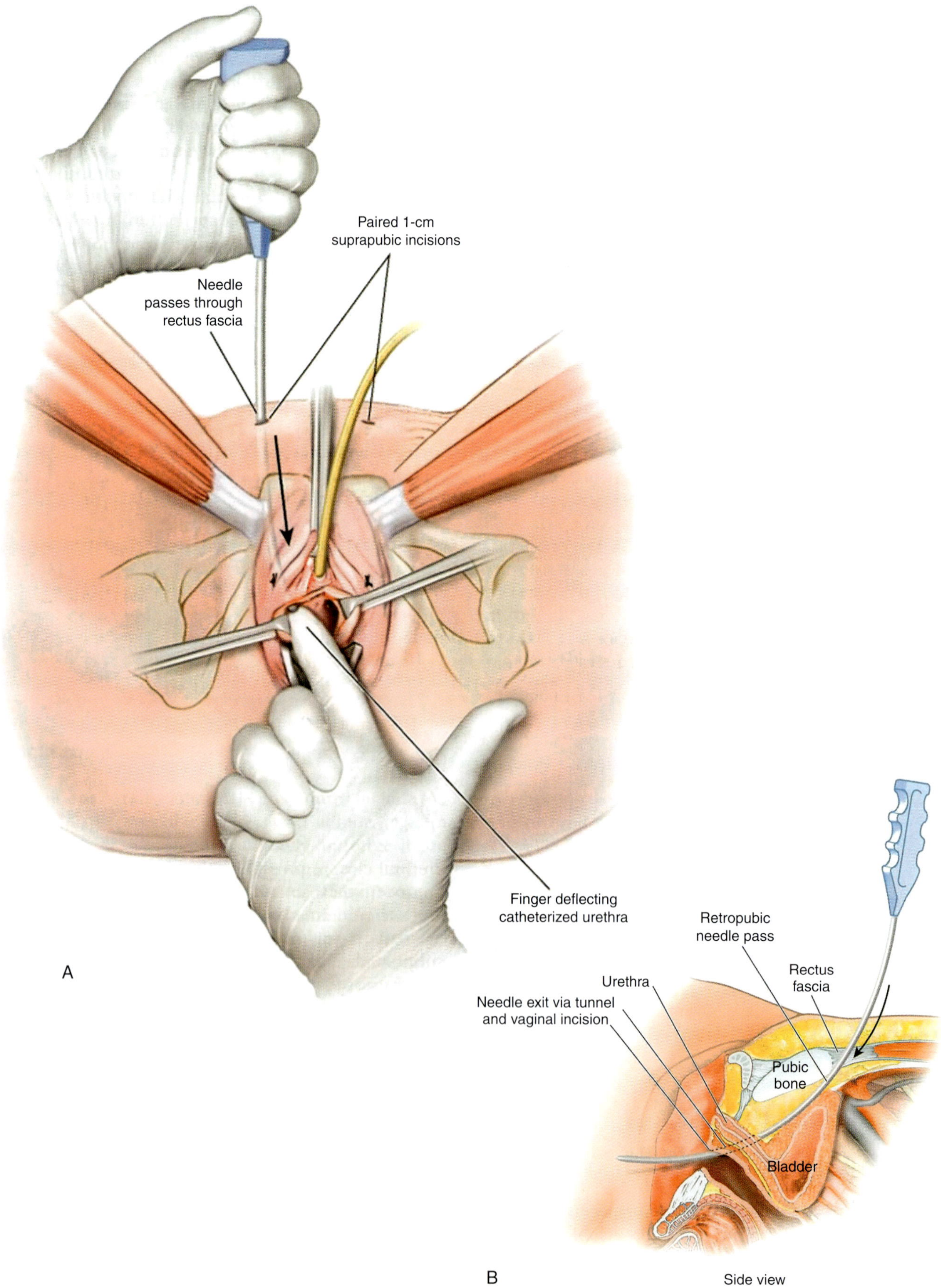

Fig. 17.7 **A**, Technique for passage of top-to-bottom trocar through vaginal incision. **B**, Side view illustrating how a top-to-bottom trocar should hug the back of pubic bone.

3. Anesthesia. Although we prefer to perform these procedures using a general anesthetic, they can be performed using intravenous sedation with local infiltration of the vaginal and groin tissue, which allows the use of a cough test to assist in appropriate tensioning of the sling.
4. The exit site of the needle is marked. It should be 2 cm above the level of the urethra and 2 cm lateral to the labial fold (Fig. 17.8).
5. Vaginal incision. Anterior retraction of the vaginal mucosa with an Allis clamp facilitates visualization. We prefer to hydrodistend the anterior vaginal wall with either a combination of epinephrine and lidocaine or injectable-grade saline. A scalpel is used to make a distal incision in the anterior vaginal wall under the midurethra.
6. Vaginal dissection. Sharp dissection is used to mobilize the anterior vaginal wall off the underlying urethra. Some physicians prefer to hydrodissect the trocar trajectory bilaterally before placing the sling and its trocar.
7. Trocar passage. The trocar tip is inserted into the previously dissected vaginal incision lateral to the urethra and advanced gently while rotating the trocar handle. This insertion is done while hugging the pubic rami, knowing that the obturator canal, which houses both the obturator nerve and vessels, is at the opposite anterolateral margin of the foramen. The tip should emerge at the exit site generated previously at the level of the clitoris. The vaginal sulcus is inspected to ensure that no perforation or mucosal damage has occurred. Certain TOT sling kits (TVT-Transobturator [TVT-O] and TVT-Abbrevo; Ethicon, Somerville, NJ) have a winged guide introducer that helps facilitate appropriate passage of the needle through the obturator membrane, easily guiding the trocar into position (Fig. 17.9). Some surgeons prefer perforating the membrane with Metzenbaum scissors before passing the trocar. Once the membrane is penetrated with the tip of the trocar, the surgeon's hand is lowered or dropped toward the patient to allow the helical passer to rotate around the ischiopubic ramus and exit in the inner thigh (Fig. 17.10A and B).
8. Cystourethroscopy. Careful cystoscopy of the urethra and the bladder should be performed to visualize any damage. If the trocar were to perforate the bladder, it would generally be visualized in the anterolateral aspect of the bladder (usually the area between 3 o'clock and 5 o'clock on the left side and 7 o'clock and 9 o'clock on the right side). If not detached yet, the offending trocar can be withdrawn and reinserted. Occurrence of bladder or urethral perforation or injury is extremely rare during TOT placement.
9. Tensioning. The sling should lay flat against the urethra (without a gap at rest), easily allowing a right-angled clamp

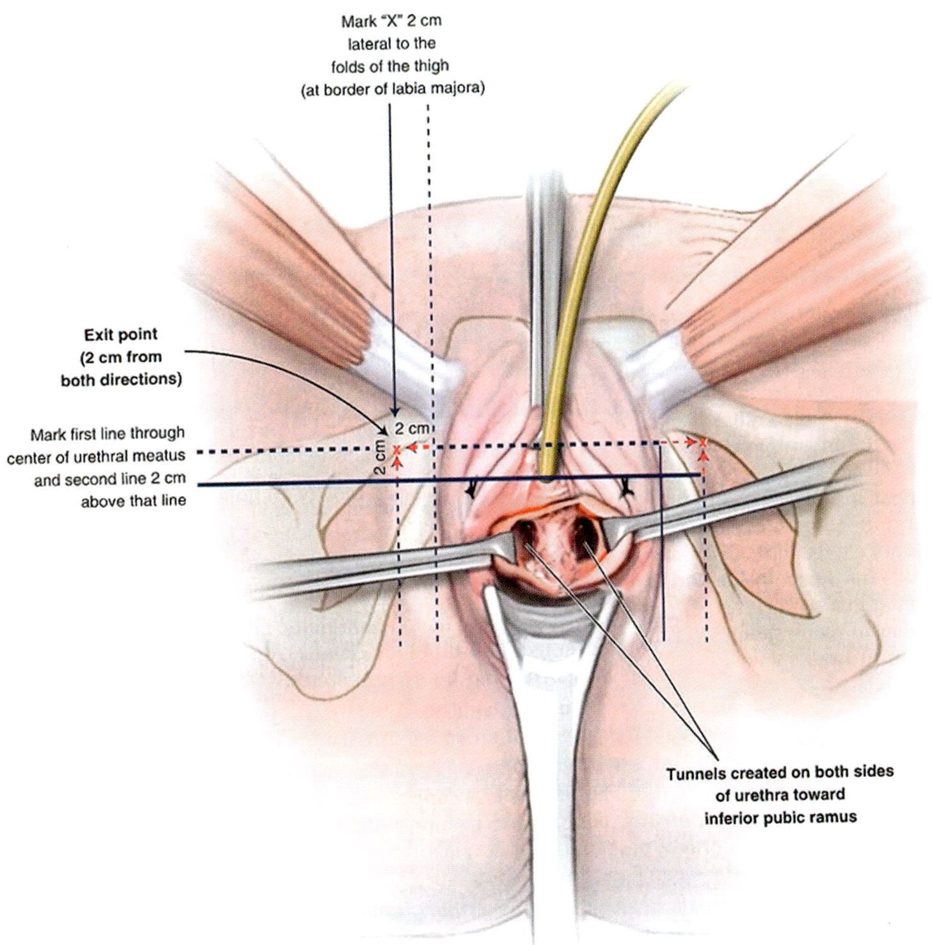

Fig. 17.8 Vaginal incision and exit point for the inside-out transobturator sling.

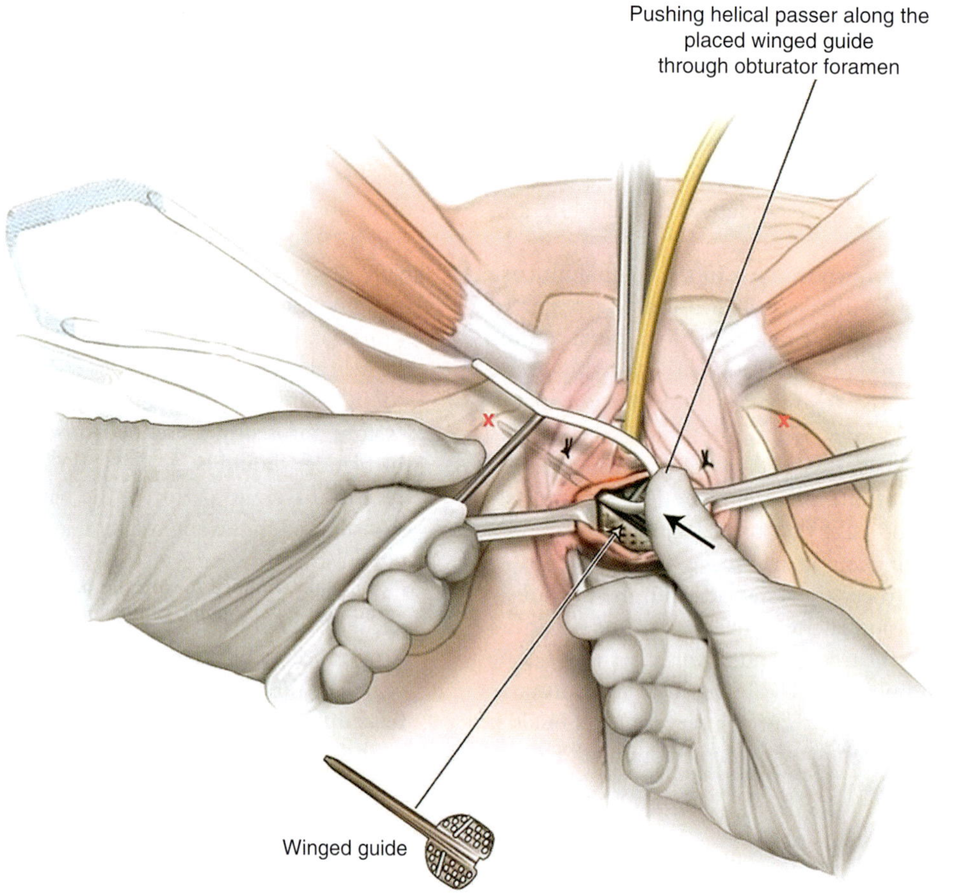

Fig. 17.9 Technique for passage of the tension-free vaginal tape-obturator trocar from the vaginal incision into the inner groin using a vaginal guide.

to be passed between the sling and the posterior urethra. We prefer to tension TOT slings slightly tighter than retropubic MUSs (Fig. 17.11). The plastic sheaths covering the mesh, if present, are removed, and tension of the mesh is rechecked. The mesh at the groin incisions is resected flush with the skin, making sure the skin is mobilized away from the mesh ends before skin closure.

10. The vaginal wound is copiously irrigated and closed with a running 3-0 polyglycolic acid suture. The groin stab wounds are closed with an absorbable suture or covered with liquid tissue adhesive.
11. The catheter may be removed in the recovery room, and the patient is discharged after documenting voiding efficiency. If unable to void, the patient is taught intermittent self-catheterization, or an indwelling Foley catheter is placed.

The TVT-Abbrevo is a more recent version of the inside-out TOT sling. It differs from earlier slings in that the sling is only 12 cm long (versus the traditional 18- to 19-cm–long TOT sling). The shorter mesh traverses only the obturator internus, obturator membrane, and obturator externus, avoiding all the other inner groin muscles. Nonabsorbable polypropylene sutures are attached to the lateral edges of the mesh to allow for adjustments in mesh tensioning. Also, a midline placement loop serves as a visual aid to help center the mesh. Both the loop and the polypropylene sutures are removed after the sling is tensioned to the surgeon's satisfaction (Video 17.3).

Outside-In (See Video 17.4)

1. Preoperative considerations, patient positioning, and anesthesia are similar to the inside-out technique.
2. The penetration site for the trocar is marked in the inner groin, which should be just below the adductor longus tendon, lateral to the clitoris (Fig. 17.12). Placing the index finger in the vaginal fornix and the thumb in the inner groin facilitates identification of the appropriate location for needle penetration.
3. Vaginal incision. The incision is similar to the inside-out technique.
4. Vaginal dissection. The dissection is carried laterally on both sides of the urethra, aiming toward the obturator membrane. We prefer to make the incision slightly longer for TOT (outside-in) and single-incision slings than the incision required for a retropubic MUS. We prefer to mobilize the distal anterior vaginal wall completely off the posterior urethra, allowing the surgeon's finger to be placed into the periurethral space for palpation of the inferior pubic ramus. For the outside-in TOT, the surgeon's index finger should guide the trocar as it rotates around the ischiopubic ramus.
5. Trocar passage. A stab wound is made with the scalpel at the previously marked puncture sites in the groin region, and

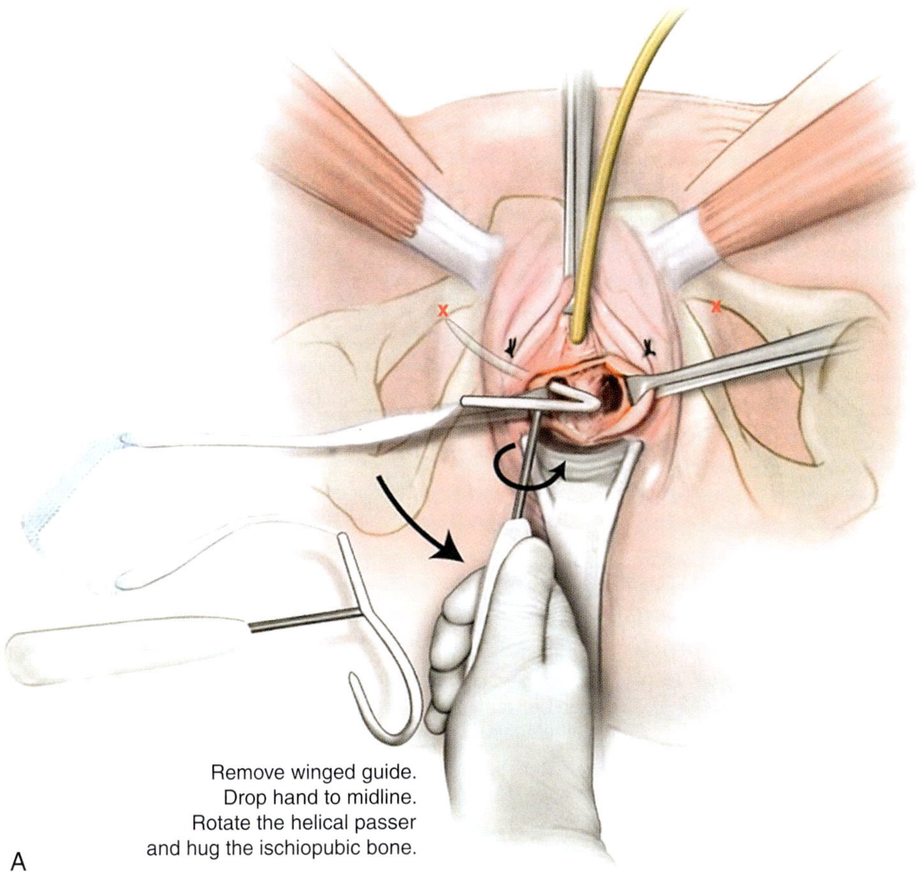

A

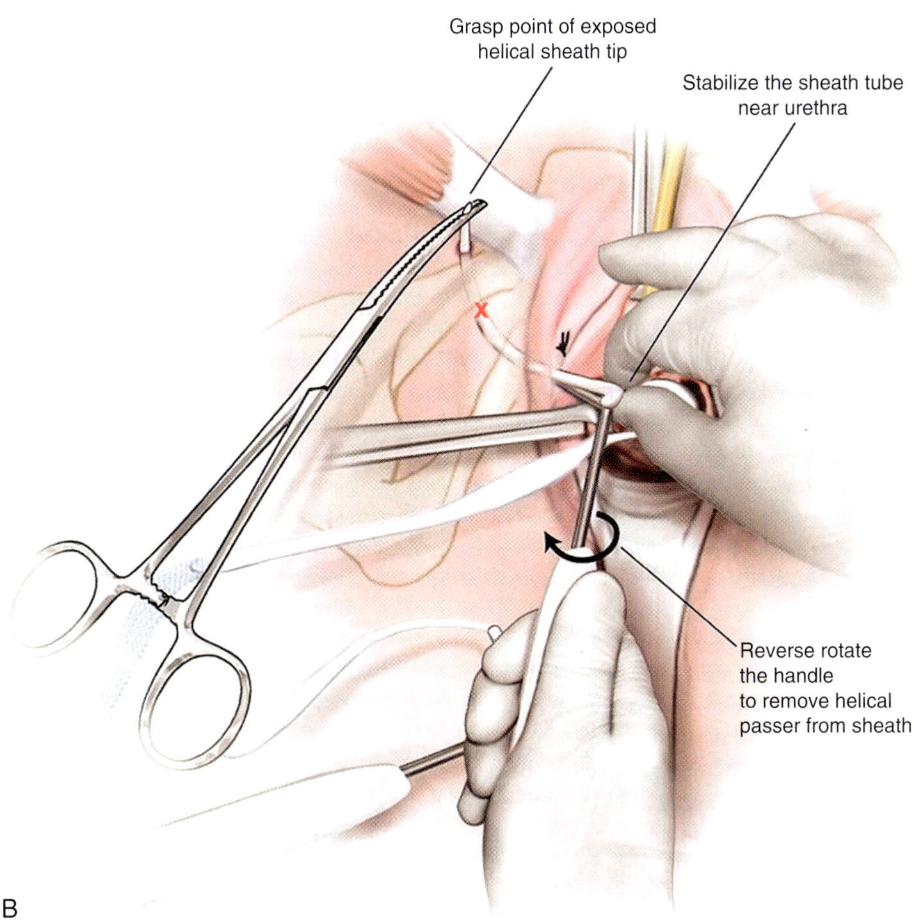

B

Fig. 17.10 **A**, Technique of how to rotate inside-out the tension-free vaginal tape-obturator (TVT-O) trocar handle through the obturator membrane and around the ischiopubic ramus. **B**, Technique of how best to remove the helical trocar from sheath during the inside-out technique for a TVT-O sling.

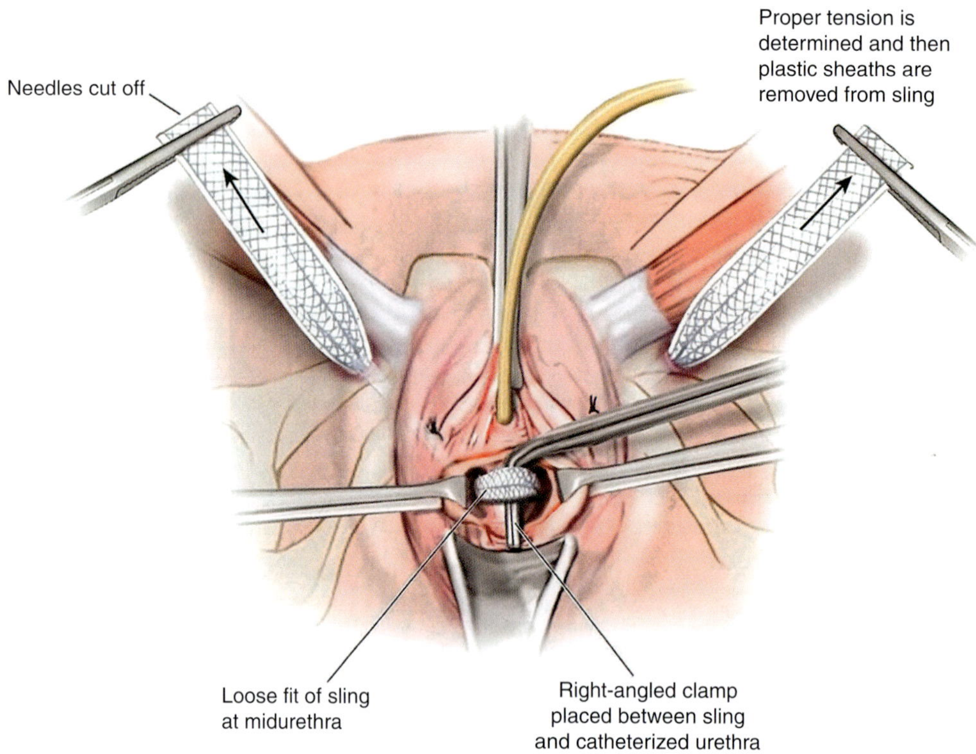

Fig. 17.11 Technique of how best to tension a transobturator sling.

the trocar is inserted carefully, with the handle nearly horizontal or parallel to the floor. The obturator membrane is carefully pierced, and the trocar handle is rotated and advanced along the ischiopubic ramus, with the needle exiting into the previously created vaginal space. The initial rotation should be to drop the handle of the trocar so that it becomes perpendicular to the floor. At the same time, the trocar handle is dropped from the initial near-horizontal starting position to the nearly vertical position; careful angling and "walking off" the bone allows for appropriate passage around the ischiopubic ramus (Fig. 17.13).

6. Cystoscopy. Cystourethroscopy is performed as previously described for the inside-out technique.
7. Loading the mesh. The mesh is attached to the trocar, and the needles are withdrawn, pulling the sling and the plastic sheath, when present, through the groin incision.
8. Tensioning. Tensioning is as described in the inside-out section, using a right-angled clamp (see Fig. 17.11). Excess mesh at the groin incisions is trimmed as previously described.
9. The wound is irrigated, and the mucosal edges are approximated using a running 3-0 polyglycolic acid suture. The groin stab wounds are closed with an absorbable suture or liquid tissue adhesive.
10. The catheter may be removed in the recovery room, and the patient is discharged after documenting voiding efficiency. If the patient is unable to void spontaneously, either intermittent self-catheterization is taught, or the patient is discharged with an indwelling Foley catheter.

SINGLE-INCISION MINISLINGS

In 2006, the single-incision "minisling" was introduced as a modification of traditional retropubic and TOT MUS. These slings were designed to require less dissection in the midurethral area without the need to make additional incisions suprapubically or in the groin. They are placed entirely through an incision in the vagina and have no exit point. They were also designed to minimize the risk of bladder perforation associated with traditional retropubic MUS and the risk of groin discomfort or other issues related to the inner thigh associated with passage of TOT slings. Single-incision minislings are anchored into the obturator internus muscle or connective tissue of the endopelvic fascia of the retropubic space behind the pubic bone, depending on the configuration of the sling chosen by the surgeon. A survey of US urologists in 2009 found that 10% had adopted this technology for regular use in patients with primary SUI. In 2012 the US Food and Drug Administration (FDA) required manufacturers of single-incision slings to pursue additional studies (522 postmarket surveillance studies) to document long-term efficacy and safety. A number of single-incision slings, including the TVT-Secur (Ethicon, Somerville, NJ) and Mini-Arc (American Medical Systems, Minneapolis, MN), were subsequently removed from the market. However, others continued to be marketed while conducting the FDA-mandated studies. Several of these studies have now been published and suggest similar safety and efficacy, at least in the short-term, to full-length slings (Erickson et al., 2020; Nambiar et al., 2017; White et al., 2020).

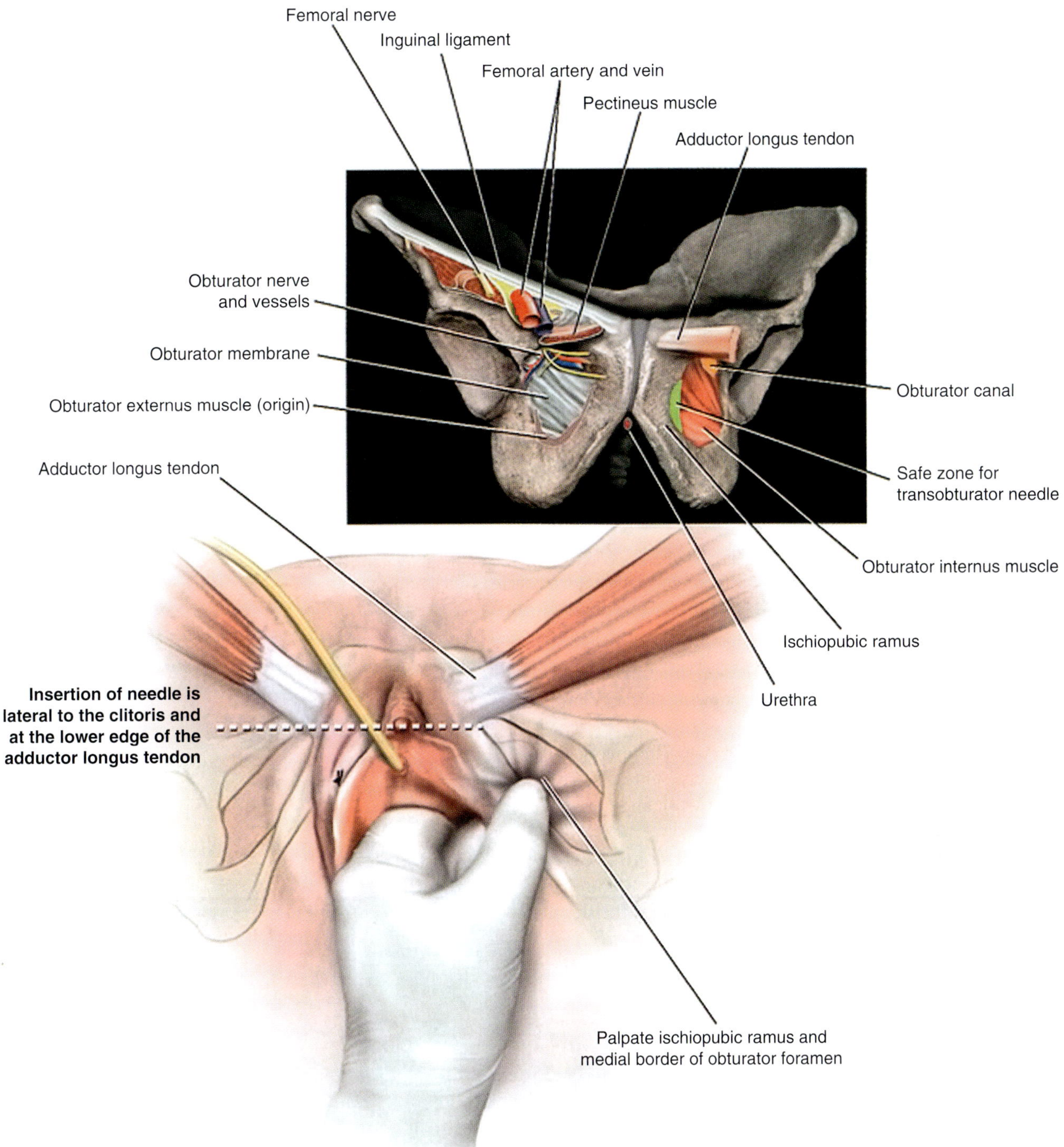

Fig. 17.12 Penetration site for outside-in transobturator tape. The trocar should be at the level of the clitoris, which is just below the insertion of the adductor longus tendon. Placing an index finger in the anterior vaginal fornix and the thumb in the inner groin allows this location to be palpated.

Indications, Patient Selection, and Types of Slings

Indications for the single-incision minisling are similar to indications for the more traditional MUS. It can be offered as an initial, definitive treatment for SUI. Because the minisling is less invasive than a retropubic or TOT MUS, it may be desired for use in some special patient populations. Because it avoids the retropubic space, the minisling may be considered specifically for patients who have undergone previous retropubic and abdominal surgeries and may be at higher risk for significant pelvic adhesions. Because it does not entail complete passage of trocars to the skin level, it may be considered in patients with significant soft tissue mass or morbid obesity in the traditional sites of MUS trocar site (i.e., truncal or intertrigonal obesity) that may surpass the length of the trocar. Because single-incision minisling procedures can be done using local anesthesia, they can also be considered in patients with significant comorbidities in whom general anesthesia

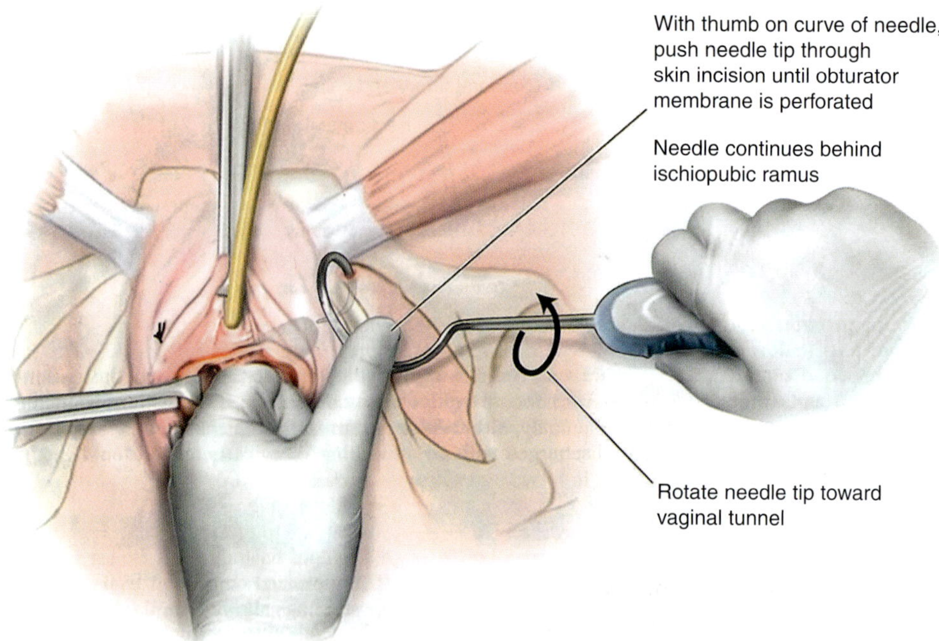

Fig. 17.13 Technique for passage of outside-in trocar through the obturator membrane. Once the obturator membrane is penetrated, appropriate rotation of the handle is required for the needle to hug the back of the ischiopubic ramus and to enter the periurethral tunnel.

is contraindicated. We rarely use single-incision slings in patients with primary SUI, because long-term data showing efficacy comparable to retropubic or TOT MUS are lacking (Table 17.1).

Three single-incision minislings are currently commercially available in the United States: Solyx SIS (Boston Scientific Corp, Natick, MA); Altis (Coloplast., Minneapolis, MN); and Desara One (Caldara Medical, Agoura Hills, CA).

The Solyx SIS system includes a polypropylene mesh tape (9 cm in length) with permanent barbed self-fixating tips and a metal and plastic delivery device or trocar. Each tip of the sling is sequentially attached to the end of the delivery device for mesh placement, and the delivery device is removed after insertion of the mesh. The edges of the center 4 cm of the mesh (advertised as the suburethral portion) are bonded together to reduce irritation and the possibility of mesh erosion or extrusion. The Altis sling also uses self-fixing barbed anchors but has helical trocars much like an inside-out TOT sling. Unique to the Altis sling is a "dynamic" tensioning suture that allows the tension of the sling to be adjusted after both ends of the sling have been fixed into the obturator tissues bilaterally. The Desara One sling is similar to the Solyx device.

Surgical Technique (See Video 17.5)

1. Preoperative considerations. A minisling may be inserted using many different types of anesthesia, including general, spinal or epidural, regional, and local. Perioperative antibiotics (e.g., fluoroquinolone or first-generation cephalosporin) are generally administered before the incision. Antiembolic prophylaxis is given as indicated.
2. Patient positioning. The patient is positioned in the dorsal lithotomy position, with legs in stirrups. The perineum and vagina are prepared and draped to exclude the anus. A weighted

TABLE 17.1 Outcomes of Retropubic Versus Transobturator Midurethral Slings: Summary of 2017 Cochrane Review[a]

No Difference in Objective or Subjective Cure	
Objective cure	RR 0.98, 95% CI 0.96-1.00
Subjective cure	
<1 year	RR 0.98, 95% CI 0.96-1.00
1–5 years	RR 0.97, 95% CI 0.82-1.03
>5 years	RR 0.95, 95% CI 0.87-1.04
Adverse Events	
Transobturator	**Retropubic[b]**
More groin pain–short-term RR 4.62 (6.6% vs. 1.4%)	Greater bladder or urethral perforation. RR 8.0 (4.9% vs. 0.6%)
Greater repeat SUI surgery >5 years[c]	More voiding dysfunction RR 2.0 (7.2% vs. 3.8%)
	Major vascular/visceral injury RR 3.0 (2% vs. 0.4%)
	More suprapubic pain–short term RR 3.4 (2.9% vs. 0.8%)
	Higher cost ($2500 by 5 years)
	Lower cost-effectiveness
No Difference	
Mesh exposure/erosion	
Urgency incontinence (at 1 year)	
Reoperations (at 1 year)	

[a]Data summarized from Ford et al., 2017, which included 55 clinical trials and 8652 participants.
[b]Retropubic slings associated with longer operating time (mean difference 7.5 minutes) and greater blood loss (mean difference 6.5 mL) that are likely not clinically significant.
[c]Long-term reoperations analysis based on limited data that Cochrane reviewers note that should be "interpreted with caution."
RR, Relative risk; *CI*, confidence interval; *SUI*, stress urinary incontinence.

vaginal speculum is placed, and the bladder is drained using a Foley catheter.

3. Vaginal incision. A 1- to 1.5-cm midline incision is marked starting 1 cm below the urethral meatus, and the area is infiltrated with injectable-grade saline or 1% lidocaine with epinephrine for hydrodissection of the periurethral tissues. An Allis clamp may be placed distal to the incision to facilitate visualization; care must be taken not to traumatize the urethral meatus. An incision is made sharply with a scalpel.
4. Vaginal flap dissection. Dissection of lateral vaginal flaps proceeds in a standard fashion, with attention paid to developing an appropriately robust and well-vascularized vaginal flap while not jeopardizing the thickness of the periurethral tissue. This flap is carried laterally and anteriorly until the endopelvic fascia is encountered, but the retropubic space is not entered.
5. Preparation of the sling. The sling is prepared by inserting the tip of the delivery device or needle into the self-affixing end of the mesh apparatus, ensuring that the mesh is orientated on the outside of the bend of the delivery needle.
6. Insertion of sling. To place the Solyx SIS, the tip of the delivery needle (with the mesh assembly attached) is inserted into the previously dissected vaginal space and aimed along a path 45 degrees from the midline. Placement should be immediately posterior to the ischiopubic ramus; the needle can be "walked off" the posterior aspect of the bone, as described previously, maintaining close proximity to the posterior surface of the bone. The tip should be advanced until the midline marking on the mesh is situated under the middle of the urethra (Fig. 17.14). The needle is removed from the mesh, attached to the other end of the mesh device, and inserted on the contralateral side in a similar manner, ensuring the mesh lies flat under the urethra, until the proper degree of desired tension is achieved. The delivery device is disengaged and removed.
7. In general, single-incision slings are tensioned tighter than TOT or retropubic synthetic MUSs, with the tape lying directly against the urethra. For the Altis sling, the "static" anchor should be placed first, followed by the "dynamic" anchor. To tension the Altis sling, the suture loop on the "dynamic" side is pulled across the patient's midline until desired support is achieved. The sling can be loosened by putting a blunt instrument between the urethra and sling and gently pulling down on the sling.
8. Cystoscopy. Cystourethroscopy should be performed to evaluate for bladder or urethral injury.
9. Vaginal closure. The vaginal incision is closed in the same way as described previously.

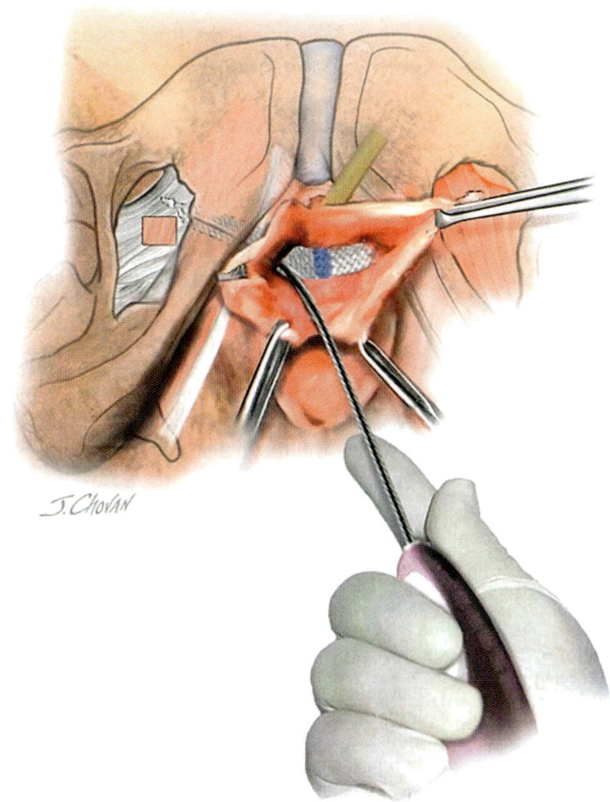

Fig. 17.14 Technique for placement of a single-incision sling. The sling is placed directly into the obturator internus muscle. The square cutout in the obturator fascia shows the obturator internus muscle underneath.

OUTCOMES

The MUS procedure is the most extensively studied antiincontinence surgery to date, with over 2000 peer-reviewed publications and 80 randomized clinical trials. Multiple randomized controlled trials have consistently demonstrated its clinical effectiveness (Fusco et al., 2017; Novara et al., 2010; Ogah et al., 2009) and patient satisfaction (Richter et al., 2010). As such, it has become the most popular surgical treatment for SUI in the United States and the developed world. Compared with older effective procedures such as the Burch colposuspension and fascial sling, the MUS has similar short- and long-term efficacy but less pain, shorter hospitalization, faster return to usual activities, and reduced costs (Ogah et al., 2009). As such, the MUS, particularly full-length retropubic and TOT slings, has been endorsed by multiple professional societies, including the American Urogynecologic Society (AUGS), Society of Urodynamics, Female Pelvic Medicine & Urogenital Reconstruction (SUFU), American College of Obstetricians and Gynecologists, International Urogynecologic Association (IUGA), and Society of Gynecologic Surgeons (SGS) as the current gold standard treatment for SUI (AUGS/SUFU Position Statement, 2018).

A Cochrane review meta-analysis compared MUS to other surgical treatments for SUI; overall, 62 randomized studies involving 7101 women were included (Ogah et al., 2009). Short-term cure rates for retropubic MUS were between 73% and 82%, and the quality of evidence was moderate for most trials. A number of important conclusions came from this Cochrane review:

- Minimally invasive synthetic suburethral sling operations seemed to be as effective as traditional suburethral fascial slings (8 trials, $n = 599$, risk ratio [RR] 1.03, 95% confidence interval [CI] 0.94–1.13), but had shorter operating times and less postoperative voiding dysfunction and *de novo* symptoms of urgency.

- Minimally invasive synthetic suburethral sling operations seemed to be as effective as open retropubic colposuspension (subjective cure rate at 12 months: RR 0.96, 95% CI 0.90–1.03; at 5 years: RR 0.91, 95% CI 0.74–1.12), with fewer perioperative complications, less postoperative voiding dysfunction, shorter operative time, and shorter hospital stay, but significantly more bladder perforations (6% vs. 1%; RR 4.24, 95% CI 1.71–10.52).
- There was conflicting evidence about the effectiveness of minimally invasive synthetic suburethral sling operations compared with laparoscopic colposuspension in the short term (objective cure: RR 1.15, 95% CI 1.06–1.24; subjective cure: RR 1.11, 95% CI 0.99–1.24). Minimally invasive synthetic suburethral sling operations had significantly less *de novo* urgency and urgency incontinence and shorter operating time, hospital stay, and time to return to daily activities.
- A retropubic bottom-to-top route was more effective than top-to-bottom route (RR 1.10, 95% CI 1.01–1.20) and incurred significantly less voiding dysfunction and fewer bladder perforations and tape erosions.
- Monofilament tapes had significantly higher objective cure rates (RR 1.15, 95% CI 1.02–1.30) compared with multifilament tapes, and fewer tape erosions (1.3% vs. 6%; RR 0.25, 95% CI 0.06–1.00).

Retropubic Versus Transobturator Midurethral Slings

Many studies have shown consistent and reliably good effectiveness of both retropubic and TOT MUS for treating SUI. Although the retropubic sling is more popular in many US academic centers, a survey of IUGA members in 2017 found that the TOT approach was the preferred approach worldwide for the treatment of uncomplicated SUI, while the retropubic approach was preferred for recurrent SUI. The largest randomized controlled study comparing retropubic and TOT slings (Trial of Mid-Urethral Slings [TOMUS], $n = 565$) with a strict definition of cure, showed retropubic sling subjective and objective cure rates of 62% and 81%, respectively (Richter et al., 2010). Two years after surgery, the TOT sling was found to have an equivalent objective cure rate to the retropubic sling. Subjective cure rates were similar and not significantly different but did not meet the trial's formal definition of "equivalent." The TOT approach was associated with 50% fewer serious adverse events than the retropubic approach, including fewer urinary tract infections (10% vs. 17%), fewer bladder perforations (0% vs. 5%), less voiding dysfunction requiring surgical correction (0% vs. 3%), but more postoperative neurologic symptoms (9.7% vs. 5.4%) (Richter et al., 2010). Treatment success decreased over 5 years for both retropubic and TOT slings and did not meet the trial's prespecified criteria for equivalence, with retropubic demonstrating a slight benefit (Kenton et al., 2015). However, 5 years after surgery women with a retropubic sling reported greater urinary urgency ($P = .001$), more negative impact on quality of life ($P = .02$), and worse sexual function ($P = .001$) than those who received the TOT sling. Satisfaction remained high in both arms (Kenton et al., 2015).

In 2017, a Cochrane review meta-analysis (55 trials, 8652 women) compared MUS approaches, including the retropubic and TOT approaches (Ford et al., 2017). Table 17.1 summarizes the findings of this review. The review concluded that MUS is the most extensively researched surgical treatment for SUI in women and has a good safety profile. Irrespective of the routes traversed, MUS procedures are highly effective in the short and medium term, and accruing evidence demonstrates their effectiveness in the long term. The authors found similar subjective and objective cure rates between the retropubic and TOT approaches through 5 years after surgery. Like the results of the TOMUS trial, the TOT approach was associated with fewer adverse events, including voiding dysfunction, bladder or urethral perforation, and major vascular/visceral injury (Ford et al., 2017). Rates of repeat surgery for SUI were similar between the two techniques at 1 year, but favored the retropubic approach beyond 5 years, although data for this long-term follow-up were weak. TOT slings were associated with greater groin pain, while retropubic slings were associated with greater suprapubic pain. No differences were noted in postoperative urinary urgency or mesh exposure/erosion between the two approaches. Three trials in the review suggested that the TOT approach may be more cost-effective than the retropubic approach (Ford et al., 2017).

Short-and medium-term subjective cure rates between TOT tapes passed using inside-out and outside-in techniques appear to be similar (RR 1.00, 95% CI 0.96–1.06 for six trials involving 759 women; and RR 1.06, 95% CI 0.91–1.23 for two trials involving 235 women) (Ford et al., 2017). However, voiding dysfunction is more frequent with the inside-out approach (RR 1.74, 95% CI 1.06–2.88; 8 trials, 1121 women), while vaginal perforation was less frequent (RR 0.25, 95% CI 0.12–0.53; three trials, 541 women).

Despite differences in technique, brand of mesh used, and study design, treatment success rates for uncomplicated primary SUI seem to be similar for the retropubic and TOT MUS. The percentage of patients treated successfully ranges from 60% to 96% (depending on how "cure" is defined). When the definition of success is restricted to SUI symptoms, especially over a short time, the reported effectiveness is high. In contrast, when the definition of success includes incontinence of any type, the reported effectiveness is lower. In studies that reported lower effectiveness, "success" was usually strictly defined as no incontinence symptoms of any type, a negative cough stress test, and no subsequent retreatment for SUI or postoperative urinary retention. Thus, it is important to counsel patients before surgery that improvement in SUI symptoms and general satisfaction is highly likely, but perfect bladder function is not. See Table 17.2 for our recommendations for surgical correction of SUI in different clinical situations.

Single-Incision Slings

Compared with TOT and retropubic slings, long-term outcomes of single-incision slings vary depending on the study, and probably device. Barber et al. (2012), De Ridder et al. (2010), Neuman et al. (2011), and Bianchi-Ferraro et al. (2013) showed similar cure rates, whereas Walsh et al. (2011) and Hinoul et al. (2011) showed higher long-term cure rates for retropubic or TOT MUS. In particular, the TVT-Secur device (Ethicon, Somerville, NJ), which relied on absorbable "fleece"

TABLE 17.2 **Authors' Recommendations for Surgical Correction of Stress Urinary Incontinence Based on Different Clinical Situations**

Clinical Problem and Patient Characteristics	Surgery	Rationale
Primary SUI with urethral hypermobility—young patient	TOT or TVT	Similar efficacy; TVT may result in less sexual pain than TOT; TOT has fewer intraoperative complications and less voiding dysfunction
Primary SUI with urethral hypermobility—older patient; leak point pressure >60 cm H_2O	TOT	Similar effectiveness; fewer complications with TOT
Recurrent SUI with urethral hypermobility—any age; leak point pressure >60 cm H_2O	TVT	Limited data suggest effectiveness of TVT after TOT failure; TVT has higher cure rate for recurrent SUI
Recurrent SUI with urethral hypermobility—leak point pressure <60 cm H_2O (ISD)	TVT or pubovaginal fascial sling	Some but not all data indicate that TVT is more effective for ISD; fascial slings in expert hands are effective, based on cohort studies
Recurrent SUI with nonmobile bladder neck; any leak point pressure	Urethral bulking or pubovaginal fascial sling with urethrolysis	All sling procedures have lowered effectiveness when the bladder neck is immobile
SUI mixed with dominant urgency or voiding dysfunction	TOT	TOT improves or does not exacerbate mixed urinary symptoms to the extent that TVT might
SUI with prolapse and planned vaginal prolapse repair	TVT or TOT	Limited data support similar effectiveness for either approach; TOT has less voiding dysfunction
"Occult" SUI with prolapse reduced and planned vaginal prolapse repair	TOT or wait-and-see approach	TOT has a lower chance of creating new retention and irritative voiding symptoms; wait-and-see approach allows treatment of SUI if it develops after prolapse repair, but second surgery would be needed
Recurrent SUI with previous synthetic sling mesh complication (or patients who desire treatment without mesh)	Pubovaginal fascial sling or Burch colposuspension (assuming the urethra is mobile)	These nonmesh options are effective for recurrent SUI, but have higher surgical morbidity

Single-incision slings, or minislings, are not mentioned in this table because currently insufficient long-term outcome data exist to recommend them on a regular basis.

ISD, Intrinsic sphincter deficiency; *TVT*, tension-free vaginal tape or similar retropubic midurethral sling; *TOT*, transobturator sling placed either by outside-in or inside-out approach; *SUI*, stress urinary incontinence.

material on its ends, purportedly to enhance tissue fixation, appears to have lower efficacy than standard full-length slings; this device has been removed from the market (Nambiar et al., 2017). A meta-analysis by Abdel-Fattah et al. (2011a) involving 758 women showed inferior subjective and objective cure rates over 6- and 12-month periods for single-incision slings relative to TOT and retropubic slings. The need for repeat incontinence surgery for patients with prior single-incision slings was significantly greater (RR 6.72, 95% CI 2.39–18.89), and there was increased *de novo* urgency (RR 2.08, 95% CI 1.01–4.28). This study also found that single-incision slings were associated with shorter operative times and lower pain scores immediately postoperatively.

The 2017 Cochrane review comparing single-incision to full-length retropubic or TOT slings included 31 trials involving 3290 women and concluded:

- TVT-Secur is inferior to standard midurethral slings for treatment of SUI.
- Not enough evidence has been found on other single-inclusion slings compared with retropubic or TOT slings to allow for reliable comparisons.
- The duration of the operation was slightly shorter for single-incision slings, but there was a higher risk of *de novo* urgency.

Since the publication of this Cochrane review, several of the 522 postmarket surveillance studies involving currently marketed single-incision slings have been published. White et al. (2020) reported on a nonrandomized parallel cohort study of 281 patients receiving either the Solyx single-incision sling (Boston Scientific Corp, Boston, MA) or a TOT sling and concluded that the single-incision sling was noninferior to the TOT approach. At 36 months, treatment success was 90.4% in the single-incision sling group and 88.9% in the TOT sling group (P = .93). At 36 months, mesh-related complications were similar between groups (mesh exposure: 2.8% vs. 5.0%, P = .38), as were serious adverse events, including pain during intercourse (0.7% vs. 0%, P = 1.00), pelvic pain (0.7% vs. 0%, P = 1.00), and urinary retention (2.8% vs. 4.3%, P = .54). Erickson et al. (2020) reported 12-month follow-up of a multicenter, nonrandomized cohort study comparing the Altis single-incision sling (Coloplast, Minneapolis, MN) with standard TOT or retropubic slings and found similar safety and efficacy between the single-incision and full-length devices. As of the writing of this chapter, the postmarket surveillance study for the Desara One single-incision sling (Caldera Medical, Agoura Hills, CA) has not been completed.

At the present time, data on single-incision slings are maturing. In spite of their original intent, no clear safety benefit has been demonstrated thus far. Given the proven safety and efficacy of standard retropubic and TOT slings, we currently see little role for the single-incision devices. However, if the data eventually demonstrate acceptable long-term durability, particularly if there is also improved safety, increased indications for their use are likely.

Intrinsic Sphincter Deficiency and Recurrent Incontinence

Although there is no standardized definition, ISD has been defined in the literature based on urodynamics findings of Valsalva leak point pressure of less than 60 cm H_2O or maximum urethral closure pressure of less than 20 cm H_2O. Women with ISD usually have more severe incontinence symptoms with higher risk of treatment failure, and before the development of synthetic sling kits, biologic bladder neck slings had been recommended in such cases, with cure rates of 80% to 85%. Numerous studies to date have reported good success with retropubic MUS in women with ISD. Rezapour et al. (2001) first reported their favorable and durable results using TVT in 49 women with ISD (defined as maximum urethral closure pressure under 20 cm H_2O, not Valsalva leak point pressure), with a cure rate of 74% and significant improvement in 12% of cases. Only eight patients did not have urethral hypermobility (as defined by Q-tip test >30 degrees), and of the seven failures, five had fixed urethras. Although the numbers were small, the authors suggested that lack of hypermobility may be a risk factor for failure.

Numerous subsequent studies compared retropubic with TOT approaches in patients with ISD using the previously mentioned urodynamic criteria. Jeon et al. (2008) retrospectively compared TVT, TOT, and pubovaginal sling in women with ISD followed for 2 years. Patients with TVT had a cure rate of 86.9%, which was similar to the cure rate of 87.3% seen with the pubovaginal sling; in contrast, the TOT group had a cure rate of only 34.9% ($P < .0001$). At 31 months, Gungorduk et al. (2009) found cure rates of 78.3% using TVT versus 52.5% using TOT, and reported that TOT was five times more likely than TVT to fail in women with ISD. In a prospective, randomized study addressing this issue, Schierlitz et al. (2008) randomly assigned 164 women with ISD to TVT or TOT, with the primary outcome of urodynamic SUI at 6 months. At postoperative testing, 21% of the TVT group versus 45% of the TOT group had urodynamic SUI ($P = .004$). At 3 years, 20% of women in the TOT group underwent repeat surgery to correct SUI compared with only 1.4% in the TVT group (Schierlitz et al., 2012). A systematic review of eight randomized trials that included women with ISD found that, while both retropubic and TOT slings were effective in women with ISD and improved overall quality of life, the retropubic route resulted in higher subjective cure (Ford & Ogah, 2016). Importantly, Nager et al. (2011) showed that lower Valsalva leak point pressure or maximum urethral closure pressure resulted in a nearly two-fold increased risk of SUI 1 year after either retropubic or TOT MUS.

Regarding the effectiveness of MUS in recurrent SUI, Pradhan et al. (2012) reviewed the literature and found that the overall subjective cure rate following MUS for recurrent SUI after any previous surgery was 78.5% after 30-month follow-up. There seems to be a lower cure rate with TOT compared with retropubic sling for recurrent SUI (Kim et al., 2019; Pradhan et al., 2012).

Urethral Mobility

The studies noted earlier suggest that retropubic slings work relatively well for patients with ISD, whereas TOT slings may not work as well. In contrast, a retrospective study by Rapp et al. (2009) found no difference between retropubic and TOT slings in women with ISD, with success rates of 76% and 77%, respectively. Constantini et al. (2008) also reported no difference between TVT and TOT in women with ISD; they used a subset analysis of their randomized controlled trial, in which all of their patients had urethral hypermobility ranging from 43 to 90 degrees as measured by the Q-tip test. They found no difference in outcomes between 45 patients with TVT and 50 patients with TOT at 35 months (68% vs. 76%, respectively). Although this was a *post hoc* analysis that was underpowered to detect a difference, it does suggest that patients with ISD who have concurrent hypermobility may show similar outcomes with both TVT and TOT slings.

A study by Haliloglu et al. (2010) examined the effect of ISD and urethral hypermobility in 65 patients with TOT by dividing them into three groups: ISD with hypermobility ($n = 18$), ISD with fixed urethra ($n = 16$), and hypermobility without ISD ($n = 31$). At 24 months, the two groups with hypermobility with and without ISD had similar cure rates (87.5% and 96.4%, respectively). However, patients with no hypermobility had a significantly lower cure rate (66.7%).

Hypermobility was also a predictive factor of treatment failure in patients undergoing TVT in studies by Fritel et al. (2002) (success rates of 92% with Q-tip test >30 degrees vs. 70% for Q-tip test <30 degrees) and Richter et al. (2011) (Q-tip test <30 degrees had an odds ratio [OR] of 1.89 for treatment failure). ISD, defined in this study as maximum urethral closure pressure less than 20 cm H_2O, had no effect on success rate. The literature seems to indicate that hypomobility is a risk factor for failure and decreased efficacy for MUS, whether retropubic or TOT.

Mixed Stress and Urgency Incontinence

Up to 50% of women with urinary incontinence suffer from a mixture of both SUI and urgency urinary incontinence or mixed urinary incontinence. In a systematic review of the effectiveness of MUS in mixed urinary incontinence, Jain et al. (2011) found that there was a persistent and good cure of the stress component (85%–97%), but a variable and lower cure of the urgency and urgency incontinence component (30%–85%). Retropubic and TOT MUS had similar subjective cure of mixed incontinence. Several studies have shown that overactive bladder (OAB) with urgency incontinence symptoms may actually improve in 30% to 85% after MUS (Barber et al., 2008; Palva & Nilsson, 2011; Richter et al., 2011). The ESTEEM trial found significant improvements in OAB symptom severity and OAB-related quality of life after MUS in patients with mixed urinary incontinence (Sung et al., 2019). Less than 5% of patients in this trial reported worsening urgency after MUS.

Current evidence suggests that the overall incidence of *de novo* OAB following MUS procedures is approximately 9%. A systematic review of 31 studies concluded that there is not enough evidence to support differences in the effects of the different types of sling on this outcome (Pergialotis et al., 2017).

Obesity

Both safety and effectiveness are important when assessing surgical procedures. Multiple studies reported no significant difference in outcomes in obese patients undergoing long-term follow-up. However, a meta-analysis in 2008 showed a statistically significant difference in SUI cure rates: 81% in obese patients versus 85% in nonobese patients. *De novo* urgency incontinence did not vary between the two groups, but the rate of persistent urgency incontinence was significantly higher in obese patients. When comparing safety, the same meta-analysis showed that obese patients had a statistically significant lower rate of bladder perforation. Having severe or morbid obesity (BMI $\geq$40 kg/m^2) may increase the rate of failure after MUS as much as twice as high as normal weight women, however (Dykes et al., 2020; Elshatanoufy et al., 2019).

AVOIDING AND MANAGING COMPLICATIONS

Complications of retropubic MUS procedures include bladder perforation, pelvic visceral injuries, vascular injuries and hemorrhage, mesh erosion and exposure, *de novo* development of urgency and urgency incontinence, bladder outlet obstruction, pelvic pain, and urinary tract infection. Retropubic MUS have a higher rate of morbidity than TOT slings, although the overall rate of adverse events with either is low. In particular, retropubic slings are associated with a higher frequency of bladder perforation, postoperative voiding dysfunction requiring surgical intervention, and urinary tract infections than TOT MUS (Ford et al., 2017; Richter et al., 2010). Overall, the risk of sling excision for a complication such as pain, mesh exposure, or voiding dysfunction is approximately 2.2%, and this occurs at a median of 0.9 years after the initial surgery (interquartile range 0.35–2.5 years) (Welk et al., 2015). The cumulative risk of sling excision for a mesh complication at 9 to 10 years in several very large population-based cohorts ranged from 1.1% to 5.3% (Berger et al., 2019; Brennand et al., 2019; Gurol-Urganci et al., 2018; Welk et al., 2015). The cumulative risk of reoperation for SUI through 9 years after surgery is approximately 5%, with a total cumulative rate of reoperation for complication or recurrent SUI of 6% to 7% at 9 years (Berger et al., 2019; Gurol-Urganci et al., 2018).

Bladder Perforation

Bladder perforation occurs in 3% to 5% of cases after retropubic and 0.6% after TOT MUS. The risk of perforation with retropubic slings appears to be particularly high when surgeons are early in their learning curve, as high 30% to 40% in the first 10 cases (McLennan & Melick, 2005). Use of simulation as part of a surgeon's early training in sling placement appears to mitigate this risk (Rosen et al., 2019). Careful intraoperative cystoscopy with the bladder fully distended is essential for diagnosing this complication, regardless of route. For retropubic slings, perforation typically occurs in the upper lateral portion of the bladder dome. Perforation during the TOT sling procedure is rare, but typically is located lateral to the trigone. When perforation occurs, it is simply managed by removing and carefully reinserting the trocar. However, if a large injury has been encountered in a dependent portion of the bladder (trigone or bladder base), prolonged drainage or, rarely, aborting the procedure is recommended. Mesh immediately adjacent to a bladder injury can result in erosion into the urinary tract. If urethral injury is noted, the procedure is preferably abandoned until complete healing has occurred to reduce the likelihood of erosions of mesh into the urethra.

Voiding Dysfunction

Of women undergoing retropubic sling procedures, 4% to 8% develop some form of temporary voiding dysfunction postoperatively. TOT slings have approximately half this risk (Ford et al., 2017). *De novo* development of urgency and urgency incontinence occurs in approximately 6% of women undergoing sling procedures. Initial postoperative management of urinary retention includes catheterization; however, if this persists beyond several weeks, the option of sling lysis is contemplated. Urethral dilation is typically not recommended, because of fear of predisposing the patient to erosion of the sling material into the urethra. Some have described tape "loosening" rather than lysis if done within the first 10 to 14 days postoperatively before tissue ingrowth has occurred. See Chapter 34 for a more detailed discussion of how best to manage voiding dysfunction after sling placement.

Vascular Injury

Depending on the amount, bleeding may indicate trocar-induced injury to pelvic vessels, including paravesical veins, accessory obturator vessels, obturator vessels, superficial or inferior epigastric vessels, and, in rare situations, external iliac or femoral vessels. Cadaver studies have shown that major vascular structures are as close as 3.2 cm cephalad and lateral to the retropubic MUS trocar (Muir et al., 2003; Fig. 17.15). Sometimes this bleeding may be concealed and result in a large hematoma, with the only indications being a subjective feeling of discomfort, pressure, frequent urination, or orthostatic changes from the anemia. The rate of significant vascular injury or pelvic hematoma is less than 1% and is significantly less frequent with the transobuturator versus retropubic approach (RR 0.33) (Ford et al., 2017). Objective indicators of vascular injury include patient vital signs, oliguria, a palpable suprapubic mass and/or ecchymosis, and loss of consciousness in extreme cases. Most retropubic hematomas are self-limiting and can be managed conservatively. One study showed a correlation between hematoma size and symptoms; patients were in severe discomfort if the collection was larger than 300 mL, compared with minimal to absent symptoms at volumes less than 100 mL. Persistent bleeding refractory to passive actions such as compression and fluid resuscitation may require angiographic management with vascular surgical consultation or surgical exploration.

Groin and Suprapubic Pain

Surgical pain after both retropubic and TOT sling procedures is uncommon, and, when it occurs, typically resolves quickly. According to the Cochrane review, overall rates of groin pain are higher with the TOT approach (6.4% vs. 1.3%), while suprapubic pain is more common with the retropubic approach (2.9% vs. 0.8%), with both being of short duration (Ford et al., 2017). In TOMUS, the rate of bothersome pain at or beyond 6 weeks was low (retropubic 2.3% vs. TOT 2.0%) (Richter et al., 2010). In a secondary analysis of TOMUS, Thomas et al. (2017), analyzing

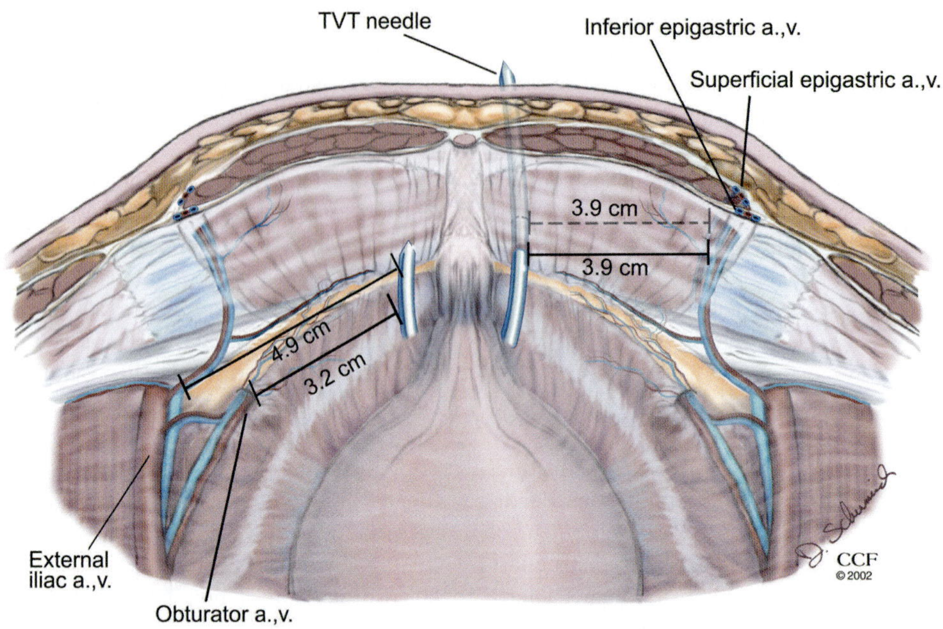

Fig. 17.15 The relationship of the tension-free vaginal tape (*TVT*) needle to the vascular anatomy of the anterior abdominal wall and retropubic space. Numbers represent the mean distance from the lateral aspect of the TVT needle to the medial edge of the vessels. *a*, Artery; *v*, vein. (From Cleveland Clinic, with permission.)

prospectively-collected daily pain diaries, pain maps, and pain severity scales, found no difference in the prevalence of overall surgical pain, pain severity, or pain medication use between the two approaches. At 2 weeks after surgery, retropubic slings were associated with greater suprapubic pain, whereas TOT slings were associated with more groin pain at 2 weeks and 6 weeks. However, there were no differences between groups by 6 months postoperatively, and overall rates were low.

In most cases, surgical pain after an MUS procedure will resolve by 6 weeks after surgery. When it does not, nonsurgical treatment including nonsteroidal antiinflammatory medications, trigger point injections, and/or physical therapy should be attempted, and usually results in pain relief. If suprapubic pain continues despite aggressive nonsurgical management in patients who have received a retropubic sling, then retropubic excision of the sling arms through laparotomy or laparoscopy should be performed. In patients with persistent groin pain after a TOT sling procedure that is not responsive to nonsurgical treatment, transvaginal excision of the sling to release the tension on the sling arms can be considered. Rarely is removal of the entire sling in the inner thigh necessary; this should only be done if the sling is infected, and as a last resort, because of its difficulty and relative morbidity. Excision of the suburethral portion of the sling will result in resolved or improved pain, whether vaginal, groin, or suprapubic, in 50% to 70% of patients.

Sexual Function/Dyspareunia

Sexual function usually improves after both retropubic and TOT MUS, mainly because of resolution of SUI (De Souza et al., 2012). However, dyspareunia can occur, and often is related to superficial mesh location or mesh exposure in the vagina. Although application of topical vaginal estrogen and observation have been advocated for this problem, many patients require mesh removal for symptom resolution.

Dyspareunia can occur if the sling tape is exposed or erodes into the vaginal lumen. Also, unique to TOT MUS, the sling may be palpable or tender in the vaginal fornix. This can lead to sexual pain in the patient or in her male partner. A randomized controlled trial by Ross et al. (2009) mentioned the concerning fact that the sling tape may be frequently palpable postoperatively in patients with TOT slings. In addition to the risk for dyspareunia, palpable sling tape may predispose to vaginal exposure. One study found a higher frequency of *de novo* sexual dysfunction secondary to a palpable and tender sling after the outside-in approach, causing penile pain in the male partner during intercourse (Scheiner et al., 2012). However, this complication has not been observed in all studies (Sentilhes et al., 2009). If sexual pain persists after MUS and is not responsive to conservative measures, surgical resection of the offending section of the sling is usually necessary.

Vaginal Mesh Exposure

Vaginal mesh exposure after MUS occurs in approximately 1% of patients in the first year after surgery, with a 9- to 10-year cumulative risk of requiring surgery for mesh exposure of 1.1% to 5.3% (Berger et al., 2019; Brennand et al., 2019; Gurol-Urganci et al., 2018; Welk et al., 2015). Common symptoms include vaginal discomfort, vaginal discharge, spotting, and dyspareunia, although many patients will be asymptomatic. Treatment options consist of observation, office excision, and excision in the operating room. If the patient is asymptomatic and not sexually active, and the erosion is very small (<3 mm), observation alone can be considered. Although the exposure will not often heal spontaneously, it rarely progresses. Many authors advocate the use of vaginal estrogen in these patients, although there are few data documenting an improved rate of healing with vaginal estrogen over observation alone. If conservative treatment is unsuccessful, applicable surgical options include mobilization and reapproximation of vaginal epithelium, excision of the exposed mesh, or extensive or complete removal of the suburethral portion of the mesh with vaginal closure. The mesh should be removed only after adequate patient counseling regarding the likelihood of recurrence of SUI.

Vaginal mesh exposure is a known complication associated with all types of synthetic slings, and is discussed in detail in Chapter 25.

Single-Incision Slings

Complications that can occur related to single-incision slings are similar to the complications previously discussed in regard to retropubic and TOT MUS; these include bladder or urethral injury or perforation, bleeding, vaginal mesh exposure, urinary tract mesh erosion, voiding dysfunction, urinary retention, and urinary tract infection. Organ damage and major vessel injury still may occur, but should be much less common, because the design of the minisling enables a significantly more truncated needle/trocar trajectory through the retropubic or obturator space.

Bladder perforation may occur during dissection or at the time during sling insertion; the self-affixing points of many single-incision slings may make removal and reinsertion of the device difficult, because these slings are not designed to be removed. If bladder perforation occurs and is discovered during cystoscopy, the sling should be immediately removed. A secondary insertion should not be attempted at that operative time. In our opinion, cystourethroscopy should be routinely performed when a single-incision sling is placed.

PERIOPERATIVE PELVIC MUSCLE EXERCISES

As noted in *Chapter 14*, pelvic muscle exercise programs and other behavioral interventions are effective nonsurgical treatments for women with urinary incontinence. It is unclear, however, if these behavioral treatments conducted perioperatively as an adjunct to surgery for SUI improve outcomes beyond surgery alone. Jarvis et al. (2005) conducted a small, single-center randomized trial evaluating the impact of perioperative pelvic floor physiotherapy in women undergoing surgery for pelvic organ prolapse or SUI. Although those who received perioperative physiotherapy had improved daytime urinary frequency compared to those who received surgery alone, there were no differences in other urinary symptoms or quality of life between the two groups. Similarly, the OPTIMAL trial investigated a standardized perioperative behavioral therapy program that included pelvic muscle exercises in women undergoing vaginal reconstructive surgery and a retropubic sling for pelvic organ prolapse and SUI and found no improvement in urinary symptoms or quality of life at 6 months or 2 years after surgery related to the behavioral therapy (Barber et al., 2014). More recently, the ESTEEM trial investigated the effect of behavioral and pelvic floor muscle therapy combined with MUS surgery versus surgery alone in patients with mixed urinary incontinence (Sung et al., 2019). One year after surgery, those who received the perioperative behavioral therapy demonstrated improved urinary symptoms as measured by the Urinary Distress Inventory; however, while statistically significant, the magnitude of effect did not meet the trial's predefined threshold of clinically meaningful difference. That said, at 12 months the combined behavioral therapy plus surgery group was significantly less likely to receive additional treatment for lower urinary tract symptoms than was the sling-only group (8.5% vs. 15.7%, adjusted OR, 0.47; 95% CI, 0.26-0.85). The combined therapy group also had fewer urgency and total incontinence episodes as recorded in bladder diaries and greater improvement in Incontinence Impact Questionnaire scores. In summary, there is currently insufficient evidence to recommend perioperative pelvic muscle exercises and other behavioral therapies as an adjunct to MUS in women with SUI. There may be some benefit in women with mixed urinary incontinence, however.

PREGNANCY AFTER MIDURETHRAL SLINGS

In our opinion, whenever possible, SUI surgery should be delayed until a woman's childbearing is completed. If a synthetic sling is placed in a woman who eventually becomes pregnant, there are few studies available to guide decisions about mode of delivery. Because of the stretch and pressure generated during labor and pregnancy itself, there is concern that the support offered by synthetic slings may be negatively affected, with subsequent loss of adequate urinary control postpartum. The limited data available suggest no difference in the rate of recurrent SUI between women who undergo cesarean versus vaginal delivery. A review on this topic by the AUGS Guidelines Committee concludes that, given the small number of cases reported and the absence of any randomized trials, it is impossible to draw any firm conclusions about whether recurrent SUI differs by route of delivery (Wieslander et al., 2020). On this basis, several authors concur that the mode of delivery for women who have undergone surgery for SUI should be decided on a case-by-case basis. A systematic review of pregnancy outcomes following surgery for SUI suggested that any increase in risks for pregnancy after surgery for stress incontinence is likely small (Pollard et al., 2012). A low risk of urinary retention during pregnancy does appear to exist. Similarly, women with a prior sling who undergo childbirth, whether by vaginal delivery or cesarean section, are at risk of recurrence of SUI, although the limited data available suggest that the risk is low.

CONCLUSION

Most urogynecologists and urologists currently consider synthetic MUS to be the primary surgical treatment for women with SUI. Data indicate that similar long-term efficacy can be obtained in most patients with a retropubic or TOT approach. However, patients with more severe or recurrent SUI, or ISD, may be better served with a retropubic approach, whereas those with mixed symptoms and/or less severe SUI may be better served with a TOT approach (see Table 17.2). More long-term data on single-incision slings are needed.

BIBLIOGRAPHY

Abouassaly R, Steinberg JR, Lemieux M, et al. Complications of tension-free vaginal tape surgery: multi-institutional review. *BJU Int.* 2004;94:110.

Abdel-Fattah M, Ramsay I, Pringle S, et al. Randomised prospective single-blinded study comparing 'inside-out' versus 'outside-in' transobturator tapes in the management of urodynamic stress incontinence: 1-year outcomes from the E-TOT study. *BJOG.* 2010;117:870.

Abdel-Fattah M, Mostafa A, Young D, Ramsay I. Evaluation of transobturator tension-free vaginal tapes in the management of women with mixed urinary incontinence: one-year outcomes. *Am J Obstet Gynecol.* 2011a;205:150.e1.

Abdel-Fattah M, Ford JA, Lim CP, Madhuvrata P. Single-incision mini-slings versus standard midurethral slings in surgical management of female stress urinary incontinence: a meta-analysis of effectiveness and complications. *Eur Urol.* 2011b;60:468.

American College of Obstetricians and Gynecologists. Urinary incontinence in women, ACOG Practice Bulletin No. 63. *Obstet Gynecol.* 2005;105:1533.

Anger JT, Weinberg AE, Albo ME, et al. Trends in surgical management of stress urinary incontinence among female Medicare beneficiaries. *Urology.* 2009;74:283.

AUGS/SUFU Position Statement: Mesh midurethral slings for stress urinary incontinence. Updated February 2018. Available at: https://www.augs.org/assets/1/6/AUGS-SUFU_MUS_Position_Statement.pdf. Accessed July 19, 2020.

Austin PF, Westney OL, Leng WW, et al. Advantages of rectus fascial slings for urinary incontinence in children with neuropathic bladders. *J Urol.* 2001;165:2369.

Barber MD. Surgical techniques for removing problematic mesh. *Clin Obstet Gynecol.* 2013;56:289.

Barber MD, Brubaker L, Burgio KL, et al. Comparison of 2 transvaginal surgical approaches and perioperative behavioral therapy for apical vaginal prolapse: the OPTIMAL randomized trial. *JAMA.* 2014;311:1023.

Barber MD, Kleeman S, Karram MM, et al. Transobturator tape compared with tension-free vaginal tape for the treatment of stress urinary incontinence: a randomized controlled trial. *Obstet Gynecol.* 2008;111:611.

Barber MD, Weidner AC, Sokol AI, et al. Single-incision mini-sling compared with tension-free vaginal tape for the treatment of stress urinary incontinence: a randomized controlled trial. *Obstet Gynecol.* 2012;119:328.

Basu M, Duckett J. A randomised trial of a retropubic tension-free vaginal tape versus a mini-sling for stress incontinence. *BJOG.* 2010;117:730.

Berger AA, Tan-Kim J, Menefee SA. Long-term risk of reoperation after synthetic mesh midurethral sling surgery for stress urinary incontinence. *Obstet Gynecol.* 2019;134:1047.

Bezerra CA, Bruschini H. Suburethral sling operations for urinary incontinence in women. *Cochrane Database Syst Rev.* 2001;3:CD001754. [Update in *Cochrane Database Syst Rev.* 2005;(3):CD001754].

Bianchi-Ferraro AM, Jarmy-Di Bella ZI, Castro Rde A, et al. Single-incision sling compared with transobturator sling for treating stress urinary incontinence: a randomized controlled trial. *Int Urogynecol J.* 2013;24:1459.

Blaivas JG, Sandhu J. Urethral reconstruction after erosion of slings in women. *Curr Opin Urol.* 2004;14:335.

Bodelsson G, Henriksson L, Osser S, Stjernquist M. Short term complications of the tension free vaginal tape operation for stress urinary incontinence in women. *Br J Obstet Gynaecol.* 2002;109:566.

Brennand EA, Quan H. Evaluation of the effect of surgeon's operative volume and specialty on likelihood of revision after mesh midurethral sling placement. *Obstet Gynecol.* 2019;133:1099.

Brubaker L, Cundiff GW, Fine P, et al. Abdominal sacrocolpopexy with Burch colposuspension to reduce urinary stress incontinence. *N Engl J Med.* 2006;354:1557.

Brubaker L, Norton PA, Albo ME, et al. Adverse events over two years after retropubic or transobturator midurethral sling surgery: findings from the Trial of Midurethral Slings (TOMUS) study. *Am J Obstet Gynecol.* 2011;205:498.e1.

But I, Faganelj M. Complications and short-term results of two different transobturator techniques for surgical treatment of women with urinary incontinence: a randomized study. *Int Urogynecol J.* 2008;19:857.

Carey MP, Goh JT, Fynes MM, Murray CJ. Stress urinary incontinence after delayed primary closure of genitourinary fistula: a technique for surgical management. *Am J Obstet Gynecol.* 2002;186:948.

Cholhan HJ, Hutchings TB, Rooney KE. Dyspareunia associated with paraurethral banding in the transobturator sling. *Am J Obstet Gynecol.* 2010;202:481.e1.

Constantini E, Lazzeri M, Giannantoni A, et al. Preoperative Valsalva leak point pressure may not predict outcome of mid-urethral slings: analysis from a randomized controlled trial of retropubic versus transobturator mid-urethral slings. *Int Braz J Urol.* 2008;34:73.

Cornu JN, Sebe P, Peyrat L, et al. Midterm prospective evaluation of TVT-Secur reveals high failure rate. *Eur Urol.* 2010;58:157.

Dargent D, Bretones S, George P, Mellier G. Insertion of a sub-urethral sling through the obturating membrane for treatment of female urinary incontinence [Article in French]. *Gynecol Obstet Fertil.* 2002;30:576.

Deffieux X, Daher N, Mansoor A, et al. Transobturator TVT-O versus retropubic TVT: results of a multicenter randomized controlled trial at 24 months follow-up. *Int Urogynecol J.* 2010;21:1337.

De Ridder D, Berkers J, Deprest J, et al. Single incision mini-sling versus a transobutaror sling: a comparative study on MiniArc and Monarc slings. *Int Urogynecol J.* 2010;21:773.

De Souza A, Dwyer PL, Rosamilia A, et al. Sexual function following retropubic TVT and transobturator Monarc sling in women with intrinsic sphincter deficiency: a multicentre prospective study. *Int Urogynecol J.* 2012;23:153.

Duckett JR, Patil A, Papanikolaou NS. Predicting early voiding dysfunction after tension-free vaginal tape. *J Obstet Gynaecol.* 2008;28:89.

Dursun M, Otunctemur A, Ozbek E, et al. Impact of the transobturator tape procedure on sexual function in women with stress urinary incontinence. *J Obstet Gynaecol Res.* 2013;39:831.

Dykes N, Hayward L, Coomarasamy C. Impact of severe obesity on long-term success and complications of the retropubic midurethral sling. *Int Urogynecol J.* 2021;32:57.

Elshatanoufy S, Matthews A, Yousif M, et al. Effect of morbid obesity on midurethral sling efficacy for the management of stress urinary incontinence. *Female Pelvic Med Reconstr Surg.* 2019;25:448.

Erickson T, Roovers JP, Gheiler E, et al. A multicenter prospective study evaluating efficacy and safety of a single-incision sling procedure for stress urinary incontinence. *J Minim Invasive Gynecol.* 2020;19:S1553.

Flock F, Reich A, Muche R, et al. Hemorrhagic complications associated with tension-free vaginal tape procedure. *Obstet Gynecol.* 2004;104:989.

Fong ED, Nitti VW. Review article: mid-urethral synthetic slings for female stress urinary incontinence. *BJU Int.* 2010;106:596.

Ford AA, Ogah JA. Retropubic or transobturator mid-urethral slings for intrinsic sphincter deficiency-related stress urinary incontinence in women: a systematic review and meta-analysis. *Int Urogynecol J*. 2016;27:19.

Ford AA, Rogerson L, Cody JD, et al. Mid-urethral sling operations for stress urinary incontinence in women. *Cochrane Database Syst Rev*. 2017;7:CD006375.

Fusco F, Abdel-Fattah M, Chapple CR, et al. Updated systematic review and meta-analysis of the comparative data on colposuspensions, pubovaginal slings, and midurethral tapes in the surgical treatment of female stress urinary incontinence. *Eur Urol*. 2017;72:567.

Fritel X, Zabak K, Pigne A, et al. Predictive value of urethral mobility before suburethral tape procedure for urinary stress incontinence in women. *J Urol*. 2002;168:2472.

Gauruder-Burmester A, Popken G. The MiniArc sling system in the treatment of female stress urinary incontinence. *Int Braz J Urol*. 2009;35:334.

Greer WJ, Richter HE, Bartolucci AA, Burgio KL. Obesity and pelvic floor disorders: a systematic review. *Obstet Gynecol*. 2008;112:341.

Groenen R, Vos MC, Willekes C, Vervest HA. Pregnancy and delivery after mid-urethral sling procedures for stress urinary incontinence: case reports and a review of literature. *Int Urogynecol J Pelvic Floor Dysfunct*. 2008;19:441.

Gungorduk K, Celebi I, Ark C, et al. Which type of mid-urethral sling procedure should be chosen for treatment of stress urinary incontinence with intrinsic sphincter deficiency? Tension-free vaginal tape or transobturator tape. *Acta Obstet Gynecol Scand*. 2009;88:920.

Gurol-Urganci I, Geary RS, Mamza JB, et al. Long-term rate of mesh sling removal following midurethral mesh sling insertion among women with stress urinary incontinence. *JAMA*. 2018;320:1659.

Haliloglu B, Karateke A, Coksuer H, et al. The role of urethral hypermobility and intrinsic sphincteric deficiency on the outcome of transobturator tape procedure: a prospective study with 2-year follow-up. *Int Urogynecol J*. 2010;21:173.

Hengel AR, Carlson KV, Baverstock RJ. Prevention, diagnosis, and management of midurethral mesh sling complications. *Can Urol Assoc J*. 2017;11:S135.

Hinoul P, Vervest HA, den Boon J, et al. A randomized, controlled trial comparing an innovative single incision sling with an established transobturator sling to treat female stress urinary incontinence. *J Urol*. 2011;185:1356.

Jain P, Jirschele K, Botros SM, Latthe PM. Effectiveness of midurethral slings in mixed urinary incontinence: a systematic review and meta-analysis. *Int Urogynecol J*. 2011;22:923.

Jang HC, Jeon JH, Kim DY. Changes in sexual function after the midurethral sling procedure for stress urinary incontinence: long-term follow-up. *Int Neurourol J*. 2010;14:170.

Jarvis SK, Hallam TK, Lujic S, et al. Peri-operative physiotherapy improves outcomes for women undergoing incontinence and or prolapse surgery: results of a randomised controlled trial. *Aust N Z J Obstet Gynaecol*. 2005;45:300.

Jeffry L, Deval B, Birsan A, et al. Objective and subjective cure rates after tension-free vaginal tape for treatment of urinary incontinence. *Urology*. 2001;58:702.

Jeon MJ, Jung HJ, Chung SM, et al. Comparison of the treatment outcome of pubovaginal sling, tension-free vaginal tape, and transobturator tape for stress urinary incontinence with intrinsic sphincter deficiency. *Am J Obstet Gynecol*. 2008;199:76.e1.

Kaelin-Gambirasio I, Jacob S, Boulvain M, et al. Complications associated with transobturator sling procedures: analysis of 233 consecutive cases with a 27 month follow-up. *BMC Women's Health*. 2009;9:28.

Kenton K, Stoddard AM, Zyczynski H, et al. 5-Year longitudinal followup after retropubic and transobturator mid urethral slings. *J Urol*. 2015;193:203.

Kim A, Kim MS, Park YJ, et al. Retropubic versus transobturator mid urethral slings in patients at high risk for recurrent stress incontinence: a systematic review and meta-analysis. *J Urol*. 2019;202:132.

Koops SE, Bisseling TM, van Brummen HJ, et al. What determines a successful tension-free vaginal tape? A prospective multicenter cohort study: results from The Netherlands TVT database. *Am J Obstet Gynecol*. 2006;194:65.

Lapitan MC, Cody JD. Open retropubic colposuspension for urinary incontinence in women. *Cochrane Database Syst Rev*. 2012;6:CD002912.

Latthe PM, Singh P, Foon R, Toozs-Hobson P. Two routes of transobturator tape procedures in stress urinary incontinence: a meta-analysis with direct and indirect comparison of randomized trials. *BJU Int*. 2010;106:68.

de Leval J. Novel surgical technique for the treatment of female stress urinary incontinence: transobturator vaginal tape inside-out. *Eur Urol*. 2003;44:724.

Liapis A, Bakas P, Creatsas G. Monarc vs TVT-O for the treatment of primary stress incontinence: a randomized study. *Int Urogynecol J*. 2008;19:185.

Liapis A, Bakas P, Creatsas G. Tension-free vaginal tape in the management of recurrent urodynamic stress incontinence after previous failed midurethral tape. *Eur Urol*. 2009;55:1450.

Lim JL, de Cuyper EM, Cornish A, Frazer M. Short-term clinical and quality-of-life outcomes in women treated by the TVT-Secur procedure. *Aust N Z J Obstet Gynaecol*. 2010;50:168.

Lovatsis D, Easton W, Wilkie D. Guidelines for the evaluation and treatment of recurrent urinary incontinence following pelvic floor surgery, Society of Obstetricians and Gynaecologists of Canada Urogynaecology Committee. *J Obstet Gynaecol Can*. 2010;32:893.

Madhuvrata P, Riad M, Ammembal MK, et al. Systematic review and meta-analysis of "inside-out" versus "outside-in" transobturator tapes in management of stress urinary incontinence in women. *Eur J Obstet Gynecol Reprod Biol*. 2012;162:1.

McLennan MT, Melick CF. Bladder perforation during tension-free vaginal tape procedures: analysis of learning curve and risk factors. *Obstet Gynecol*. 2005;106:1000.

Meschia M, Barbacini P, Baccichet R, et al. Short term outcomes with the Ajust system: a new single incision sling for the treatment of stress urinary incontinence. *Int Urogynecol J*. 2011;22:177.

Meschia M, Bertozzi R, Pifarotti P, et al. Perioperative morbidity and early results of a randomised trial comparing TVT and TVT-O. *Int Urogynecol J*. 2007;18:1257.

Miller JJ, Botros SM, Akl MN, et al. Is transobturator tape as effective as tension-free vaginal tape in patients with borderline maximum urethral closure pressure? *Am J Obstet Gynecol*. 2006;195:1799.

Minassian VA, Stewart WF, Wood GC. Urinary incontinence in women: variation in prevalence estimates and risk factors. *Obstet Gynecol*. 2008;111:324.

Moore RD, Mitchell GK, Miklos JR. Single-center retrospective study of the technique, safety, and 12-month efficacy of the MiniArc single-incision sling: a new minimally invasive procedure for treatment of female SUI. *Surg Technol Int*. 2009;18:175.

Morgan JE, Farrow GA, Stewart FE. The Marlex sling operation for the treatment of recurrent stress urinary incontinence: a 16-year review. *Am J Obstet Gynecol*. 1985;151:224.

Morton HC, Hilton P. Urethral injury associated with minimally invasive mid-urethral sling procedures for the treatment of stress urinary incontinence: a case series and systematic literature search. *Br J Obstet Gynaecol.* 2009;116:1120.

Muir TW, Tulikangas PK, Paraiso MF, Walters MD. The relationship of tension-free vaginal tape insertion to the vascular anatomy of the retropubic space and anterior abdominal wall. *Obstet Gynecol.* 2003;101:933.

Nager CW, Sirls L, Litman HJ. Baseline urodynamic predictors of treatment failure 1 year after mid urethral sling surgery. *J Urol.* 2011;186:597.

Nambiar A, Cody JD, Jeffery ST, Aluko P. Single-incision sling operations for urinary incontinence in women. *Cochrane Database Syst Rev.* 2017;7:CD008709.

Neuman M. TVT-obturator: short-term data on an operative procedure for the cure of female stress urinary incontinence performed on 300 patients. *Eur Urol.* 2007;51:1083.

Neuman M, Sosnovski V, Kais M, et al. Transobturator vs single-incision suburethral mini-slings for treatment of female stress urinary incontinence: early postoperative pain and 3-year follow-up. *J Minim Invasive Gynecol.* 2011;18:769.

Nilsson CG, Palva K, Rezapour M, Falconer C. Eleven years prospective follow-up of the tension-free vaginal tape procedure for treatment of stress urinary incontinence. *Int Urogynecol J Pelvic Floor Dysfunct.* 2008;19:1043.

North CE, Hilton P, Ali-Ross NS, Smith AR. A 2-year observational study to determine the efficacy of a novel single incision sling procedure (Minitape) for female stress urinary incontinence. *BJOG.* 2010;117:356.

Novara G, Artibani W, Barber MD, et al. Updated systematic review and meta-analysis of the comparative data on colposuspensions, pubovaginal slings, and midurethral tapes in the surgical treatment of female stress urinary incontinence. *Eur Urol.* 2010;58:218.

Ogah J, Cody JD, Rogerson L. Minimally invasive synthetic suburethral sling operations for stress urinary incontinence in women. *Cochrane Database Syst Rev.* 2009;4:CD006375.

Ogah J, Cody DJ, Rogerson L. Minimally invasive synthetic suburethral sling operations for stress urinary incontinence in women: a short version Cochrane review. *Neurourol Urodyn.* 2011;30:284.

Palva K, Nilsson CG. Prevalence of urinary urgency symptoms decreases by mid-urethral sling procedures for treatment of stress incontinence. *Int Urogynecol J.* 2011;22:1241.

Panel L, Triopon G, Courtieu C, et al. How to advise a woman who wants to get pregnant after a sub-urethral tape placement? *Int Urogynecol J Pelvic Floor Dysfunct.* 2008;19:347.

Pergialotis V, Mudiaga Z, Perrea DN, Doumouchtsis SK. De novo overactive bladder following midurethral sling procedures: a systematic review of the literature and meta-analysis. *Int Urogynecol J.* 2017;28:1631.

Pollard ME, Morrisroe S, Anger JT. Outcomes of pregnancy following surgery for stress urinary incontinence: a systematic review. *J Urol.* 2012;187:1966.

Pradhan A, Jain P, Latthe PM. Effectiveness of midurethral slings in recurrent stress urinary incontinence: a systematic review and meta-analysis. *Int Urogynecol J.* 2012;23:831.

Rafii A, Daraï E, Haab F, et al. Body mass index and outcome of tension-free vaginal tape. *Eur Urol.* 2003;43:288.

Rapp DE, Govier FE, Kobashi KC. Outcomes following mid-urethral sling placement in patients with intrinsic sphincteric deficiency: comparison of SPARC and MONARC slings. *Int Braz J Urol.* 2009;35:68.

Rehman H, Bezerra CC, Bruschini H, Cody JD. Traditional suburethral sling operations for urinary incontinence in women. *Cochrane Database Syst Rev.* 2011;1:CD001754.

Reyna JA, Terry PJ. Transobturator versus transabdominal mid urethral slings: a multi-institutional comparison of obstructive voiding complications. *J Urol.* 2006;175:1014.

Rezapour M, Falconer C, Ulmsten U. Tension-free vaginal tape (TVT) in stress incontinent women with intrinsic sphincter deficiency (ISD)—a long term follow-up. *Int Urogynecol J Pelvic Floor Dysfunct.* 2001;12:S12.

Richter HE, Albo ME, Zyczynski HM, et al. Retropubic versus transobturator midurethral slings for stress incontinence. *N Engl J Med.* 2010;362:2066.

Richter HE, Litman HJ, Lukacz ES, et al. Demographic and clinical predictors of treatment failure one year after midurethral sling surgery. *Obstet Gynecol.* 2011;117:913.

Rigaud J, Pothin P, Labat JJ, et al. Functional results after tape removal for chronic pelvic pain following tension-free vaginal tape or transobturator tape. *J Urol.* 2010;184:610.

Rosen L, Jacobson N, Weinberg A, Ascher-Walsh C. Resident simulation training improves operative time of the retropubic midurethral sling procedure for stress incontinence. *Int Urogynecol J.* 2019;30:1359.

Ross S, Robert M, Swaby C, et al. Transobturator tape compared with tension-free vaginal tape for stress incontinence: a randomized controlled trial. *Obstet Gynecol.* 2009;114:1287.

Scheiner DA, Betschart C, Wiederkehr S, et al. Twelve months effect on voiding function of retropubic compared with outside-in and inside-out transobturator midurethral slings. *Int Urogynecol J.* 2012;23:197.

Schierlitz L, Dwyer PL, Rosamilia A, et al. Effectiveness of tension-free vaginal tape compared with transobturator tape in women with stress urinary incontinence and intrinsic sphincter deficiency: a randomized controlled trial. *Obstet Gynecol.* 2008;112:1253.

Schierlitz L, Dwyer PL, Rosamilia A, et al. Three-year follow-up of tension-free vaginal tape compared with transobturator tape in women with stress urinary incontinence and intrinsic sphincter deficiency. *Obstet Gynecol.* 2012;119:321.

Sentilhes L, Berthier A, Loisel C, et al. Female sexual function following surgery for stress urinary incontinence: tension-free vaginal versus transobturator tape procedure. *Int Urogynecol J.* 2009;20:393.

Serels S, Douso M, Short G. Preliminary findings with the Solyx single-incision sling system in female stress urinary incontinence. *Int Urogynecol J.* 2010;21:557.

Smith AL, Karp DR, Aguilar VC, Davila GW. Repeat versus primary slings in patients with intrinsic sphincter deficiency. *Int Urogynecol J.* 2013;24:963.

Stav K, Dwyer PL, Rosamilia A, et al. Risk factors of treatment failure of midurethral sling procedures for women with urinary stress incontinence. *Int Urogynecol J.* 2010;21:149.

Sung VW, Borello-France D, Newman DK, et al. Effect of behavioral and pelvic floor muscle therapy combined with surgery vs surgery alone on incontinence symptoms among women with mixed urinary incontinence: The ESTEEM Randomized Clinical Trial. *JAMA.* 2019;322:1066.

Thomas TN, Siff LN, Jelovsek JE, Barber M. Surgical pain after transobturator and retropubic midurethral sling placement. *Obstet Gynecol.* 2017;130:118.

Ulmsten U, Petros P. Intravaginal slingplasty (IVS): an ambulatory surgical procedure for treatment of female urinary incontinence. *Scand J Urol Nephrol.* 1995;29:75.

Walsh CA. TVT-Secur mini-sling for stress urinary incontinence: a review of outcomes at 12 months. *BJU Int.* 2011;108:652.

Wang AC. The techniques of trocar insertion and intraoperative urethrocystoscopy in tension-free vaginal taping: an experience of 600 cases. *Acta Obstet Gynecol Scand.* 2004;83:293.

Ward KL, Hilton P, UK and Ireland TVT Trial Group. Tension-free vaginal tape versus colposuspension for primary urodynamic stress incontinence: 5-year follow up. *Br J Obstet Gynaecol.* 2008;115:226.

Wang YJ, Li FP, Wang Q, et al. Comparison of three mid-urethral tension-free tapes (TVT, TVT-O, and TVT-Secur) in the treatment of female stress urinary incontinence: 1-year follow-up. *Int Urogynecol J.* 2011;22:1369.

Welk B, Al-Hothi H, Winick-Ng J. Removal or revision of vaginal mesh used for the treatment of stress urinary incontinence. *JAMA Surg.* 2015;150:1167.

Wieslander CK, Weinstein MM, Handa VL, Collins SA. Pregnancy in women with prior treatments for pelvic floor disorders. *Female Pelvic Med Reconstr Surg.* 2020;26:299.

White AB, Kahn BS, Gonzalez RR, et al. Prospective study of a single-incision sling versus a transobturator sling in women with stress urinary incontinence: 3-year results. *Am J Obstet Gynecol.* 2020;223:545.e1.

Whiteside JL, Walters MD. Anatomy of the obturator region: relations to a transobturator sling. *Int Urogynecol J.* 2004;15:223.

Yoshizawa T, Yamaguchi K, Obinata D, et al. Laparoscopic transvesical removal of erosive mesh after transobturator tape procedure. *Int J Urol.* 2011;18:861.

Zahn CM, Siddique S, Hernandez S, Lockrow EG. Anatomic comparison of two transobturator tape procedures. *Obstet Gynecol.* 2007;109:701.

18

Urethral Injection of Bulking Agents for Intrinsic Sphincter Deficiency

Tamara Grisales and Amy Rosenman

CHAPTER OUTLINE

INTRODUCTION

In 1938 Murless reported the use of morrhuate sodium for injection management of urinary incontinence. In the early 1990s, transurethral and periurethral injection of bovine collagen was introduced for the treatment of stress urinary incontinence and was the gold standard with which all later studies have been compared, although production of this material ceased in 2011. Since the 1990s, several urethral bulking agents have been introduced for this purpose, although some have been removed from the market because of a high rate of adverse events, difficulties with injection, or expense. The ideal urethral bulking material is biocompatible, nonimmunological, and hypoallergenic. It should retain its bulking characteristics for a prolonged interval and therefore should not biodegrade, nor should it migrate (particle size should be >80 μm). The material should be easy to prepare and easy to inject. The ideal material is safe, readily obtainable, inexpensive, efficacious, and durable and induces minimal tissue reaction. Bulking agent injection is thought to treat stress incontinence by mucosal coaptation of the bladder neck and proximal urethra, with subsequent increased urethral resistance to outflow of urine. Although transmission of pressure to the urethra during increased intraabdominal pressure may not change in patients treated with urethral bulking injections, the pressure forcing the urine from the bladder through the urethra is resisted by the bulking of the mucosa in the immediate proximal urethra; this essentially prevents involuntary bladder neck opening.

INDICATIONS AND CONTRAINDICATIONS

The ideal patient for urethral bulking has both limited mobility of the urethra and bladder and a compromised urethral sphincter. More often she is older because repeat injections are often necessary, and a younger patient could be facing decades of treatment over time to maintain effect. Exceptions would include patients who are surgical candidates but who have not completed their family, or others who are putting off surgery for other reasons. In this new era of concern over permanent mesh implants, and possibly reduced availability, many women are seeking solutions without mesh, and bulking agents provide an option.

The most common indications for urethral bulking agents are: (1) intrinsic sphincter deficiency with or without urethral hypermobility, (2) persistent stress urinary incontinence after a urethral sling or urethropexy, (3) stress urinary incontinence in women who cannot undergo surgery because of multiple comorbidities (e.g., poor surgical candidate and/or cannot discontinue anticoagulation), and (4) stress urinary incontinence in women who do not desire a more invasive antiincontinence surgery (e.g., prefer to avoid mesh material, desire future fertility, require treatment for occult stress incontinence after successful pessary placement, etc.). Relative contraindications to the use of urethral bulking injections include active urinary tract infection, high postvoid residual urine (>100 mL), urinary stricture/obstruction, severe detrusor overactivity, and fragile urethral mucosa.

Midurethral slings work poorly in women with a fixed (nonhypermobile) urethra and intrinsic sphincter deficiency. Urethral hypermobility is diagnosed when the angle of the urethra with the patient supine exceeds 30 to 40 degrees from horizontal during straining efforts (Valsalva or cough). In classic teaching, intrinsic sphincter deficiency is diagnosed when (1) the maximal urethral closure pressure is less than 20 to 25 cm H_2O, and/or (2) the abdominal (Valsalva) leak point pressure is less than 60 cm H_2O when the bladder is filled to 150 to 250 mL.

Certain patients respond better to urethral bulking injections. Should the procedure provide no relief after two or three injections, it is usually futile to attempt subsequent injections. Incontinence surgery, whether sling or retropubic urethropexy, can be performed before or after urethral bulking injections. Theoretically, in a woman with a previous urethral bulking injection, there is a risk of encountering the bulking material during the dissection for a urethral sling. Conversely, in a woman with a previous urethral sling, there may be difficulty placing the bulking material in the correct space, because the sling may compress the urethra and not allow sufficient room for tissue expansion. If stress incontinence persists or recurs after a urethral sling or other pelvic reconstructive surgery, a urethral bulking agent may be used, and often it is very effective. This may be done as early as 6 weeks after surgery, except for Macroplastique, which is not recommended until after 12 weeks.

Bulking agents generally are not the first-line treatment for patients with urethral hypermobility and stress urinary incontinence because the midurethral sling is highly effective. However, there are situations in high-risk patients who are poor surgical candidates with pelvic organ prolapse and stress incontinence when a pessary has provided excellent control of prolapse and has provided temporary stabilization of bladder neck mobility. Urethral bulking may be used in these patients to treat occult stress incontinence that was unmasked after the prolapse was reduced. Similarly, in patients who develop *de novo* stress urinary incontinence after prolapse surgery, urethral bulking agent injection gives patients an office-based option that can be performed as soon as 6 weeks after surgery that may temporize their new urinary complaint. In addition, treatment of stress urinary incontinence in women who have not completed childbearing is a difficult situation in which urethral bulking may be considered as an alternative to physical therapy, midurethral sling, or expectant management. Some women may require or prefer nonmesh alternatives, and some may choose bulking after discussion of all options.

EVALUATION

Evaluation before therapy consists of a history and physical examination to include a postvoid residual urine determination and urinalysis and/or urine culture. This is sometimes complemented by a bladder diary and urodynamic evaluation to establish the diagnosis of intrinsic sphincter deficiency. Multichannel urodynamic studies that include abdominal (Valsalva) leak point pressure determination and/or a urethral pressure profile to assess maximum urethral closure pressure can aid in the diagnosis of intrinsic sphincter deficiency. Another evaluation technique that may aid in diagnosis of intrinsic sphincter deficiency is direct urethroscopic visualization of the bladder neck and proximal urethra to evaluate for urethral coaptation/open bladder neck at rest and during Valsalva or cough.

MATERIALS

All currently available materials are nonbiodegradable and nonimmunological, do not require refrigeration, and do not require skin testing (Table 18.1).

Durasphere was initially approved by the US Food and Drug Administration (FDA) in 1999. The second-generation material, Durasphere EXP (Coloplast Corporation, Minneapolis, MN), consists of pyrolytic carbon–coated graphite beads suspended in a water-based carrier gel containing 3% β-glucan. β-glucan is a simple polysaccharide that causes a subtle inflammatory response. The current preparation has a particle size of 90 to 212 μm and is injected through a 20-gauge needle. The material is nonbiodegradable. According to the manufacturer, it should not migrate because the particle size is greater than 80 μm and thus theoretically cannot be engulfed by macrophages. The product is versatile and is the only material that is approved for periurethral methods, as well as transurethral methods. It is available in 1- and 3-mL syringes. Typically, 2 to 4 mL is injected at the 4 and 8 o'clock positions. Importantly, for women with "fragile urethral mucosa" (possibly from prior radiation therapy or prior urethral surgery), Durasphere EXP is the only material that is not contraindicated.

Coaptite (Boston Scientific Corporation, Natick, MA) was approved by the FDA in 2005. It consists of 75- to 125-μm (average 100-μm) calcium hydroxylapatite spheres suspended in an aqueous gel of sodium carboxylmethylcellulose. This synthetic material is a natural constituent of bones and teeth and has been used in dental and orthopedic applications for many years. In the urethra, it does not encapsulate but allows for ingrowth of native tissues with time as the gel carrier dissolves. It has not been shown to induce heterotopic bone formation. It is biocompatible, nonbiodegradable, and radiopaque; is injected through a 21-gauge needle; and is available in 1-mL syringes. Typically, 2 to 4 mL is injected at the 4 and 8 o'clock positions. According to the manufacturer's instructions for use, Coaptite is contraindicated in patients with a "fragile urethral mucosal lining."

Macroplastique (Uroplasty, Geleen, the Netherlands, and Minnetonka, MN) has been approved for use in Europe since 1991 and was approved by the FDA in 2006 for use in the United States. It is made from highly textured polydimethylsiloxane macroparticles suspended in a bioexcretable carrier hydrogel of polyvinylpyrrolidone. It consists of silicone microimplants of 120 to 600 μm (average 140 μm) and is prepared in 2.5-mL syringes injected through an 18- or 20-gauge needle. Typically, two syringes are required, with 2.5 mL delivered to the 6 o'clock position and 1.25 mL each delivered to the 2 and 1 o'clock positions, for a total of 5 mL. It requires a special administration device for transurethral injection (Fig. 18.1). According to the manufacturer's instructions for use, Macroplastique is contraindicated in patients (1) with "fragile urethral mucosal lining" (e.g., postradiation therapy or postsurgery to the bladder neck) or (2) within 12 weeks of previous Macroplastique injection or a minimally invasive sling procedure.

Bulkamid (Contura International, Soeborg, Denmark, and Ethicon, Somerville, NJ) is newly FDA approved in 2020 in the United States. It is a nonparticulate, nonresorbable

TABLE 18.1 Injectable Agents in Use in North America

Trade Name	Bulking Material	Company	Approval	Carrier Media	Syringe	Needle Gauge/Type	Approach	Ancillary Components
Contigen	Bovine dermal collagen cross-linked with glutaraldehyde	Bard, Inc., Covington, GA	1993 (off market in 2011)	Phosphate-buffered physiological saline	2.5 mL	22- to 23-gauge, rigid or flexible needle	Transurethral or periurethral	None
Durasphere EXP	Pyrolytic carbon–coated graphite beads	Coloplast Corporation, Minneapolis, MN	1999	β-glucan and water gel	1.0 and 3.0 mL	18- or 20-gauge, pencil-point tip, rigid needle, bent spiral-tip needle	Transurethral or periurethral	None
Coaptite	Calcium hydroxylapatite	Boston Scientific Corporation, Natick, MA	2005	Sodium carboxymethyl cellulose, sterile water, and glycerine	1.0 mL	21-gauge, side-kick rigid needle	Transurethral	None
Macroplastique	Polydimethylsiloxane macroparticle	Uroplasty, Geleen, The Netherlands, and Minnetonka, MN	2006	Polyvinylpyrrolidone gel	2.5 mL	18- or 20-gauge, rigid needle	Transurethral	Administration device/pressure gun
Bulkamid	Polyacrylamid hydrogel	Contura International, Soeburg, Denmark	2020	None	1.0 mL	23-gauge needle or Bulkamid device	Transurethral	Bulkamid Urethral Bulking system—specially designed urethroscopic instrument

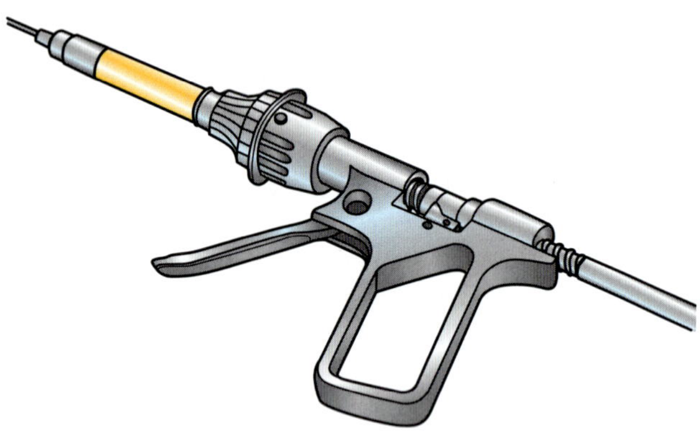

Fig. 18.1 Macroplastique administration device.

polyacrylamide hydrogel made of cross-linked polyacrylamide and water. Bulkamid is the only FDA-approved material that contains no solid particles (crystals or particulates), theoretically abolishing the risk of migration. Being a gel, it can be injected through the operative channel of a regular cystourethroscope using a special 23-gauge needle or the Bulkamid Urethral Bulking System—a specially designed lightweight urethroscopic instrument that facilitates injection (Fig. 18.2 and Video 18.1).

Permacol (Tissue Science Laboratories PLC, Aldershot, Hampshire, UK) is approved for use in Europe but is not currently under study protocol in the Unites States. It is a sterile, injectable suspension of acellular cross-linked porcine collagen matrix. It is available in 2.5-mL syringes and is injected through a 19-gauge needle.

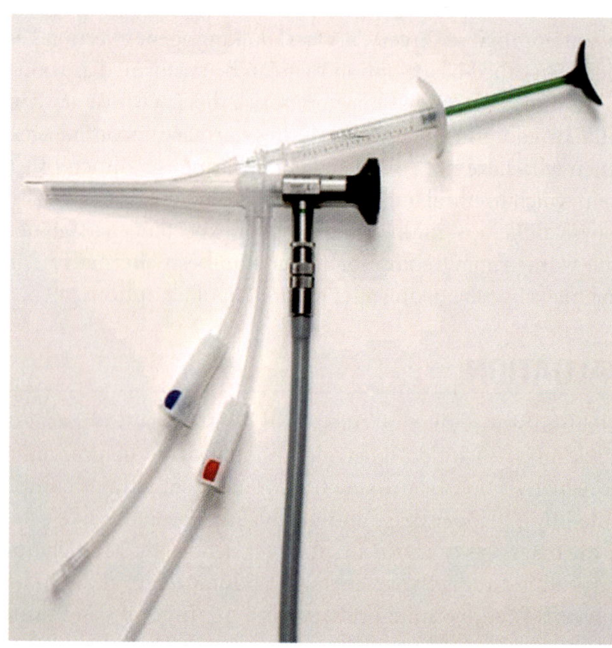

Fig. 18.2 Bulkamid urethroscopic system.

Urethral bulking materials no longer available for clinical use include: Contigen, Zuidex, and Uryx or Tegress. Approved by the FDA in 1993, Contigen (Bard Inc., Covington, GA) was the primary urethral injectable agent until 1999. It consists of glutaraldehyde cross-linking of bovine dermal collagen. The manufacturing of bovine collagen was halted in June 2011. Of note, this was the only material that was biodegradable and not permanent. Additionally, this was the only material that required skin testing, as allergic reactions occurred in 2% to 5% of women. All currently marketed urethral bulking materials have used bovine collagen as the control material in their representative comparative studies.

Zuidex gel (Q-Med AB, Uppsala, Sweden) was a combination of dextranomer (cross-linked polysaccharides) and hyaluronic acid. Dextranomer has been used in wound treatment for many years. Biotechnological (nonanimal) stabilized hyaluronic acid is similar to natural hyaluronic acid found in the body. The material is prepared in 0.7-mL syringes; it is used periurethrally with an implantation device (Implacer) and requires the injection of four syringes of material. The Implacer allows transurethral injection without visualization of the injection site. The material was FDA-approved in the United States in 2001 for ureterovesical reflux and is marketed as Deflux. Zuidex has been available in Europe for urethral bulking since 2002. The FDA initially approved the use of Zuidex for clinical trials in the United States in 2003, although the results were not superior to those with bovine collagen. Also, granuloma/abscess formation rates as high as 14% to 28% were found in case series; thus, it is not FDA approved and has been withdrawn from the market.

Uryx or Tegress (Bard Medical, Covington, GA) was an ethylene vinyl copolymer dissolved in dimethylsulfoxide. It was discontinued in 2007 owing to more than 200 adverse events being reported to the FDA, mostly related to urethral erosion.

Future injectable materials may come from tissue engineering and autologous cellular therapy, using myoblasts, fibroblasts, or stem cells. Another possibility is the use of transplanted stem cells that may differentiate and regenerate the urethral sphincter. This was briefly studied in the past by the use of autologous ear cartilage and *in vitro* expansion of cells for implant. The technology was not advanced, because of the ready availability of less expensive products.

TECHNIQUES

The procedure must be fully explained to the patient, including the predicted effectiveness and the possible need for repeat injections. Patients should have a basic understanding that all currently marketed bulking procedures involve the injection of nonbiodegradable material. Despite good initial subjective success by the patient and coaptation of the proximal urethra noted by the surgeon, the improvements may be short-lived, as the carrier medium is absorbed over time, leaving behind the permanent implant. The permanent material volume may be less than the volume of the material plus the carrier medium, leading to reduced coaptation in the initial few weeks after surgery. Thus, setting the expectation that additional bulking procedures may be required is essential.

Transurethral and Periurethral Injection

In most cases, the materials are injected transurethrally through disposable injection needles, which fit through the operating channel of a cystoscope sheath, or through a special channel in an operating sheath and bridge set. There are a variety of injection sites, including the 4 and 8 o'clock positions (as recommended for Coaptite and Durasphere EXP); the 4, 8, and 6 o'clock positions (as recommended by Bulkamid); and the 2, 6, and 1 o'clock positions (as recommended for Macroplastique), or the circumferential technique, with injection of material at the 3, 6, 9, and 12 o'clock positions. The bulking materials are intended for injection between the urethral submucosa and the superficial urethral muscle and between the bladder neck and the midurethra. Higher success rates have been demonstrated if the bulking material is injected circumferentially and at the proximal urethra, although the needle enters in the midurethra and advances to the proximal urethra for injection.

The transurethral method uses a cystourethroscope with a 0- to 30-degree lens with the appropriate sheath (20- or 21-French with no fenestration). The operating channel allows the passage of a beveled disposable injection needle. A built-in needle delivery system is found in most products. The various materials for injection may dictate injection systems, such as the pressure gun administration device required for the injection of Macroplastique. Bulkamid has an optional disposable cystoscope and delivery system.

The procedure typically begins with placement of 2% lidocaine gel in the urethra for 5 to 10 minutes. This can be performed by inserting 5- to 15-mL in a prefilled coned delivery system (UroJet, International Medication Systems, El Monte, CA). The disposable injection needle is then primed with bulking material before or after insertion of the cystourethroscope, until the material is seen at the needle tip. The optimal implant site is between 0.5 and 2 cm distal to the bladder neck. Once a proper injection site is located, the cystourethroscope is angled so that the injection needle enters the urethra at a 30- to 45-degree angle, and the needle inserted 1.5 to 2 cm from the urethrovesicle junction until the bevel cannot be seen (approximately 1 cm). The scope is then realigned parallel to the urethra, and the needle is advanced to the level of the proximal urethra. The injection should gradually cause distention of the urethral mucosa, and this is observed by appropriate parallel angling of the cystourethroscope during the injection (Fig. 18.3). The urethral mucosa should swell with the injection material, and gradually the urethral mucosa meets in the midline. If the injection is too superficial, there will be blanching or superficial appearance of the injection material under the urethral mucosa, and the needle must be repositioned. Coaptation of the proximal urethral mucosa when fluids are running and/or a negative cough stress test are commonly used to determine when the procedure is complete. If needed, another syringe of bulking agent can be attached, and the injection at the second site is performed. There are different techniques regarding whether the needle bevel should turn toward the urethral lumen, or away from it, while injecting, depending on the material used (Video 18.2).

Periurethral injection is a less commonly used technique. The sites for injection of local anesthesia are selected at the level of Skene's glands on either side of the urethra. Using a 25-gauge

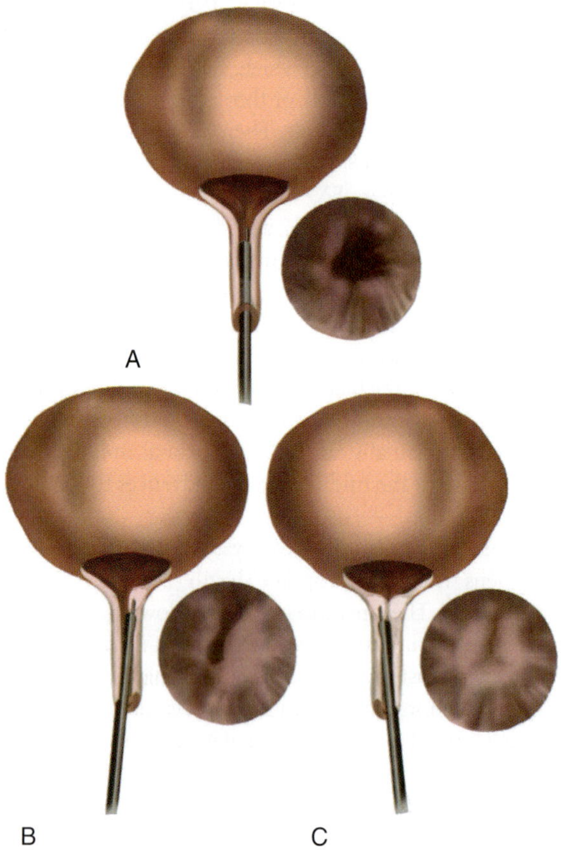

Fig. 18.3 Transurethral method of urethral bulking injection. **A**, Bladder neck is open. **B**, Submucosal placement of material results in partial closure of bladder neck. **C**, Injection is complete, and bladder neck is closed.

needle, 1 mL of 1% lidocaine solution is injected 0.5 to 1 cm lateral to the urethral meatus. Lidocaine 2% gel is also placed in the urethra at the start of the procedure. The cystourethroscope with a 0- to 30-degree lens is inserted to the urethrovesical junction and then withdrawn to observe the proximal urethra. A syringe with 1% lidocaine solution, with or without a small amount of indigo carmine to stain the tissues, may be inserted and guided almost parallel to the urethra at a very slight inward angle, directing the needle bevel medially toward the urethral lumen. This allows the injection material to be viewed more easily as the position of the needle is determined. The cystourethroscope is used to observe the advancing needle, and the syringe is moved in short strokes to allow the needle tip to be seen under the tissue at the proximal urethra until the desired location is found. The syringe is replaced with a syringe of bulking agent, and the material is injected until the entire syringe has been injected or there has been adequate effect noted with urethral bulking. The process is repeated on the opposite site; the second side may be more difficult because of distortion of the proximal urethra caused by the initial injection. Durasphere EXP comes with a periurethral injection needle, which is 20-gauge, short, and angled so as to aid in accurate submucosal placement (Fig. 18.4, second row of diagrams). Patients may experience pain during the procedure. Therefore, these procedures are often done under sedation at an ambulatory surgery center, although some patients tolerate the procedure in the outpatient clinic setting.

Postinjection Management and Follow-Up

Immediately after injection, the patient should have minimal to no pain. She may have urethral burning and mild hematuria

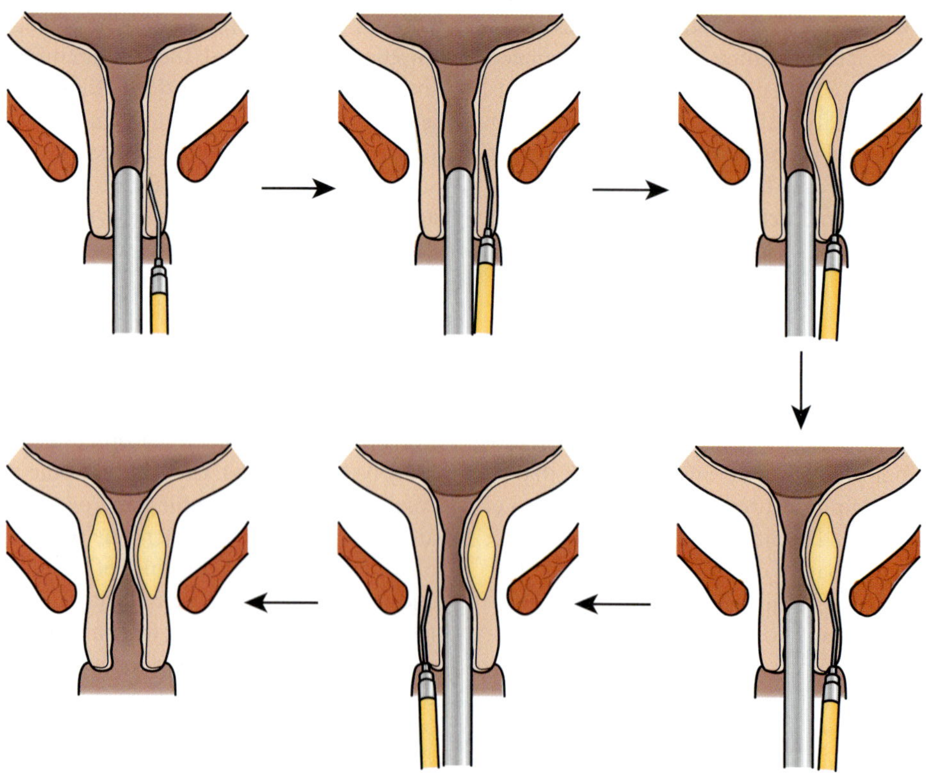

Fig. 18.4 Periurethral method of Durasphere EXP urethral bulking injection.

with urination, which should last less than 48 hours. Antibiotics are commonly given immediately before and/or 1 or 2 days after injection, because the rate of urinary tract infection is lower if prophylactic antibiotics are administered. The patient may experience transient urinary retention for 24 to 72 hours. If she is not able to void after the procedure, then the patient should be instructed in self-catheterization. Some providers prefer teaching women self-catheterization before the injection. Alternatively, a pediatric (8- to 10-French) Foley catheter may be placed, but this is less desirable, because there is a theoretic risk of molding around the catheter leading to persistent stress urinary incontinence symptoms. If a pediatric Foley catheter is placed, the patient should return in 24 to 72 hours for another voiding assessment. There is no need to continue to perform self-catheterization after voiding commences and residual urine amounts are less than 100 to 150 mL or less than 25% to 50% of voided volumes that are greater than 100 mL. At follow-up, symptoms of persistent urinary incontinence, voiding dysfunction, overactive bladder symptoms, and urinary tract infection should be assessed. Repeat injections can be scheduled every 6 to 12 weeks as needed for persistent symptoms of stress incontinence.

COMPLICATIONS AND SAFETY

The most common adverse events with urethral bulking are mild pain, urinary retention, dysuria, hematuria, and urinary tract infection. Rarely, urethral erosion may result. The main advantage of this procedure is that it is the least invasive procedure for stress urinary incontinence and can be used in women who are poor surgical candidates or who are using anticoagulants. Most women are taken off their anticoagulants temporarily. They may resume anticoagulation immediately postoperation. The most common complication during the injection is pain. Another complication is extrusion of material from the injection site. This can be avoided or decreased by submucosal placement of the needle approximately 1 to 1.5 cm from the desired implant site and by holding the needle in place for several seconds (up to 30 seconds) to allow the pressure to dissipate. Most materials are injected through a 20-gauge needle or smaller; thus, the extrusion of a large amount of material is seldom a problem.

The most common adverse events immediately after the injection are urinary retention and voiding dysfunction. It is important to assess voiding after the injection is complete, and this can be accomplished by comparing the amount voided with the amount of fluid infused during the procedure using a bladder scanner, or by performing a straight catheterization with a pediatric 8- to 10-French catheter. Usually, if 200 mL is placed during the procedure and the patient is able to void 100 mL or greater within the hour after injection, there is little concern regarding retention. In a 2001 study by Lightner et al., urinary retention resolved in all patients within 7 days of the urethral bulking injection.

Urinary tract infection occurs in 10% to 25% of cases; thus, antibiotic treatment should be considered after the injection, and/or the urine should be checked for infection at the initial postoperative visit. Pain with urination occurs in some patients but is self-limited, as previously discussed. Macroplastique has been associated with a high incidence of dysuria lasting up to 48 hours.

Delayed complications are uncommon but can include suburethral abscess and urethral prolapse. An abscess may be associated with increasing voiding dysfunction with or without pain. Cystourethroscopy may be required to be certain there is no abscess present. If suspected, magnetic resonance imaging or urethral ultrasound imaging is recommended for further evaluation.

Overall, the currently available products used for urethral bulking are safe. The most common event is urinary tract infection, which often occurs remote from the injection procedure. There appears to be little risk of obstructive uropathy. Suburethral abscess has been reported, but the incidence is less than 1%. Other rare events include tissue necrosis at the injection site, urethral prolapse, and urethrovaginal fistula. Migration of Durasphere particles has been reported, but the clinical significance is unknown.

Effectiveness

There is no standardized manner to evaluate the effectiveness of urethral bulking injections. Most of the FDA-approved trials use voiding diaries, pad tests, and subjective data such as Stamey Continence Grading and validated questionnaires. Postprocedural urodynamic testing has not been proved to be useful in evaluating effectiveness. Definitions of "cure," "improvement," and "failure" vary in the literature. Additionally, the optimal volume of urethral bulking material injected and number of injections that classifies as "failure" have not been defined. Moreover, there is limited evidence in the literature regarding the optimal injection location, although the available data support proximal and/or midurethral placement.

A Cochrane review from 2017 reported that randomized trials suggest, but do not prove, that urethral bulking injections result in objective and subjective short-term improvement of symptomatic stress incontinence in females (Kirchin et al., 2017). Historically, many of the study reports on Contigen included patients with severe incontinence (leak point pressures <65 cm H_2O) and minimal urethral mobility precluding operative intervention other than potentially obstructive slings. A number of these patients were significantly improved, and, although injection therapy may only last 12 months, repeat injections were generally reproducible.

According to the 2017 Cochrane review, the use of Macroplastique, Coaptite, and Durasphere (as well as Tegress and Zuidex) resulted in improvements that were not shown to be more or less efficacious than Contigen (Kirchin et al., 2017). A comparison of periurethral and transurethral methods of injection found similar outcomes but a higher (although not statistically significant) rate of early complications in the periurethral group.

Cure or improvement occurs in 70% to 80% of patients, with total continence achieved in around 40%. Repeat injections may be required at varying intervals to maintain the effect. If there is no improvement after two or three injections, then success with repeated injections is unlikely; however, the maximum number of treatments that defines failure has not been demonstrated in the literature. Table 18.2 shows the results of the recent randomized controlled trials on urethral bulking injection for stress incontinence.

TABLE 18.2 **Results of Studies of US Food and Drug Administration–Approved Urethral Bulking Agents**[a]

Investigators	Agent	Study Design	Follow-Up (Months)	Volume of Injections (mL)	Dry/Improved
Lightner et al. (2001)	Durasphere	RCT	12	4.8	–/80%[b]
Mayer et al. (2007)	Coaptite	RCT	12	4.0	39%/63%[b]
Ghoniem et al. (2009)	Macroplastique	RCT	12	5.0	37%/62%[b]
Sokol et al. (2014)	Bulkmid	RCT	12	3.3	47%/77%[c]

[a]All randomized controlled trials used Contigen as the active control group for comparison.
[b]Defined as ≥1-point improvement on Stamey Continence Grading, which is a 4-level scale of incontinence severity ranging from 0 = continent-dry to 3 = total incontinence, regardless of activity.
[c]As defined by patient-reported outcomes.
RCT, Randomized controlled trial.

Durasphere

The effectiveness of Durasphere at 1, 2, and 3 years was reported in a randomized study in which it was compared with Contigen (Chrouser et al., 2004). Overall effectiveness was similar but diminished over time. The Durasphere group exhibited 63%, 33%, and 21% cure or improvement rates at 1, 2, and 3 years, respectively, compared with the Contigen group, which exhibited 63%, 19%, and 9% cure or improvement rates at 1, 2, and 3 years, respectively. Despite diminished effectiveness over time, one-third of patients in each group believed that their treatment was a success.

Macroplastique

A systematic review of Macroplastique by Ghoneim and Miller in 2013 demonstrated improvement rates of 73% at 6 to 18 months and 64% at longer than 18 months. Cure rates were 37% and 36% over the same respective follow-up periods. Higher study reinjection rates were associated with improved long-term outcomes. Hegde et al. (2013) evaluated the efficacy of Macroplastique based on the location of injection, with statistically higher success rates noted with proximal location and circumferential distribution of material, as measured with transvaginal ultrasound.

Coaptite

A single randomized study by Mayer et al. (2007) that compared Coaptite with Contigen demonstrated similar rates of efficacy and adverse events. At 12 months, 63% of Coaptite patients compared with 57% of Contigen patients showed improvement in urinary incontinence symptoms. Fewer patients in the Coaptite group required reinjection (62% vs. 74%, $P = .03$).

Bulkamid

In a single-blind, randomized, multicenter study in which 229 women were randomized to Bulkamid and 116 women to Contigen, Bulkamid was demonstrated to be equally efficacious to Contigen. At 12 months, 77.1% of women treated with Bulkamid compared with 79% of women treated with Contigen considered themselves cured or improved, while 47.2% versus 50%, respectively, reported zero episodes of stress incontinence, and the 24-hour pad test was completely dry in 24.0% versus 24.4% of patients, respectively (Sokol et al., 2014). In a *post hoc* analysis of the same study, age greater than 60 years and fewer than 2.5 stress incontinence episodes per day were identified as predictors of cure (Elmelund et al., 2019). In a 2016 review of eight Bulkamid studies involving 767 patients, seven studies reported a statistically significant improvement in stress incontinence. The overall rate of repeat injection was 24.3% (186/767) and ranged from 12% to 35% (Kasi et al., 2016). Lastly, a randomized, controlled, noninferiority trial comparing tension-free vaginal tape and Bulkamid urethral injection demonstrated higher rates of both satisfaction (95% versus 60%) and negative cough stress test (95% vs. 66.4%) after sling compared with Bulkamid urethral injection, although postoperative complications and reoperations were significantly lower after bulking (Itkonen Freitas et al., 2020).

Urethral Bulking Before, After, and Compared With Surgery for Stress Urinary Incontinence

Urethral bulking has been studied in various specific patient populations, including before and after sling procedures and in comparison with other procedures. A multicenter randomized trial comparing collagen injection with surgery (six needle suspensions, 19 Burch procedures, and 29 pubovaginal slings) demonstrated higher efficacy in the surgery group (72%) versus the collagen group (51%), although a higher complication rate was demonstrated in the surgery group (Corcos et al., 2005). Koski et al. (2011) demonstrated the safety and efficacy of sling placement for persistent stress urinary incontinence after urethral bulking injection (including Durasphere, Coaptite, and Contigen). The mean number of previous urethral bulking injections was three. Thirty pubovaginal slings and 13 synthetic midurethral slings were placed, with an 18.6% complication rate, mostly urinary retention and urinary tract infection. In an observational study of 60 patients with recurrent stress incontinence after a midurethral sling procedure, Bulkamid resulted in cure/improvement in 83.6% at 12 months (Zivanovic et al., 2017). These studies may require reinvestigation with other available bulking agents.

FUTURE CONSIDERATIONS

Durasphere EXP, Coaptite, and Macroplastique are the most popular urethral bulking agents in the United States now that Contigen is no longer available. Soon, Bulkamid will also be available in the United States. The ideal bulking material has not been found, and, despite a prolonged search, nothing financially feasible as yet appears to be better than the available bulking agents. However, adult stem cell injection therapy using autologous muscle-derived stem cells for the regenerative repair of an impaired sphincter is currently at the forefront of incontinence research. The implanted cells fuse with muscle and release trophic factors, promoting nerve and muscle integration. Small pilot studies have suggested restoration of the urethral sphincter over several months' time.

BIBLIOGRAPHY

Bent AE, Tutrone RT, McLennan MT, et al. Treatment of intrinsic sphincter deficiency using autologous ear chondrocytes as a bulking agent. *Neurourol Urodyn.* 2001;20:157.

Bridges MD, Petrou SP, Lightner DJ. Urethral bulking agents: imaging review. *AJR Am J Roentgenol.* 2005;185:257.

Carr LK, Steele D, Steele S, et al. 1-year follow-up of autologous muscle derived stem cell injection pilot study to treat stress urinary incontinence. *Int Urogynecol J.* 2008;19:881.

Chrouser KL, Fick F, Goel A, et al. Carbon coated zirconium beads in beta-glucan gel and bovine glutaraldehyde cross-linked collagen injections for intrinsic sphincter deficiency: continence and satisfaction after extended followup. *J Urol.* 2004;171:1152.

Clemons JL, LaSala CA. The tension-free vaginal tape in women with a non-hypermobile urethra and low maximum urethral closure pressure. *Int Urogynecol J.* 2007;18:727.

Corcos J, Collet JP, Shapiro S, et al. Multicenter randomized clinical trial comparing surgery and collagen injections for treatment of female stress urinary incontinence. *Urology.* 2005;65:898.

Elmelund M, Sokol ER, Karram MM, et al. Patient characteristics that may influence the effect of urethral injection therapy for female stress incontinence. *J Urol.* 2019;202:125.

Gaddi A, Guaderrama N, Bassiouni N, et al. Repeat midurethral sling compared with urethral bulking for recurrent stress urinary incontinence. *Obstet Gynecol.* 2014;123:1207.

Ghoniem GM, Khater U. Urethral prolapse after durasphere injection. *Int Urogynecol J Pelvic Floor Dysfunct.* 2006;17:297.

Ghoniem G, Corcos J, Comiter C, et al. Cross-linked polydimethylsiloxane injection for female stress urinary incontinence: results of a multicenter, randomized, controlled, single-blind study. *J Urol.* 2009;181:204.

Ghoniem G, Corcos J, Comiter C, et al. Durability of urethral bulking agent injection for female stress urinary incontinence: 2-year multicenter study results. *J Urol.* 2010;183:444.

Ghoniem GM, Miller CJ. A systematic review and meta-analysis of Macroplastique for treating female stress urinary incontinence. *Int Urogynecol J.* 2013;24:27.

Hegde A, Smith AL, Aguilar VC, Davila GW. Three-dimensional endovaginal ultrasound examination following injection of Macroplastique for stress urinary incontinence: outcomes based on location and periurethral distribution of the bulking agent. *Int Urogynecol J.* 2013;24:1151.

Isom-Batz G, Zimmern PE. Collagen injection for female urinary incontinence after urethral or periurethral surgery. *J Urol.* 2009;181:701.

Itkonen Freitas AM, Mentula M, Mikkola TS et al. Tension-free vaginal tape surgery versus polyacrylamide hydrogel injection for primary stress urinary incontinence: a randomized clinical trial. *J Urol.* 2020;203:372.

Kasi AD, Pergialiotis V, Perrea DN, Khunda A. Polyacrylamide hydrogel (Bulkamid®) for stress urinary incontinence in women: a systematic review of the literature. *Int Urogyncol J.* 2016;27:367.

Kim BS, Chun SY, Lee JK, et al. Human amniotic fluid stem cell injection therapy for urethral sphincter regeneration in an animal model. *BMC Med.* 2012;10:94.

Kirchin V, Page T, Aluko P, et al. Urethral injection therapy for urinary incontinence in women. *Cochrane Database Syst Rev.* 2017;7:CD003881.

Koski ME, Enemchukwu EA, Padmanabhan P, et al. Safety and efficacy of sling for persistent stress urinary incontinence after bulking injection. *Urology* 2011;77:1076.

Lightner D, Calvosa C, Andersen R, et al. A new injectable bulking agent for treatment of stress urinary incontinence: results of a multicenter, randomized, controlled, double-blind study of Durasphere. *Urology.* 2001;58:12.

Lightner D, Rovner E, Corcos J, et al. Randomized controlled multisite trial of injected bulking agents for women with intrinsic sphincter deficiency: midurethral injection of Zuidex via the Implacer versus proximal urethral injection of Contigen cystoscopically. *Urology* 2009;74:771.

Mayer RD, Dmochowski RR, Appell RA, et al. Multicenter prospective randomized 52-week trial of calcium hydroxylapatite versus bovine dermal collagen for treatment of stress urinary incontinence. *Urology* 2007;69:876.

McCrery RJ, Appell RA. Safety of carbon bead injection for incontinence in patients taking warfarin. *Urology.* 2006;67:97.

Mohr S, Siegenthaler M, Mueller MD, Kuhn A. Bulking agents: an analysis of 500 cases and review of the literature. *Int Urogynecol J.* 2013;24:241.

Murless BC. The injection treatment of stress incontinence. *J Obstet Gynaecol Br Emp.* 1938;45:521.

Pannek J, Brands FH, Senge T. Particle migration after transurethral injection of carbon coated beads for stress urinary incontinence. *J Urol.* 2001;166:1350.

Pickard R, Reaper J, Wyness L, et al. Periurethral injection therapy for urinary incontinence in women. *Cochrane Database Syst Rev.* 2003;2:CD003881.

Rovner ES, Goudelock CM. Which injectable to use in the treatment of intrinsic sphincter deficiency? *Curr Opin Urol.* 2010;20:29.

Schulz JA, Nager CW, Stanton SL, Baessler K. Bulking agents for stress urinary incontinence: short-term results and complications in a randomized comparison of periurethral and transurethral injections. *Int Urogynecol J.* 2004;15:261.

Sokol ER, Karram MM, Dmochowski R. Efficacy and safety of polyacrylamide hydrogel for the treatment of female stress incontinence: a randomized prospective multicenter North American Study. *J Urol.* 2014;192:843.

Steele AC, Kohli N, Karram MM. Periurethral collagen injection for stress incontinence with and without urethral hypermobility. *Obstet Gynecol.* 2000;95:327.

Sweat SD, Lightner DJ. Complications of sterile abscess formation and pulmonary embolism following periurethral bulking agents. *J Urol.* 1999;161:93.

Toozs-Hobson P, Al-Singary W, Fynes M, et al. Two-year follow-up of an open-label multicenter study of polyacrylamide hydrogel (Bulkamid®) for female stress and stress-predominant mixed incontinence. *Int Urogynecol J.* 2012;23:1373.

Von Heland M, Mantovani F, Zanetti G, et al. Urethral implantation of collagen in the treatment of urinary incontinence. Comparison of transurethral and periurethral approach. *Minerva Urol Nefrol.* 1998;50:213.

Wang HJ, Chuang YC, Chancellor MB. Development of cellular therapy for the treatment of stress urinary incontinence. *Int Urogynecol J.* 2011;22:1075.

Zivanovic I, Ratenberg O, Lobodasch K, et al. Urethral bulking for recurrent stress urinary incontinence after midurethral sling failure. *Neurourol Urodyn.* 2017;36:722.

19

Surgical Treatment of Anterior Vaginal Wall Prolapse

Matthew D. Barber and Mark D. Walters

CHAPTER OUTLINE

INTRODUCTION

Anterior vaginal prolapse occurs commonly and may coexist with disorders of micturition. Mild anterior vaginal prolapse often occurs in parous women, but usually presents few problems. As the prolapse progresses, symptoms may develop and worsen, and treatment becomes indicated. The anterior vaginal wall is the most common segment of the vagina to prolapse and the segment that is most likely to fail long-term after surgical correction. Over 80% of the more than 300,000 vaginal prolapse surgeries performed annually in the United States include correction of anterior compartment prolapse. This chapter reviews the anatomy and pathology of anterior vaginal prolapse, with and without stress urinary incontinence, and describes methods of surgical repair.

ANATOMY AND PATHOLOGY

Anterior vaginal prolapse (cystocele) is defined as pathologic descent of the anterior vaginal wall and overlying bladder base. According to the International Continence Society standardized terminology for prolapse grading (Bump et al., 1996), the term anterior vaginal prolapse is preferred over cystocele. This is because information obtained during the physical examination does not allow the exact identification of structures behind the anterior vaginal wall, although it usually is, in fact, the bladder. The Pelvic Organ Prolapse Quantification (POPQ) system for grading and describing prolapse is discussed in detail in Chapter 8.

The etiology of anterior vaginal prolapse is not completely understood, but it is probably multifactorial, with different factors implicated in prolapse in individual patients. Although age is the most significant factor, other factors include pregnancy, childbirth, connective tissue defects, pelvic floor muscle weakness from denervation or avulsion, hysterectomy, and conditions such as chronic cough or straining associated with elevated intraabdominal pressure (see Chapter 5). Normal support for the vagina and adjacent pelvic organs is provided by the interaction of the pelvic muscles and connective tissue. The upper vagina rests on the levator plate and is stabilized by superior (level 1) and lateral (level 2) connective tissue attachments. The midvagina is attached to the arcus tendineus fasciae pelvis ([ATFP], "white lines") on each side (level 2 attachments), and the apical portion of the anterior vagina is attached to the web of endopelvic fascia, including pubocervical fascia, and the cardinal and uterosacral ligaments. Pathologic loss of lateral and/or apical support (levels 1 and 2) may occur with damage to or impairment of the pelvic muscles, connective tissue attachments, or both, leading to anterior vaginal prolapse.

Nichols and Randall (1996) described two types of anterior vaginal prolapse: distension and displacement. Distension was thought to result from overstretching and attenuation of the anterior vaginal wall, caused by overdistension of the vagina associated with vaginal delivery or atrophic changes associated with aging and menopause. The distinguishing physical feature of this type was described as diminished or absent rugal folds of the anterior vaginal epithelium caused by thinning or loss of midline vaginal fascia. The other type of anterior vaginal prolapse—displacement—was attributed to pathologic detachment or elongation of the anterolateral vaginal supports to the ATFP. This may occur unilaterally or bilaterally, and often coexists with some degree of distension cystocele, with urethral hypermobility, or with apical prolapse. Rugal folds may or may not be preserved.

Another theory ascribes most cases of anterior vaginal prolapse to disruption or detachment of the lateral connective tissue attachments at the ATFP, resulting in a paravaginal defect and corresponding to the displacement type discussed earlier. This was first described by White in 1909 and 1912 but was disregarded until reported by Richardson in 1976. Richardson et al. (1976) described transverse defects, midline defects, and defects involving isolated loss of integrity of pubourethral ligaments. Transverse defects were said to occur when the "pubocervical" fascia separated from its insertion around the cervix, whereas midline defects represented an anteroposterior separation of the fascia between the bladder and vagina. A contemporary conceptual representation of vaginal and paravaginal defects is shown in Fig. 19.1.

Improvements in pelvic imaging are leading to a greater understanding of normal pelvic anatomy and the structural and functional abnormalities associated with prolapse. Magnetic resonance imaging (MRI) holds great promise, with its excellent ability to differentiate soft tissues and its capacity for multiplanar imaging. The pelvic organs, pelvic muscles, and connective tissues can be identified easily with MRI. Various measurements can be made that may be associated with anterior vaginal prolapse or urinary incontinence, such as the urethrovesical angle, the descent of the bladder base, the quality of the levator muscles, and the relationship between the vagina and its lateral and apical connective tissue attachments. Aronson et al. (1995) used an endoluminal surface coil placed in the vagina to image pelvic anatomy with MRI and compared four continent nulliparous women with four incontinent women with anterior vaginal prolapse. Lateral vaginal attachments were identified in all continent women. In Fig. 19.2 the "posterior pubourethral ligaments" (bilateral attachment of the ATFP to the posterior aspect of the pubic symphyses) are clearly seen. In the two subjects with clinically apparent paravaginal defects, lateral detachments were evident (Fig. 19.3). More recent studies based on MRI analysis and computer modeling suggest that apical support abnormalities are at least as important as, if not more important than, paravaginal defects; the degree of apical decent can explain about half of anterior wall descent (Summers et al., 2006). Similarly, the size of the genital hiatus (level 3 support) appears important for anterior prolapse recurrence after surgical repair. Other factors, such as levator muscle impairment, levator avulsion, greater anterior wall length, and widened levator hiatus, also contribute to anterior vaginal prolapse. The mean length of the anterior vagina is approximately 6 cm. Women with anterior vaginal wall prolapse have, on average, a 23% longer anterior vaginal wall than women without prolapse, suggesting that anterior vaginal lengthening is one component of the pathophysiology of anterior prolapse.

Anterior vaginal prolapse commonly coexists with urodynamic stress incontinence. Some features of pathophysiology may overlap, such as loss of anterior vaginal support with bladder-base descent and urethral hypermobility; other features, such as sphincteric dysfunction, may occur independent of vaginal and urethral support. The pathophysiology of stress incontinence is covered more fully in Chapter 5.

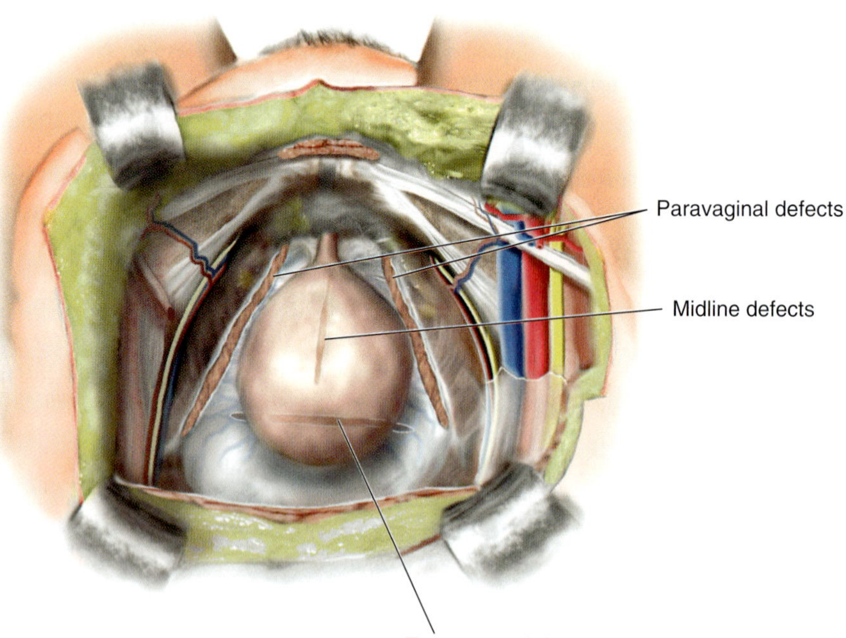

Fig. 19.1 Three different defects can result in anterior vaginal wall prolapse. Lateral or paravaginal defects occur when there is a separation of the pubocervical fascia from the arcus tendineus fasciae pelvis, midline defects occur secondary to attenuation of fascia supporting the bladder base, and transverse defects occur when the pubocervical fascia separates from the vaginal cuff or uterosacral ligaments. (From Maher CF, Karram MM. Surgical management of anterior vaginal wall prolapse. In Karram MM, Maher CF, eds. *Surgical Management of Pelvic Organ Prolapse.* Philadelphia: Saunders, 2013. With permission.)

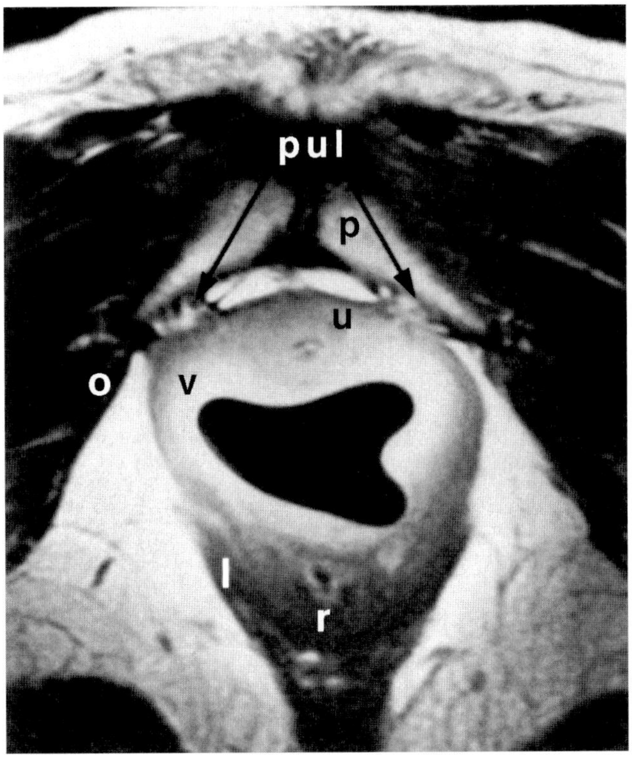

Fig. 19.2 Axial T1-weighted image from a continent 38-year-old nulliparous woman that shows the connection of the anterior vaginal wall (*v*) to the posterior pubic symphysis (*p*) by the pubourethral ligaments (*pul*). The anterior vaginal wall and endopelvic fascia function as a sling, or hammock, for support of the urethra (*u*). *l*, Levator ani musculature; *o*, obturator internus muscle; *r*, rectum. (From Aronson MP, Bates SM, Jacoby AF, et al. Periurethral and paravaginal anatomy: an endovaginal magnetic resonance imaging study. *Am J Obstet Gynecol.* 1995;173:1702. With permission.)

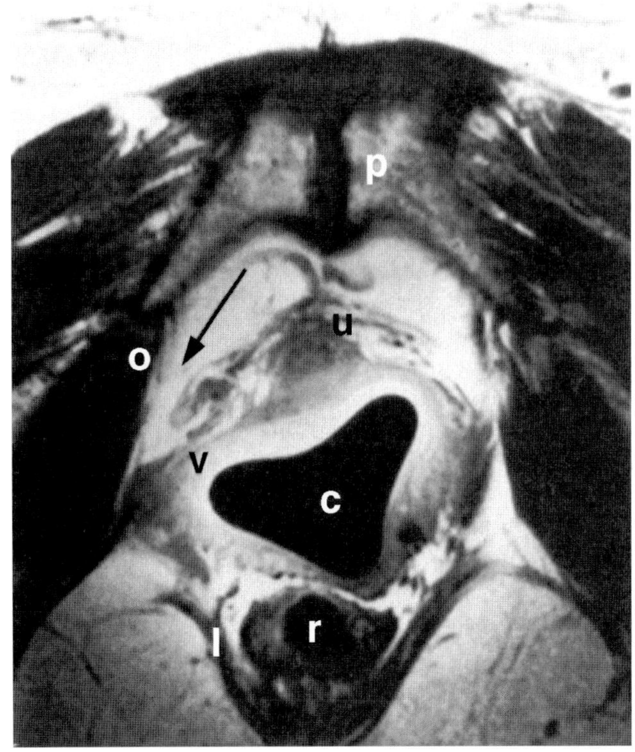

Fig. 19.3 Axial T1-weighted image from a 57-year-old woman, para 5, with stress urinary incontinence. The paravaginal detachment (*arrow*) is seen at the level of the urethrovesical junction. *c*, Endovaginal coil; *r*, rectum; *l*, levator ani musculature; *o*, obturator internus muscle; *p*, posterior pubic symphysis; *u*, urethra; *v*, anterior vaginal wall. (From Aronson MP, Bates SM, Jacoby AF, et al. Periurethral and paravaginal anatomy: an endovaginal magnetic resonance imaging study. *Am J Obstet Gynecol.* 1995;173:1702. With permission.)

EVALUATION

History

When evaluating women with pelvic organ prolapse or urinary or fecal incontinence, attention should be paid to all aspects of pelvic organ support. The reconstructive surgeon must determine the specific sites of damage for each patient, with the ultimate goal of restoring both anatomy and function.

Patients with anterior vaginal prolapse complain of symptoms related directly to vaginal protrusion, or associated symptoms such as urinary incontinence or voiding difficulty. Symptoms related to prolapse may include the sensation of a vaginal mass or bulge, pelvic pressure, low back pain, and sexual difficulty. Stress urinary incontinence commonly occurs in association with anterior vaginal prolapse, particularly when it is mild. In contrast, women with anterior vaginal prolapse that extends beyond the hymen are less likely to complain of stress incontinence and are more likely to have obstructed voiding symptoms such as urinary hesitancy, intermittent flow, weak or prolonged stream, a feeling of incomplete emptying, the need to reduce (splint) the prolapse manually to initiate or complete urination, and, in rare cases, urinary retention. The mechanism for this appears to be mechanical obstruction resulting from urethral kinking that occurs with progressively worsening anterior vaginal prolapse.

Physical Examination

The physical examination should be conducted with the patient in the lithotomy position, as for a routine pelvic examination. The examination is first performed with the patient supine. If physical findings do not correspond to symptoms, or if the maximum extent of the prolapse cannot be confirmed, the woman is reexamined in the standing position.

The genitalia are inspected, and, if no displacement is apparent, the labia are gently spread to expose the vestibule and hymen. The integrity of the perineal body is evaluated, and the approximate size of all prolapsed parts is assessed. A retractor or vaginal speculum can be used to depress the posterior vagina to aid in visualizing the anterior vagina. After the resting examination, the patient is instructed to strain down forcefully or to cough vigorously. During this maneuver, the order of descent of the pelvic organs is noted, as is the relationship of the pelvic organs at the peak of straining.

It may be possible to differentiate lateral defects, identified as detachment or effacement of the lateral vaginal sulci, from central defects, seen as midline protrusion but with preservation of the lateral sulci, by using a curved forceps placed in the anterolateral vaginal sulci directed toward the ischial spines. Bulging of the anterior vaginal wall in the midline between the forceps blades implies a midline defect; blunting or descent of the vaginal fornices on either side with straining suggest lateral paravaginal defects. Studies have shown that the physical examination technique to detect paravaginal defects is not particularly reliable or accurate. In a study by Barber et al. (1999) of 117 women with prolapse, the sensitivity of clinical examination to detect paravaginal defects was good (92%), yet the specificity was poor (52%), and, despite an unexpectedly high prevalence of paravaginal defects, the positive predictive value was poor (61%). Less than two-thirds of women believed to have a paravaginal defect on physical examination were confirmed to have the same at surgery. Another study by Whiteside et al. (2004) demonstrated poor reproducibility of clinical examination in detecting specific anterior vaginal wall defects. Thus, the clinical value of determining the location of midline, apical, and lateral paravaginal defects remains unknown.

Anterior vaginal wall descent usually represents bladder descent with or without concomitant urethral hypermobility. In 1.6% of women with anterior vaginal prolapse, an anterior enterocele mimics a cystocele on physical examination (Tulikangas et al., 2004). Other uncommon conditions, such as anterior vaginal cysts or myomas, can also mimic anterior vaginal prolapse.

Diagnostic Tests

After a careful history and physical examination, few diagnostic tests are needed to evaluate patients with anterior vaginal prolapse. A urinalysis should be performed to evaluate for urinary tract infection if the patient complains of any lower urinary tract dysfunction. Hydronephrosis occurs in a small proportion of women with severe prolapse; however, even if identified, it usually does not change management in women for whom surgical repair is planned. Therefore, routine imaging of the kidneys and ureters is not necessary.

If urinary incontinence is present, further diagnostic testing is indicated to determine the cause of the incontinence. Urodynamic (simple or complex), endoscopic, or radiologic assessments of filling and voiding function are generally indicated only when symptoms of incontinence, voiding dysfunction, or other bothersome lower urinary tract symptoms are present. Even if no urologic symptoms are noted, voiding function should be assessed to evaluate for completeness of bladder emptying. This procedure usually involves a timed, measured void, followed by urethral catheterization or bladder ultrasound to measure postvoid residual urine volume.

In women with severe prolapse, it is important to check urethral function after the prolapse is repositioned. Women with severe prolapse may be paradoxically continent because of urethral kinking; when the prolapse is reduced, urethral dysfunction may be unmasked, with occurrence of incontinence (occult stress incontinence). A pessary, vaginal retractor, or vaginal packing can be used to reduce the prolapse before office bladder filling or electronic urodynamic testing. If urinary leaking occurs with coughing or Valsalva maneuvers after reduction of the prolapse, the urethral sphincter may be incompetent, even if the patient is normally continent. This is reported to occur in 17% to 69% of women with stage III or IV prolapse. In this situation, the surgeon may recommend an antiincontinence procedure in conjunction with anterior vaginal prolapse repair. If stress incontinence is not present even after reduction of the prolapse, an antiincontinence procedure probably is not indicated, although this is a subject of ongoing research. Additional discussion about the decision to perform a concurrent incontinence procedure at the time of vaginal prolapse repair can be found in Chapter 11; see also the Complications section later in this chapter.

SURGICAL REPAIR TECHNIQUES

In this chapter, we describe surgical techniques to address prolapse in the anterior vaginal compartment. Importantly, concomitant apical support procedures at the time of anterior compartment repair increase the success rate compared with isolated anterior repair. An apical prolapse suspension (see Chapter 21) should be performed concurrently for most patients with anterior vaginal prolapse that is beyond the hymen.

Anterior Colporrhaphy

The objective of anterior colporrhaphy is to plicate the layers of vaginal muscularis and adventitia overlying the bladder ("pubocervical fascia") or to plicate and reattach the paravaginal tissue in such a way as to reduce the protrusion of the bladder and vagina. Modifications of the technique depend on how lateral the dissection is carried, where the plicating sutures are placed, and whether additional layers (natural or synthetic grafts) are placed in the anterior vagina for extra support (Videos 19.1 and 19.2).

The operative procedure begins with the patient supine, with the legs elevated and abducted and the buttocks placed just past the edge of the operating table. Antibiotics should be given within 60 minutes of incision to achieve minimal inhibitory concentrations in the skin and tissues by the time the incision is made. This typically means a first-generation cephalosporin (cefazolin), or combination regimens (metronidazole or clindamycin plus gentamicin or aztreonam) if the patient has an allergy to penicillin (ACOG Practice Bulletin No. 195, 2018). In general, all patients undergoing apical prolapse surgery are at moderate risk for thromboembolic events and require a prevention strategy (Clarke-Pearson et al., 2012). Low-dose unfractionated heparin (5000 units every 12 hours) or low-molecular-weight heparins (e.g., 40 mg enoxaparin or 2500 units of dalteparin), an intermittent pneumatic compression device, or a combination of these are recommended. Either form of heparin should be started 2 hours before surgery, and the compression stockings should be placed on the patient in the operating room before incision. These treatment approaches should be continued until the patient is ambulatory.

The abdomen, vagina, and perineum are prepped sterilely and draped, and a 16-French Foley catheter with a 10-mL balloon is inserted for easy identification of the bladder neck. A weighted speculum is placed into the vagina. Hemostatic solution (such as 0.5% lidocaine with 1:200,000 epinephrine) or saline may be injected below the epithelium along the midline of the anterior vaginal wall to decrease bleeding and to aid in dissection. If a vaginal hysterectomy has been performed, the incised apex of the anterior vaginal wall is grasped transversely with two Allis clamps and elevated. Otherwise, a transverse or diamond-shaped incision is made in the vaginal epithelium near the apex. A third Allis clamp is placed about 2 cm below the posterior margin of the urethral meatus and pulled up. If a midurethral sling procedure is to be done, then the incision is made to the bladder neck only. Additional Allis clamps may be placed in the midline between the urethra and apex. A scalpel is used to open the anterior wall in the midline (Fig. 19.4A). Alternatively, the points of a pair of curved Mayo scissors are inserted between the vaginal epithelium and the vaginal muscularis, or between the layers of the vaginal muscularis, and gently forced upward while being kept half open/half closed (Fig. 19.4B). Countertraction during this maneuver is important to minimize the chance of perforation of the bladder. The vagina is incised in the midline, and the incision is continued to the level of the midurethra (or bladder neck, if a sling procedure is being done). As the vagina is incised, the edges are grasped with Allis or T-clamps and drawn laterally for further mobilization. Dissection of the vaginal flaps is then accomplished by turning the clamps back across the forefinger and incising the vaginal muscularis with a scalpel or Metzenbaum scissors, as shown in Fig. 19.4C. An assistant maintains constant traction medially on the remaining vaginal muscularis and underlying vesicovaginal adventitia. This procedure is performed bilaterally until the entire extent of the anterior vaginal prolapse has been dissected; in general, the dissection should be carried farther laterally with more advanced prolapse. The spaces lateral to the urethrovesical junction are sharply dissected toward the ischiopubic rami. It is also important to use sharp dissection to mobilize the bladder base from the vaginal apex, if necessary.

Some surgeons routinely perform a bladder neck plication (Kelly–Kennedy plication) at the time of anterior colporrhaphy, particularly when a concurrent midurethral sling is not planned. Vesical neck plication was used to treat mild stress urinary incontinence in the past, but it is no longer done for that indication. It may, however, help to prevent the later development of stress incontinence in the patient. After the vaginal flaps have been completely developed, the urethrovesical junction can be identified visually or by pulling the Foley catheter downward until the bulb obstructs the vesical neck. Repair should begin at the urethrovesical junction, using No. 2-0 or 0 delayed absorbable sutures. The first plicating stitch is placed into the periurethral endopelvic fascia and tied (Fig. 19.5A). One or two additional stitches are placed to support the length of the urethra and urethrovesical junction.

In a standard anterior colporrhaphy, stitches using No. 2-0 or 0 delayed absorbable sutures are placed in the vaginal tissue (muscularis and adventitia) medial to the vaginal flaps and plicated in the midline without excessive tension. Depending on the severity of the prolapse, one or two rows of plication sutures or a purse-string suture followed by plication sutures are placed (Fig. 19.4E–G). Excess vaginal epithelium is then trimmed from the flaps bilaterally, and the remaining anterior vaginal wall is closed with a running No. 2-0 subcuticular or locking suture (Fig. 19.4H).

Antiincontinence operations are often performed at the same time as anterior vaginal prolapse repair to treat coexisting stress incontinence; suburethral bladder neck sling placement may also improve the cure rate of the prolapse. Bladder neck suspension procedures (sling procedures or retropubic colposuspension) treat effectively mild anterior vaginal prolapse associated with urethral hypermobility and stress incontinence. More advanced anterior vaginal prolapse will not be treated adequately, and in these cases anterior colporrhaphy or anterior vaginal mesh repair should be performed, often in conjunction with a colpopexy procedure and a midurethral sling. Surgical judgment is required to perform the bladder plication tightly enough to reduce the anterior vaginal prolapse sufficiently yet preserve some mobility of the anterior vagina. If anterior colporrhaphy is combined with a sling procedure (midurethral or bladder neck), the cystocele should be repaired before the final tension is set for the sling. A midurethral sling procedure, whether retropubic or transobturator, is best done through a separate midurethral incision after the cystocele repair is complete.

Anterior Prolapse Repair With Grafts

A prosthetic material can be used to provide support in the anterior vagina. This can be done in a number of ways, and the surgical techniques continue to evolve. Graft materials may include synthetic absorbable grafts (e.g., polyglactin 910 mesh), synthetic permanent meshes (e.g., polypropylene), and biologic materials (see Chapter 7). Biologic materials that have been used include autografts of harvested rectus fascia and fascia lata; human allografts including fascia lata and dura mater; and xenografts such as porcine dermis, porcine small intestinal submucosa, and bovine pericardium.

In 2010, approximately 25% of surgeries for pelvic organ prolapse in the United States included transvaginal placement of biologic or synthetic mesh. Many surgeons used transvaginal graft placement in an attempt to increase the efficacy and durability of their surgical repair. For anterior prolapse, studies demonstrate improved anatomic outcomes after transvaginal placement of permanent synthetic mesh compared with anterior colporrhaphy without mesh ("native-tissue repair"). However, this comes at the expense of an increased rate of complications unique to synthetic mesh placement, including vaginal mesh exposure or extrusion, mesh erosion or perforation into an adjacent organ (bladder, urethra, or rectum), and vaginal mesh contraction with associated pain and dyspareunia. Concerns about increased adverse events from transvaginal mesh placement led the US Food and Drug Administration (FDA) to issue two consecutive public health notifications warning of complications associated with transvaginal meshes (2008, 2011) and to upgrade them from class II to class III devices in 2018. As class III devices, industry is now required to perform small clinical trials before bringing new products to the market. In April 2019, the FDA mandated that manufacturers of transvaginal prolapse meshes stop the sale and distribution of their products, citing a failure to demonstrate reasonable assurance of safety and effectiveness. In a joint Committee Opinion published in December 2011, the American Urogynecologic Society and the American College of Obstetrics and Gynecology recommended that pelvic organ prolapse vaginal mesh repair should be reserved for high-risk individuals in whom the benefit

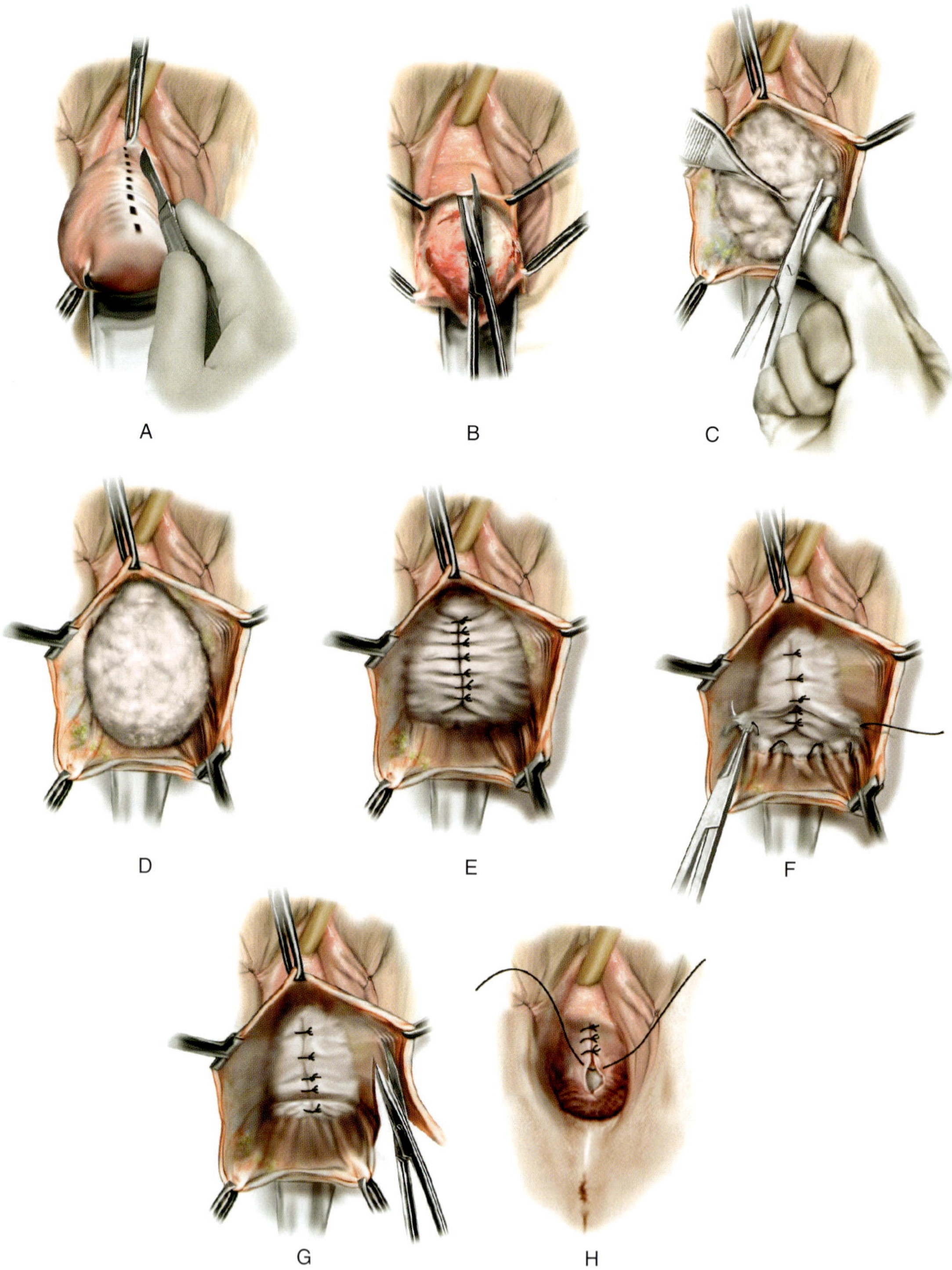

Fig. 19.4 Classic anterior colporrhaphy. **A**, The initial midline anterior vaginal wall incision is demonstrated. **B**, The midline incision is extended using scissors. **C**, Sharp dissection of the bladder off the vaginal wall should be lateral to the superior pubic ramus, and the base of the bladder should be dissected off the vaginal cuff or cervix to the level of the preperitoneal space of the anterior cul-de-sac. **D**, The bladder has been completely mobilized off the vagina. **E**, The initial plication layer is placed. **F**, The second plication layer is placed, which commonly requires further mobilization of vaginal muscularis off the vaginal epithelium. The most proximal stitch involves plication of the inside of the vaginal wall at the level of the vaginal apex or upper portion of the cervix. **G**, The completed second plication layer and trimming of excess vaginal mucosa are demonstrated. **H**, Closure of vaginal mucosa is demonstrated. (From Maher CF, Karram MM. Surgical management of anterior vaginal wall prolapse. In Karram MM, Maher CF, eds. *Surgical Management of Pelvic Organ Prolapse*. Philadelphia: Saunders, 2013. With permission.)

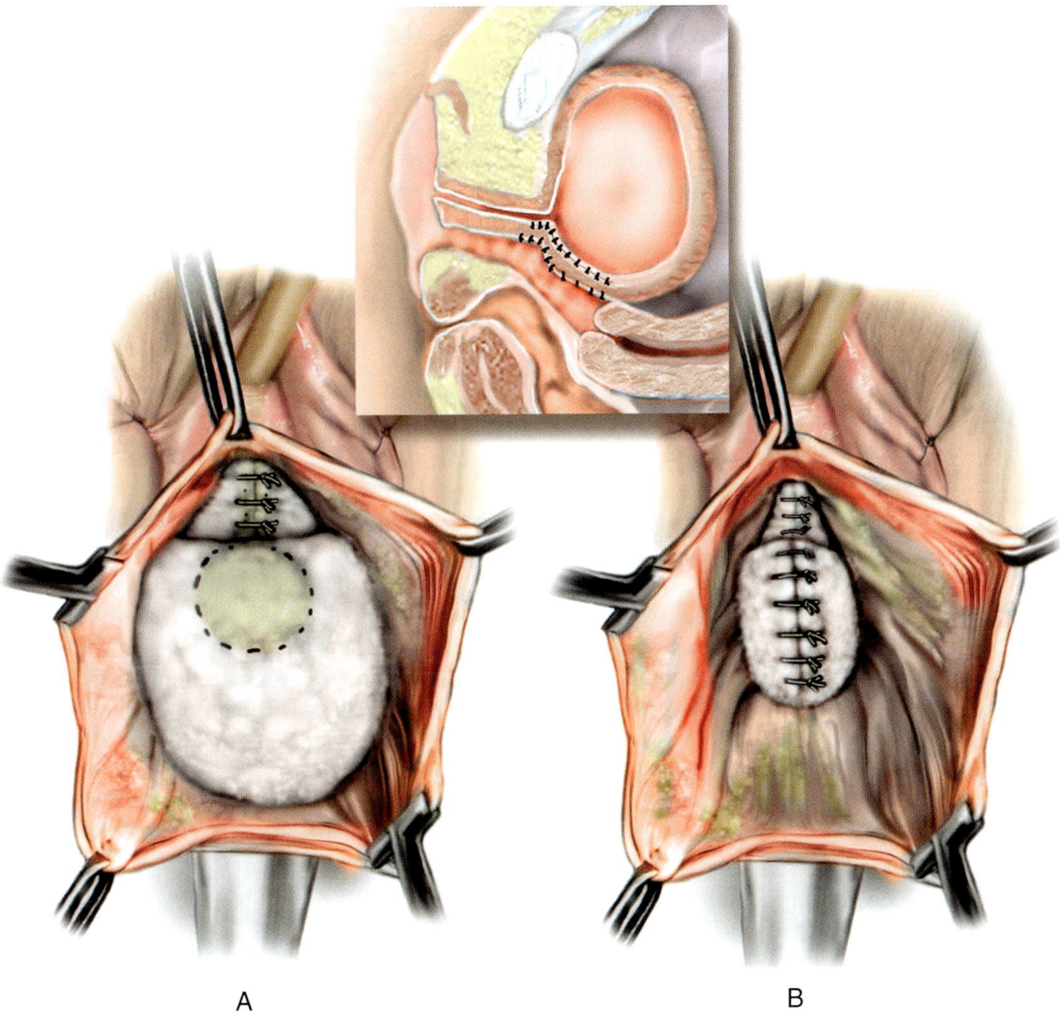

Fig. 19.5 Anterior colporrhaphy with Kelly–Kennedy plication. **A**, The vaginal mucosa is opened, and interrupted sutures are started under the urethra. **B**, The completed colporrhaphy uses midline plication with interrupted sutures. Preferential support is provided to the proximal urethra over that provided to the bladder. (From Maher CF, Karram MM. Surgical management of anterior vaginal wall prolapse. In Karram MM, Maher CF, eds. *Surgical Management of Pelvic Organ Prolapse*. Philadelphia: Saunders, 2013. With permission.)

of mesh placement may justify the risk, such as individuals with recurrent anterior prolapse or with medical comorbidities that preclude more invasive and lengthier open and endoscopic procedures. This Committee Opinion was retracted by both Societies after the FDA's 2019 mandate to stop sale and distribution of transvaginal mesh products. Thus, as of the writing of this chapter, any use of a synthetic or biologic graft or mesh transvaginally to augment anterior vaginal prolapse repair is considered "off-label" use and should be undertaken with caution. Careful and thorough informed consent is required. See Chapter 7 and Chapter 25 for further details of synthetic mesh/grafts and management of their complications.

Before treating anterior vaginal prolapse with graft or mesh, patients should undergo a thorough informed consent process, including discussion of risks, benefits, and both surgical and nonsurgical alternative treatments. There are several situations when mesh use is specifically contraindicated. Many surgeons would not consider the use of mesh in a patient who has had a previous mesh complication. Mesh augmentations should not be used in pregnant women or women who are contemplating future pregnancy, because the mesh does not stretch significantly. In patients who have had pelvic radiation, mesh placement is not recommended, because of the risk of poor wound healing. Similarly, preexisting local or systemic infection is a contraindication for the placement of vaginal mesh, particularly nonabsorbable synthetic mesh. Many surgeons would not recommend the use of nonabsorbable synthetic mesh if colorectal surgery is being performed concurrently. Chronic steroid use, smoking, uncontrolled diabetes mellitus, or other causes of a compromised immune system can impair wound healing, and many would consider these conditions to be relative contraindications to vaginal mesh placement. Pelvic pain syndromes such as endometriosis, vulvodynia, interstitial cystitis, fibromyalgia, and dyspareunia should be evaluated preoperatively to allow for comprehensive counseling regarding the best surgical and nonsurgical form of treatment.

Historically, there have been three general categories of transvaginal mesh or graft placement options for the management of anterior vaginal prolapse: (1) self-tailored mesh, (2) commercially available trocar-guided mesh kits that use a transobturator approach, and (3) commercially available mesh kits that use a transvaginal fixation method rather than a trocar (nontrocar kits). Today, only "off-label" use of self-tailored mesh/graft is available. Regardless of the placement option used, the general surgical approach to treat anterior vaginal wall prolapse is fixation of mesh to the ATFP or the coccygeus muscle/sacrospinous ligament. The initial incision for anterior vaginal mesh placement involves significant hydrodissection and a deeper colpotomy incision than is usually performed for a traditional native-tissue anterior colporrhaphy, so that the perivesical space is entered. The mesh is spread laterally toward the ATFP proximally and distally and, in many of the nontrocar kits, attached apically to the sacrospinous ligament. Despite the lack of evidence that any one placement technique is best in managing a patient's symptoms, most experts would agree on some basic perioperative tenets:

- The bladder should be drained with a transurethral catheter.
- A well-estrogenized vaginal wall is preferred before surgery. (We use intravaginal estrogen cream daily [0.5–1.0 g/day] for 2 to 3 weeks preoperatively.) A vaginal pessary should be removed 1 to 2 weeks before surgery to limit vaginal epithelium irritation.
- All patients require perioperative prophylactic antibiotics and efforts to prevent venous thromboembolic events, as noted earlier.
- Avoid making inverted "T-shaped" incisions from a concurrent hysterectomy and colporrhaphy, if possible.
- Exposure of the correct vesicovaginal space is performed with hydrodissection of 20 to 80 mL of 0.5% lidocaine with 1:200,000 epinephrine, dilute pitressin (20 U in 60–100 mL saline) or normal saline. The correct space for dissection is found using a "loss-of-resistance" technique similar to that used by an anesthesiologist placing an epidural. A wheal or blanching illustrates incorrect intraepithelial placement of the fluid. Hydrodissection in the correct plane will create a fluid bubble in the avascular vesicovaginal space.
- As opposed to an anterior colporrhaphy, in which the vaginal epithelium and muscularis are split for plication, mesh should be placed underneath the vaginal muscularis. It is vital that the surgeon perform a full-thickness dissection deep into the vesicovaginal space to avoid vaginal exposure of the mesh postoperatively. Proper hydrodissection, as described earlier, facilitates the identification of the proper dissection plane.
- It is unknown whether the bladder wall should be plicated in the midline before placing the graft.
- Place the graft loosely, because mesh can contract by up to 20% after placement, compromising vaginal length and caliber. Allow enough room for Mayo scissors to be placed easily between the mesh and the vagina. Also, ensuring that the mesh or graft is placed flat and has minimal tension will improve fibroblast growth and will minimize complications of pain or erosion.
- The vaginal epithelium should not be trimmed. Trimming the vaginal epithelium can lead to discomfort, and possibly contraction. The colpotomy incision is closed using a nonlocking, continuous, absorbable suture.
- Cystourethroscopy with intravenous indigo carmine (or other) dye should be performed routinely after anterior mesh placement to identify potential urethral, bladder, or ureteral injury.
- Vaginal packing is typically recommended.

Below we describe the technique for self-tailored mesh placement and, for historical context, placement of trocar and nontrocar-based mesh kits.

Self-Tailored Mesh Placement

Self-tailored mesh can be customized by the surgeon to match the size and shape of each patient's individual pelvic anatomy. Mesh is cut into a trapezoid multiarm shape for compartment augmentation and is fixed to the sacrospinous ligaments, obturator fascia, ATFP, and/or the distal bladder neck (Fig. 19.6). This type of surgery requires a strong set of vaginal surgical skills, because it involves dissections similar to sacrospinous ligament fixation, iliococcygeus suspension, uterosacral suspension, and vaginal paravaginal defect repair. No studies have compared standard repair techniques using self-tailored mesh with other mesh placement techniques. Concurrent procedures, such as a midurethral sling, should be done through a separate vaginal incision at this time. See Video 19.3.

Trocar-Based Mesh Kits

Trocar-guided devices were used to suspend mesh by passing needles through the transobturator and/or ischiorectal fossa. Trocar-based mesh kits were the first commercially available transvaginal mesh products and included Anterior Prolift (Ethicon, Somerville, NJ), Perigee (American Medical Systems, Minnetonka, MN), Avaulta (CR Bard, Murray Hill, NJ), and Exair (Coloplast, Minneapolis, MN). In general, the technique for placement of these products is similar. First, a weighted speculum, self-retaining retractor, or Deaver retractors are placed in the vagina. Allis clamps are positioned at the urethrovesical junction for traction and 1 cm distal to the vaginal apex. The bladder is palpated between the two Allis clamps. As opposed to an anterior colporrhaphy, in which the vaginal epithelium and muscularis are split for plication, the mesh is placed underneath the muscularis to maintain a thickened vascularized epithelium to minimize mesh exposure or erosion. To enter this potential space, the surgeons inject a dilute vasopressin solution or 0.5% lidocaine with 1:200,000 epinephrine underneath the vaginal muscularis to facilitate dissection and minimize blood loss. A sagittal colpotomy incision is made between the Allis clamps long enough to admit two fingers comfortably. Next, countertraction along the entire incision line is achieved with either serial Allis clamps or a self-retaining retractor. The vaginal epithelium and full-thickness muscularis are dissected away from the bladder defect. Sharp and blunt dissection of the bladder are then performed, while keeping the muscularis and epithelium on the vaginal flaps. As this dissection plane is advanced superiorly, loose areolar tissue is encountered until the ischial spine, the ATFP, and, depending on the kit, the sacrospinous ligaments are exposed.

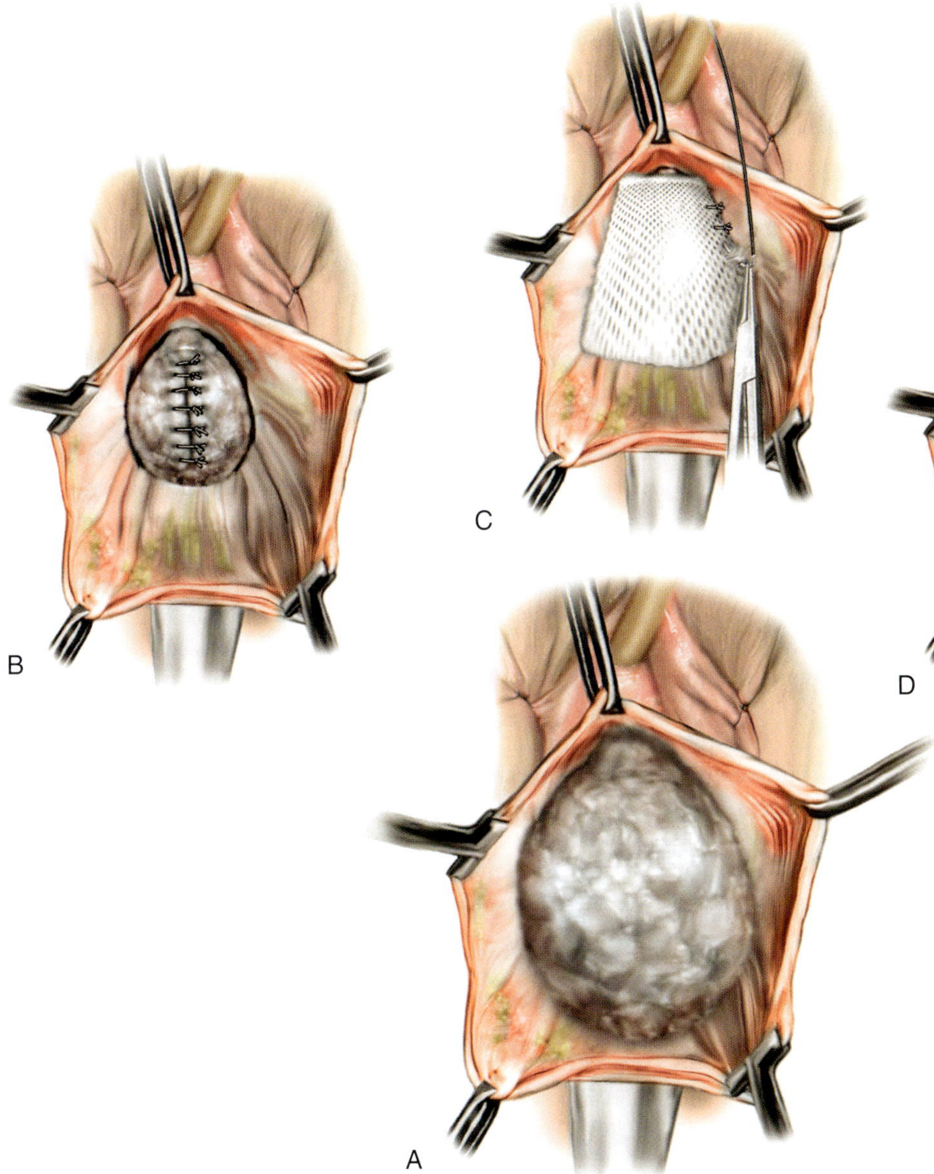

Fig. 19.6 Cystocele repair with mesh. **A**, The bladder is dissected bilaterally and off the vaginal apex. **B**, Midline plication is completed. **C**, After entering the left paravaginal space and exposing the arcus tendineus fasciae pelvis (white line) if desired, the self-styled prosthetic mesh is sewn in place. **D**, The mesh is attached bilaterally, and all sutures are tied, supporting the bladder. (From Maher CF, Karram MM. Surgical management of anterior vaginal wall prolapse. In Karram MM, Maher CF, eds. *Surgical Management of Pelvic Organ Prolapse*. Philadelphia: Saunders, 2013. With permission.)

A number of different trocar types were available, including helical-shaped trocars similar to those for transobturator slings and flexible straight trocars. Cutaneous incisions that are 4 to 7 mm in length are made over the appropriate locations for the obturator foramen trocars. When placing multiple mesh arms through the transobturator space, the superior and inferior puncture sites should be at least 3 cm apart so the mesh can lay flat. Two fingers placed into the vagina can retract the colon, elevate the bladder, and minimize deviation of the trocar tip with direct palpation. For anterior compartment mesh, the surgeon immediately identifies the incoming trocar passing through the ATFP. The prosthesis is loosely placed in a "tension-free" manner, because, as mentioned earlier, mesh can contract by up to 20% after placement, creating tension and compromising vaginal length and caliber. Stay sutures can be used to help the mesh lay flat against the vagina. If the surgeon conserves the uterus, then permanent sutures can be placed into the cervical stroma to stabilize the mesh and prevent enterocele. When adequate hemostasis is obtained, the vaginal epithelium is closed with a continuous nonlocking stitch of delayed absorbable suture. After desired tensioning, all ends of the mesh arms should be trimmed below the surface of the skin, and the incisions closed.

Nontrocar Mesh Kits

The nontrocar or "single-incision" mesh kits avoided the potential complications associated with blind trocar passage through the transobturator space and ischiorectal fossa and allowed mesh fixation via direct visualization. In addition, most nontrocar kits provided apical fixation to the sacrospinous ligaments bilaterally, as well as anterior vaginal support. The technique for the nontrocar kits begins similarly to the technique for trocar-guided kit placement. After the vesicovaginal space is dissected, pertinent fixation points are identified, including the ischial spines, ATFP, and sacrospinous ligaments. For apical fixation, the surgeon palpates the location of interest then identifies the sacrospinous ligament at least one fingerbreadth medial to the ischial spine. The ligament is penetrated using the surgeon's device of choice. The Pinnacle and Uphold kits used the Capio Transvaginal Suture Capturing Device (all from Boston Scientific, Natick, MA) to suture the mesh arms to the sacrospinous ligaments and ATFP. Alternatively, the Elevate system (American Medical Systems, Minnetonka, MN) used self-fixating appendage tips delivered by vaginal trocars to the same site. The ATFP mesh arms provide lateral fixation. The mesh can be passed through the upper-third of the ATFP using the same fixation methods. With the Uphold device, there are no ATFP arms to implant, and a sutured anterior colporrhaphy is often performed before mesh placement. The mesh arms are adjusted slowly and individually to a loose tension, then the mesh is sutured flat. Cystoscopy with intravenous indigo carmine dye is performed to ensure integrity of the bladder and ureters. The colpotomy is closed, and the vagina packed as described earlier.

Paravaginal Defect Repair

The aim of paravaginal defect repair for anterior vaginal prolapse is to reattach the detached lateral vagina to its normal place of attachment at the level of the ATFP. This can be accomplished using a vaginal, open, or laparoscopic retropubic approach. Retropubic paravaginal defect repair is discussed in Chapter 15, along with other retropubic procedures, such as the Burch colposuspension. (See Videos 19.4 and 19.5.)

The preparation for vaginal paravaginal repair begins similar to an anterior colporrhaphy. Marking sutures are placed on the anterior vaginal wall on each side of the urethrovesical junction, identified by the location of the Foley balloon after gentle traction is placed on the catheter. In patients who have had a hysterectomy, marking sutures are also placed at the vaginal apex. If a culdoplasty or apical suspension procedure is being performed, the stitches are placed, but not tied until completion of the paravaginal repair and closure of the anterior vaginal wall. As for anterior colporrhaphy, vaginal flaps are developed by incising the vagina in the midline and dissecting the vaginal muscularis laterally. The dissection is performed bilaterally until a space—the paravaginal space—is developed between the vaginal wall and obturator internus muscle. Blunt dissection using an index finger is used to extend the space anteriorly along the ischiopubic rami, medially to the pubic symphysis, and laterally toward the ischial spine. If the defect is present, and dissection is occurring in the appropriate plane, one should enter the retropubic space easily, visualizing retropubic and paravaginal adipose tissue. The ischial spine can then be palpated on each side. The ATFP coming off the spine can be followed to the back of the symphysis pubis (Fig. 19.7A). After dissection is complete, midline plication of the bladder adventitia is usually performed, either at this point or after placement and tying of the paravaginal sutures.

On the lateral pelvic sidewall, the obturator internus muscle and the ATFP are identified by palpation and then visualization. Retraction of the bladder and urethra medially is best accomplished with a Breisky–Navratil retractor, and posterior retraction could be provided with a lighted right-angle retractor. Using No. 0 nonabsorbable or delayed absorbable sutures, the first stitch is placed around the tissue of the white line just anterior to the ischial spine. A Capio device (Boston Scientific, Natick, MA) works well to facilitate suture placement. If the white line is detached from the pelvic sidewall or clinically not felt to be durable, then the attachment should be to the fascia overlying the obturator internus muscle. The placement of subsequent sutures is aided by placing tension on the first suture. A series of three to six stitches is placed and held, working anteriorly along the white line from the ischial spine to the level of the urethrovesical junction (Fig. 19.7A). Starting with the most anterior stitch, the surgeon picks up the edge of the periurethral tissue (vaginal muscularis or pubocervical fascia) at the level of the urethrovesical junction, and then tissue from the undersurface of the vaginal flap at the previously marked sites. Subsequent stitches move posteriorly until the last stitch closest to the ischial spine is attached to the vagina nearest the apex, again using the previously placed marking sutures for guidance. Stitches in the vaginal wall must be placed carefully to allow adequate tissue for subsequent midline vaginal closure. After all the stitches are placed on one side, the same procedure is carried out on the other side. The stitches are then tied in order from the urethra to the apex, alternating from one side to the other. This repair is a three-point closure involving the vaginal epithelium, vaginal muscularis and endopelvic fascia (pubocervical fascia), and lateral pelvic sidewall at the level of the ATFP (Fig. 19.7B and C). There must be tissue-to-tissue approximation between these structures. Suture bridges must be avoided by careful planning of suture placement. Vaginal tissue should not be trimmed until all the stitches are tied. The vaginal flaps are trimmed and closed with a running subcuticular or interlocking delayed absorbable suture.

Cystoscopy

Cystoscopy to evaluate bladder integrity and ureteral patency is usually performed after cystocele repair, especially if slings or apical suspension procedures are also being performed. Intravenous indigo carmine or fluorescein, preoperative oral pyridium, or transurethral infusion of 5% or 10% dextrose can aid in evaluating for urethral patency. The rate of ureteral obstruction after simple anterior colporrhaphy is only 0.4%, but the rate increases with the addition of some types of apical suspension. Intraoperative release of the offending sutures almost always releases the ureteral obstruction without further sequelae.

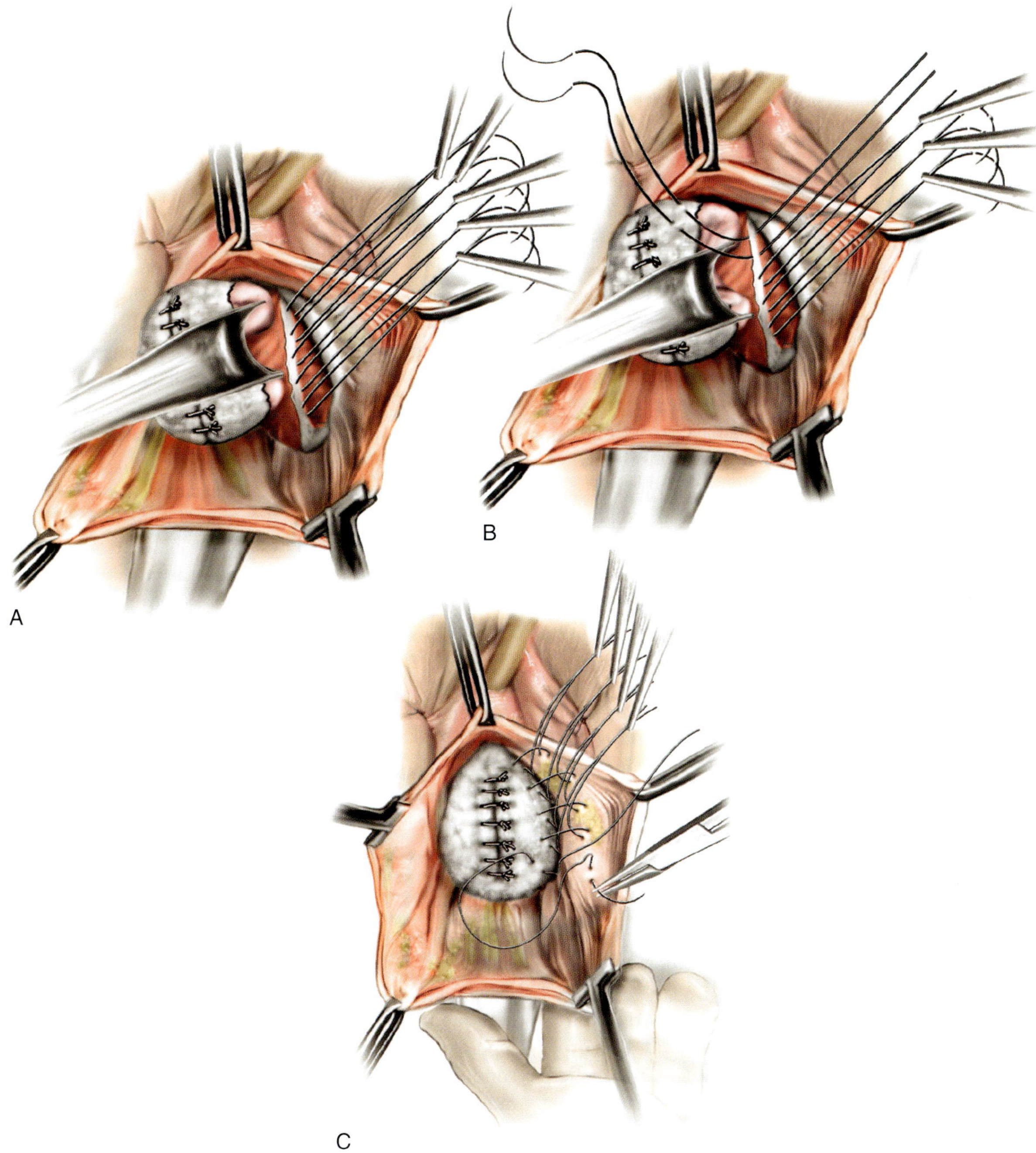

Fig. 19.7 Surgical steps for vaginal paravaginal (three-point) repair. **A**, Numerous sutures are passed through the white line on the fascia over the obturator internus muscle (point 1). **B**, Each suture is passed through the lateral edge of the detached fascia (point 2). **C**, Each suture is passed through the full thickness of the vaginal wall, excluding the epithelium (point 3). (From Maher CF, Karram MM. Surgical management of anterior vaginal wall prolapse. In Karram MM, Maher CF, eds. *Surgical Management of Pelvic Organ Prolapse*. Philadelphia: Saunders, 2013. With permission.)

RESULTS

The main indication for surgical repair of anterior vaginal prolapse is to relieve symptoms when they exist, or as part of a comprehensive pelvic reconstructive procedure for multiple sites of pelvic organ prolapse with or without stress urinary incontinence. Few studies have addressed the long-term success of surgical treatments for anterior vaginal prolapse. Although the majority of studies evaluating anterior vaginal prolapse repairs are uncontrolled series, an increasing number of randomized surgical trials have been conducted in recent years. Success rates vary considerably, depending on the outcome measure used to define success. Historically, most studies evaluating the treatment of pelvic organ prolapse have focused exclusively on anatomic success, without considering other important areas such as symptoms, vaginal compliance, quality of life, or economic outcomes. For an individual patient, the most important outcome of a surgical procedure is the relief of her symptoms and improvement in her quality of life, yet until recently these areas have largely been ignored. Reported anatomic success rates for native-tissue anterior colporrhaphy range from 37% to 100%, with most cohorts reporting success rates greater than 80%. Importantly, the anterior compartment appears to be at the highest risk of surgical failure relative to the apical and posterior compartments.

Weber et al. (2001) studied three variations of anterior colporrhaphy using a prospective, randomized study design and a strict definition of success (Aa and Ba points at –3 or –2 cm; stage 0 or I). Standard anterior colporrhaphy resulted in 30% of patients with an optimal or satisfactory anatomic result, anterior colporrhaphy with polyglactin 910 mesh overlay had a 42% optimal or satisfactory result, and ultralateral plication under tension had a 46% optimal or satisfactory result. No difference was seen in anatomic or functional outcomes, and most patients reported satisfaction with their symptom improvement. The low success rates found in the trial are used as evidence that anterior colporrhaphy should be augmented by synthetic mesh, or that another approach (e.g., sacrocolpopexy) should be used for treatment of anterior vaginal prolapse. More recently, Chmielewski et al. (2011) reanalyzed the data from this trial using more clinically relevant definitions of success and reported considerably better outcomes, with only 10% of subjects developing anatomic recurrence beyond the hymen, 5% of subjects developing symptomatic recurrence, and less than 1% having another surgery for prolapse at 23 months of follow-up. In general, it appears that native-tissue anterior colporrhaphy commonly results in asymptomatic anterior vaginal descent to within 1 cm of the hymen (POPQ stage II); however, prolapse beyond the hymen, development of symptomatic prolapse (e.g., vaginal bulging symptoms), and reoperation for recurrent prolapse are uncommon events in the first 2 to 3 years after surgery.

Long-term results of anterior colporrhaphy are largely unknown, although Gotthart et al. (2012) reported only 13 reoperations for prolapse (2.9%) after 10 years in 456 patients who had vaginal hysterectomy and colporrhaphy. The median interval from the first surgery to the second was 5.5 years. Lavelle et al. (2016) reported outcomes of isolated anterior native tissue repair for women with surgery from a single institution over an 18-year period and defined failure as stage 2 or greater anatomic recurrence or surgery for recurrent prolapse symptoms. Patients with concurrent apical or posterior prolapse surgery were excluded. With a mean follow-up of 5.8 years, they found a 7.4% rate of recurrent isolated anterior compartment prolapse, a 10.7% rate of apical prolapse, an 8.3% rate of posterior prolapse, and a 19% rate of multicompartment prolapse with low morbidity. Overall 33% required a repeat surgery 0.6 to 13 years after their initial surgery.

As previously noted, apical support can correct more than half of anterior wall prolapse. Similarly, higher prolapse recurrence has been demonstrated among women who do not undergo apical repair. A 2013 study of over 2700 women undergoing isolated anterior repair or combined anterior and apical repair found that the 10-year reoperation rates were lower in the combined anterior and apical repair group, at 11.6% versus 20.2% (Eilber et al., 2013).

No randomized trials have been performed to evaluate the efficacy of paravaginal defect repair for the treatment of anterior vaginal prolapse. Single-center uncontrolled case series suggest good anatomic results for both open retropubic (success rate, 75%–97%) and vaginal (success rate, 67%–100%) approaches. However, the vaginal approach appears to be associated with a high risk of hemorrhage, with one series reporting a 21% blood transfusion rate (Young et al., 2001). Few data are available on the efficacy or safety of laparoscopic or robotic paravaginal defect repair. Two studies evaluated the use of absorbable polyglactin 910 mesh to augment anterior colporrhaphy, and reported mixed results. The trial by Weber et al. (2001) described earlier found no benefit, whereas a randomized trial by Sand et al. (2001) found a 75% success rate 1 year after surgery in those receiving absorbable mesh compared with a 57% success in those who underwent native-tissue anterior colporrhaphy.

The PROlapse Surgery: Pragmatic Evaluation and randomised Controlled Trials (PROSPECT) study included two parallel-group pragmatic randomized controlled trials investigating augmentation of transvaginal anterior and posterior prolapse surgery with synthetic nonabsorbable (type 1 monofilament microporous polypropylene) or biologic grafts (porcine acellular collagen matrix, porcine small intestinal submucosa, or bovine dermal) (Glazener et al., 2017). These trials involved 65 surgeons across 35 UK sites. A total of 865 women were included in the mesh trial (430 were randomized to standard repair alone, and 435 to mesh augmentation) and 735 in the graft trial (367 were randomized to standard repair alone, and 368 to graft augmentation), and all were followed for 2 years, making these the largest prolapse trials evaluating mesh/graft augmentation to date. Mesh/grafts were self-tailored ("inserted below the facial layer if possible and secured with peripheral sutures"), and surgeons were allowed to choose any synthetic or biologic graft that was available to them, depending upon the group assignment, consistent with a pragmatic approach. The primary outcomes of the trials were patient-reported prolapse symptoms (via validated questionnaire) and condition-specific quality of life. No difference was found in these outcomes between native-tissue (standard) repair and biologic or synthetic graft augmentation at 1 or 2 years after surgery. Prolapse beyond the hymen was noted in 14% to 18% of patients at 1 year, and, overall, 5% of patients underwent surgery for recurrent prolapse at 2 years, with no differences between groups. There were no differences in non–mesh-related complications between treatment groups; however, those who received synthetic mesh had a cumulative rate of mesh complications of 12% by 2 years, with 9% requiring surgical removal. In the biologic graft arm, only four patients had a mesh complication, and all had received concomitant synthetic mesh (i.e., midurethral sling).

Similar to the results of the PROSPECT study, the currently available evidence does not demonstrate benefit for biologic graft augmentation for anterior prolapse surgery. The Society of Gynecologic Surgeons (SGS) Systematic Review Group identified seven randomized clinical trials and two retrospective cohort studies with a minimum of 1-year follow-up comparing native tissue anterior colporrhaphy with biologic graft augmentation for anterior vaginal wall prolapse (Schimpf et al., 2016). They found that, overall, high-quality evidence suggests no difference in anatomic or quality-of-life outcomes when biologic grafts are used compared with native tissue repair. Two of the seven available trials did find an anatomic benefit over native tissue repair, but no difference in symptoms or quality of life. There was variability in biologic grafts used in these studies, including cadaveric dermis, porcine dermis, bovine pericardium, and porcine small intestinal submucosa. Given the different characteristics of many of the biologic grafts, it seems likely that results may depend on the specific biologic graft used; however, no head-to-head comparisons have been performed. The most common graft used in these studies, Pelvicol (porcine dermis; CR Bard, Murray Hill, NJ), is no longer available in the United States. Less than 1% of patients in these studies required reoperation for graft complication. The 2016 Cochrane review on surgery for women with anterior compartment prolapse concurred with the SGS Systematic Review Group, concluding that biological graft repair or absorbable mesh provides minimal advantage compared with native tissue repair (Maher et al., 2016). Results showed no evidence of differences between biological graft and native tissue repair in rates of awareness of prolapse or repeat surgery for prolapse. However, in contrast to the SGS review, the Cochrane review concluded that the recurrent anterior prolapse rate was higher after native tissue repair than after any biological graft. They attempted to quantify this difference, noting that the data "[suggest] that if awareness of prolapse after biological graft occurs in 12% of women, 7% to 23% would be aware of prolapse after native tissue repair."

The SGS Systematic Review Group identified 20 studies (13 randomized clinical trials and seven cohort studies) comparing outcomes of native tissue anterior colporrhaphy to permanent synthetic mesh (type 1 wide-pore polypropylene) (Schimpf et al., 2016). In approximately half of the studies, the mesh was placed using a trocar-based kit, with the remainder being self-tailored mesh. In these studies, use of mesh consistently resulted in improved anatomic outcomes compared with native tissue repair. This meta-analysis confirmed that mesh repairs also provided superior relief of subjective bulge symptoms. However, there was also high-quality evidence to suggest no difference for other subjective outcomes, including quality of life and urinary and sexual function. Mesh exposure/erosion rates ranged from 1.4% to 19%, with most of these treated in the office. Operative mesh revision rates in the identified studies ranged from 3% to 8% across studies. The 2016 Cochrane review, in a meta-analysis of 16 clinical trials, concluded that permanent mesh resulted in lower rates of awareness of prolapse, recurrent anterior wall prolapse, and repeat surgery for prolapse compared with native tissue repair (Maher et al., 2016). However, native tissue repair was associated with reduced risk of new stress urinary incontinence, reduced bladder injury, fewer blood transfusions, shorter operative time, and reduced rates of any repeat surgery (prolapse, stress urinary incontinence, and mesh exposure combined). The rate of mesh exposure in those receiving permanent mesh was 11.3%, with 7.3% requiring surgery for a mesh complication at 1 to 3 years. Of note, the differences in improved outcomes noted between mesh kits and native tissue repair were not large. For instance, the Cochrane review authors stated "if 19% of women are aware of prolapse after native tissue repair, between 10 and 15% will be aware of prolapse after permanent mesh repair" (Maher et al., 2016). As noted, in the FDA's view these benefits do not outweigh the risks associated with transvaginal mesh implantation.

Risk factors for failure of anterior vaginal prolapse repair have not been specifically studied separate from studies of multicompartment prolapse. Vaginal prolapse in general recurs with increasing age and length of follow-up, but the actual frequency is unknown and tends to vary with different definitions of prolapse. Recurrence of anterior prolapse is more likely to occur with more severe initial prolapse and probably with transvaginal, compared with abdominal, repairs. Recurrence may represent a failure to identify and repair all support defects, or weakening, stretching, or breaking of patients' tissues, as occurs with advancing age and after menopause. Sacrospinous ligament suspension of the vaginal apex, with exaggerated retrosuspension of the vagina, may predispose patients to recurrence of anterior vaginal prolapse. Other characteristics that may increase chances of recurrence are genetic predisposition, subsequent pregnancy, heavy lifting, chronic pulmonary disease, chronic straining at stool, smoking, and obesity.

COMPLICATIONS

Intraoperative complications are uncommon with native-tissue anterior vaginal prolapse repair. Excessive blood loss may occur, requiring blood transfusion, or a hematoma may develop in the anterior vagina; this is probably more common after vaginal paravaginal repair than anterior colporrhaphy. The lumen of the bladder or urethra may be entered in the course of dissection. Accidental cystotomy should be repaired in layers at the time of the injury. After repair of cystotomy, the bladder is generally drained for 7 to 14 days to allow adequate healing. Ureteral damage or obstruction occurs rarely (0%–2%), usually with very large cystoceles or with apical prolapse. Other rare complications include intravesical or urethral suture placement (and associated urologic problems) and fistulae, either urethrovaginal or vesicovaginal.

Complications unique to synthetic mesh use in the vagina include vaginal mesh exposure or extrusion; mesh erosion or perforation into an adjacent organ, including the bladder, urethra, and rectum; and vaginal mesh contraction with associated pain and dyspareunia. Complications that can occur with any pelvic reconstructive surgery but that can be made more severe or complicated by the presence of synthetic mesh include bleeding, infection, fistulas, pelvic pain, sexual dysfunction, and dysfunction of the lower urinary and lower gastrointestinal tracts. Although many of these complications can be managed nonsurgically, a significant proportion require surgical excision of some or all of the mesh. The incidence of these complications varies from 3% to 39%. A systematic review of 110 studies by Abed et al. (2011) found the average rate of graft erosion or exposure to be 10.3% with permanent synthetic grafts, and 10.1% after biologic grafts. Wound granulation was seen in 7.8%. Approximately two-thirds of women with a mesh exposure after permanent synthetic mesh placement require some surgery to correct the exposure; in some cases, multiple procedures are required. In contrast, the rate of mesh exposures with biologic grafts in the SGS Systematic Review Group review was less than 1% (Schimpf et al., 2016). For a more detailed discussion of incidence and management of mesh or graft complications, see Chapter 25.

De novo stress urinary incontinence occurs in 15% to 59% of women after anterior vaginal prolapse repair. This risk is greater in women who demonstrate a positive cough stress test with prolapse reduction before surgery than those who do not. However, performance of an antiincontinence procedure such as a midurethral sling or Burch colposuspension decreases this risk, regardless of whether the preoperative stress test is positive (Brubaker et al., 2006; Wei et al., 2012). Jelovsek et al. (2014) developed and validated a clinical prediction model, available publicly as an online calculator (https://riskcalc.org/FemalePelvicMedicineandReconstructiveSurgery/), to determine a woman's personal risk of developing *de novo* stress urinary incontinence after prolapse surgery, to help guide patients and surgeons about the risks and benefits of performing a concurrent incontinence procedure at the time of prolapse repair. This prediction calculator has been shown to outperform the use of preoperative cough stress testing and predictions by experts. This model was developed using data from the Outcomes Following Vaginal Prolapse Repair and Midurethral Sling (OPUS) trial and externally validated using data from the Colpopexy And Urinary Reduction Efforts (CARE) trial, as well as two other 14-center clinical trials from the Netherlands (Jelovsek et al., 2014; Jelovsek et al., 2019).

Voiding difficulty can occur after anterior vaginal prolapse repair. This problem may occur more often in women with subclinical preoperative voiding dysfunction, especially if suburethral plication is done. Treatment is bladder drainage or intermittent self-catheterization until spontaneous voiding resumes, usually within 6 weeks. Urinary tract infections are common (especially with concurrent catheter use), but other infections such as pelvic or vaginal abscesses are uncommon.

Sexual function may be affected positively or negatively by vaginal operations for anterior vaginal prolapse. Most prospective studies demonstrate that sexual function either does not change or improves in the majority of women after vaginal reconstructive surgery for pelvic organ prolapse; however, worsening sexual function is seen in some patients. As many as 50% of patients with advanced prolapse report dyspareunia before surgery. In general, dyspareunia rates decrease after prolapse surgery; however, *de novo* dyspareunia can be seen in as many as 18%, especially if a posterior colporrhaphy is also performed. Vaginal length and caliber appear to have little relationship with postoperative sexual satisfaction. In a comprehensive study by Kuhn et al. (2009) of male and female sexual function within heterosexual couples after primary repair of vaginal prolapse without the use of mesh, female patients reported improvement in sexual desire, arousal, lubrication, pain, and overall satisfaction, but not orgasm. *De novo* dyspareunia occurred in only two of 70 women. Male partner function improved as well in domains of interest, sexual desire, and overall satisfaction. One prospective comparison of patients undergoing vaginal versus nonvaginal (open or robotic) prolapse repair found that sexual function improved overall after surgery, with no difference between groups. Comparisons of sexual outcomes between native-tissue and mesh-augmented repairs have had mixed results, with some showing worse sexual function after mesh repairs and others showing no difference between the groups. The Cochrane reviewers found no difference in postoperative *de novo* dyspareunia between native-tissue prolapse repair and those augmented with synthetic or biologic grafts (Maher et al., 2016).

BIBLIOGRAPHY

Abed H, Rahn DD, Lowenstein L, et al. Incidence and management of graft erosion, wound granulation, and dyspareunia following vaginal prolapse repair with graft materials: a systematic review. *Int Urogynecol J*. 2011;22:789.

ACOG Practice Bulletin No. 195. Prevention of infection after gynecologic procedures. *Obstet Gynecol*. 2018;131:e172.

ACOG Committee on Gynecologic Practice Committee Opinion No 513. Vaginal placement of synthetic mesh for pelvic organ prolapse. *Obstet Gynecol*. 2011;118:1459.

Altman D, Vayrynen T, Engh ME, et al. Anterior colporrhaphy versus transvaginal mesh for pelvic-organ prolapse. *N Engl J Med*. 2011;364:1826.

Aronson MP, Bates SM, Jacoby AF, et al. Periurethral and paravaginal anatomy: an endovaginal magnetic resonance imaging study. *Am J Obstet Gynecol*. 1995;173:1702.

Barber MD. Symptoms and outcome measures of pelvic organ prolapse. *Clin Obstet Gynecol*. 2005;48:648.

Barber MD, Brubaker L, Nygaard I, et al. Defining success after surgery for pelvic organ prolapse. *Obstet Gynecol*. 2009;114:600.

Barber MD, Cundiff GW, Weidner AC, et al. Accuracy of clinical assessment of paravaginal defects in women with anterior vaginal wall prolapse. *Am J Obstet Gynecol*. 1999;181:87.

Beverly CJ, Walters MD, Weber AM, et al. Prevalence of hydronephrosis in women undergoing surgery for pelvic organ prolapse. *Obstet Gynecol*. 1997;90:37.

Brubaker L, Cundiff GW, Fine P et al. Abdominal sacrocolpopexy with Burch colposuspension to reduce urinary stress incontinence. *N Engl J Med*. 2006;354:1557.

Bump RC, Fantl JA, Hurt WG. The mechanism of urinary continence in women with severe uterovaginal prolapse: results of barrier studies. *Obstet Gynecol*. 1988;72:291.

Bump RC, Mattiasson A, Bo K, et al. The standardization of terminology of female pelvic organ prolapse and pelvic floor dysfunction. *Am J Obstet Gynecol*. 1996;175:10.

Carey M, Higgs P, Goh J, et al. Vaginal repair with mesh versus colporrhaphy for prolapse: a randomized controlled trial. *BJOG*. 2009;116:1380.

Chen CH, Wu WY, Sheu BC, et al. Comparison of recurrence rates after anterior colporrhaphy for cystocele using three different surgical techniques. *Gynecol Obstet Invest*. 2007;63:214.

Chen L, Ashton-Miller JA, DeLancey JOL. A 3D finite element model of anterior vaginal wall support to evaluate mechanisms underlying cystocele formation. *J Biomech*. 2009;42:1371.

Chmielewski L, Walters MD, Weber AM, Barber MD. Reanalysis of a randomized trial of 3 techniques of anterior colporrhaphy using clinically relevant definitions of success. *Am J Obstet Gynecol*. 2011;205:69.

Clarke-Pearson DL, Abaid LN. Prevention of venous thromboembolic events after gynecologic surgery. *Obstet Gynecol*. 2012;119:155.

Colombo M, Vitobello D, Proietti F, Milani R. Randomised comparison of Burch colposuspension versus anterior colporrhaphy in women with stress urinary incontinence and anterior vaginal wall prolapse. *BJOG*. 2000;107:544.

DeLancey JO. Fascial and muscular abnormalities in women with urethral hypermobility and anterior vaginal wall prolapse. *Am J Obstet Gynecol*. 2002;187:93.

DeLancey JOL. Anatomic aspects of vaginal eversion after hysterectomy. *Am J Obstet Gynecol*. 1992;166:1717.

Eilber KS, Alperin M, Khan A, et al. Outcomes of vaginal prolapse surgery among female Medicare beneficiaries: the role of apical support. *Obstet Gynecol*. 2013;122:981.

Feldner Jr PC, Castro RA, Cipolotti LA, et al. Anterior vaginal wall prolapse: a randomized controlled trial of SIS graft versus traditional colporrhaphy. *Int Urogynecol*. 2010;J 21:1057.

Gandhi S, Goldberg RP, Kwon C, et al. A prospective randomized trial using solvent dehydrated fascia lata for the prevention of recurrent anterior vaginal wall prolapse. *Am J Obstet Gynecol*. 2005;192:1649.

Ganj FA, Okechukwu AI, Bedestani A, et al. Complications of transvaginal monofilament polypropylene mesh in pelvic organ prolapse repair. *Int Urogynecol J*. 2009;20:919.

Glazener C, Breeman S, Elders A, et al. Mesh, graft or standard repair for women having primary transvaginal anterior or posterior compartment prolapse surgery: two parallel-group, multicenter, randomized, controlled trials (PROSPECT). *Lancet*. 2017;389:381.

Goldberg RP, Koduri S, Lobel RW, et al. Protective effect of suburethral slings on postoperative cystocele recurrence after reconstructive pelvic operation. *Am J Obstet Gynecol*. 2001;185:1307.

Gotthart PT, Aigmueller T, Lang PF, et al. Reoperation for pelvic organ prolapse within 10 years of primary surgery for prolapse. *Int Urogynecol J*. 2012;23:1221.

Gustilo-Ashby AM, Jelovsek JE, Barber MD, et al. The incidence of ureteral obstruction and the value of intraoperative cystoscopy during vaginal surgery for pelvic organ prolapse. *Am J Obstet Gynecol*. 2006;194:1478.

Haase P, Skibsted L. Influence of operations for stress incontinence and/or genital descensus on sexual life. *Acta Obstet Gynecol Scand*. 1988;67:659.

Hsu Y, Chen L, Summers A, et al. Anterior vaginal wall length and degree of anterior compartment prolapse seen on dynamic MRI. *Int Urogynecol J*. 2008;19:137.

Hviid U, Hviid TV, Rudnicki M. Porcine skin collagen implants for anterior vaginal wall prolapse: a randomised prospective controlled study. *Int Urogynecol J*. 2010;21:529.

Jelovsek JE, Chagin K, Brubaker L, et al. A model for predicting the risk of de novo stress urinary incontinence in women undergoing pelvic organ prolapse surgery. *Obstet Gynecol*. 2014;123:279.

Jelovsek JE, van der Ploeg JM, Roovers JM, Barber MD. Validation of a model predicting de novo stress urinary incontinence in women undergoing pelvic organ prolapse surgery. *Obstet Gynecol*. 2019;133:683.

Jia X, Glazener C, Mowatt G, et al. Efficacy and safety of using mesh or grafts in surgery for anterior and/or posterior vaginal wall prolapse: systematic review and meta-analysis. *BJOG*. 2008;115:1350.

Kapoor DS, Nemcova M, Pantazis K, et al. Reoperation rate for traditional anterior vaginal repair: analysis of 207 cases with a median 4-year follow-up. *Int Urogynecol J*. 2010;21:27.

Karp DR, Peterson TV, Mahdy A, et al. Biologic grafts for cystocele repair: does concomitant midline fascial plication improve surgical outcomes? *Int Urogynecol J*. 2011;22:985.

Karram MM. Vaginal operations for prolapse. In: Baggish MS, Karram MM, eds. *Atlas of Pelvic Anatomy and Gynecologic Surgery*. Philadelphia: Saunders; 2001.

Kobak WH, Walters MD, Piedmonte MR. Determinants of voiding after three types of incontinence surgery. *Obstet Gynecol*. 2001;97:86.

Kuhn A, Brunnmayr G, Stadimayr W, et al. Male and female sexual function after surgical repair of female organ prolapse. *J Sex Med*. 2009;6:1324.

Kwon CH, Goldberg RP, Koduri S, et al. The use of intraoperative cystoscopy in major vaginal and urogynecologic surgeries. *Am J Obstet Gynecol*. 2002;187:1466.

Lang P, Whiteside JL. Anterior compartment prolapse: what's new? *Curr Opin Obstet Gynecol*. 2017;29:337.

Lavelle RS, Christie AL, Alhalabi F, et al. Risk of prolapse recurrence after native tissue anterior vaginal suspension procedure with intermediate to long-term follow-up. *J Urol*. 2016;195:1014.

Macer GA. Transabdominal repair of cystocele, a 20-year experience, compared with the traditional vaginal approach. *Am J Obstet Gynecol*. 1978;131:203.

Maher C. Anterior vaginal compartment surgery. *Int Urogynecol J*. 2013;24:1791.

Maher C, Baessler K, Barber M, et al. Surgery for pelvic organ prolapse. In: Abrams P, Brubaker L, Cardozo C, Wein A, eds. *5th International Consultation on Incontinence*. Paris: Health Publications, Ltd.; 2013.

Maher C, Feiner B, Baessler K, Schmid C. Surgical management of pelvic organ prolapse in women. *Cochrane Database Syst Rev*. 2013;4:CD004014.

Maher C, Feiner B, Baessler K, et al. Surgery for women with anterior compartment prolapse. *Cochrane Database Syst Rev*. 2016;11:CD004014.

Maher CF, Karram MM. Surgical management of anterior vaginal wall prolapse. In Karram MM, Maher CF, eds. *Surgical Management of Pelvic Organ Prolapse*. Philadelphia, Saunders, 2013.

Mallipeddi PK, Steele AC, Hohli N, et al. Anatomic and functional outcome of vaginal paravaginal repair in the correction of anterior vaginal prolapse. *Int Urogynecol J*. 2001;12:83.

Medina CA, Candiotti K, Takacs P. Wide genital hiatus risk factor for recurrence following anterior vaginal repair. *Int J Gynaecol Obstet*. 2008;101:184.

Menefee SA, Dyer KY, Lukacz ES, et al. Colporrhaphy compared with mesh or graft-reinforced vaginal paravaginal repair for anterior vaginal wall prolapse: a randomized controlled trial. *Obstet Gynecol*. 2011;118:1337.

Meschia M, Pifarotti P, Bernasconi F, et al. Porcine skin collagen implants to prevent anterior vaginal wall prolapse recurrence: a multicenter, randomized study. *J Urol*. 2007;177:192.

Meschia M, Pifarotti P, Spennacchio M, et al. A randomized comparison of tension-free vaginal tape and endopelvic fascia plication in women with genital prolapse and occult stress urinary incontinence. *Am J Obstet Gynecol*. 2004;190:609.

Morse AN, O'dell KK, Howard AE, Baker SP, Aronson MP, Young SB. Midline anterior repair alone vs anterior repair plus vaginal paravaginal repair: a comparison of anatomic and quality of life outcomes. *Int Urogynecol J Pelvic Floor Dysfunct*. 2007;18:245.

Muffly TM, Barber MD. Insertion and removal of vaginal mesh for pelvic organ prolapse. *Clin Obstet Gynecol*. 2010;53:99.

Natale F, La Penna C, Padoa A, et al. A prospective, randomized, controlled study comparing Gynemesh, a synthetic mesh, and Pelvicol, a biologic graft, in the surgical treatment of recurrent cystocele. *Int Urogynecol J Pelvic Floor Dysfunct*. 2009;20:75.

Nguyen JN, Burchette RJ. Outcome after anterior vaginal prolapse repair: a randomized controlled trial. *Obstet Gynecol.* 2008;111:891.

Nichols DH, Randall CL. *Vaginal Surgery.* 4th ed. Baltimore: Williams and Wilkins; 1996.

Nieminen K, Hiltunen R, Takala T, et al. Outcomes after anterior vaginal wall repair with mesh: a randomized, controlled trial with a 3 year follow-up. *Am J Obstet Gynecol.* 2010;203:235.

Nüssler EK, Greisen S, Kesmodel US, et al. Operation for recurrent cystocele with anterior colporrhaphy or non-absorbable mesh: patient reported outcomes. *Int Urogynecol J.* 2013;24:1925.

Richardson AC, Lyon JB, Williams NL. A new look at pelvic relaxation. *Am J Obstet Gynecol.* 1976;126:568.

Ridgeway B, Walters MD, Paraiso MF, et al. Early experience with mesh excision for adverse outcomes after transvaginal mesh placement using prolapse kits. *Am J Obstet Gynecol.* 2008;199:703.

Sand PK, Koduri S, Lobel RW, et al. Prospective randomized trial of polyglactin 910 mesh to prevent recurrence of cystoceles and rectoceles. *Am J Obstet Gynecol.* 2001;184:1357.

Schimpf MO, Abed H, Sanses T, et al. Graft and mesh use in transvaginal prolapse repair: a systematic review. *Obstet Gynecol.* 2016;128:81.

Shull BL, Benn SJ, Kuehl TJ. Surgical management of prolapse of the anterior vaginal segment: an analysis of support defects, operative morbidity, and anatomic outcome. *Am J Obstet Gynecol.* 1994;171:1429.

Siddiqui NY, Fulton RG, Kuchibhatla M, Wu JM. Sexual function after vaginal versus nonvaginal prolapse surgery. *Fem Pelvic Med Reconstruct Surg.* 2012;18:238.

Sivaslioglu AA, Unlubilgin E, Dolen I. A randomized comparison of polypropylene mesh surgery with site-specific surgery in the treatment of cystocoele. *Int Urogynecol J Pelvic Floor Dysfunct.* 2008;19:467.

Summers A, Winkel LA, Hussain HK, DeLancey JOL. The relationship between anterior and apical compartment support. *Am J Obstet Gynecol.* 2006;194:1438.

Tulikangas PK, Lukban JC, Walters MD. Anterior enterocele: a report of three cases. *Int Urogynecol J.* 2004;15:350.

Vollebregt A, Fischer K, Gietelink D, van der Vaart CH. Primary surgical repair of anterior vaginal prolapse: a randomised trial comparing anatomical and functional outcome between anterior colporrhaphy and trocar-guided transobturator anterior mesh. *BJOG.* 2011;118:1518.

Weber AM, Walters MD, Piedmonte MA, et al. Anterior colporrhaphy: a randomized trial of three surgical techniques. *Am J Obstet Gynecol.* 2001;185:1299.

Weber AM, Walters MD. Anterior vaginal prolapse: review of anatomy and techniques of surgical repair. *Obstet Gynecol.* 1997;89:311.

Wei JT, Nygaard I, Richter HE, et al. A midurethral sling to reduce incontinence after vaginal prolapse repair. *N Engl J Med.* 2012;366:2358.

White GR. A radical cure by suturing lateral sulci of vagina to white line of pelvic fascia. *JAMA.* 1909;21:1707.

White GR. An anatomical operation for the cure of cystocele. *Am J Obstet Dis Women Child.* 1912;65:286.

Whiteside JL, Barber MD, Paraiso MF, et al. Clinical evaluation of anterior vaginal wall support defect: interexaminer and intraexaminer reliability. *Am J Obstet Gynecol.* 2004;191:100.

Whiteside JL, Weber AM, Meyn LA, et al. Risk factors for prolapse recurrence after vaginal repair. *Am J Obstet Gynecol.* 2004;191:1533.

Young SB, Daman JJ, Bony LG. Vaginal paravaginal repair: one-year outcomes. *Am J Obstet Gynecol.* 2001;185:1360.

20

Surgical Treatment of Posterior Vaginal Wall Prolapse

Mark D. Walters and Tristi W. Muir

CHAPTER OUTLINE

One-third to one-half of all surgeries for pelvic organ prolapse involve the posterior vaginal wall. Although rectocele repair has been commonly performed for over a century, the long-term functional and anatomic outcomes and ideal surgical technique have not been determined. This chapter will review the anatomy, pathophysiology, evaluation techniques, and surgical management of posterior vaginal wall prolapse and perineal body defects.

ANATOMY AND PATHOPHYSIOLOGY

The histology of the apical portion of the posterior vaginal wall consists of mucosa (which includes the epithelium of the posterior wall and the lamina propria), a superficial and deep muscularis layer, and adventitia. This fibromuscular layer has been named rectovaginal fascia and perirectal fascia, perhaps giving the surgeon an illusion of more sturdy tissue than is actually present. Comparisons of the histology of women with and without vaginal prolapse have shown that the smooth muscle content of the posterior vaginal wall of women with prolapse is disorganized and significantly reduced in comparison to women without prolapse.

Prolapse of the posterior vaginal wall may be secondary to the presence of an enterocele, sigmoidocele, rectocele, or a combination of these entities. A rectocele is an anterior protrusion of the rectal wall to the posterior vaginal wall. The rectovaginal space exists between the vaginal tube and the rectum. This potential space, occupied by areolar tissue, allows the vagina and rectum to function independent of each other. Support of the posterior vaginal wall is provided by a complex interaction of the integrity of the vaginal tube, the connective tissue support, and muscular support of the pelvic floor. DeLancey (1996) divided the connective tissue support of the vagina into three levels. All three levels of support should be evaluated and addressed during surgical management of the posterior vaginal wall.

At level I, the apical portion of the posterior vaginal wall is suspended and supported primarily by the cardinal–uterosacral ligaments. This mesentery-like endopelvic fascia originates at the sacrum and the pelvic sidewalls and inserts onto the posterior cervix and upper vagina. With normal support, the apical posterior wall of the vagina is dorsally directed to lie upon the rectum in a horizontal fashion overlying the levator ani muscles. With increases in abdominal pressure, the vaginal tube is closed top to bottom and supported by the pelvic floor muscles.

Level II includes the support for the middle half of the vagina. This support is provided by the endopelvic fascia attaching the lateral posterior vaginal wall to the aponeurosis of the levator ani on the pelvic sidewall. Most of the fibers of the endopelvic fascia connect the lateral edge of the vaginal tube to the pelvic sidewall. Very few of the fibers actually run like a sheet from sidewall to sidewall. The sidewall attachment of the apical half of the posterior vaginal wall is convergent with the anterior vaginal wall at the arcus tendineus fasciae pelvis (ATFP), giving the vagina a flat profile. The distal sidewall attachment of the posterior vaginal wall, the arcus tendineus fasciae rectovaginalis (ATFR), deviates dorsally from the anterior vaginal wall, giving the vagina an "H" appearance at the introitus (Fig. 20.1).

The role of the perineal body is to resist forces directed caudally by the rectum and to provide a physical barrier between the vagina and rectum. The perineal body is thicker (approximately 3 cm in length) and more defined in women than in men. It includes interlacing muscle fibers of the bulbospongiosus, transverse perinei, and external anal sphincter. Larson et al. (2010)

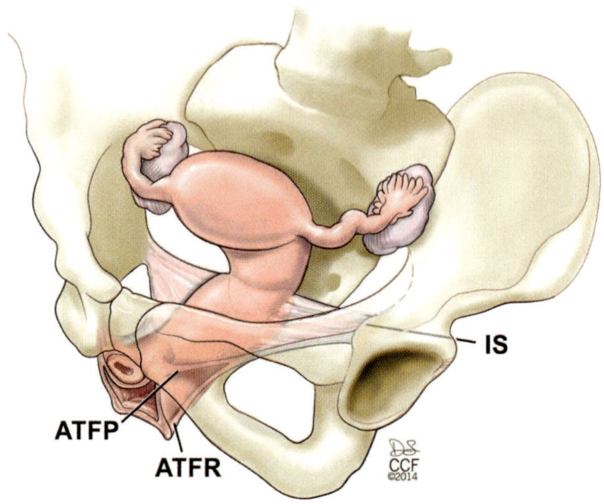

Fig. 20.1 Level II support of the posterior vaginal wall includes attachment to the pelvic sidewall from the arcus tendineus fasciae rectovaginalis (*ATFR*) in the distal half of the vagina, and from the arcus tendineus fasciae pelvis (*ATFP*) proximally, which is attached to the ischial spine (*IS*) near the apex.

reconstructed the perineal body into three distinct regions (superficial, mid, and deep) with three-dimensional analysis of thin-slice magnetic resonance imaging (MRI). The superficial region of the perineal body is at the level of the vestibular bulb. The bulbospongiosus muscle inserts into the lateral margins of the perineal body, whereas caudally the transverse perinei muscle and external anal sphincter comprise the bulk of the superficial component. The perineal body extends cranially in the posterior wall of the vagina to approximately 2 to 3 cm proximal to the hymenal ring. The puborectalis loops around the rectum and lateral vagina but does not send fibers to the perineal body. Laterally, the perineal body is attached to the ischiopubic rami through the superficial transverse perinei muscles and the perineal membrane. The perineal membrane spans the anterior half of the pelvic outlet and is comprised of dense fibromuscular tissue. This dense, fused level of support represents level III. Interruption in the support of the perineal body allows the posterior vaginal wall, the perineal body, and the distal portion of the anterior rectal wall to descend with increased rectal pressure (allowing for perineal body hypermobility).

The pelvic floor muscles, of which the levator ani are a major contributor, provide substantial support of the pelvic organs. In a woman with an intact pelvic floor, the puborectalis and remaining levator ani muscles maintain constant tone. This contraction closes the vaginal canal, and the anterior and posterior vaginal walls are in direct apposition. With defecation, the increased pressure placed on the posterior vaginal wall is equilibrated by the opposing anterior vaginal wall, and there is minimal stress placed on the endopelvic fascial attachments (Fig. 20.2A). The puborectalis also provides a sling of support for the vaginal tube. This sling leads to an angulation of the midposterior wall of approximately 45 degrees from vertical. The proximal portion of the vagina lies upon (and is supported by) the pubococcygeus and iliococcygeus muscles. The puborectalis helps to close the potential space of the vagina and close the levator hiatus. With a healthy pelvic floor, little stress or strain is placed on the connective tissue support system.

The levator hiatus has been shown to be larger in women with prolapse than in women with normal pelvic support. If there is muscular and/or neurologic damage to the puborectalis, the levator hiatus widens, and the vaginal canal opens. The increased rectal pressure and distension associated with defecation place strain on the endopelvic fascial attachments and the fibromuscularis of the posterior vaginal wall and can result in rectocele and perineal descent (Fig. 20.2B and C).

A description and understanding of normal anatomy guides us in identifying areas of loss of support and challenges us to return the vagina to its "normal position" during prolapse surgery. However, static anatomy does not give us insight into the complexities of the pathophysiology of posterior vaginal wall prolapse. Luo et al. (2012) compared MR images at rest and maximal Valsalva between women with predominant rectocele and those without prolapse (controls). As the women with posterior vaginal wall prolapse strained, all 10 experienced descent of the apical two-thirds of posterior vaginal wall, resulting in a folding—"kneeling fashion"—that obstructed the rectum in the process. A proportion (but not all) of the women with a rectocele also had widening of the genital hiatus and descent of the distal posterior wall and perineal body. Therefore, identifying and repairing apical posterior wall support is critical to restoring normal anatomy.

A dynamic and complex interplay of the bony pelvis and connective tissue support with the tonically and actively contracted pelvic floor muscles allow the vagina to maintain its anatomic position. Disruption of support leading to herniation of the vagina and surrounding organs (pelvic organ prolapse) can impact urinary, defecatory, and sexual function. Prolapse is most likely attributed to an accumulation of injuries. Risk factors for the development of prolapse may begin at conception and continue to accrue until death. Table 20.1 shows various risk factors for development of posterior vaginal wall prolapse. Lince et al. (2012) performed a meta-analysis of the family history of prolapse and concluded that there is strong evidence that women with at least one family member with pelvic organ prolapse have a significantly higher risk of developing prolapse than those without a family history of prolapse. In families with many members affected by pelvic organ prolapse, chromosomal linkage analysis has identified an area on the long arm of chromosome 9 (9q21) that is associated with the development of prolapse. This area of chromosome 9 houses genes involved with the development of connective tissue and muscle in the pelvic floor. It is apparent that abnormalities of connective tissue development (e.g., Ehlers–Danlos syndrome and Marfan syndrome) are related to early development of pelvic organ prolapse. Women with less pronounced connective tissue disorders often have hyperextensible skin and joints. Women with joint hypermobility are more likely to have defecatory evacuation disorders and develop a rectocele.

Vaginal delivery, particularly in the occiput-posterior position, is associated with an increased risk for posterior vaginal wall and perineal body trauma and is one of the greatest risk

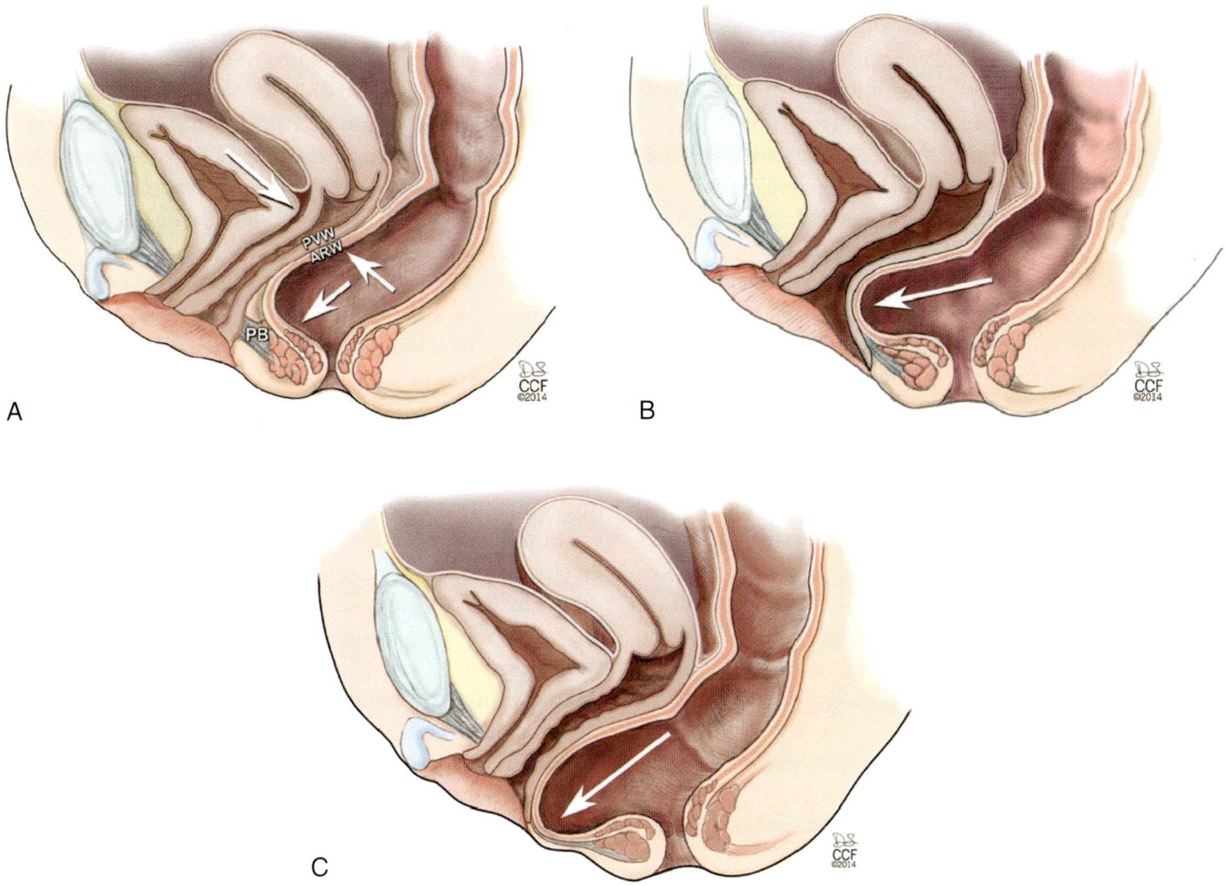

Fig. 20.2 Pathophysiology of rectocele. **A**, Normal posterior wall support provided by the levator ani muscles holds the vagina closed. When abdominal pressure is increased, pressure on the posterior vaginal wall is equilibrated by pressure on the anterior vaginal wall. Stress on the connective tissue supports is avoided. Distally, the pressure in the rectum is resisted by the perineal body. **B**, When the levator ani no longer holds the vagina closed, the anterior wall pressure no longer balances the posterior wall pressure. The pressure in the rectum is not counterbalanced by atmospheric pressure in the open vagina and stress is placed on the connective tissue support. As this gives way (or in the presence of a connective tissue defect), a rectocele may develop. **C**, Increased abdominal pressure distally on a damaged perineal body may result in severe rectocele and perineal descent. *ARW*, Anterior rectal wall; *PB*, perineal body; *PVW*, posterior vaginal wall.

factors for pelvic organ prolapse development. The greatest risk is caused by the first vaginal delivery, with subsequent deliveries likely increasing the risk. MR images in the postpartum period show changes in intensity within the levator ani muscle. These changes likely reflect the recovery process following neurologic or muscular damage related to childbirth. Additionally, aging may impact the levator ani muscles, leading to muscle atrophy and devascularization. Vaginal delivery, age, and size of the genital hiatus (>2 cm often associated with levator injury) have been associated with the development and progression of prolapse in parous women.

Table 20.1 Risk Factors for the Development of Posterior Vaginal Wall Prolapse

Inheritable	Trauma	Promotional
Genetic	Vaginal delivery	Aging
	Pelvic surgery	Defecatory dysfunction/chronic straining
	Hysterectomy	Obesity
		Hormonal
		Smoking
		Chronic disease

Chronic strain and constipation are often found in women with rectocele, perineal descent, and fecal incontinence. It is suggested that, with chronic straining, there is a stretch placed on the pudendal nerve and the nerve to the levator ani muscle; this stretch is amplified in the setting of rectocele and perineal body descent. Meschia et al. (2002) found that fecal incontinence was more prevalent in women with a rectocele that extended beyond the hymen (31%) than in women with less severe prolapse (19%). Increasing body mass index has been strongly associated with incident rectocele, but not with prolapse of other areas of the vagina (anterior or apical vaginal wall).

Pelvic surgery can predispose a woman to develop prolapse. Alterations of the connective tissue support and injury to the innervation and vascularization to the pelvic floor muscles can occur with pelvic surgery. However, the indication for the pelvic surgery contributes to the risk of subsequent prolapse surgery. In a large case–control study, Dällenbach et al. (2007) found that the primary risk factor for development of prolapse after hysterectomy was the degree of prolapse before the hysterectomy. The risk of subsequent prolapse repair in a woman with prolapse to the hymen at the time of hysterectomy was eight times that in women without prolapse, regardless of the route of surgery. The performance of a hysterectomy outside of the setting of prolapse also is a risk for prolapse development. Shalom et al. (2012) retrospectively evaluated women who presented with primary prolapse. When matched for age and parity, women who underwent a prior hysterectomy were more likely to present with stage 2 or greater posterior vaginal wall prolapse as compared with women without prior hysterectomy (46.5% vs. 25.3%, respectively; $P = .01$). Additionally, surgical procedures in the pelvis may alter the axis of the vagina, increasing the forces placed on the connective tissue supports. Overelevation of the anterior vaginal wall, as with anterior vaginal mesh or retropubic urethropexy, alters the distribution of force on the vaginal walls and can open the posterior wall to the development of an enterocele and/or rectocele.

EVALUATION

History

Many women with a rectocele or a perineal body defect are asymptomatic or unaware of the loss of support. However, most women electing to undergo surgical management of a rectocele report a sense of bulging and/or symptoms relating to sexual, defecatory, or urinary function.

Women with prolapse often describe bulging of the vagina and pressure (particularly if the prolapse extends beyond the hymen), which worsens by the end of the day and improves when lying down. Sexual function is multifaceted in women. Sexual dysfunction may occur in the setting of prolapse through discomfort, loss of sensation, alteration in body image, or incontinence. Vulvovaginal atrophy from lack of estrogen can exacerbate this problem. Women with a perineal body defect, which leads to a widened genital hiatus, may describe loss of sensation for her and her partner during intercourse. If stool is trapped in the rectocele, intercourse may lead to fecal incontinence or instill the fear of fecal incontinence, leading to the avoidance of sex.

Defecatory dysfunction is common in women with a symptomatic rectocele. Women with a large rectocele may trap stool within this rectal pocket, leading to feeling of incomplete emptying, which can result in soiling. Splinting, or placing manual pressure in the vagina or rectum or on the perineum to reduce the prolapse and facilitate emptying of the rectum, is commonly described. Sung et al. (2012) prospectively evaluated 160 women undergoing rectocele repair; 87% had bowel symptoms preoperatively. The most common symptom was incomplete evacuation (85%), followed by straining (74%), sensation of obstructed defecation (66%), anal incontinence (63%), and manual splinting (56%). In most studies splinting is the symptom most reliably associated with posterior vaginal prolapse. Defecatory dysfunction of various types is common in women with and without posterior wall prolapse and may be resolved by increasing fiber and water in a woman's diet. It also may be impacted by a multitude of medical factors and medication use (see Table 20.2).

Infrequent defecation, diarrhea, and irritable bowel are not likely related to a rectocele and may require additional evaluation. Further, appropriate screening for colorectal cancer should be followed. Anal incontinence to some degree is commonly seen in patients with posterior wall and perineal body defects. Many women are reluctant to initiate the conversation about anal incontinence, because of embarrassment, so it is crucial to ask about accidental loss of solid or liquid stool.

An important part of the history to obtain from your patient is an understanding of what her management desires are. If the patient requires and is willing to undergo surgical management, having her verbally express her expectations of surgery can be illuminating.

Physical Examination

The patient is typically examined in the dorsal lithotomy or semirecumbent position. There is excellent correlation in the evaluation of prolapse between the supine and standing positions in women performing maximal Valsalva maneuver. If the prolapse observed in the lithotomy position does not recreate the degree of prolapse that the patient described, a standing examination should be performed. However, it is physically more difficult to perform measurements of the prolapse in this position.

To stage the severity of prolapse, the posterior vaginal wall is visualized with the posterior blade of a bivalve speculum or a Sims speculum. The retractor elevates the anterior wall and

Table 20.2 Medical Factors Impacting Defecatory Function

Systemic Illness	Mechanical Bowel Obstruction	Medications (Common Culprits)	Psychiatric Conditions
Diabetes mellitus	Hirschsprung disease	Aluminum antacids	Abuse (psychologic, physical, and sexual)
Metabolic disorders	Malignancy	Anticholinergics	Eating disorders
Thyroid disorders	Inflammatory bowel disease	Antidepressants	Pelvic pain
Neuromuscular disorders	Rectal intussusception	Antiinflammatory medications	
Autonomic neuropathy	Pelvic organ prolapse	β blockers	
		Calcium channel blockers	
		Iron sulfate	
		Opiates	

reduces any uterine or apical prolapse. The patient is asked to increase abdominal pressure with a Valsalva maneuver or cough. The Pelvic Organ Prolapse Quantification (POPQ) system is a standardized, validated tool for measuring and staging pelvic organ prolapse and is described in detail in Chapter 8. Measurements of the posterior vaginal wall are documented at maximal strain, 3 cm proximal to the hymen (Ap), at the most dependent portion of the posterior vaginal wall proximal to this mark (Bp), and at the vaginal cuff (C) or cul-de-sac, if the uterus is present (D). The genital hiatus (gh) and perineal body (pb) are measured with the patient straining. Evaluation for and staging of concurrent anterior wall and apical prolapse should be performed.

A rectovaginal examination can facilitate evaluation of the support and descent of the perineal body, as well as evaluate the protrusion of the anterior rectum into the posterior vaginal wall. Palpation of loops of small bowel or sigmoid colon in the rectovaginal space with straining confirms an enterocele or sigmoidocele, respectively. Performing a rectovaginal examination in the standing position may increase the detection of an enterocele by allowing the bowel to enter the rectovaginal space. Pressure on the posterior wall of the vagina, directed downward toward the rectum, may facilitate identification of rectal prolapse or intussusception. If you suspect rectal prolapse, allowing a woman to Valsalva in privacy with a handheld mirror to guide her may allow you to see what she is describing.

The perineal body should be evaluated for length (POPQ measurement of pb), strength (including anal sphincter), and descent. It may be difficult to measure perineal descent, but documentation of its presence or absence can be helpful in planning your surgery. Descent of the perineal body occurs with a lack of continuity of the suspensory support at the apex (level I) to the perineal body (level III). It may occur also because of a mass effect of the rectum or small bowel herniating into the perineal body, a perineocele. Perineal descent has been associated with fecal incontinence, possibly related to concurrent damage to the integrity of or stretch and damage to the innervation of the anal sphincter.

Because anal incontinence commonly coexists with rectocele, assessment of the anal sphincter should be performed. This includes evaluation of anal tone, squeeze, and symmetry. If a symptomatic woman is found (or suspected) to have a disrupted anal sphincter on examination, further testing is indicated (see Chapter 27).

A focused neurologic examination includes evaluation of sensation, motor function, and reflexes of sacral nerves 2 to 4. The patient is asked to discriminate between sharp and dull on the perineum. Pelvic floor muscle strength can be assessed by asking the patient to contract and relax the pelvic floor muscles around the examiner's fingers. Reflex testing includes the bulbocavernosus reflex and anal wink.

Diagnostic Tests

A woman with defecatory dysfunction and rectocele may benefit from further testing. Defecography provides a two-dimensional view of the efficiency of rectal emptying and quantification of rectal parameters. Evaluation includes rest, squeeze, strain, and evacuation. Contrast in the small and large bowel may also reveal the presence of an enterocele, sigmoidocele, or perineocele. Rectocele, enterocele, and rectal intussusception can be graded based on anatomic evaluation obtained with defecography (Table 20.3). Rectal intussusception, perineal descent, and spastic pelvic floor (pelvic floor dyssynergia) may be apparent during strain. The dynamic nature of the study allows for insight into the defecation process. Retention of more than 10% of the barium following defecation is referred to as barium trapping. It should be recognized that this examination is done in an artificial environment, which may make the patient more prone to incomplete emptying.

Defecation occurs through the coordination of relaxation of the levator ani and external anal sphincter and contraction of the colon. If the puborectalis and/or external anal sphincter is paradoxically contracted during defecation, defecatory dysfunction with straining and incomplete emptying may result. A balloon expulsion test and manometry can indirectly measure the function of the pelvic floor muscles. A woman with a normally functioning pelvic floor should easily be able to expel a 60-mL balloon. Failure to expel the balloon suggests a functional abnormality. Physical therapy with biofeedback can promote coordinated defecation. Resolution of paroxysmal contraction of the pelvic floor muscles before any surgery is imperative to address the woman's symptoms and to decrease the strain that would be placed on the surgically repaired posterior vaginal wall.

Rectoceles that retain contrast tend to be larger than those that do not. However, fluoroscopic evidence of barium trapping does not relate to patient symptoms. In a symptomatic elderly population, Savoye-Collet et al. (2003) found no association between the abnormalities demonstrated by defecography and symptoms. Defecography performed following surgical management of posterior wall prolapse generally has shown reduction in the size of the rectocele and improvement in emptying. The limitations of defecography include the requirement for special equipment, radiation exposure of the patient, inability to show the rectum and adjacent soft tissue structures simultaneously, and that it is uncomfortable and poorly accepted by patients.

Dynamic MRI provides high-quality images of the pelvic soft tissues and viscera (see Chapter 13). It is noninvasive and does not require ionizing radiation or significant patient preparation. However, there is poor correlation between MR grading of prolapse and clinical staging. Because of limited availability of open MR imaging facilities, most facilities perform dynamic MR imaging in the dorsal supine position with a woman's legs together. Images are obtained at rest, while performing a Valsalva maneuver, and with evacuation. However, during a Valsalva maneuver in this position, the true extent of the prolapse may not be exhibited

Table 20.3 Grading of Posterior Wall Prolapse by Defecography

	Grade 1	Grade 2	Grade 3
Rectocele	<2 cm	2–4 cm	>4 cm
Enterocele	Proximal third of vagina	Middle third of vagina	Distal third of vagina
Intussusception	Above puborectalis	At puborectalis	In anal canal

and may not simulate that woman's ability to defecate. The limitations of this method of imaging include a lack of standardization of grading of prolapse, high cost, and limited availability of open MRI.

Translabial, perineal, and three-dimensional endoanal ultrasound have been used to evaluate the pelvic organs at rest, with contraction, and with Valsalva (see Chapter 13). Ultrasound compares favorably to defecography in identification of rectocele, enterocele, paroxysmal contraction of puborectalis, and rectal intussusception. An endoanal ultrasound provides anatomic detail of the integrity of the external and internal anal sphincters. The advantages of a dynamic ultrasound evaluation of the pelvic floor are avoidance of ionizing radiation, decreased expense, real-time visualization of dynamic maneuvers, and avoidance of asking a woman to defecate in public.

At this time there is a lack of a standardized method of establishing a radiologic diagnosis of a rectocele. Clinical examination has good sensitivity for the detection of a rectocele; therefore radiologic confirmation of the presence or absence of a rectocele is not worthwhile. Although defecatory dysfunction is common in women with prolapse, the extent of the prolapse does not necessarily correlate with the extent of bowel symptoms. If the woman's primary complaint is defecatory dysfunction or fecal incontinence, rather than a bulge and/or splinting, surgical correction of a rectocele or perineal body defect may not correct her symptoms. Sung et al. (2012) evaluated bowel symptoms before and 12 months after rectocele repair and found that, although defecatory dysfunction improved in all categories (incomplete evacuation, straining, sensation of obstructed defecation, anal incontinence, and manual splinting), nearly one-half of women continued to have some defecatory complaint after surgery.

Thus, ancillary testing is pursued based on the woman's complaints. Validated functional and quality-of-life questionnaires are available and may be administered preoperatively and postoperatively to provide a standardized method of evaluating the surgical outcomes. The patient's preoperative symptoms and surgical goals will guide the provider in selecting additional testing. A woman who describes lifelong infrequent bowel movements (less than one per week) and an absence of a daily urge to defecate is unlikely to be cured of her constipation with a rectocele repair. A colon transit study may be helpful in identifying patients with slow-transit constipation. Dietary modifications including fiber and laxatives should be encouraged in any woman whose main complaint is constipation (see Chapter 28).

Urodynamic testing with prolapse reduction may be useful in women with stage III or stage IV posterior wall prolapse. With retraction of the posterior wall prolapse (simulating correction of the prolapse), women may "develop" stress incontinence or have an increase in leak volumes. If occult stress urinary incontinence is uncovered, then this observation should be factored into preoperative surgical recommendations and planning.

SURGICAL REPAIR TECHNIQUES

The decision to undergo surgical repair of pelvic organ prolapse is influenced by the stage and degree of bother from the prolapse, satisfaction with nonsurgical options, and various surgeon- and patient-specific factors. The social context in which a patient lives can greatly impact her decision to pursue surgery. Typically, severity of prolapse symptoms, medical comorbidities, and socioeconomic status play a role in the physician's and patient's treatment plan. The decision to perform an isolated posterior repair versus a concurrent posterior repair at the time of other prolapse surgery is influenced by all of the aforementioned factors, but also has some nuances that are important to consider. First, is the patient bothered primarily by bulge symptoms, or does she also have outlet defecation symptoms that need to be addressed? Second, it is important to assess whether or not she is sexually active, and consideration needs to be given to approaching the repair in such a way that sexual functioning will not be affected. The risks and benefits of performing the procedure must be carefully weighed, and the decision to proceed should be shared between the patient and her surgeon.

Current repair techniques address connective tissue defects. A dysfunctional levator ani, which usually widens the levator hiatus, increases the stress and strain on the connective tissues. This is likely a key contributor to the development of pelvic organ prolapse in general. Currently, pelvic floor muscle exercises (with or without biofeedback) are our primary method of strengthening the remaining innervated pelvic floor muscles, but this approach does not address denervated or damaged muscle.

The goals of rectocele repair are to provide anatomic correction, relieve prolapse symptoms, and restore normal bowel and sexual function without creating new symptoms. Understanding the patient's goals for surgical correction and providing realistic expectations of outcomes are essential components of preoperative management and counseling. Evaluation of prolapsed posterior vaginal wall in the office and then in the operating room should include careful inspection for an enterocele or sigmoidocele and for associated apical support defects.

It is difficult to compare various techniques for repair of posterior vaginal wall prolapse and anterior rectal wall prolapse, because the indications for surgery, exact surgical steps, and standardized definitions of bowel function symptoms usually are incompletely reported. The definitions of anatomic or functional cure also vary from study to study. There are few appropriately powered, prospective randomized studies comparing surgical procedures to correct posterior wall prolapse.

The gynecologist typically approaches repair of a rectocele through a transvaginal incision. The patient is placed in the dorsal lithotomy position with her legs in high leg holders. The colorectal surgeon usually performs an endoanal repair of the rectocele with the patient in the prone position. Patients are given appropriate perioperative prophylactic antibiotics and antiembolic prophylaxis. Mechanical bowel preparation is optional.

Posterior Colporrhaphy

The posterior colporrhaphy is a plication of the vaginal wall muscularis (or so-called rectovaginal fascia) in the midline, decreasing the width of the posterior vaginal wall and increasing the fibromuscularis in the midline. Traditionally, a perineorrhaphy is included in this repair, purposely narrowing the vaginal tube and levator hiatus. Estimation of adequate vaginal caliber is not standardized. It will vary depending upon physician training and experience, the patient's current and future desire for sexual activity, and partner factors (e.g., men with erectile dysfunction may have a difficult time penetrating a smaller-caliber vagina).

To begin the procedure (shown in Video 20.1), subepithelial injection of saline or local anesthetic with dilute epinephrine may be done to aid dissection. A midline or triangular-shaped incision is made into the perineal skin, with the base of the triangle at the hymen (Fig. 20.3A). The skin is dissected away from the perineal body. The vaginal epithelium is opened in the midline extending the incision toward the vaginal apex (Fig. 20.3B). The posterior vaginal epithelium is dissected bilaterally away from the underlying fibromuscularis and extended to the pelvic sidewall (Fig. 20.3C). It is important to remain in a plane close to the epithelium to avoid injury to the rectum. The fibromuscularis of the posterior vaginal wall, stripped of its epithelium, is plicated in the midline with interrupted vertically or transversely placed lateral sutures. Plication begins proximally and progresses toward the hymenal ring (Fig. 20.4). Care should be taken to ensure that each plication suture is in continuity with the previous one. If continuity is not maintained, ridging of the posterior vaginal wall may occur and be a source of dyspareunia. The vaginal epithelium is trimmed if necessary and closed with a running absorbable suture. Care should be taken to avoid trimming too much vaginal epithelium, particularly in women with atrophy. The caliber of the vagina at the conclusion of the vaginal reconstruction should be approximately three fingerbreadths in sexually active women.

The posterior colporrhaphy can include plication of the levator ani muscles. Interrupted sutures are placed in the muscular sidewall of the posterior wall and brought to the midline. This provides a sturdy posterior shelf but may further constrict the vaginal caliber and be a source of postoperative pain and/or dyspareunia. However, this may be considered for elderly women with a wide levator hiatus who do not expect to be sexually active, and it is especially useful in combination with a colpocleisis procedure.

Site-Specific Defect Repair

The site-specific defect repair relies upon the theory that herniation of the rectum into the vagina is the result of identifiable defects in the fibromuscularis (rectovaginal fascia). Defects may occur as an isolated defect in the lateral, distal, midline, or superior portions of the posterior vaginal wall, or as a combination of defects (Fig. 20.5). (See Video 20.2.)

The vaginal epithelium is opened with a transverse incision at the posterior fourchette (Fig. 20.6A). The posterior vaginal epithelium is incised in the midline to a level proximal to the bulge and dissected away from the underlying fibromuscularis (Fig. 20.6B). The dissection is extended laterally to the endopelvic fascial attachment of the posterior vaginal wall to the ATFP and ATFR. The fibromuscularis is carefully inspected to identify breaks. Irrigation and a rectal examination may accentuate the defects to aid identification (Fig. 20.7). Defects are individually isolated and repaired with delayed-absorbable or nonabsorbable suture (Fig. 20.8A–G). If a distal defect is present, such as a separation of the fibromuscularis from the perineal body, repair with absorbable suture is done. Repair of perineal body defects is also addressed with interrupted sutures. A levator plication is not performed. Repeating the rectal examination should confirm repair of the rectocele. Plication of the reattached fibromuscularis may be performed if a rectocele persists, or to further correct a widened genital hiatus.

Inspection of apical support is a critical part of correcting posterior wall support. Reattaching the apical posterior wall to the apex or performing an additional apical support procedure, such as a sacrospinous colpopexy, may improve anatomic and functional outcomes and reduce the chance of recurrence. The vaginal epithelium is closed with a running absorbable suture.

Graft Augmentation

Based on current understanding, approximately one-third of women who have had surgery for pelvic organ prolapse and/or urinary incontinence will undergo a subsequent procedure for recurrence. Graft augmentation procedures attempted to capitalize on the durability and efficacy of the abdominal sacrocolpopexy while maintaining the advantages of a vaginal approach. Placement of transvaginal graft augmentation, particularly in the form of a tension-free vaginal mesh kits, was becoming more common in the United States until 2011, when the US Food and Drug Administration (FDA) published an update on serious complications associated with transvaginal mesh placement for pelvic organ prolapse. The notification stated that, compared with nonmesh repairs, there was no evidence that mesh placement added benefit. Additionally, transvaginal mesh placement was associated with more risks, including mesh erosion and the development of *de novo* pelvic pain. In 2019, all commercially available transvaginal mesh augmentation kits for surgical management of pelvic organ prolapse (synthetic and biologic) were removed from the US market by the FDA because of lack of assurance of safety and efficacy.

The rectovaginal septum can be reinforced with mesh through an abdominal, vaginal, or perineal body incision (or combination of these approaches). Of note, as of the writing of this chapter, any use of a synthetic or biologic graft or mesh transvaginally to augment prolapse repair is "off-label" use and requires careful and thorough informed consent. With biologic graft augmentation, the graft may be placed through a vaginal incision as another layer of support upon completion of the rectocele repair or serve as a scaffolding for ingrowth of a woman's own connective tissue (Fig. 20.9 and Video 20.3). The graft is attached to the pelvic sidewall (levator fascia) bilaterally. If the patient is concurrently undergoing an apical suspension procedure (with or without mesh), the apical portion of the graft can be attached to the apical support sutures. Delayed-absorbable or permanent sutures are used. The graft is trimmed, and the distal portion of the graft is attached to the perineal body with interrupted, absorbable suture. The vaginal epithelium is closed, and a perineorrhaphy is performed if needed.

Tension-free placement of vaginal mesh requires a plane of dissection that is deeper than that used for traditional native tissue repairs. The rectovaginal space is injected with a dilute vasoconstrictive agent or normal saline. The plane of dissection is under the vaginal wall, rather than splitting the thickness of

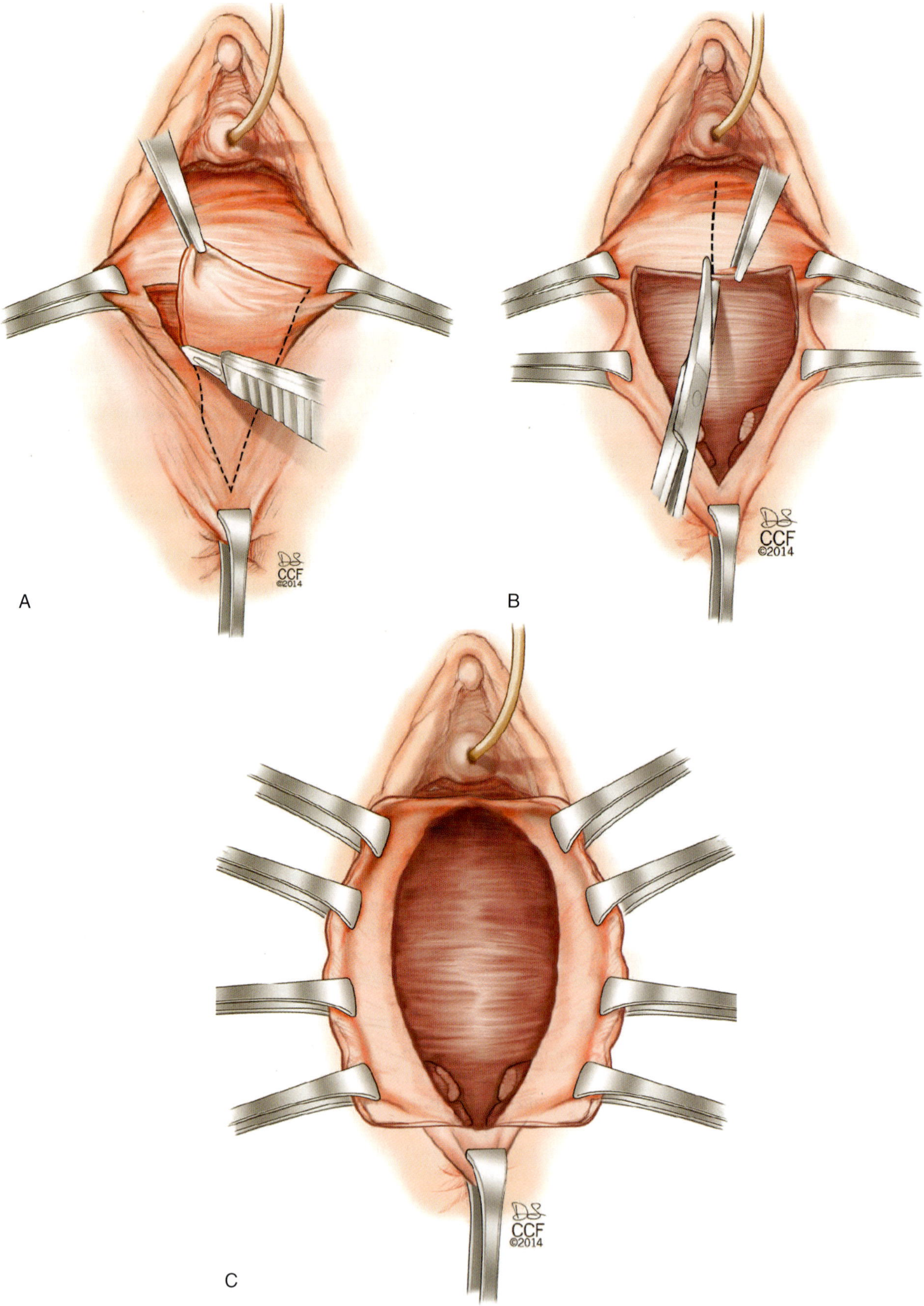

Fig. 20.3 Surgical repair of rectocele. **A**, A triangular incision is made in the epithelium of the overlying posterior fourchette and perineal body. **B**, The vaginal epithelium is opened in the midline. **C**, Dissection of the posterior vaginal wall is completed bilaterally exposing the fibromuscularis from sidewall to sidewall.

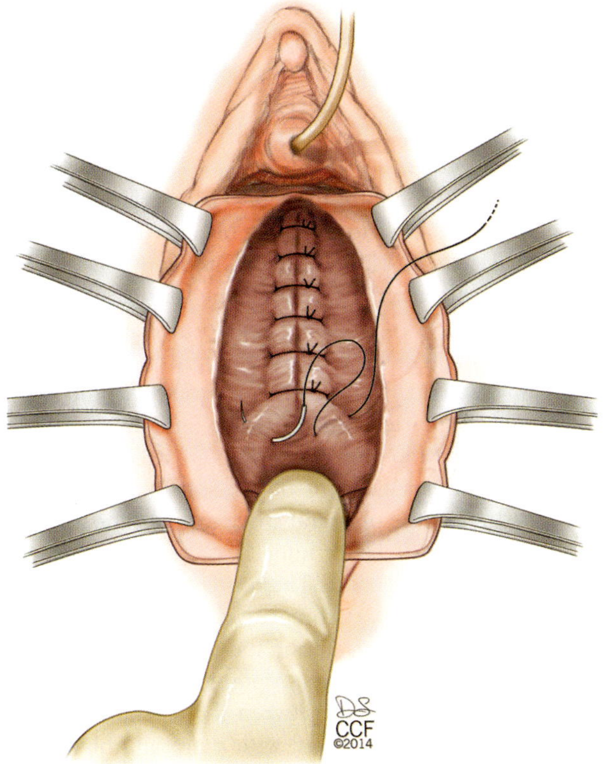

Fig. 20.4 Posterior colporrhaphy includes midline plication of the vaginal fibromuscularis over the rectum.

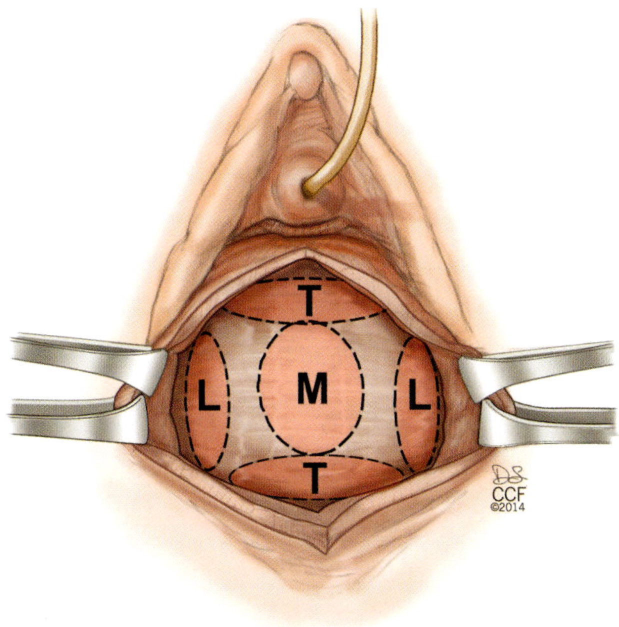

Fig. 20.5 Locations of site-specific defects in the posterior vaginal wall. Defects in the posterior wall fibromuscularis may be found in the lateral sidewalls (*L*), midline (*M*), or in a transverse orientation (*T*) at the apex or distally near the perineal body. Combinations of defects may be identified.

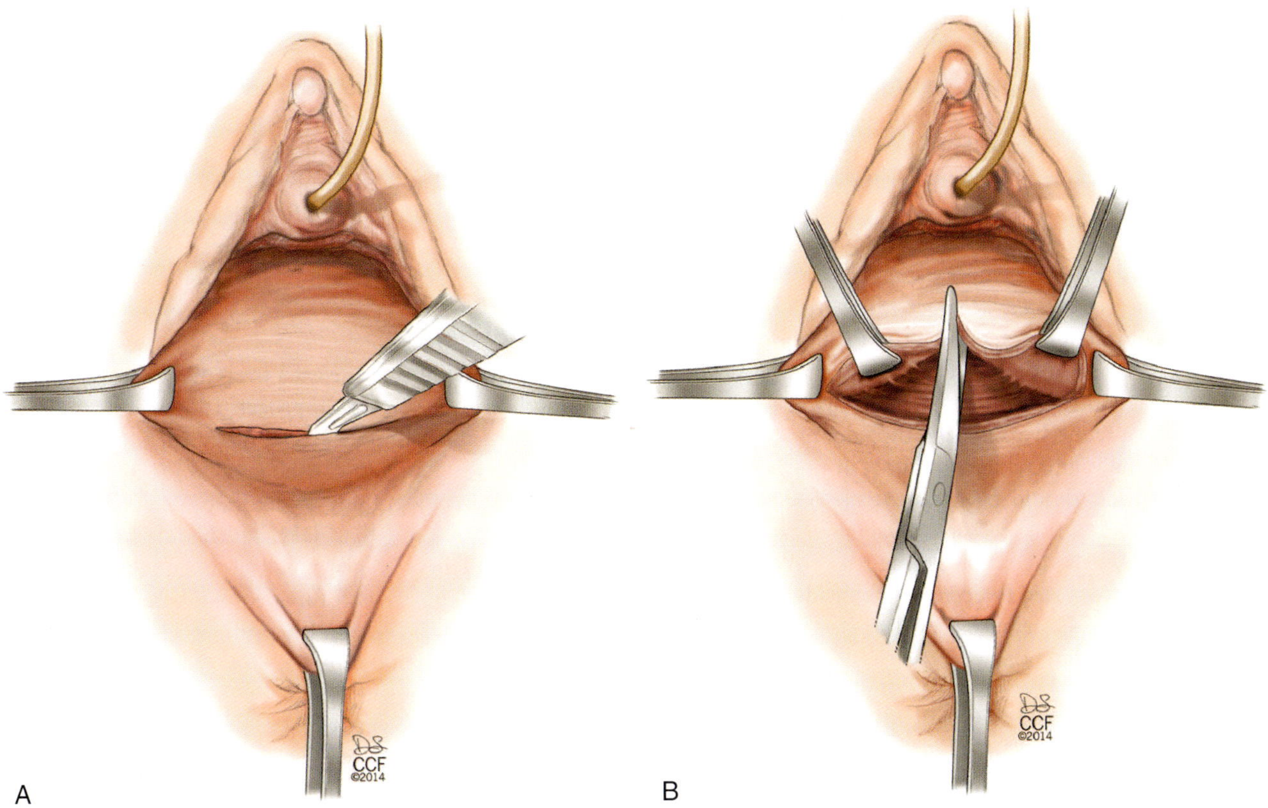

Fig. 20.6 Opening the posterior vaginal epithelium for a site-specific defect repair. **A**, A transverse incision at the level of the hymen can be done if there is not a perineal body defect. **B**, The epithelium is opened in the midline. The dissection is extended proximal to the defect.

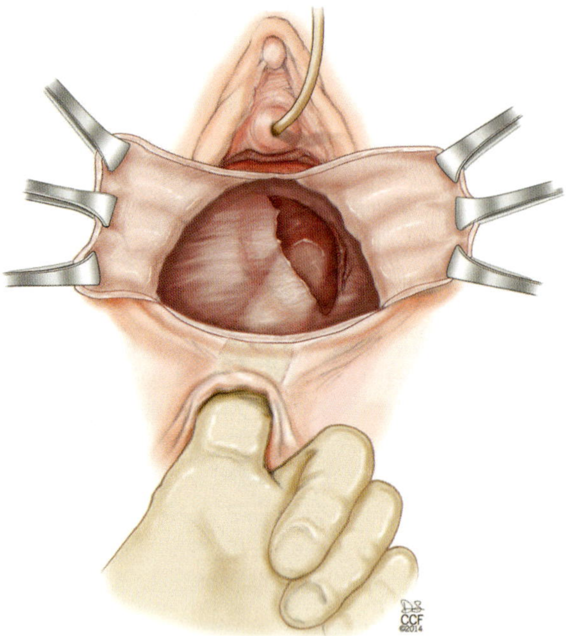

Fig. 20.7 A finger is placed in the rectum to elevate the anterior rectal wall toward the posterior vaginal wall. Areas of weakness or defects in the fibromuscularis can be identified, as shown here on the left.

the vaginal wall as in a colporrhaphy or site-specific repair. An incision is made through the entire vaginal wall, most commonly in a vertical fashion. Sharp and blunt dissection are performed from the perineal body to the ischial spines and sacrospinous ligaments (the apical anchoring points for most vaginal mesh procedures). Various methods are employed to bilaterally suspend the mesh without tension to the sacrospinous ligaments. The mesh is additionally attached with absorbable sutures to the vaginal apex or cervix near the internal os and to the perineal body. Tacking sutures to the vaginal sidewall may be performed in an attempt to prevent the mesh from bunching up. During mesh placement, the surgeon must be cognizant that contraction of the mesh (up to 20%) may occur. If mesh tension results, complications such as mesh exposure, vaginal pain that worsens with movement, focal tenderness (particularly over the mesh arms), and dyspareunia may result.

Trimming of the vaginal skin is minimal or not performed. A rectal examination should be done to rule out a palpable rectal injury or suture in the rectum. A vaginal pack is placed. Pre- and postsurgical treatment of the vaginal epithelium with topical estrogen is advocated to decrease the incidence of mesh erosion. Cessation of pessary use 2 weeks before surgery may decrease vaginal inflammation.

Abdominal Sacrocolpopexy (Colpoperineopexy)

An abdominal, laparoscopic, or robotic approach to rectocele repair can be performed when the rectocele is accompanied by apical prolapse (see also Chapter 21). Suspension of the posterior vaginal wall is accomplished through a sacrocolpopexy, or through a sacral colpoperineopexy in the case that the posterior support defect continues to the level of the perineal body. Mesh is placed on the posterior vaginal wall posterior to the vaginal tube and bridged to the anterior longitudinal ligament of the sacrum. A variety of meshes have been used in sacral colpopexy procedures, but most evidence supports the use of lightweight large-pore polypropylene.

To perform the procedure, the patient is placed in low leg holders with a Foley catheter to drain the bladder. The procedure is accomplished laparoscopically, with or without robotic assistance, or through a Pfannenstiel incision into the peritoneal cavity.

The surgical steps are the same if performed laparoscopically or through an open incision. The right ureter is identified. The peritoneum is opened from the sacral promontory to the cul-de-sac lateral to the right side of the colon and medial to the right ureter. Sharp and blunt dissection are used to expose the anterior longitudinal ligament of the sacrum over S1 to S2. Hydrodissection of the presacral space may also be performed by placing a suction-irrigator underneath the peritoneum and inserting water into the space. The rectovaginal space is identified with an end-to-end anastomosis sizer in the vagina (elevating the vagina toward the anterior abdominal wall) and one in the rectum (deflecting the rectum posteriorly). The rectovaginal space is entered sharply between the vagina and rectum. This avascular space is dissected with sharp and blunt dissection. The dissection proceeds to the perineal body for correction of a distal rectocele or significant perineal descent. Cautery is used sparingly in this dissection to preserve vascularization of the vagina (and potentially decrease the risk of mesh erosion). Laparoscopically, the posterior mesh (~3 × 15 cm in length) is introduced into the abdomen through a lower quadrant port. The mesh is attached to the posterior vaginal wall with a series of three to five pairs of delayed absorbable sutures. The posterior mesh is then laid over the sacrum to determine the length of the mesh bridge. The mesh should provide support of the posterior vaginal wall without tension. The mesh is then attached to the anterior longitudinal ligament with two to three nonabsorbable sutures or surgical tacks. The excess mesh is trimmed, and the peritoneum is closed with absorbable suture.

Endorectal Repair

Colorectal surgeons often select a transanal approach to correct a rectocele. An endorectal approach allows for simultaneous correction of other anorectal pathology such as hemorrhoids and mucosal rectal prolapse. Ayabaca et al. (2002) reported that 53% of women undergoing a rectocele repair also had rectal mucosa prolapse, and that 41% had hemorrhoids. However, repair of a proximal (high) rectocele is difficult with the endorectal approach because of inadequate exposure.

This procedure is done in the prone jackknife position with the buttocks spread and taped. An anal retractor is inserted to expose the anterior rectal wall. A transverse incision is made in the rectal mucosa at or proximal to the dentate line. Two vertical incisions are made in parallel. A flap is developed including a portion of the muscular wall of the rectum to a level proximal to the rectocele (usually approximately 7 cm in length). Vertical plication sutures are placed with No. 3-0 polyglycolic acid suture. One or two transverse sutures are placed to buttress the vertically plicated area. Levator ani plication also can be done with the endorectal approach, but care must be taken to avoid constricting the vagina. The rectal mucosal flap is trimmed, and the rectal mucosa is closed with a running No. 5-0 polyglycolic acid suture. The use of the circular stapler for closure of the rectocele and treatment of the redundant rectal mucosa also has been described.

Perineorrhaphy

A perineorrhaphy, when indicated, completes the vaginal approach to a rectocele repair. Allis clamps are placed on the posterior hymen and brought together in the midline. Preservation of an appropriate vaginal caliber is important for comfortable future coital activity. A midline or triangular incision is made medial to the Allis clamps, extending to the midline of the perineal skin with the base of the triangle at the posterior hymen. The bulbospongiosus muscles are plicated in the midline of the perineal body with an interrupted absorbable suture. To provide continuity with the posterior repair (and avoid a step down in support to the posterior repair), the bulbospongiosus plication suture should incorporate the distal rectocele repair. The transverse perinei muscles are plicated (Fig. 20.10). An anal sphincteroplasty may be performed as indicated for fecal incontinence and an external/internal anal sphincter defect. The skin is closed with a running absorbable suture.

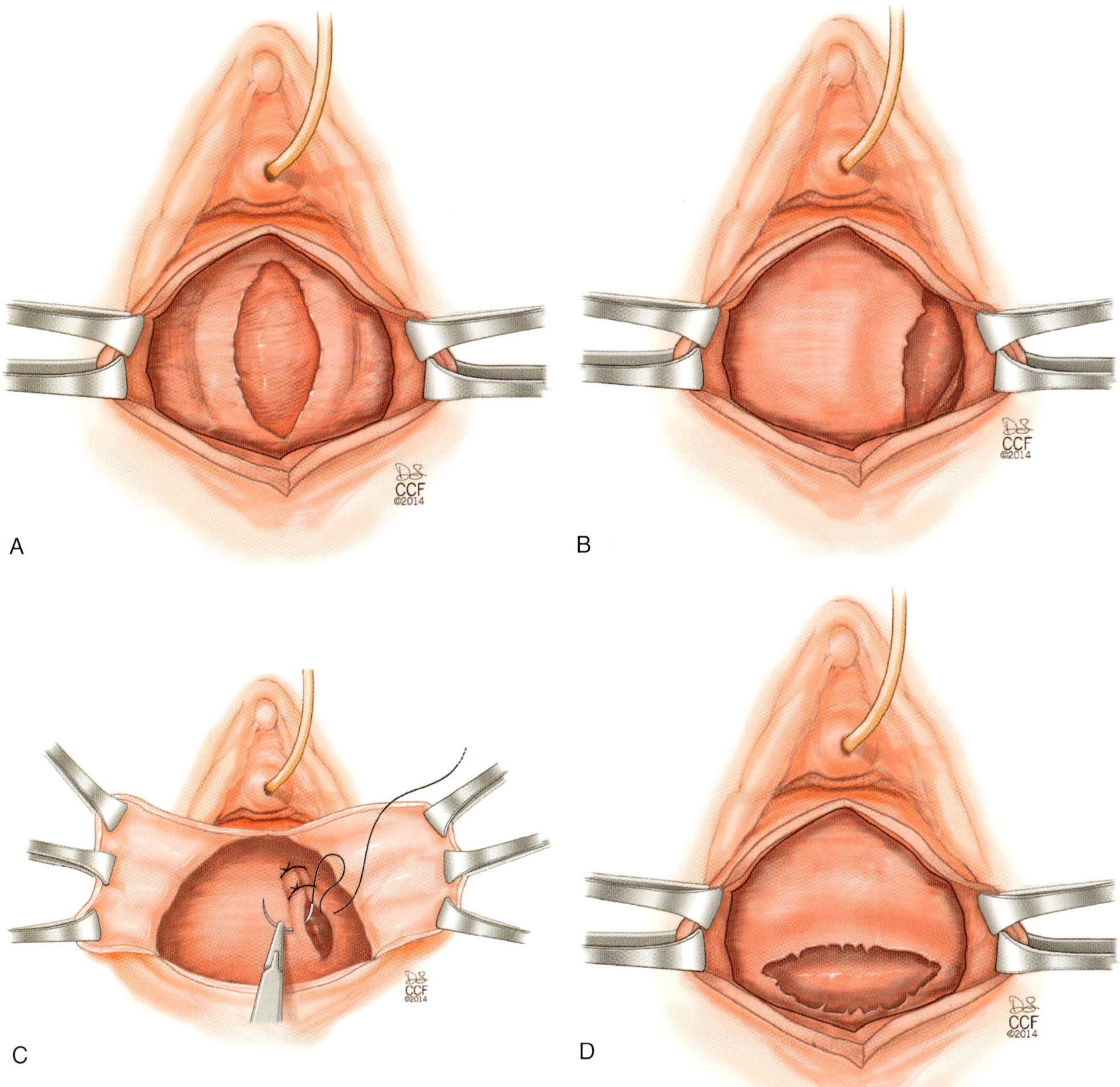

Fig. 20.8 Site-specific rectocele defects: before and after repair. **A**, Midline defect of the fibromuscularis. **B**, Left lateral defect of the fibromuscularis. **C**, Repair of left lateral defect with interrupted sutures. **D**, Distal transverse defect, separating the fibromuscularis of the posterior wall from the perineal body.

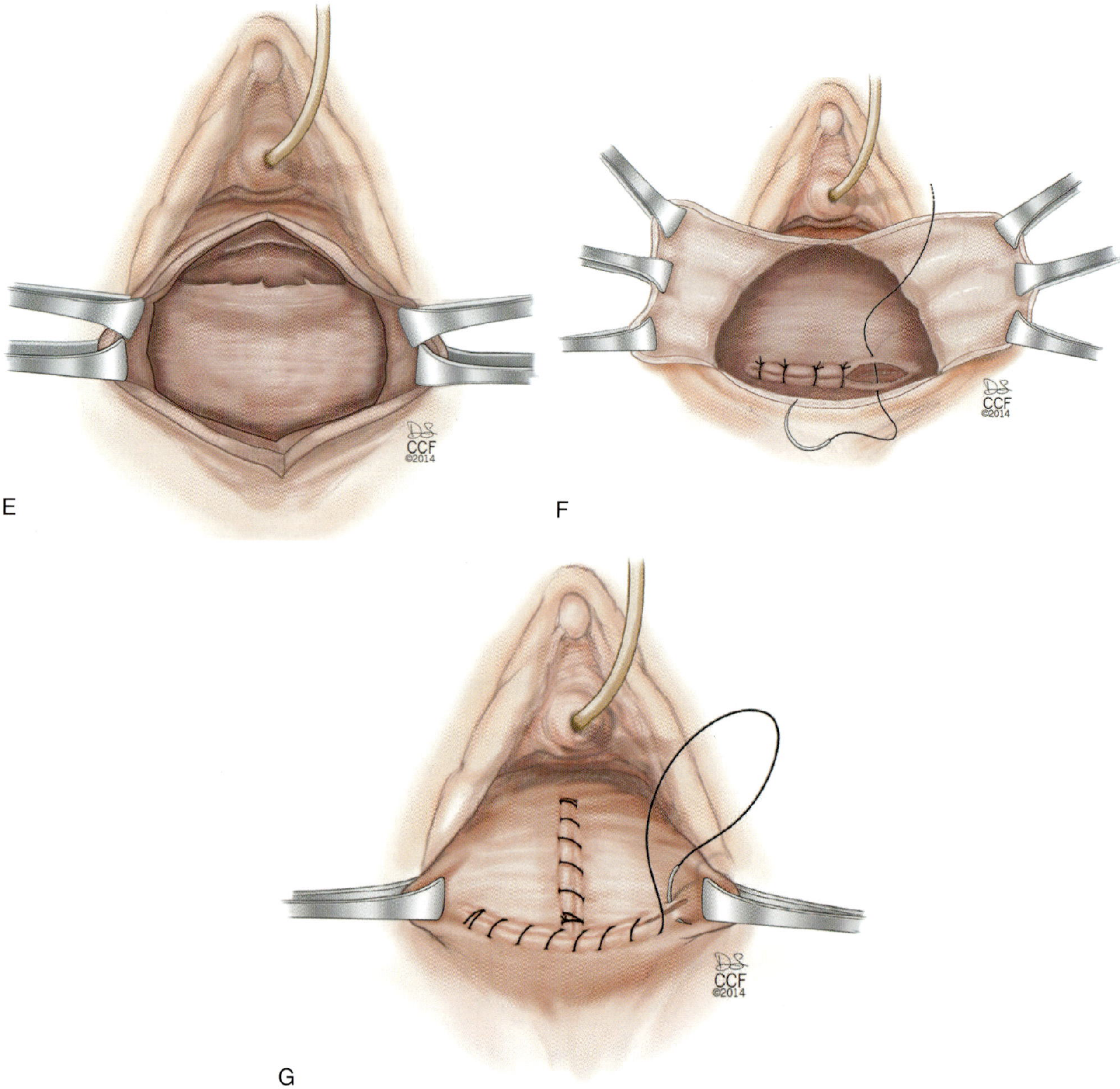

Fig. 20.8 cont'd **E**, Proximal transverse defect in the fibromuscularis near the apex. Repair of the proximal transverse defect is done as with a distal defect. If a level I vaginal vault suspension procedure is done, the distal portion of the break in the fibromuscularis may be incorporated in the apical repair. **F**, The distal defect is repaired with interrupted sutures. These sutures should reestablish continuity of the vaginal fibromuscularis with the perineal body. **G**, The epithelium of the posterior vagina and perineum are closed with running absorbable suture.

Extensive dissection and repair are required for women with an absent perineal body, most commonly as a result of difficult vaginal delivery or surgical trauma. A transverse semicircular incision is made in the layer separating the posterior vaginal wall and the anterior rectal wall. Dissection is extended laterally and proximally. To facilitate proximal dissection in the rectovaginal space without injury to the rectal mucosa, the surgeon may insert a finger of the nondominant hand into the rectum. The internal anal sphincter is plicated in the midline with No. 3-0 absorbable suture. The rectal mucosa is reapproximated, as needed, with a running absorbable No. 3-0 suture and extending to the skin overlying the external anal sphincter. Dissection of the anus is performed to identify the retracted ends of the external anal sphincter. Care should be taken with this step to avoid extensive lateral and posterior dissection and injury to the inferior hemorrhoidal nerves and vessels. The scarred ends of the external anal sphincter are identified and reapproximated in an overlapping fashion with vertical mattress sutures with delayed absorbable suture. The scar tissue on the two ends of the external anal sphincter is left intact and used for suture placement. The transversus perinei and bulbospongiosus muscles are plicated in the midline. With midline construction of the perineal

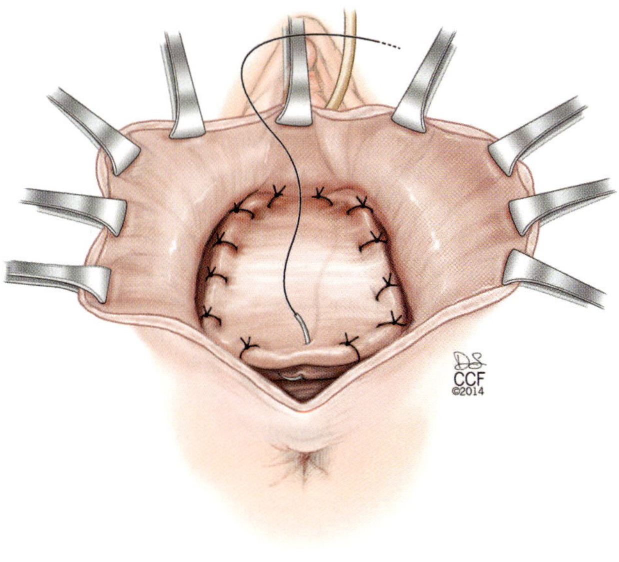

Fig. 20.9 Graft-augmented rectocele repair. A graft is trimmed and placed over a posterior colporrhaphy or site-specific defect repair.

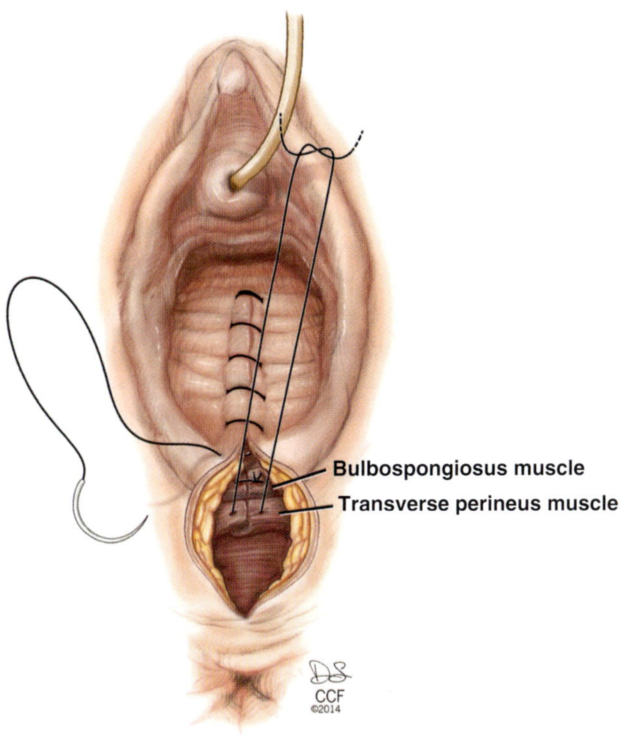

Fig. 20.10 Perineorrhaphy. Following the completion of the repair of the rectocele, the perineal body may need to be reconstructed. The bulbospongiosus and the superficial transverse perineus muscles are plicated in the midline with absorbable sutures.

body, the transverse portion of the initial incision becomes vertically oriented. The vaginal epithelium is closed with an absorbable suture. The skin of the perineal body is closed in an inverted Y shape with interrupted absorbable sutures. The patient is instructed that superficial wound breakdown on the perineum may occur. In most cases, this superficial wound breakdown will respond to conservative management rather than require aggressive debridement. See Chapter 27 for expanded description of anal sphincter repair.

The use of fine absorbable sutures in the perineal body and distal vagina may decrease the incidence of entrance dyspareunia, but care should be taken to avoid ridging the introitus with a tight plication of the bulbocavernosus muscles and/or overtrimming of the distal vaginal and vulvar skin. A perineorrhaphy will increase slightly the functional length of the posterior vaginal wall.

Postoperative Instructions

A vaginal pack and Foley catheter are placed after the surgery, if desired, and removed later that day or the following morning. The patients are discharged with stool softeners to be used for several months and with instructions to avoid heavy lifting or abdominal straining for 3 months and to avoid constipation in the future. Pelvic rest (avoiding the use of tampons, douching, or sexual intercourse) is recommended for at least 6 weeks.

ANALYSIS OF OUTCOMES

The majority of the published literature on surgical outcomes includes small case control series with varying definitions of cure (level III evidence). The 2018 Cochrane systematic review on surgery for posterior vaginal prolapse (Mowat et al., 2018) reported on 10 randomized controlled trials published on rectocele repair. Three trials compared native tissue repair to graft augmentation: Sand et al. (2001) compared posterior colporrhaphy to posterior colporrhaphy augmented with absorbable mesh; Paraiso et al. (2006) compared posterior colporrhaphy to site-specific repair to site-specific repair augmented with cross-linked porcine small intestine submucosa (SIS) graft; and Sung et al. (2012) compared native tissue repair (posterior colporrhaphy or site-specific repair dependent upon surgeon discretion) with native tissue repair augmented with non–cross-linked SIS graft.

Anatomic cure rates ranged from 76% to 96% for posterior colporrhaphy and from 69% to 100% for site-specific defect repair. Evidence is insufficient to permit any conclusions about the relative effectiveness of the different transvaginal rectocele repairs. In these surgeries, the sensation of a vaginal bulge was generally relieved, as was splinting to assist emptying, but disorders of defecation, such as constipation and fecal incontinence, were often not significantly improved. There are insufficient data on the overall effects of surgery on bowel symptoms and on whether one variation of vaginal repair (posterior colporrhaphy versus site-specific defect repair versus graft augmentation) is superior to others.

Gustilo-Ashby et al. (2007) performed an ancillary analysis of the data from the Paraiso et al. (2006) randomized trial of three rectocele repair techniques. Regardless of route of repair, most women had improvement of defecatory symptoms. Women with postoperative stage 0/1 posterior wall support had reduced risk of postoperative straining (adjusted odds ratio [OR] 0.17; 95% confidence interval [CI] 0.03–0.9) and feeling of incomplete emptying (adjusted OR 0.1; 95% CI 0.01–0.52). New bothersome defecatory complaints occurred postoperatively in 11/99 (11%)

women, including incomplete emptying 2/43 (5%), fecal urgency 3/65 (5%), anal incontinence-solid 2/87 (2%), anal incontinence-gas 5/49 (10%), straining 1/49 (2%), and pain with defecation 2/82 (2%).

Evaluation of the outcomes of the use of transvaginal mesh is difficult. The avenue of approach, mesh of choice (synthetic versus biologic), anchoring points (and kit systems), type of suture, and surgeon experience can vary depending upon the surgeon. The Cochrane review of the evidence of graft augmentation of posterior wall prolapse found that this augmentation did not improve outcomes of rectocele repair. Unique to synthetic graft placement (versus native tissue repair), vaginal mesh exposure occurs in 7% of women. Randomized trials of synthetic mesh and posterior colporrhaphy are lacking. As was noted earlier, allografts and xenografts have been used in rectocele repair; however, lack of uniform graft composition, decreasing tensile strength, and unpredictable tissue incorporation limit the success of these repairs. Nevertheless, there may be a future role of graft augmentation in selected high-risk patients in the setting of clinical trials.

There have been four randomized trials comparing vaginal and endoanal approaches to posterior wall prolapse. The transvaginal repair had lower recurrence rates on examination and on defecography and fewer recurrent prolapse symptoms, with no differences in rates of complications or dyspareunia.

Our understanding of factors associated with surgical failure of pelvic organ prolapse is still in its infancy. Younger age, advanced preoperative prolapse stage, and high body mass index have been associated with recurrence in some studies but not in others. Dällenbach et al. (2012) found in a case-control series (including all recurrent prolapse surgeries from 1988 to 2007) that the most important risk factors for recurrent prolapse requiring surgical management were sexual activity (adjusted OR 2.0; 95% CI 1.0–2.7; $P = .022$), presence of prolapse in more than two vaginal segments (adjusted OR 5.2; 95% CI 2.8–9.7; $P < .001$), history of surgery for pelvic organ prolapse and/or urinary incontinence (adjusted OR 3.02; 95% CI 1.4–6.3; $P = .003$), and the *absence* of posterior repair at initial surgery (adjusted OR 2.9; 95% CI 2.8–9.7; $P < .001$).

The development of recurrent prolapse is probably related to both surgeon and patient factors. Surgeon factors might include failure to do an appropriate concurrent apical suspension at rectocele repair, or even choosing to not repair a small rectocele during a multicompartment prolapse repair if it is not symptomatic. Many of the patient's initial risk factors may persist after the initial surgery, including genetic predisposition, estrogen deficiency, occupational exposures, chronic defecatory dysfunction with straining, and/or injured pelvic floor muscles. Identification of modifiable risk factors for recurrence should prompt targeted therapies for management of these factors, including weight loss, smoking cessation, and aggressive management of chronic lung disease and constipation.

COMPLICATIONS

Short-term complications associated with rectocele repair include pain, temporary urinary retention, and constipation. Hematoma, infection, fecal impaction, and injury to the rectum with the development of a rectovaginal fistula may occur but are uncommon.

Anal incontinence has been reported to occur after rectocele repair, and there is a significant association between fecal incontinence and more than one prior posterior colporrhaphy. A rectocele may be associated with altered rectal sensation and/or anal sphincter defect related to trauma or prolonged straining. Anal sphincter function may be improved if identified preoperatively and corrected at the time of rectocele repair. However, anal sphincter function may be damaged by a rectocele repair, particularly with the dilation associated with an endoanal repair. It is important to determine if a woman with recurrent posterior wall prolapse has a history of fecal incontinence and to consider ancillary testing (endoanal ultrasonography with possible electromyography testing) to evaluate the anal sphincter.

Rectocele repairs that include biologic or synthetic mesh have complications related to the specific mesh material that is used. The potential complications that have been described with the use of graft material are pain, infection, erosion into the surrounding tissue (in this case the vagina and rectum), fistula, scarring (which may increase the occurrence of dyspareunia), allergic reaction to the material used, and failure. It is important to have a thorough understanding of the mesh material that you may use.

Postoperative sexual dysfunction has been of significant concern for a number of decades with the surgical management of women with posterior wall prolapse. Francis and Jeffcoate (1961) observed a high rate of sexual dysfunction following prolapse surgery. Some 70 of 140 (50%) sexually active women reported apareunia or dyspareunia after an anterior and posterior colporrhaphy and perineorrhaphy. On postoperative examination, 43 of the 70 women were found to have a significantly narrowed vagina that would only admit one finger. It is likely that these surgeons had performed tight levator plications as part of their prolapse repairs.

With attention to preserving vaginal caliber, nearly 40 years later Weber et al. (2000) evaluated pre- and postoperative sexual function and vaginal caliber and length in 165 women. In this prospective, observational study, the performance of a posterior colporrhaphy (especially a posterior colporrhaphy with Burch colposuspension) was the only variable that predicted postoperative dyspareunia. Vaginal dimensions in general did not predict dyspareunia, and pain was often caused by ridging in the posterior vaginal wall. Even though dyspareunia increased with prolapse surgery, the satisfaction with sexual function improved from 82% preoperatively to 89% postoperatively. Jeong et al. (2010) found a similar improvement in sexual function in women who had undergone a midurethral sling procedure with and without a posterior colporrhaphy. Interestingly, there was no difference in the pain component of sexual function between women who had undergone a midurethral sling procedure alone or in combination with a posterior colporrhaphy. Abramov et al. (2005) compared site-specific defect repair and posterior colporrhaphy and found similar dyspareunia rates (16% vs 17%). Paraiso et al. (2006) found no significant difference in rates of postoperative dyspareunia when randomizing women to posterior colporrhaphy, site-specific defect repair, or graft-augmented site-specific repair. In general, avoidance of sutures that constrict vagina or genital hiatus and cause ridging of the posterior wall, as well as taking care to not overtrim the vaginal epithelium before closing, will help keep postoperative dyspareunia to a minimum.

Correction of prolapse and concomitant improvement of body image may be a dominant factor in postoperative sexual function, despite postoperative dyspareunia. Azar et al. (2008) found that sexual function significantly improved following anterior and posterior colporrhaphy. The domains of desire, arousal, lubrication, orgasm, and satisfaction were all significantly improved 3 months postoperatively. Unfortunately, pain with intercourse did increase in this immediate postoperative period; in this study, three levator plication sutures were included in the posterior colporrhaphy. Levator ani plication has been implicated as a possible cause of postoperative dyspareunia.

Levator myalgia (pain in the pelvic floor muscles) is an often unrecognized etiology or contributor to postoperative pelvic pain and dyspareunia. A woman who has vaginal pain following surgery may tighten the pelvic floor muscles in anticipation of pain with sexual activity. This can lead to chronic spasm and pain in the muscles surrounding the vagina. Physical therapy to relieve the spasm of the muscles is key to resolution of the pain.

Correction of posterior wall prolapse by other methods is also related to dyspareunia, including the transanal route. Arnold et al. (1990) found similar rates of dyspareunia among women who had undergone a transvaginal approach (23%) versus an endoanal approach (21%).

Graft placement can have a negative effect on sexual function. The severity of the pain can vary widely and may lead to severe chronic pelvic pain. However, in the majority of women with pain, it is described as mild or moderate. Mesh erosion can contribute to the development of pain for both partners during intercourse. Even if erosion does not occur, the "behavior" of the graft under the epithelium of the vagina after it is placed may be a cause of discomfort with intercourse. The graft may shrink or have been placed under tension, leading to chronic pain that is particularly evident at the connection points with the pelvic sidewall (mesh arms or sutures) or sacrospinous ligament. The graft may become encapsulated and fibrotic, or completely disappear. These factors may have profound effects on the function of the vagina as a sexual organ.

CONCLUSION

Correction of anatomy does not always result in symptomatic cure or patient satisfaction. In general, though, anatomic correction, overall satisfaction, and relief of symptoms occur in most women after surgery for posterior vaginal prolapse. However, correction of function is more complicated because of multiple confounding factors, such as coexisting bowel and sexual dysfunction. High-quality randomized controlled trials (RTCs) comparing different procedures and different clinical scenarios are needed.

The demand for the treatment of prolapse is predicted to double over the next 40 years. Further understanding of the etiology of prolapse, avoidance of obstetric trauma, early identification of women at risk for development, and treatment options for repair of injured nerves and muscles would be ideal. It is imperative that we obtain level I evidence (RTCs) in women with posterior wall prolapse to determine when a procedure should be done and what the most efficacious procedure is from an anatomic and functional standpoint. Further focus on understanding the complications associated with each procedure and ways to minimize and effectively resolve these problems when they arise is warranted.

BIBLIOGRAPHY

Anatomy and Pathophysiology

Boreham MK, Wai CY, Miller RT, et al. Morphometric properties of the posterior vaginal wall in women with pelvic organ prolapse. *Am J Obstet Gynecol.* 2002;187:1501.

Boyles SH, Weber AM, Meyn L. Procedures for pelvic organ prolapse in the United States, 1979–1997, *Am J Obstet Gynecol.* 2003;188:108.

Brown JS, Waetjen LE, Subak LL, et al. Pelvic organ prolapse surgery in the United States, 1997. *Am J Obstet Gynecol.* 2002;186:712.

Buchsbaum GM, Duecy EE, Kerr LA, et al. Pelvic organ prolapse in nulliparous women and their parous sisters. *Obstet Gynecol.* 2006;108:1388.

Carley ME, Schaffer J. Urinary incontinence and pelvic organ prolapse in women with Marfan or Ehlers–Danlos syndrome. *Am J Obstet Gynecol.* 2000;182:1021.

Cundiff GW, Fenner D. Evaluation and treatment of women with rectocele: focus on associated defecatory and sexual dysfunction. *Obstet Gynecol.* 2004;104:1403.

Dällenbach P, Kaelin-Gambirasio I, Dubuisson JB, Boulvain M. Risk factors for pelvic organ prolapse repair after hysterectomy. *Obstet Gynecol.* 2007;110:625.

Dällenbach P, Jungo Nancoz C, Eperon I, et al. Incidence and risk factors for reoperation of surgically treated pelvic organ prolapse. *Int Urogynecol J.* 2012;23:35.

DeLancey JOL. Standing anatomy of the pelvic floor. *J Pelvic Surg.* 1996;2:260.

DeLancey JOL. Structural anatomy of the posterior pelvic compartment as it relates to rectocele. *Am J Obstet Gynecol.* 1999;180:815.

DeLancey JOL, Hurd WW. Size of the urogenital hiatus in the levator ani muscles in normal women and women with pelvic organ prolapse. *Obstet Gynecol.* 1998;91:364.

Dietz HP, Gomez M, Atan IK, Ferreira CS. Association between vaginal parity and rectocele. *Int Urogynecol J.* 2018;29:1479.

Gyhagen M, Bullarbo M, Nielsen TF, Milsom I. Prevalence and risk factors for pelvic organ prolapse 20 years after childbirth: a national cohort study in singleton primiparae after vaginal or cesarean delivery. *BJOG.* 2013;120:152.

Handa VL, Garrett E, Hendrix S, et al. Progression and remission of pelvic organ prolapse: a longitudinal study of menopausal women. *Am J Obstet Gynecol.* 2004;190:27.

Hudson CN, Sohaib SA, Shulver HM, Reznek RH. The anatomy of the perineal membrane: its relationship to injury in childbirth and episiotomy. *Aust N Z J Obstet Gynaecol.* 2002;42:193.

Larson KA, Yousuf A, Leicky-Gaupp C, et al. Perineal body anatomy in living women: 3-dimensional analysis using thin-slice magnetic resonance imaging. *Am J Obstet Gynecol.* 2010;203:494.

Lince SL, van Kempen LC, Vierhout ME, Kluivers KB. A systematic review of clinical studies on hereditary factors in pelvic organ prolapse. *Int Urogynecol J.* 2012;23:1327.

Leffler KS, Thompson JR, Cundiff GW, et al. Attachment of the rectovaginal septum to the pelvic sidewall. *Am J Obstet Gynecol.* 2001;185:41.

Luo J, Larson KA, Fenner DE, et al. Posterior vaginal prolapse shape and position changes at maximal Valsalva seen in 3-D MRI-based models. *Int Urogynecol J.* 2012;23:1301.

Meschia M, Buonaguidi A, Pifarotti P, et al. Prevalence of anal incontinence in women with symptoms of urinary incontinence and genital prolapse. *Obstet Gynecol.* 2002;100:719.

Mohammed SD, Lunniss PJ, Zarte N, et al. Joint hypermobility and rectal evacuatory dysfunction: an etiological link in abnormal connective tissue? *Neurogastrenterol Motil.* 2010;22:1085.

Morren GL, Beets-Tan RGH, van Engelshoven JMA. Anatomy of the anal canal and perianal structures as defined by phased-array magnetic resonance imaging. *Br J Surg.* 2001;88:1506.

Nygaard I, Barber MD, Burgio KL, et al. Prevalence of symptomatic pelvic floor disorders in US women. *JAMA.* 2008;300:1311.

Oh C, Kark AE. Anatomy of the perineal body. *Dis Colon Rectum.* 1973;16:444.

Oladokun A, Babarinsa IA, Adewole IF. The deficient perineum: oblique presentation of a clinically obvious anomaly. *Afr J Med Sci.* 2002;31:267.

Pierce CB, Hallock JL, Bloomquist JL, Handa VL. Longitudinal changes in pelvic organ support among parous women. *Female Pelvic Med Reconstr Surg.* 2012;18:227.

Shah AD, Kohli N, Rajan SS, Hoyte L. The age distribution, rates, and types of surgery for pelvic organ prolapse in the USA. *Int Urogynecol J Pelvic Floor Dysfunct.* 2008;19:421.

Shalom DF, Lin SN, O'Shaughnessy DO, Lind LR, Winkler HA. Effect of prior hysterectomy on the anterior and posterior vaginal compartments of women presenting with pelvic organ prolapse. *Int J Gynecol Obstet.* 2012;119:274.

Stern R, Bernstein P, Sherer DM. Spontaneous delivery through the rectovaginal septum and perineal body: an unusual complication of persistent occiput posterior position. *J Matern-Fetal Med.* 1998;7:194.

Subak LL, Waetjen LE, van den Eeden S, et al. Cost of pelvic organ prolapse surgery in the United States. *Obstet Gynecol.* 2001;98:646.

Woodman PJ, Graney DO. Anatomy and physiology of the female perineal body with relevance to obstetrical injury and repair. *Clin Anat.* 2002;15:321.

Evaluation

Agildere AM, Tarhan NC, Ergeneli MH, et al. MR rectography evaluation of rectoceles with oral gadopentetate dimeglumine and polyethylene glycol solution. *Abdom Imaging.* 2003;28:28.

Burrows LJ, Sewell C, Leffler KS, Cundiff GW. The accuracy of clinical evaluation of posterior vaginal wall defects. *Int Urogynecol J.* 2003;14:160.

Cortes E, Reid WMN, Singh K, Berger L. Clinical examination and dynamic magnetic resonance imaging in vaginal vault prolapse. *Obstet Gynecol.* 2004;103:41.

Henry MM, Parks AG, Swash M. The pelvic floor musculature in the descending perineum syndrome. *Br J Surg.* 1982;69:470.

Hullfish KL, Bovbjerg VE, Gibson J, Steers WD. Patient-centered goals for pelvic floor dysfunction surgery: what is success, and is it achieved? *Am J Obstet Gynecol.* 2002;187:88.

Ganeshan A, Anderson EM, Upponi S, et al. Imaging of obstructed defecation. *Clin Radiol.* 2008;14:160.

Johansson C, Nilsson BY, Holmström B, et al. Association between rectocele and paradoxical sphincter response. *Dis Colon Rectum.* 1992;35:503.

Kenton K, Shott S, Brubaker L. The anatomic and functional variability of rectoceles in women. *Int Urogynecol J Pelvic Floor Dysfunct.* 1999;10:96.

Martellucci J, Naldini G. Clinical relevance of transperineal ultrasound compared with evacuation proctography for the evaluation of patients with obstructed defecation. *Colorectal Dis.* 2011;13:1167.

Mimura T, Roy AJ, Storrie JB, Kamm MA. Treatment of impaired defecation associated with rectocele by behavioral retraining (biofeedback). *Dis Colon Rectum.* 2000;43:1267.

Murad-Regadas SM, Regadas FS, Rodrigues LV, et al. A novel three-dimensional dynamic anorectal ultrasonography technique (echodefecography) to assess obstructed defecation, a comparison with defecography. *Surg Endosc.* 2008;22:974.

Olsen AL, Smith VJ, Bergstrom JO, et al. Epidemiology of surgically managed pelvic organ prolapse and urinary incontinence. *Obstet Gynecol.* 1997;89:501.

Rentsch M, Paetzel C, Lenhart M, et al. Dynamic magnetic resonance imaging defecography. *Dis Colon Rectum.* 2001;44:999.

Ridgeway BM, Weinstein MM, Tunitsky-Bitton E. American Urogynecologic Society best-practice statement on evaluation of obstructed defecation. *Female Pelvic Med Reconstr Surg.* 2018;24:383.

Roos AM, Thakar R, Sultan AH, et al. Pelvic floor dysfunction: women's sexual concerns unraveled. *J Sex Med.* 2014;11:743.

Savoye-Collet C, Savoye G, Koning E, et al. Defecography in symptomatic older women living at home. *Age Ageing.* 2003;32:347.

Steiner RA, Healy JC. Patterns of prolapse in women with symptoms of pelvic floor weakness: magnetic resonance imaging and laparoscopic treatment. *Curr Opin Obstet Gynecol.* 1998;10:295.

Sung VW, Rardin CR, Raker CA, et al. Changes in bowel symptoms 1 year after rectocele repair. *Am J Obstet Gynecol.* 2012;207:423.

Swift SE, Herring M. Comparison of pelvic organ prolapse in the dorsal lithotomy compared with the standing position. *Obstet Gynecol.* 1998;91:961.

Swift SE, Tate SB, Nicholas J. Correlation of symptoms with degree of pelvic organ support in a general population of women: what is pelvic organ prolapse? *Am J Obstet Gynecol.* 2003;189:372.

Tunn R, DeLancey JOL, Howard D, et al. MR imaging of levator ani muscle recovery following vaginal delivery. *Int Urogynecol J.* 1999;10:3001999.

Wallace SL, Torosis M, Rogo-Gupta L. Does rectocele on defecography equate to rectocele on physical examination in patients with defecatory symptoms? *Female Pelvic Med Reconst Surg.* 2021;27:18.

Weber AM, Walters MD, Ballard LA, et al. Posterior vaginal prolapse and bowel function. *Am J Obstet Gynecol.* 1998;179:1446.

Surgical Techniques, Complications, and Recurrence

Abramov Y, Gandhi S, Goldberg RP, et al. Site-specific rectocele repair compared with standard posterior colporrhaphy. *Obstet Gynecol.* 2005;105:314.

Altman D, Zetterström J, López A, et al. Functional and anatomic outcome after transvaginal rectocele repair using collagen mesh: a prospective study. *Dis Colon Rectum.* 2005;48:1.

Altomare DF, Rinaldi M, Veglia A, et al. Combined perineal and endorectal repair of rectocele by circular stapler. *Dis Colon Rectum.* 2002;45:1549.

Arnold MW, Stewart WR, Aguilar PS. Rectocele repair: four years' experience. *Dis Colon Rectum.* 1990;33:684.

Ayabaca SM, Zbar AP, Pescatori M. Anal continence after rectocele repair. *Dis Colon Rectum.* 2002;45:63.

Azar M, Noohi S, Radfar S, et al. Sexual function and vaginal anatomy in women before and after surgery for pelvic organ prolapse. *Int Urogynecol J Pelvic Floor Dysfunct.* 2008;19:53.

Chang OH, Davidson ER, Thomas TN, et al. Does concurrent posterior repair for an asymptomatic rectocele reduce the risk of surgical failure in patients undergoing sacrocolpopexy? *Int Urogynecol J.* 2020;31:2075.

Clark AL, Gregory T, Smith VJ, Edwards R. Epidemiologic evaluation of reoperation for surgically treated pelvic organ prolapse and urinary incontinence. *Am J Obstet Gynecol.* 2003;189:1261.

Cundiff GW, Harris RL, Coates K, et al. Abdominal sacral colpoperineopexy: a new approach for correction of posterior compartment defects and perineal descent associated with vaginal vault prolapse. *Am J Obstet Gynecol.* 1997;177:1345.

Cundiff GW, Weidner AC, Visco AG, et al. An anatomic and functional assessment of the discrete defect rectocele repair. *Am J Obstet Gynecol.* 1998;179:1451.

Diez-Itza I, Aizpitarte I, Becerro A. Risk factors for the recurrence of pelvic organ prolapse after vaginal surgery: a review at 5 years after surgery. *Int Urogynecol J Pelvic Floor Dysfunct.* 2007;18:1317.

Doumouchtsis SK, Raheem AA, Haddad JM, et al. An update of a former FIGO Working Group report on management of posterior compartment prolapse. *Int J Gynecol Obstet.* 2020;148:135.

Dua A, Radley S, Brown S, Jha S, Jones G. The effect of posterior colporrhaphy on anorectal function, *Int Urogynecol J.* 2012;23:749.

Farid M, Madbouly KM, Hussein A, et al. Randomized controlled trial between perineal and anal repairs of rectocele in obstructed defecation. *World J Surg.* 2010;34:822.

Fox SD, Stanton SL. Vault prolapse and rectocele: assessment of repair using sacrocolpopexy with mesh interposition. *Br J Obstet Gynaecol.* 2000;107:1371.

Francis WJA, Jeffcoate TNA. Dyspareunia following vaginal operations. *J Obstet Gynaecol Br Commonwealth.* 1961;68:1.

Glavind K, Madsen H. A prospective study of the discrete fascial defect rectocele repair. *Acta Obstet Gynecol Scand.* 2000;79:145.

Grimes CL, Schimpf MO, Wieslander CK, et al. Surgical interventions for posterior compartment prolapse and obstructed defecation symptoms: a systematic review with clinical practice recommendations. *Int Urogynecol J.* 2019;30:1433.

Gustilo-Ashby AM, Paraiso MF, Jelovsek JE, et al. Bowel symptoms 1 year after surgery for prolapse: further analysis of a randomized trial of rectocele repair. *Am J Obstet Gynecol.* 2007;197:76.

Haase P, Skibsted L. Influence of operations for stress incontinence and/or genital descensus on sexual life. *Acta Obstet Gynecol Scand.* 1988;67:659.

Hakelius L. Reconstruction of the perineal body as treatment for anal incontinence. *Brit J Plastic Surg.* 1979;32:245.

Jeffcoate TNA. Posterior colpoperineorrhaphy. *Am J Obstet Gynecol.* 1959;77:490.

Jeong TY, Yang SA, Seo JT. The effect of posterior colporrhaphy performed concurrently with midurethral sling surgery on the sexual function of women with stress urinary incontinence. *Int Neurourol J.* 2010;14:177.

Kahn MA, Stanton SL. Posterior colporrhaphy: its effects on bowel and sexual function. *Brit J Obstet Gynaecol.* 1997;104:82.

Kenton K, Shott S, Brubaker L. Outcome after rectovaginal fascia reattachment for rectocele repair. *Am J Obstet Gynecol.* 1999;181:1360.

Kenton KS, Woods MP, Brubaker L. Uncomplicated erosion of polytetrafluoroethylene grafts into the rectum. *Am J Obstet Gynecol.* 2002;187:233.

Khubchandani IT, Clancy JP, Rosen L, et al. Endorectal repair of rectocele revisited. *Brit J Surg.* 1997;84:89.

Kohli N, Miklos JR. Dermal graft-augmented rectocele repair. *Int Urogynecol J.* 2003;14:146.

van Laarhoven CJHM, Kamm MA, Bartram CI, et al. Relationship between anatomic and symptomatic long-term results after rectocele repair for impaired defecation. *Dis Colon Rectum.* 1999;42:204.

Lim YN, Muller R, Corstiaans A, et al. A long-term review of posterior colporrhaphy with Vypro 2 mesh. *Int Urogynecol J Pelvic Floor Dysfunct.* 2007;18:1053.

López A, Anzén B, Bremmer S, et al. Cystodefecoperitoneography in patients with genital prolapse. *Int Urogynecol J.* 2002;13:22.

Maher CF, Qatawneh AM, Baessler K, Schluter PJ. Midline rectovaginal fascial plication for repair of rectocele and obstructed defecation. *Obstet Gynecol.* 2004;104:685.

Mellgren A, Anzén B, Nilsson B, et al. Results of rectocele repair: a prospective study. *Dis Colon Rectum.* 1995;38:7.

Mohammed N, Hoda MR, Fornara P. Prolapse surgery in octogenarians: are we pushing the limits too far? *World J Urol.* 2013;31:623.

Mowat A, Maher D, Baessler K, et al. Surgery for women with posterior compartment prolapse. *Cochrane Database Syst Rev.* 2018;2018:CD 012975.

Nichols DH. Posterior colporrhaphy and perineorrhaphy: separate and distinct operations. *Am J Obstet Gynecol.* 1991;164:714.

Nieminen K, Hiltunen KM, Laitinen J, et al. Transanal or vaginal approach to rectocele repair: a prospective, randomized pilot study. *Dis Colon Rectum.* 2004;47:1636.

Nygaard I, Brubaker L, Zyczynski HM, et al. Long-term outcomes following abdominal sacrocolpopexy for pelvic organ prolapse. *JAMA.* 2013;309:2016.

Paraiso MF, Barber MD, Muir TW, Walters MD. Rectocele repair: a randomized trial of three surgical techniques including graft augmentation. *Am J Obstet Gynecol.* 2006;195:1762.

Pierce LM, Rao A, Hou Y, et al. Long-term histological response to synthetic and biologic graft materials implanted in the vagina and abdomen of a rabbit model. *Am J Obstet Gynecol.* 2009;200:546.

Polin MR, Gleason JL, Szychowski JM, et al. Effects of transvaginal repair of symptomatic rectocele on symptom-specific distress and impact on quality of life. *Int J Gynaecol Obstet.* 2012;117:224.

Porter WE, Steele A, Walsh P, et al. The anatomic and functional outcomes of defect-specific rectocele repairs. *Am J Obstet Gynecol.* 1999;181:1353.

Rovner ES, Ginsberg DA. Posterior vaginal wall prolapse: transvaginal repair of pelvic floor relaxation, rectocele, and perineal laxity. *Tech Urology.* 2001;7:161.

Sand K, Koduri S, Lobel RW, et al. Prospective randomized trial of polyglactin 910 mesh to prevent recurrence of cystoceles and rectoceles. *Am J Obstet Gynecol.* 2001;184:1357.

Sardeli C, Axelsen SM, Kjaer D, Bek KM. Outcome of site-specific fascia repair for rectocele. *Acta Obstet Gynecol Scand.* 2007;86:973.

Singh K, Cortes E, Reid WMN. Evaluation of the fascial technique for surgical repair of isolated posterior vaginal wall prolapse. *Obstet Gynecol.* 2003;101:320.

Sullivan ES, Leaverton GH, Hardwick CE. Transrectal perineal repair: an adjunct to improved function after anorectal surgery. *Dis Colon Rectum.* 1968;11:106.

Sung VW, Rardin CR, Raker CA, et al. Porcine subintestinal submucousal graft augmentation for rectocele repair: a randomized controlled trial. *Obstet Gynecol.* 2012;119:125.

Tegerstedt G, Maehle-Schmidt M, Nyrén O, Hammarström M. Prevalence of symptomatic pelvic organ prolapse in a Swedish population. *Int Urogynecol J.* 2005;16:497.

van Dam JH, Hop WCJ, Schouten WR. Analysis of patients with poor outcome of rectocele repair. *Dis Colon Rectum.* 2000;43:1556.

Venkatesh KS, Ramanujam P. Surgical treatment of traumatic cloaca. *Dis Colon Rectum.* 1996;39:811.

Visco AG, Weidner AC, Barber MD, et al. Vaginal mesh erosion after abdominal sacral colpopexy. *Am J Obstet Gynecol.* 2001;184:297.

Weber AM, Walters MD, Piedmonte MA. Sexual function and vaginal anatomy in women before and after surgery for pelvic organ prolapse and urinary incontinence. *Am J Obstet Gynecol.* 2000;182:1610.

21 Surgical Treatment of Vaginal Apex Prolapse

Matthew D. Barber, Anthony G. Visco, and Mark D. Walters

CHAPTER OUTLINE

INTRODUCTION

Although anterior vaginal prolapse is most common, loss of apical support is usually present in women with prolapse that extends beyond the hymen. There is growing recognition that adequate support for the vaginal apex is an essential component of a durable surgical repair for women with advanced prolapse (Shull et al., 1999; Toozs-Hobson et al., 1998). At least half of the observed variation in anterior compartment support may be explained by apical support (Summers et al., 2006). Because of the significant contribution of the apex to anterior vaginal support, the best surgical correction of the anterior and posterior walls may fail unless the apex is adequately supported. Recognition of apical defects is one of the biggest challenges in the preoperative evaluation of pelvic support defects; however, surgical correction of the apex has several good options with relatively high success rates. Apical suspension procedures can broadly be separated into those performed tranvaginally and those performed abdominally. Abdominal procedures can be performed via laparotomy or using conventional laparoscopic or robotically-assisted laparoscopic techniques. Although precise estimates are not available, most studies suggest that the vaginal approach is most common with over 80% of procedures using this approach. This chapter reviews the indications, surgical techniques, outcomes, and complications associated with a variety of apical support procedures performed vaginally or abdominally, often through minimally invasive techniques.

ANATOMIC CONSIDERATIONS

The vaginal axis in an erect woman normally is nearly horizontal in the upper half of the vagina, with the uterus and upper 3 to 4 cm of the vagina lying over the levator plate in the hollow of the sacrum (Fig. 21.1). Funt et al. (1978) found that the vagina is directed toward the S3 and S4 vertebrae and extends approximately 3 cm past the ischial spines in most nulliparous women. Distortion of the normal vaginal axis during reconstructive pelvic surgery predisposes women to the development of pelvic organ prolapse at an anatomic site opposite to where the repair was performed. Examples of this are the development of posterior vaginal wall prolapse after colposuspension procedures for stress incontinence and the development of anterior vaginal wall prolapse after suspension of the vaginal apex to the sacrospinous ligament.

When planning an effective surgical approach to pelvic organ prolapse, a surgeon must keep in mind the three levels of support of the vagina. The proximal or upper fourth of the vagina (level I) is suspended by the cardinal/uterosacral complex, the middle half (level II) is attached laterally to the arcus tendineus fasciae pelvis and the medial aspect of the levator ani muscles, and the distal or lower fourth (level III) is fused to the perineal body. See Chapter 1 for more details. The goals of pelvic reconstructive surgery are to correct all defects, thus reestablishing vaginal support at all three levels, and to maintain or restore normal visceral and sexual function.

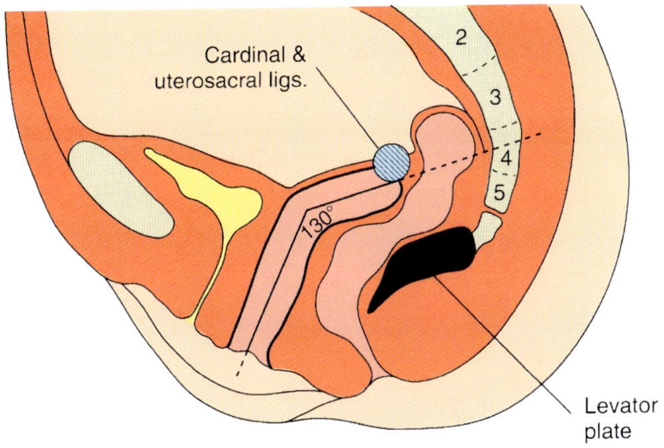

Fig. 21.1 Normal vaginal axis of nulliparous woman in the standing position. Note that the upper third of the vagina is nearly horizontal and is directed toward the S3 and S4 sacral vertebrae. (From Funt MI, Thompson JD, Birch H. Normal vaginal axis. *South Med J.* 1978;71:1534. With permission.)

TRANSVAGINAL NATIVE TISSUE SUTURE REPAIRS

The uterosacral ligament suspension (ULS) and sacrospinous ligament suspension (SSLS) are the two most common and widely studied transvaginal native tissue vaginal apical procedures. The iliococcygeus suspension offers an alternative vaginal extraperitoneal approach that can be useful in women with foreshortened vaginas and/or apical-posterior prolapse.

Uterosacral Ligament Suspension

A popular transvaginal approach to the management of apical prolapse is bilateral ULS. This approach was first described by Miller in 1927 and later popularized by Shull in the late 1990s (Miller, 1927; Shull et al., 2000). The ULS suspends the vaginal apex to the proximal remnants of the uterosacral ligaments using an intraperitoneal surgical approach. This procedure restores the vagina to its normal axis, avoiding the retroflexion that is associated with the SSLS. The procedure requires intraperitoneal access and can be easily accomplished at the time of a vaginal hysterectomy to treat concurrent uterine/apical prolapse. The location of the sutures along the uterosacral ligament can be tailored to the amount of prolapse present, with more advanced amounts of prolapse requiring higher placement of sutures (Fig. 21.2). Whereas surgeons frequently "reattach" the distal uterosacral ligaments to the vaginal cuff with the intention of preventing future prolapse, a ULS performed to treat prolapse of the apex includes sutures placed proximal to the level of the ischial spines. The procedure suspends the apex of the vagina into the hollow of the sacrum and thus maintains the midline orientation of the vaginal axis. A ULS procedure can be performed abdominally or laparoscopically, but the transvaginal route is most common. The technique for the intraperitoneal transvaginal approach is described below. Also, Video 21.1 provides a description of the surgical anatomy and steps of the ULS.

1. The peritoneal cavity has already been accessed if performed after a vaginal hysterectomy. For vaginal vault prolapse, the vaginal apex is grasped with two Allis clamps (Fig. 21.3A) and incised with a scalpel. The vaginal epithelium is dissected off the enterocele sac, the enterocele is opened, and the hernia sac is excised (Fig. 21.3B). See Video 21.2 for a demonstration of techniques for vaginal entry into the peritoneal cavity in posthysterectomy prolapse patients. If intraperitoneal access cannot be obtained, we prefer to proceed with a sacrospinous suspension.
2. Several moist tail sponges are placed in the posterior cul-de-sac. A wide Deaver retractor is used to elevate the packs and the intestines out of the operative field. A Breisky–Navratil detractor is often a valuable tool.
3. The ischial spines are palpated transperitoneally. The remnants of the uterosacral ligaments are found posterior and medial to the ischial spine, and the ureter can sometimes be palpated or visualized along the pelvic side wall, anywhere from 2 to 5 cm ventral and lateral to the ischial spine.
4. Traction on long Allis clamps placed at approximately the 5 o'clock and 7 o'clock positions allows palpation of the uterosacral ligament complex (Fig. 21.3C).
5. Usually, two to three delayed absorbable sutures are passed through the ligament on each side. Some prefer a combination of delayed absorbable and permanent sutures. To ensure adequate vaginal suspension, the highest (most proximal) suture should be 1 to 3 cm proximal to the level of the ischial spine (Fig. 21.3D). We have found that grasping the proximal uterosacral ligament at the position where the suspension sutures will be placed facilitates placement and minimizes the risk of entrapping underlying structures like nerves (Fig. 21.4A–C).
6. The delayed absorbable sutures that had been passed high up through the uterosacral ligaments then are passed either through the full thickness of the posterior vaginal wall (Fig. 21.3E) or, as is our usual practice, through the full thickness of both the anterior and posterior vaginal walls (Fig 21.4B). To assess ureteral patency we place the uterosacral sutures under moderate tension and perform cystoscopy after administration of intravenous indigo carmine. If ureteral spill is not present on either side, the suture can easily be replaced, typically more medially, and cystoscopy repeated until bilateral ureteral patency is confirmed. Cystoscopy can also be performed at the end of the procedure, but should be performed concomitantly given the risk of ureteral stricture.
7. If necessary, an anterior colporrhaphy or posterior colporrhaphy can be performed. The vagina is trimmed and closed with a No. 3-0 delayed absorbable suture (Fig. 21.3F and G).
8. Next, the vault suspension sutures are tied elevating the vagina high up into the hollow of the sacrum (Fig. 21.3H).

With the exception of the Operations and Pelvic Muscle Training in the Management of Apical Support Loss (OPTIMAL) trial (Barber et al., 2014), the current evidence supporting the use of ULS is limited primarily to uncontrolled cohorts or case series, and evaluation of these data suggest a mean objective success rate of 85% (range 48%–96%) and mean reoperation rate for prolapse of 5.8% (range 0%–12%) (Maher et al., 2016a). A metaanalysis performed by Margulies et al. (2010)

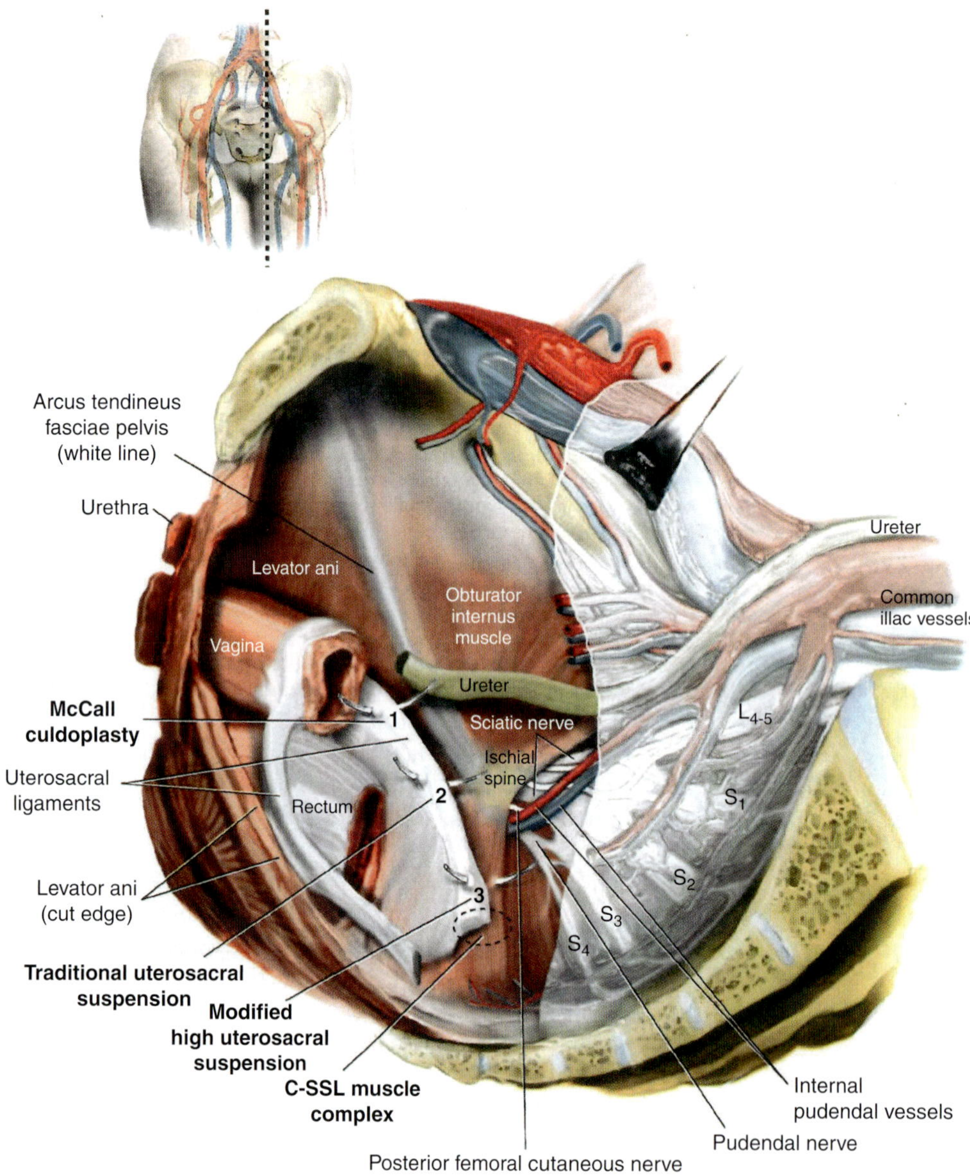

Fig. 21.2 Cross-section of the pelvic floor demonstrating intraperitoneal placement of sutures for (1) McCall culdoplasty, (2) traditional reattachment of the uterosacral ligaments to the vaginal cuff after hysterectomy, and (3) uterosacral ligament suspension, with sutures placed through the ligaments proximal to the ischial spines. Note that uterosacral ligament suspension may involve passage of the suture through the coccygeus muscle–sacrospinous ligament (*C-SSL*) complex, because a portion of the uterosacral ligament inserts into this structure.

found pooled rates of anatomic success (Pelvic Organ Prolapse Quantification [POPQ] stage 0–1) of 81.2% (95% confidence interval [CI] 67.5–94.5) for the anterior segment, 98.3% (95% CI 95.7–100) for the apical segment, and 87.4% (95% CI, 67.5–94.5) for the posterior segment. Postoperative prolapse symptoms were relieved in 82% to 100% of patients. These promising results are balanced by ureteral kinking/injury rate of 4% to 6%. A review of 700 consecutive vaginal prolapse surgeries found intraoperative ureteral kinking/injury in 5.9% of patients that was directly attributable to ULS. However, 87% of these cases of ureteral kinking/injury were identified at cystoscopy before the completion of the index surgery and were relieved by removing suspension sutures intraoperatively, with no long-term consequence to the patient (Gustilo-Ashby et al., 2006). Only three of 355 ULS procedures (0.9%) performed in this series required additional procedures to relieve or correct ureteral obstruction or injury. A retrospective review of over 900 patients receiving ULS found an overall adverse event rate of 31.2%, with 20.3% being attributed to postoperative urinary tract infection (Unger et al., 2015). Rates of pulmonary and cardiac events were 2.3%, whereas the rate of ileus and small bowel obstruction (SBO) was less than 0.5%. The intraoperative bladder injury rate was 1%. There were no intraoperative ureteral injuries; however, 4.5% of cases were complicated by ureteral kinking, all of which were resolved without subsequent sequelae by intraoperative suture removal with or without

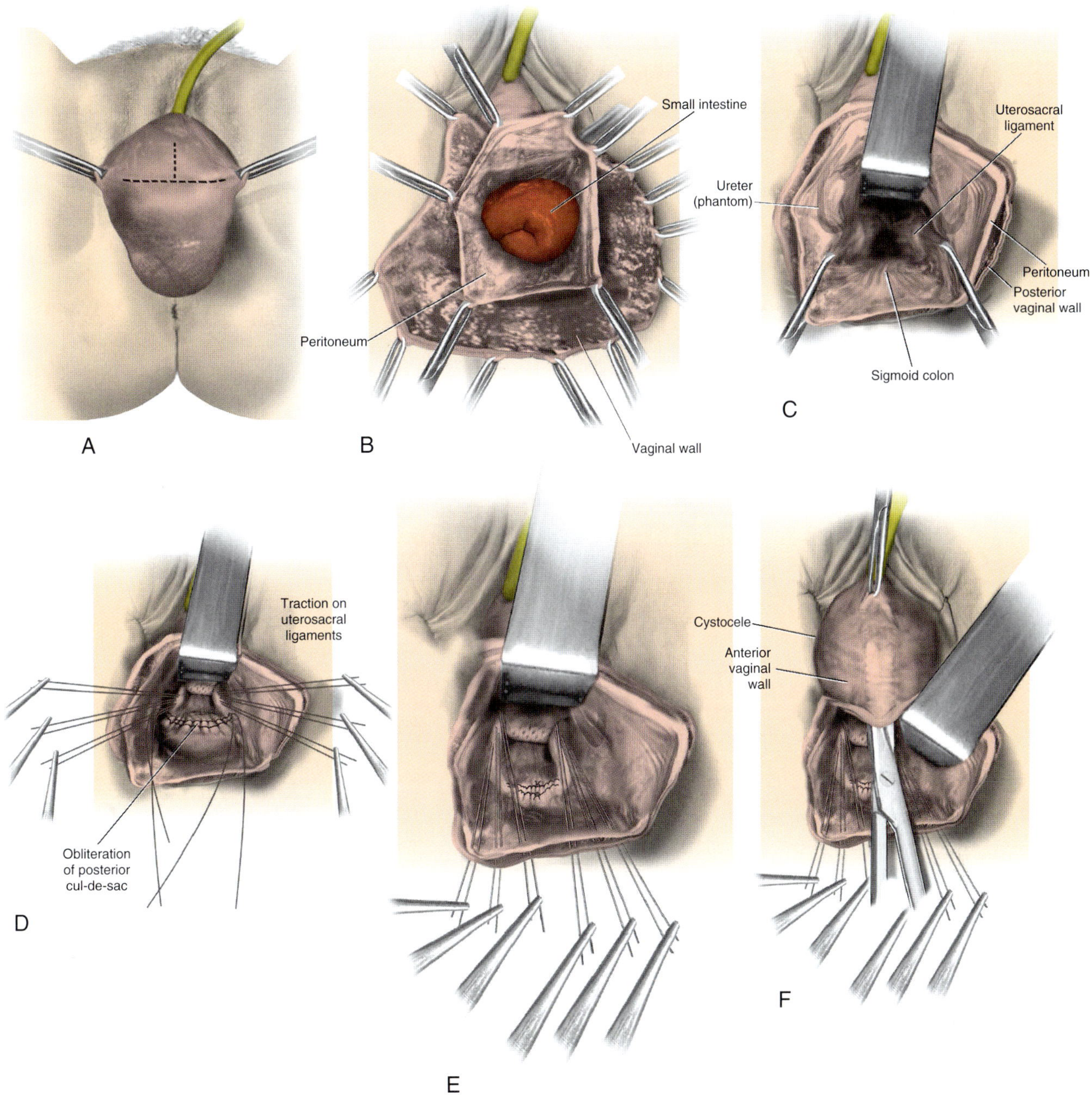

Fig. 21.3 Technique for uterosacral ligament suspension of the vaginal vault. **A**, The most prominent portion of the prolapsed vaginal vault is grasped with Allis clamps. **B**, The vaginal wall is opened, and the enterocele sac is identified and entered. **C**, The bowel is packed high up into the pelvis using laparotomy sponges. The retractor lifts the sponges up out of the lower pelvis, thus completely exposing the cul-de-sac. When appropriate downward traction is applied on the uterosacral ligaments with an Allis clamp, the uterosacral ligaments are easily palpated bilaterally. **D**, Delayed absorbable sutures are passed through the uppermost portion of the uterosacral ligaments (proximal to the spines) on each side and are individually tagged. **E**, Each end of the previously passed sutures is brought out through the posterior peritoneum and the posterior vaginal wall (or separate ends passed through the anterior and posterior vaginal walls, not shown). A free needle is used to pass both ends of these delayed absorbable sutures through the full thickness of the vaginal wall. **F**, The anterior colporrhaphy is begun by initiating a dissection between the prolapsed bladder and the anterior vaginal wall. **G**, The anterior colporrhaphy has been completed. **H**, The vagina has been appropriately trimmed and closed with interrupted or continuous delayed absorbable sutures. After closing the vagina, the delayed absorbable sutures that were previously brought out through the full thickness of the posterior (or anterior and posterior) vaginal wall(s) are tied, thereby elevating the prolapsed vaginal vault high up into the hollow of the sacrum. (From Baggish MS, Karram MM. Vaginal repair of vaginal vault prolapse. In: *Atlas of Pelvic Anatomy and Gynecologic Surgery*. 3rd ed. Saunders: St. Louis; 2011:713-714.)

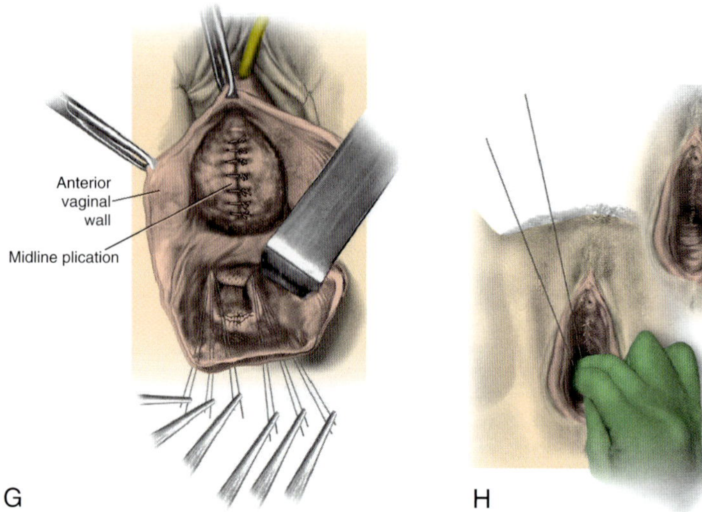

Fig. 21.3 cont'd

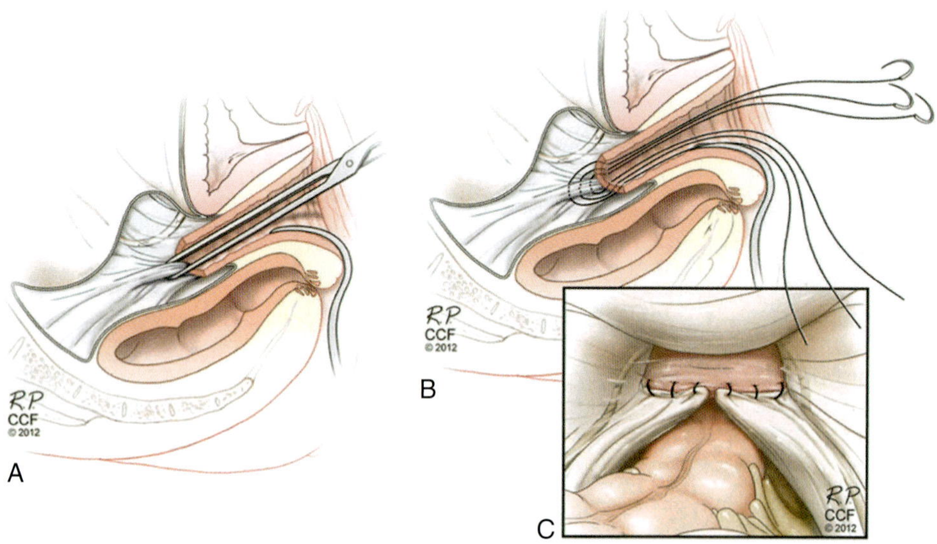

Fig. 21.4 Uterosacral ligament suspension. **A**, The uterosacral ligament proximal to the level of the ischial spine is grasped with an Allis clamp. **B**, Three sutures are placed through the ipsilateral uterosacral ligament and then through the vaginal apex. **C**, Sutures are placed bilaterally and tied, suspending the apex. (Illustration by Ross Papalardo. Reprinted with permission, Cleveland Clinic Center for Medical Art and Photography © 2012–2013. All rights reserved; From Walters MD, Ridgeway BM. Surgical treatment of vaginal apex prolapse. *Obstet Gynecol.* 2013;121:354.)

replacement of the vault suspension stitches. Margulies et al. (2010) identified 10 studies including a total of 820 women that reported on perioperative complications of ULS. The ureteral reimplantation rate in this series was only 0.6%. Blood transfusions were reported in 1.3%, cystotomy in 0.1%, and bowel injury in 0.2%.

Abdominal and laparoscopic ULS techniques have also been described. Lowenstein et al. (2009) reported a retrospective review of 107 women who underwent prolapse surgery that included an abdominal ULS. In the 75 patients who completed 1-year follow-up, 12% reported recurrent or persistent prolapse symptoms, and 7% had an anatomic failure (POPQ stage 2 or greater). Complications were relatively few; however, exposure of the apical sutures (expanded polytetrafluorethylene) occurred in 9% at an average of 56 months postsurgery (range 3–75 months). Two retrospective comparisons between vaginal and laparoscopic ULS procedures found no significant difference in perioperative morbidity or anatomic or subjective outcomes (Rardin et al., 2009; Turner et al., 2016).

Sacrospinous Ligament Suspension

One of the most popular and widely reported native tissue transvaginal procedures for correcting apical prolapse is the SSLS. First described in 1958, this procedure suspends the vaginal apex to the sacrospinous ligament either unilaterally or bilaterally, typically using an extraperitoneal approach (Sederl, 1958). The SSLS is often performed for moderate to severe apical uterine prolapse or for vaginal vault prolapse after hysterectomy. To perform SSLS, the surgeon must be familiar with pararectal anatomy, as well as the anatomy of the ischial spine, ileococcygeus and coccygeus muscles, sacrospinous ligament, and the surrounding structures (Fig. 21.5). The sacrospinous ligaments extend from the ischial spines on each side to the lower portion of the sacrum and coccyx. The fibromuscular coccygeus muscle closely overlies the sacrospinous ligament, and thus these structures are often referred to as the sacrospinous ligament complex (C-SSL). We usually perform the apical suspension unilateral to the right C-SSL, but surgeons occasionally use the left C-SSL or perform a bilateral suspension. The C-SSL is identified by palpating the ischial spine and tracing the flat triangular thickening medial and posterior to the sacrum. The pudendal nerves and vessels lie directly posterior to the ischial spine. The sciatic nerve lies superior and lateral to the C-SSL. Also, an abundant vascular supply that includes inferior gluteal vessels and hypogastric venous plexus lies superiorly.

The ischial spines and C-SSL should be palpated preoperatively during pelvic examination. This operation usually requires

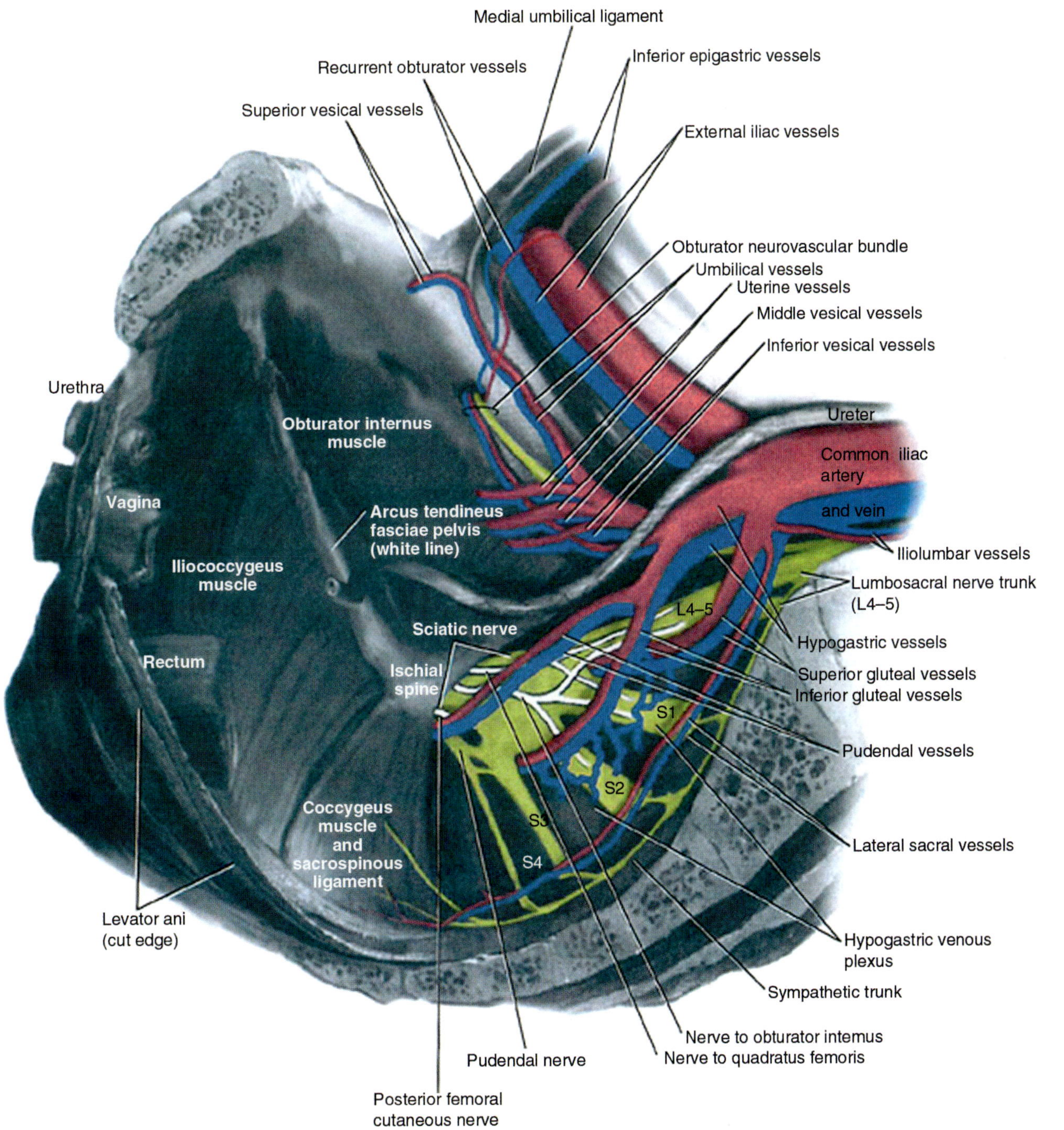

Fig. 21.5 Anatomy surrounding the coccygeus muscle–sacrospinous ligament complex.

simultaneous correction of the anterior and posterior vaginal walls and an enterocele repair. Placing the prolapsed vaginal apex to the sacrospinous ligament to see whether the vagina is long enough to complete the repair and whether the anterior and posterior vaginal wall prolapse is corrected by apical suspension helps to determine whether cystocele and rectocele repairs are needed. Patient consent to these possible repairs should be routinely obtained, because it is frequently difficult to discern the extent of the various defects in the office. The technique of unilateral SSLS is described below. Also, see Video 21.3 for a demonstration of the procedure.

1. If the uterus is present, a vaginal hysterectomy is done, and the peritoneum is closed, as previously described. Sacrospinous cervicopexy or hysteropexy could also be done using similar technique, if desired. (See Chapter 22.)
2. The apex of the vagina is grasped with two Allis clamps, and downward traction is used to determine the extent of the vaginal prolapse and associated vaginal support defects. The vaginal apex then is reduced to the sacrospinous ligament intended to be used. At times the true apex of the vagina at the hysterectomy scar is foreshortened and will not reach the intended area of fixation, as with a shortened anterior vaginal wall and a prominent posterior enterocele. The "new" apex should be moved to a portion of the vaginal wall over the most severe prolapse, thus allowing sufficient vaginal length for suspension to the C-SSL and the even and optimal suspension of the anterior and posterior vaginal walls. The intended apex is tagged with two sutures for later identification.
3. The C-SSL can be accessed via a posterior vaginal dissection, through the apex, or by an anterior approach dissecting at the base of a paravaginal dissection. In the posterior approach a proximal midline posterior vaginal wall incision is made just short of the apex of the vagina, leaving a small vaginal bridge approximately 3 or 4 cm wide. If an enterocele sac is encountered, it is dissected off the rectum and posterior vaginal wall and apex and closed with a high purse string suture.
4. The pararectal space or the space along the peritoneum near the apex then is entered by breaking through the fibroareolar tissue just lateral to the enterocele sac at the level of the ischial spine. This can usually be accomplished with blunt dissection after mobilizing the rectum medially. At times, however, the use of gauze on the index finger or a tonsil clamp is necessary to break into this space.
5. Once the pararectal space is entered, the ischial spine is identified, and, with dorsal and medial movement of the fingers, the C-SSL is palpated. Blunt dissection is used to further remove tissue from this area. The surgeon should take great care to ensure that the rectum is adequately retracted medially. At this time, we recommend performing a rectal examination to ensure that no inadvertent rectal injury has occurred.
6. Several techniques are used for the actual passage of sutures through the ligament. Our preferred technique for passing the sutures through the C-SSL uses a device that places and captures transvaginal sutures (Fig. 21.6A). This technique is safer and easier than other techniques because the device enters the C-SSL under direct palpation of distinct landmarks, proceeding top to bottom, and then is pulled down into the safe pararectal space below. Alternative options for placing the C-SSL sutures are the long-handled Deschamps ligature carrier and nerve hook, the Miya hook, and even direct suturing. To perform this technique on the right, the left middle or index fingertip is placed on the C-SSL just below its superior margin, approximately 2 to 3 cm medial to the ischial spine or in the midposition of the C-SSL. A long retractor such as a Briesky–Navratil retractor can be placed medially to mobilize and protect the rectum if needed. Great care should be taken when dissecting and retracting in this area to prevent bleeding, as well as nerve and rectal damage. The suture-capturing device, held in the right hand in a closed position, is slid along the palmar surface of the left hand. With the tip of the middle finger, the suture-capturing device notch is placed 2 to 3 cm medial to the ischial spine, approximately 0.5 cm below the superior edge. With the middle and index fingers, firm downward pressure is applied, and the device is engaged at the handle, so the needle passer penetrates the C-SSL (Fig. 21.6A). The handle is released, the device is removed with the suture, and the suture is tagged. Depending on the size of the ligament, most surgeons place between two and four sutures through the C-SSL to attach it to the vaginal apex (Fig. 21.6B). There is no consensus about suture type; a combination of delayed absorbable and nonabsorbable monofilament sutures is commonly used.
7. If the patient requires an anterior vaginal wall repair, we prefer performing an anterior colporrhaphy at this point in the operation and before tying the apical support sutures.
8. The surgeon then brings the stitches out to the apex of the vagina, either with the use of a pulley stitch for permanent sutures or by simply passing each pair of sutures through the apex for delayed absorbable sutures (Fig. 21.6B). After the sutures have been brought out through the vagina, the upper portion of the posterior vaginal wall is closed with continuous absorbable No. 2-0 sutures. The vaginal apex suspension stitches then are tied, thus elevating the apex of the vagina to the C-SSL (Fig. 21.6C). It is important that the vagina comes into contact with the C-SSL and that no suture bridge exists, especially if delayed absorbable sutures are being used. While tying these sutures, it may be useful to perform a rectal examination to detect any suture bridges.
9. After these sutures are tied, an anti-incontinence procedure and a posterior colpoperineorrhaphy are completed, as needed. The vagina can be packed with moist gauze for 24 hours, if desired.
10. The risk of ureteral obstruction or kinking is extremely low with sacrospinous ligament fixation. However, we still recommend cystourethroscopy, particularly if a concomitant enterocele repair, anterior colporrhaphy, or anti-incontinence procedure is performed, to confirm ureteral patency and absence of suture in the bladder.

Observational series and clinical trials suggest that, while apical recurrence after SSLS is uncommon (0.6%–19%), recurrence of anterior vaginal prolapse is more problematic (3.7%–28.5%) (Maher et al., 2016a). A meta-analysis by Morgan et al. (2007) found an overall failure rate at any site

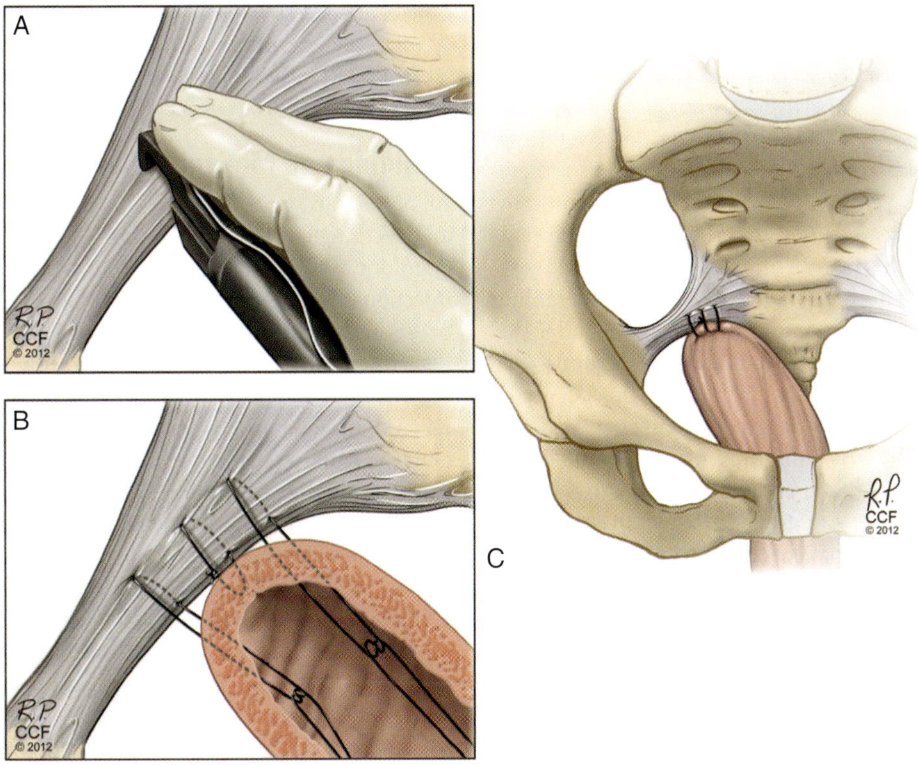

Fig. 21.6 Sacrospinous ligament suspension. **A**, Placement of the suture-capturing device with suture against the coccygeus muscle–sacrospinous ligament complex (C-SSL). Note that needle tip is passed downward from above. **B**, Three sutures are placed through the C-SSL; in this figure, the middle suture is nonabsorbable, so it is passed through the muscularis, and the knot buried. **C**, Final attachment of the vagina to the C-SSL. (Illustration by Ross Papalardo. Reprinted with permission, Cleveland Clinic Center for Medical Art & Photography © 2012–2013. All rights reserved; From Walters MD, Ridgeway BM. Surgical treatment of vaginal apex prolapse. *Obstet Gynecol.* 2013;121:354.)

of 28.8% (95% CI 18.4–36.3) with failure of the anterior segment seen in 21.3% (95% CI 17.3–25.3), apical segment 7.2% (95% CI 4.0–10.4), and posterior segment 6.3% (95% CI 4.2–8.4). Whether the relatively high rate of anterior vaginal prolapse recurrence seen with SSLS is caused by the posterior deflection of the vaginal axis or simply represents a general predilection of anterior support to fail after pelvic reconstructive surgery remains unknown. Reoperation rates after SSLS range from 1.3% to 37%, with the majority of studies reporting rates less than 9% (Maher et al., 2016a).

Maher et al. (2004) demonstrated significant improvements in condition-specific and generic quality of life after SSLS, similar to those seen after abdominal sacral colpopexy. A meta-analysis of randomized and observational studies found a pooled average for failure to provide relief of prolapse symptoms after SSLS of 10.3% (95% CI 4.4–16.2) (Morgan et al., 2007). The pooled average for failure to provide patient satisfaction after SSLS in this analysis was 13% (95% CI 7.4–18.6). Although infrequent, serious complications associated with SSLS include buttock pain and sacral/pudendal neurovascular injury. Unilateral buttock/gluteal pain occurs in 3% to 15% of patients and typically resolves within 6 weeks after surgery. In one multicenter trial, neurologic pain requiring medical or surgical intervention occurred in 12.4% immediately after SSLS and persisted in 4.3% at 4 to 6 weeks after surgery. In a review of 22 studies that included 1229 SSLS procedures, three patients (0.2%) had life-threatening hemorrhage from sacral or pudendal vascular injury, and the overall transfusion rate was 2% (Sze & Karram, 1997).

Comparing Uterosacral and Sacrospinous Ligament Suspensions. In 2014, the National Institutes of Health–funded Pelvic Floor Disorders Network reported the results of the OPTIMAL trial, whose primary objective was to compare the safety and efficacy of the SSLS to ULS in women with uterine or posthysterectomy apical prolapse (Barber et al., 2014). The original trial reported outcomes at 2 years, but 5-year outcomes have now been reported (Jelovsek et al., 2018). To date, this is the only randomized trial to compare these two commonly performed procedures. Success was defined as a composite outcome measurement and included the absence of: (1) descent of the vaginal apex more than one-third of the vaginal canal; (2) anterior or posterior vaginal wall descent beyond the hymen; (3) bothersome vaginal bulge symptoms as reported by the Pelvic Floor Distress Inventory; and (4) retreatment with surgery or a pessary. A total of 374 patients were randomized (188 ULS and 186 SSLS) from nine US centers. Two years after surgery, there was no statistical difference between the two groups for the composite outcome (ULS 64.5% versus SSLS 63.1%; adjusted odds ratio [OR] 1.1; 95% CI 0.7–1.7).

Additionally, bothersome vaginal bulge symptoms were seen in 18%, anterior or posterior prolapse beyond the hymen in 17.5%, and retreatment with pessary or surgery in 5.1% 2 years postoperatively, with no differences between groups. By 5 years, although surgical success rates continued to decline over time (61.5% in the ULS group and 70.3% in the SSLS group), there were no differences between groups, and pelvic floor symptom improvements and quality of life remained clinically relevant and similar to the results from 1 and 2 years after surgery (Jelovsek et al., 2018). The proportion of women undergoing retreatment for prolapse by 5 years was 11.9% for ULS and 8.1% for SSLS, with no significant difference between the groups.

Almost all surgical adverse events in both groups occurred within the first 2 years. Neurological pain requiring medical, behavioral, or surgical intervention was higher in the SSLS group (12.4% vs. 6.9%, $P = .049$) and persisted to 4 to 6 weeks in more participants (4.3% vs. 0.5%). Intraoperative ureteral obstruction was noted in five patients (3.2%) in the ULS group and none in the SSLS. Granulation tissue at the postsurgical vaginal cuff was higher in the ULS group than in the SSLS group.

Iliococcygeus Fascia Suspension

In women for whom the surgeon is unable to enter the peritoneal cavity safely or whose vaginal length does not allow the apex to reach the sacrospinous ligament, an iliococcygeus fascia suspension can be considered. This procedure has not undergone as rigorous an evaluation of safety and efficacy as either SSLS or ULS. Bilateral fixation of the prolapsed vaginal apex to the iliococcygeus fascia just below the ischial spines is a useful and effective technique in such circumstances. It can also be considered if the vagina is somewhat foreshortened, but the posterior apex needs additional support during a rectocele repair. The technique of this repair is as follows:

1. The posterior vaginal wall is opened in the midline as for a posterior colporrhaphy, and the rectovaginal spaces are dissected widely to the bilateral levator muscles.
2. The dissection is extended bluntly toward the ischial spines.
3. With the surgeon's nondominant hand depressing the rectum downward and medially, an area 1 to 2 cm caudad and posterior to the ischial spine in the iliococcygeus muscle and fascia is exposed (Fig. 21.7). A single No. 0 delayed absorbable suture is placed deep into the levator muscle and fascia. Both ends of the suture are then passed through the ipsilateral posterior vaginal apex and held with a hemostat. This is repeated on the opposite side.
4. The posterior colporrhaphy is completed, and the vagina is closed. Both sutures are tied, elevating the posterior vaginal apices.

There are no randomized trials that support the use of this procedure. Several case series have provided some information. In a retrospective case-control study, Maher and colleagues (2001) reported similar subjective (91% vs. 94%) and objective (53% vs. 67%) cure rates with iliococcygeus suspension ($n = 50$) compared with SSLS ($n = 78$). A prospective cohort of 44 subjects receiving iliococcygeus suspension followed for a median of 68.8 (range 60–92) months provides the longest-term data on this procedure (Serati et al., 2015). The rates of objective success (POPQ stage 0 or 1) and subjective success (patient global impression of improvement <2) were both 84%. Preoperative stage 4 vault prolapse was an independent predictor of failure (OR 8.8; 95% CI 1.3–9.4).

Avoiding and Managing Complications

All of the transvaginal surgeries involve dissection of vesicovaginal and rectovaginal spaces, and thus have small risks of bleeding, cystotomy, and proctotomy. Postoperative vaginal or pelvic infections, voiding difficulties, and urinary tract infections can occasionally occur but are short-lived. The most worrisome complication with ULS is ureteral compromise. The risk of ureteral obstruction is approximately 2% to 4%, and most obstructions are relieved intraoperatively if recognized during cystoscopy. It is imperative that intraoperative cystoscopy be done after tying the suspension sutures to ensure ureteral patency. If ureteral spill is not observed, then the sutures on that side should be cut and removed, and the ureter reevaluated. Often, the suture can be replaced using a more medial placement into the uterosacral ligament complex.

Unique but serious intraoperative complications can occur, especially with SSLS. Potential complications of the procedure include hemorrhage, nerve injury, and rectal injury. Video 21.4 discusses the prevention and management of complications associated with SSLS. Severe hemorrhage with blood transfusion can result from overzealous dissection superior to the coccygeus muscle or ischial spine. This can result in hemorrhage from the inferior gluteal vessels, hypogastric venous plexus, or pudendal vessels. Hemorrhage from these vessels can be difficult to control. For this reason, we prefer limited, careful dissection on top of (but not behind) the C-SSL. We also use the transvaginal suture-capturing technique, in which the needle tip is passed downward toward the muscle, rather than the technique using the Deschamps ligature carrier, in which the needle tip is passed superiorly toward the vasculature. If severe bleeding occurs in the area around the coccygeus muscle, we recommend initially packing the area. If this does not control the bleeding, then visualization, attempted ligation with clips or sutures, and use of thrombin products should be performed. This area is difficult to approach transabdominally or with selective embolization, so bleeding should be controlled vaginally, if possible.

Moderate to severe buttock pain on the side on which the sacrospinous suspension was performed can occur; this also has been reported after uterosacral suspension. This is probably caused by compression or injury of a small nerve that runs through the C-SSL or, in cases of USL, the sacral plexus (Siddiqui et al., 2006). The buttock pain is almost always self-limiting and should resolve completely by 6 weeks postoperatively. Reassurance and antiinflammatory agents usually are all that is necessary. Because of the close proximity of the pudendal nerves (and vessels) lateral to the C-SSL, the potential for injury is present, so dissection and suturing should avoid the ischial spine. If pudendal nerve injury occurs with postoperative symptoms of unilateral vulvar pain and/or numbness, immediate reoperation with removal of the offending suture material may be necessary.

Rectal examination should be performed frequently during all transvaginal repairs because of the close proximity of the rectum to vaginal dissection and colpopexy sutures. Rectal injury can

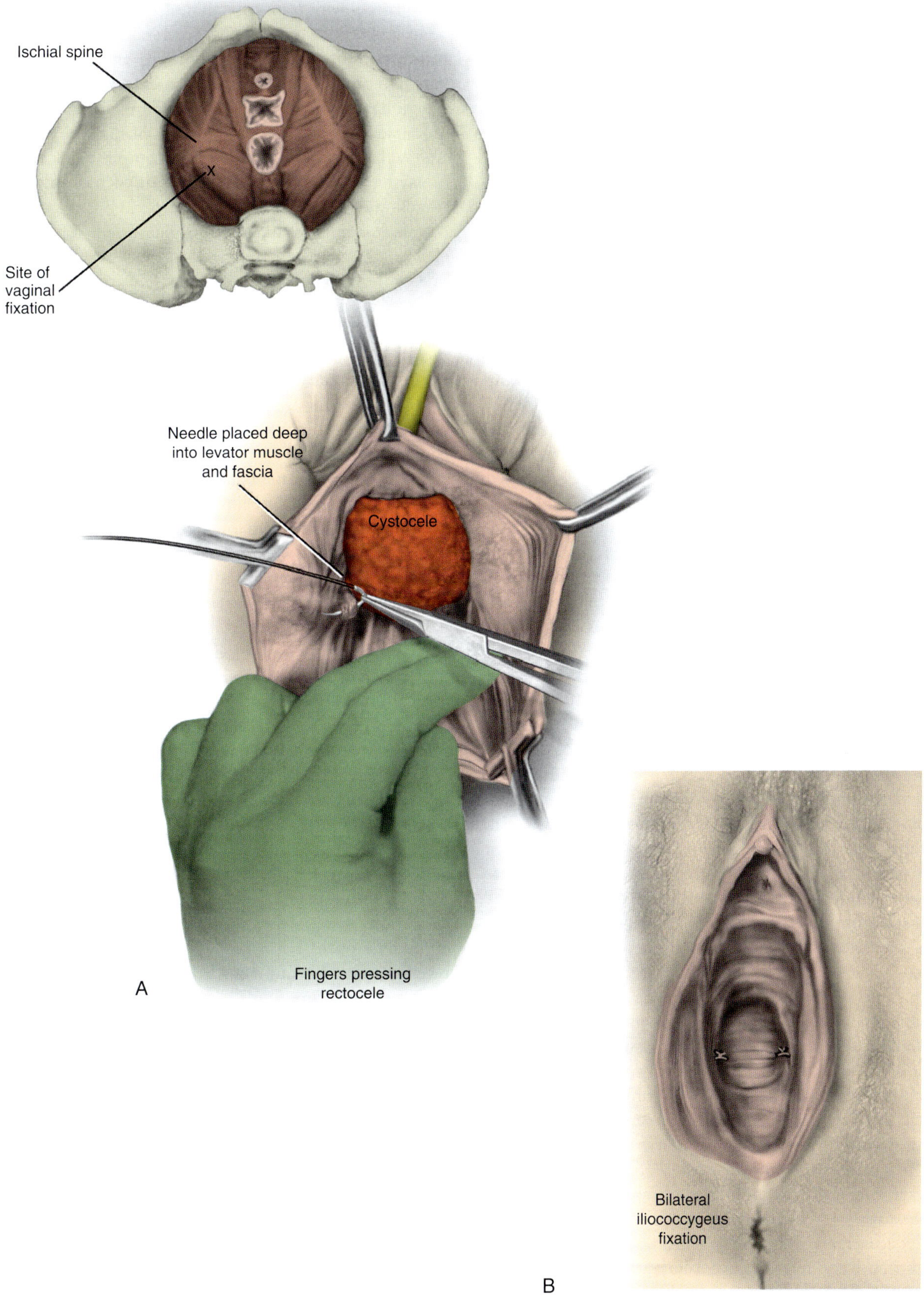

Fig. 21.7 Iliococcygeus fascia suspension. **A**, With the surgeon's finger pressing the rectum downward, the right iliococcygeus fascia suture is placed. Approximate location of the iliococcygeus fascia sutures (*inset*). **B**, Bilateral iliococcygeus fascia suspension.

occur when entering the pararectal space, as well as during mobilization of tissue off of the C-SSL. If a rectal injury is identified, it can usually be repaired primarily transvaginally by conventional techniques. Small-bowel obstruction also has been reported after transvaginal colpopexy, but is rare.

Vaginal stenosis and dyspareunia can occur if too much anterior and posterior vaginal wall tissue is trimmed, if the vagina is left too short, or if a tight posterior colporrhaphy is performed. We recommend postoperative use of estrogen vaginal cream and vaginal dilators in these patients in the hope of preventing or decreasing the incidence of this problem.

TRANSVAGINAL MESH PROCEDURES

In 2004, prepackaged kits to place mesh transvaginally were introduced, initially using longitudinal midline incisions in the vaginal epithelium and trocars to attach mesh or graft bilaterally to the arcus tendineus fasciae pelvis or sacrospinous ligaments. Later modifications allowed for smaller vaginal incisions not overlying the mesh and used direct suturing to the sacrospinous ligament rather than trocars. These procedures were advocated to allow the advantages of a transvaginal approach while augmenting the native tissue, with the goal of reducing prolapse recurrence and improving the durability of the repair. The majority of mesh kits have been marketed and used for anterior vaginal prolapse or anterior and apical prolapse. For more details of their use and outcomes for the anterior compartment, see Chapter 19.

The vaginal mesh kits were introduced to market through the US Food and Drug Administration (FDA)'s 510K process that allows manufacturers to reference a predicate device and describe how their product is "substantially equivalent" to the previously cleared device. This process specifically did not require premarket approval (PMA), whereby the device companies would need to demonstrate, typically in a randomized trial, both safety and efficacy. The majority of published research studies, particularly in the first 10 years after introduction, were case series and retrospective studies. There were, however, some notable randomized trials comparing various vaginal mesh products to native tissue repair.

The Cochrane Collaboration identified six randomized trials comparing native tissue vaginal repairs with transvaginal polypropylene mesh for apical prolapse in 589 women (Maher et al., 2016b). In all six of these trials, the native tissue repair included an SSLS or ULS, and the mesh was polypropylene (four trials of monofilament weave and two trials of multifilament weave). No significant differences in anatomic outcomes, vaginal bulge symptoms, repeat surgery for prolapse, dyspareunia, or postoperative stress urinary incontinence were noted between groups. The average rate of mesh exposure after transvaginal mesh was 18%, and surgery for mesh exposure was required in 9.5% of patients. Success rates of transvaginal meshes for apical prolapse from prospective and retrospective cohorts ranges from 87% to 100% for monofilament polypropylene meshes, with mesh exposure rates varying from 0% to 15% (Maher et al., 2016a). A systematic review by Schimpf et al. (2016) identified only three comparative studies that focused specifically on apical prolapse (as opposed to anterior prolapse), and found no improvement in outcomes with transvaginal mesh.

In addition to the complications inherent to all transvaginal prolapse repairs, unique complications can occur for transvaginal mesh procedures related to the mesh or trocars. Mesh-related functional complications such as chronic pelvic pain, leg and groin pain, vaginal pain, and dyspareunia have all been reported. A systematic review that evaluated complications and reoperations after vaginal apex surgical repair demonstrated that the overall rate of reoperation (for complications and for recurrent prolapse) is highest after transvaginal mesh repair (Diwadkar et al., 2009). Exposure of mesh through the vaginal epithelium is one of the most common complications; the Cochrane review reported an overall exposure rate of 10%. At least half of mesh exposures are symptomatic and require reoperation for treatment. Notably, mesh exposure rates for nontrocar mesh devices, introduced after 2008 (Elevate, American Medical Systems, Minnetonka, MN; Uphold, Boston Scientific, Natick, MA), were generally lower than those noted with older devices (0%–5.7%) based on the limited data available.

Long-term outcome data after mesh-augmented and native tissue vaginal repairs are limited. Adequately powered randomized controlled trials with long-term outcomes that include prolapse symptoms, as well as anatomic and functional outcomes, are required. Nager et al. (2019) performed a randomized trial comparing Uphold Lite (Boston Scientific) hysteropexy to vaginal hysterectomy with ULS. Of the 183 randomized participants, 169 completed the 3-year follow-up. After 3 years of follow-up, they concluded that vaginal mesh hysteropexy compared with vaginal hysterectomy with ULS did not result in a significantly lower rate of the composite prolapse outcome after 3 years. However, results from the extended follow-up of this trial showed fewer failures for hysteropexy compared to hysterectomy and USLS through 5 years (adjusted hazard ratio, 0.58 [95% CI, 0.36–0.94], $P = .03$) with failure rates of 37% versus 54%, respectively, resulting in a difference of –18% (95% CI, –33% to –3%) at 5 years (Nager et al., 2021). Hysteropexy mesh exposure rate was 8%, and, remarkably, no participant required reoperation for mesh exposure.

Because of the type of FDA approval transvaginal mesh kits received, the high number of complications encountered in a relatively short time, and the lack of superior clinically significant prolapse symptom outcomes, the FDA issued a Public Health Notice in 2008 and a Safety Communication in 2011. The 2008 document reported that "serious complications associated with surgical mesh for transvaginal repair of (pelvic organ prolapse) were rare," but the 2011 Safety Communication described these complications as "not rare" and stated that "it is not clear that transvaginal (pelvic organ prolapse) repair with mesh is more effective than traditional non-mesh repair" and made recommendations for physicians to explicitly disclose to patients a variety of risks.

In 2012, the FDA issued a series of 522 orders requiring manufacturers to perform additional postmarket surveillance studies that included mandatory deadlines. In 2016 the FDA upclassified vaginal mesh for prolapse repair to a class III medical device requiring PMA. In April 2019, the FDA ordered manufacturers of vaginal mesh products to stop selling and distributing their products in the United States because the results from the 522 mandated research studies were not available by the predetermined deadline, partially because of slower than expected recruitment. The future of transvaginal mesh is uncertain. In a joint Committee Opinion published in December 2011, the American Urogynecologic Society and the American College of Obstetricians and Gynecologists recommended that pelvic organ prolapse vaginal mesh repair should be reserved for high-risk individuals in whom the benefit of mesh placement may justify the risk, such as individuals with recurrent anterior prolapse or with medical comorbidities that preclude more invasive and lengthier open and endoscopic procedures. This Committee Opinion was retracted by both Societies after the FDA's 2019 mandate to stop sale and distribution of transvaginal mesh products. Although the manufacturers could choose to resubmit the results of the 522 studies when completed under the same PMA, their intentions are unclear. Thus, as of the writing of this chapter, any use of a synthetic or biologic graft or mesh transvaginally for apical vaginal prolapse repair is considered "off-label" use and should be carried out with caution. Careful and thorough informed consent is required. See Chapters 7 and 25 for further details of synthetic mesh/grafts and management of their complications.

SACROCOLPOPEXY

In 2010, approximately 34,000 sacrocolpopexies were performed in the United States, representing 11% of all prolapse surgeries performed during that time period. Sacrocolpopexy can be performed through laparotomy or by laparoscopy with or without robotic assistance. Although the surgical approach may be different, the steps of the procedure should remain fundamentally the same. Sacrocolpopexy, the suspension of the vagina using a bridging graft to the anterior longitudinal ligament, distal and inferior to the sacral promontory, is an effective treatment for uterovaginal and vaginal apex prolapse. Many different materials have been used as sacrocolpopexy graft, including biologic materials (fascia lata, rectus fascia, dura mater) and synthetic materials (polypropylene mesh, polyester fiber mesh, polytetrafluorethylene mesh, Dacron mesh, and Silastic silicone rubber). Large-pore, lightweight polypropylene mesh is most commonly used and likely causes fewer complications compared with other synthetics because of its monofilament and macroporous characteristics.

Randomized trials comparing objective anatomic outcomes after sacrocolpopexy demonstrated that polypropylene mesh was superior to cadaveric fascia lata in terms of objective POPQ measurements, prolapse stage, and objective anatomic failure rates at 1 and 5 years after surgery (Culligan et al., 2005; Tate et al., 2011).

Abdominal Sacrocolpopexy

The technique of abdominal sacrocolpopexy (ASC) using graft placement is as follows:

1. The patient should be placed in low lithotomy position using Allen stirrups so that the surgeon has access to the vagina during the operation. A uterine manipulator, sponge stick, or end-to-end anastomosis (EEA) sizer can be placed in the vagina for manipulation of the apex. A Foley catheter is placed into the bladder for drainage.
2. Intraperitoneal access is gained using either an open incision or laparoscopic or robotic cannula placement. Small bowel is placed or packed into the upper abdomen, and the sigmoid colon is deviated to the left pelvis as much as possible. The ureters are identified bilaterally. A supracervical or total hysterectomy may be performed first in the case of uterovaginal prolapse.
3. Elevation of the vaginally placed EEA sizer nicely identifies the prolapsed vaginal vault (Fig. 21.8A). We perform the vaginal dissection next. The vagina is elevated cephalad using an EEA sizer, and the bladder is dissected sharply off the anterior vaginal wall for approximately 4 to 8 cm. To avoid a cystotomy, care should be taken to identify the location of the proximal edge of the bladder, as the bladder can occasionally be adherent over the vaginal apex and to the posterior vaginal wall. If this plane is difficult to establish, the bladder can be retrograde-filled with fluid to delineate its border, or the Foley bulb proximally can be manipulated to help designate the bladder/vagina interface.
4. We next dissect the posterior vaginal wall, starting at the reflection of the rectum, and create a U-shaped incision in the posterior peritoneum. Removal of the peritoneum over the posterior vagina is unnecessary and may weaken the posterior vaginal wall. We extend the peritoneal dissection bilaterally to create flaps that will later be used to retroperitonealize the mesh. We expose the posterior peritoneum for 6 to 8 cm to create adequate attachment of the mesh along the posterior vaginal wall toward the perineal body. Some experts recommend dissecting to the perineal body. We prefer to reserve this for women with rectal prolapse or severe defecatory dysfunction, because a permanent graft in the distal vagina can be problematic and does not increase symptomatic improvement for the average patient. We routinely evaluate the distal posterior vagina after sacrocolpopexy and use a native tissue repair if indicated. In the rare situation where delineation of the rectum is difficult, a second EEA sizer can be placed in the rectum. Manipulating the two EEA sizers in the vagina and rectum so that the tips are apart can define the rectovaginal septum.
5. Attention is turned to the sacrum. The aortic bifurcation, the common and internal iliac vessels, the sigmoid colon, and the right ureter are identified so that these structures can be avoided (Fig. 21.8B). The left common iliac vein is medial to the left common iliac artery and is particularly vulnerable to damage during this portion of the surgery. A longitudinal incision is made in the peritoneum just distal to the sacral promontory.
6. The L5/S1 disc is present at the sacral promontory, so we purposefully dissect the anterior longitudinal ligament distally for approximately 4 cm using blunt and sharp dissection. It is preferable to dissect deep and posterior to the subperitoneal fat pad overlying the sacrum. Special care should be taken to avoid the delicate plexus of presacral veins that often are present, especially as one dissects more caudally. The middle sacral artery and vein should be identified (Fig. 21.8B) and avoided or coagulated using bipolar energy.

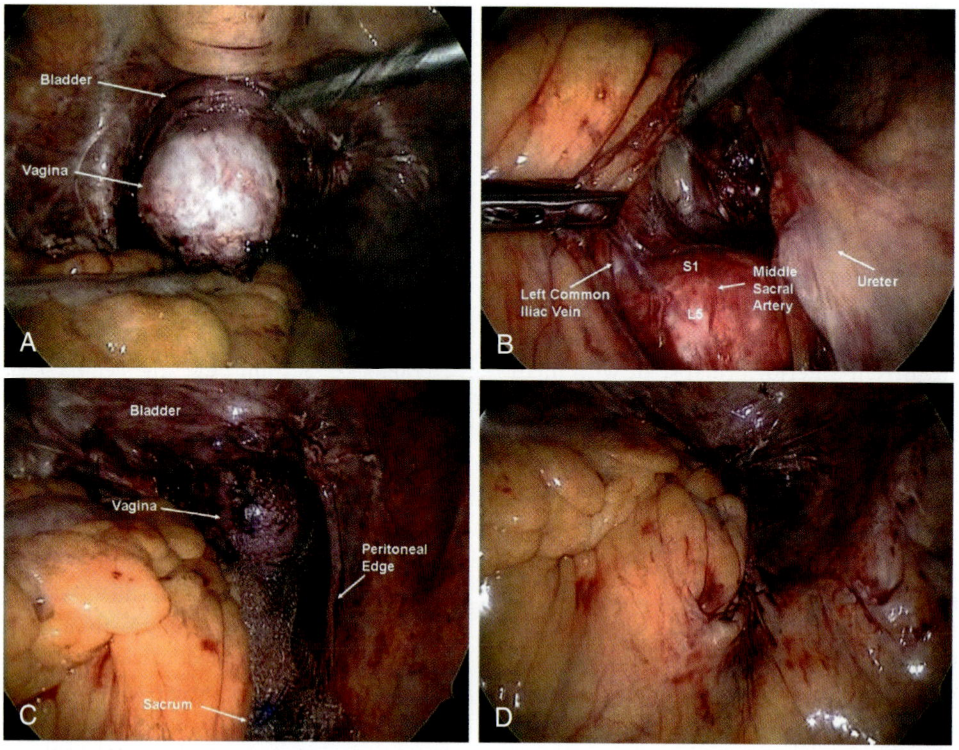

Fig. 21.8 Steps of sacrocolpopexy. **A**, The bladder and rectum have been dissected from the vagina. A probe provides shape and stability to the vagina during this process. **B**, This view of the sacral promontory demonstrates where the mesh will be attached and the proximity to vital structures. **C**, The polypropylene mesh has been attached to the anterior and posterior vaginal walls as well as the sacral promontory. **D**, The peritoneum is closed over the graft. (From Walters MD, Ridgeway BM. Surgical treatment of vaginal apex prolapse. *Obstet Gynecol.* 2013;121:354.)

7. The peritoneal incision overlying the sacrum is extended distally to create a space to retroperitonealize the mesh to reduce the risk of SBO. Some recommend the creation of a subperitoneal tunnel, but this practice has been associated with large bowel injury. During these processes, the rectum and right ureter are visualized at all times, and the course of the dissection is located between these structures.
8. A graft is prepared. We recommend a lightweight polypropylene mesh. If this comes in a sheet, two strips measuring 4 × 15 cm can be created. Alternatively, a prefabricated "Y mesh" can be used. The graft is cut to 6 to 8 cm in length anteriorly and 6 to 9 cm in length posteriorly. The mesh is attached to the anterior vaginal wall with five to eight nonabsorbable No. 0 or 2-0 sutures 1 to 2 cm apart. Sutures are placed through the full fibromuscular thickness of the vagina but not into the vaginal epithelium. The graft should extend approximately halfway down the length of the anterior vaginal wall (Figs. 21.8C and 21.9).
9. The posterior mesh is then attached in a similar fashion.
10. Some recommend using delayed absorbable sutures to attach the mesh to vagina to reduce the risk of mesh or suture exposure, assuming that the long-term strength of this repair is primarily dependent on scarring of the mesh to the vaginal walls.
11. The vagina is elevated with the EEA sizer and deviated toward the sacral promontory. The appropriate amount of vaginal elevation is determined that provides gentle mesh tension without undue traction on the vagina. The graft should be trimmed to the appropriate length, allowing ample mesh to attach all sacral sutures to the anterior longitudinal ligament of the sacrum. Using a stiff but small half-curved tapered needle with a permanent No. 0 suture, two to four sutures are used to attach the mesh to the anterior longitudinal ligament of the sacrum (Fig. 21.9).
12. The peritoneum then is closed over the exposed graft with absorbable sutures (Fig. 21.8D).
13. An antiincontinence procedure, if planned, is performed. Cystoscopy is performed after the administration of indigo carmine to evaluate bladder integrity and to confirm ureteral patency.
14. Posterior colporrhaphy, perineoplasty, and, rarely, anterior colporrhaphy are performed as needed to treat any remaining vaginal defect.

Minimally Invasive Sacrocolpopexy: Laparoscopic and Robotic-Assisted Approaches

Operative Setup and Instrumentation. Patent positioning is particularly important for laparoscopic and robotic cases that place the patient in Trendelenburg to prevent patients from sliding toward the head of the bed and avoid nerve injuries. A variety of products are available that pad or cushion the patient's

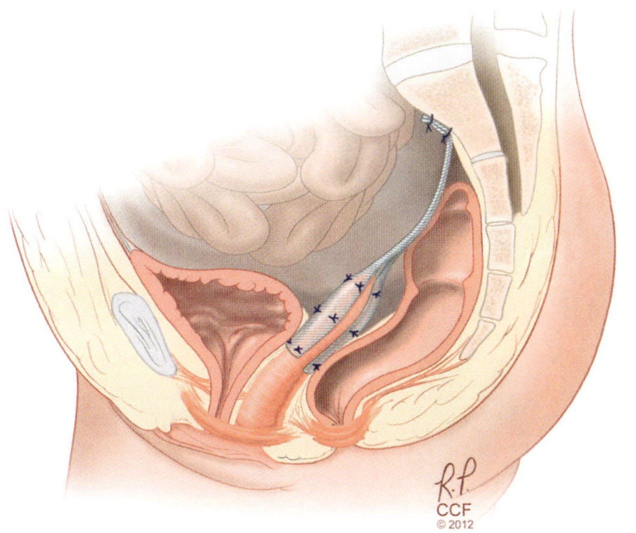

Fig. 21.9 Lateral view of completed sacrocolpopexy with graft attaching the anterior and posterior vagina to the sacral promontory. (Illustration by Ross Papalardo. Reprinted with permission, Cleveland Clinic Center for Medical Art & Photography © 2012–2013. All rights reserved; From Walters MD, Ridgeway BM. Surgical treatment of vaginal apex prolapse. *Obstet Gynecol.* 2013;121:354.)

arms with gel pads or foam. Some are available as kits or all-in-one solutions. Shoulder braces are another option, but we do not recommend these, as they have been associated with brachial plexus injuries. Careful attention is paid to extremity positioning to prevent peripheral nerve injuries. Regardless of product used, the minimum amount of Trendelenburg necessary to allow the bowel to move and remain in the upper abdomen should be used. Repositioning during robotic procedures, specifically after docking, has been prohibited, because the robot and the operating room table were not synced. However, the newest da Vinci Xi robot (Intuitive, Sunnyvale, CA) has an option that allows it to be paired with a Trumpf operating room table (Trumpf Medical, Saalfeld, Germany). This allows the surgeon to adjust the operating room table during a surgical procedure because the operating room table and the robot move in sync using this particular setup.

Consistent with Association of periOperative Registered Nurses (AORN) guidelines, the patient's hands and arms are typically tucked with the wrist in a neutral, thumbs-up position. Ideal stirrups for combined laparoscopic/vaginal cases are the Allen stirrups and Yellofins (Allen Medical Systems, Acton, MA), which have levers that can quickly adjust the degree of lithotomy positioning, while preserving the sterility of the field. Attention should be paid to avoiding compression of the lower extremity, including the lateral knee near the fibular prominence, to minimize risk of nerve injury.

The umbilicus is approximately at the L3 to L4 level, and the aortic bifurcation is at L4 to L5. In obese women, the umbilicus is caudal to the bifurcation. Thus, for maximal safety, the intraumbilical trocar should be introduced at a more acute angle toward the pelvis in thin women and closer to 90 degrees in obese women. It is important not to track when placing trocars, particularly with obese patients. The inferior epigastric artery branches from the external iliac artery at the medial border of the inguinal ligament and runs laterally to and below the rectus sheath at the level of the arcuate line. Inferior epigastric veins accompany the artery. Computed tomography studies of abdominal wall vasculature show that, above the pubic symphysis, the inferior and superficial epigastric vessels are 5.6 $\pm$ 1.0 cm and 5.5 $\pm$ 2.0 cm from the midline, respectively (Hurd et al., 1994). The inferior epigastric vessels course along the parietal peritoneum proximally and anastomose with the superior epigastric vessels, the terminal branches of the internal mammary vessels. Given the anatomic anastomoses, if these vessels are compromised and bleeding ensues, it is often necessary to ligate the vessels superior to and inferior to the vessel injury.

The operating room setup for laparoscopic pelvic surgery is shown in Fig. 21.10. The monitor screens should be placed laterally to the legs in direct view of the bedside surgeons standing on the opposite side of the table. The scrub nurse should have an unobstructed view of a monitor screen as well. A sterile pouch attached to each thigh is equipped with commonly used instruments, such as monopolar scissors, bipolar cautery or vessel sealing device, graspers, and laparoscopic blunt-tipped dissectors. The irrigation should be set up before making incisions for trocars in the event hemorrhage is encountered during the placement of the initial trocars. Incisions are made depending on the anatomy of the umbilicus and if any previous abdominal wall surgeries have been performed, particularly if abdominal wall mesh was placed. After the insertion of the camera laparoscope (0 or 30 degrees) through the umbilical trocar, intraperitoneal insufflation is commenced, and a thorough inspection of the peritoneal cavity is performed, delineating the inferior epigastric vessels just lateral to the medial umbilical folds, abdominal and pelvic organs, pelvic adhesions, and coexisting abdominal or pelvic pathology.

Laparoscopic Sacrocolpopexy (See Video 21.5). Many variations of the accessory trocar sites have been described. We use two additional trocars: a 5/12-mm disposable trocar with reducer in the right lower quadrant (if knot-tying from the right) lateral to the right inferior epigastric vessels and a 5-mm port or an additional 5/12-mm disposable trocar, with reducer in the left lower quadrant lateral to the left inferior epigastric vessels. We close the fascia of all trocars 10 mm or greater regardless of location. Trocars are placed laterally to the rectus muscle, approximately 3 cm medial to and above the anterior superior iliac spine. One or two additional 5-mm ports are placed at the level of the umbilicus, lateral to the rectus muscle for simultaneous suturing and/or retraction (Fig. 21.11A).

An additional 5-mm port may be placed on the principal surgeon's side so that he or she can operate with two hands. Both reusable and disposable ports may be secured with circumferential screws to prevent port slippage. In addition, both 5- and 10-mm balloon ports exist (Kii Fios First Entry with Advanced Fixation Cannula, Applied Medical, Rancho Santa Margarita, CA), where insufflation of a circumferential

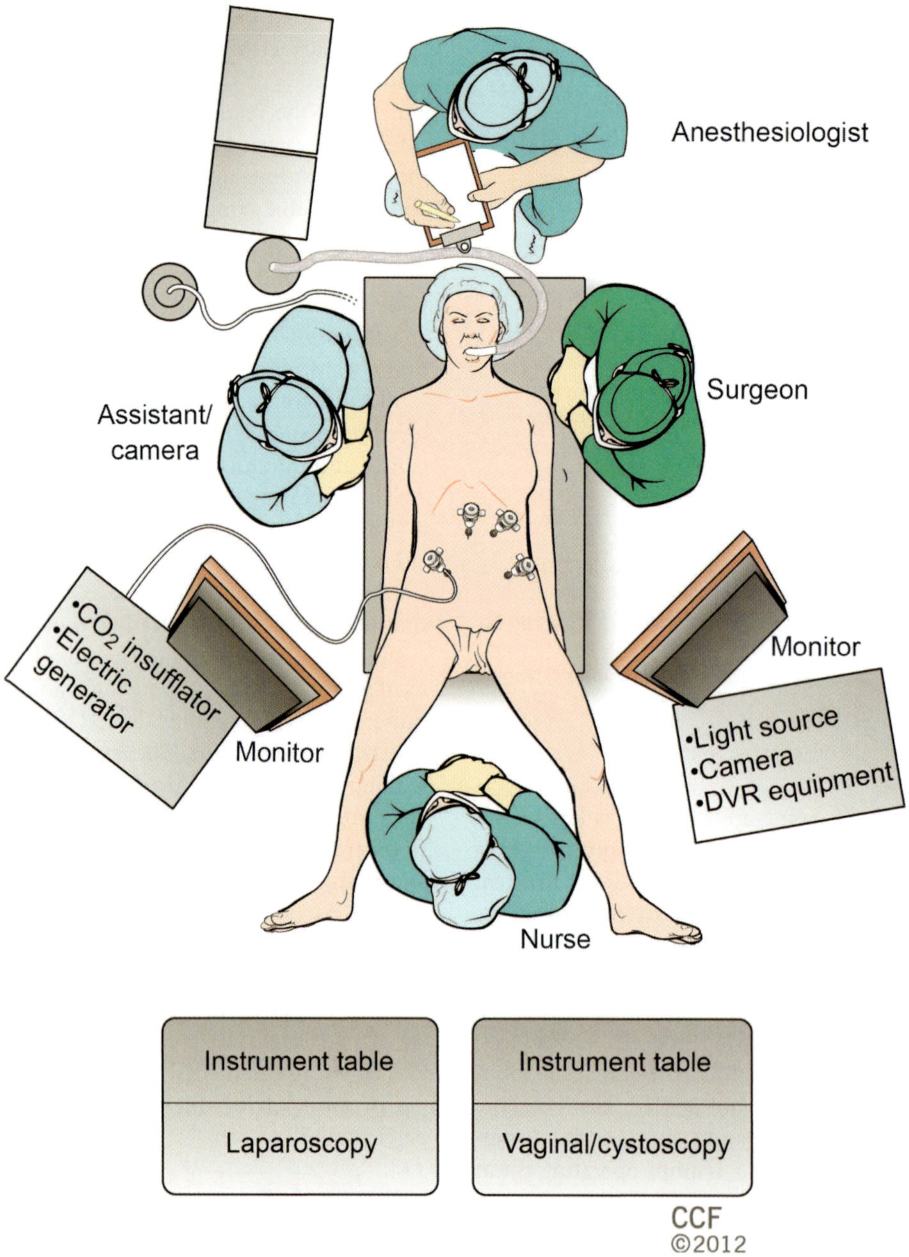

Fig. 21.10 Operating room setup for operative laparoscopy. *DVR*, Digital video recording.

intraperitoneal balloon helps to maintain the port's intraperitoneal location with port manipulation and instrument exchanges. Port placement is shown in (Fig. 21.11A).

For the standard suturing technique, the needle holder preference is determined by comfort of the surgeon. Conventional and 90-degree self-righting German needle holders (Ethicon Endo-Surgery, Inc., Cincinnati, OH) have ratchet spring handles. The Storz Scarfi needle holder and notched assistant needle holder (Karl Storz Endoscopy, El Segundo, CA) are similar to conventional needle holders used during laparotomy. However, the handles can be difficult to maintain and may pop open after extended use. The needle holder tips may become magnetized, which hampers needle grasping. Disposable suturing devices, such as the Endo-stitch (Covidien Surgical, Dublin, Ireland), have been introduced, but its needle is short and straight and does not allow for the same degree of tissue purchase as a curved surgical needle. Extracorporeal knot-tying is generally preferred because of technical ease and the ability to maintain tension on the suture. The choice of an open-ended or close-ended knot pusher for extracorporeal knot-tying depends on surgeon preference. Other options for knot-tying include various premade knots, such as clinch knots that do not require knot pushers and intracorporeal knots.

Some surgeons have chosen to avoid knot-tying altogether by securing the mesh with a barbed suture (Quill by Angiotech, Vancouver, BC and V-Loc by Covidien, Boulder, CO) and using a tacking device to tack the mesh into the anterior longitudinal ligament. Although the use of barbed suture could greatly improve efficiency, there are potential risks of bowel obstruction with the use of barbed suture to close the peritoneum and

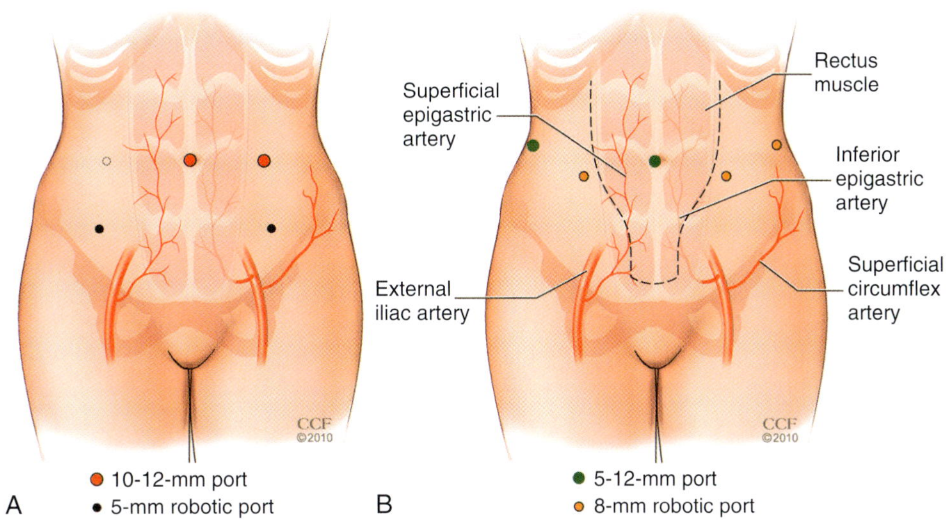

Fig. 21.11 Anatomy of the anterior abdominal wall and relationship to suggested laparoscopic (**A**) and robotic (**B**) port sites.

vaginal cuff. Lumbosacral osteomyelitis and spondylodiscitis are rare but devastating complications of sacrocolpopexy. Fewer than 40 cases have been reported in the literature, and most are related to sutures, not tacks, placed in the presacral space (Grimes et al., 2012; Roth & Reight, 2012; Collins et al., 2011; Muffly et al., 2010; Gungor Ugurlucan et al., 2019). If placed at or proximal to the sacral promontory, bone tacks or curved needles may penetrate the intervertebral disc or disc space and could increase the risk of lumbosacral osteomyelitis and spondylodiscitis.

If exposure of the sacral promontory and presacral space is not adequate, the bed should be airplaned to the left, and a reusable triangle retractor (Snowden Pencer, Tucker, GA) or fan retractor (Origin Medsystems, Menlo Park, CA) can be placed through an ancillary port. Suture can also be passed through several sigmoid epiploica and brought through the left lower quadrant lateral to the left lower quadrant port site with a Carter Thomason suture carrier. Both suture ends are secured with minimal tension at the skin surface with a Kelly clamp, retracting the sigmoid laterally. Once the sigmoid is adequately retracted, the peritoneum overlying the sacral promontory is incised longitudinally with laparoscopic scissors and extended to the cul-de-sac. Some surgeons prefer to first dissect the presacral space, thus first focusing on the most technically difficult portion of the procedure. If blood vessels are encountered during the dissection, coagulation or clip placement is used to achieve hemostasis. The need for or efficacy of a culdoplasty is controversial, because review of the literature shows no improved cure or decreased risk of recurrence with concomitant culdoplasty at the time of sacrocolpopexy (Nygaard et al., 2004).

The bladder is sharply dissected off the anterior vaginal wall, and the rectum is dissected off the posterior vagina to allow for an adequate attachment of both the anterior and posterior mesh. Sponge sticks can be placed in the vagina and rectum, respectively, to assist with this dissection (Fig. 21.12).

A variety of lightweight, macroporous, polypropylene mesh options are available, some prefashioned in a Y-shape. The mesh

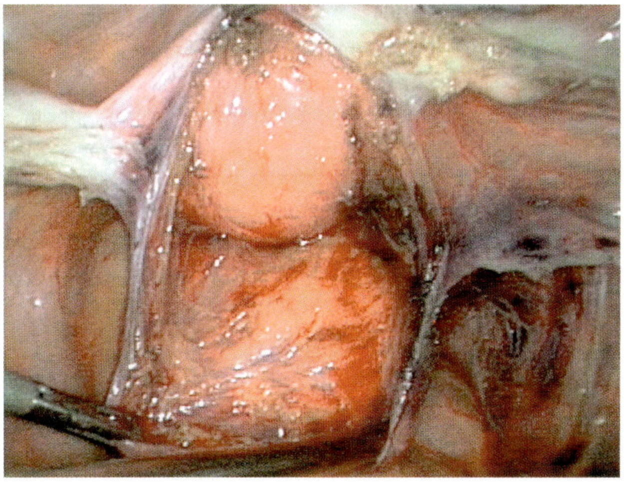

Fig. 21.12 Rectovaginal dissection. Sponge sticks have been placed in the vagina (superiorly) and rectum (inferiorly).

is sutured anteriorly to the anterior vaginal wall and apex with two to three pairs of sutures. Efficiency of mesh arm placement may be improved by first placing the suture and then back-threading the mesh through the suture. There is controversy whether permanent (polypropylene) suture or delayed absorbable (polydioxanone) is preferable for mesh attachment to the vagina.

The posterior mesh is attached to the posterior vaginal wall with three to four similar rows of No. 2-0 polypropylene. Alternatively, some surgeons like to place the posterior mesh first. When we do this, we first place the most distal posterior suture, thread the mesh, and tie down these sutures. We then place the posterior apical sutures, which helps to retract the mesh out of the visual field and facilitates placement of the additional, more distal, posterior sutures. When a Y-shaped mesh is used, it is easier to first suture the anterior portion so that the cephalad portion of the mesh may be retracted anteriorly while the posterior rows of sutures are being placed.

The sutures are tied extracorporeally as they are placed. Care is taken to place the stitches through the entire thickness of the vaginal wall, excluding the epithelium. The surgeon sutures the mesh to the longitudinal ligament of the sacrum at the level of S1 to S2 in one or two rows, purposefully suturing the anterior longitudinal ligament to obtain purchase of different longitudinal fibers. We use CV-2 polytetrafluoroethylene suture (Gore-tex, W. L. Gore & Associates, Flagstaff, AZ). As an alternative, No. 0 or 2-0 polypropylene sutures can be used. A vaginal examination is performed, assuring that no undue tension has been placed on the mesh. Titanium tacks or hernia staples may also be used to attach the mesh to the anterior longitudinal ligament of the sacrum. The redundant portion of the mesh is excised, and the peritoneum is reapproximated over the mesh with a No. 2-0 polyglactin suture. If the mesh remains exposed, sigmoid epiploic fat may be sutured over it.

Robotic Sacrocolpopexy. The robotic sacrocolpopexy is performed using a technique similar to the laparoscopic sacrocolpopexy. The da Vinci Surgical System (Intuitive Surgical, Inc., Sunnyvale, CA) is currently the only widely used robotic surgical system in the United States. The da Vinci Surgical System has three components: the patient cart (operative robot), the surgeon console, and the vision cart. The first da Vinci that was introduced was the Standard system, which has since been replaced by the S system and the Si system. The four-armed da Vinci Si system and the da Vinci Xi system are currently the most commonly used. The Xi system provides significant advantages that include improved ease of docking, the ability to place the robotically controlled 8-mm camera in any of the trocars, and an additional vessel sealing option. If using the da Vinci Xi robot, the patient cart position is flexible, as the rotating boom allows the robotic arms significant flexibility and movement independent of where the base of the patient cart is in relation to the operating room table. An example of robotic operative room arrangement is depicted in Fig. 21.13.

The robotic approach to sacrocolpopexy differs from the laparoscopic approach in a few parameters: trocar locations, docking the robotic patient cart, and use of intracorporeal knot-tying. Five trocars are placed in a shallow "W" or arc configuration (Fig. 21.11B). If using the da Vinci Xi robot, all trocars can be 8 mm, including the umbilical camera trocar and the bedside assistant/accessory port. Two of the 8-mm robotic ports are placed bilaterally, 10 to 11 cm lateral and inferior from the umbilicus, and the third robotic trocar is placed in the left lower quadrant, 10 cm lateral and superior to the more medial left-sided port. A 12-mm umbilical port is required if using the Si, given the size of the robotic camera, but an 8-mm umbilical trocar can be used if using the da Vinci Xi, given its smaller camera. Finally, an 8-mm assistant trocar is placed 9 cm lateral and superior to the right-sided robotic trocar. This trocar size allows introduction and removal of suture with SH and THX-22 needles and does not require fascial closure, thus decreasing the risk of postoperative pain. We have been performing robotic sacrocolpopexy since 2006, and initially we placed a 12-mm accessory trocar laterally and closed the fascia with a needle device. Despite placing the 12-mm trocar at least 2 cm cephalad to the anterior superior iliac spines, as recommended by the anatomic study by Whiteside et al. (2003), a few patients experienced ilioinguinal or iliohypogastric nerve entrapment during fascial closure of the 12-mm right lateral trocar that required release. This has been eliminated since transitioning to an

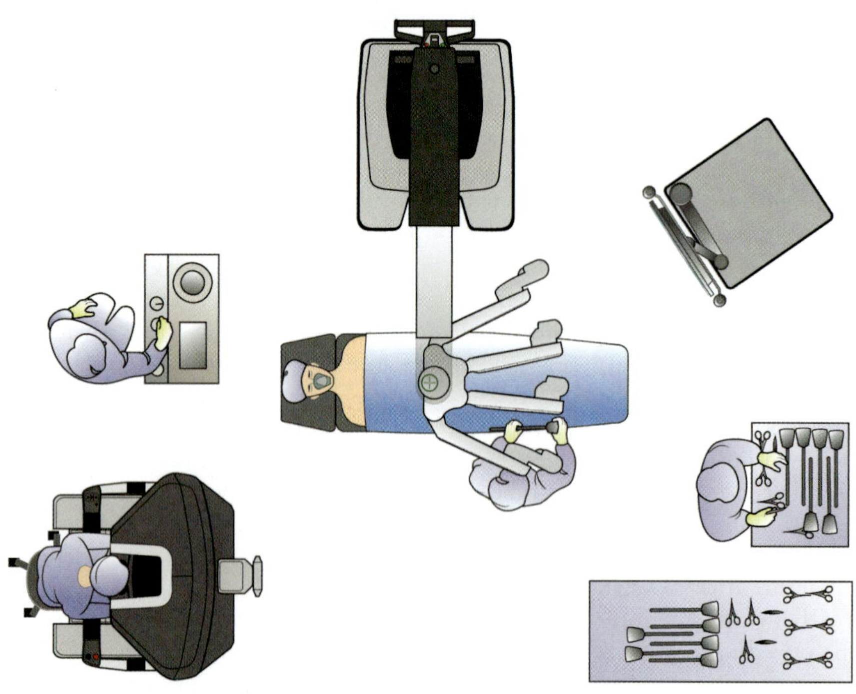

Fig. 21.13 Robotic sacrocolpopexy operating room setup—overhead view, side-docking.

8-mm lateral accessory trocar. The reduced pain has also allowed us to routinely perform robotic sacrocolpopexy as an outpatient procedure.

The robotic trocars should be placed approximately 10 cm apart to minimize risk of internal or external robotic arm collision. If this happens during a robotic surgery, it is natural for the console surgeon to move the robotic instruments in a manner that avoids collision. However, we suggest that the console surgeon temporarily leave the robotic instruments in the collided location and, with them in this orientation, walk to the bedside and observe the location of robotic arms. This often allows the robotic surgeon to make adjustments to the orientation or perhaps identify suboptimal trocar placement that will facilitate improved efficiency in subsequent surgeries.

We used to start with a 0-degree scope and switch to a 30-degree–down scope at the point of sacral dissection. To improve efficiency, we now start with a 30-degree scope and use it for the entire surgery. In addition, care should be taken to assure that the robotic trocars' black remote center, a fixed point around which the robotic arm articulates, is at or just above the peritoneum. After the robotic trocars are safely placed, the patient is placed in Trendelenburg position (about 25–30 degrees), and the small bowel is moved out of the pelvis. In the rare situation that Trendelenburg positioning and gentle movement of the small bowel fails to keep it positioned in the upper abdomen, a RayTec gauze sponge can be placed through the assistant port and carefully opened in a parachute-like fashion to drape over the small intestines to help keep them positioned. This is performed laparoscopically with the surgeon at the bedside, but is challenging and requires advanced laparoscopic skills. Next, the key anatomic landmarks of sacrocolpopexy are noted: the middle sacral artery and vein; the sacral promontory with anterior longitudinal ligament; the aortic bifurcation and the vena cava (at the L4–L5 level); the right common iliac vessels and right ureter (at the right margin of the presacral space); and the sigmoid colon, which is at the left margin. The left common iliac vein is medial to the left common iliac artery and can be damaged during dissection or retraction.

The technique of robotic sacrocolpopexy is shown in Video 21.6 (short version) and Video 21.7 (full-length). The steps are as follows:

1. If a hysterectomy is performed before sacrocolpopexy, a supracervical hysterectomy is advised to minimize risk of mesh exposure (Cundiff et al., 2008; Warner et al., 2012; Tan-Kim et al., 2011). If contraindications for supracervical hysterectomy exist, a double layered closure of the vaginal apex is recommended. In addition, care should be taken to avoid affixing the mesh to the apical suture line to decrease risk of mesh exposure. We use a disposable uterine manipulator (V-Care, ConMed, Utica, NY) to delineate the cervical vaginal junction and allow the dissection to help move the ureters laterally to avoid injury.
2. Anterior dissection: We begin the robotic sacrocolpopexy with a Tip-Up instrument in the left lateral position, a bipolar Maryland in the left hand, and monopolar HotShears in the right hand. We first perform the anterior dissection by placing a rounded EEA sizer (31–33 mm) in the vagina and elevating the vaginal apex (Fig. 21.14A). We provide some gentle upward traction on the bladder and, using the monopolar scissors, dissect the bladder off the anterior vaginal wall for 6 to 8 cm. Care is taken to avoid a cystotomy or vaginotomy, given the risk of mesh erosion/exposure or vesicovaginal fistula formation. Cystotomy should be rare, but can be closed in a double-layer closure with delayed absorbable suture. The mesh may still be placed, but we recommend attempting to orient the repair so mesh is not directly overlying the cystotomy site. The goal is to identify the avascular plane between the bladder and the anterior vaginal wall. This generally can be accomplished easily using a combination of sharp and blunt dissection. Retrograde filling of the bladder or pushing the Foley bulb and catheter into the bladder can help identify the plane between bladder and vaginal wall.
3. Posterior dissection: With the EEA sizer still in the vagina, we look for the peritoneal reflection of the rectum and posterior vaginal wall. There is typically a yellowish line that can be identified. An incision is made at this point and carried laterally in a U shape creating wide peritoneal edges bilaterally that will be used after mesh attachment to retroperitonealize the mesh to reduce the risk of SBO (Fig. 21.14B). For difficult dissections, a rectal EEA sizer (29 mm) may be helpful to identify the rectovaginal septum. If posterior visualization is limited, rotating the camera to 30 degrees up is helpful. We do not recommend a midline peritoneal incision along the posterior cervix or vaginal apex. Rather, making a U-shaped incision along the posterior vaginal wall or cervix will result in an easier dissection and may avoid creating a vaginal apical

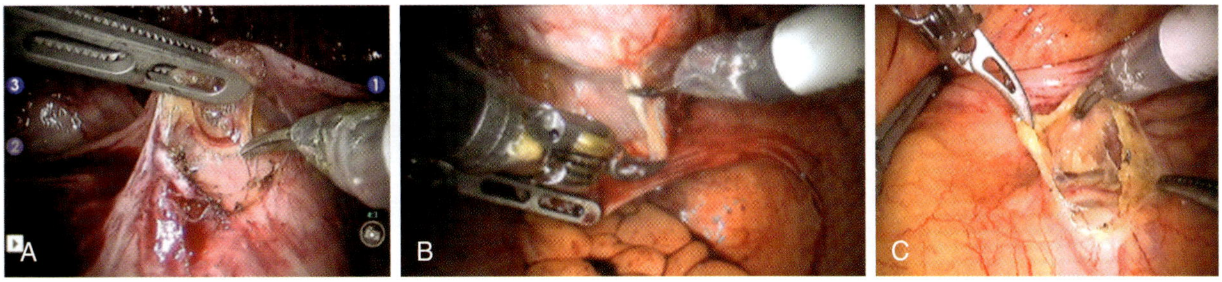

Fig. 21.14 Robotic sacrocolpopexy. **A**, Bladder dissection off the anterior vaginal wall. **B**, Dissection of rectum off the posterior vaginal wall. **C**, Presacral dissection, avoiding the middle sacral vessels and presacral venous plexus while identifying the anterior longitudinal ligament.

dissection that is too thin and that could promote mesh exposure. We typically dissect the posterior vaginal wall for approximately 8 cm. During a sacral colpoperineopexy, the dissection is carried down to the perineum and bilateral levator ani muscles, to which the inferior and lateral segments of posterior mesh are attached.

4. Develop the presacral space and expose the anterior longitudinal ligament: We recommend performing the presacral dissection with a 30-degree–down camera to maximize visualization over the sacral promontory. We gently retract the sigmoid using the Tip-Up instrument in the #1 robotic arm. We confirm that our camera orientation is midline. We tent the peritoneum during the initial incision to avoid injuring a vessel/ureter. We purposefully dissect the avascular plane under the fat pad overlying the sacrum and lift it gently to expose the anterior longitudinal ligament (Fig. 21.14C). We often coagulate the middle sacral vessels using bipolar coagulation. We then extend the presacral peritoneal dissection inferiorly to the vagina in a curvilinear fashion, purposefully creating peritoneal flaps that we later use to retroperitonealize the proximal portion of the mesh. It is important to not only make the peritoneal incision, but to also separate the two edges to allow for easier closure over the mesh.
   If bleeding at the sacrum is encountered:
   - Apply pressure.
   - If bleeding occurs during suturing, it may be necessary to swap the left needle driver for a Maryland Bipolar Forceps or other bipolar instrument.
   - Communicate effectively with the bedside team and anesthesia staff.
   - For significant bleeding, consider applying pressure with the x-ray–detectable sponge and applying a hemostatic matrix with laparoscopic applicator.
   - Although rarely needed, the robotic surgeon should be familiar with emergency undocking procedures specific to the robotic platform and model being utilized in case laparotomy is required.
5. Attach mesh to the anterior vaginal wall: See Fig. 21.15A. The authors prefer Y-shaped, polypropylene mesh, although two separate strips of mesh (anterior and posterior) can also be used. We attach the mesh to the anterior and posterior vagina using monofilament permanent polypropylene suture. Some advocate using a monofilament, delayed absorbable suture, and others utilize a barbed suture to decrease the need for tying surgical knots. The authors use an 18-inch suture anteriorly and another 18-inch suture posteriorly. This minimizes the need for multiple needle passes. We typically use a Large Needle Driver and Large SutureCut, a device that allows the console surgeon increased autonomy by placing the suture and cutting it after the surgical knot is tied. We typically attach the right and left distal corners of the mesh first. A total of six to ten sutures are typically placed anteriorly, depending on the degree of prolapse.
6. Attach mesh to the posterior vaginal wall: We orient the tip of the EEA sizer anteriorly and confirm that the connection between the anterior and posterior mesh arms is at the apex

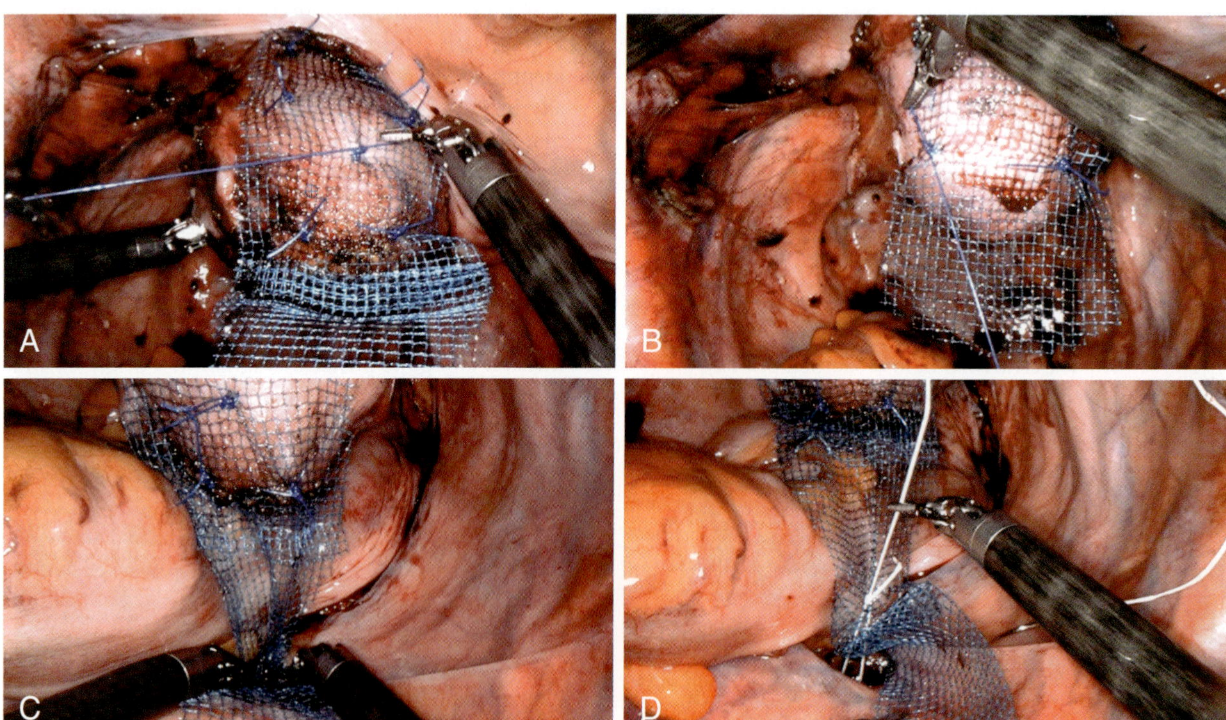

Fig. 21.15 Robotic sacrocolpopexy. **A**, Attachment of the anterior mesh to the anterior vaginal wall. **B**, Attachment of the posterior mesh to the posterior vaginal wall. **C**, Assessing the appropriate amount of tension on the sacral tail of the sacrocolpopexy mesh. **D**, Robotic slip knot at sacrum for first sacral stitch.

of the vagina. On the right side of the patient, we place the sutures by backhanding the needle. On the left side of patient, we use an overhand motion with the right hand to drive the needle from the patient's left side toward the midline. We secure the mesh with four to eight sutures (Fig. 21.15B). We typically place sutures closest to the vaginal apex first and then work our way distally. The posterior arm of the Y-shaped mesh is continuous with mesh that ultimately is attached to the sacrum. Once the first two posterior sutures are placed, the sacral end of the mesh can be lifted more to help facilitate exposure of the posterior vaginal wall. For subsequent sutures, the EEA sizer should pull back successively and assume a slightly downward-facing orientation. This will help to expose the posterior vaginal wall and facilitate mesh attachment. If visualization is still limited, one can switch to a 30-degree–up orientation of the scope.

7. Adjust mesh tension: The robotic surgeon estimates the appropriate tension by grasping the lateral edges of the sacral mesh, holding it against the planned location of the distal/inferior sacral suture, and then removing his or her head from the console locking the instruments in place. The surgeon then scrubs back in to check the proposed tension on the mesh. Generally, the width of the mesh is equal to the distance between the vaginal apex or cervix and the distal sacral suture (Fig. 21.15C).
8. Attaching mesh to the sacrum: With some gentle pressure on the EEA sizer to relieve tension on the sacral edge of the mesh, the distal suture is brought through the mesh, then through the distal aspect of the anterior longitudinal dissection and back through the mesh. We prefer to use a slip knot (Fig. 21.15D). We place the needle through anterior longitudinal ligament, using several small motions to avoid placing increased pressure on the needle that can result in the needle driver slipping or sliding off the needle in the presacral space. We fold the mesh longitudinally and place additional sutures superiorly through the double layer of mesh. This allows for a narrower attachment, keeping the mesh away from the iliac vessels and ureters but not trimming the mesh, which may impact strength. The excess proximal portion of the mesh is trimmed at the superior aspect and removed.
9. Closing the peritoneum: We always retroperitonealize the mesh to help prevent SBO. Some surgeons feel that this step is not necessary, but we would feel uncomfortable leaving mesh exposed intraabdominally. We purposefully dissect the peritoneum and create full-length peritoneal flaps that facilitate efficient closure. The peritoneum is closed with a running suture of No. 2-0 polyglactin 910 on an SH needle cut to a 14-inch length. The bedside assistant follows along holding tension on the suture using a Maryland laparoscopic grasper.

There are a few points of caution for robotic-assisted laparoscopic surgery: (1) there is no haptic feedback with the robotic system, so the surgeon has to pay close attention to visual cues when placing tension on tissues or suture; (2) unless using the Xi system is paired with a special compatible operating room table, the patient operating room table position should not be changed once the robotic system is docked; (3) the tip of the older robotic endoscopic camera may become very hot, so the end of the camera should not be cleaned by rubbing against bowel or other intraperitoneal surfaces; (4) the ability to clutch, exchange instruments, focus the camera, and use monopolar and bipolar energy modalities differs between the different generations of da Vinci Robotic Surgical Systems. Consequently, a surgeon should be comfortable with the features of the particular robotic system before its use.

A concomitant midurethral sling or laparoscopic Burch colposuspension can be performed if the patient has urethral hypermobility with urodynamic stress incontinence. If concurrent rectal prolapse is present, a rectopexy with or without sigmoid resection can be performed laparoscopically, with or without robotic assistance.

Most surgeons prefer a vaginal posterior colporrhaphy for patients with concurrent distal rectocele. After we perform a minimally invasive sacrocolpopexy with mesh extending down the posterior vaginal wall, we assess the posterior vaginal support and make an intraoperative determination as to whether a posterior repair is indicated. It is important to consider that recurrent posterior compartment prolapse is common, whether a concomitant posterior repair is performed (12%) or not (9%) (Grimes et al., 2014).

Sacro Colpoperineopexy

Some surgeons skilled in minimally invasive sacrocolpopexy perform sacral colpoperineopexy for patients with a rectocele and perineal descent. The original approach for this surgery was a combined vaginal and open abdominal approach, described by Cundiff et al. (1997), in which the posterior vaginal mesh was placed in the rectovaginal septum, anchored to the perineal body vaginally, passed through a colpotomy incision, and then affixed to the posterior vagina and anterior longitudinal ligament abdominally.

This technique has been used laparoscopically. A retrospective cohort study compared abdominal (n = 17) versus vaginal (n = 51) introduction of posterior polypropylene mesh overlaid with a biologic porcine dermis graft (Pelvicol, Bard, Murray Hill, NJ) with attachment to the perineal body and rectovaginal septum for colpoperineopexy, followed by laparoscopic attachment of a second mesh to the anterior vagina with laparoscopic affixation of both meshes to the anterior longitudinal ligament (McDermott et al., 2011). At 6 months of follow-up, there were no significant differences in perioperative outcomes and objective anatomic cure. Four patients in the abdominal group had symptoms of recurrent prolapse, compared with one in the vaginal group (P = .01). Although there were no patients with mesh exposure in the abdominal group, the vaginal group had four (P = .6), with one being apical and three noted at the posterior, distal vagina; all required surgical excision. Although often used for patients with apical prolapse with defecatory symptoms, Ramanah et al. (2012) found no improvement in bowel symptoms after laparoscopic colpoperineopexy. Mesh exposure rates have been estimated to be approximately 6% with sacral colpoperineopexy (Nosti et al., 2009), and there are conflicting data regarding mesh exposure associated with sacral colpoperineopexy and sacral colpoperineopexy with concomitant hysterectomy (Cundiff et al., 2008; Nosti et al., 2009; Visco et al., 2001).

Outcomes

The 2016 Cochrane review identified six randomized trials comparing sacrocolpopexy to vaginal prolapse repair, including three trials comparing ASC to SSLS, one trial comparing ASC to ULS, one trial comparing laparoscopic sacrocolpopexy to transvaginal mesh repair, and one trial comparing abdominal or laparoscopic sacrocolpopexy to ULS with mesh augmentation (Maher et al., 2016b). On meta-analysis, the authors concluded that, overall, sacrocolpopexy is associated with lower risk of awareness of prolapse, recurrent prolapse on examination, repeat surgery for prolapse, postoperative stress urinary incontinence, and dyspareunia when compared broadly with vaginal prolapse repairs with and without mesh augmentation. A systematic review by the Society of Gynecologic Surgeons Systematic Review Group that included both randomized trials and cohort studies comparing sacrocolpopexy with native tissue (nonmesh) vaginal repairs found improved anatomic outcomes with sacrocolpopexy and no difference in reoperation rates or postoperative sexual function (Siddiqui et al., 2015). Adverse event data compiled from 79 studies found sacrocolpopexy associated with a higher rate of ileus or SBO (2.7% vs. 0.2%, $P < .01$), mesh or suture complications (4.2% vs. 0.4%, $P < .01$), and thromboembolic disease (0.6% vs. 0.1%, $P = .03$).

A systematic review of the literature and international expert consensus using a Delphi process drew the following conclusions about specific technical aspects of sacrocolpopexy (Costantini et al., 2016):

- Monofilament polypropylene mesh is the graft of choice (grade B).
- Laparoscopy is the preferred approach for sacrocolpopexy (grade B).
- Uterus/cervix preservation at the time of sacrocolpopexy reduces mesh exposure rate (grade B). However, there are insufficient or conflicting data on hysterectomy (total or subtotal) or uterus preservation regarding efficacy during sacrocolpopexy (grade D).
- Either permanent or delayed sutures may be used for securing the mesh to the vagina (grade C).
- Either permanent tacks or sutures may be used to secure the mesh to the sacral promontory (grade C).
- The peritoneum should be closed (grade C).
- No conclusion could be reached about the number of sutures that should be placed in the vagina to secure the mesh (grade D).

Abdominal. Observational studies and clinical trials suggest that ASC is a highly effective procedure for apical prolapse. The success rate of ASC, when defined as lack of apical prolapse, ranges from 78% to 100% (Maher et al., 2016a). A systematic review of ASC performed by Nygaard et al. (2004) reported a median reoperation rate for recurrent prolapse of 4.4% (range 0%–18.2%) and for postoperative stress incontinence of 4.9% (range 1.2%–30.9%) and a mesh exposure rate of 3.4%. Wound complications occurred in 4.6% (range 0.4%–19.8%), hemorrhage or transfusion in 4.4% (0.2%–16.9%), cystotomy in 3.1% (0.4%–15.8%), ureteral injury in 1.0% (0.8%–1.9%), and bowel injury in 1.6% (0.4%–2.5%). Long-term follow-up shows a substantial decline in anatomic and subjective outcomes and an increase in mesh exposure, however. Subjects enrolled in the long-term follow-up (5–7 years) branch of the Colpopexy and Urinary Reduction Efforts (CARE) trial demonstrated objective failure rates of 24% to 48%, depending upon the definition of failure and a cumulative mesh exposure rate of 10.5% by 7 years (Nygaard et al., 2013). Clinical trials demonstrate significant improvements in prolapse symptoms, urinary function, and quality of life after ASC. There is level 1 evidence that ASC has superior anatomic outcomes when compared to SSLS, but this is balanced by longer operating time, longer recovery, and higher cost. A single trial has compared ASC (n = 63) to ULS (n = 61) and found that ASC was associated with greater anatomic success, fewer reoperations, and greater postoperative complications, but that there was no difference in improvement in symptoms or quality of life (Rondini et al., 2015).

Minimally Invasive. Multiple prospective and retrospective case series demonstrate good short- to midterm success rates with laparoscopic sacrocolpopexy, with a mean objective success rate of 90.5% (range 60%–100%), subjective success rates of 79% to 98%, and mean reoperation rate of 5.9% (Maher et al., 2016a). Although there are few direct comparisons of ASC with the laparoscopic approach, available studies suggest no difference in objective or subjective cure rates, with the laparoscopic approach associated with lower blood loss, longer operating time, and shorter hospital stay (Maher et al., 2016a; Maher et al., 2016b). Despite the clinical advantages of a laparoscopic approach, its adoption has been relatively limited, probably because of the steep learning curve associated with attaining laparoscopic suturing and knot-tying skills required to attach the mesh to the vagina and sacrum. Various studies have estimated a decrease in operative time and/or improved efficacy after 15 to 60 cases (Maher et al., 2020).

Because of the relatively long learning curve required for the laparoscopic approach, many surgeons have turned to robotic-assisted surgery to offer patients a minimally invasive approach to sacrocolpopexy. Robotic surgical systems have been developed with the goal of facilitating technically difficult procedures by improving the surgeon's vision, dexterity. and ergonomics. Limited data suggest that operating time and efficiency improve significantly after performing 20 robotic sacrocolpopexy procedures (Geller et al., 2013). A systematic review of 27 studies including 1488 cases found that the robotic approach to sacrocolpopexy is associated with objective cure rates of 84% to 100% and subjective cure rates of 92% to 95%, with mesh exposure rates of 2% (range 0%–8%) (Serati et al., 2014). Overall, the postoperative complication rate in this meta-analysis was 11%, with severe complications occurring in 2% of cases. Conversion to the open approach occurred in less than 1% of cases (range 0%–5%).

To date, two randomized trials have compared robotic to laparoscopic sacrocolpopexy. Paraiso et al. (2011) reported a single-center, blinded, randomized trial comparing robotic (n = 40) to laparoscopic (n = 38) sacrocolpopexy in women with stage 2 to 4 posthysterectomy vaginal prolapse. Patients undergoing the robotic approach experienced longer operating time (mean difference +67 minutes; 95% CI 43–89), had increased postoperative pain up to 6 weeks following surgery, and required longer use of nonsteroidal antiinflammatory medications (20 vs. 11 days) compared with the laparoscopic approach. At 1 year, there were no differences in anatomic and quality-of-life measures between the two groups. Additionally, the cost of robotic sacrocolpopexy was significantly higher (mean difference +$1936; 95% CI 417–3454). In 2014, Anger et al. conducted a multicenter trial comparing 78 women with stage 2 or greater pelvic organ prolapse undergoing robotic (n = 40) or laparoscopic (n = 38) sacrocolpopexy with a primary outcome of cost. The robotic sacrocolpopexy group had higher initial hospital costs ($19,616 compared with $11,573; $P < .001$) and, over 6 weeks, hospital costs remained higher for robotic sacrocolpopexy ($20,898 compared with $12,170; $P < .001$). However, when excluding costs of robot purchase and maintenance, there was no difference in hospital costs over 6 weeks ($13,867 compared with $12,170; $P = .06$). The robotic group had longer operating room times (202.8 minutes compared with 178.4 minutes; $P = .03$) and higher pain scores 1 week after surgery (3.5 ± 2.1 compared with 2.6 ± 2.2; $P = .04$). At 1 year, there were significant improvements in sexual activity, quality of life, and symptoms in both groups, with no differences between groups (Kenton et al., 2016). No reoperations for mesh complications occurred in either group.

Avoiding and Managing Complications

Intraoperative complications during sacrocolpopexy are uncommon but can be life-threatening. Most complications reported after sacrocolpopexy tend to be similar to those of other abdominal operations, including hemorrhage, enterotomy, ureteral damage, cystotomy, proctotomy, hernias, and extrafascial wound infections. Postoperative complications unique to operative laparoscopy and robotic surgery also can occur. Life-threatening bleeding from the presacral space is one of the most feared complications of sacrocolpopexy. When there is bleeding from presacral vessels, hemostasis can be difficult to achieve because of the complex interlacing venous plexus on the surface of the periosteum. When these veins have been damaged, they can retract beneath the bony surface of the anterior sacrum and recede into the underlying channels of cancellous bone. Communications with adjacent pelvic veins, especially the left common iliac vein, can be particularly troublesome. Packing the presacral space may control bleeding temporarily, but it often recurs when the pack is removed, and packing may further lacerate delicate veins. We have found that the most effective way to manage presacral bleeding refractory to simple bipolar coagulation is to apply pressure immediately, alert and focus the entire operating room including anesthesia, urgently place up to 5 mL of FloSeal (Baxter, Dearfield, IL), and continue to hold pressure for up to 5 minutes. Others suggest sutures, metallic clips, cautery, and bone wax, but we have found these to be minimally effective. Before minimally invasive approaches, some have reported the use of sterilized stainless-steel thumbtacks placed into the sacrum at the site of the retracted bleeding presacral vein to treat life-threatening hemorrhage that has not responded to other measures.

Longer-term postoperative complications include SBO, hernia, and erosion/exposure of implanted materials. The median rate of SBO requiring surgery has been reported as 1.1% (range 0.6%–8.6%), which is similar to the rate of SBO encountered in prospective studies. Although rare, nerve injuries and sacral osteomyelitis have been reported (Nygaard et al., 2004). With the exception of wound infection, it is unclear if minimally invasive approaches significantly reduce these complications relative to the abdominal approach.

The most common long-term complication is exposure of synthetic mesh or suture through the vagina, which occurs in 6% of cases at 2-year follow-up (Brubaker et al., 2008) and was noted to increase to 10.5% at 7-year follow-up (Nygaard et al., 2013). Of note, these data come from the CARE trial, which was a randomized trial of Burch urethropexy versus no continence procedure at the time of sacrocolpopexy. As such, the technique for sacrocolpopexy was not standardized, and there was wide variety in technique, as well as mesh and suture material used. Cigarette smoking and concurrent hysterectomy each increase the risk of mesh exposure by an odds ratio of five (Cundiff et al., 2008). In patients with uterine prolapse, preserving the uterus (see Chapter 22) or performing a subtotal hysterectomy with sacrocervicopexy appears to reduce the risk of mesh exposure. When mesh exposures are encountered, conservative treatment with vaginal estrogen should be a first-line treatment. If the patient is asymptomatic, observation can be considered. However, most patients with this complication require partial removal of the mesh and closure of the defect in the vagina. (See Chapter 25.)

CHOOSING APPROACH OF SURGERY

Surgery is indicated in women with symptomatic apical or uterine prolapse who have failed or declined conservative therapies such as pessary and pelvic muscle therapy. To date, there is incomplete evidence on which to base the decision about which surgery to perform for advanced uterovaginal or posthysterectomy vaginal vault prolapse. The Apical Suspension Repair for Vault Prolapse In a Three-Arm Randomized Trial Design (ASPIRe) (Clinicaltrials.gov NCT02676973) comparing vaginal native tissue repair, vaginal mesh (Uphold Lite; Boston Scientific, Boston, MA), and sacrocolpopexy for posthysterectomy vault prolapse has completed enrollment, but the study findings have not been reported as of the writing of this chapter. Extent and type of prolapse, surgical history, concurrent pathology (e.g., ovarian mass, rectal prolapse), age, health status, sexual status, surgeon experience, and patient preference are important to consider when making this decision. Individual surgeon experience, especially for vaginal, laparoscopic, and robotic surgery, is an important predictor of successful outcome. For example, less-experienced surgeons have higher rates of recurrent prolapse after transvaginal surgery and, in general, low-volume surgeons have an increased rate of complications compared to high-volume surgeons (Maher et al., 2020). The increase in the use of robots to assist in prolapse surgery has increased the number of minimally invasive sacrocolpopexies available to patients. The long-term efficacy and cost-effectiveness of this option need further study. When deciding between native tissue transvaginal approaches, transvaginal mesh, and sacrocolpopexy, each of these factors must be considered to balance the efficacy and safety of the options. Ultimately, the choice should be made as part of a shared decision-making process between the surgeon and patient after a careful informed consent discussion.

In 2017, the International Consultation on Incontinence (ICI) Surgical Management of Prolapse Committee developed an evidence-based clinical pathway to guide appropriate route and approach for prolapse surgery (Maher et al., 2020) (Fig. 21.16). Importantly, this pathway is meant as guidance and is only as

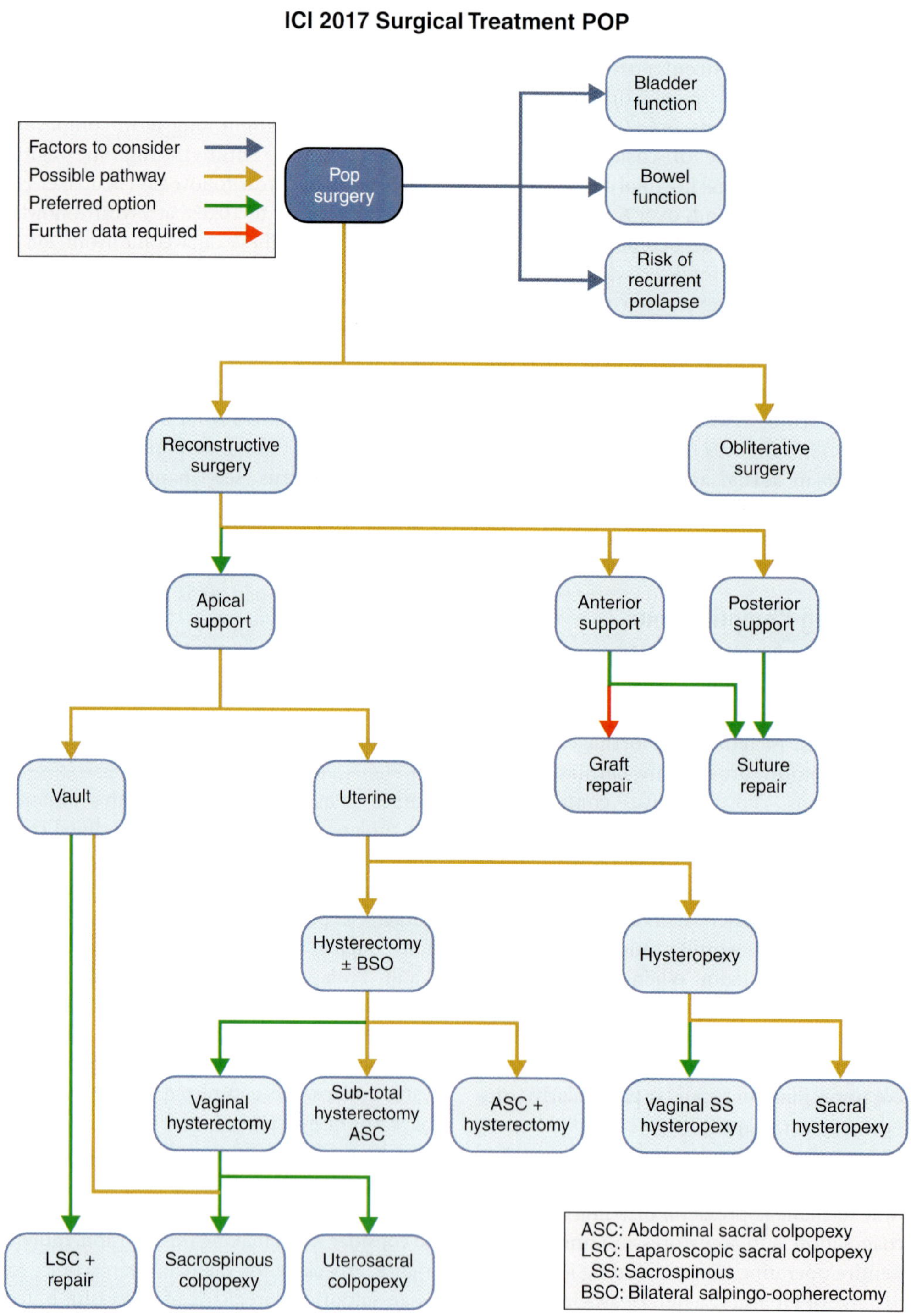

Fig. 21.16 The 6th International Consultation on Incontinence Clinical Pathway for Surgical Treatment of Pelvic Organ Prolapse (*POP*). (From Maher CF, Baessler KK, Barber MD, et al. Summary: 2017 International Consultation on Incontinence Evidence-Based Surgical Pathway for Pelvic Organ Prolapse. *Female Pelvic Med Reconstr Surg*. 2020;26:30. With permission.)

good as the currently available evidence, which is incomplete. For posthysterectomy vault prolapse, the pathway suggests sacrocolpopexy as the preferred apical suspending procedure over transvaginal native tissue and mesh repairs for vaginal vault prolapse, given the superiority of anatomic and subjective outcomes seen in the Cochrane review (grade A). As not all women are suitable for sacrocolpopexy (i.e., multiple prior laparotomies, prior radiation, the very obese or frail), vaginal uterosacral and sacrospinous colpopexy are also acceptable alternatives, given their superior safety profile. The pathway suggests that the laparoscopic approach to sacrocolpopexy has some advantages over both the open and robotic approaches, while also acknowledging the longer learning curve of the laparoscopic route (grade B). For uterine prolapse, the pathway separates between uterine preservation and hysterectomy. Relative contraindications to uterine preservation including uterine abnormalities (fibroids, adenomyosis, endometrial pathology, abnormal cervical cytology, uterine or postmenopausal bleeding) or factors that increase the risk of gynecological cancer (*BRCA1* and *BRCA2* variants associated with familial cancer, Lynch syndrome, tamoxifen therapy, obesity, and patients who are not compliant with gynecological surveillance). Indications, contraindications, and techniques for hysteropexy are discussed in Chapter 22. In patients with uterine prolapse in whom hysterectomy is chosen, vaginal hysterectomy with native tissue vaginal vault suspension is the recommended approach. This recommendation is based on evidence from meta-analysis that vaginal hysterectomy with apical suspension has a lower reoperation rate for prolapse than abdominal sacrohysteropexy (grade B), sacrocolopexy with hysterectomy has a relatively high rate of mesh exposure postoperatively (grade C), and supracervical hysterectomy with sacrocolpopexy has an increased rate of recurrent POP compared with sacrocolpopexy and hysterectomy (grade C) (Maher et al., 2020). Importantly, hysterectomy and subtotal hysterectomy with sacrocolpopexy is also an acceptable option in these patients.

The ICI pathway also identified risk factors for recurrent prolapse that should be considered when choosing route of prolapse surgery, including age less than 60 years (grade C) and stage 3 or 4 prolapse (grade B) (Maher et al., 2020). Some studies suggest that widened genital hiatus and levator ani defects identified by ultrasound may increase the risk of failure, but these data are inconsistent. Another factor that should be considered when choosing route of surgery is vaginal length. As SSLS and ULS both require sufficient vaginal length to attach the vaginal apex to their respective ligaments without undue tension, a sacrocolpopexy may be necessary in women with prolapse who have a shortened vagina.

Efforts to decrease recurrence after prolapse surgeries are paramount to improving patient care. In spite of the ICI pathway guidance, the question of whether transvaginal apical repair or minimally invasive sacrocolpopexy is best for older patients, those with primary and less severe prolapse, and those with comorbidities that might increase surgical risk remains controversial, and is dependent on the surgeon's experience and ability to perform each procedure in a safe and efficient manner. Many surgeons offer younger women, women with more severe prolapse or recurrences after vaginal surgery, and women with prolapsed, short vaginas a mesh sacrocolpopexy, preferably through a minimally invasive route. The traditional paradigm of vaginal versus abdominal prolapse repair has shifted because a large laparotomy incision and long hospital stay and postoperative recovery have been obviated with the increase in minimally invasive sacrocolpopexy. However, improved anatomic outcomes seen with sacrocolpopexy have not necessarily translated into improved quality of life or decreased symptom burden, and must be balanced with increased risk of complications and cost, particularly in older patients with comorbidities.

The use of hysterectomy during prolapse surgery is not always necessary, and attitudes about this are changing slowly among patients and surgeons (see Chapter 22). Consideration of hysteropexy procedures is reasonable after reviewing the pros and cons of this surgery with the patient. Further research is necessary before this can be routinely recommended.

More education and research into the anatomy of pelvic support, the pathogenesis of prolapse, and the principles of pelvic and vaginal reconstructive surgery is needed to improve care for all affected women. More high-quality comparative surgical trials are greatly needed, as is more information about the pros and cons of surgical innovations such as vaginal grafts and the use of surgical robots.

BIBLIOGRAPHY

Joint Report on Terminology for Surgical Procedures to Treat Pelvic Organ Prolapse. *Female Pelvic Med Reconstr Surg*. 2020;26:173.

ACOG Committee on Gynecologic Practice. ACOG committee opinion no. 513: vaginal placement of synthetic mesh for pelvic organ prolapse. *Obstet Gynecol*. 2011;118:1459.

Addison WA, Livengood CH, Sutton GP, et al. Abdominal sacral colpopexy with Mersilene mesh in the retroperitoneal position in the management of posthysterectomy vaginal vault prolapse and enterocele. *Am J Obstet Gynecol*. 1985;153:140.

Addison WA, Livengood CH, Parker RT. Posthysterectomy vaginal vault prolapse with emphasis on management by transabdominal sacral colpopexy. *Postgrad Obstet Gynecol*. 1988;8:1.

Addison WA, Timmons CM, Wall LL, et al. Failed abdominal sacral colpopexy: observations and recommendations. *Obstet Gynecol*. 1989;74:480.

Altman D, Väyrynen T, Engh ME, et al. Anterior colporrhaphy versus transvaginal mesh for pelvic-organ prolapse. *N Engl J Med*. 2011;364:1826.

Amreich I. Atiologie und operation des scheiden stump prolapses. *Wien Klin Wochenschr*. 1951;65:74.

Angulo A, Ligman I. Retroperitoneal sacrocolpopexy for correction of prolapse of vaginal vault. *Surg Gynecol Obstet*. 1989;169:319.

Anger J, Mueller E, Tarnay C, et al. Robotic compared with laparoscopic sacrocolpopexy: a randomized controlled trial. *Obstet Gynecol*. 2014;23:5.

Backer MH. Success with sacrospinous suspension of the prolapsed vaginal vault. *Surg Gynecol Obstet*. 1992;175:419.

Baggish MS, Karram MM. Vaginal repair of vaginal vault prolapse. In: *Atlas of Pelvic Anatomy and Gynecologic Surgery*. 3rd ed. Saunders: St. Louis; 2011:713.

Bai SW, Kim EH, Shin JS. A comparison of different pelvic reconstruction surgeries using mesh for pelvic organ prolapse patients. *Yonsei Med J*. 2005;46:112.

Baker KR, Beresford JM, Campbell C. Colposacropexy with Prolene mesh. *Surg Gynecol Obstet.* 1990;171:51.

Barber MD, Visco AG, Weidner AC, et al. Bilateral uterosacral ligament vaginal vault suspension with site specific endopelvic fascia defect repair for treatment of pelvic organ prolapse. *Am J Obstet Gynecol.* 2000;183:1402.

Barber MD, Maher C. Apical prolapse. *Int Urogynecol J.* 2013;24:1815.

Barber MD, Brubaker L, Burgio KL, et al. Comparison of 2 transvaginal surgical approaches and perioperative behavioral therapy for apical vaginal prolapse: the OPTIMAL randomized trial. *JAMA.* 2014;311:1023.

Benson JT, Lucente V, McClellan E. Vaginal versus abdominal reconstructive surgery for the treatment of pelvic support defects: a prospective randomized study with long-term outcome evaluation. *Am J Obstet Gynecol.* 1996;175:1418.

Boyles SH, Weber AM, Meyn L. Procedures for pelvic organ prolapse in the United States, 1979–1997. *Am J Obstet Gynecol.* 2003;188:108.

Brown WE, Hoffman MS, Bouis PJ, et al. Management of vaginal vault prolapse: retrospective comparison of abdominal versus vaginal approach. *J Fla Med Assoc.* 1989;76:249.

Brown JS, Waetjen LE, Subak LL, et al. Pelvic organ prolapse surgery in the United States, 1997. *Am J Obstet Gynecol.* 2002;186:712.

Brubaker L, Cundiff GW, Fine P, et al. Abdominal sacrocolpopexy with Burch colposuspension to reduce urinary stress incontinence. *N Engl J Med.* 2006;354:1557.

Brubaker L, Nygaard I, Richter HE, et al. Two-year outcomes after sacrocolpopexy with and without Burch to prevent stress urinary incontinence. *Obstet Gynecol.* 2008;112:49.

Bump RC, Norton PA. Epidemiology and natural history of pelvic floor dysfunction. *Obstet Gynecol Clin North Am.* 1998;25:723.

Bump RC, Mattiasson A, Bo K, et al. The standardization of terminology of female pelvic organ prolapse and pelvic floor dysfunction. *Am J Obstet Gynecol.* 2004;175:10.

Carey MP, Slack MC. Transvaginal sacrospinous colpopexy for vault and marked uterovaginal prolapse. *Br J Obstet Gynaecol.* 1994;101:536.

Carey MP, Dwyer PL. Genital prolapse: vaginal versus abdominal route of repair. *Curr Opin Obstet Gynecol.* 2001;13:499.

Chen L, Ashton-Miller JA, Hsu Y, DeLancey JO. Interaction among apical support, levator ani impairment, and anterior vaginal wall prolapse. *Obstet Gynecol.* 2006;108:324.

Collins SA, Tulikangas PK, LaSala CA, Lind LR. Complex sacral abscess 8 years after abdominal sacral colpopexy. *Obstet Gynecol.* 2011;118:451.

Costantini E, Brubaker L, Cervigni M, et al. Sacrocolpopexy for pelvic organ prolapse: evidence-based review and recommendations. *Eur J Obstet Gynecol Reprod Biol.* 2016;205:60.

Cowan W, Morgan HR. Abdominal sacral colpopexy. *Am J Obstet Gynecol.* 1980;138:348.

Creighton SM, Stanton SL. The surgical management of vaginal vault prolapse. *Br J Obstet Gynaecol.* 1991;98:1150.

Cruikshank SH, Cox IN. Sacrospinous fixation at the time of vaginal hysterectomy. *Am J Obstet Gynecol.* 1990;162:1611.

Cruikshank SH. Sacrospinous fixation: should this be performed at the time of vaginal hysterectomy? *Am J Obstet Gynecol.* 1991;164:1072.

Cruikshank SH, Kovac SR. Randomized comparison of three surgical methods used at the time of vaginal hysterectomy to prevent posterior enterocele. *Am J Obstet Gynecol.* 1999;180:859.

Culligan PJ, Blackwell L, Goldsmith LJ. A randomized controlled trial comparing fascia lata and synthetic mesh for sacral colpopexy. *Obstet Gynecol.* 2005;106:29.

Cundiff GW, Harris RL, Coates K, et al. Abdominal sacral colpoperineopexy: a new approach for correction of posterior compartment defects and perineal descent associated with vaginal vault prolapse. *Am J Obstet Gynecol.* 1997;177:1345.

Cundiff GW, Varner E, Visco AG, et al. Risk factors for mesh/suture erosion following sacral colpopexy. *Am J Obstet Gynecol.* 2008;199:688.e1.

DeLancey JO. Anatomic aspects of vaginal eversion after hysterectomy. *Am J Obstet Gynecol.* 1992;166:1717.

Diwadkar GB, Barber MD, Feiner B, et al. Complication and reoperation rates after apical vaginal prolapse surgical repair: a systematic review. *Obstet Gynecol.* 2009;113:367.

Diwan A, Rardin CR, Kohli N. Uterine preservation during surgery for uterovaginal prolapse: a review. *Int J Urogynecol.* 2004;15:286.

Drutz HP, Cha LS. Massive genital and vaginal vault prolapse treated with abdominal-vaginal sacropexy with use of Marlex mesh: review of the literature. *Am J Obstet Gynecol.* 1987;156:387.

Elkins TE, Hopper JB, Goodfellow K, et al. Initial report of anatomic and clinical comparison of the sacrospinous ligament fixation to the high McCall culdoplasty for vaginal cuff fixation at hysterectomy for uterine prolapse. *J Pelvic Surg.* 1995;1:12.

Farnsworth BN. Posterior intravaginal slingplasty (infracoccygealsacropexy) for severe posthysterectomy vaginal vault prolapse—a preliminary report on efficacy and safety. *Int Urogynecol J Pelvic Floor Dysfunct.* 2002;13:4.

Farrell SA, Scotti RJ, Ostergard DR, et al. Massive evisceration: a complication following sacrospinous vaginal vault fixation. *Obstet Gynecol.* 1991;78:560.

Feldman GB, Birnbaum SJ. Sacral colpopexy for vaginal vault prolapse. *Obstet Gynecol.* 1979;53:399.

Funt MI, Thompson JD, Birch H. Normal vaginal axis. *South Med J.* 1978;71:1534.

Geller EJ, Parnell BA, Dunivan GC. Robotic vs abdominal sacrocolpopexy: 44-month pelvic floor outcomes. *Urology.* 2012;79:532.

Geller EJ, Lin FC, Matthews CA. Analysis of robotic performance times to improve operative efficiency. *J Min Invasiv Gynecol Surg.* 2013;20:43.

Given FY, Muhlendorf TK, Browning GM. Vaginal length and sexual function after colpopexy for complete uterovaginal eversion. *Am J Obstet Gynecol.* 1993;169:284.

Grimes CL, Tan-Kim J, Garfin SR, Nager CW. Sacral colpopexy followed by refractory Candida albicans osteomyelitis and discitis requiring extensive spinal surgery. *Obstet Gynecol.* 2012;120:464.

Grimes CL, Lukacz ES, Gantz MG, et al. What happens to the posterior compartment and bowel symptoms after sacrocolpopexy? evaluation of 5-year outcomes from E-CARE. *Female Pelvic Med Reconstr Surg.* 2014;20:261.

Grunberger W, Grunberger V, Wierrani F. Pelvic promontory fixation of the vaginal vault in sixty-two patients with prolapse after hysterectomy. *Surg Gynecol Obstet.* 1994;178:69.

Gungor Ugurlucan F, Yasa C, Demir O, et al. Long-term follow-up of a patient with spondylodiscitis after laparoscopic sacrocolpopexy: an unusual complication with review of the literature. *Urol Int.* 2019;103:364-368.

Gustilo-Ashby AM, Jelovsek JE, Barber MD, et al. The incidence of ureteral obstruction and the value of intraoperative cystoscopy during vaginal surgery for pelvic organ prolapse. *Am J Obstet Gynecol.* 2006;194:1478.

Handa VL, Garrett E, Hendrix S, et al. Progression and remission of pelvic organ prolapse: a longitudinal study of menopausal women. *Am J Obstet Gynecol.* 2004;190:27.

Harrison JE, McDonagh JE. Hernia of Douglas pouch and high rectocele. *Am J Obstet Gynecol.* 1950;60:83.

Haylen BT, de Ridder D, Freeman RM, et al. An International Urogynecological Association (IUGA)/International Continence

Society (ICS) joint report on the terminology for female pelvic floor dysfunction. *Neurourol Urodyn.* 2010;29:4.

Heinonen PK. Transvaginal sacrospinous colpopexy for vaginal vault and complete genital prolapse in aged women. *Acta Obstet Gynecol Scand.* 1992;71:377.

Heit M, Rosenquist C, Culligan P, et al. Predicting treatment choice for patients with pelvic organ prolapse. *Obstet Gynecol.* 2001;101:1279.

Hendrix SL, Clark A, Nygaard I, et al. Pelvic organ prolapse in the Women's Health Initiative: gravity and gravidity. *Am J Obstet Gynecol.* 2002;186:1160.

Hilger WS, Poulson M, Norton PA. Long-term results of abdominal sacrocolpopexy. *Am J Obstet Gynecol.* 2003;189:1606.

Hsu Y, Chen L, Summers A, et al. Anterior vaginal wall length and degree of anterior compartment prolapse seen on dynamic MRI. *Int Urogynecol J.* 2008;19:137.

Hurd WW, Bude RO, DeLancey JO, Newman JS. The location of abdominal wall blood vessels in relationship to abdominal landmarks apparent at laparoscopy. *Am J Obstet Gynecol.* 1994;171:642.

Inmon WB. Pelvic relaxation and repair including prolapse of vagina following hysterectomy. *South Med J.* 1963;56:577.

Iosif CS. Abdominal sacral colpopexy with use of synthetic mesh. *Acta Obstet Gynecol Scand.* 1993;72:214.

Jelovsek JE, Maher C, Barber MD. Pelvic organ prolapse. *Lancet.* 2007;369:1027.

Jelovsek JE, Barber MD, Brubaker L, et al. Effect of uterosacral ligament suspension vs sacrospinous ligament fixation with or without perioperative behavioral therapy for pelvic organ vaginal prolapse on surgical outcomes and prolapse symptoms at 5 years in the OPTIMAL randomized clinical trial. *JAMA.* 2018;319:1554.

Kaminski PF, Sorosky JI, Pees RC, et al. Correction of massive vaginal prolapse: an older population. *J Am Geriatr Soc.* 1993;41:42.

Karram MM, Goldwasser S, Kleeman S, et al. High uterosacral vaginal vault suspension with fascial reconstruction for vaginal repair of enterocele and vaginal vault prolapse. *Am J Obstet Gynecol.* 2001;185:1339.

Karram MM, Ridgeway BM, Walters MD. Surgical treatment of vaginal apex prolapse. In: Walters MD, Karram MM, eds. *Urogynecology and Reconstructive Pelvic Surgery.* 4th ed. Philadelphia: Elsevier; 2015.

Kasturi S, Bentley-Taylor M, Woodman PJ, et al. High uterosacral ligament vaginal vault suspension: comparison of absorbable vs. permanent suture for apical fixation. *Int Urogynecol J.* 2012;23:941.

Keetel LM, Hebertson RM. An anatomic evaluation of the sacrospinous ligament colpopexy. *Surg Gynecol Obstet.* 1989;168:318.

Kenton K, Mueller ER, Tarney C, et al. One-year outcomes after minimally invasive sacrocolpopexy. *Female Pelvic Med Reconstr Surg.* 2016;22:382.

Kohle N, Walsh P, Roat TW, et al. Mesh erosion following abdominal sacral colpopexy. *Obstet Gynecol.* 1998;92:999.

Kovac SR, Cruikshank SH. Successful pregnancies and vaginal deliveries after sacrospinous uterosacral fixation in five of 19 patients. *Am J Obstet Gynecol.* 1993;168:1778.

Krause HG, Groh JT, Sloane K, et al. Laparoscopic sacral suture hysteropexy for uterine prolapse. *Int Urogynecol J.* 2006;17:378.

Kuhn RJ, Hollyock MD. Observations on the anatomy of the rectovaginal pouch and septum. *Obstet Gynecol.* 1982;59:445.

Lansman HH. Posthysterectomy vault prolapse: sacral colpopexy with dura mater graft. *Obstet Gynecol.* 1984;63:577.

Lee RA, Symmonds RE. Surgical repair of posthysterectomy vault prolapse. *Am J Obstet Gynecol.* 1972;112:953.

Lo TS, Wang AL. Abdominal colposacropexy and sacrospinous ligament suspension for severe uterovaginal prolapse: a comparison. *J Gynecol Surg.* 1998;14:59.

Lowenstein L, Fitz A, Kenton K, et al. Transabdominal uterosacral suspension: outcomes and complications. *Am J Obstet Gynecol.* 2009;200:656.e1.

Mädakinen J, Soderstrom K, Kiilholma P, et al. Histologic changes in the vaginal connective tissue of patients with and without uterine prolapse. *Arch Gynecol.* 1986;239:17.

Mädakinen J, Kähäri V, Soderstrom K, et al. Collagen synthesis in the vaginal connective tissue of patients with and without uterine prolapse. *Eur J Obstet Gynecol Reprod Biol.* 1987;24:319.

Maher CF, Carey MP, Murray CJ. Laparoscopic suture hysteropexy for uterine prolapse. *Obstet Gynecol.* 2001;97:1010.

Maher CF, Murray CJ, Carey MP, et al. Iliococcygeus or sacrospinous fixation for vaginal vault prolapse. *Obstet Gynecol.* 2001;98:40.

Maher CF, Qatawney AM, Dwyer PL, et al. Abdominal sacral colpopexy or vaginal sacrospinous colpopexy for vaginal vault prolapse: a prospective randomized study. *Am J Obstet Gynecol.* 2004;190:20.

Maher C, Feiner B, Baessler K, Schmid C. Surgical management of pelvic organ prolapse in women. *Cochrane Database Syst Rev.* 2013;4:CD004014.

Maher C, Baessler K, Barber M, et al. Pelvic organ prolapse surgery. In: Abrams P, Cardozo L, Wagg A, Wein A. eds. *Incontinence.* 6th ed. ICI-ICS. International Continence Society, Bristol UK. 2017.

Maher C, Feiner B, Baessler K, et al. Surgery for women with apical vaginal prolapse. *Cochrane Database Syst Rev.* 2016;10:CD012376.

Maher CF, Baessler KK, Barber MD, et al. Surgical management of pelvic organ prolapse. *Climacteric.* 2019;22:229.

Maher CF, Baessler KK, Barber MD, et al. Summary: 2017 International Consultation on Incontinence Evidence-Based Surgical Pathway for Pelvic Organ Prolapse. *Female Pelvic Med Reconstr Surg.* 2020;26:30.

Maloney JC, Dunton CJ, Smith K. Repair of vaginal vault prolapse with abdominal sacropexy. *J Reprod Med.* 1990;35:6.

Mant J, Painter R, Vessey M. Epidemiology of genital prolapse: observations from the Oxford Family Planning Association Study. *Br J Obstet Gynaecol.* 1997;104:579.

Margulies RU, Rogers MA, Morgan DM. Outcomes of transvaginal uterosacral ligament suspension: systematic review and metanalysis. *Am J Obstet Gynecol.* 2010;202:124.

McDermott CD, Park J, Terr CL, et al. Laparoscopic sacral colpoperineopexy: abdominal versus abdominal-vaginal posterior graft attachment. *Int Urogynecol J.* 2011;22:469.

Meeks GR, Washburne JF, McGeher RP, et al. Repair of vaginal vault prolapse by suspension of the vagina to iliococcygeus (prespinous) fascia. *Am J Obstet Gynecol.* 1994;171:1444.

Miller N. A new method of correcting complete inversion of the vagina. *Surg Gynecol Obstet.* 1927;44:550.

Milley PS, Nichols DH. A correlative investigation of the human rectovaginal septum. *Anat Rec.* 1969;163:443.

Miyazaki FS. Miya hook ligature carrier for sacrospinous ligament suspension. *Obstet Gynecol.* 1987;70:286.

Monk BJ, Ramp JF, Montz FJ, et al. Sacrospinous fixation for vaginal vault prolapse. Complications and results. *J Gynecol Surg.* 1991;7:87.

Morgan DM, Rogers MA, Huebner M, et al. Heterogeneity in anatomic outcome of sacrospinous ligament fixation for prolapse: a systematic review. *Obstet Gynecol.* 2007;109:1424.

Morley G, DeLancey JO. Sacrospinous ligament fixation for eversion of the vagina. *Am J Obstet Gynecol.* 1988;158:872.

Muffly TM, Diwadkar GB, Paraiso MF. Lumbosacral osteomyelitis after robotic-assisted total laparsocopic hysterectomy and sacral colpopexy. *Int Urogynecol J.* 2010;21:1569.

Nagata I, Kato K. Sacrospinous ligament fixation of vaginal apex for repair operation of uterine prolapse: operative procedure and postoperative outcome evaluated with score system and X-ray subtraction colpography. *Acta Obstet Gynacol Jpn*. 1986;38:29.

Nager CW, Visco AG, Richter HE, et al. Effect of vaginal mesh hysteropexy vs vaginal hysterectomy with uterosacral ligament suspension on treatment failure in women with uterovaginal prolapse: a randomized clinical trial. *JAMA*. 2019;322:1054.

Nager CW, Visco AG, Richter HE, et al. Effect of sacrospinous hysteropexy with graft vs vaginal hysterectomy with uterosacral ligament suspension on treatment failure in women with uterovaginal prolapse: 5-year results of a randomized clinical trial. *Am J Obstet Gynecol*. 2021 epub ahead of print.

Nichols DH. Fertility retention in the patient with genital prolapse. *Am J Obstet Gynecol*. 1991;164:1155.

Nichols D. Massive eversion of the vagina. In: *Gynecologic and Obstetric Surgery*. St. Louis: Mosby; 1993.

Nichols DH, Randall CL. *Vaginal Surgery*. 3rd ed. Baltimore: Williams & Wilkins; 1989.

Nosti PA, Lowman JK, Zollinger TW, et al. Risk of mesh erosion after abdominal sacral colpoperineopexy with concomitant hysterectomy. *Am J Obstet Gynecol*. 2009;201:541.

Nygaard IE, McCreery R, Brubaker L, et al. Abdominal sacrocolpopexy: a comprehensive review. *Obstet Gynecol*. 2004;104:805.

Nygaard IE, Brubaker L, Zyczynski HM, et al. Long-term outcomes following abdominal sacrocolpopexy for pelvic organ prolapse. *JAMA*. 2013;309:2016.

Olsen AL, Smith VJ, Bergstrom JO, et al. Epidemiology of surgically managed pelvic organ prolapse and urinary incontinence. *Obstet Gynecol*. 1997;89:501.

Paraiso MFR, Ballard LA, Walters MD, et al. Pelvic support defects and visceral and sexual function in women treated with sacrospinous ligament suspension and pelvic reconstruction. *Obstet Gynecol*. 1996;175:1423.

Paraiso MF, Walters MD, Rackley RR, et al. Laparoscopic and abdominal sacral colpopexies: a comparative cohort study. *Am J Obstet Gynecol*. 2005;192:1752.

Paraiso MF, Jelovsek JE, Frick A, et al. Laparoscopic compared with robotic sacrocolpopexy for vaginal prolapse: a randomized controlled trial. *Obstet Gynecol*. 2011;118:1005.

Peters WA, Christenson ML. Fixation of the vaginal apex to the coccygeus fascia during repair of vaginal vault eversion with enterocele. *Am J Obstet Gynecol*. 1995;172:1894.

Phaneuf TE. Inversion of the vagina and prolapse of the cervix following suprapubic hysterectomy and inversion of the vagina following total hysterectomy. *Am J Obstet Gynecol*. 1952;64:739.

Quiroz LH, Gutman RE, Shippey S, et al. Abdominal sacrocolpopexy: anatomic outcomes and complications with Pelvicol, autologous and synthetic graft materials. *Am J Obstet Gynecol*. 2008;198:557.e1.

Ramanah R, Ballester M, Chereau E, et al. Anorectal symptoms before and after laparoscopic sacrocolpoperineopexy for pelvic organ prolapse. *Int Urogynecol J*. 2012;23:779.

Randall C, Nichols D. Surgical treatment of vaginal inversion. *Obstet Gynecol*. 1971;38:327.

Rardin CR, Erekson EA, Sung VW, et al. Uterosacral colpopexy at the time of vaginal hysterectomy: comparison of laparoscopic and vaginal approaches. *J Reprod Med*. 2009;54:273.

Richardson AC, Lyon JB, Williams NL. A new look at pelvic relaxation. *Am J Obstet Gynecol*. 1976;126:568.

Richardson DA, Scotti RJ, Ostergard DR. Surgical management of uterine prolapse in young women. *J Reprod Med*. 1989;34:388.

Richardson AC. The anatomic defects in rectocele and enterocele. *J Pelvic Surg*. 1995;1:215.

Richter K. Massive eversion of the vagina: pathogenesis, diagnosis, and therapy of the "true" prolapse of the vaginal stump. *Clin Obstet Gynecol*. 1982;25:897.

Ridley JH. A composite vaginal vault suspension using fascia lata. *Am J Obstet Gynecol*. 1976;126:590.

Rondini C, Braun H, Alvarez J, et al. High uterosacral vault suspension vs sacrocolpopexy for treating apical defects: a randomized controlled trial with twelve months follow-up. *Int Urogynecol J*. 2015;26:1131.

Roovers JP, van der Vaart CH, van der Bom JG, et al. A randomized controlled trial comparing abdominal and vaginal prolapse surgery: effects for urogenital function. *Br J Obstet Gynaecol*. 2004;111:50.

Roth TM, Reight I. Laparoscopic mesh explantation and drainage of sacral abscess remote from transvaginal excision of exposed sacral colpopexy mesh. *Int Urogynecol J*. 2012;23:953.

Rust JA, Botte JM, Howlett RJ. Prolapse of the vaginal vault. Improved techniques for management of the abdominal approach or vaginal approach. *Am J Obstet Gynecol*. 1976;125:768.

Sauer HA, Klutke CG. Transvaginal sacrospinous ligament fixation for treatment of vaginal prolapse. *J Urol*. 1995;154:1008.

Schimpf MO, Abed H, Sanses T, et al. Graft and mesh use in transvaginal prolapse repair: a systematic review. *Obstet Gynecol*. 2016;128:81.

Sederl J. Zur operation des prolapses der blind endigendensheiden. *Geburtshilfe Frauenheilkd*. 1958;18:824.

Serati M, Bogani G, Sorice P, et al. Robot-assisted sacrocolpopexy for pelvic organ prolapse: a systematic review and meta-analysis of comparative studies. *Eur Urol*. 2014;66:303.

Serati M, Braga A, Bogani G, et al. Iliococcygeus fixation for the treatment of apical vaginal prolapse: efficacy and safety at 5 years of follow-up. *Int Urogynecol J*. 2015;26:1007.

Sharp TR. Sacrospinous suspension made easy. *Obstet Gynecol*. 1993;82:873.

Shull BL, Capen CV, Riggs MW, et al. Preoperative analysis of site-specific pelvic support defects in 81 women treated with sacrospinous ligament suspension and pelvic reconstruction. *Am J Obstet Gynecol*. 1992;166:1764.

Shull BT, Capen CV, Riggs MW, et al. Bilateral attachment of the vaginal cuff to ileococcygeus fascia: an effective method of cuff suspension. *Am J Obstet Gynecol*. 1993;168:1669.

Shull BL. Pelvic organ prolapse: anterior, superior, and posterior vaginal segment defects. *Am J Obstet Gynecol*. 1999;181:6.

Shull BL, Bachofen C, Coates KW, Kuehl TJ. A transvaginal approach to repair of apical and other associated sites of pelvic organ prolapse with uterosacral ligaments. *Am J Obstet Gynecol*. 2000;183:1365.

Siddiqui SA, Gutman RE, Schön Ybarra MA, et al. Relationship of the uterosacral ligament to the sacral plexus and to the pudendal nerve. *Int Urogynecol J*. 2006;17:642.

Siddiqui NY, Fulton RG, Kuchibhatla M, Wu JM. Sexual function after vaginal versus nonvaginal prolapse surgery. *Female Pelvic Med Reconstr Surg*. 2012;18:239.

Siddiqui NY, Geller EJ, Visco AG. Symptomatic and anatomic 1-year outcomes after robotic and abdominal sacrocolpopexy. *Am J Obstet Gynecol*. 2012;206:435.e1.

Siddiqui NY, Grimes CL, Casiano ER, et al. Mesh sacrocolpopexy compared with native tissue vaginal repair: a systematic review and meta-analysis. *Obstet Gynecol*. 2015;25:44.

Snyder TE, Krantz KE. Abdominal-retroperitoneal sacral colpopexy for the correction of vaginal prolapse. *Obstet Gynecol*. 1991;77:944.

Subak LL, Waetjen LE, van den Eeden S, et al. Cost of pelvic organ prolapse surgery in the United States. *Obstet Gynecol.* 2001;98:646.

Summers A, Winkel LA, Hussain HK, DeLancey JO. The relationship between anterior and apical compartment support. *Am J Obstet Gynecol.* 2006;194:1438.

Sutton GP, Addison WA, Livengood CH, et al. Life-threatening hemorrhage complicating sacral colpopexy. *Am J Obstet Gynecol.* 1981;140:836.

Swift SE. The distribution of pelvic organ support in a population of female subjects seen for routine gynecologic health care. *Am J Obstet Gynecol.* 2000;183:277.

Sze EH, Karram MM. Transvaginal repair of vault prolapse: a review. *Obstet Gynecol.* 1997;89:466.

Tan-Kim J, Menefee SA, Luber KM, et al. Prevalence and risk factors for mesh erosion after laparoscopic-assisted sacrocolpopexy. *Int Urogynecol J.* 2011;22:205.

Tancer ML, Fleischer M, Berkowitz BJ. Simultaneous colpo-recto-sacropexy. *Obstet Gynecol.* 1987;70:951.

Tarr ME, Paraiso MFR. Laparoscopic and robotic surgery for pelvic organ prolapse and stress urinary incontinence. In: Walters MD, Karram MM, eds. *Urogynecology and Reconstructive Pelvic Surgery.* 4th ed. Philadelphia: Elsevier; 2015.

Tate SB, Blackwell L, Lorenz DJ, et al. Randomized trial of fascia lata and polypropylene mesh for abdominal sacrocolpopexy: 5-year follow-up. *Int Urogynecol J.* 2011;22:137.

Timmons MC, Kohler MF, Addison WA. Thumbtack use for control of presacral bleeding, with description of an instrument for thumbtack application. *Obstet Gynecol.* 1991;78:313.

Timmons MC, Addison WA, Addison SB, et al. Abdominal sacral colpopexy in 163 women with posthysterectomy vaginal vault prolapse and enterocele. *J Reprod Med.* 1992;37:323.

Todd JW. Mesh suspension for vaginal prolapse. *Int Surg.* 1978;63:91.

Toozs-Hobson P, Boos K, Cardozo L. Management of vaginal vault prolapse. *Br J Obstet Gynaecol.* 1998;105:13.

Traiman P, De Lucia LA, Silva AA, et al. Abdominal colpopexy for complete prolapse of the vagina. *Int Surg.* 1992;77:91.

Turner LC, Lavelle ES, Shepherd JP. Comparison of complications and prolapse recurrence between laparoscopic and vaginal uterosacral ligament suspension for the treatment of vaginal prolapse. *Int Urogynecol J.* 2016;27:797.

Twijnstra AR, Blikkendaal MD, van Zwet EW, et al. Predictors of successful surgical outcome in laparoscopic hysterectomy, *Obstet Gynecol.* 2012;119:700.

Ulmsten U, Ekman G, Giertz G, et al. Different biochemical composition of connective tissue in continent and stress incontinent women. *Acta Obstet Gynecol Scand.* 1987;66:455.

Unger CA, Walters MD, Ridgeway B, et al. Incidence of adverse events after uterosacral colpopexy for uterovaginal and posthysterectomy vault prolapse. *Am J Obstet Gynecol.* 2015;212:603.e1.

US. Food and Drug Administration. *Urogynecologic Surgical Mesh Implants.* Available at: http://www.fda.gov/MedicalDevices/ProductsandMedicalProcedures/ImplantsandProsthetics/UroGynSurgicalMesh/default.htm. Accessed November 02, 2020.

van Brummen HJ, van de Pol, Aulders CI, et al. Sacrospinous hysteropexy compared to vaginal hysterectomy as primary surgical treatment for a descensus uteri: effects on urinary symptoms. *Int J Urogynecol.* 2003;14:350.

van Lindert AC, Groenendijk AG, Scholten PC, et al. Surgical support and suspension of genital prolapse, including preservation of the uterus, using Gore-Tex soft tissue patch. *Eur J Obstet Gynecol Reprod Biol.* 1996;50:133.

Visco AG, Weidner AC, Barber MD, et al. Vaginal mesh erosion after abdominal sacral colpopexy. *Am J Obstet Gynecol.* 2001;184:297.

Vitranen H, Hirvonen T, Makinen J, et al. Outcome of thirty patients who underwent repair of posthysterectomy prolapse of the vaginal vault with abdominal sacral colpopexy. *J Am Coll Surg.* 1994;178:283.

Wallenstein MR, Ananth CV, Kim JH, et al. Effect of surgical volume on outcomes for laparoscopic hysterectomy for benign indications. *Obstet Gynecol.* 2012;119:709.

Walters MD, Ridgeway BM. Surgical treatment of vaginal apex prolapse. *Obstet Gynecol.* 2013;121:354.

Warner WB, Vora S, Hurtado EA, et al. Effect of operative technique on mesh exposure in laparoscopic sacrocolpopexy. *Female Pelvic Med Reconstr Surg.* 2012;18:113.

Webb MJ, Aronson MP, Ferguson LK, et al. Posthysterectomy vaginal vault prolapse: primary repair in 693 patients. *Obstet Gynecol.* 1998;92:281.

Wei JT, Nygaard I, Richter HE, et al. A midurethral sling to reduce incontinence after vaginal prolapse repair. *N Engl J Med.* 2012;366:2358.

Whiteside JL, Barber MD, Walters MD, Falcone T. Anatomy of ilioinguinal and iliohypogastric nerves in relation to trocar placement and low transverse incisions. *Am J Obstet Gynecol.* 2003;198:1574.

Wu JM, Hundley AF, Fulton RG, Myers ER. Forecasting the prevalence of pelvic floor disorders in US Women: 2010 to 2050. *Obstet Gynecol.* 2009;114:1278.

Wu JM, Vaughan CP, Goode PS, et al. Prevalence and trends of symptomatic pelvic floor disorders in US women. *Obstet Gynecol.* 2014;123:141.

22

Uterine Preservation in Pelvic Organ Prolapse Surgery

Beri M. Ridgeway and Kate V. Meriwether

CHAPTER OUTLINE

INTRODUCTION

Uterine prolapse is a common disorder in women. It represents the third leading cause of hysterectomy for benign disease and is responsible for approximately 70,000 hysterectomies annually in the United States, double the operation rate on women posed by mastectomies with reconstruction for breast cancer (Sisco et al., 2016). Given this large surgical volume, measures to increase the efficiency and safety of prolapse surgeries are paramount. Traditionally, operations to treat uterine and uterovaginal prolapse include a hysterectomy, even when no specific uterine disease is present. It is known from anatomical studies that the uterus is not the cause of prolapse, and that hysterectomy itself is a risk factor for prolapse formation (DeLancey, 1992; Forsgren et al., 2012). A recent systematic review that included a dozen randomized trials and 41 nonrandomized trials comparing prolapse surgery with hysterectomy to prolapse surgery with uterine preservation found no differences in prolapse outcomes in the short to medium term and found that the morbidity of some procedures (such as blood loss and operative time) decreased with preservation of the uterus (Meriwether et al., 2018).

The surgical treatment of uterovaginal prolapse using uterine-sparing techniques has evolved from vaginal procedures using native tissue to laparoscopic and robotic procedures using polypropylene mesh. Although many of these operations use the same techniques and principles as those used to treat vaginal vault prolapse, the outcome data are fewer, and direct comparisons lack rigorous or long-term follow-up. The interest in uterine conservation among patients and physicians is growing worldwide, despite some data from a large population study indicating that hysterectomy may be protective against repeat prolapse surgery (Dallas et al., 2018). Overall, there are limited guidelines regarding the choice of uterine preservation in prolapse surgery. The objective of this chapter is to review and summarize the medical literature describing the role of uterine preservation during the surgical management of uterovaginal prolapse.

HISTORICAL PERSPECTIVE

The origins of the vaginal hysteropexy date back to the late 1800s when techniques were developed to treat uterine retroversion. Initial accounts describe a procedure that delivered the fundus of the uterus through an anterior colpotomy and sutured the anterior fundus to the anterior vaginal wall. Various modifications to this technique were made, although no modification obtained published endorsement. Despite this, vaginal fixation of the uterus had taken hold, and outcomes were endorsed by Mackenrodt's numerous publications and a comprehensive report by Duhrssen in 1894 detailing 207 operations. These techniques were later translated into treatment for vesicovaginal fistula (using the fundus as a plug) and later, in 1896, as treatment for prolapse (Eastman, 1897).

In 1899, Thomas Watkins was the first to publish descriptions of what came to be known as a uterine interposition operation (Watkins, 1899). The uterus was separated from the vagina using a circumferential incision, and the bladder was separated from the uterus using blunt dissection. The fundus of the uterus was grasped and anteverted through the anterior colpotomy and sutured to the proximal 2 inches of the anterior vaginal wall. The posterior vaginal wall was opened to 1 inch distal to the cervix to allow the cervix to be displaced upward and backward by this inversion. Although outcomes were only reported for one patient, this procedure was quite popular during the early twentieth century. However, as theoretical concerns developed regarding potential pregnancy in younger patients and difficult endometrial access in older patients, the interposition operation gradually became less popular and was largely supplanted by the Manchester procedure.

The Manchester procedure was first performed in 1888 by Archibald Donald of Manchester, England, with several modifications introduced by W.E. Fothergill. The procedure was first described for uterovaginal prolapse in patients with cervical elongation and intact uterosacral-cardinal ligaments. This procedure begins by making a circumferential incision around the cervix, dissecting the vaginal epithelium cephalad similar to during performance of a vaginal hysterectomy, and clamping and transecting the cardinal ligaments bilaterally. The distal, elongated cervix is then amputated, and the remaining proximal cervix is retracted downward while the cardinal ligament pedicles are sutured to the anterior cervix. This serves to retract the cervix posteriorly and elevate the uterus anteriorly. The transformation zone is then recreated with the invagination of vaginal epithelium into the cervical os.

The largest study on the Manchester procedure (and the largest study on hysteropexy to date), by Conger and Keettel (1958), reported on 960 patients. Based on a review of medical records and a mailed questionnaire with a 52% response rate, the prolapse recurrence rate was determined to be 4.3%. Other studies note a reoperation rate of 21%, including reoperation for prolapse, as well as abnormal bleeding and cervical carcinoma. More recent data include a retrospective chart review by Thomas et al. (1995) that compared the outcomes of 88 consecutive patients who underwent Manchester procedures with the outcomes of 105 randomly selected patients who underwent vaginal hysterectomy with anterior and posterior repair as indicated. The Manchester group was older and had worse uterovaginal prolapse compared with the hysterectomy group. The Manchester procedure was noted to be quicker (30 minutes shorter) and to have less blood loss (200 vs. 300 mL). Follow-up consisted of questionnaires mailed to the surgeons who performed the operations. With a mean follow-up of 2.5 years, and a 76% response rate, only 6% of patients were noted to have recurrent prolapse after the Manchester procedure, with time to recurrence ranging from 8 weeks to 5.5 years, but no follow-up data for the vaginal hysterectomy group were reported. Despite relatively limited outcomes data, the Manchester procedure is still considered a safe option for treating uterovaginal prolapse without requiring hysterectomy. In fact, a recent study that analyzed data from a nationwide database in Denmark reported that the Manchester procedure had less than a fourth of the risk for anterior recurrence of prolapse compared with sacrospinous hysteropexy and a much lower reoperation for prolapse, bringing into question the relatively low utilization of this procedure in modern practice (Husby et al., 2019).

Complications of the Manchester procedure need to be taken in the context of when the procedures were performed. In the series describing 960 patients (Conger & Keettel, 1958), the procedures were performed from 1936 to 1955, and the following complications were reported: cystotomy and proctotomy less than 0.5%; blood transfusion 20%; febrile morbidity 63%; urinary retention 15.2%; and mortality 0.7%. Clearly, the high rates of some complications are related more to medical and surgical practices of the era than directly to the Manchester procedure itself. In another series, complications were not noted to be significantly different when compared with vaginal hysterectomy with anterior and posterior repair, with the exception of decreased cuff abscess and cellulitis in the Manchester procedure (Thomas et al., 1995). Other complications noted in these series include abnormal uterine bleeding and carcinoma, both of which are of a concern for all uterine-sparing procedures. Furthermore, cervical amputation is related to infertility, miscarriage, and preterm delivery. Tipton and Atkin (1970) specifically examined uterine disease 6 to 12 years after the Manchester procedure in 82 patients, finding that 35% of women complained of menorrhagia and dysmenorrhea, and over half of these patients required treatment. Additionally, 2.4% of patients developed adenocarcinoma of the uterus, and 4% of patients experienced unplanned pregnancies. Interestingly, 27% of patients stated that they would have welcomed hysterectomy at the time of the operation, and many patients stated that contraception was unsatisfactory. Vaginal hysterectomy has become more popular since that time, as antibiotics and improved surgical technique have led to decreased morbidity and mortality related to pelvic reconstructive surgery. In the twenty-first century, the patients who are optimal candidates for the Manchester procedure must weigh this against good safety data for other approaches to hysteropexy, as well as hysterectomy with vault suspension. In the recent large Danish study, the 5-year reoperation rates for vaginal hysterectomy and the Manchester procedure were comparable (11% and 7%, respectively) (Husby et al., 2019).

In the 1950s, as the abdominal approach to hysterectomy became popular, cases describing an abdominal approach to hysteropexy were published. Sacrocervicopexy, in this instance indicating suspension of the cervix as still attached to a preserved uterine body, was first described by Stoesser in 1955 as the attachment of a band of external oblique fascia from the cervix to the sacral periosteum. The case series of 22 patients reported "good" results but provided limited information on methodology and outcome measurement. A combined vaginal-abdominal procedure targeting both uterovaginal prolapse and stress urinary incontinence was described by Nesbitt (1989) in a case series of 16 patients. The procedure involved vaginal mobilization of the bladder neck, periurethral tissue, uterine, isthmus, and uterosacral-cardinal ligament complex, followed by a Moschcowitz culdoplasty and transabdominal suspension of the periurethral endopelvic fascia and uterosacral ligaments to Cooper's ligament. There were no complications or failures noted at a follow-up interval of over 5 years, although the study was limited by its size and lack of control group. Joshi (1993) published a case series of 20 patients who underwent a transabdominal Cooper's ligament uterine suspension using Mersilene tape. There were no complications reported, nor were there any cases of recurrent prolapse. However, the follow-up was limited to a range of 6 to 30 months, and postoperative examination findings were not described. Notably, seven women conceived within 6 months of the operation, five of whom delivered vaginally at term. Procedures using Cooper's ligament suspension are no longer routinely used for uterine preservation and have been replaced by transvaginal native tissue or minimally invasive approaches to sacrohysteropexy using polypropylene mesh.

CONSIDERATIONS FOR UTERINE PRESERVATION

With the advent of antibiotics and improved surgical techniques, the morbidity and mortality related to hysterectomy were greatly reduced, and the rates of uterine removal increased in the later part of the twentieth century. Additionally, hysterectomy was considered favorable, given the potential to reduce endometrial and cervical cancer risks. Since that time, improved conservative treatment for abnormal bleeding and symptomatic leiomyoma, effective strategies for cervical cancer screening, the human papilloma virus (HPV) vaccine, and an emphasis on quality of life have led physicians and patients to modify their thoughts on hysterectomy. Please see Box 22.1 for perceived and studied advantages and disadvantages of uterine preservation at the time of prolapse surgery.

Patient Interest

A study by Frick et al. (2013) investigated attitudes towards hysterectomy in women undergoing evaluation for uterovaginal prolapse. Patients who were scheduled for evaluation were sent a questionnaire in the mail that queried their perceptions of the impact of hysterectomy on health, social life, and emotional well-being. It also presented hypothetical situations. Of the 100 women who completed the questionnaire, 60% indicated they would decline a hysterectomy if presented with an equally efficacious prolapse repair that preserved the uterus. In a scenario in which the prolapse repair after hysterectomy was considered "probably more successful," 54% preferred a hysterectomy if it offered any benefit, while 32% desired hysterectomy for "substantial benefit," and 14% did not desire hysterectomy in this situation. Those patients who were younger and who were considered active decision-makers were more likely to decline hysterectomy. Additionally, those with family and friends who had had a negative experience after hysterectomy were more likely to decline a hysterectomy-based procedure.

This perception of hysterectomy is also gaining significant media attention. Although not scientific journals, well-read publications for the lay public such as *Health Magazine* and the *American Association of Retired People* magazine have recently published articles citing hysterectomy as a "surgery to avoid."

The American College of Obstetrics and Gynecology acknowledged the importance of patient autonomy and the increased access to information in a Committee Opinion published in 2013. Although urging that decision-making should be guided by the ethical principles of respect for patient autonomy, beneficence, nonmaleficence, veracity, and justice, they recommend that it is important to take a broad view of the consequences of surgical treatment and to acknowledge the lack of firm evidence for the benefit of one approach over the other.

Lack of Data Supporting Hysterectomy to Treat Prolapse

The need for hysterectomy at the time of prolapse repair has never been proven. Removing the uterus fails to address the underlying deficiency causing prolapse. Additionally, removal of the uterus disrupts the uterosacral-cardinal ligament complex, which may further weaken support. This is not a novel concept, as Bonney in the 1930s stated that the uterus only has a passive role in prolapse. Uterine preservation at the time of prolapse repair avoids an unnecessary procedure and has been associated with faster operative times and less blood loss. Now that a systematic review has investigated the utility of hysterectomy in prolapse repair and found no notable differences in outcomes and decreased morbidity in some surgeries (such as lower mesh exposure following mesh surgeries), there still appears to be no

BOX 22.1 Perceived and Studied Advantages and Disadvantages of Uterine Preservation at the Time of Prolapse Surgery

Advantages	Disadvantages
Reduction in surgical time and blood loss	Fewer surgical outcome data available
Maintenance of fertility	Maintenance of fertility
Natural menopausal timing	Small, ongoing risk for cervical or endometrial cancer
Avoidance of an unnecessary procedure	Subsequent hysterectomy may be difficult
Perceived role of the uterus and cervix in pelvic stability and sexual satisfaction	Continuation of menses
Less invasive	Ongoing surveillance of cervix and endometrium (which may be difficult)
Association with a quicker recovery	Colpopexy may be easier for surgeon after hysterectomy
Decreased blood loss	Worse POPQ C point
Decreased risk of mesh exposure	
Similar short-term outcomes	
Patient preference	
Longer total vaginal length on POPQ	

POPQ, Pelvic Organ Prolapse Questionnaire.

good evidence that hysterectomy improves incomes for women seeking surgery with prolapse (Meriweather et al., 2018).

Role of Hysterectomy in Menopause Timing and Sexual Function

There may be additional benefits to avoiding hysterectomy, including ovarian and sexual function. Even in women who undergo ovarian-sparing hysterectomies, ovarian function is affected. Two studies (Farquhar et al., 2005; Moorman et al., 2011) compared ovarian function after ovarian-sparing hysterectomies with a nonsurgical control group basing menopause on follicle-stimulating hormone levels of 40 IU/L or higher. In these cohorts, approximately twice as many women who underwent hysterectomy compared with the control group became menopausal during the 5-year study period. The difference persists even when preoperative anti-Mullerian hormone levels are similar (Trabuco et al., 2016). Sexual function is also often cited as a reason to avoid hysterectomy. Jeng et al. (2005) compared sexual function after randomizing women with uterovaginal prolapse to transvaginal hysterectomy or transvaginal sacrospinous uterine suspension for uterine prolapse, and found no significant difference between groups in sexual scores, sexual interest, and orgasm frequency. Costantini et al. (2013) compared women who underwent hysterectomy and sacral colpopexy to those who underwent a uterine-sparing procedure, noting that, although both groups had improved scores on a validated questionnaire, the uterine-sparing group was associated with a greater improvement.

Unanticipated Uterine Pathology

One concern about uterine-sparing procedures is that the rate of abnormal uterine pathology may be high, and that preserving the uterus may confer an increased cancer risk to women. Despite a large body of data on uterine preservation surgery, there are little data on occult uterine malignancy or risk of later development of malignancy in preserved uteri. In a recent systematic review on uterine preservation prolapse surgery that included 94 studies (with 53 comparing uterine preservation with hysterectomy for prolapse), only two studies, one randomized and one nonrandomized, reported clearly on uterine pathology. Cvach et al. reported that 1/18 (5.5%) patients needed subsequent surgery owing to uterine pathology (hysteroscopy and curettage with benign findings), and 4/18 (22%) needed some type of workup because of abnormal bleeding, with all having benign findings on workup. Rahmanou et al. reported that 1/50 (2%) patients randomized to vaginal hysterectomy had an incidental finding of uterine malignancy, but no subsequent findings of uterine malignancy were seen in patients randomized to uterine preservation.

The risk of cervical carcinoma has not been well studied in hysteropexy, but data from studies evaluating supracervical hysterectomy can be extrapolated to hysteropexy. Even in studies that predated modern cytologic and viral screening techniques, the rate of cervical carcinoma was low (<0.3%). With improved cytologic and viral screening, as well as the HPV vaccine, the true number is likely to be even lower. Studies evaluating uterine pathology also demonstrate a low risk for endometrial cancer. Renganathan et al. (2013) studied pathologic specimens from 517 women who underwent vaginal hysterectomy for prolapse and found the rate of endometrial cancer to be 0.8%. Frick et al. (2010) also evaluated the risk of unanticipated pathology at the time of hysterectomy for uterovaginal prolapse. Of 681 pathologic specimens, 2.6% had unanticipated premalignant or malignant uterine pathology, including 0.3% with low-grade cervical dysplasia, 0.8% with simple hyperplasia, 0.5% with complex hyperplasia, 1.1% with complex hyperplasia with atypia, and 0.3% with endometrial carcinoma. Interestingly, none of the premenopausal women had premalignant or malignant pathology, even those with preoperative bleeding concerns. In contrast, postmenopausal women with abnormal bleeding had a very high rate (13.3%) of unanticipated endometrial pathology, even though all had had negative diagnostic evaluations.

Contraindications to uterine-sparing prolapse procedures are listed in Box 22.2.

BOX 22.2 Contraindications for Uterine Preservation

- Pregnancy
- Postmenopausal bleeding
- Current or recent cervical dysplasia
- Familial cancer syndrome (*BRCA1* and *BRCA2* mutations, HNPCC, etc.)
- Tamoxifen therapy
- Symptomatic uterine abnormalities
- Fibroids, adenomyosis, abnormal endometrial sampling
- Abnormal uterine bleeding
- Inability to comply with routine gynecologic surveillance
- Cervical elongation (relative contraindication)

HNPCC, Hereditary nonpolyposis colorectal cancer.

VAGINAL APPROACH

The vaginal approach to hysteropexy has a long history dating back to 1888. Vaginal surgery was highly preferable because of the high morbidity and mortality related to abdominal surgery, and hysterectomy by any route added further morbidity. Current data continue to support this, as vaginal hysteropexy is associated with less operative time, less blood loss, faster recovery, and better cosmesis than other approaches (Meriwether et al., 2019). Vaginal hysteropexy using native tissue consists of four surgical procedures: the Watkins interposition surgery, the Manchester procedure, the transvaginal uterosacral ligament suspension/plication, and the sacrospinous hysteropexy. Of these procedures, the sacrospinous hysteropexy is the most popular, and data are available supporting satisfactory anatomic, subjective, and functional outcomes. Prepackaged mesh prolapse kits were used in the past to correct uterovaginal prolapse without requiring hysterectomy, but these kits are no longer available. For this reason, interest in mesh-free uterine preservation procedures by the least invasive route (vaginally) is currently reemerging.

Transvaginal Uterosacral Ligament Suspension/Plication

This procedure was first reported in 1966 and was described as entering the peritoneal cavity via a posterior colpotomy, dividing the uterosacral ligaments from the cervix, plicating them across the midline, and then reinserting them into the cervix. Following this, a transverse incision was made at the junction of the bladder reflection and cervix, and the cardinal ligaments were plicated across the midline anteriorly, drawing the cervix upward. Follow-up data for this procedure are limited (Romanzi & Tyagi, 2012). A case series by Williams (1966) of 20 women aged 21 to 37 years, all of whom had uterovaginal prolapse at least to the introitus, noted a failure rate of 15.5%; all of these cases were treated with vaginal hysterectomy within 6 months of the original surgery. Three additional patients (15%) required subsequent hysterectomy for continued vaginal bleeding. Although length of follow-up is not clearly reported, six women subsequently had full-term pregnancies with no recurrence of prolapse. A more recent study by Romanzi and Tyagi (2012) compared 100 cases of vaginal hysterectomy and uterosacral ligament suspension with uterosacral ligament hysteropexy. In this series, the surgeon performed a colpotomy, identified the high uterosacral ligament, and placed two delayed-absorbable sutures through each ligament, attaching them to the posterior vaginal cuff and lower uterine wall. Culdoplasty, trachelorrhaphy, and concomitant repairs were performed at the discretion of the surgeon. Anatomic success was defined as grade 2 (or less) prolapse using the Baden–Walker system, and average follow-up was 1.5 years. In the hysteropexy group, apical success was noted to be 96%, anterior wall success was noted to be 86.8%, and posterior wall success was noted to be 97.8%, all statistically similar to the hysterectomy group.

Video 22.1 demonstrates the surgical technique for a uterosacral hysteropexy.

Complications related to the transvaginal uterosacral ligament suspension/plication include genitourinary tract infection, pelvic cellulitis, and atonic bladder symptoms. The overall complication rate in the Williams study was 20%. In this series, three patients required hysterectomies for abnormal uterine bleeding. In the Romanzi study, the complication rate was much lower (6%). In this series, three women required hysterectomy for various, unrelated reasons (breast cancer, *BRCA1/2* mutation carrier, enlarging fibroid). One pregnancy was reported.

Sacrospinous Ligament Hysteropexy

The sacrospinous hysteropexy is the best-studied native tissue vaginal approach to uterine-sparing prolapse repair. The literature contains anatomic outcomes data with a larger number of patients, as well as functional, reproductive, and sexual outcomes. This procedure typically consists of performing an extraperitoneal dissection until the right sacrospinous ligament is identified and exposed. The right sacrospinous ligament is then attached to the posterior cervix or uterosacral ligaments and vagina using a combination of permanent and delayed absorbable sutures (Fig. 22.1 and 22.2). Placing suture in the sacrospinous ligament can be achieved with free suturing, with the aid of reusable ligature carriers, such as the Miyazaki hook or the Deschamps needle ligature carrier, or with disposable suture-capturing devices. In many cases, an anterior and/or posterior colporrhaphy are performed as indicated. In patients wishing to maintain fertility, this procedure has advantages over the Manchester procedure, as it does not require cervical amputation, which has been associated with infertility, miscarriage, and preterm birth. Furthermore, it may provide higher suspension compared with the transvaginal uterosacral ligament suspension/plication. Video 22.2 demonstrates the surgical technique of a sacrospinous hysteropexy.

Results of this procedure were first presented in a 1989 case series by Richardson et al. Five patients ranging in age from 24 to 31 years underwent this procedure to treat uterovaginal prolapse and had follow-up ranging from 6 to 24 months. No recurrences or pregnancies were reported. These data, however, lack descriptions of preoperative prolapse and definitions of success.

The first descriptions of pregnancy following this procedure were reported by Kovac and Cruikshank (1993). The authors detailed 19 patients with a mean age of 27 years with uterovaginal prolapse at least to the hymen with Valsalva who wished to maintain childbearing capacity. Four patients underwent unilateral fixation of the uterosacral ligaments to the right sacrospinous ligament, with the remainder undergoing bilateral fixation. At a mean follow-up of 3.1 years, the majority of patients were doing well. Of the patients not attempting pregnancy, 11 of 12 had good objective results with excellent uterovaginal support. One patient with unilateral fixation presented with recurrent prolapse 6 weeks following surgery and underwent bilateral fixation with good anatomic results. Over the 3 years, slight cervical descensus was generally noted; however, no patient had prolapse past the midvagina. Five of the nineteen patients became pregnant, with all having uncomplicated vaginal deliveries. Of these patients, only one noted moderate uterovaginal prolapse after her delivery and, subsequent to a second delivery, underwent vaginal hysterectomy and sacrospinous ligament fixation of the vaginal vault.

Additional data using medical records, patient surveys, validated questionnaires, and follow-up Pelvic Organ Prolapse Quantification (POPQ) exams confirm these positive outcomes. A study published by Dietz et al. in 2007 described 133 women who underwent unilateral sacrospinous hysteropexy and anterior/posterior repair as indicated. Ninety-nine women responded to the postal questionnaire, and 60 followed up for detailed POPQ examination. At a mean follow-up time of 22.8 months, 6% of the 133 women were diagnosed with recurrent uterovaginal prolapse to at least 1 cm above the hymen. Of women undergoing gynecologic examination with POPQ measurements, 30% had a stage II cystocele, and 8% had a stage III cystocele. Of all patients, only three (2.8%) women required surgical treatment of recurrent prolapse. The great majority of patients were very satisfied with the results of the surgery, and 91% would recommend the procedure to other women.

The first comparison of sacrospinous hysteropexy to hysterectomy with sacrospinous vaginal vault suspension was reported by Carey and Slack (1994). This small, nonrandomized study of 11 women with sacrospinous hysteropexy and 13 with vaginal hysterectomy and sacrospinous vaginal vault suspension demonstrated that 3/11 women with uterine preservation had "marked cervical elongation," and 1/11 had "dependent ulceration of the cervix" at a mean follow-up of 4 months. There were 3/11 women in the hysteropexy group and 1/13 women in the

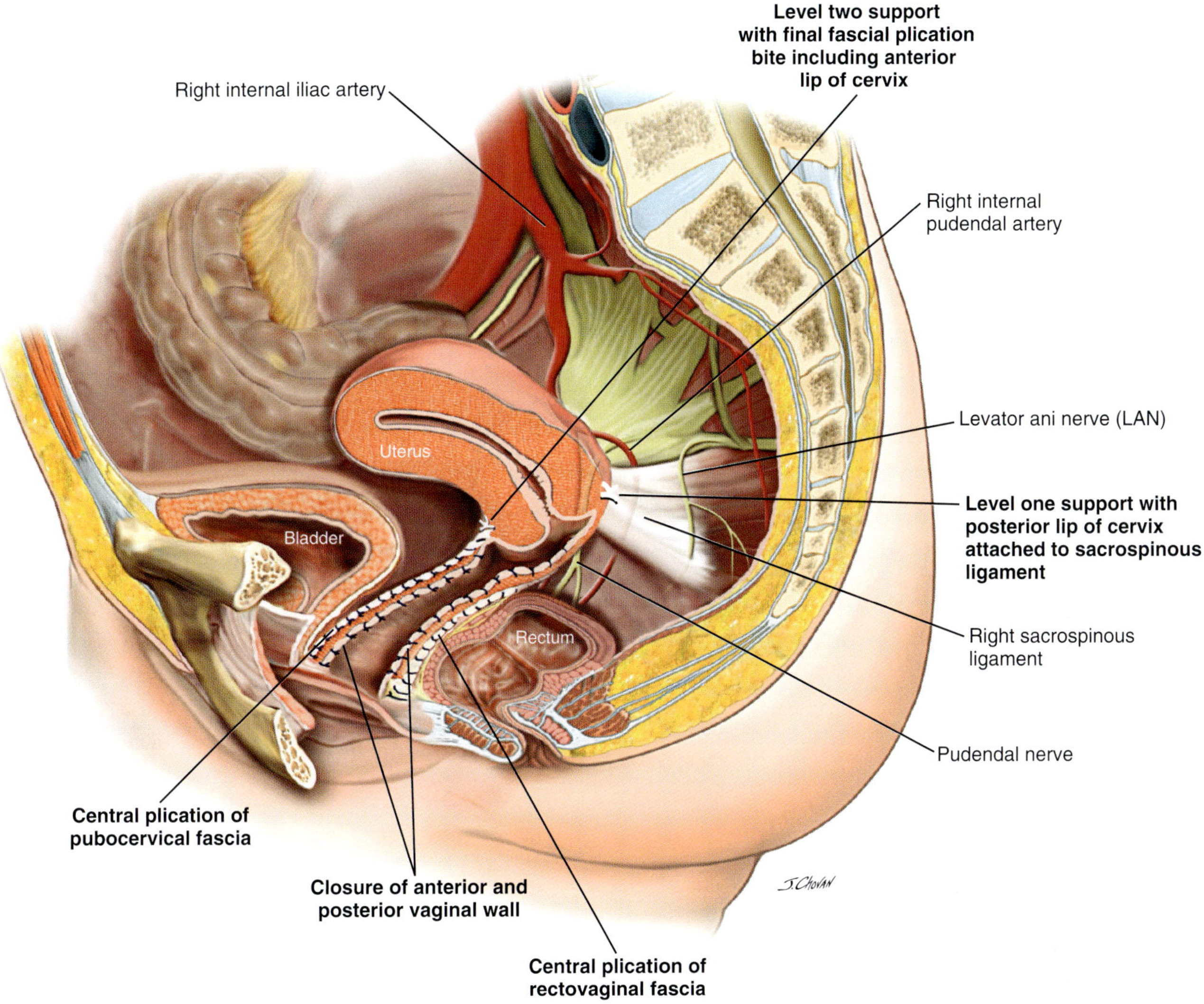

Fig. 22.1 Native tissue sacrospinous hysteropexy with the distal posterior cervix attached to the right sacrospinous ligament and anterior and posterior colporrhaphy.

hysterectomy group who had "small asymptomatic cystocele" in this short time period. A larger subsequent study by Maher et al. (2001) also showed promising results. Seventy women with uterovaginal prolapse at or beyond the vaginal introitus self-selected to hysterectomy with sacrospinous ligament fixation or sacrospinous hysteropexy. Although not randomized, the groups were similar with regard to demographics, grade of vault prolapse, history of previous surgery for prolapse or incontinence, sexual activity, and length of follow-up. The operative time and intraoperative blood loss were significantly less for the hysteropexy group. With a mean follow-up of 33 months for the hysterectomy group and 26 months for the hysteropexy group, subjective and objective outcomes were similar between groups. The subjective success rate (no awareness of prolapse) was 86% in the hysterectomy group and 78% in the hysteropexy group (P = .70), while the objective success rate (no prolapse beyond the midvagina) was also similar between groups, at 72% and 74% respectively (P = 1.00). Only two women became pregnant in this cohort, both delivering by cesarean section, with one requiring additional surgery for prolapse postdelivery. This study collected specific outcomes, used a blinded evaluator, and had a control group, lending credibility to these findings.

Subsequent randomized trials by Jeng et al. (2005), Dietz et al. (2010), and Detollenaere et al. (2015) compared sacrospinous hysteropexy to transvaginal hysterectomy and uterosacral ligament colpopexy. The largest, by Detollenaere et al., included 208 women, 103 randomized to sacrospinous hysteropexy. There were apical compartment recurrences to stage 2 in none of the hysteropexy patients and 4% of the hysterectomy patients, and this difference was not significant. At 12 months' follow-up, overall anatomic recurrences, function outcomes, quality of life, sexual function, and recovery parameters were all similar between groups. Dietz et al. randomized 71 women to one of the procedures described earlier, with return to activities at home and work as the primary outcome. They also looked at complications, anatomic outcomes, functional outcomes, and quality of life as secondary outcomes. Women who were assigned to hysteropexy returned to work 23 days earlier compared with those who underwent hysterectomy and prolapse repair. There were very few complications in both groups.

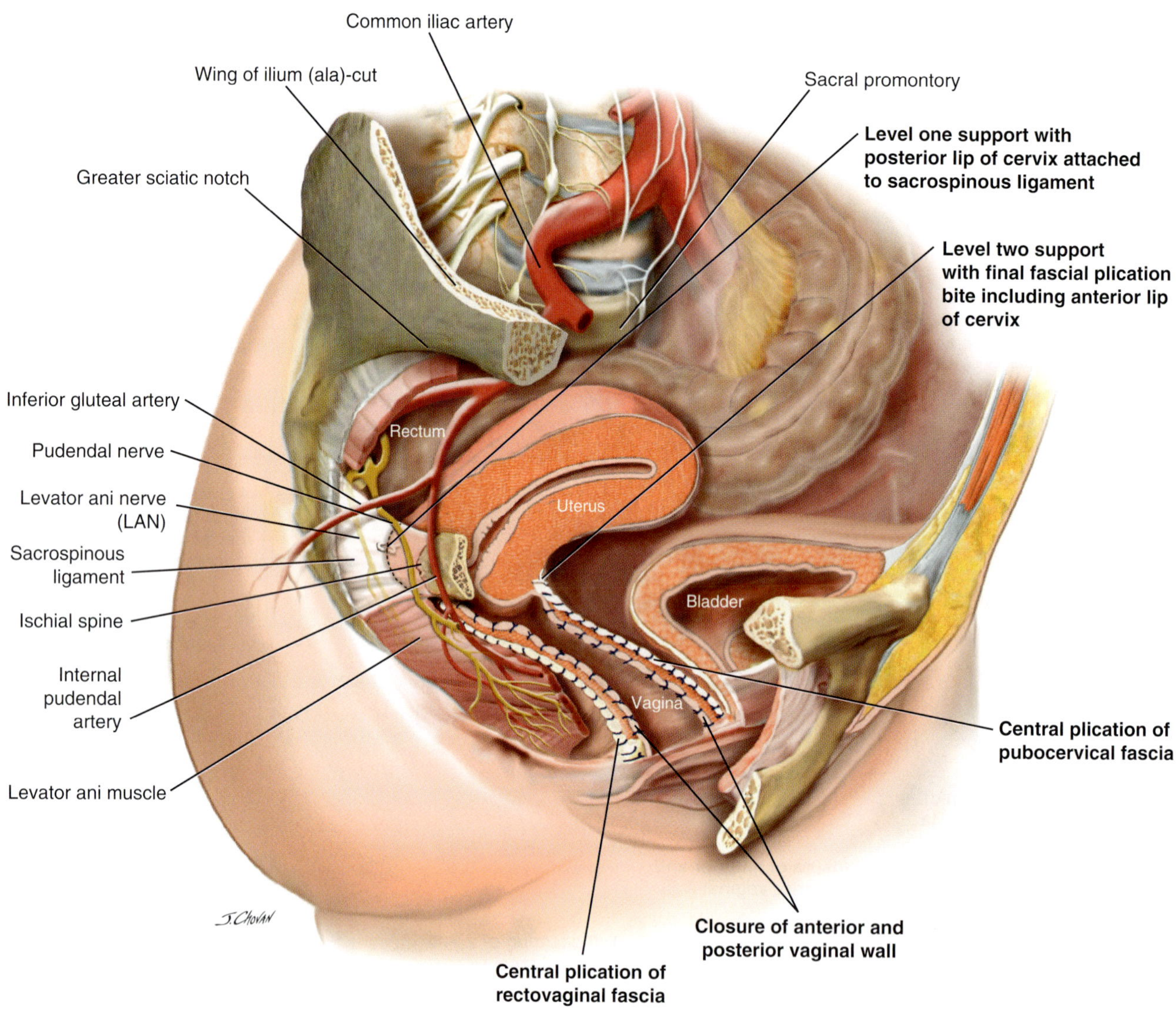

Fig. 22.2 Lateral view of the pelvis demonstrating the relationship of sacrospinous hysteropexy suspension to vessels and nerves.

At 1 year, 27% of women who underwent hysteropexy had uterine descensus of POPQ stage II or greater, with about half of these women electing repeat surgery. This was a statistically significant difference compared with those who underwent hysterectomy and prolapse repair (11%). Of women with stage IV prolapse who underwent hysteropexy, all recurred within a year. Between groups, there were no differences in validated questionnaires for prolapse symptoms, incontinence symptoms, or quality of life. The Jeng et al. study randomized 80 of 158 total patients to sacrospinous hysteropexy, and although this trial only investigated sexual function outcomes (see later), the safety of the two procedures were similar, with neither group experiencing major complications.

Additional studies have concentrated on functional outcomes, including effects on urinary symptoms and sexual function. van Brummen et al. (2003) sent postal questionnaires to 103 women who had undergone either vaginal hysterectomy or sacrospinous hysteropexy and possible anterior and posterior colporrhaphy for greater or equal to grade 2 pelvic organ prolapse according to the Baden–Walker system. The recurrence rate of grade 2 or higher vaginal prolapse was 6.7% after vaginal hysterectomy and 11.4% after sacrospinous hysteropexy (this difference was not significant). Recovery was faster ($P = .04$), and fewer patients complained of urge incontinence ($P = .05$) postprocedure following hysteropexy compared with vaginal hysterectomy. Dietz et al. (2008) prospectively followed 72 patients undergoing sacrospinous hysteropexy using validated questionnaires and the POPQ exam pre- and postoperatively. At an average follow-up of 12.7 months, 22.2% of women had recurrent prolapse in one of the compartments, with the great majority having stage II prolapse. Quality-of-life questionnaires, including the Urogenital Distress Inventory, Incontinence Impact Questionnaire, and the Defecatory Distress Inventory, demonstrated improvement in all urogenital and quality-of-life domains, as well as constipation and obstructive defecation domains. Large effect sizes were noted on pain, genital prolapse, physical functioning, and emotional health. These studies provide additional data that demonstrate that, in addition to improving anatomic outcomes, sacrospinous hysteropexy leads to functional improvement and positive changes in quality of life.

Given that unilateral sacrospinous hysteropexy deviates and somewhat changes the axis of the vagina, dyspareunia and sexual function are concerns. Sexual functioning was evaluated using face-to-face interviews after vaginal hysterectomy and sacrospinous ligament hysteropexy by Jeng et al. (2005). Patients younger than 50 years of age who were sexually active were randomly assigned to hysterectomy or sacrospinous ligament hysteropexy to treat grade 2 or 3 uterine prolapse. Before surgical intervention and 6 months after surgery women were interviewed by a trained gynecologic nurse specialist using portions of Rosen's Female Sexual Function Index. With the exception of orgasm frequency, which was slightly decreased postoperatively, sexual interest, frequency of sexual intercourse, and sexual satisfaction were not different pre- and postoperatively in either group or between groups. Neither group had changes in vaginal dryness or dyspareunia between pre- and postoperative data, and these outcomes showed no difference between groups. Although this study has some methodological flaws and did not investigate prolapse outcomes, it provides important data describing sexual function and supports that sexual function is not negatively affected by sacrospinous hysteropexy.

Now that sacrospinous hysteropexy has been established as an effective and long-lasting treatment for uterovaginal prolapse, researchers are looking for risk factors for those cases with less than ideal outcomes. A study by Lin et al. (2005b) with follow-up of at least 5 years demonstrated that cervical elongation ($P = .007$) and grade 3 uterine prolapse ($P = .007$) are significant risk factors for failure, after sacrospinous hysteropexy. Using these findings to modify the surgical practice, the authors reported that concomitant partial trachelectomy for those with an elongated cervix significantly reduced the failure rate from 75% to 0% ($P = .024$). No other risk factors were identified.

Complications of sacrospinous hysteropexy are much better documented than those for the other vaginal approaches to hysteropexy. The earliest reports note one case of proctotomy during the initial dissection that was recognized, repaired, and had no subsequent sequelae. Buttock pain has also been reported, with a rate of 5%. The most complete information on complications related to sacrospinous hysteropexy comes from data collected by van Brummen et al. (2003) from 133 consecutive women. Intraoperative complications included excessive blood loss (>500 mL) in 8% of patients and rectal injury in 0.8% of women. Postoperative complications included: buttock pain in 15%, buttock pain lasting greater than 2 weeks in 4%, urinary tract infections in 13%, and urinary retention in 27%. Of note, several patients experienced specific neurologic symptoms, including one patient with severe buttock pain based on nerve entrapment that required suture release and replacement, and another patient with introital numbness. The high proportion of right buttock pain (side of the suspension) was also seen in 12/80 women (15%) in the Jeng et al. study. Prospective data from Deitz et al. (2008) found similar rates and types of complications: reoperation for hemorrhage in 1.4%, buttock pain in 18.1%, vaginal hematoma in 2.8%, urinary tract infection in 9.7%, urinary retention in 27.8%, and vaginal adhesion 4.2%. This complication profile seems acceptable compared with other treatment options for uterovaginal prolapse.

Prolapse Mesh Kits

From 2001 to 2008, there was a growing popularity of mesh kits for the correction of pelvic organ prolapse. One advantage of these kits was that they easily accommodated uterine preservation. The majority of these kits involved the blind passage of insertion needles through small perineal incisions into the obturator foramen and ischiorectal fossa to facilitate the tension-free vaginal placement of mesh or graft. Others used suturing devices to assist with the attachment of mesh to anatomic landmarks. The US Food and Drug Administration (FDA) noted adverse events and safety concerns in 2006. An investigation of these issues led to a 2008 Public Health Notification regarding the safety and efficacy of mesh kits for prolapse and incontinence. Over the last 12 years, the notification has been updated twice regarding the safety of the mesh kits used to treat prolapse, as well as the lack of clear evidence demonstrating superior prolapse outcomes compared with native tissue repair. The companies who manufacture the trocar-based mesh kits voluntarily removed the devices from the market. The mesh kits were reclassified to "high risk" by the FDA in 2016, requiring preapproval studies. Data did not demonstrate reasonable assurance of safety and effectiveness, and the FDA required that the companies stop selling and distributing the devices. Despite this, it is worth noting that, when vaginal mesh kits were available, systematic review evidence supported that uterine preservation with these kits had a lower risk for mesh exposure [17/337 (5%) uterine preservation vs. 29/192 (15%) hysterectomy, odds ratio (OR) 0.34, 95% confidence interval (CI) 0.18–0.67] and reoperation for mesh exposure [5/378 (1.3%) preservation vs. 12/154 (7.3%) hysterectomy, OR 0.16, 95% CI 0.05–0.46] than mesh kits placed with concurrent hysterectomy (Meriwether et al., 2018).

One of the last vaginal mesh kits to leave the marketplace was the Uphold Vaginal Support System (Boston Scientific, Natick, MA). A retrospective study by Vu et al. (2012) followed 115 women, including 53 women who elected hysteropexy for a median of 11.8 months. Anatomic outcomes demonstrated a recurrence rate, defined as POPQ of −1 or more in any segment, of 1.89%. There was one mesh exposure noted in this group, and self-reported dyspareunia rates decreased from preoperative rates. Ironically, although vaginal mesh kits are no longer in the marketplace, this is the largest group of studies describing uterine preservation procedures and comparing them to procedures with hysterectomy (18 studies, including five randomized trials) (Meriwether et al., 2018; Meriwether et al., 2019). In fact, over 30 other studies looking at outcomes from formerly available mesh kits detail hysteropexy outcomes, but most involve older kits that have long left the market, and many of these studies did not include a comparison group.

ABDOMINAL APPROACH

The abdominal approach to uterovaginal prolapse includes open, laparoscopic, and robotic procedures. Open abdominal approaches to uterovaginal prolapse with uterine preservation include combined vaginal-abdominal retropubic uterine suspension, pectineal ligament uterine suspension, abdominal uterosacral hysteropexy, and sacrohysteropexy. Outcome data for these procedures are limited, with small, retrospective studies representing the bulk of the existing literature. Although the earliest reports describe procedures using autologous grafts and retropubic suspensions, more contemporary literature focuses on sacrohysteropexy using synthetic mesh.

A laparoscopic or robotic approach to uterovaginal prolapse with uterine preservation presents potential benefits, including improved visualization of pelvic anatomy, decreased postoperative pain, and a shorter hospital stay and recovery period compared with the open abdominal approach. Numerous small studies published over the past 20 years have examined outcomes in laparoscopic and robotic approaches to uterovaginal prolapse with uterine preservation. Procedures described include uterine suspension to the round ligaments, plication of the uterosacral ligaments, and sacrohysteropexy.

Open Abdominal Sacrohysteropexy

The evidence supporting sacrohysteropexy is more robust compared to other open abdominal uterine conservation procedures. However, variations in the operative technique, including sites of mesh attachment and type, size, and shape of mesh make comparison difficult. All authors describe placing synthetic mesh between the vagina and/or cervico-uterine junction and the sacral promontory after mobilization of the bladder, rectum, and peritoneum. The distal mesh attachment site is described as either the vaginal wall or the uterus at the level of the uterosacral ligament. The type, size, and shape of mesh are not consistent across studies, and Teflon, polyester, and polypropylene systems are described. Although no authors elaborate on the size, shape, and configuration of mesh in detail, several studies describe placing the body of a Y-shaped mesh anteriorly with the arms passing through the broad ligament, followed by placement of a rectangular piece of mesh posteriorly (Figs. 22.3 and 22.4). Finally, both are affixed to the sacral promontory. Each procedure includes peritoneal closure after mesh placement.

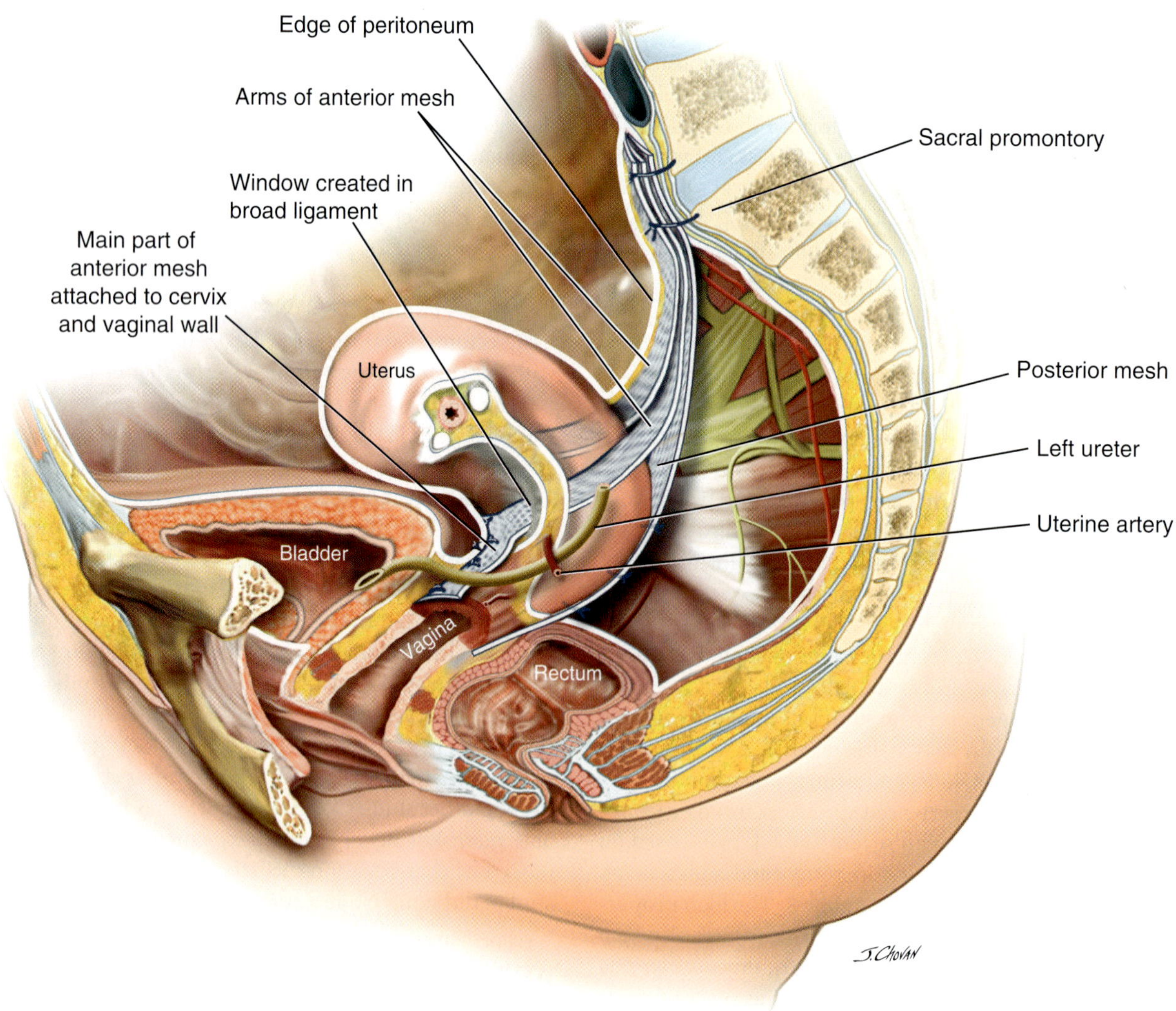

Fig. 22.3 Dual-leaf sacral colpohysteropexy.

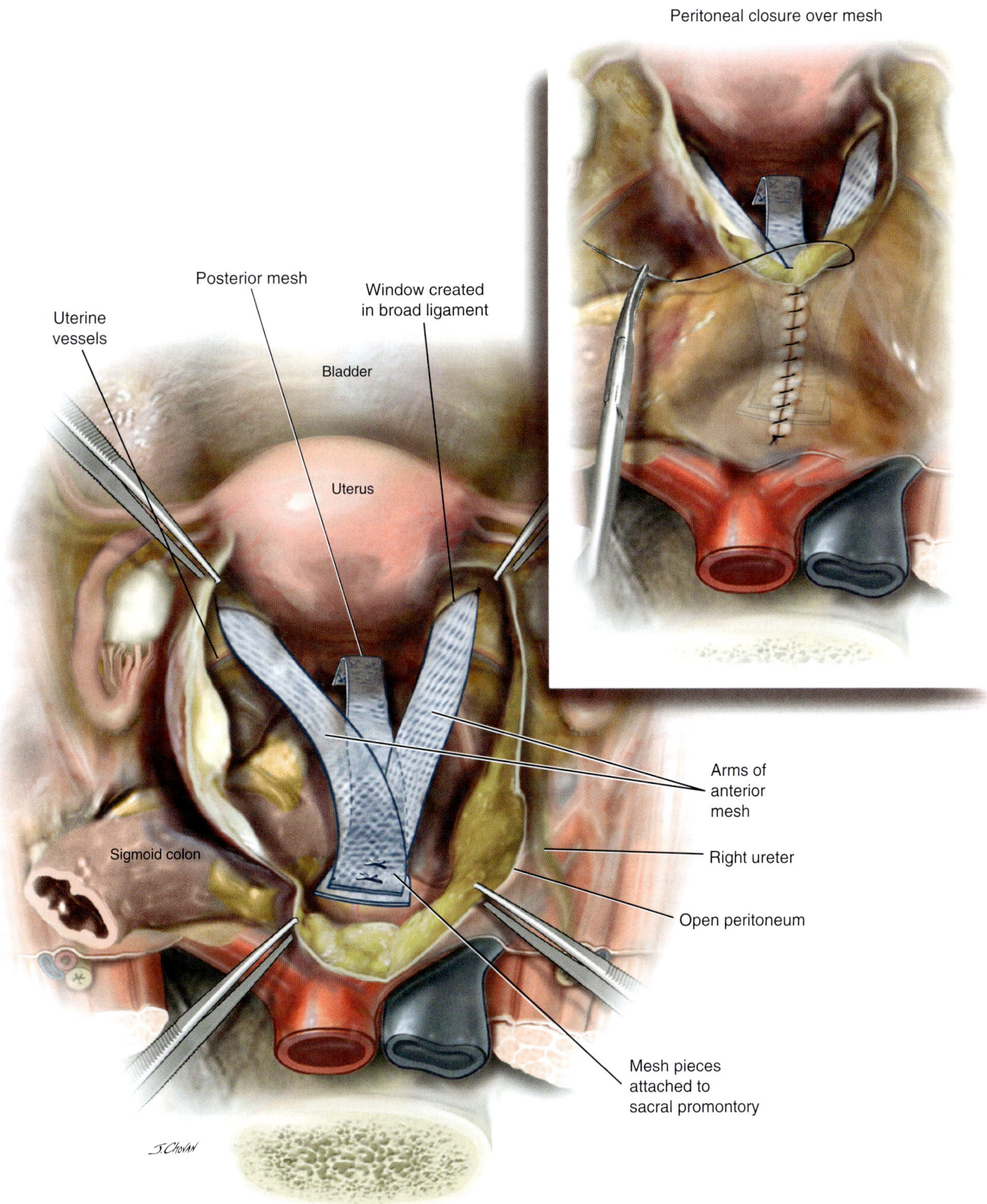

Fig. 22.4 The two arms of the anterior leaf of mesh exit the broad ligament. They are secured with the posterior mesh leaf to the sacral promontory. In the insert, the retroperitoneal space is closed over the mesh arms.

Published studies reflect relatively good success rates with sacrohysteropexy. One randomized controlled trial compared open sacrohysteropexy and vaginal hysterectomy with uterosacral suspension and found that, although patients in the hysteropexy group had more pain and slower recovery, as expected for open abdominal surgery, only 5% of patients in both groups had prolapse to stage II or greater, and reoperation did not differ at 8 years. There are four studies on open sacrohysteropexy, with follow-up ranging from 12 to 84 months, and repeat surgery rates ranged from 0% to 22%, with recurrent prolapse rates ranging from 0% to 14%. A retrospective comparative study found that open and laparoscopic techniques for sacrohysteropexy both had high objective success rates (96% robotic and 98% open) and greater than 90% satisfaction.

Constantini et al. (2005) prospectively compared abdominal sacrohysteropexy to abdominal hysterectomy with sacral colpopexy. Some 72 consecutive patients with symptomatic grade 3 to 4 prolapse self-selected to either sacrohysteropexy or hysterectomy with abdominal sacral colpopexy. The sacrohysteropexy ($n = 34$) group had shorter mean operative times (89 vs. 115 minutes), less mean estimated blood loss (200 vs. 325 mL), and a shorter mean hospital stay (each $P < .05$) compared with the hysterectomy and sacral colpopexy group. At a mean follow-up of 51 months, there were no statistically significant differences in anatomic outcomes. Subjective follow-up was also encouraging, with similar proportions of patients free of prolapse symptoms (sacrocervicopexy 87% vs. sacrohysteropexy 97%, not significant). Other prospective trials comparing open sacrohysteropexy to open sacrocolpopexy with abdominal hysterectomy by the same Italian group of surgeons, Costantini et al. (2013) and Zucchi et al. (2008), showed that women postoperatively had good sexual function, good quality of life, and no prolapse recurrence at 12 months.

Abdominal sacrohysteropexy appears to be a relatively safe procedure. Similar to sacral colpopexy, complications reported include dyspareunia and persistent pain, *de novo* incontinence or urinary urgency, mesh erosion, presacral vessel hemorrhage, wound infection, small bowel obstruction, and hernia. Studies describe new-onset dyspareunia in 7% to 15% of subjects. Voiding dysfunction was described in 5% to 12% of patients. Additionally, with 4 years of follow-up, the mesh erosion rate was noted to be 3%, which is comparable to that reported after sacral colpopexy. There were no pregnancy outcomes reported among these data.

Laparoscopic Ventrosuspension

This approach to hysteropexy involves either laparoscopic plication of the round ligaments to the rectus sheath or attachment of the uterus or cervix via sutures or mesh to the pectineal or Cooper's ligament. An early case series by O'Brien and Ibrahim (1994) of nine postmenopausal women with "moderate or marked" uterovaginal prolapse who underwent laparoscopic ventrosuspension using the round ligaments yielded discouraging results, with 89% of women experiencing complete recurrence within 3 months, all of whom required additional surgery. Since then, more rigorous studies and methods have shown improved results. Joshi et al. (2015) followed 194 women who had pectineal ligament suspension either laparoscopically or with open incision with a polypropylene tap attached to the cervix. Of these women, 10 (5.1%) had prolapse recurrence, and in seven of these 10 it followed a vaginal delivery after the procedure. Mean follow-up was over 6 years, and the overall reoperation rate was 15% in all women for any reason. A small study of 23 women with "butterfly mesh" hysteropexy (Li et al., 2015) showed equal Pelvic Floor Distress Inventory (PFDI) and Pelvic Floor Impact Questionnaire (PFIQ) scores between this surgery and laparoscopic sacrocervicopexy, and patients with the butterfly suspension had better sexual function. Various other large case series of ventrosuspension techniques (round ligament plication through the inguinal ring, suspension with mesh to the anterior superior iliac spine, etc.) with uterine preservation have shown overall recurrence rates of 0% to 18% and reoperation rates from 0% to 28%, with most prevalence rates around 10%. It is possible that ventrosuspension with mesh is more durable than that without, although no trials have directly compared these techniques (Meriwether et al., 2019).

Laparoscopic Uterosacral Ligament Uterine Suspension

Although wide variation exists in approaches to uterosacral ligament uterine suspension, each procedure attaches the uterus to a more proximal portion of the uterosacral ligament. Advocates of the procedure tout the uterosacral ligament's role in physiologic uterine support and creation of an anatomically correct repair among its advantages. The ligament also has a high tensile strength, with studies indicating that it can withstand pressures up to 37 pounds. Multiple authors advocate initiating the procedure with a peritoneal ureteral releasing incision to avoid ureteral kinking, whereas others recommend completing this step as indicated after placing the suspension sutures. All procedure descriptions employ permanent suture for the suspension, although the exact location, number of sutures placed, and additional steps vary between studies.

Evidence suggests that laparoscopic uterosacral ligament uterine suspension is relatively safe and effective, although the existing literature is limited by a lack of adequately powered randomized, prospective trials. Three nonrandomized comparative trials that compare the procedure to prolapse surgeries with hysterectomy report prolapse recurrence rates of 8% to 27%. In the largest of these trials (Bedford et al., 2013), the recurrence was greater (27% vs. 11%, $P < .02$) than with uterine removal in a retrospective comparison of 103 women who underwent uterosacral suspension to 160 who underwent laparoscopic hysterectomy with uterosacral suspension. The one prospective comparative study of these investigations was by Rosen et al. (2008), which compared laparoscopic uterosacral ligament suspension of the uterus with laparoscopic hysterectomy and uterosacral suspension of the vaginal vault, and concluded that the hysterectomy adds 35 minutes to procedures without any change in complications or prolapse outcomes.

One study of these comparative investigations was performed by Diwan et al. (2006), who retrospectively compared 25 women who underwent laparoscopic uterosacral ligament uterine suspension with 25 who underwent uterosacral vaginal vault suspension with total vaginal hysterectomy. They concluded that uterine suspension is a safe, effective treatment in selected patients with uterovaginal prolapse, and noted no repeat surgery (0/25) for prolapse in the laparoscopic hysteropexy group at 26 weeks' mean follow-up and 3/25 in the vaginal group at 46 weeks' mean follow-up. All vaginal hysterectomy patients underwent a concomitant vault suspension including a McCall culdoplasty, a sacrospinous ligament suspension, or a laparoscopic uterosacral ligament suspension. Pairs were age-matched, with 25 subjects in each arm, and did not differ significantly by preoperative POPQ point C or symptoms. When controlling for preoperative POPQ values, uterine conservation patients exhibited better vault support postoperatively ($P = .001$). The uterine preservation group also had fewer reoperations for failures (one vs. three). The authors are the first to compare laparoscopic uterine suspension to the conventional standard of hysterectomy with vault suspension. However, their conclusions are limited by the study size, retrospective design, and short, variable follow-up intervals between the two groups.

The largest prospective study of laparoscopic uterosacral hysteropexy to date, conducted by Maher et al. (2001), reported outcomes of 43 nonobese patients undergoing laparoscopic uterosacral ligament uterine suspension. At a mean follow-up of 12 months, 81% had no prolapse symptoms, while 79% had no objective evidence of recurrence. Seven patients (16%) had reoperations for failure. There were no significant differences in preoperative examination, age, body mass index, or parity between successful and failed cases. Although the study is small, lacks a comparison group, excludes obese women who are at a high risk of failure, and does not include detailed examination findings, it offers the best prospective data available regarding uterosacral ligament uterine suspension. A smaller prospective study presented similar findings in 10 patients with greater than or equal to stage 2 symptomatic pelvic organ prolapse (Uccella et al., 2007). At a median follow-up of 21 months, 80% of patients were objectively cured, defined as stage 1 or less prolapse, with only two patients requiring reoperation for recurrent prolapse.

These studies also support that laparoscopic uterosacral ligament suspension is safe. When compared to hysterectomy with vault suspension, laparoscopic uterosacral ligament suspension resulted in less blood loss ($P < .0001$) and shorter hospital stay ($P = .002$) in Diwan's retrospective cohort study comparing to vaginal hysterectomy and lower operating room time (–20 min, $P < .01$) in the two other cohort studies comparing to laparoscopic hysterectomy (–20 minutes and –35 minutes for Bedford et al. and Rosen et al., respectively). Mean reported operating times are less than an hour. Complications reported are few and include a uterine artery laceration resulting in a broad ligament hematoma that necessitated laparotomy and transfusion and two cases involving ureteral kinking remedied by a peritoneal ureteral releasing incision.

Laparoscopic Sacrohysteropexy

The term laparoscopic sacrohysteropexy encompasses many different techniques. Past approaches were varied, such as creation of new uterosacral ligaments by attaching two 5-mm Mersilene tapes from the cervix and bilateral uterosacral ligaments to the sacral promontory or suture plication of the uterosacral ligament to the anterior longitudinal ligament. Most modern techniques describe a technique similar to sacral colpopexy, with a polypropylene mesh attached to the cervix and vagina distally and the anterior longitudinal ligament proximally. This can be performed either with a posterior mesh alone or with the addition of two anterior arms passing through the broad ligament to the anterior cervix and vagina. See Video 22.3 demonstrating the surgical technique of laparoscopic sacrohysteropexy using the dual anterior/posterior mesh approach.

Outcome data are increasing on laparoscopic sacrohysteropexy. Early case series, such as Krause et al. (2006), who followed 81 women prospectively after laparoscopic sacral suture hysteropexy for a mean of 20.3 months with 95% success and Rosenblatt et al. (2008), who followed 23 women undergoing laparoscopic hysteropexy for 12 months with a follow-up mean POPQ point C score of –5, had shorter follow-up, smaller sample sizes, and lacked comparison groups. More recently, Kupelian et al. (2016) described a large, 113-woman cohort with laparoscopic "wrap-around" mesh for sacrohysteropexy and found 96% satisfaction at a mean follow-up of 2.6 years. As interest increased in this procedure, however, higher-quality comparative studies emerged. In 2012, Bojahr et al. retrospectively compared 30 women having laparoscopic sacrohysteropexy to a larger number of women who had laparoscopic hysterectomy and sacrocolpopexy and found that, at 7 to 9 months, prolapse outcomes were comparable, but the uterine preservation patients had less rectocele formation. Gracia et al. (2015) prospectively compared 15 women having laparoscopic sacrohysteropexy to 30 women undergoing supracervical hysterectomy and sacrocervicopexy, and at 12 months' follow-up unfortunately found less apical success in the hysterectomy group, but found no difference in the subjective primary outcome (100% success as assessed by question #35 of the Epidemiology of Prolapse and Incontinence Questionnaire). In 2016, Paek et al. compared laparoscopic mesh sacrohysteropexy to hysterectomy with mesh sacrocolpopexy and found similar rates of anatomic cure. Although patient satisfaction was higher with hysterectomy in this cohort study, high satisfaction was noted for both cohorts (94% and 100%, respectively). Most recently, Gutman and colleagues (2016) prospectively compared laparoscopic mesh sacrohysteropexy ($n = 74$) to vaginal mesh hysteropexy ($n = 76$) and found that both arms of the study had greater than 75% anatomic success and greater than 90% subjective success at 1 year.

Robotic-assisted laparoscopic sacrohysteropexy has been described in a small case series by Vitobello et al. (2012) and a prospective cohort study by Mourik et al. (2012). The cohort study included 50 women and reported that, at up to 29 months, women undergoing robotic-assisted laparoscopic sacrohysteropexy had significant improvement in quality of life (Mourik et al., 2012). Multiple case reports of a single-port laparoscopic sacrohysteropexies have been published, documenting the feasibility of this approach, and one indicated that the patient had no subjective prolapse at 18 months postoperatively.

Although minimally invasive sacrohysteropexy may result in lower blood loss than an open procedure, it requires advanced surgical skills and can complicate future hysterectomy should it become necessary. Little data about intraoperative complications exist, although reported postoperative complications include a small bowel obstruction that required a bowel resection and reanastomosis (Nightengale et al., 2020). There were two reported cases of mesh erosion in the open sacrohysteropexy group of one study that compared open to laparoscopic hysteropexy (Paek et al., 2015), and another series comparing laparoscopic sacrohysteropexy to vaginal mesh found three mesh erosions and two sutures erosions in the sacrohysteropexy group (Gutman et al., 2017). Furthermore, the Gutman et al. study noted two small bowel injuries, one deep venous thrombosis, and one small bowel obstruction in the sacrohysteropexy group. It should be noted here, however, that many comparative cohort studies of sacrohysteropexy report no mesh erosions at all in the hysteropexy groups, but did find such erosions in the hysterectomy groups (Bai et al., 2005; Cvach et al., 2012; Bojahr et al., 2012; Costantini et al., 2005; Gracia et al., 2015; Pan et al., 2016). A more serious complication involving an rectal injury necessitating a proximal proctectomy, mesh removal, small bowel resection, left colectomy, and temporary colostomy demonstrates that serious complications can occur with any of these techniques (Khan et al., 2016).

COMPARING APPROACHES TO HYSTEROPEXY

There are limited data comparing one type of hysteropexy to another, but those studies that do tend to be either prospective or have longer follow-up. Gutman et al. (2016) compared vaginal mesh hysteropexy with the Uphold device to laparoscopic mesh sacrohysteropexy and found that, although the procedures had similar 1-year anatomic results and high patient satisfaction, the laparoscopic approach was significantly longer and universally required general anesthesia, but resulted in a higher POPQ point D, a longer vaginal length, and better quality of life scores on the PFDI. This seems consistent with other studies indicating that a laparoscopic approach is generally longer and more morbid but may result in some improved results. Another study by Kow et al. (2016) compared many different approaches to hysteropexy, including open abdominal, laparoscopic/robotic sacrohysteropexy, open abdominal and laparoscopic/robotic native tissue uterosacral plication, and vaginal approach with both native tissue or mesh, and had mean follow-up of 6 to 23 months (shortest in the robotic group and longest in the laparoscopic group). This study concluded that all approaches had similar complication rates, and that mesh repairs in general were not significantly less likely to have recurrence.

Studies by Paek et al. (2016) and Joshi et al. (2015) compared open and minimally invasive approaches of sacrohysteropexy and pectineal ligament suspension, respectively. Both concluded that the minimally invasive approach had differing operating times (shorter robotic times than open for sacrohysteropexy and longer laparoscopic versus open times for pectineal ligament suspension) with similar anatomic outcomes. Paek et al. found improved morbidity (less blood loss and hemoglobin drop) and improved recovery (less postoperative symptoms) with the robotic approach to sacrohysteropexy.

A systematic review incorporating these comparative studies concluded that the least invasive approach is preferred with mesh hysteropexy; vaginal appears to have advantages over laparoscopic/robotic, and laparoscopic/robotic appears to have advantages over open abdominal surgery. The reasons for this are no apparent differences in anatomical outcomes or bothersome complications such as mesh exposure based on approach but improved operating times and less blood loss (Meriwether et al., 2019).

SUMMARY AND FUTURE QUESTIONS

For the treatment of uterovaginal prolapse, most long-term studies describe vaginal vault suspension with hysterectomy. However, uterine-sparing procedures to treat uterovaginal prolapse have a long history and are becoming more popular worldwide. Several techniques with vaginal, open abdominal, and laparoscopic/robotic approaches have been described, with varying success rates. Of vaginal native tissue techniques, the sacrospinous hysteropexy is the most studied. Data support its medium-term cure of prolapse, with newer studies demonstrating favorable results in comparison to uterosacral ligament vaginal vault suspension. Quality-of-life and sexual function outcomes appear good after sacrospinous hysteropexy. Abdominally, both open and laparoscopic sacrohysteropexy have promising findings, with well-measured prolapse outcomes from comparative trials that are similar to hysterectomy concurrent with sacrocolpopexy.

Because of the inherent risks of hysterectomy and its possible effect on quality of life, strategies to avoid a hysterectomy as part of a prolapse repair should lower the surgical times and potentially decrease surgical morbidity such as bleeding, infectious complications, and damage to the lower urinary tract. It could also make laparoscopic and robotic prolapse surgeries less time-consuming and thus more attractive to gynecologic surgeons.

It is important to select patients carefully for uterus-sparing prolapse repairs. Women with prolapse who also have disease specific to the uterus, such as postmenopausal bleeding, endometrial hyperplasia, or cervical dysplasia, should have a concurrent hysterectomy as part of their surgery. Women at high risk for future gynecologic cancers, such as those with strong positive family histories or high-risk HPV exposure to the cervix may consider having hysterectomy as well. However, women with a normal uterus, as documented by a pelvic examination, Pap smear, and perhaps endometrial biopsy or transvaginal ultrasound, can undergo conservation of the uterus as part of the prolapse repair, assuming the risks and benefits of hysterectomy versus uterine preservation have been carefully reviewed by the physician and patient and the patient gives informed consent. Likewise, women with prolapse who desire future fertility would be motivated toward uterine conservation. The risk-benefit profile thus changes with the age, malignancy risks, and family planning goals of the patient.

Although the overall risks of hysterectomy are well described in the literature, relatively few studies address unique morbidities added by hysterectomy during a prolapse repair or delayed morbidity that may arise from uterine conservation. A recent systematic review has synthesized the data to quantify the increase in operating time and surgical blood loss, as well as mesh exposure, with addition of hysterectomy. Data indicate quicker recovery and less pain with well-studied, minimally invasive hysteropexy procedures as compared to prolapse repair with hysterectomy. Other long-term factors, including the risk of future gynecologic pathology and effects on quality of life and sexual satisfaction, have not been well-studied in this population, because of the small number of studies that both had long-term follow-up and measured this outcome. In clinical practice, strong feelings by patients and physicians are commonly seen, in favor of both hysterectomy and of uterine conservation, but opinions are often not supported by substantial evidence.

One benefit of removing the uterus at the time of prolapse repair is facilitation of peritoneal access if required for the apical suspension. Long-term benefits include lowering the lifetime risks of (and tests for) uterine disease such as dysplasia, postmenopausal bleeding, and endometrial and cervical cancer. Since the relative long-term cure rates of various colpopexy procedures with or without hysterectomy have not been compared, it is unknown whether one option would require more future surgeries to correct recurrent prolapse and/or stress incontinence.

The cervix is a unique structure that raises several interesting issues. Removal of the cervix as part of the hysterectomy would minimize the risk of future cervical dysplasia or cancer and the need for future evaluations for this. However, bleeding from the cervix after supracervical hysterectomy occurs in 2% to 14% of cases and sometimes requires a trachelectomy for cure. Some believe that retaining the cervix provides continued sexual response and satisfaction that would be diminished if the cervix was removed. The literature on this remains controversial, and addressing this question would require more careful, randomized surgical trials studying sexual outcomes. Women who have a long cervix may sometimes feel continued symptoms of cervical prolapse or sexual discomfort if a uterine-sparing hysteropexy is performed. Such patients may require a trachelectomy at the time of hysteropexy to help provide more normal anatomy and function, and some procedure types such as the Manchester or transvaginal native tissue repairs either already include this step or make it easy to perform a trachelectomy concurrently with suspension.

Uterine-sparing procedures seem to be safe and, in some cases, faster and associated with less blood loss than procedures that require hysterectomy. Many questions still exist surrounding hysteropexy. Will the durability of the prolapse repair be as good as (or better than) vaginal vault suspension in the long term? Will these repairs reliably hold up to the strains related to pregnancy, labor, and delivery? How often will reoperations related to uterine pathology be required? Who is the ideal candidate to undergo hysteropexy? Will uterine preservation save costs and resources for the medical system if used in more patients? As these procedures regain popularity, it is our hope that these issues will be addressed, ideally in the form of prospective, randomized, controlled trials.

BIBLIOGRAPHY

AARP The Magazine. *Conditions and Treatment*. Updated August 2014. Available at: https://www.aarp.org/health/conditions-treatments/info-05-2011/4-surgeries-to-avoid.html#slide1. Accessed June 11, 2021.

American College of Obstetricians and Gynecologists. ACOG Committee Opinion No. 388 November 2007: supracervical hysterectomy. *Obstet Gynecol*. 2007;110:1215.

American College of Obstetricians and Gynecologists. ACOG Committee Opinion No. 395. Surgery and patient choice. *Obstet Gynecol*. 2013;122:1134.

Bai SW, Kim EH, Shin JS, Kim SK, Park KH, Lee DH. A comparison of different pelvic reconstruction surgeries using mesh for pelvic organ prolapse patients. *Yonsei Med J*. 2005;46(1):112–118. doi:10.3349/ymj.2005.46.1.112.

Barranger E, Fritel X, Pigne A. Abdominal sacrohysteropexy in young women with uterovaginal prolapse: long-term follow-up. *Am J Obstet Gynecol*. 2003;189:1245.

Bedford ND, Seman EI, O'Shea RT, Keirse MJ. Effect of uterine preservation on outcome of laparoscopic uterosacral suspension. *J Minim Invasive Gynecol*. 2013;20:172.

Behnia-Willison F, Garg A, Keirse MJ. A laparoendoscopic single-site surgery approach to mesh sacrohysteropexy. *Case Rep Med*. 2013;2013:641.

Bojahr B, Tchartchian G, Waldschmidt M, et al. Laparoscopic sacropexy: a retrospective analysis of perioperative complications and anatomical outcomes. *JSLS*. 2012;16(3):428–436. doi:10.4293/108680812X13462882736132.

Carey MP, Slack MC. Transvaginal sacrospinous colpopexy for vault and marked uterovaginal prolapse. *Br J Obstet Gynaecol*. 1994;101:536.

Conger GT, Keettel WC. The Manchester-Fothergill operation, its place in gynecology; a review of 960 cases at University Hospitals, Iowa City, Iowa. *Am J Obstet Gynecol*. 1958;76:634.

Costantini E, Mearini L, Bini V, et al. Uterus preservation in surgical correction of urogenital prolapse. *Eur Urol*. 2005;48(4):642–649. doi:10.1016/j.eururo.2005.04.022.

Costantini E, Porena M, Lazzeri M, et al. Changes in female sexual function after pelvic organ prolapse repair: role of hysterectomy. *Int Urogynecol J*. 2013;24:1481.

Cutner A, Kearney R, Vashisht A. Laparoscopic uterine sling suspension: a new technique of uterine suspension in women desiring surgical management of uterine prolapse with uterine conservation. *BJOG*. 2007;114:1159.

Cvach K, Geoffrion R, Cundiff GW. Abdominal sacral hysteropexy: a pilot study comparing sacral hysteropexy to sacral colpopexy with hysterectomy. *Female Pelvic Med Reconstr Surg*. 2012;18(5):286–290. doi: 10.1097/SPV.0b013e3182673772.

Dallas K, Elliott CS, Syan R, et al. Association Between Concomitant Hysterectomy and Repeat Surgery for Pelvic Organ Prolapse Repair in a Cohort of Nearly 100,000 Women. *Obstet Gynecol*. 2018;132:1328.

DeLancey JO. Anatomic aspects of vaginal eversion after hysterectomy. *Am J Obstet Gynecol*. 1992;166:1717.

Demirci F, Ozdemir I, Somunkiran A, et al. Abdominal sacrohysteropexy in young women with uterovaginal prolapse: results of 20 cases. *J Reprod Med*. 2006;51:539.

Detollenaere RJ, den Boon J, Stekelenburg J, et al. Sacrospinous hysteropexy versus vaginal hysterectomy with suspension of the uterosacral ligaments in women with uterine prolapse stage 2 or higher: multicentre randomised non-inferiority trial. *BMJ*. 2015;351:h3717.

Dietz V, de Jong J, Huisman M, et al. The effectiveness of the sacrospinous hysteropexy for the primary treatment of uterovaginal prolapse. *Int Urogynecol J Pelvic Floor Dysfunct*. 2007;18:1271.

Dietz V, Huisman M, de Jong JM, et al. Functional outcome after sacrospinous hysteropexy for uterine descensus. *Int Urogynecol J Pelvic Floor Dysfunct*. 2008;19:747.

Dietz V, van der Vaart CH, van der Graaf Y, et al. One-year follow-up after sacrospinous hysteropexy and vaginal hysterectomy for uterine descent: a randomized study. *Int Urogynecol J*. 2010;21:209.

Diwan A, Rardin CR, Kohli N. Uterine preservation during surgery for uterovaginal prolapse: a review. *Int Urogynecol J Pelvic Floor Dysfunct*. 2004;15:286.

Diwan A, Rardin CR, Strohsnitter WC, et al. Laparoscopic uterosacral ligament uterine suspension compared with vaginal hysterectomy with vaginal vault suspension for uterovaginal prolapse. *Int Urogynecol J Pelvic Floor Dysfunct*. 2006;17:79.

Duhrssen A. Ueber die operative Heilung der mobilen und fixirten Retroflexio uteri auf vaginalem Wege an der hand von 207 eigenen Operationsfallen, mit besonderer Berucksichtigung der Dauerfolge. *Arch f Gynak*. 1894;47:284.

Eastman JR. Gynecology in Berlin. A. Mackenrodt. *JAMA*. 1897;XXIX(15):737–738. doi:10.1001/jama.1897.02440410025002j.

Falcone T, Walters MD. Hysterectomy for benign disease. *Obstet Gynecol.* 2008;111:753.

Farquhar CM, Sadler L, Harvey SA, Stewart AW. The association of hysterectomy and menopause: a prospective cohort study. *BJOG.* 2005;112:956.

Frick AC, Barber MD, Paraiso MF, et al. Attitudes toward hysterectomy in women undergoing evaluation for uterovaginal prolapse. *Female Pelvic Med Reconstr Surg.* 2013;19:103.

Frick AC, Walters MD, Larkin KS, Barber MD. Risk of unanticipated abnormal gynecologic pathology at the time of hysterectomy for uterovaginal prolapse. *Am J Obstet Gynecol.* 2010;202:507.e1.

Forsgren C, Lundholm C, Johansson AL, et al. Vaginal hysterectomy and risk of pelvic organ prolapse and stress urinary incontinence surgery. *Int Urogynecol J.* 2012;23:43.

Gracia M, Perello M, Bataller E, et al. Comparison between laparoscopic sacral hysteropexy and subtotal hysterectomy plus cervicopexy in pelvic organ prolapse: a pilot study. *Neurourol Urodyn.* 2015;34(7):654–658. doi:10.1002/nau.22641.

Gutman RE, Rardin CR, Sokol ER, et al. Vaginal and laparoscopic mesh hysteropexy for uterovaginal prolapse: a parallel cohort study. *Am J Obstet Gynecol.* 2017;216:38.e31.

Health Magazine. *Mind & Body.* Updated September 2001. Available at: https://www.health.com/mind-body/surgery-to-avoid-1-hysterectomy. Accessed June 11, 2021.

Husby KR, Larsen MD, Lose G, Klarskov N. Surgical treatment of primary uterine prolapse: a comparison of vaginal native tissue surgical techniques. *Int Urogynecol J.* 2019;30:1887.

Ingber MS, Colton MD, Zimmerman GE. Laparoendoscopic single-site (LESS) hysteropexy. *Updates Surg.* 2012;64:53.

Jeng CJ, Yang YC, Tzeng CR, et al. Sexual functioning after vaginal hysterectomy or transvaginal sacrospinous uterine suspension for uterine prolapse: a comparison. *J Reprod Med.* 2005;50:669.

Jeng CJ, Yang YC, Tzeng CR, et al. Sexual functioning after vaginal hysterectomy or transvaginal sacrospinous uterine suspension for uterine prolapse: a comparison. *J Reprod Med.* 2005;50:669.

Joshi VM. A new technique of uterine suspension to pectineal ligaments in the management of uterovaginal prolapse. *Obstet Gynecol.* 1993;81:790.

Joshi VM, Otiv SR, Dagade VB, et al. Pectineal ligament hysteropexy for uterine prolapse in premenopausal women by open and laparoscopic approach in indian urban and rural centers. *Female Pelvic Med Reconstr Surg.* 2015;21:215.

Khan A, Jaleel R, Nasrullah FD. Sacrohysteropexy performed as uterus conserving surgery for pelvic organ prolapse: Review of case files. *Pak J Med Sci.* 2016;32(5):1174–1178.

Kilkku P, Grönroos M. Peroperative electrocoagulation of endocervical mucosa and later carcinoma of the cervical stump. *Acta Obstet Gynecol Scand.* 1982;61:265.

Kovac SR, Cruikshank SH. Successful pregnancies and vaginal deliveries after sacrospinous uterosacral fixation in five of nineteen patients. *Am J Obstet Gynecol.* 1993;168:1778.

Kow N, Goldman HB, Ridgeway B. Uterine Conservation During Prolapse Repair: 9-Year Experience at a Single Institution. *Female Pelvic Med Reconstr Surg.* 2016;22:126.

Krause HG, Goh JT, Sloane K, et al. Laparoscopic sacral suture hysteropexy for uterine prolapse. *Int Urogynecol J Pelvic Floor Dysfunct.* 2006;17:378.

Kupelian AS, Vashisht A, Sambandan N, Cutner A. Laparoscopic wrap round mesh sacrohysteropexy for the management of apical prolapse. *Int Urogynecol J.* 2016;27:1889.

Leron E, Stanton SL. Sacrohysteropexy with synthetic mesh for the management of uterovaginal prolapse. *BJOG.* 2001;108:629.

Li S, Ji M, Zhao Z. The effectiveness of two different laparoscopic surgeries for apical support of pelvic organ prolapse. *Eur J Obstet Gynecol Reprod Biol.* 2015;188:74.

Lin LL, Ho MH, Haessler AL, et al. A review of laparoscopic uterine suspension procedures for uterine preservation. *Curr Opin Obstet Gynecol.* 2005;17:541.

Lin TY, Su TH, Wang YL, et al. Risk factors for failure of transvaginal sacrospinous uterine suspension in the treatment of uterovaginal prolapse. *J Formos Med Assoc.* 2005;104:249.

Maher CF, Carey MP, Murray CJ. Laparoscopic suture hysteropexy for uterine prolapse. *Obstet Gynecol.* 2001;97:1010.

Maher CF, Cary MP, Slack MC, et al. Uterine preservation or hysterectomy at sacrospinous colpopexy for uterovaginal prolapse? *Int Urogynecol J Pelvic Floor Dysfunct.* 2001;12:381.

Marcus-Braun N, von Theobald P. Single port laparoscopic sacrohysteropexy in a young patient presenting with grade III uterine prolapse and rectocele. *Int Urogynecol J.* 2013;24:1445.

Medina C, Takacs P. Laparoscopic uterosacral uterine suspension: a minimally invasive technique for treating pelvic organ prolapse. *J Minim Invasive Gynecol.* 2006;13:472.

Meriwether KV, Antosh DD, Olivera CK, et al. Uterine preservation vs hysterectomy in pelvic organ prolapse surgery: a systematic review with meta-analysis and clinical practice guidelines. *Am J Obstet Gynecol.* 2018;219(2):129–146.e2. doi:10.1016/j.ajog.2018.01.018.

Meriwether KV, Balk EM, Antosh DD, et al. Uterine-preserving surgeries for the repair of pelvic organ prolapse: a systematic review with meta-analysis and clinical practice guidelines. *Int Urogynecol J.* 2019;30:505.

Moiety FM, Hegah HM, Ghanema IA, et al. Abdominal sacrohysteropexy for uterovaginal prolapse: a prospective study on 33 cases. *Arch Gynecol Obstet.* 2010;281:631.

Moorman PG, Myers ER, Schildkraut JM, et al. Effect of hysterectomy with ovarian preservation on ovarian function. *Obstet Gynecol.* 2011;118:1271.

Mourik SL, Martens JE, Aktas M. Uterine preservation in pelvic organ prolapse using robot assisted laparoscopic sacrohysteropexy: quality of life and technique. *Eur J Obstet Gynecol Reprod Biol.* 2012;165:122.

Nesbitt Jr RE. Uterine preservation in the surgical management of genuine stress urinary incontinence associated with uterovaginal prolapse. *Surg Gynecol Obstet.* 1989;168:143.

Nightingale G, Phillips C. Long-term safety and efficacy of laparoscopically placed mesh for apical prolapse. *Int Urogynecol J.* 2021 Apr;32(4):871–877. doi:10.1007/s00192-020-04374-6.

O'Brien PM, Ibrahim J. Failure of laparoscopic uterine suspension to provide a lasting cure for uterovaginal prolapse. *Br J Obstet Gynaecol.* 1994;101:707.

Paek J, Lee M, Kim BW, Kwon Y. Robotic or laparoscopic sacrohysteropexy versus open sacrohysteropexy for uterus preservation in pelvic organ prolapse. *Int Urogynecol J.* 2016;27:593.

Pan K, Cao L, Ryan NA, Wang Y, Xu H. Laparoscopic sacral hysteropexy versus laparoscopic sacrocolpopexy with hysterectomy for pelvic organ prolapse. *Int Urogynecol J.* 2016;27(1):93–101. doi:10.1007/s00192-015-2775-9.

Price N, Slack A, Jackson SR. Laparoscopic hysteropexy: the initial results of a uterine suspension procedure for uterovaginal prolapse. *BJOG.* 2010;117:62.

Rabenau Fv. Ueber eine neue operative Behandlung der Retroflexio uteri. *Berl klin Wehnschr.* 1886;23:232.

Rahmanou P, Price N, Jackson SR. Laparoscopic hysteropexy versus vaginal hysterectomy for the treatment of uterovaginal prolapse: a prospective randomized pilot study. *Int Urogynecol J.* 2015;26:1687.

Renganathan A, Edwards R, Duckett JR. Uterus conserving prolapse surgery—what is the chance of missing a malignancy? *Int Urogynecol J.* 2010;21:819.

Richardson DA, Scotti RJ, Ostergard DR. Surgical management of uterine prolapse in young women. *J Reprod Med.* 1989;34:388.

Romanzi LJ, Tyagi R. Hysteropexy compared to hysterectomy for uterine prolapse surgery: does durability differ? *Int Urogynecol J.* 2012;23:625.

Roovers JP, van der Bom JG, van der Vaart CH, et al. A randomized comparison of post-operative pain, quality of life, and physical performance during the first 6 weeks after abdominal or vaginal surgical correction of descensus uteri. *Neurourol Urodyn.* 2005;24:334.

Roovers JP, van der Vaart CH, van der Bom JG, et al. A randomised controlled trial comparing abdominal and vaginal prolapse surgery: effects on urogenital function. *BJOG.* 2004;111:50.

Roovers J, Bleijenberg E, Schagen van Leeuwen JH, et al. Long term follow-up of a randomized controlled trial comparing abdominal and vaginal surgical correction of uterine prolapse. *Int Urogynecol J.* 2008;19:S1.

Rosen DM, Shukla A, Cario GM, et al. Is hysterectomy necessary for laparoscopic pelvic floor repair? A prospective study. *J Minim Invasive Gynecol.* 2008;15:729.

Rosenblatt PL, Chelmow D, Ferzandi TR. Laparoscopic sacrocervicopexy for the treatment of uterine prolapse: a retrospective case series report. *J Minim Invasive Gynecol.* 2008;15:268.

Sisco M, Kyrillos AM, Lapin BR, et al. Trends and variation in the use of nipple-sparing mastectomy for breast cancer in the United States. *Breast Cancer Res Treat.* 2016;160:111.

Skiadas CC, Goldstein DP, Laufer MR. The Manchester-Fothergill procedure as a fertility sparing alternative for pelvic organ prolapse in young women. *J Pediatr Adolesc Gynecol.* 2006;19:89.

Stoesser FG. Construction of a sacrocervical ligament for uterine suspension. *Surg Gynecol Obstet.* 1955;101:638.

Storm HH, Clemmensen IH, Manders T, Brinton LA. Supravaginal uterine amputation in Denmark 1978-1988 and risk of cancer. *Gynecol Oncol.* 1992;45:198.

Thomas AG, Brodman ML, Dottino PR, et al. Manchester procedure vs. vaginal hysterectomy for uterine prolapse: a comparison. *J Reprod Med.* 1995;40:299.

Tipton RH, Atkin PF. Uterine disease after the Manchester repair operation. *J Obstet Gynaecol Br Commonw.* 1970;77:852.

Trabuco EC, Moorman PG, Algeciras-Schimnich A, et al. Association of ovary-sparing hysterectomy with ovarian reserve. *Obstet Gynecol.* 2016;127:819.

Uccella S, Ghezzi F, Bergamini V, et al. Laparoscopic uterosacral ligaments plication for the treatment of uterine prolapse. *Arch Gynecol Obstet.* 2007;276:225.

van Brummen HJ, van de Pol G, Aalders CI, et al. Sacrospinous hysteropexy compared to vaginal hysterectomy as primary surgical treatment for a descensus uteri: effects on urinary symptoms. *Int Urogynecol J Pelvic Floor Dysfunct.* 2003;14:350.

Vitobello D, Siesto G, Bulletti C. Robotic sacral hysteropexy for pelvic organ prolapse. *Int J Med Robot.* 2012;8:114.

Vu MK, Letko J, Jirschele K, et al. Minimal mesh repair for apical and anterior prolapse: initial anatomical and subjective outcomes. *Int Urogynecol J.* 2012;23:1753.

Watkins TJ. The treatment of cystocele and uterine prolapse after the menopause. *Am Gynaec Obst J.* 1899;15:420.

Williams BF. Surgical treatment for uterine prolapse in young women. *Am J Obstet Gynecol.* 1966;95:967.

Wright JD, Herzog TJ, Tsui J, et al. Nationwide trends in the performance of inpatient hysterectomy in the United States. *Obstet Gynecol.* 2013;122:233.

Wu MP. Laparoscopic uterine suspension for the treatment of uterovaginal prolapse. *Int J Gynaecol Obstet.* 1997;59:259.

Zucchi A, Costantini E, Mearini L, et al. Female sexual dysfunction in urogenital prolapse surgery: colposacropexy vs. hysterocolposacropexy. *J Sex Med.* 2008;5:139.

23

Obliterative Procedures for Pelvic Organ Prolapse

Mickey M. Karram and Hoi Tik Hyde Yuen

CHAPTER OUTLINE

INTRODUCTION

As our population ages, pelvic floor disorders are becoming more prevalent and increasingly important health and social issues. Approximately 63 million women will be 45 years old or older by 2030, and 33% of the population will be postmenopausal by 2050. In the United States, the fastest growing segment in the population is women above 60 years of age. Approximately 11% of women will undergo surgery at some point for pelvic organ prolapse (POP) or incontinence, with some studies quoting a reoperation rate for failures of up to 30%, the majority of which occur in the anterior compartment.

Obliterative surgery or colpocleisis is undertaken in approximately 5% of women in the United States undergoing surgery for POP. The surgery is usually undertaken in the elderly or medically compromised who are happy to sacrifice vaginal intercourse and is an effective procedure with quick recovery and low morbidity. As more women enter the eighth and ninth decades of life, many develop symptomatic primary or recurrent POP, often after unsuccessful attempts at pessary therapy or surgery, owing to the inherent limits on the longevity of repairs, as well as many other factors. In addition, elderly women frequently have concomitant medical issues and are not sexually active, making extensive surgery less than ideal. Both the Le Fort partial colpocleisis, which is uterine sparing, and a partial or complete colpectomy and colpocleisis performed posthysterectomy are viable options for vaginal obliteration. This chapter discusses the indications and techniques for these procedures.

HISTORICAL PERSPECTIVES

Before the advent of surgical procedures for severe prolapse, women were treated with obstructing foreign bodies such as vaginal packing or pessaries, being hung upside down to invert the prolapse, or with caustic substances that were introduced into the vaginal canal to promote scarring. Early surgical procedures then arose that described the reapproximation of denuded vaginal mucosa to obliterate the vaginal canal (Gerardin of Metz, 1823). Gerardin never performed the procedure himself, but it served as a basic concept for several other techniques. This hypothesized procedure was further elaborated by in 1867 by Neugebauer, who removed a 3 × 6 cm area of vaginal epithelium anteriorly and posteriorly and sutured the edges of the removed area together. Neugebauer published this technique in 1881 after Leon Le Fort described a similar procedure. Some descriptions also incorporate partial closure of the labia with suture. In 1877, Le Fort described what we now term the Le Fort partial colpocleisis, whereby a narrow rectangle of the anterior and posterior walls is denuded and then sutured to replace the prolapse and leave channels for cervical drainage at the lateral fornices. He then coupled this procedure with a delayed colpoperineorrhaphy to narrow the genital hiatus. Rubovits and Litt (1935) ultimately described a Le Fort partial colpocleisis in conjunction with a levator muscle plication and perineorrhaphy to further narrow the introitus and build up the perineum.

Early literature from the twentieth century further modified these descriptions and, by the 1920s, a series of outcomes data began to arise. In 1928, Baer and Reis reported a series of 14 women who underwent the Le Fort procedure with 100% success. Adair and DaSef (1936) published a series of 38 women, of whom one had a recurrent prolapse through the Le Fort drainage channel and two others had recurrent cystocele. In 1948, Mazer and Isral showed a 97% success rate in 38 women using the Le Fort technique. In a larger series of 288 patients,

Hanson and Keettel (1969) described excellent results, with only 1% of patients experiencing complete recurrence within the first year and 5% of patients experiencing some degree of recurrence. Overall, 92% of these patients believed that they had good or excellent support as a result of their colpocleisis.

Total colpectomy and colpocleisis with levator plication at the time of hysterectomy or posthysterectomy was first described by Martin (1898). Masson and Knepper (1938) described excellent success in a case series of 23 patients who underwent complete vaginectomy with purse-string closure and levator plication. Williams (1950) also described success with no recorded recurrences in a series of 60 patients undergoing vaginal hysterectomy and vaginectomy with levator plication.

PREOPERATIVE EVALUATION

The most important first step when considering obliterative prolapse surgery is proper patient selection. In-depth discussion of a patient's current and future sexual desires is essential, as is an understanding of the patient's comorbidities and perioperative risk. The risks and benefits of and alternatives to obliterative versus reconstructive procedures and pessary should be included as part of a shared decision-making process. As with most urogynecologic complaints, choice of imaging and testing before treatment options is contingent on a thorough history and physical examination. Pelvic floor complaints may vary widely between patients and are associated with a variety of both anatomic and functional derangements that must be elucidated to determine whether ancillary testing will assist in determining the best treatment options. In addition, thorough counseling regarding sexual function and desire to preserve a functional vagina should guide selection of surgical intervention, regardless of age and baseline functional status.

Urodynamic testing prior to obliterative procedures is widely performed, but there is a lack of evidence regarding its necessity in an elderly population with medical comorbidities. Since occult stress urinary incontinence (SUI) may be masked in cases of obstructive prolapse in which the urethra may kink because of anatomic distortion, use of a simple office cough stress test is often helpful. This is performed by asking a patient to perform a Valsalva maneuver with her prolapse reduced; this will reveal stress incontinence without the need to perform formal urodynamics.

Von Pechmann et al. (2003) illustrated the high prevalence of occult SUI in patients with advanced prolapse. In this study, 75 of 92 subjects underwent urodynamic testing, 48% had stress incontinence, 17% had detrusor instability, and 21.3% had mixed incontinence. Another study in 2003 by Fitzgerald and Brubaker showed a 27% *de novo* stress incontinence rate after surgery. However, in a randomized controlled trial of 91 women who underwent vaginal POP surgery with occult SUI, only 48% of patients who did not receive a concomitant midurethral sling (MUS) experienced SUI postoperatively, and only 13% of those patients subsequently underwent a secondary antiincontinence procedure for SUI (Van der Ploeg et al., 2018). Whereas some argue that placement of an MUS at the time of colpocleisis increases the rate of voiding dysfunction at a higher rate in elderly individuals, Abbasy et al. (2009) evaluated a series of 38 elderly women with SUI diagnosed preoperatively who underwent concomitant MUS with colpocleisis and found low rates of urinary retention and voiding dysfunction postoperatively, regardless of preoperative postvoid residual (PVR) volumes.

Radiologic imaging may be helpful in revealing hydronephrosis or hydroureter as a result of obstruction from severe POP. Beverly et al. (1997) showed that the presence of hydronephrosis increases with increasing prolapse, and that knowledge of poor function may be helpful in evaluating changes in renal status postoperatively. Radiologic evidence of hydronephrosis, however, does not generally change the surgical management plan.

Voiding diaries, although recommended in some populations, may be difficult in extremely elderly patients due to both cognitive disability and compliance, as well as the potential for mobility and dexterity issues.

An additional preoperative consideration for Le Fort partial colpocleisis includes endometrial and cervical assessment, especially in patients with symptoms of abnormal uterine bleeding or a history of abnormal Pap smears. Because the uterus is retained, evaluating any future uterine bleeding or cervical pathology is difficult. A study by Jones et al. (2017) based on an anonymous web-based survey of 322 physicians reported that the preferred first-line endometrial evaluation is a transvaginal ultrasound (81%), whereas a minority of physicians (14%) perform dilatation and curettage with or without hysteroscopy. Although it is commonly performed, there is a lack of consensus regarding the optimal workup modality or the clinical utility of preoperative endometrial evaluation to rule out uterine cancer before obliterative POP surgeries in asymptomatic patients. Endometrial evaluation may be of limited clinical value because of the low prevalence (0.5% of 786 patients) of occult uterine malignancy in asymptomatic, low-risk patients who undergo POP surgeries (Kandadai et al., 2014; Vallabh-Patel et al., 2016). In contrast, a study by Hill et al. (2014) reported pathologic endometrial findings in 3.17% (2 of 63) patients who underwent morcellation during benign robotic-assisted supracervical hysterectomy and cervicosacropexy. Similarly, a retrospective evaluation of 644 women undergoing surgery for uterovaginal prolapse by Frick et al. (2010) found that the rate of unanticipated uterine pathology was 2.6%. In postmenopausal women without bleeding, the risk of unanticipated uterine pathology is 2.6%. Importantly, in women with a history of postmenopausal bleeding who had negative endometrial evaluation, the risk of unanticipated endometrial hyperplasia or cancer was 13%. As such, these authors do not recommend uterine preservation at the time of prolapse surgery, including Le Fort colpocleisis, in women with postmenopausal bleeding, even in the face of a negative endometrial evaluation.

LE FORT PARTIAL COLPOCLEISIS

A Le Fort partial colpocleisis is an option if the patient with prolapse has her uterus, is no longer sexually active, and does not have postmenopausal bleeding (see earlier). This procedure can be performed under local anesthesia or with a pudendal block (Buchsbaum & Lee, 2017), but is typically performed using regional or general anesthesia, depending upon the patient's comorbidities. The ideal candidate for a Le Fort partial colpocleisis is the patient who has uterine procidentia with symmetric eversion of the anterior and posterior vaginal walls who no longer desires sexual activity (Fig. 23.1).

Surgical Technique and Outcomes

1. The procedure is begun by placing the cervix on traction to evert the vagina. A Foley catheter with a 5- to 10-mL balloon is placed in the bladder to aide in identification of the bladder neck.
2. The rectangular areas to be denuded are marked anteriorly and posteriorly. The area should extend from approximately 2 cm from the tip of the cervix to 4 to 5 cm below the external urethral meatus. A mirror image on the posterior aspect of the cervix and vagina is also identified. The vaginal epithelium is injected with 0.025% bupivacaine or 2% lidocaine with 1:200,000 epinephrine just below the vaginal epithelium.
3. The previously outlined areas are removed by sharp dissection (Fig. 23.1A and B). The surgeon should leave the maximum amount of muscularis behind on the bladder and rectum. Hemostasis is an absolute must. While removing the posterior vaginal flap, one should not attempt to enter the peritoneum. If the peritoneum is inadvertently entered, the defect should be closed with an interrupted delayed absorbable suture.
4. The cut edges of the anterior and posterior vaginal walls are sewn together with interrupted delayed absorbable sutures (Fig. 23.1C). The knots are turned into the epithelium-lined tunnels, which have been created bilaterally (see Fig. 23.1C). After the uterus and vagina have been inverted, the superior and inferior margins of the rectangle can be sutured together (Fig. 23.1D).
5. In the authors' opinion, plication of the bladder neck (see Fig. 23.1A) or a synthetic MUS procedure should be routinely performed in the hope of avoiding postoperative stress incontinence. In addition, an aggressive perineorrhaphy with a distal levator plication should be performed to decrease the caliber of the genital hiatus and to build up the perineum. For the technique of levatorplasty, the reader is referred to a discussion described later in this chapter (Fig. 23.3). (See Video 23.1: LeFort Partial Colpocleisis.)

According to the literature, 90% to 95% of patients achieve good anatomic results, with relief of many of their symptoms and low risk of regret (Zebede et al., 2013). Recent long-term follow-up studies reported satisfaction rates at 75% with a mean follow-up of 6.4 years and 94.3% with a median follow-up of 5 years (Song et al., 2016; Winkelman & Elkadry 2018). Partial recurrence or breakdown of the repair is seen in 2% to 5% and is thought to be due to poor hemostasis with hematoma formation or infectious morbidity (Goldman et al., 1981). In a retrospective cohort study of 107 patients who underwent colpocleisis for stage 3 or 4 POP, a longer duration from prolapse occurrence to surgery (24.6 ± 22.8 years vs. 8.0 ± 12.9 years, $P = .021$) was associated with recurrence (Cho et al., 2017).

Several studies have looked at complication rates after partial colpocleisis, which is generally quoted at 5% for significant complications and 15% for minor complications. These are mostly due to multiple comorbidities and the frailty of the population being considered. Quantified frailty using the National Surgical Quality Improvement Program – Frailty Index (NSQIP-FI) shows that age is strongly correlated with an increased risk of complication (NSQIP-FI 0.18 vs. 0.0, odds ratio 2.8, 95% confidence interval 1.8–3.0) in a retrospective cohort study by Suskind et al. comparing obliterative and reconstructive POP surgery (2017). Sung et al. (2006), in a population-based study, showed that, although complications increase in subjects over 80 years of age, obliterative procedures had fewer major adverse events than reconstructive procedures. In contrast, Erekson et al. (2017) reported more postoperative complications (5%) in patients who undergo vaginal obliterative surgery in comparison to other vaginal or abdominal procedures (3.0% vs. 3.0%; $P = .71$). The trends noted in this NSQIP database analysis of 33,416 patients are likely the result of increased age and morbidity in patients who undergo obliterative procedures.

TOTAL COLPECTOMY AND COLPOCLEISIS

In patients with posthysterectomy prolapse with near complete vaginal eversion and who are not interested in further sexual function, a total colpectomy and colpocleisis provides a minimally invasive durable option to correct their prolapse. However, if there is significant prolapse of just one segment of the pelvic floor, for example the anterior vaginal wall, then an aggressive repair of the compartment with a narrowing of the genital hiatus will accomplish the same result without requiring complete removal of all vaginal epithelium.

Total colpectomy may also be performed at the same time as vaginal hysterectomy if desired, although the total blood loss tends to be greater with the addition of this procedure (Von Pechmann et al., 2003). A study by Hill et al. (2016) reported higher preoperative and postoperative risks in patients who underwent colpocleisis with concomitant vaginal hysterectomy. The retrospective chart review used Current Procedural Terminology codes to categorize patients into three groups: partial or complete vaginectomy/colpectomy, vaginal hysterectomy with total or partial colpectomy, and Le Fort colpocleisis. Concomitant vaginal hysterectomy was associated with longer mean operating times (144 vs. 108 vs. 111 minutes, $P = .0001$) and higher estimated blood loss (253 vs. 135 vs. 146 mL, $P = .0001$), independent of age, body mass index, or comorbidities.

The rationale for performing a hysterectomy at the time of colpocleisis is to eliminate the risk of endometrial or cervical malignancy. It also eliminates the risk of development of pyometra, a rare but serious complication that can occur if the lateral canals become obstructed after a Le Fort procedure (Kohli et al., 1996; Yasa et al., 2016).

Surgical Technique and Outcomes

1. The most prominent portion of the prolapse is grasped with two Allis clamps. The vaginal epithelium is injected with a 1% or 2% lidocaine with epinephrine solution as previously mentioned for the Le Fort partial colpocleisis.

A

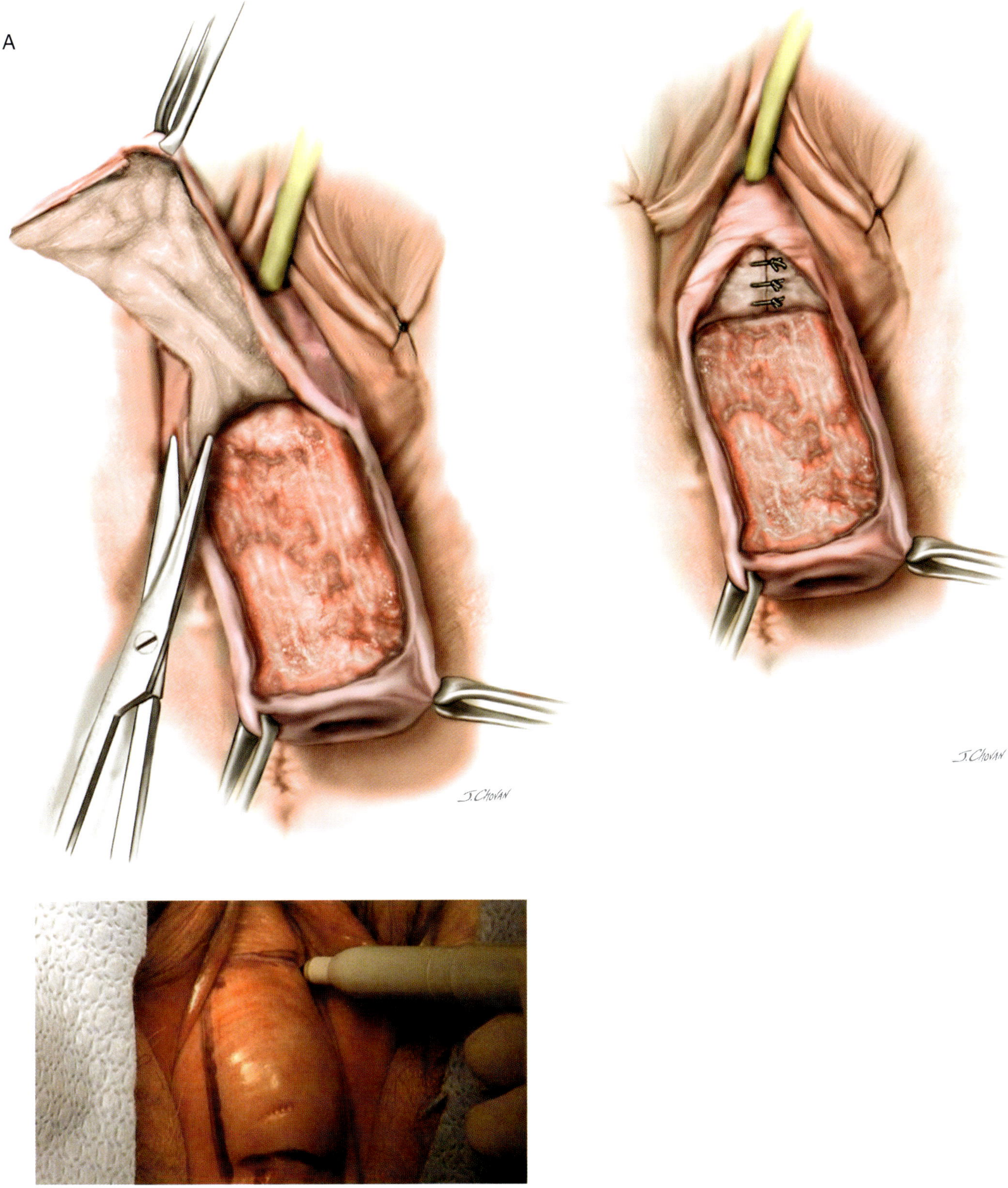

Fig. 23.1 Le Fort partial colpocleisis. **A**, A rectangular piece of anterior vaginal wall has been removed. Note in the *inset* that the dissection has been extended laterally at the level of the proximal urethra to perform a Kelly–Kennedy plication in the hope of providing preferential support to the bladder neck and thus preventing any occult or potential stress incontinence.

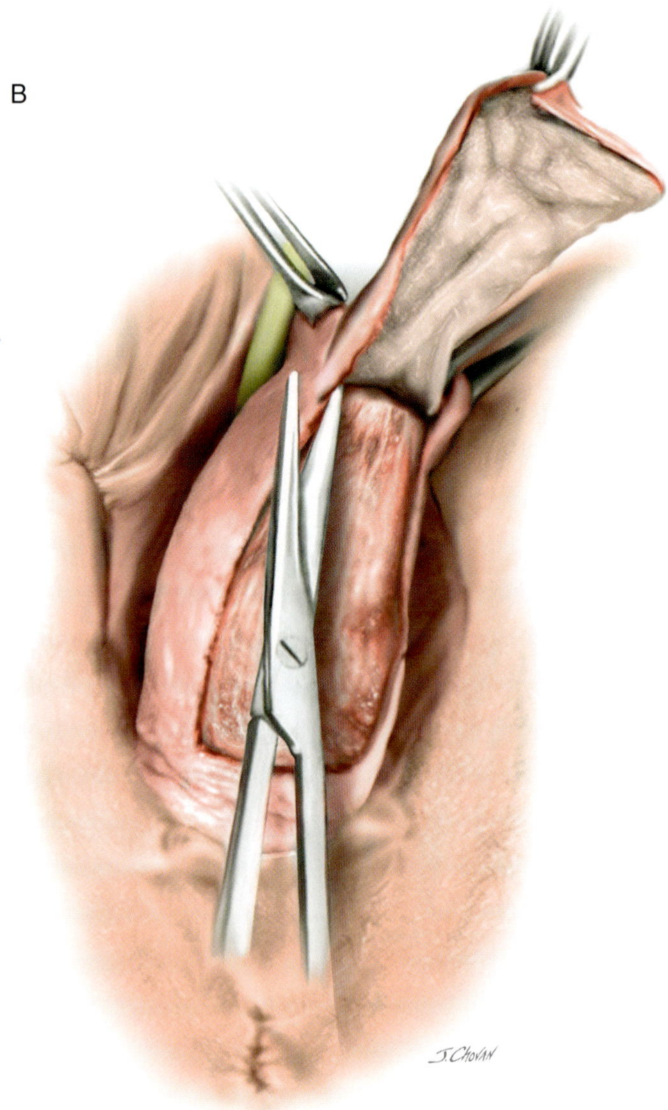

Fig. 23.1 cont'd **B**, A similar rectangular piece of posterior vaginal wall is removed. A portion of the posterior vaginal wall will usually lie over an enterocele, and the surgeon should attempt to avoid entering the peritoneal cavity if at all possible.

2. The vagina is circumscribed by an incision several centimeters from the hymen at the base of the prolapse. A marking pencil is then used to mark rectangular portions of the vagina that will be removed sharply. The vaginal epithelium is completely removed. An effort is made to avoid entering the peritoneal cavity (Fig. 23.2A and B).
3. A series of purse-string sutures is placed, sequentially inverting the vagina by tying the sutures (Fig. 23.2C). The apex of the soft tissue is inverted by the tip of a forceps as each purse-string suture is tied. A variation of this procedure can involve performing a separate anterior and posterior colporrhaphy with two purse-string sutures to close the anterior and posterior segments together and to obliterate any dead space between compartments.
4. Levatorplasty is then performed; the genital hiatus is invariably widened in this patient population. The puborectalis and pubococcygeus muscles are reapproximated in the midline with delayed absorbable sutures (see Fig. 23.3), creating a shelf above the rectum as a barrier to visceral descent.
5. As with Le Fort partial colpocleisis, a Kelly plication at the bladder neck or a MUS should be considered to avoid the development of SUI. (See Video 23.2: Technique of complete colpectomy and Colpocleisis and Video 23.3: Technique of complete colpectomy in a patient who had failed two prior obliterative procedures.)

Complications of total colpectomy are comparable to those of Le Fort partial colpocleisis, most of which are related to medical complications rather than surgical sequelae. Retrospective cohort studies report urinary tract infection as the most common postoperative complication, ranging from 4.3% to 6.4% (Bochenska et al., 2017; Catanzarite et al., 2014). However, Hill et al. (2016) reported urinary tract infection rates as high as 34.7%. Stepp et al. (2005) reported that most postoperative complications in women over age 75 years, regardless of

C

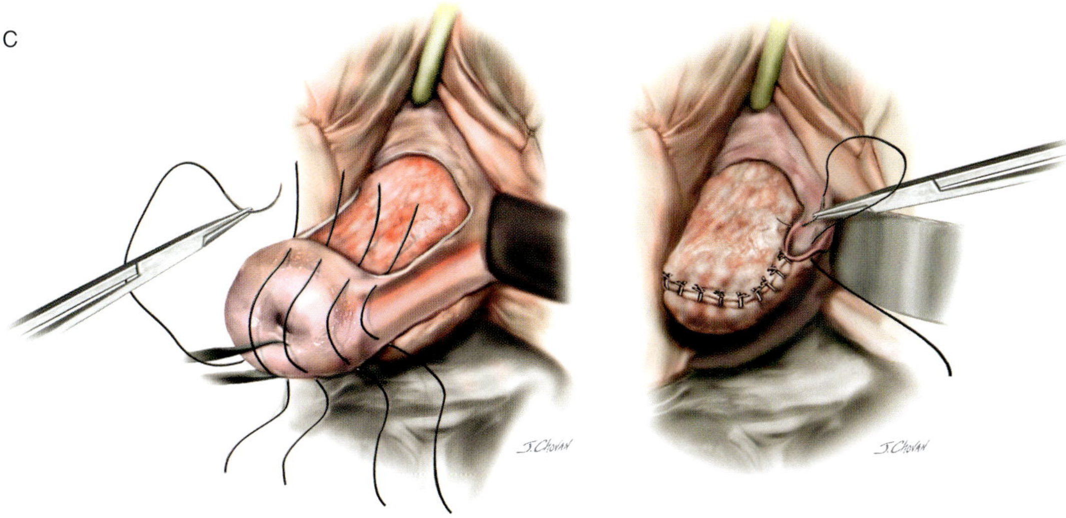

D

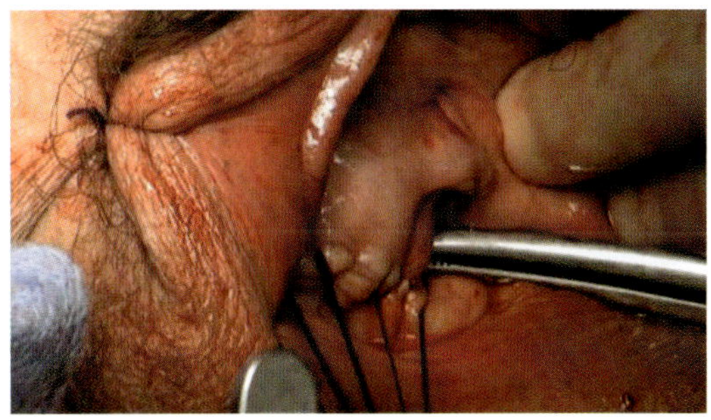

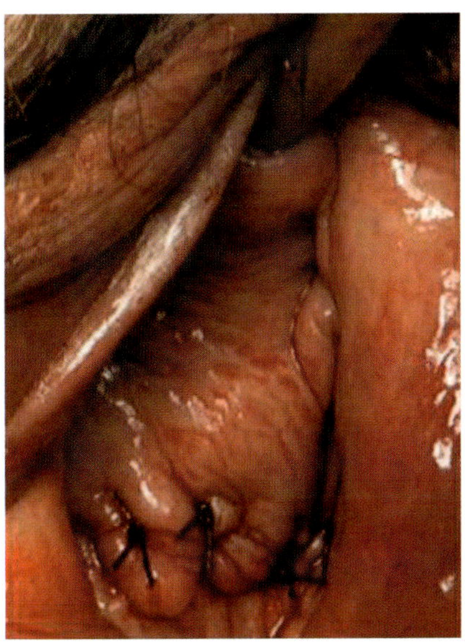

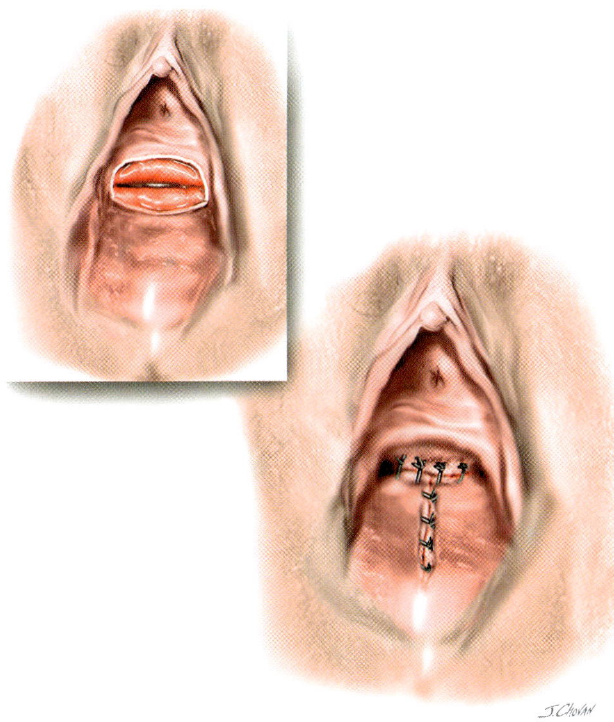

Fig. 23.1 cont'd **C**, The cut edge of the anterior incision at the level of the cervix is sewn to the distal cut edge of the posterior incision with interrupted No. 2-0 delayed absorbable sutures. (*inset*) Once the cervix is inverted, the interrupted sutures are taken through the cut edges of the lateral portions of the incision. **D**, Once the entire vagina has been inverted, the superior and inferior margins over the rectangle can be sutured horizontally, thus completely obliterating the midportion of the vagina. Note: draining channels are left in the lateral portions of the vagina to facilitate drainage of any cervical discharge. A levatoroplasty is commonly performed to increase posterior pelvic muscle support and narrow the introitus. (See Fig. 23.3 for technique of levatoroplasty.)

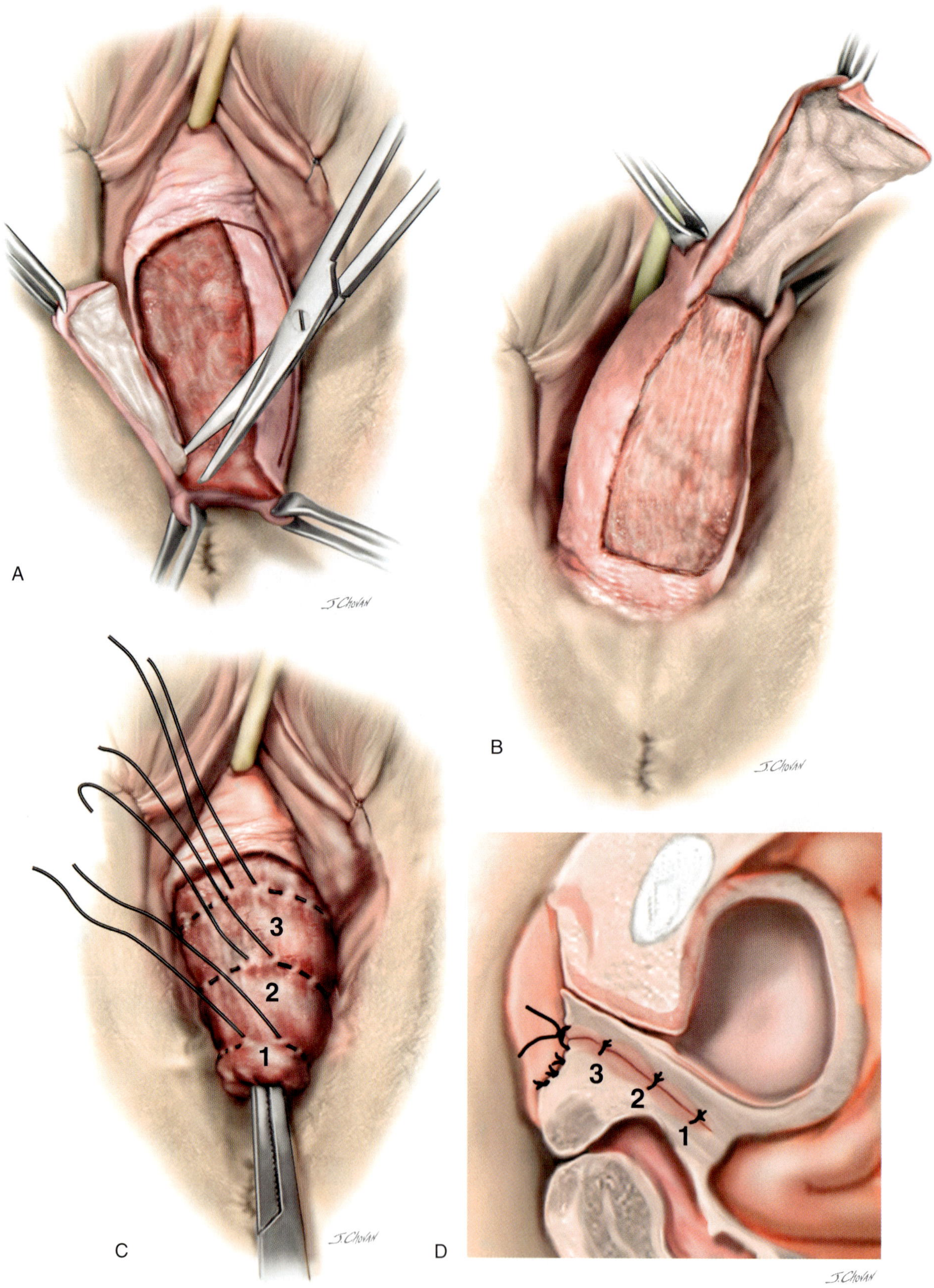

Fig. 23.2 Colpectomy and complete colpocleisis. **A** and **B**, The vagina is circumscribed by an incision at the site of the hymen and is marked into quadrants. Each quadrant is removed by sharp dissection. **C**, Purse-string delayed absorbable sutures are placed. The leading edge of the soft tissue is inverted by the tip of the forceps. Purse-string sutures are tied 1 before 2 and 2 before 3, with progressive inversion of the soft tissue before tying of each suture. **D**, The final relationship is shown in a cross-section. A perineorrhaphy is also usually performed.

the type of prolapse surgery performed, are related to medical problems. Risk factors for complications included length of surgery and a history of cardiac or peripheral vascular disease.

Ureteral injury, resulting from kinking of the ureter by a purse-string stitch, occurs in about 2% of cases. The majority of ureteral obstructions resolve with removal of the occluding stitch. For this reason, the authors endorse routine cystoscopy with all obliterative surgical procedures.

Colpocleisis literature reports high anatomic success and satisfaction rates. Koski et al. (2012) studied 53 patients with Pelvic Organ Prolapse Quantification stage III or greater or Baden–Walker grade 3. Total colpocleisis or Le Fort partial colpocleisis was performed in 73.6% and 26.4%, respectively. Concomitant slings were inserted in 60.4%. There was no recurrence of prolapse at a mean follow-up of 9.3 months.

LEVATOR PLICATION AND PERINEORRHAPHY

Several studies have shown benefit to incorporating a levator muscle plication across the midline along with aggressive extended perineorrhaphy to narrow the genital hiatus and essentially build a wall of perineal support after obliterative procedures. The addition of this procedure is advocated by the authors.

1. Two Allis clamps are placed superiorly on the genital hiatus to demarcate the lateral edges of tissue removal from the posterior fourchette (see Fig. 23.3).
2. A diamond-shaped flap of epithelium is marked over the distal posterior vaginal wall proximally and perineal skin distally. The marked perineal skin and vaginal epithelium is sharply removed (Fig. 23.3B).
3. The distal posterior vaginal wall is mobilized laterally to allow access to the distal levator ani muscle. Two to three No. 0 Vicryl sutures on a CT-1 needle are used to plicate the levator muscles across the midline, thus significantly decreasing the caliber of the distal vaginal canal (see Fig. 23.3B and C).
4. The perineal body is reconstructed using a series of No. 2-0 Vicryl sutures, greatly reducing the size of the genital hiatus. The vaginal and perineal skins are then closed with interrupted or running No. 3-0 Vicryl sutures (see Fig. 23.3C).

(See Videos 23.1–23.3.)

The addition of levator plication and high perineorrhaphy at the time of colpocleisis significantly reduces the size of the genital hiatus, which may prevent recurrent prolapse. In addition, some surgeons believe that building up the posterior wall may also support the vaginal vault and urethra and prevent stress incontinence.

URINARY AND BOWEL FUNCTION FOLLOWING OBLITERATIVE PROCEDURES

It is difficult to predict urinary function after correction of severe POP. *De novo* stress incontinence is a frequent and bothersome issue following obliterative surgery. In the elderly population, however, there may be a risk of worsening any preexisting voiding dysfunction if an antiincontinence procedure is used at the time of colpocleisis. Conversely, it is also possible to improve voiding dysfunction and retention by correction of an obstructive prolapse, oftentimes resulting in a normalization of elevated preoperative PVRs.

Although use of MUSs at the time of prolapse repair has become common practice for many, there has been significant debate regarding routine placement of an MUS or other antiincontinence procedure at the time of colpocleisis. Sling lysis rates attributed to voiding dysfunction postoperatively are 2.5% to 7%. As an alternative to MUS for primary or occult stress incontinence, urethral bulking agents may also be considered. In a study by Isom-Batz and Zimmern (2009) involving 31 subjects, 93% reported improvement or resolution of their symptoms following bulking agent injection.

Some recent studies have described the effect of obliterative surgery with or without antiincontinence procedures on urge urinary incontinence and voiding dysfunction symptoms. Fitzgerald and Brubaker (2003) reported a retrospective series focused on perioperative incontinence and found that 36% of patients choosing an obliterative option had elevated PVR volumes, and 78% had stress incontinence on examination (33% occult). Autologous fascial slings were placed in one-third of the patients, and 19% had Kelly plication. Interestingly, 34 of 36 patients with elevated PVR preoperatively had normal PVR following colpocleisis, although three patients required midline sling lysis for retention. In all, 27% of patients still developed *de novo* stress incontinence.

Moore and Miklos (2003) described excellent results when placing an MUS at the time of colpocleisis. At nearly 20 months, 94% of patients considered themselves "cured" of their stress incontinence. They concluded from this study that placement of a retropubic synthetic MUS at the time of obliterative procedure is effective; however, they could not comment on other types of MUSs.

Abbasy and Brubaker (2009) described a retrospective cohort of 38 women who had an MUS (tension-free vaginal transobturator tape in 40% vs. tension-free vaginal tape in 60% of patients) placed at the time of colpocleisis. They found that, although 30% of the patients had a PVR greater than 100 mL preoperatively, only two of the 38 continued to have elevated PVR after the prolapse was corrected. Median prolapse and incontinence scores on the Pelvic Floor Distress Inventory significantly improved in all patients. Fitzgerald et al. (2008) reported objective and subjective data on 152 patients after colpocleisis and found that 15% had bothersome urgency/frequency.

Koski et al. (2012) observed no postoperative *de novo* urgency or urinary retention in 53 patients who underwent total colpectomy or Le Fort partial colpocleisis. Frequency and urgency were the most common and bothersome complaints on the Urogenital Distress Inventory, Short Form (UDI-6) (33.3%), but most of these patients had these same complaints preoperatively.

Another study by Smith et al. (2011) evaluated the risk of voiding dysfunction and sling placement in 210 patients undergoing Le Fort partial colpocleisis. Median follow-up was 22 weeks, with a total of 161 patients having a concurrent sling placed. Overall, sling placement resulted in a 92.5% subjective cure of stress incontinence. Of the 56 patients who had preoperative voiding dysfunction, there was complete resolution of symptoms postoperatively in 51 (91%) patients. *De novo* voiding dysfunction

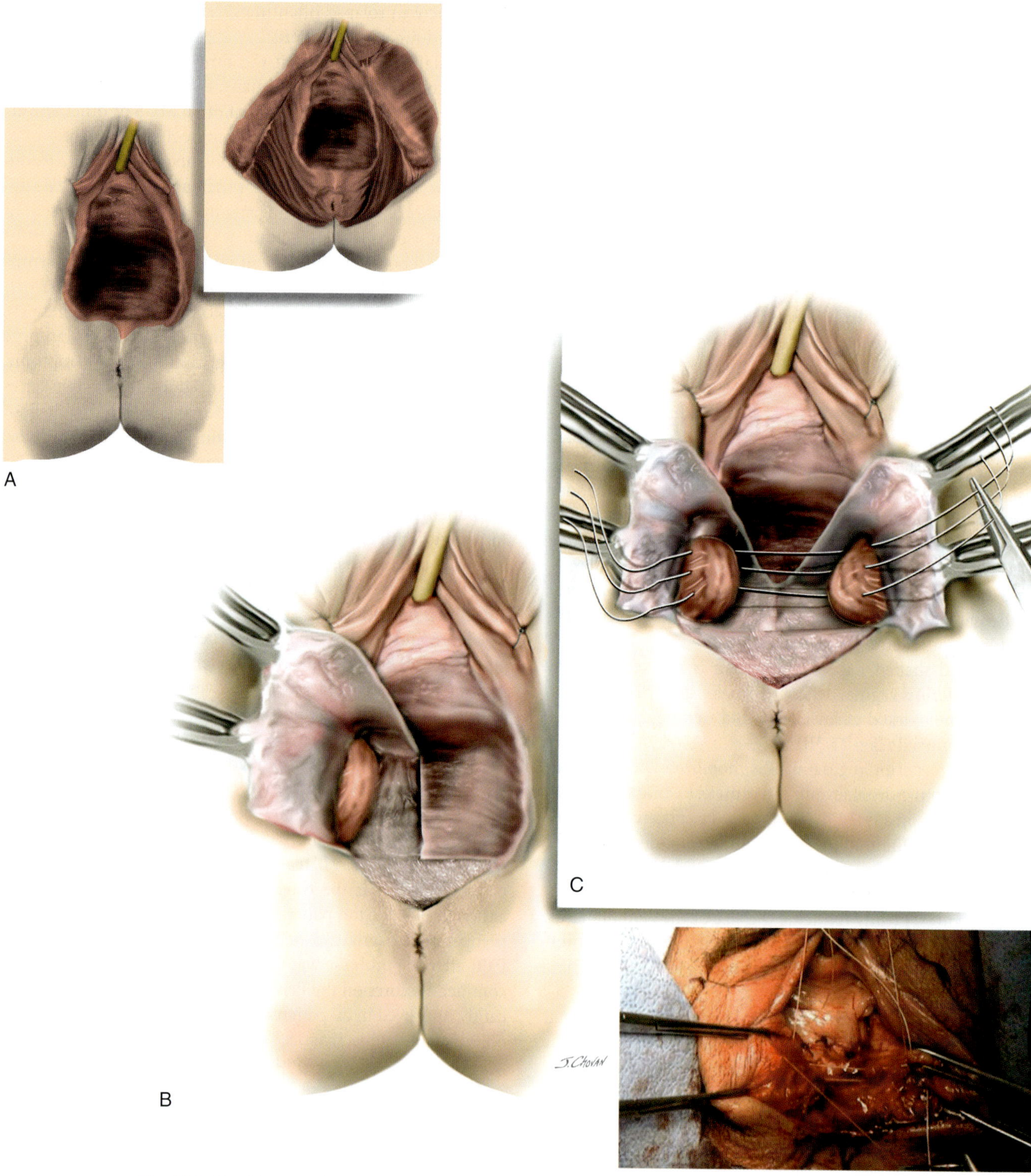

Fig. 23.3 Distal levatoroplasty and perineorrhaphy. **A**, Widened genital hiatus with levator muscle shown in a lateral position. **B**, Perineal and midline vaginal incision is used to expose medial edge of levator muscle. (*inset*) Distal portions of levator muscle are plicated across the midline. **C**, Plication sutures are placed and tied, and perineorrhaphy is performed.

occurred in two patients (1.9%), and one patient (0.6%) required sling revision. The authors concluded that sling placement at the time of colpocleisis was associated with high continence rates with minimal risk of postoperative voiding dysfunction.

Oliphant et al. (2012) constructed a computer model to compare staged and concomitant MUSs and found that both approaches had similar overall utilities. They suggested that surgical decision-making should be tailored to individual patient needs and preferences, and, in their model, a staged approach greatly reduced the number of urethral slings performed. Catanzarite el al. (2014) reported no increase in postoperative complications with MUS placement within the first 30 days postoperatively. With extreme variations of findings, it remains important to judge surgical strategy on a patient-by-patient basis.

Gutman et al. (2010) performed an ancillary analysis to assess bowel symptoms in a prospective cohort of 152 women who underwent total and partial colpocleisis, using the Colorectal-Anal Distress Inventory and Colorectal-Anal Impact Questionnaire. The majority of patients (77%) reported bothersome bowel symptoms at baseline, categorized as: obstruction (17%–26%), incontinence (12%–35%), and pain/irritation (3%–34%). At 1 year, 50% to 100% of the baseline bothersome bowel symptoms resolved, with a *de novo* bowel symptom rate of 0% to 14%.

QUALITY OF LIFE AND REGRET OF LOSS OF SEXUAL FUNCTION

Given that obliterative surgery relies on patient willingness to forego sexual intercourse, proper counseling and information must be provided for patients to make an appropriate decision. Preoperative counseling should include a discussion and documentation regarding sexual consequences of vaginal obliteration. In general, however, overall satisfaction rates with obliterative procedures are very high, with a low overall sense of regret.

Choosing patients appropriately for obliterative procedures is based on age, medical comorbidities, desire for sexual function, and patient preference. For example, an older patient may be more amenable to an obliterative procedure, given that overall sexual activity decreases over time, with only 40% of 65- to 74-year-old women and 17% of women 75 years and older reporting sexual activity (Lindau et al., 2007). Comorbidities or desire to avoid general anesthesia may also contribute to this decision.

The Pelvic Floor Disorder Network (Fitzgerald et al., 2008) followed a cohort of 152 patients after colpocleisis and measured both objective and subjective outcomes at 3 and 12 months postoperatively. They found that 82% of patients at 3 months and 73% at 12 months had prolapse stage 1 or less. All pelvic symptom scores on standardized questionnaires improved. The satisfaction rate was 95% among this cohort. Fitzgerald et al. (2008) studied 132 women 1 year after colpocleisis. All Pelvic Floor Distress Inventory (PFDI) and Pelvic Floor Impact Questionnaire (PFIQ) scores showed significant improvement at 3 and 12 months. In all, 125 (95%) patients said they were either "very satisfied" or "satisfied" with the outcome of their surgery.

Hullfish et al. (2007) assessed patients 2.75 years ($\pm$ 1.90 years) after colpocleisis. Of the 40 patients who returned questionnaires, most agreed or strongly agreed that their goals were met for vaginal pressure (100%), urinary incontinence (84.9%), bladder emptying (76.4%), urinary frequency/urgency (91.2%), physical activity (88.6%), restoration of normal anatomy (95%), colorectal symptoms (65.0%), and self-image (96.9%). UDI-6 (39.9 ± 24.9 vs. 21.0 ± 20.3, $P < .01$) and Incontinence Impact Questionnaire, Short Form (IIQ-7; 35.4 ± 29.3 vs. 17.3 ± 24.6, $P < .01$) scores improved. Of the patients studied, 95% were either "very satisfied" or "satisfied," whereas 5% reported postoperative regret.

In a retrospective cohort study of 90 women with stage III or IV prolapse, Murphy et al. (2008) compared preoperative and postoperative responses to the UDI-6 and IIQ-7. Vaginal reconstructive and obliterative surgery was performed in 45 women per group. Improvements in the IIQ-7 and UDI-6 were comparable, as were postoperative Surgical Satisfaction Questionnaire scores.

Barber et al. (2007) conducted a prospective study in which women underwent either obliterative or reconstructive vaginal surgery based on their personal preference and sexual expectations. Of 79 subjects, 70 completed follow-up 6 and 12 months after surgery. Both groups demonstrated significant improvements in the POP, urinary, and colorectal scales of the PFDI and PFIQ, as well as the various scales of the 36-Item Short Form Health Survey (bodily pain, vitality, social functioning, role-emotional, and mental health) at 6 and 12 months postoperatively. Of the women, 90% said that they would choose the obliterative surgery again.

A prospective, seven-site, multicenter study through the Society of Gynecologic Surgeons Fellows' Pelvic Research Network by Crisp et al. (2013) reported improved body image and pelvic floor symptoms with low regret and high satisfaction after colpocleisis. A total of 87 patients reported a decrease in mean modified Body Image Scale score from 4.8 to 1.2 ($P < .001$), which corresponds to improved body image, and a decrease in PFIQ and PFDI scores at 6 weeks. A low rate of *de novo* urgency urinary incontinence requiring medication (1.4%) and *de novo* SUI were noted.

In contrast, a recent retrospective cohort study of patients who underwent colpocleisis showed a decline in satisfaction rates (75%) over time, with a mean follow-up of 6.4 years (Winkelman & Elkadry, 2018). Regret was reported in 19% of patients, with reasons including urgency urinary incontinence, loss of sexual function, and insufficient preoperative counseling. Over half of the patients reported urinary urgency (63%) and urge incontinence (56%), whereas 32% of patients reported a PFDI score of zero.

CONCLUSION

Obliterative surgery for advanced-stage POP remains an excellent option for patients who would like to avoid an extensive reconstructive procedure or who have medical problems that preclude such an option, or in patients who no longer desire sexual activity. Le Fort partial colpocleisis and colpectomy/colpocleisis have very high rates of cure and satisfaction among properly selected patients. As with any surgical procedure, patients and providers must discuss the disease process and expectations of any surgery in order to determine which procedure is most amenable for the individual case.

BIBLIOGRAPHY

Historical Perspectives

Adair F, DaSef L. The Le Fort colpocleisis. *Am J Obstet Gynecol.* 1936;32:218.

Adams HD. Total colpocleisis for pelvic eventration. *Surg Gynecol Obstet.* 1951;2:321.

Anderson GV, Deasy PP. Hysterocolpectomy. *Obstet Gynecol.* 1960;16:344.

Baer J, Reis R. Immediate and remote results in two hundred twelve cases of prolapse of the uterus. *Am J Obstet Gynecol.* 1928;16:646.

Berlin F. Three cases of complete prolapsus uteri operated upon according to the method of Leon Le Fort. *Am J Obstet Gynecol.* 1881;14:866.

Bradbury WC. Subtotal vaginectomy. Present status in treating uterovaginal prolapse, with modified technique. *Am J Obstet Gynecol.* 1963;86:663.

Collins C, Lock F. The Le Fort colpocleisis. *Am J Surg.* 1941;53:202.

Edebohls GM. Panhysterocolpectomy: a new prolapsus operation. *Med Rec N Y.* 1901;60:561.

Gerardin R. Memoire presente a la Societe Medicale de Metz en 1823. *Arch Gen Med.* 1825;8.

Hanson GE, Keettel WC. The Neugebauer-Le Fort operation. A review of 288 colpocleises. *Obstet Gynecol.* 1969;34:352.

LeFort L. Nouveau procede pour la guerlson, du prolapsus utérin. *Bul Gen Ther.* 1877;92:337.

Martin A. Ueber estirpatio vaginae. *Berl Klin Wschr.* 1898;35:910.

Masson JC, Knepper PA. Vaginectomy. *Am J Obstet Gynecol.* 1938;36:94.

Mazer C, Isral SL. The Le Fort colpocleisis: an analysis of 43 operations. *Am J Obstet Gynecol.* 1948;56:944.

Neugebauer JA. Einige worte uber die mediane vaginalnaht als mittel zur beseitgung des gebarmuttervorfalls. *Zentralbl Gynaekol.* 1881;5:3.

Phaneuf L. The place of colpectomy in the treatment of uterine and vaginal prolapse. *Am J Obstet Gynecol.* 1935;30:544.

Pratt J, Baker R. Urinary incontinence following the Le Fort operation: report of a case. *Obstet Gynecol.* 1960;16:722.

Ridley JF. Evaluation of the colpocleisis: a report of fifty-eight cases. *Am J Obstet Gynecol.* 1972;113:1114.

Rubovits W, Litt S. Colpocleisis in the treatment of uterine and vaginal prolapse. *Am J Obstet Gynecol.* 1935;29:222.

Taft C. Le Fort's operation for complete procidentia of the uterus, with a report of a case. *Am J Med Sci.* 1889;98:128.

Tauber R. The modern technique of the Le Fort operation. *Ann Surg.* 1947;125:334.

Thomsen H. Vaginal evisceration trods kolpokleise og kolpoperineoplastik. *Ugeskr Laeger.* 1988;150:867.

Ubachs JM, Van Sante TJ, Schellekens LA. Partial colpocleisis by a modification of Le Fort's operation. *Obstet Gynecol.* 1973;42:415.

Williams JT. Vaginal hysterectomy and colpectomy for prolapse of the uterus and bladder. *Am J Obstet Gynecol.* 1950;59:365.

Evaluation, Surgical Treatment, and Complications

Abbasy S, Kenton K. Obliterative procedures for pelvic organ prolapse. *Clin Obstet Gynecol.* 2010;53:86.

Abbasy S, Lowenstein L, Pham T, et al. Urinary retention is uncommon after colpocleisis with concomitant mid-urethral sling. *Int Urogynecol J Pelvic Floor Dysfunct.* 2009;20:213.

Barber MD, Amundsen CL, Paraiso MF, et al. Quality of life after surgery for genital prolapse in elderly women: obliterative and reconstructive surgery. *Int Urogynecol J Pelvic Floor Dysfunct.* 2007;18:799.

Beverly C, Walters MD, Weber AM, et al. Prevalence of hydronephrosis in patients undergoing surgery for pelvic organ prolapse. *Obstet Gynecol.* 1997;90:37.

Bochenska K, Leader-Cramer A, Mueller M, et al. Perioperative complications following colpocleisis with and without concomitant vaginal hysterectomy. *Int Urogynecol J.* 2017;28:1671.

Buchsbaum GM, Lee TG. Vaginal obliterative procedures for pelvic organ prolapse: a systematic review. *Obstet Gynecol Surv.* 2017;72:175.

Catanzarite T, Rambachan A, Mueller MG, et al. Risk factors for 30-day perioperative complications after Le Fort colpocleisis. *J Urol.* 2014;192:788.

Cespedes RD, Winters JC, Ferguson KN. Colpocleisis for the treatment of vaginal vault prolapse. *Tech Urol.* 2001;7:152.

Cho MK, Moon JH, Kim CH. Factors associated with recurrence after colpocleisis for pelvic organ prolapse in elderly women. *Int J Surg.* 2017;44:274.

Crisp CC, Book NM, Cunkelman JA, et al. Body image, regret, and satisfaction 24 weeks after colpocleisis: a multicenter study. *Female Pelvic Med Reconstr Surg.* 2016;22:132.

DeLancey JO, Morley GW. Total colpocleisis for vaginal eversion. *Am J Obstet Gynecol.* 1997;176:1228.

Erekson E, Murchison RL, Gerjevic KA, et al. Major postoperative complications following surgical procedures for pelvic organ prolapse: a secondary database analysis of the American College of Surgeons National Surgical Quality Improvement Program. *Am J Obstet Gynecol.* 2017;217:608.e1.

Falk HC, Kaufman SA. Partial colpocleisis: the effort procedure. *Obstet Gynecol.* 1955;5:617.

Fitzgerald MP, Brubaker L. Colpocleisis and urinary incontinence. *Am J Obstet Gynecol.* 2003;189:1241.

Fitzgerald MP, Richter HE, Bradley CS, et al. Pelvic support, pelvic symptoms, and patient satisfaction after colpocleisis. *Int Urogynecol J Pelvic Floor Dysfunct.* 2008;19:1603.

Fitzgerald MP, Richter HE, Siddique S, et al. Colpocleisis: a review. *Int Urogynecol J Pelvic Floor Dysfunct.* 2006;17:261.

Frick AC, Walters MD, Larkin KS, Barber MD. Risk of unanticipated abnormal gynecologic pathology at the time of hysterectomy for uterovaginal prolapse. *Am J Obstet Gynecol.* 2010;202:507.e1.

Goldman J, Ovadia J, Feldberg D. The Neugebauer-Le Fort operation: a review of 118 partial colpocleisis. *Eur J Obstet Gynecol Reprod Biol.* 1981;12:31.

Gutman RE, Bradley CS, Ye W, et al. Pelvic Floor Disorders Network. Effects of colpocleisis on bowel symptoms among women with severe pelvic organ prolapse. *Int Urogynecol J.* 2010;21:461.

Hanson GE, Keettel WC. The Neugebauer-Le Fort operation: a review of 288 colpocleisis. *Obstet Gynecol.* 1969;34:352.

Harmanli OH, Dandolu V, Chatwani AJ, Grody MT. Total colpocleisis for severe pelvic organ prolapse. *J Reprod Med.* 2003;48:703.

Hill AJ, Carroll AW, Matthews CA. Unanticipated uterine pathologic finding after morcellation during robotic-assisted supracervical hysterectomy and cervicosacropexy for uterine prolapse. *Female Pelvic Med Reconstr Surg.* 2014;20:113.

Hill AJ, Walters MD, Unger CA. Perioperative adverse events associated with colpocleisis for uterovaginal and posthysterectomy vaginal vault prolapse. *Am J Obstet Gynecol.* 2016;214:501.e1.

Hullfish KL, Bovbjerg VE, Steers WD. Colpocleisis for pelvic organ prolapse: patient goals, quality of life, and satisfaction. *Obstet Gynecol.* 2007;110:341.

Isom-Batz G, Zimmern PE. Collagen injection for female urinary incontinence after urethral or periurethral surgery. *J Urol.* 2009;181:701.

Jones K, Wang G, Romano R, et al. Colpocleisis: a survey of current practice patterns. *Female Pelvic Med Reconstr Surg.* 2017;23:276.

Kandadai P, Flynn M, Zweizig S, et al. Cost-utility of routine endometrial evaluation before Le Fort colpocleisis. *Female Pelvic Med Reconstr Surg.* 2014;20:168.

Kohli N, Sze E, Karram M. Pyometra following Le Fort colpocleisis. *Int Urogynecol J.* 1996;7:264.

Koski ME, Chow D, Bedestani A, et al. Colpocleisis for advanced pelvic organ prolapse. *Urology.* 2012;80:542.

Lindau ST, Schumm LP, Laumann EO, et al. A study of sexuality and health among older adults in the United States. *N Engl J Med.* 2007;357:762.

McIntyre A, Blumenthal N, Merkur H. Vaginal evisceration following colpocleisis and sacrocolpopexy. *J Gynaecol Womens Healthcare.* 2018;1:105.

Moore RD, Miklos JR. Colpocleisis and tension-free vaginal tape sling for severe uterine and vaginal prolapse and stress urinary incontinence under local anesthesia. *J Am Assoc Gynecol Laparosc.* 2003;10:276.

Murphy M, Sternschuss G, Haff R, et al. Quality of life and surgical satisfaction after vaginal reconstructive vs obliterative surgery for the treatment of advanced pelvic organ prolapse. *Am J Obstet Gynecol.* 2008;198:573.

Nichols DH, Randall CL. *Vaginal Surgery.* 3rd ed. Baltimore: Williams & Wilkins; 1989.

Oliphant SS, Shepherd JP, Lowder JL. Midurethral sling for treatment of occult stress urinary incontinence at the time of colpocleisis: a decision analysis. *Female Pelvic Med Reconstr Surg.* 2012;18:216.

Olsen AL, Smith VJ, Bergstrom JO, et al. Epidemiology of surgically managed pelvic organ prolapse and urinary incontinence. *Obstet Gynecol.* 1997;89:501.

Smith AL, Karp DR, Lefevre R, et al. LeFort colpocleisis and stress incontinence: weighing the risk of voiding dysfunction with sling placement. *Int Urogynecol J.* 2011;22:1357.

Sokol AI, Jelovsek JE, Walters MD, et al. Incidence and predictors of prolonged urinary retention after TVT with and without concurrent prolapse surgery. *Am J Obstet Gynecol.* 2005;192:1537.

Song X, Zhu L, Ding J, et al. Long-term follow-up after LeFort colpocleisis: patient satisfaction, regret rate, and pelvic symptoms. *Menopause.* 2016;23:621.

Stepp KJ, Barber MD, Yoo EH, et al. Prevalence of perioperative complications of urogynecologic surgery in elderly women. *Am J Obstet Gynecol.* 2005;192:1630.

Sung VW, Weitzen S, Sokol ER, et al. Effect of patient age on increasing morbidity and mortality following urogynecologic surgery. *Am J Obstet Gynecol.* 2006;194:1411.

Suskind AM, Jin C, Walter LC, Finlayson E. Frailty and the role of obliterative versus reconstructive surgery for pelvic organ prolapse: A National Study. *J Urol.* 2017;197:1502.

Vallabh-Patel V, Saiz C, Salamon C, et al. Prevalence of occult malignancy within morcellated specimens removed during laparoscopic sacrocolpopexy. *Female Pelvic Med Reconstr Surg.* 2016;22:190.

Van der Ploeg JM, van der Steen A, Zwolsman S, et al. Prolapse surgery with or without incontinence procedure: a systematic review and meta-analysis. *BJOG.* 2018;125:289.

Von Pechmann WS, Mutone M, Fyffe J, Hale DS. Total colpocleisis with high levator plication for the treatment of advanced pelvic organ prolapse. *Am J Obstet Gynecol.* 2003;189:121.

Wheeler TL, Gerten KA, Garris J. Obliterative vaginal surgery for pelvic organ prolapse. *Obstet Gynecol Clin North Am.* 2009;36:637.

Wheeler TL, Richter HE, Burgio KL, et al. Regret, satisfaction, and symptom improvement: analysis of the impact of partial colpocleisis for the management of severe pelvic organ prolapse. *Am J Obstet Gynecol.* 2005;193:2067.

Winkelman WD, Elkadry EA. Colpocleisis: long-term outcomes. *Am J Obstet Gynecol.* 2018;218:S932.

Yasa C, Ugurlucan FG, Yalcin O. Management of pyometra after LeFort colpocleisis resistant to drainage. *Int Urogynecol J.* 2016;27:645.

Zebede S, Smith AL, Plowright LN, et al. Obliterative LeFort colpocleisis in a large group of elderly women. *Obstet Gynecol.* 2013;121:279.

Zhang YH, Lu YX, Liu X, et al. Impact of colpocleisis on body image in women with severe pelvic organ prolapse. *Zhonghua Fu Chan Ke Za Zhi.* 2011;46:431.

PART 4

Surgical Complications and their Management

24

Avoiding and Managing Lower Urinary Tract Injuries During Pelvic Surgery

Catherine A. Matthews and John B. Gebhart

CHAPTER OUTLINE

INTRODUCTION

Lower urinary tract injury is one of the most serious complications of gynecologic surgery and, in addition to causing significant patient morbidity, is a common cause of litigation. Between 50% and 90% of all lower urinary tract injuries occur during gynecologic surgery because of the intimate anatomic relationship that exists between the female genital and lower urinary tracts.

Review of the surgical literature reveals two disturbing facts: most injuries occur during gynecologic surgery performed for benign and otherwise uncomplicated conditions, and most lower urinary tract injuries are not recognized during the operative procedure in which they occur. For these reasons, we emphasize prevention and recognition of lower urinary tract injuries during gynecologic surgery.

INCIDENCE

Historically, the reported rates for injuries during pelvic surgery range from 0.2% to 1.8% for bladder injury and from 0.03% to 1.5% for ureteral injury. The true figures are thought to exceed these numbers, given the number of unreported cases, the spontaneous resolution of partial ureteral obstructions, and the loss of some renal systems. When universal cystoscopy was performed in a large cohort of women undergoing hysterectomy for benign disease, the rate of bladder injury was 2.9%, and the rate of ureteral injury was 1.8%, with a cumulative injury rate of 4.3% (Ibeanu et al., 2009). As 600,000 hysterectomies are performed annually in the United States, an estimated 25,800 women could experience a bladder or ureter injury each year in this country as a result of this procedure. Laparoscopic and vaginal hysterectomy have been associated with higher rates of bladder injury in the United States than abdominal hysterectomy. Ureteral injury is also more commonly observed after laparoscopic (and robotic) hysterectomy. High-volume surgeons have demonstrated lower rates of urinary tract injury regardless of mode of hysterectomy than low-volume surgeons.

Surgery for prolapse or incontinence increases the risk of urinary tract injury. Vaginal surgery for anterior and/or apical pelvic organ prolapse is associated with an intraoperative ureteral obstruction rate of approximately 5%; most of these injuries are sustained during high uterosacral ligament suspension, proximal McCall culdoplasty, and colpocleisis. Anterior colporrhaphy is associated with a 0.5% to 2% risk of ureteral obstruction, prompting consideration for routine cystoscopy after this procedure as well. Retropubic slings result in a 3% to 5% rate of bladder perforation when performed by experienced surgeons but can occur in up to 34% of cases performed by resident trainees, whereas transobturator slings result in bladder perforation in less than 1% of cases. If these injuries are recognized during surgery, no long-term sequelae are sustained.

Studies of genitourinary fistulas reveal that the ratio of bladder injury to ureteral injury resulting in fistula is approximately 5:1. Most injuries that result in the formation of genitourinary fistulas are not recognized during surgery.

PREVENTION OF INJURIES

In over 40% of all ureteric injuries, no predisposing factors are identified, and the surgery that is performed is described as routine. Familiarity with the course of the ureter, and maintaining ureteric consciousness during each gynecologic procedure, are critical. Contributing factors that have been identified in ureteral injuries include bleeding, enlarged uterus, endometriosis, adhesions, obesity, and pelvic organ prolapse. An awareness of these risk factors, and an attempt to optimize surgical planning and execution, are paramount. The liberal use of cystoscopy after the injection of indigo carmine or similar dye is strongly endorsed.

Preoperative Assessment

The patient's history, physical examination, and preoperative laboratory evaluation may suggest abnormal function of the urinary tract. Ureteral kinking and obstruction should be considered in women who present with massive prolapse. Sonographic imaging of the urinary tract is useful in determining kidney size, detecting ureteral obstruction, and estimating urinary residual volumes. A computed tomography (CT) urogram documents anatomic abnormalities, further defines renal function, and localizes ureteric obstruction; it is important in the evaluation of complex genitourinary fistulas. A retrograde pyelogram may be useful intraoperatively to determine the site of ureteral obstruction. Routine preoperative imaging studies have not been shown to reduce the incidence of operative injuries to the lower urinary tract.

Cystourethroscopy is indicated in the preoperative evaluation of hematuria, abnormal urine cytology, persistent or recurrent urinary tract infections, lower urinary tract fistulas, urethral or bladder diverticula, urethral and bladder pain, selected cases of urinary incontinence, certain vaginal mesh and sling complications, and staging of gynecologic malignancies.

Preoperative retrograde ureteral stent or catheter placement has not been shown to reduce the incidence of surgical injury to the ureter. The procedure itself may cause bleeding, edema, and perforation of the ureter. The stent is often difficult to feel within an area of fibrosis, and it may predispose the ureter to damage as a result of the immobility that it imparts to the ureter.

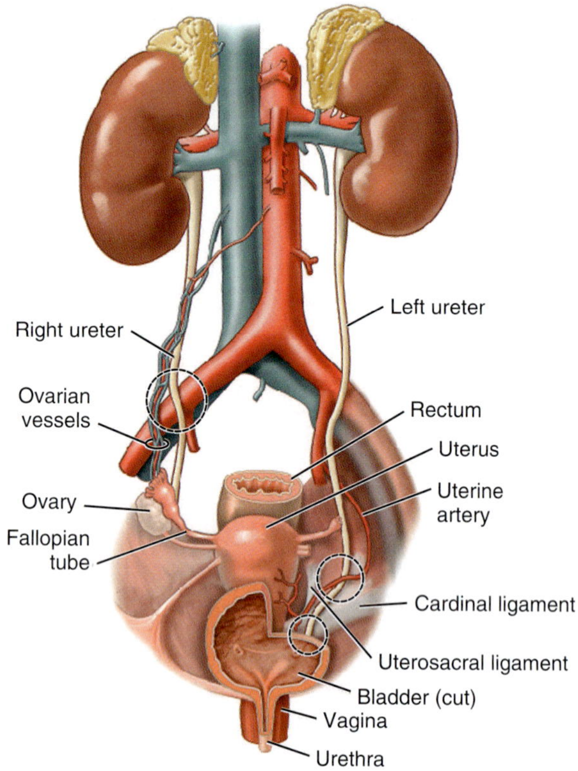

Fig. 24.1 Course of the ureter. Locations of potential sources of ureteral injury during gynecologic surgery are noted (*dotted circles*). (From Walters MD, Barber MD. *Hysterectomy for Benign Disease (with CD)*. Philadelphia: Elsevier Inc.; 2010.)

Intraoperative Care

The pelvic surgeon should always be ureter-conscious. Full knowledge of the anatomic location and course of the ureters is paramount to injury prevention. Visualization of ureteric peristalsis may not be adequate evidence of ureteral patency. One can always find the ureter on the medial leaf of the broad ligament after opening the roof of the pararectal space and dissecting medial to the iliac vessels.

The most common location of ureteral injury during hysterectomy is in the distal 3 to 4 cm of the ureter where the ureter crosses under the uterine artery in the cardinal ligament, and then across the lateral vaginal fornix to enter into the bladder. Potential sources of ureteric injury are demonstrated in Fig. 24.1. One must recognize that the close anatomic relationship between the uterine artery and ureter in the cardinal ligament puts the ureter at risk during each hysterectomy, but it is especially vulnerable to lateral thermal spread when electrocautery is used for vessel ligation. Familiarity with the specific properties of the vessel-sealing instrument that is selected may assist with injury prevention. The ureters may also be kinked during obliteration of the cul-de-sac, plication of the uterosacral ligaments, or suspension of the vaginal apex.

In the operating room there are no substitutes for appropriate case selection, good lighting, proper patient preparation and positioning, adequate exposure, and strict adherence to sterile techniques. Lighting can be improved by the use of headlamps, light-containing suction irrigators, or fiberoptic lighted retractors. During complicated cases, abdominal–perineal–vaginal preparation, drapes that permit access to the abdominal and vaginal areas, positioning of the patient in universal stirrups, and a transurethral three-way continuous irrigation balloon catheter (16 or 18 French) for emptying and filling the bladder are recommended. These measures give the surgeon the flexibility to operate abdominally or vaginally, to perform endoscopy, and to detect and repair lower urinary tract injuries if they occur.

During all surgical procedures, sharp dissection is preferable to blunt dissection, and taking small pedicles is preferred to taking large pedicles. When hemostasis is a problem, pressure should be applied with a sponge stick until the bleeding vessel can be identified and selectively clamped. Many ureters are damaged by the application of clamps in a frantic effort to control pelvic hemorrhage.

Abdominal Approach

Abdominal incisions should allow adequate exposure of the entire pelvis. Entry into the peritoneal cavity should be as cephalad as possible to avoid direct cystotomy. The surgeon should be aware that the bladder may be pulled up beneath the anterior abdominal wall by its peritoneal reflection as a result of incomplete emptying, tumor, or previous surgery, especially cesarean section. If a cystotomy is sustained in the extraperitoneal portion of the bladder, single-layer closure without prolonged catheter drainage is adequate.

Entry into the peritoneal cavity is followed by exploration of its contents, restoration of normal anatomic relationships, and exposure of the operative site. Attention is given to the location and size of each kidney. With the patient in the Trendelenburg position, the bowel may be packed into the upper abdomen and retained by a retractor.

At this point, an effort should be made to identify both ureters and to trace their pelvic courses. The ureters are most easily identified as they descend into the pelvis over the bifurcation of the common iliac arteries. They then follow the posterior boundaries of the ovarian fossae to pass beneath the uterine arteries and to course anteriorly and laterally about the cervix and upper vagina. Each ureter enters a separate tunnel within the base of the bladder. Although palpation of the ureter between the forefinger and thumb imparts a "clicking" sensation and sound, these characteristics can also be obtained by palpating other retroperitoneal structures. To positively identify the ureter, it is best to observe its distinctive periodic peristalsis directly.

The ureter usually can be dissected away from or out of a gynecologic disease process. The aim is to do so with the least possible ureteral trauma. Placing the tips of a right-angle or tonsil forceps between the adventitial sheath of the ureter and the adjacent tissue to guide the dissection is helpful. If at all possible, the ureter should not be separated from its overlying peritoneum. This attachment protects the ureter's blood supply, elevates it out of the depths of the pelvis (where it might be surrounded by blood and serum), and assists its peristalsis. If a portion of the ureter is invaded by endometriosis or cancer, it may have to be resected and a ureteroneocystostomy or ureteroureterostomy performed.

Likewise, determining the location and extent of the outer wall of the bladder is important. Sharply dissecting the bladder from adjacent pathologic conditions is usually possible. Rarely, in some cases of endometriosis or cancer, resecting a portion of the bladder wall is necessary. The presence of hematuria may indicate that a full- or partial-thickness bladder injury has been sustained and demands further investigation.

Increasingly, urogynecologists and reconstructive pelvic surgeons are encountering dense adherence of the bladder to the posterior symphysis when performing repeat retropubic procedures, or to the lower uterine segment in cases of prior cesarean section. Sharp dissection of the bladder from the lower uterine segment is always recommended (Fig. 24.2). When dense adhesions are encountered, perform an extraperitoneal cystotomy in the dome of the bladder, then dissect the bladder and upper urethra from the surrounding tissues under direct vision. Experience has shown that this procedure reduces the extent of damage to both organs.

Vaginal Approach

In preparing the patient for vaginal surgery, we drain the bladder with a transurethral catheter, and then we sometimes instill undiluted indigo carmine (5 mL) into the bladder. After this is done, the catheter is clamped or removed to keep the dye within the bladder. During surgery, if the bladder is partially or completely incised, the blue color of the indigo carmine is recognized, alerting the surgeon to the bladder injury. If this step has been omitted, and fluid is encountered during dissection, the bladder can be retrograde-filled with either saline mixed with methylene blue or indigo carmine, and one can look for extravasation of dye. This likely is more helpful than cystoscopy.

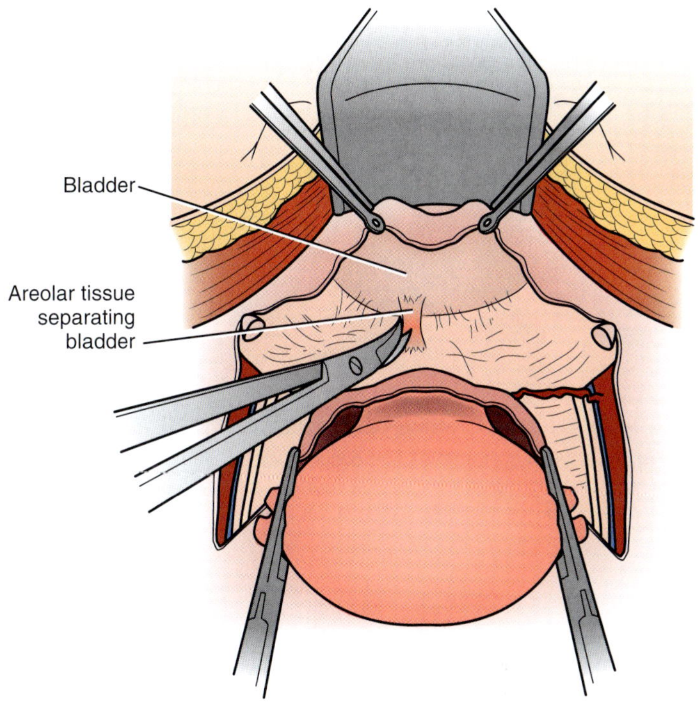

Fig. 24.2 Sharp dissection of the bladder flap reduces the risk of bladder injury. (Modified from Lee RA, Hagen JV. *Atlas of Gynecologic Surgery*. Philadelphia: WB Saunders; 1992. Copyrighted by and used with the permission of Mayo Foundation for Medical Education.)

During vaginal operations, the surgeon should avoid a cystotomy by identifying the trigone and base of the bladder. Unlike an extraperitoneal cystotomy that can occur during entry into the abdominal cavity during laparotomy, a cystotomy that is sustained during attempted entry into the anterior cul-de-sac during vaginal hysterectomy is in the supratrigonal, intraperitoneal portion of the bladder and carries an increased risk for fistula formation if not repaired correctly (Fig. 24.3). Helpful tips for correct bladder identification include palpating the balloon of a transurethral catheter, inserting a probe or Kelly clamp and palpating its tip, or reaching through a posterior colpotomy incision around and in front of the lower uterine segment with a finger or curved retractor and seeing the tip between the bladder and the lower uterine segment. If one can successfully accomplish entry into the anterior cul-de-sac and place a vaginal retractor to deviate the bladder and ureters out of the surgical field before clamping the cardinal ligaments, the risk of ureteral injury is minimized (Fig. 24.4). If a cystotomy is sustained during attempted entry into the anterior cul-de-sac, the edges should be tagged with sutures, and the cystotomy used as a guide for the correct dissection plane. The cystotomy should be closed after completing the hysterectomy.

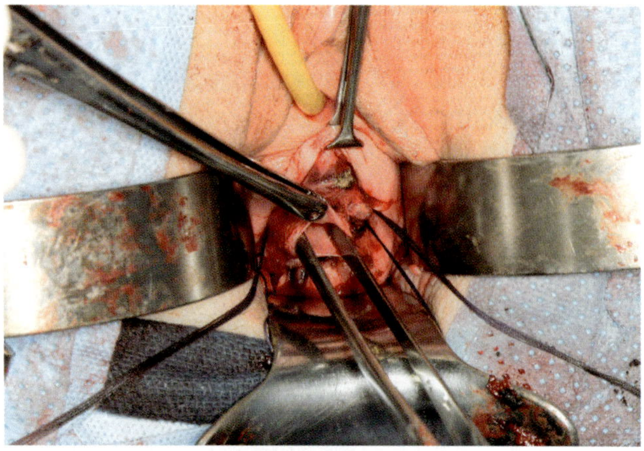

Fig. 24.3 Most cystotomies that occur during vaginal hysterectomy are in the supratrigonal, transperitoneal portion of the bladder and carry an increased risk for fistula formation if not repaired correctly.

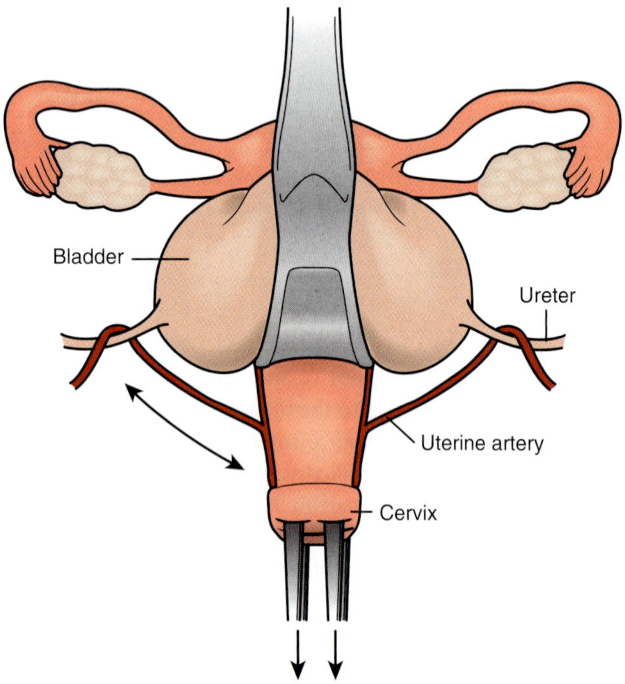

Fig. 24.4 Ureter anatomy in relation to the uterus at total vaginal hysterectomy. Upward traction of the bladder during vaginal hysterectomy increases the distance of the ureter away from the area of clamp placement. (From Walters MD, Barber MD. *Hysterectomy for Benign Disease (with CD)*. Philadelphia: Elsevier Inc.; 2010.)

During vaginal surgery, visualization of the ureter is difficult and somewhat hazardous. When the pelvic cavity has been opened, it is possible, with experience, to palpate the ureters against an appropriately placed vaginal sidewall retractor. This is a very important maneuver when operating on patients with prolapse and when performing extensive culdoplasties. If there is any question about the integrity of the ureters or bladder, cystoscopy should be performed.

Dissection of the anterior vaginal wall exposes the urethra and the bladder trigone to injury. Most urethral injuries result from diverticulum repair, anterior colporrhaphy, urethropexy, or instrumentation of the urethra. Increasingly, urethral injuries are caused by midurethral sling procedures, either during the initial dissection or following trocar placement. Urethral injuries, both direct and indirect, may damage the organ's sphincter mechanism and cause stress urinary incontinence.

Removal of vaginal mesh may result in bladder and unrecognized ureteral injury. Based on reports of severe delayed morbidity from unilateral and bilateral ureteral injury following vaginal mesh removal, routine performance of cystoscopy with these procedures is recommended.

Laparoscopic Approach

Increasing numbers of urinary tract injuries have been reported since the introduction of laparoscopic surgery. In a study where intraoperative cystoscopy following the injection of indigo carmine was routinely performed after total laparoscopic hysterectomy, the incidence of injury was 4%. Laparoscopically-assisted vaginal hysterectomy has demonstrated consistently higher rates of lower urinary tract injury than either abdominal or vaginal hysterectomy. The incidence of urinary tract complications appears to increase with the complexity of the procedure, likely because of adhesions caused by endometriosis, pelvic inflammatory disease, or previous surgery. Alternatively, ureteral injuries may be increased because of instrumentation that is used for vessel sealing, or because ureteral identification is more challenging when the ureter cannot be directly palpated.

Most bladder injuries result from sharp dissection, with or without cautery, during laparoscopically-assisted vaginal hysterectomy. Many surgeons believe that the incidence of bladder injuries associated with laparoscopically-assisted vaginal hysterectomy can be reduced if the bladder dissection is done vaginally instead of laparoscopically. Most series of laparoscopic urinary continence and pelvic support procedures report some bladder and urethral injuries. The incidence of these injuries appears to be related directly to the surgeon's experience with these procedures.

Comparative studies of laparoscopic versus robotic-assisted hysterectomy are currently not large enough to delineate any difference in urinary tract injury. The absence of haptic feedback with robotic surgery could potentially increase the risk of injury. Rates of bladder injury during robotic sacrocolpopexy, however, have not been higher than during laparoscopic or open sacrocolpopexy. Anecdotal reports of extensive bladder and ureteral injury with complex vesicovaginal fistulae following robotic-assisted hysterectomy exist.

A surgical technique that may reduce the risk of ureteral injury during any type of laparoscopic hysterectomy is the use of a uterine manipulator with either a cervical ring or cup that fits tightly into the vaginal fornices. Upward traction on the ring during uterine artery ligation and colpotomy places the ureters more lateral and decreases the risk of lateral thermal spread and ureteral injury.

During laparoscopy, urinary tract injury may be revealed by direct observation, injection of dye solution, presence of gas in the catheter bag, and detection of bubbles during cystoscopy. If urinary tract injury is suspected, cystoscopy should be performed and sometimes repeated. If ureteral injury is suspected, a ureteral catheter should be inserted.

RECOGNITION AND MANAGEMENT OF INJURIES

Several general principles apply to the management and repair of all lower urinary tract injuries. The administration of prophylactic antibiotics is indicated. The extent of the damage to the urinary tract must be explored. Devitalized tissues must be excised. Urinary tract repairs should be performed with small-caliber delayed absorbable (polyglactin or polyglycolic acid) or absorbable (chromic) suture. Absolutely no tension should be placed on the repair site. Extraperitoneal suction drainage should be placed adjacent to, but not in contact with, all retroperitoneal repairs. Bladder drainage is important to reduce tension within the wall of the bladder during the healing phase.

Recognition of Ureteral Injury

All pelvic surgeons should have a clear algorithm for the recognition and management of ureteral injury. Although the use of intraoperative cystoscopy does not usually prevent urinary tract injury, it does allow for the early diagnosis and repair of injuries and avoids the need for additional surgery and/or the potential loss of renal function. Box 24.1 describes the recommended sequence of steps, which are described in detail later.

Intravenous Dye Injection. Intravenous injection of indigo carmine (slow infusion of 5 mL) or sodium fluorescein (10% preparation, 0.25–1 mL) normally results in the excretion of blue or green urine, respectively, within 5 to 10 minutes. If the dye injection is accompanied by an increase in intravenous fluids or the administration of a diuretic, dye excretion may be enhanced. In women with intrinsic renal disease or in those who are diuretic-dependent, the excretion of dye is delayed. A second dose of dye may be administered; however, indigo carmine can be vasoactive, and a third dose is not recommended. Another mechanism to enhance observation of ureteral jets is to administer oral pyridium preoperatively and look for orange hue of the urine. If no coloration agent is available intraoperatively, one may instill hypertonic glycine instead of normal saline to distend the bladder. Because of differences in specific gravity, the ureteral jets are more pronounced (oil in water effect).

BOX 24.1 Steps to Help Recognize Ureteral Injury During Gynecologic Surgery

1. Request the injection of indigo carmine dye at least 10 minutes before the anticipated start of cystoscopy to maximize surgical efficiency.
2. If >10 min and no flow of blue urine, give 10 mg furosemide IV, unless medically contraindicated.
3. In cases of uterosacral ligament suspension, high McCall culdoplasty, and anterior repair, perform cystoscopy after each step to facilitate the correct identification of any obstructing sutures. If efflux is not observed, release offending sutures (in case of uterosacral ligament suspension, release distal stitch first) and repeat cystoscopy.
4. If still no urine flow, attempt to pass a ureteral catheter—if successful, leave in place for 4 to 6 weeks to prevent postoperative ureteral stenosis.
5. Perform retrograde pyelogram to identify location of ureteral injury.

When an intravenous dye, such as indigo carmine, is administered, the passage of blue urine means that at least one renal unit is functioning. Cystoscopy (suprapubic or transurethral) or cystotomy is required for confirmation that both ureters are functioning normally. A "sluggish" ureteral jet should raise concern that the ureter in question is partially kinked and may become fully obstructed in the postoperative period. This may occur when performing high uterosacral ligament suspension, and suture replacement should be considered. If thermal injury to a ureter is suspected, observation of ureteral flow is not sufficient to ensure against subsequent development of a stricture, fistula, or ureteral blowout. In this circumstance, ureteral stenting for at least 4 to 6 weeks is required. Leakage of blue urine into the operative field is evidence of lower urinary tract injury. This requires further investigation.

Cystoscopy. Cystoscopy may be performed transurethrally or suprapubically if the patient is not in the lithotomy position. Transurethral cystoscopy is facilitated by the routine use of universal stirrups. Suprapubic cystoscopy or telescopy is typically performed with a zero-degree scope. When telescopy is completed, the cystotomy site may be used for subsequent suprapubic catheter bladder drainage.

The intravenous injection of indigo carmine (5 mL) or 10% sodium fluorescein (0.25 mL) just before cystoscopy enables the examiner to determine ureteric function, as evidenced by the excretion of colored urine. When either ureter fails to excrete dye-colored urine, the reason must be determined.

Cystotomy. A cystotomy is another method of observing the inside of the bladder. Ideally, the cystotomy should be placed in the extraperitoneal portion of the dome of the bladder. If intravenous indigo carmine is administered, the excretion of blue urine helps determine the integrity of each renal unit. This technique should be considered, for example, when cystoscopic equipment is not readily available, such as in an emergent cesarean hysterectomy.

Ureteral Catheterization. Intraoperative ureteral catheterization is usually performed by cystoscopy or cystotomy. The ureters may be catheterized using a small pediatric feeding tube, open-ended ureteral catheter, or ureteral stent (Fig. 24.5). A pediatric feeding tube may be easier to pass through the ureteral tunnels than a stent because of its flexibility. The tube is usually used intraoperatively to demonstrate ureteral patency, but it can be used for short-term postoperative ureteral drainage. If a catheter or stent is selected, placement over a flexible guidewire is recommended to avoid injury to the ureter. A deflecting bridge may facilitate placement, and the catheter or stent(s) may be brought out of the urethra or through the dome of the bladder and abdominal wall for long-term drainage. Ureteral double-J stents are ideal for longer-term ureteral drainage, because the upper J maintains the catheter within the renal pelvis, and the lower J maintains the catheter within the bladder (Fig. 24.6A and B). The appropriate ureteral catheter length varies according to patient height, but the most common size is a 6-French, 26-cm length catheter. Although

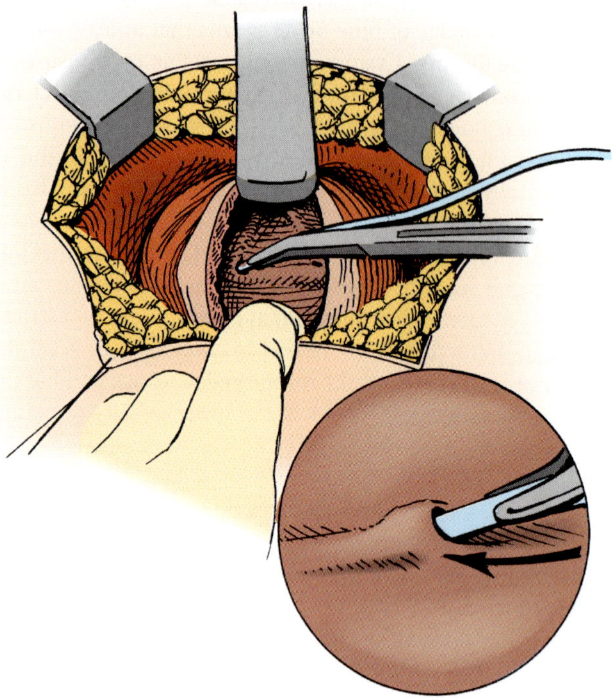

Fig. 24.5 Technique of ureteral catheter passage after cystotomy has been performed.

these catheters have the benefit of not being exposed to the external environment, they can cause significant bladder irritation and pain (see Video 24.1: Ureteral stents and Video 24.2: Retrograde ureteral stent placement).

Resistance to the passage of a ureteral catheter suggests kinking or obstruction of the ureter. The drainage of urine through the catheter documents renal function. Catheters and stents should be left in place when there are obstructions, crush injuries, or ureteral repairs to drain urine from the kidneys, to help prevent stenosis of the ureter and to facilitate healing.

See Chapter 40 for further discussion of retrograde urethrography and stent placement.

Intravenous Urography. Intravenous urography may be performed intraoperatively to determine renal function and to document the integrity of the lower urinary tracts. It requires the use of fluoroscopy. Radiologic imaging provides documentation of findings and can isolate the point of obstruction. This method of intraoperative testing is somewhat cumbersome, may miss very distal ureteral injury, and should be done in a manner that minimizes radiation exposure.

Management of Ureteral Injury

Ureteral angulations and kinks should be released if they cause obstruction. A ligated ureter should have the ligating suture removed or have a stent left in place until the offending suture has dissolved. Minor ureteral crush injuries may be managed with stenting; significant thermal or crush injuries require resection of the damaged segment and ureteroneocystostomy or ureteroureterostomy. On occasion, partial lacerations of a ureter can be repaired by appropriate placement of several fine absorbable or delayed absorbable sutures. Complete lacerations of the ureter and loss of a segment of ureter require definitive surgical repair.

In the event of delayed recognition of ureteral injury, an attempt is first made to pass a retrograde stent into the ureter. If this is unsuccessful, an attempt at antegrade stent placement is made. If this fails, the decision to proceed with nephrostomy tube placement versus proceeding with immediate surgical repair depends on the medical condition of the patient.

The surgical procedures recommended for ureteral repair vary according to the ureteral segment that is involved (see Fig. 24.1). Because most gynecologic injuries to the ureter involve its distal 4 to 5 cm, most can be repaired by ureteroneocystostomy. Injuries just below the pelvic brim may be repaired by ureteroureterostomy or ureteroneocystostomy. Ureteroneocystostomy is not recommended for injuries above the pelvic brim.

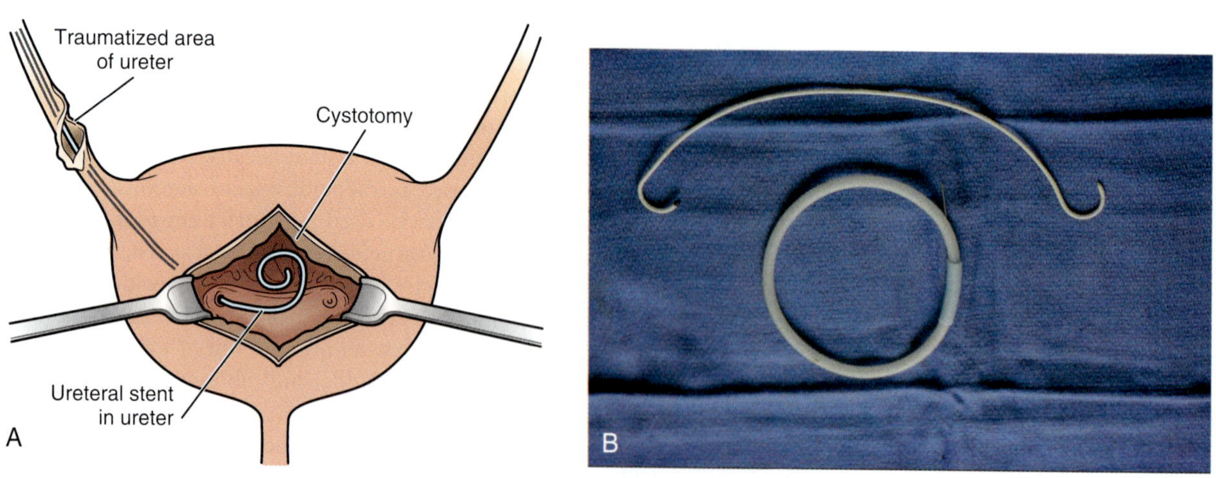

Fig. 24.6 A, Demonstration of distal right ureteral injury managed by retrograde stenting of the affected ureter via bladder dome cystotomy. Modified from Lee and Hagen (1992), copyrighted by and used with the permission of Mayo Foundation for Medical Education. B, 6-French, 26-cm double-J stent that is passed over a guidewire.

Ureteroneocystostomy. Ureteroneocystostomy is the procedure of choice for injuries involving the terminal 4 to 5 cm of either ureter (Fig. 24.7) and can be performed via laparotomy, via laparoscopy, or with robotic assistance. The distal ureteral segment is ligated with permanent suture at its entry into the bladder. If the proximal ureter has a nonviable segment, this is excised. The end of the ureter then is tagged with a long through-and-through suture. The bladder may be mobilized by the release of its attachments to the posterior surface of the pubis. An extraperitoneal cystotomy is performed in the dome of the bladder, and the base of the bladder is displaced toward the end of the injured ureter. A Kelly clamp is used to make a direct puncture through the full thickness of the base of the bladder at an appropriate location to allow the tagged distal end of the ureter to be brought into the bladder. When this is accomplished, and at least 1 cm of ureter is inside of the bladder, the end of the ureter is spatulated bilaterally, and its distal flaps are secured to the inside of the bladder with No. 3-0 chromic sutures. The adventitia of the ureter is anchored to the outside of the bladder with several No. 3-0 delayed absorbable sutures.

Most importantly, no tension should be placed on the ureter or the bladder at the site of the ureteroneocystostomy. If there is tension on the anastomosis, it should be relieved by a vesicopsoas hitch procedure (Fig. 24.8), with or without a Boari–Ockerblad flap (Fig. 24.9). If a vesicopsoas hitch is needed, it is best performed before reimplantation or reanastomosis of the ureter. Surgeons differ on the need for ureteral stenting following ureteroneocystostomy. If there is any question about the use of a stent, one should be used. The site of the anastomosis should be drained by an extraperitoneal suction drain. The cystotomy is closed, and the bladder drained continuously for at least 7 days (see Video 24.3: Ureteroneocystotomy; Video 24.4: Ureteral reimplantation with psoas hitch; and Video 24.5: Robotic ureteral reimplantation with psoas hitch).

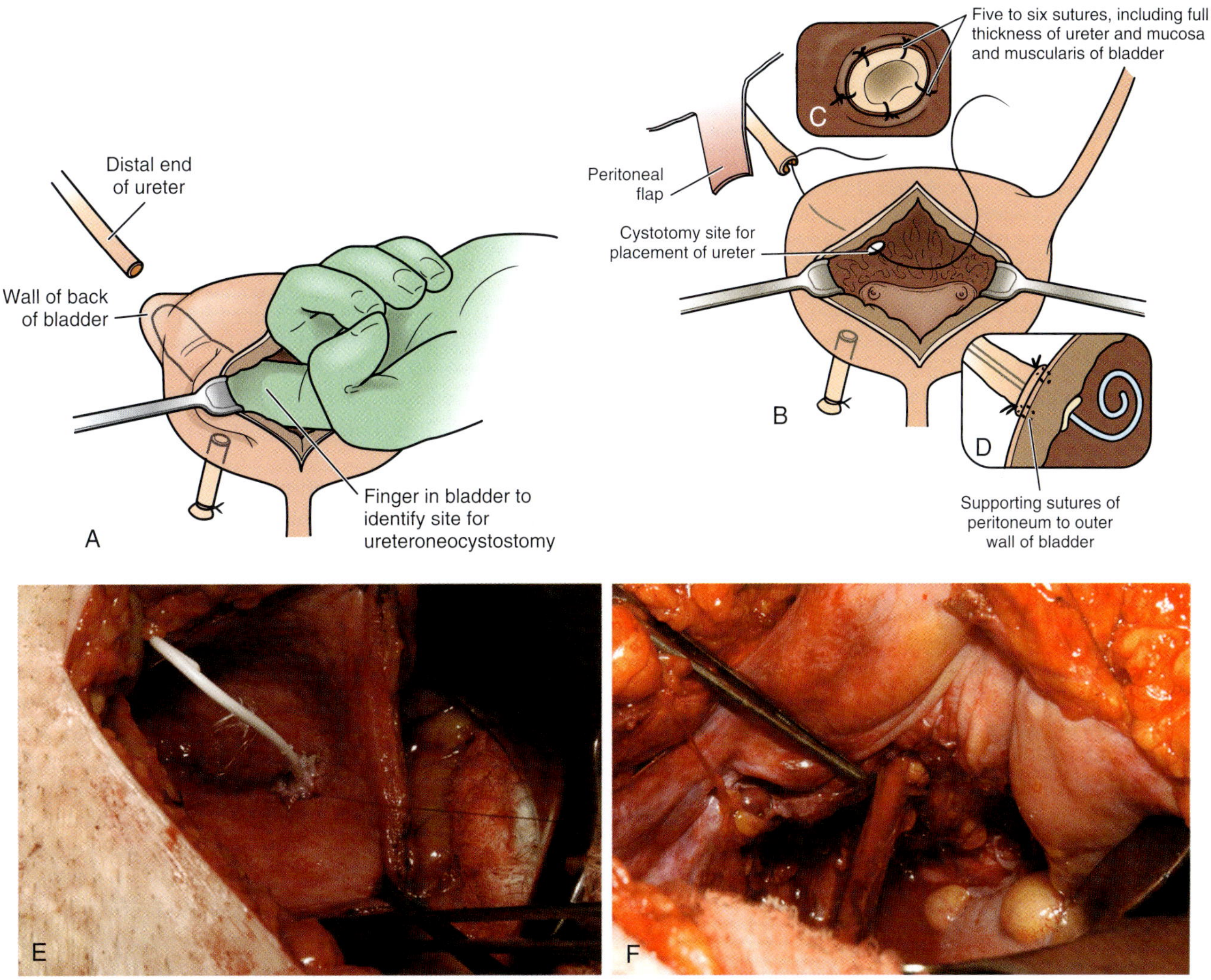

Fig. 24.7 Schematic overview of ureteroneocystostomy. **A**, Site in the bladder dome is chosen for future reimplantation of the ureter. **B**, The ureter is brought within the bladder using the previously tagged suture. **C**, Completed anastomosis. **D**, Serosa sutures further stabilize the anastomosis. **E**, Inside of bladder. **F**, Outside of bladder after completed ureteroneocystostomy. (Modified from Lee RA, Hagen JV. *Atlas of Gynecologic Surgery*. Philadelphia: WB Saunders; 1992. Copyrighted by and used with the permission of Mayo Foundation for Medical Education.)

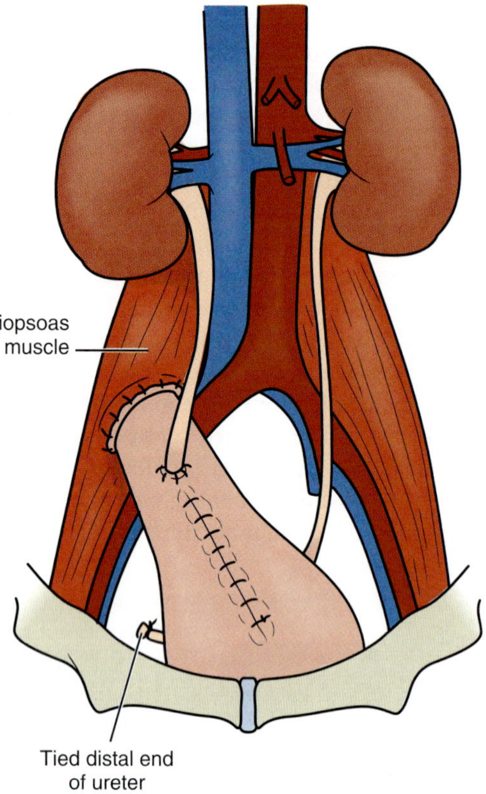

Fig. 24.8 Vesicopsoas hitch, used for distal ureteral injuries in which there is tension on a ureteroneocystostomy or ureteroureterostomy. This technique brings the bladder cephalad to relieve tension on the suture site. (Modified from Lee RA, Hagen JV. *Atlas of Gynecologic Surgery*. Philadelphia: WB Saunders; 1992. Copyrighted by and used with the permission of Mayo Foundation for Medical Education.)

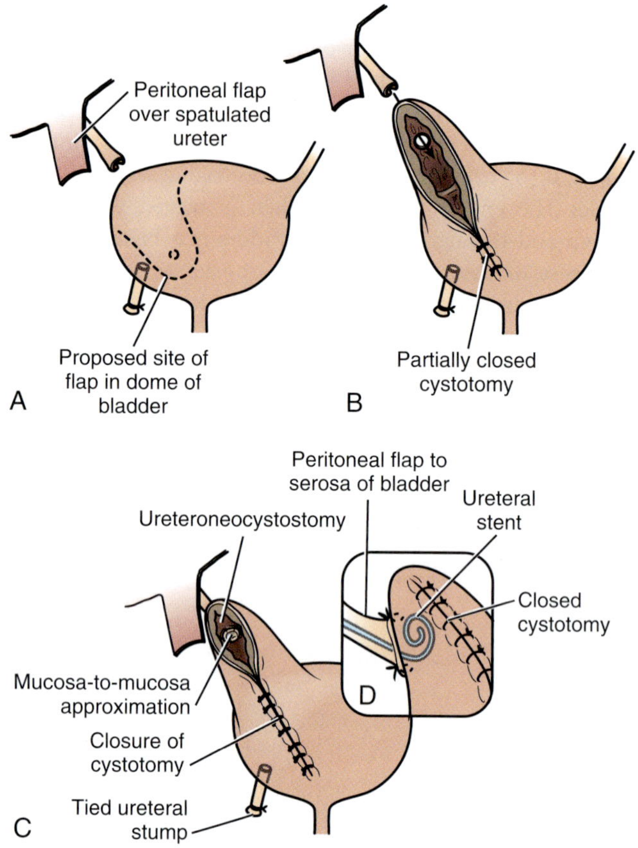

Fig. 24.9 Boari–Ockerblad bladder flap. **A**, Bladder flap is outlined on the bladder. **B**, Site of future ureteral reimplantation. **C**, End-to-side ureteral anastomosis completed and double-J ureteral stent placed. **D**, Cystotomy closure completed and (not shown) psoas hitch performed to keep anastomosis off tension. (Modified from Lee RA, Hagen JV. *Atlas of Gynecologic Surgery*. Philadelphia: WB Saunders; 1992. Copyrighted by and used with the permission of Mayo Foundation for Medical Education.)

Ureteroureterostomy. The simplest ureteroureterostomy involves the tension-free reanastomosis of two cut ends of a ureter. When there is loss of a ureteral segment, there may be a need for bladder or kidney mobilization, a bladder extension procedure, transureteroureterostomy, or the interposition of an intestinal segment.

In performing a ureteroureterostomy, the viable cut ends of each ureteral segment are spatulated for a distance of about 0.5 cm to help prevent stenosis of the anastomosis. A ureteral catheter is inserted into the ureter to bridge the anastomotic site. Four to six interrupted full-thickness No. 4-0 chromic sutures are used to perform the anastomosis. The anastomotic site is drained by an extraperitoneal suction drain to prevent the accumulation of blood, serum, or urine. This drain should remain in place until the ureteral catheter has been removed. The ureteral catheter should be left in place for at least 7 days. Postoperative bladder drainage is usually recommended (see Video 24.6: Ureteroureteroostomy).

Bladder Mobilization and Extension. When performing a ureteroneocystostomy or ureteroureterostomy, no tension should be placed on the site of the anastomosis. Dissection of the retropubic space (of Retzius) frees the bladder from its attachments to the posterior symphysis and allows it to be mobilized toward the site of the repair. If this is done and there is still some tension on the anastomosis, the surgeon should consider performing a psoas hitch or bladder extension procedure.

The vesicopsoas hitch is performed by placing one or two fingers through an extraperitoneal cystotomy and pushing the bladder toward the psoas muscle on the side of the anticipated ureteral repair (see Fig. 24.8). When it is determined that the displacement of the bladder will allow a tension-free repair, the outer muscular wall of the bladder is sutured to the psoas muscle with several interrupted No. 2-0 or 1-0 delayed absorbable sutures. The attachment of the bladder to the psoas muscle must also be tension-free to prevent pressure necrosis around the sutures and premature detachment of the bladder. Care should be taken to avoid injuring the femoral and genitofemoral nerves when anchoring the bladder to the psoas muscle.

If dissection of the retropubic space and performing a psoas hitch do not give enough mobility to the bladder to allow a satisfactory ureteral implantation or reanastomosis, the creation of a bladder flap made into a tubular structure and ureteral implantation should be considered. The Boari–Ockerblad bladder flap (see Fig. 24.9) and the Demel bladder flap differ primarily in the direction of excision of the full-thickness bladder flap. In either case, the flap must have a wide base to ensure an adequate blood supply. The flap is made tubular by suturing together its lateral margins, and the cut end of the ureter is brought near the end of the flap in much the same way as one would perform a ureteroneocystostomy.

In rare circumstances involving loss of a large portion of the ureter, bridging the gap between the cut end of a ureter and the bladder is possible by performing an ileoureteroneocystostomy. A segment of ileum of sufficient length and with adequate blood supply is isolated from the bowel. Its distal end is sutured to a cystostomy site in the dome of the bladder, and the cut end of the ureter is implanted into its proximal end. The continuity of the ileum is then reestablished.

Transureteroureterostomy. When so much of the ureter has been lost that it is impossible to perform a ureteroneocystostomy or ureteroureterostomy, a transureteroureterostomy should be considered. In performing a transureteroureterostomy, the proximal ureter is mobilized and passed retroperitoneally below the inferior mesenteric artery and in front of the great vessels to meet the opposite ureter. The recipient ureter is longitudinally incised, and an end-to-side anastomosis is performed using full-thickness No. 4-0 absorbable sutures. The anastomosis should be watertight but not ischemic. The anastomotic site should be drained by an extraperitoneal suction drain. Ureteral catheters are not usually necessary.

Cutaneous Ureterostomy. A cutaneous ureterostomy should not be considered a permanent method of urinary diversion. It may be done when the patient's chances of survival are limited or in cases in which the surgeon is not prepared to perform a more definitive repair. The procedure is performed by bringing out retroperitoneally the cut end of the ureter through the skin and performing a ureteral–skin anastomosis. Ureteral catheters are not usually necessary long-term but may help provide adequate drainage early in the wound healing process.

Follow-Up of Ureteral Repairs. Extraperitoneal suction drains should be placed to the site of, but not in contact with, all internal ureteral anastomoses. These drains should remove all blood, serum, lymph, and urine that collect near the anastomosis. They are not usually removed until all ureteral catheters and stents have been removed.

Continuous bladder catheter drainage, either transurethrally or suprapubically, should be initiated whenever there is a cystotomy, ureteroneocystostomy, or ureteroureterostomy. In the latter case, when there is no cystotomy, the bladder catheter may be removed before the ureteral catheter or stent is removed.

The repair of ureteral injuries should be followed by an intravenous urogram to determine the integrity of the repair and the presence or absence of a stenosis. This is also done to detect fistulas or conditions that might cause kidney damage.

Recognition of Bladder Injury

Bladder Dye Instillations. If surgery is performed with an indigo carmine solution inside the bladder, partial lacerations of the bladder wall reveal the underlying blue mucosa. Penetrations and lacerations of the bladder are indicated by blue dye leaking onto the surgical field. The integrity of the bladder wall cannot be tested thoroughly until the bladder is filled with 300 to 400 mL of an appropriate liquid-distending medium (sterile water or normal saline containing indigo carmine dye or sterile milk or infant's formula). The bladder can be filled using a single-channel or double-channel transurethral catheter. In difficult cases, repetitive emptying and filling of the bladder is facilitated by the placement of an indwelling three-channel transurethral balloon catheter.

Warning Signs of Bladder Injury. Hematuria signifies urinary tract injury until proven otherwise. If this is detected intraoperatively, retrograde bladder fill, as described previously, will reveal a partial- or full-thickness bladder wall injury. If a patient is found to have gross hematuria immediately following surgery, bladder injury should be immediately investigated. This is readily accomplished by retrograde filling the Foley catheter with 300 mL of sterile fluid and then carefully measuring the return once the catheter is allowed to drain. A negative return signifies extravasation of the fluid through an unrecognized cystotomy. The decision of prolonged catheter drainage versus returning to the operating room for surgical repair is case-dependent.

When performing midurethral sling procedures, immediate postoperative vaginal leakage and/or suprapubic and vulvar extravasation of fluid strongly suggest unrecognized bladder perforation that occurred during performance of the sling procedure. Identified risk factors for trocar injury to the bladder include inexperienced surgeon, local anesthesia, previous cesarean section, and previous colposuspension. Immediate cystoscopy is recommended, as sling removal is easily accomplished at this point. In the long term, intravesical mesh can cause bladder pain and other irritative symptoms, recurrent urinary tract infection, and stone formation, and should always be considered in a patient with this surgical history.

Cystoscopy. Cystoscopy may be performed transurethrally or suprapubically, as described under the section on the detection of ureteral injuries. A thorough examination of the bladder requires the use of a 70-degree lens. Detecting and removing any suture material and other foreign matter is important, as well as determining the location and extent of all bladder injuries and their relationship to each ureter and the urethra. The bladder must be distended to perform an adequate cystoscopic examination. This in itself may help identify lacerations of the bladder wall.

Cystotomy. A cystotomy may be performed in the extraperitoneal portion of the dome of the bladder, and the inside of the bladder may be examined thoroughly for injuries.

Management of Bladder Injury

Intraoperative repair of bladder injuries varies slightly according to the location of the injury. Defects should be noted and repaired once the hysterectomy and/or other gynecologic procedures are completed (Fig. 24.10). Extraperitoneal lacerations in the dome of the bladder may be closed with one

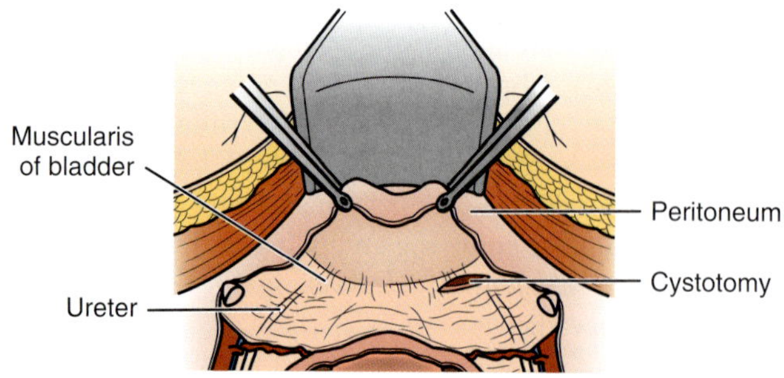

Fig. 24.10 Bladder injury during abdominal hysterectomy commonly occurs during dissection of the bladder from the cervix. Defects should be tagged and repaired once the hysterectomy is completed. (Modified from Lee RA, Hagen JV. *Atlas of Gynecologic Surgery*. Philadelphia: WB Saunders; 1992. Copyrighted by and used with the permission of Mayo Foundation for Medical Education.)

or two layers of No. 3-0 absorbable or delayed absorbable suture. The suture may be placed in an interrupted or running fashion, depending on the type and extent of the injury. Some extraperitoneal cystotomies in the dome of the bladder may be used for the insertion of a bladder catheter for postoperative suprapubic bladder drainage. If the defect in the bladder dome is small, such as in the case of bladder perforation during placement of a laparoscopic trocar, bladder drainage without surgical repair is acceptable.

Transperitoneal lacerations of the bladder and lacerations of the base of the bladder should be repaired in two layers, using No. 3-0 absorbable or delayed absorbable interrupted or running suture. Also, these lacerations should be covered by a layer of peritoneum or an omental flap (Fig. 24.11). This procedure separates the injury from adjacent structures and cushions the repair by adding bulk. An omental flap brings in new tissue with its own separate blood supply.

Significant bladder repairs should have continuous bladder drainage for at least 7 days to facilitate healing (see Video 24.7: Transvaginal cystotomy repair).

Recognition of Urethral Injury

Since the introduction of midurethral slings for the management of stress incontinence, urethral injuries have increased. They can occur with both retropubic and transobturator sling placement, and a thorough evaluation of the urethra must be included at the end of the cystoscopic portion of the case. Urethral injury may be more common in cases of undiagnosed urethral diverticula (see Video 24.8: Repair of urethrotomy).

Catheter Insertion. Intraoperatively, urethral injuries are most often diagnosed by the surgeon seeing the catheter through an incision in the wall of the urethra. Small clamps or probes may be used to confirm the injury (Fig. 24.12).

Urethroscopy. Urethroscopy is best performed with a special female urethroscope sheath and a zero-degree telescope lens. It can be used to detect suture material, foreign matter, diverticula, and lacerations of the urethra (Fig. 24.12).

Management of Urethral Injury

Lacerations of the urethra should be repaired over a transurethral catheter in layers using No. 4-0 or 3-0 absorbable or delayed absorbable sutures. If the proximal urethra is involved, it is important to buttress the urethrovesical junction in an

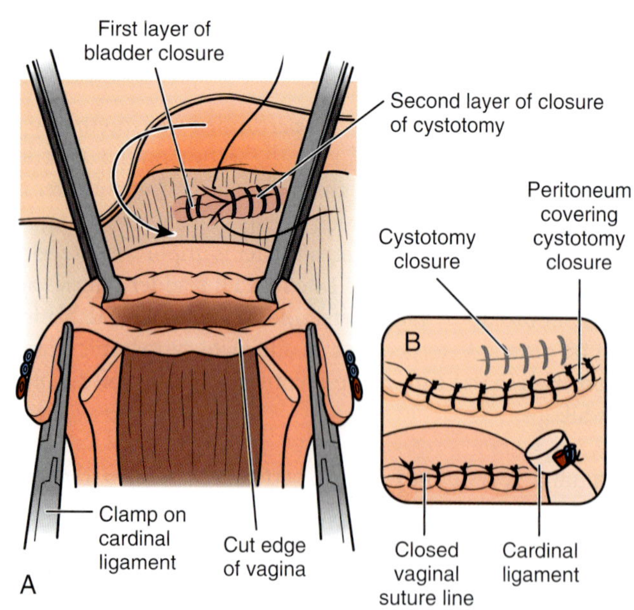

Fig. 24.11 **A**, After completing the hysterectomy, the bladder may be further mobilized and the cystotomy closed in a two-layered fashion. **B**, The peritoneum is mobilized to cover the repair, and the vaginal cuff is closed. (Modified from Lee RA, Hagen JV. *Atlas of Gynecologic Surgery*. Philadelphia: WB Saunders; 1992. Copyrighted by and used with the permission of Mayo Foundation for Medical Education.)

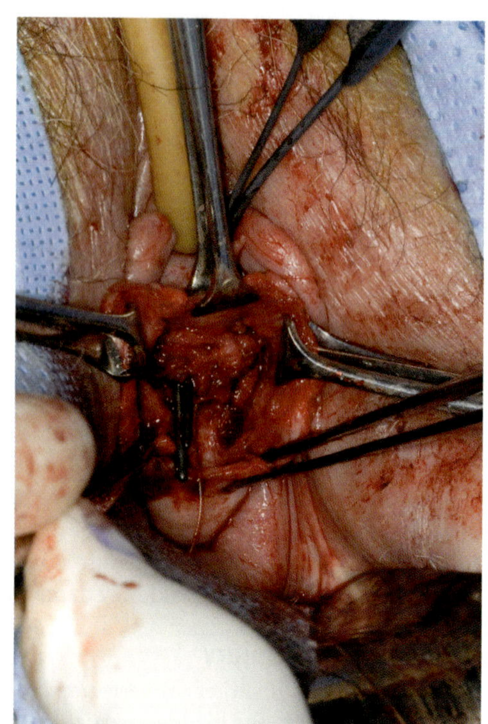

Fig. 24.12 Urethral injury demonstrated with clamp passed through urethral meatus next to catheter.

attempt to prevent the development of postoperative stress urinary incontinence. The use of a bulbocavernosus fat pad transplant should be considered if there is a need for additional tissue depth.

POSTOPERATIVE EVALUATION OF SUSPECTED GENITOURINARY FISTULAS

Postoperative genitourinary fistulas may leak urine immediately or after several weeks. Any loss of urine from the vagina should be evaluated promptly. An algorithm for bedside or office evaluation of urine leakage from the vagina is shown in Fig. 24.13. If this examination suggests that the leakage is caused by a urethrovaginal, vesicovaginal, or ureterovaginal fistula, it is important to perform endoscopy. In women with vesicovaginal or ureterovaginal fistulas, a CT urogram must be done to document the function of both renal units and to determine whether the fistula involves more than one organ. Posthysterectomy vesicovaginal fistulas are usually located just anterior to the vaginal cuff. On cystoscopy, they are usually located just above the interureteric ridge near the midline. Simple vesicovaginal fistulas that occur in the vaginal apex following an otherwise uncomplicated total hysterectomy are best treated by a partial apical colpocleisis (Latzko procedure).

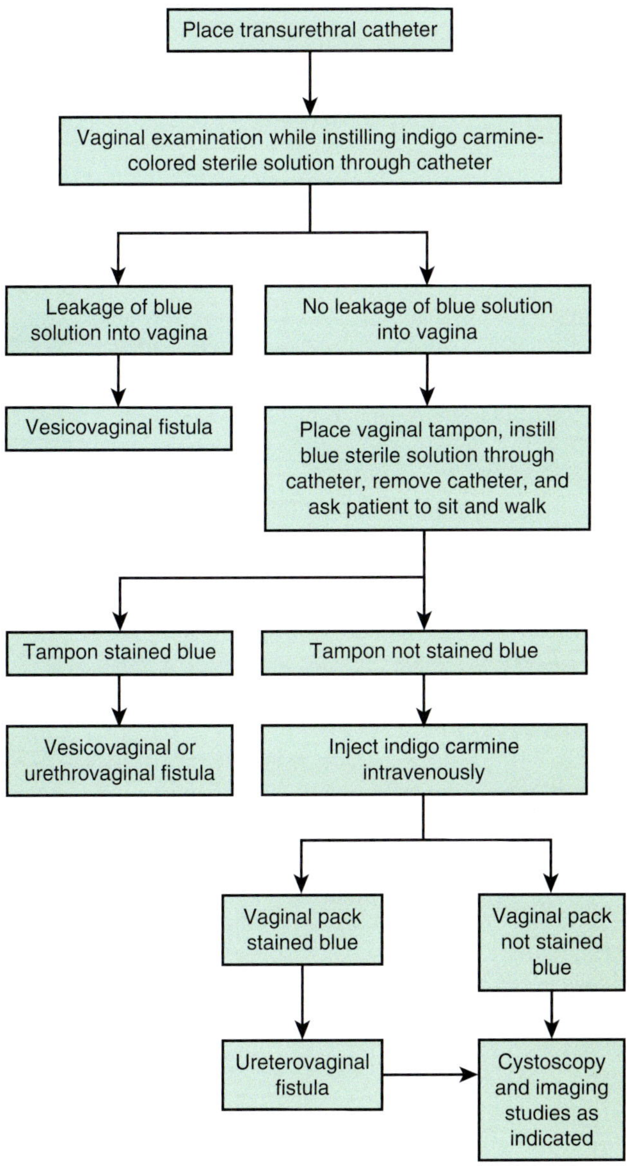

Fig. 24.13 Algorithm for the bedside or office evaluation of suspected vesicovaginal or ureterovaginal fistulas.

BIBLIOGRAPHY

American College of Obstetricians and Gynecologists. *Lower Urinary Tract Operative Injuries. ACOG Technical Bulletin 238*, Washington, DC: ACOG; 1997.

Boari A. Contributo sperimentale alla plastica dell' ureteri. *Atti Acad Sci Med Nat Ferrara.* 1894;68:149.

Brubaker LT, Wilbanks GD. Urinary tract injuries in pelvic surgery. *Surg Clin North Am.* 1991;71:968.

Chan JK, Morrow J, Manetta A. Prevention of ureteral injuries in gynecologic surgery. *Am J Obstet Gynecol.* 2003;188:1273.

Cruikshank SH. Surgical method of identifying the ureter during total vaginal hysterectomy. *Obstet Gynecol.* 1986;67:277.

Demel R. Ersatz des ureters durch eine plastik aus der harnblase (Vorlaufige Mitteilung). *Zentralbl Chir.* 1924;37:71.

Dwyer PL. Urinary tract injury: medical negligence or unavoidable complication? *Int Urogynecol J.* 2010;21:903.

Gebhart JB. *Urologic Surgery for the Gynecologist.* Philadelphia: Elsevier Saunders; 2011.

Giberti C, Germinale F, Lillo M, et al. Obstetric and gynaecological ureteric injuries: treatment and results. *Br J Urol.* 1996;77:21.

Goodno Jr JA, Powers TW, Harris VD. Ureteral injury in gynecologic surgery: a 10-year review in a community hospital. *Am J Obstet Gynecol.* 1995;172:1817.

Härkki-Siren P, Sjöberg J, Kurki T. Major complications of laparoscopy: a follow-up Finnish study. *Obstet Gynecol.* 1999;94:94.

Harkki-Siren P, Sjoberg J, Tiitinen A. Urinary tract injuries after hysterectomy. *Obstet Gynecol.* 1998;92:113.

Hurt WG, Dunn LJ. Complications of gynecologic surgery and trauma. In: Greenfield LJ, ed. *Complications in Surgery and Trauma.* 2nd ed. Philadelphia: JB Lippincott; 1990.

Hurt WG, Segreti EM. Intraoperative ureteral injuries and urinary diversion. In: Nichols DH, Clarke-Pearson D, eds. *Gynecologic and Obstetric Surgery.* 2nd ed. St. Louis: Mosby; 1999.

Ibeanu OA, Chesson RR, Echols KT, et al. Urinary tract injury during hysterectomy based on universal cystoscopy. *Obstet Gynecol.* 2009;113:6.

Jabs CF, Drutz HP. The role of intraoperative cystoscopy in prolapse and incontinence surgery. *Am J Obstet Gynecol.* 2001;185:1368.

Jelovsek JE, Chiung C, Chen G, et al. Incidence of lower urinary tract injury at the time of total laparoscopic hysterectomy. *JSLS.* 2007;11:422.

Johnson N, Barlow D, Lethaby A, et al. Surgical approach to hysterectomy for benign gynecological disease. *Cochrane Database Syst Rev.* 2006;2:CD003677.

Lee RA, Hagen JV. *Atlas of Gynecologic Surgery.* Philadelphia: WB Saunders; 1992.

Lee RA, Symmonds RE, Williams TJ. Current status of genitourinary fistulas. *Obstet Gynecol.* 1988;71:313.

Mann WJ, Arato M, Pasatner B, Stone ML. Ureteral injuries in an obstetric and gynecology training program: etiology and management. *Obstet Gynecol.* 1988;72:82.

Morton HC, Hilton P. Urethral injury associated with minimally invasive mid-urethral sling procedures for the treatment of stress urinary incontinence: a case series and systematic literature search. *BJOG.* 2009;116:1120.

Ostrzenski A, Radolinski B, Ostrzenska KM. A review of laparoscopic ureteral injury in pelvic surgery. *Obstet Gynecol Surv.* 2003;58:794.

Parpala-Spårman T, Paananen I, Santala M, et al. Increasing numbers of ureteric injuries after the introduction of laparoscopic surgery. *Scand J Urol Nephrol.* 2008;42:422.

Piscitelli JT, Simel DL, Addison WA. Who should have intravenous pyelograms before hysterectomy for benign disease? *Obstet Gynecol.* 1987;698:541.

Saidi MH, Sadler RK, Vancaillie TG, et al. Diagnosis and management of serious urinary complications after major operative laparoscopy. *Obstet Gynecol.* 1996;87:272.

Stav K, Dwyer PL, Rosamilia A, et al. Risk factors for trocar injury to the urinary bladder during mid-urethral sling procedures. *J Urol.* 2009;182:174.

Tijdink MM, Vierhout ME, Heesakkers JP, Withagen MI. Surgical management of mesh-related complications after prior pelvic floor reconstructive surgery with mesh. *Int Urogynecol J.* 2011;22:1395.

Timmons MC, Addison WA. Suprapubic telescopy: extraperitoneal intraoperative technique to demonstrate ureteral patency. *Obstet Gynecol.* 1990;75:137.

Walters MD, Barber MD. *Hysterectomy for Benign Disease (with CD).* Philadelphia: Elsevier Inc.; 2010.

25

Managing Mesh Complications After Surgeries for Urinary Incontinence and Pelvic Organ Prolapse

Mickey M. Karram and John B. Gebhart

CHAPTER OUTLINE

INTRODUCTION

Pelvic reconstructive surgery for genital prolapse and urinary stress incontinence usually results in improved quality of life (Helstrom et al., 2005). However, numerous complications from mesh-augmented prolapse repairs, as well as placement of synthetic slings, have been reported in the literature. This chapter is aimed at discussing these various complications and how best to manage them.

Pelvic organ prolapse (POP) and stress urinary incontinence (SUI) are common and often comorbid disorders in women and can greatly impact quality of life. Population-based studies report an 11% to 19% lifetime risk of women undergoing surgery for one of these conditions, with recurrence of symptoms common in both groups. In total, 6% to 29% of women who undergo a pelvic floor repair have additional surgery for recurrent prolapse, stress incontinence, or related complications (Olsen et al., 1997; Smith et al., 2010).

The success initially observed with the use of surgical mesh in general surgery combined with the perceived high failure rates for traditional native tissue suture repairs for prolapse initially led gynecologic surgeons to implement surgical approaches that use prosthetic materials. Medical device manufacturers have estimated that, in 2006 and 2007, approximately 30% of POP repair procedures and 80% of antiincontinence procedures used reconstructive materials. However, recently there have been concerns raised around the safety of transvaginal mesh and synthetic slings because of a variety of complications related to mesh erosion, pain, vaginal constriction, and other complications. Although similar types of complications have occurred with native tissue suture repairs, the perception is that graft-related complications have been more severe and difficult to manage.

Historically, loss of pelvic floor support resulting in POP has been compared with a hernia. In 1973, Dr. Stanley Birnbaum described a novel technique for treatment of vaginal prolapse in which fixation of the vaginal vault with a Teflon mesh bridge anchored the vagina to the hollow of the sacrum. This was the initial description of a sacrocolpopexy using a synthetic material. A follow-up article 6 years later noted that 20 of 21 patients treated with this technique maintained good support and vaginal function.

Over the last 15 years there has been a significant refinement and improvement in surgical mesh materials. Early on there were problems with some surgical meshes that increased erosion and infection rates. In most cases these meshes were microporous multifilament materials, which require complete explantation for symptom improvement (Occhino et al., 2012). Fortunately, the majority of these products have been taken off the market. Currently used meshes are type 1 mesh, meaning they are macroporous monofilament polypropylene with a pore size greater than 75 microns. They can further be divided by weight (heavy-, mid- or lightweight) (Amid, 1997; Sanders & Kingsnorth, 2012). (See Chapter 7 for more information on the properties and biomechanics of mesh.)

Synthetic mesh used for prolapse repairs can be placed abdominally (abdominal sacral colpopexy) or transvaginally. Transvaginal mesh can be self-fashioned, cut-to-order, or packaged in a kit. The first synthetic mesh kit for prolapse was approved by the US Food and Drug Administration (FDA) in 2001, and the first trocar-based kit was approved in 2004 (Debodinance et al., 2004). Recent changes have led to the removal of transvaginal mesh for POP from the US market (see US Food and Drug Administration Warnings). Mesh for use in sacrocolpopexy has not been affected. (See Chapter 7 for more details.)

Suburethral slings use synthetic mesh placed suburethrally for treatment of SUI and can be categorized into retropubic, transobturator, and single-incision (minisling) configurations (Chapter 17). All of the meshes used for these procedures at the present time are macroporous polypropylene with fairly low complication rates. Synthetic slings were also not affected by the recent FDA action.

Many of the complications discussed in this chapter are specific to mesh placement, while some can also occur with native tissue suture repair. This chapter will only discuss those complications specifically related to mesh procedures for POP and SUI.

US FOOD AND DRUG ADMINISTRATION WARNINGS

On October 20, 2008 the FDA issued a public health notification regarding the use of mesh in gynecologic surgery entitled "Serious Complications Associated with Transvaginal Placement of Surgical Mesh in Repair of Pelvic Organ Prolapse and SUI." This was done in response to over 1000 reports of these complications involving surgical mesh produced by nine different companies. These reports were reported through the Manufacturer and User Facility Device Experience (MAUDE) database. The most common complications reported were mesh erosion, infection, pain, and urinary symptoms. Serious injury to bowel, bladder, and blood vessels did occur, albeit rarely. Several general recommendations were made by the FDA at that time based on these reports. These included the following:

1. That physicians seek specialized training for procedures involving the use of mesh, be alert, and recognize complications early.
2. That physicians inform patients on the permanent nature of surgical mesh and that some complications associated with implanted vaginal mesh may require subsequent surgery that may or may not correct the complication.
3. That physicians inform patients about the potential for serious complications and the effect on quality of life, including pain during intercourse, scarring, and narrowing of the vagina after prolapse repairs.

The FDA continued to investigate mesh complications and, based on an updated analysis of reported adverse events and complications described in the scientific literature, released a scientific communication on July 13, 2011 entitled "Update on Serious Complications Associated with Transvaginal Placement of Synthetic Mesh for Pelvic Organ Prolapse and SUI." They noted that the use of surgical mesh for transvaginal repair of prolapse is an area of continuing serious concern and concluded that "serious complications associated with surgical mesh for transvaginal repair of prolapse are not rare." They did not find clear evidence to support increased efficacy of mesh repairs when compared with traditional native tissue repairs, and concluded that patients undergoing mesh placement may be exposed to greater risk. It was also noted that mesh placed abdominally for the treatment of POP via sacrocolpopexy had a lower rate of complications when compared with vaginally placed mesh. Lastly, mesh used to treat stress incontinence was to remain under continued investigation, with updates to come at a later date.

In the light of these FDA findings, it is important to understand the history of the FDA approval process for new materials. Mesh products were allowed to remain on the market without passing the rigorous FDA approval process that mandates premarket testing because they underwent a much more simplified regulatory process called a "510K." This process allowed new medical devices that were similar to a currently FDA-approved (or "predicate") device to be approved based on this similarity, eliminating the need for the companies to provide specific efficacy and safety data on a new product before obtaining FDA approval. Historically, transvaginal mesh kits were considered class II devices, and thus a 510K process based on a predicate device, a synthetic midurethral sling, was the approval process that was used, even though prolapse repairs involve significantly increased volumes of mesh that are placed in a different space than midurethral slings. Currently approved synthetic midurethral slings were approved by the same process based upon a prior product, the Protegen sling, which is no longer on the market because of a poor safety profile. On January 4, 2012 the FDA issued 522 orders requiring postmarket surveillance studies for transvaginal mesh devices currently being sold for use in POP, as well as single-incision (minisling) kits currently being promoted for SUI, and companies undertook these studies. In 2016 the FDA reclassified vaginal meshes from class II to class III medical devices, which require premarket approval through a scientific review to ensure safety and efficacy before going to market. In July 2018, the FDA ordered the manufacturer of the last mesh surgical products on the market for the transvaginal repair of POP in the posterior compartment (rectocele) to stop selling and distributing its products. Lastly, in April 2019, the FDA ordered all manufacturers of surgical mesh intended for transvaginal repair of anterior compartment prolapse (cystocele) and vaginal vault prolapse to stop selling and distributing their products immediately. The FDA determined that reasonable assurance of safety and effectiveness for these devices had not been demonstrated. Synthetic mesh products for the treatment of SUI and sacrocolpopexy were not affected by this FDA order.

This reflects upon recent circumstances in other countries. In the past few years, synthetic mesh has become no longer available to use in POP surgery in the United Kingdom, Scotland, New Zealand, and Australia.

PROFESSIONAL SOCIETY GUIDELINES

The American College of Obstetricians and Gynecologists (ACOG) and the American Urogynecologic Society (AUGS) issued a statement in December 2011 regarding vaginal placement of surgical mesh for POP repair. They advised that:

- Surgeons placing vaginal mesh should undergo training specific to each device and have experience with reconstructive surgical procedures and a thorough understanding of pelvic anatomy.
- Use of reconstructive materials by surgeons experienced with the specific procedure is a reasonable option for women with factors that increase the risk of prolapse recurrence (e.g., recurrent prolapse, medical comorbidities that preclude more invasive and lengthier open and endoscopic procedures). Such use should be individualized, and surgeons should counsel patients about the lack of efficacy and safety data, and about alternative treatments.
- Patients should provide their informed consent after reviewing the risks and benefits of the procedure, as well as discussing alternative repairs.

In addition, the Society of Gynecologic Surgeons (SGS) issued a statement in July 2011, advising the following:

- SGS is in agreement with the interpretations and recommendations made in the FDA Safety Communication. The general consensus is that this reservation should not apply to synthetic midurethral sling procedures or sacral colpopexies utilizing the same mesh materials, but further longer-term evaluations of all of these procedures is important.
- For now, thoughtful, discriminant use of transvaginal mesh to augment vaginal defects should be performed by trained surgeons with experience in complex reconstructive surgery, and only on patients who are perceived to have an unacceptable risk of clinical failure when other procedures are performed.
- We should all follow outcomes when we employ new procedures and should feel comfortable about benefit versus risk before employing them. It is important that patients are informed of the risks and benefits of any surgical procedure, as well as the specific potential adverse events associated with transvaginal mesh use, including outcomes that may still be unclear and require further investigation. Alternative treatments should be explained.

The International Urogynecologic Association (IUGA) convened a Grafts Roundtable regarding transvaginal graft use in 2010 (Davila et al., 2012), and advised that:

- Individual patient characteristics have to be included in the risk-benefit ratio when counseling patients regarding transvaginal mesh repair.
- Informed consent for vaginal reconstructive surgery with mesh should include verbal and written review with the patient of expected benefits, therapeutic alternatives, and potential risks.
- Manufacturers should provide detailed product description, data on biologic properties, cadaveric studies, and well-designed prospective clinical trials to support the claimed benefits of the new product.
- A process of added surgeon qualification for transvaginal mesh placement is desirable.

In the past there were minimal guidelines for this process, and physicians usually attended an industry-sponsored 1- or 2-day course to learn these procedures using cadaveric trainers. The new AUGS recommendations call for documentation of each of the following: (1) knowledge of pelvic anatomy, (2) surgical skill, (3) surgical experience, and (4) internal audits for quality assurance. Informed consent should highlight potential benefits and complications of transvaginal mesh, alternatives to mesh, including nonsurgical options and other surgical treatments, and potential complications of transvaginal mesh that may require additional interventions, as well as the fact that symptoms may not be completely resolved with mesh removal. The article addresses surgeons who are not performing transvaginal mesh repairs but would like to begin doing so, as well as those currently performing these procedures. The surgeon who approaches management of mesh complications after pelvic surgery should possess a comprehensive understanding of materials used in POP repair and pelvic floor anatomy, as well as advanced surgical skills to individualize the management of such complications specific to each patient. Patients should also understand that removal of mesh may not completely resolve all symptoms.

The American Urogynecology Society, in conjunction with the Society of Urodynamics and Female Urology, released a position statement on mesh midurethral slings for SUI in 2014, with updates in 2016 and 2018. The statement stated that "polypropylene mesh midurethral sling is the recognized worldwide standard of care for the surgical treatment of SUI. The procedure is safe, effective, and has improved the quality of life for millions of women." Justification for the position statement was as follows:

1. Polypropylene material is safe and effective as a surgical implant.
2. The monofilament polypropylene mesh midurethral sling is the most extensively studied antiincontinence procedure in history.
3. Polypropylene mesh midurethral slings are the standard of care for the surgical treatment of SUI and represent a great advance in the treatment of this condition for our patients.
4. The FDA has clearly stated that the polypropylene midurethral sling is safe and effective in the treatment of SUI.

In 2017, ACOG and AUGS issued a joint committee opinion on the management of mesh and graft complications in gynecologic surgery. They concluded that:

1. Short-term voiding dysfunction after placement of a synthetic midurethral sling is common and, if improving, can be managed expectantly for up to 6 weeks. However, retention (inability to empty the bladder) or small-volume voids with larger postvoid bladder residual volume should receive earlier intervention.
2. Asymptomatic exposures of monofilament macroporous meshes can be managed expectantly.
3. A trial of vaginal estrogen can be attempted for small (e.g., <0.5 cm) mesh exposures.
4. Persistent vaginal bleeding, vaginal discharge, or recurrent urinary tract infection after mesh placement should prompt an examination and possible further evaluation for exposure or erosion.
5. Pelvic pain (including dyspareunia), possibly related to non-exposed mesh, is complex, may not respond to mesh removal,

and should prompt referral to a clinician with appropriate training and experience, such as a female pelvic medicine and reconstructive surgery specialist.

6. Mesh removal surgery should not be performed unless there is a specific therapeutic indication.

More recently, ACOG and AUGS issued clinical guidelines for POP. The purpose is to review information on the current understanding of POP in women and to outline guidelines for diagnosis and management that are consistent with the best available scientific evidence.

Finally, the AUGS-IUGA issued a joint position statement on the management of mesh-related complications for the Female Pelvic Medicine & Reconstructive Surgery (FPMRS) specialist (2020). It has four goals:

1. Using the best and most relevant evidence available, provide guidance for the FPMRS subspecialist caring for patients who may be experiencing mesh complications.
2. Provide an algorithm to outline treatment choices for patients with mesh-related complications that can be used as a platform for shared decision making in the treatment of these complications.
3. Identify and prioritize gaps in evidence concerning specific mesh complications and their treatments.
4. Identify provider and health facility characteristics that may optimize the outcomes of treatments for these complications.

BOX 25.1 Suggestions to Decrease the Risk of Erosion or Exposure After Reconstructive Pelvic Surgeries Using Synthetic Grafts

Patient-Centered

- Stop smoking before and after surgery
- Appropriately use vaginal estrogen in postmenopausal women before and after surgery (authors' opinion)
- Have regular postoperative follow-up visits with the surgeon

Physician-Centered

Preoperative

- Understand technical aspects and surgical anatomy of the planned procedure that involves mesh placement; gain as much experience as possible with the procedure
- In a patient with uterovaginal prolapse, consider a uterine-preserving procedure or a supracervical hysterectomy
- Educate patients preoperatively on the importance of avoiding the future development of urogenital atrophy

Intraoperative

- Use lightweight large-pore polypropylene
- Use hydrodissection to facilitate the appropriate plane of dissection
- Avoid mesh bunching, taking care to make sure that the mesh lies flat
- Trim mesh appropriately to the specific prolapse repair to limit mesh load
- Consider abandoning mesh placement if excessive blood loss is encountered
- Consider abandoning mesh placement if inadvertent injury to urethra (sling placement), bladder, or bowel (mesh-augmented prolapse repairs) occurs
- Avoid overzealous trimming of vaginal mucosa

AVOIDING SYNTHETIC MESH COMPLICATIONS

In general, there are a number of modifiable risk factors that may help to diminish mesh-related complications, and these are reviewed in Box 25.1.

Patient Selection

The current consensus is that a synthetic midurethral sling procedure (via a retropubic or transobturator approach) is the gold standard for surgical correction of SUI. Similarly, use of synthetic mesh is the current standard of care when performing a sacrocolpopexy. Notably however, as of the writing of this chapter, any use of a synthetic or biologic graft or mesh transvaginally to augment vaginal prolapse repair is considered "off-label" use and should be undertaken with caution. Historically, experts argued that use of transvaginal mesh should be restricted to patients who fail native tissue suture repairs and have a higher stage of prolapse. Other commonly cited indications included patients who are not sexually active or patients who are believed to be at high risk for failure of a native tissue repair secondary to lifestyle, body habitus, or other factors. Patients who are chronically immunosuppressed (e.g., because of medication for other systemic diseases or owing to underlying disease) or who are current smokers should be similarly approached with caution. Unfortunately, there are few data to support any of these rationales.

It seems prudent to avoid or at least be cautious about performing synthetic mesh procedures in patients with underlying pelvic pain disorders, such as pelvic floor tension myalgia, interstitial cystitis, or vulvodynia. Pelvic surgeons should be aware of the high prevalence of female sexual dysfunction in the community and should preoperatively screen patients for a history of dyspareunia, pelvic pain, and sexual abuse. Abnormalities of pelvic tone or sensation should be elicited during the preoperative physical examination by palpating the levator ani muscles, obturator internus, and vaginal sulci and evaluating for signs of vulvodynia. Patients who have these findings should be referred to physical therapy in the hope of treating the underlying condition before any surgical intervention. In addition, they should be explicitly informed that surgery, if undertaken, is not meant to improve these symptoms, and may make them worse.

We believe that patients with severe atrophy and/or vaginal ulcers caused by severe prolapse or chronic pessary use should receive preoperative estrogen therapy for at least 4 weeks or until the above symptoms resolve. Ideally, these patients should continue local estrogen therapy for the foreseeable future following surgery. The optimal time to start postoperative local estrogen therapy has not been studied; however, we recommend starting about 3 weeks following surgery to avoid inadvertent disruption of any suture line during insertion of the applicator.

Surgical Technique/Mesh Selection

Expert opinion states that the key distinction between mesh and sutured repairs is the tissue plane and thickness of the dissection. In traditional plication repairs, with which most gynecologists are familiar, the vaginal epithelium is dissected from the underlying pubocervical connective tissue (fibromuscularis), which is subsequently plicated in the midline with a delayed absorbable suture. Conversely, mesh repairs require a "full-thickness" dissection. Successful full-thickness dissection requires adequate hydrodissection (not typically used with traditional repairs), and dissection is in a deeper surgical plane that leaves the pubocervical connective tissue attached to the epithelium. This allows, in theory, decreased risk of vaginal mesh exposure, maintenance of better vascular supply to the epithelium, and improved healing, with the goal of diminishing graft exposure. Local injection with lidocaine plus epinephrine at the time of mesh placement has not been shown to increase the risk of mesh erosion (Finamore et al., 2011).

Although the mesh is "suspended" tension-free via the arms, the mesh body usually needs to be trimmed, and possibly even secured to the underlying tissue, to prevent rolling or bunching, which have been observed in patients who experience mesh exposure and pain (Hurtado & Appell, 2009; Margulies et al., 2008). In general, the least amount of mesh needed to accomplish the repair should be used, as greater mesh volume is a risk factor for mesh erosion. The mesh needs to be deployed in a tension-free fashion. Excessive tension on the arms has been associated with tight vaginal bands, pain, and exposure (Feiner et al., 2009). It is unclear whether overtensioning results from mesh shrinkage (less likely, as this phenomenon has not been documented with sacrocolpopexy), inadvertent tensioning at the time of implantation (more likely), or a combination of factors. A thorough understanding by the treating surgeon of the nuances of mesh-based repairs is of the utmost importance to reduce these complications. In fact, there is evidence that complications are higher among providers with less experience.

Modifiable Risk Factors for Mesh-Related Complications

Published rates for mesh erosion range from 3% to over 30%; large reviews suggest overall rates between 10% and 15% (Abed et al., 2011; Maher et al., 2011). There are a number of modifiable patient and surgical factors that may help to diminish mesh-related complications (see Box 25.1). A major determinant is material selection. As previously discussed, type II (e.g., microporous materials) and type III (e.g., grafts with microporous components or with multifilament weave) synthetic meshes should be avoided because of increased risk of mesh-related complications. These materials undergo an encapsulation response and are more prone to erosion, sinus tract formation, and infection. A secondary analysis of the Colpopexy and Urinary Reduction Efforts (CARE) trial showed that Gore-Tex mesh use was associated with a 4.5-fold increased risk of vaginal exposure compared with macroporous polypropylene (Cundiff et al., 2008). Previous devices that used type II and type III materials have been removed from the market because of increased risk of mesh-related complications. Complications associated with these materials require complete excision of the mesh and are not the focus of this chapter.

Smoking increases the risk of mesh erosion, presumably by inhibiting wound healing. Current tobacco users had a 5.2- and 3.2-fold increased risk of mesh exposure following sacrocolpopexy and vaginal mesh, respectively (Cundiff et al., 2008; Gold et al., 2012). It would seem prudent for surgeons to recommend that patients stop smoking for at least 1 month before and after elective mesh procedures.

Increased blood loss during the index surgery greatly increased the risk of mesh exposure. In a case control study, patients who experienced excessive blood loss had a 7.3-fold increase in mesh exposure compared with patients who did not experience excessive blood loss (Gold et al., 2012). When excessive blood loss is encountered during these procedures, surgeons should consider using suture-based repairs. Tissue ischemia attributed to tobacco use or hematoma formation may lead to impaired wound healing.

MANAGING COMPLICATIONS

Mesh-Related Complications After Sacrocolpopexy

Sacrocolpopexy is an abdominal, laparoscopic, or robotic procedure that involves attaching either two grafts or a Y-shaped graft (usually synthetic mesh) to the anterior and posterior vaginal wall and securing it to the anterior longitudinal ligament of the sacrum. Mesh complications after abdominal sacrocolpopexy are fairly rare and primarily center on mesh or suture erosion (Fig. 25.1). A comprehensive review of abdominal sacrocolpopexy revealed an overall mesh erosion rate of 3.4%. Polypropylene had the lowest erosion rate at 0.5%, while Teflon had the highest rate of erosion at 5.5% (Nygaard et al., 2004). There are mixed data regarding the risk of mesh erosion when sacrocolpopexy is performed with concomitant hysterectomy. Culligan (2002) reported an increased erosion rate with concomitant hysterectomy; however, this study had a small sample size ($n = 11$). In contrast, Brizzolara (2003) reported no increased erosion rate in 60 women undergoing sacrocolpopexy with concomitant hysterectomy compared with 61 women undergoing sacrocolpopexy alone. Another study compared mesh erosion rates after sacrocolpopexy with concomitant supracervical hysterectomy as compared with sacrocolpopexy alone. A total of 277 patients were included in this study: 195 with concomitant supracervical hysterectomy with sacrocolpopexy and 82 with sacrocolpopexy alone. There were three patients with mesh erosion diagnosed at a mean follow-up of 8 months: one (0.5%) in the supracervical hysterectomy with sacrocolpopexy group and two (2.4%) in the sacrocolpopexy-only group. There was no statistical difference in mesh erosion rates among the two groups (Ginath et al., 2013).

A variety of risk factors have been identified for mesh and suture erosion after sacrocolpopexy. A secondary analysis from the CARE trial evaluated mesh and suture erosion rates among the 322 women who underwent sacrocolpopexy (Brubaker et al., 2003) and identified 20 women with mesh/suture erosion within 2 years of surgery; three were suture only, and 17 had exposed mesh. Three identifiable risk factors were found: concurrent hysterectomy, which increased the erosion rate from 4% to 14%

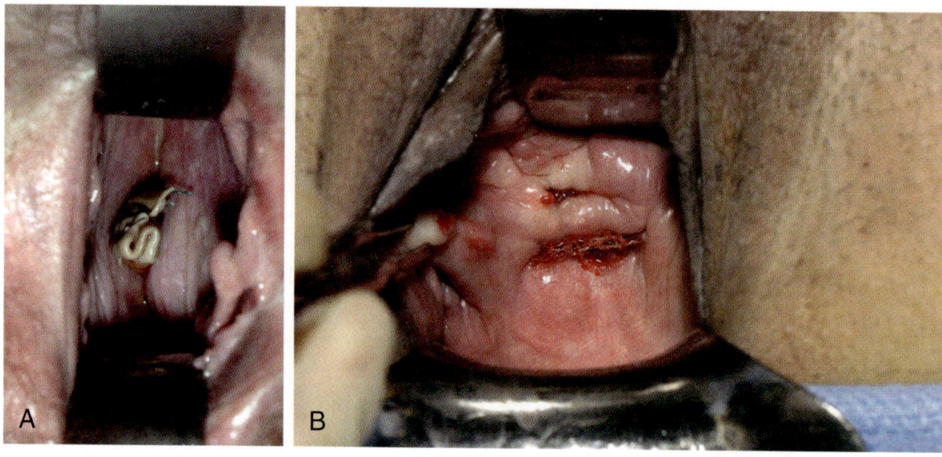

Fig. 25.1 Vaginal mesh erosion after abdominal sacrocolpopexy. **A**, Gore-Tex mesh erosion seen transvaginally after abdominal sacrocolpopexy. **B**, Polypropylene mesh erosion seen transvaginally after abdominal sacrocolpopexy.

in this study population; the use of expanded polytrafluroethylene (ePFTE; Gore-Tex; GORE Medical, Newark, NJ), which had a four-fold higher risk (19% vs. 5%) of mesh erosion compared with non-ePTFE mesh; and smoking, which was associated with a five-fold increase in the risk of mesh erosion. No other significant factors were identified as risk factors for mesh erosion, including estrogen status, diabetes, and prior surgery. The management of the three women with suture erosion included simple suture removal, and two of the three had confirmed complete healing. Four of the 17 mesh erosions were managed without surgery, and no resolution was noted in any of these four. Thirteen underwent at least one surgery, while one had two surgeries, and one had three surgeries. Of these 13, two had symptom resolution, six had persistent mesh erosion, and five were lost to follow-up. A more recent follow-up of the CARE trial noted that the probability of mesh erosion at 7 years increased to 10.5% (Nygaard et al., 2013).

Managing mesh erosion after sacrocolpopexy may only require observation and topical estrogen; however, in the authors' experience it almost always requires surgical excision. Surgical management of mesh erosion after sacrocolpopexy can be technically challenging, partially because of the usually high location within the vaginal canal, the amount of mesh used in the procedure, and the ingrowth of tissue into the mesh making surgical dissection difficult. Vaginal and abdominal routes for mesh excision have been described. In the authors' experience most mesh exposures can be successfully managed vaginally utilizing a technique of sharp dissection of the exposed mesh away from surrounding tissue, with aggressive downward traction on the mesh. The mesh is cut away as high as possible, and the vaginal defect is closed (Fig. 25.2). Vaginal entrance into the peritoneum significantly facilitates successful removal of the mesh.

South and colleagues (2007) published their experience with excision of mesh in 31 patients after sacrocolpopexy, including a novel method for endoscopic-assisted transvaginal excision of mesh. Abdominal excision of mesh was done by laparotomy; the presacral space was entered, and the mesh was detached from the sacrum and removed from the vaginal apex. Fourteen women underwent transvaginal mesh excision, and this was successful in nine, while 17 women underwent endoscopic-assisted transvaginal mesh excision, which was successful in seven. The overall success rate for vaginal excision was 53%. However, multiple attempts at vaginal excision were required in several patients for symptom resolution. Seven patients underwent abdominal excision, each having failed one of the two transvaginal excision methods. The abdominal group had two intraoperative bowel injuries during lysis of adhesions, one wound infection, and one readmission for fever requiring antibiotics. The authors concluded that complete removal of mesh may improve outcomes and decrease persistent symptoms, although significant morbidity can occur.

Albeit rare, there have been recent case reports of erosion of sacrocolpopexy mesh into the bowel (Lin et al., 2018). *De novo* vaginal apical pain has also been reported after sacrocolpopexy. This complication is uncommon but may require complete excision of the mesh to relieve symptoms (Buechel et al., 2016).

Mesh Complications After Synthetic Midurethral Sling Procedures

Vaginal Erosion/Exposure. Vaginal mesh erosion or exposure occurs in about 3% of women who undergo synthetic midurethral sling procedures (Ogah et al., 2011; Richter et al., 2010) (Fig. 25.3). Symptoms of vaginal mesh exposure can be discharge, bleeding, patient/partner dyspareunia, and recurrent urinary tract infection. Most data on the management of vaginal mesh exposure come from small case series involving both surgical and nonsurgical treatments with varying success rates. Topical estrogen is a reasonable initial treatment for women with small extrusions; however, subsequent mesh excision is often needed (Tijdink et al., 2011). Excision of exposed mesh can occur in the office setting or operating room, with the important questions being timing of excision and how much mesh to excise. Based on the authors' experience, office-based management is most often successful when the exposure is less

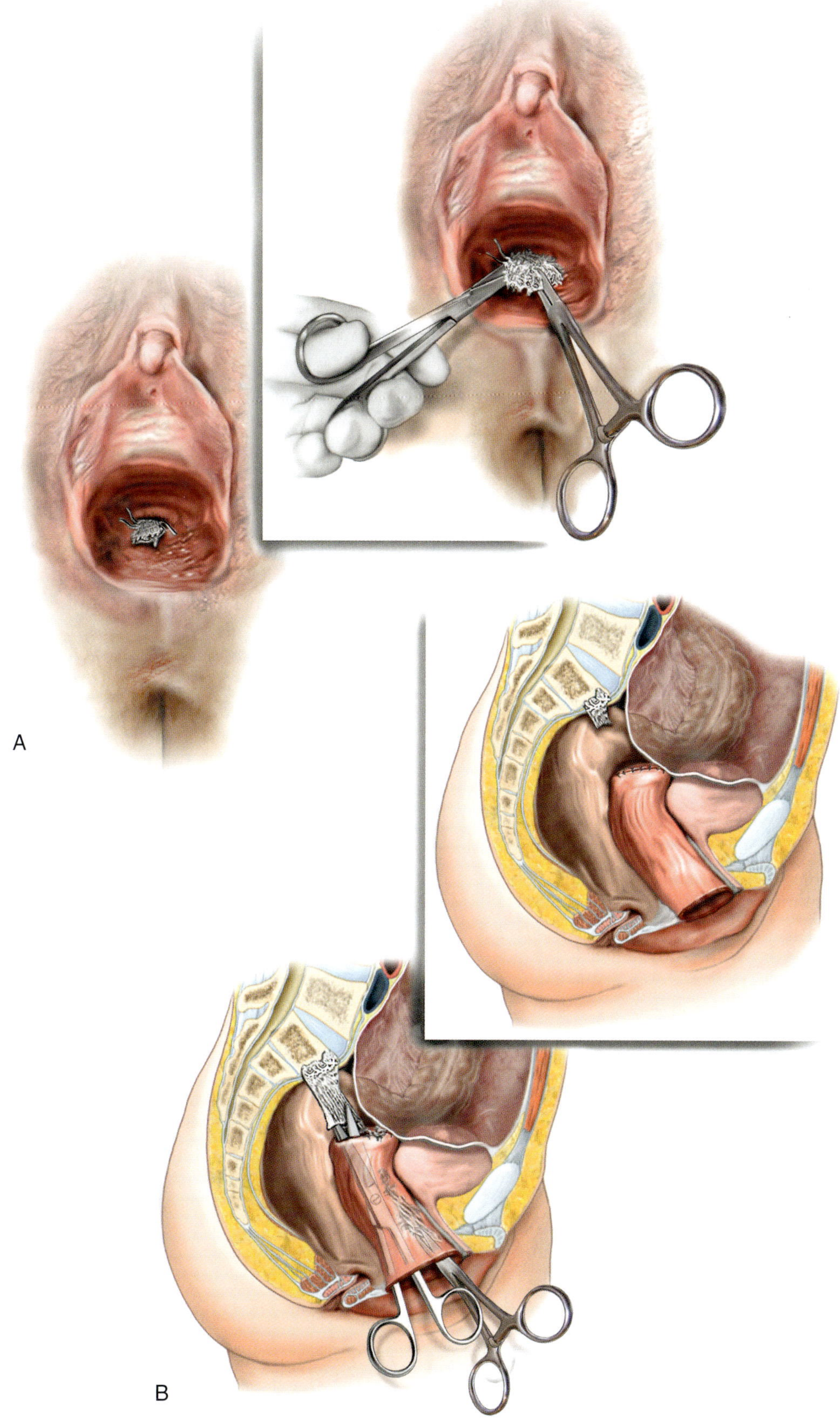

Fig. 25.2 The technique of vaginal removal of an eroded synthetic mesh after abdominal sacral colpopexy. **A**, Note that the mesh is undermined and grasped (usually with Kocher-type clamps), with aggressive downward traction applied on the mesh. **B**, The mesh is sharply dissected away from the vaginal tissue and any other tissue that it is adherent to, and, with aggressive downward traction, it is excised as high as possible. The goal is to create as much distance as possible between the closed vaginal cuff and the cut edge of the mesh (see *inset*).

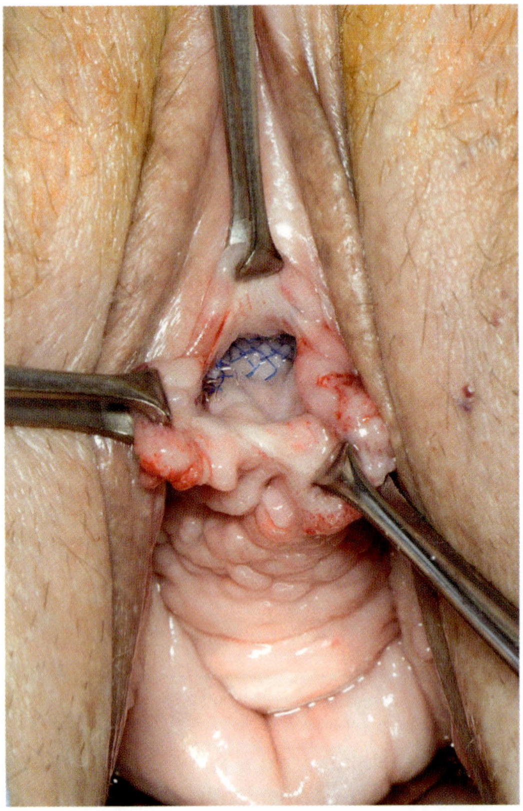

Fig. 25.3 Vaginal erosion of synthetic midurethral sling.

than 1 cm in size, when the exposure is easily visible/accessible with office instrumentation, and when the patient has healthy vaginal tissues. Local anesthesia is necessary before any attempt at office-based trimming or epithelial reapproximation. The authors prefer 1% lidocaine without epinephrine. Sterile gloves and instrumentation should be used, an assistant should be present, and instruments commonly needed include: a speculum, scissors, forceps with teeth, a needle driver, and suture. Excision of a portion of the mesh in the office can be done, but oftentimes mobilization of vaginal epithelium around the mesh with reapproximation using suture in a tension-free manner is also necessary.

Tijdink and colleagues (2011) reported recurrent SUI in 36% of women undergoing excision for mesh erosion. Fine surgical scissors (Metzenbaum) should be used to mobilize the vaginal epithelium around the area of erosion. If mesh is going to be excised, a right-angle clamp can be placed between the mesh and underlying connective tissue and gently opened to elevate the sling away from the tissue. The mesh can then be trimmed safely, and the vaginal epithelium closed in a tension-free manner (Video 25.1). There are limited clinical data to support the use of vaginal estrogen; however, the authors recommend using vaginal estrogen before and after any surgical management of mesh complications performed transvaginally.

Bladder Perforation. Inadvertent bladder perforation with a trocar during placement of synthetic midurethal sling is reported to occur in 0.3% to 8.5% of cases, with a much greater likelihood in the placement of retropubic synthetic slings versus transobturator or single-incision slings (Fig. 25.4). If this penetration goes unrecognized, synthetic mesh in the bladder will usually result in recurrent urinary tract infections, hematuria, urgency, frequency, and/or pain. Over time it is not uncommon to see a bladder stone develop on the intravesical mesh. Traditionally, removal of intravesical mesh has required an open abdominal approach through the retropubic space, in which a high deliberate cystotomy is performed, and the mesh is removed by performing a partial cystectomy with bladder reconstruction (Araco et al., 2009b; Yamada et al., 2006). Recently, to avoid increased morbidity, minimally invasive techniques such as transurethral endoscopic resection and laser ablation have been used, albeit with variable success (Doumouchtsis et al., 2011). However, a recent report of 10 patients who underwent Holmium laser excision of bladder and urethral mesh erosions reported an 80% success rate for bladder erosions and a 33% success rate for urethral erosions (Ogle et al., 2015). Techniques for vaginal extirpation of vaginal mesh have also been described, but outcome data are limited (Firoozi & Goldman, 2010).

Urethral Erosion. Rarely, synthetic mesh is identified in the urethral lumen. The surgeon placing the sling should go to great lengths to make sure the anterior vaginal wall incision is not too deep. There is no clear plane of dissection between the distal to mid anterior vaginal wall and the posterior urethra. A deep dissection plane can result in the sling being placed in the wall of the urethra, which could predispose it to eventually getting into the lumen of the urethra. One should also avoid performing a synthetic sling procedure in a patient who has received prior pelvic radiation, or at the time of repair of a urethrovaginal fistula or urethral diverticulum. Also, in the authors' opinion one should abort a planned synthetic sling placement if an inadvertent urethrotomy occurs during initial anterior vaginal wall dissection. When synthetic mesh is found in

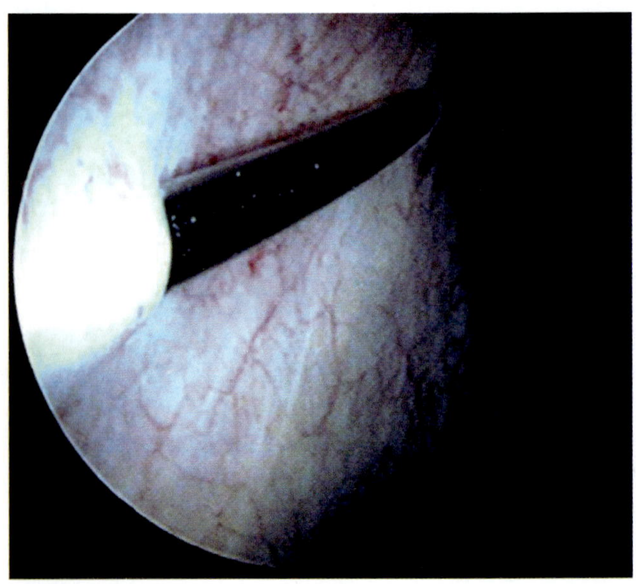

Fig. 25.4 Passage of tension-free vaginal tape needle. Note full penetration of the needle through the bladder.

the urethral lumen, it will almost always require surgical excision and urethral reconstruction. In the authors' experience transurethral resection is usually not successful. We prefer to make an inverted U-shaped incision in the anterior vaginal wall and mobilize the vagina off the posterior urethra. Next, if possible, identify the synthetic sling on either side of the urethra. Once the sling is located, it can be sharply dissected away from the urethra. The urethral defect (urethrotomy) should be closed in two layers with a fine delayed absorbable suture. If the blood supply is compromised, a Martius fat pad transposition can be performed, and if there are concerns regarding SUI, an autologous pubovaginal sling can be placed at the same time. A recent review of a series of 19 patients with urethral mesh erosion concluded that, although the surgical management is complex, most women report resolution of their pelvic pain and a high rate of satisfaction with their postoperative condition, despite high rates of incontinence (Kowalik et al., 2018).

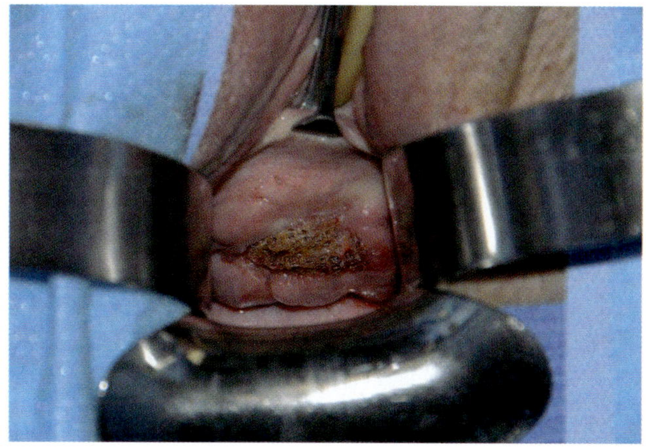

Fig. 25.5 Vaginal erosion of synthetic mesh after transvaginal mesh placement.

Complications After Transvaginal Mesh Placement for Pelvic Organ Prolapse

Between 2004 and 2019, millions of women had their POP repaired using some form of a transvaginal mesh kit. According to 2010 data from the FDA, 25% of all POP surgeries in that year used transvaginal mesh. Even though these kits are no longer commercially available in the United States, complications related to their insertion will continue to occur and require surgical intervention. Potential complications include vaginal mesh erosion, pelvic pain, and dyspareunia (Chermansky et al., 2012). Also reported, albeit very rarely, are bladder and bowel perforation and/or injury.

A complete history and examination of all patients with suspected mesh-related complications should be performed. On pelvic examination one should attempt to identify any of the following: urogenital atrophy, palpation/visualization of any exposed mesh, mesh under tension, location of mesh arms, pain with palpation of the mesh (note location), bunching of mesh or palpable abnormalities beneath the epithelium, pain with palpation of pelvic floor musculature, or evidence of fistula. Rectal examination should be performed, and cystoscopy and proctoscopy may be indicated in select cases. In patients with urogenital atrophy, the authors prefer to treat aggressively with local estrogen cream before any surgical intervention.

Mesh Erosion/Extrusion. This is the most common mesh-related complication after transvaginal placement of mesh for the management of POP (Fig. 25.5). Common presenting symptoms of women with vaginal erosion include vaginal drainage/bleeding, pelvic pain, and dyspareunia. On examination, pain with palpation of the mesh, visible mesh erosion, and vaginal shortening/tightening may be seen as well. Published rates for mesh erosion range from 3% to over 30%, with large reviews suggesting overall rates between 10% and 15% (Abed et al., 2011; Maher et al., 2011). Risk factors include concomitant hysterectomy, smoking, high total mesh volume, young patient age, early resumption of sexual activity, diabetes mellitus, and low surgeon experience. Local injection with lidocaine plus epinephrine at the time of mesh placement has not been shown to increase the risk of mesh erosion (Finamore et al., 2011). Conservative management with topical estrogen and/or topical antibiotics can be attempted; however, little evidence exists suggesting success with this treatment. Often, partial or complete excision is necessary for symptom improvement (Hurtado & Appell, 2009). Both office-based and operating-room excision are options for management. Office-based excision should be reserved for those with small exposures (usually <1 cm), adequate access to the exposed mesh, and healthy vaginal tissues. Similar to the description of office-based management of synthetic midurethral sling exposure, local anesthetic is injected around the extrusion, and the adjacent vaginal epithelium is mobilized. The mesh can be excised, and the vaginal epithelium brought together in a tension-free fashion with interrupted sutures.

The operating room affords the surgeon improved visibility, better patient anesthesia, and a wider array of instrumentation for managing mesh extrusions. The question that continues to be unanswered is: how much mesh should be excised? There seems to be a balance, with an increased risk of repeat surgery for mesh excision when partial excision is undertaken and an increased risk of recurrent prolapse, as well as more intraoperative morbidity, with complete excision (Tijdink et al., 2011). For erosions that are small and straightforward, mobilization of the surrounding epithelium to cover the mesh or simple excision of a small amount of mesh and closing the epithelium is usually all that is needed. If pain and a large-scale erosion is noted, then more aggressive resection is usually performed. Techniques for surgical excision revolve around dissection of the overlying vaginal epithelium away from the mesh, followed by the dissection of the mesh away from the adjacent organ (bladder or rectum) (Fig. 25.6). Margulies et al. (2008), Ridgeway et al. (2008), and Muffly and Barber (2010) each describe in detail surgical techniques for transvaginal mesh removal. Many mesh kits consist of a body of mesh and arms used for anchoring the mesh. After implantation and incorporation of the mesh, these arms may become vascularized. When a more complete excision is desired, and the mesh body has been mobilized satisfactorily, the authors advocate for clamping and tying of the mesh arms before

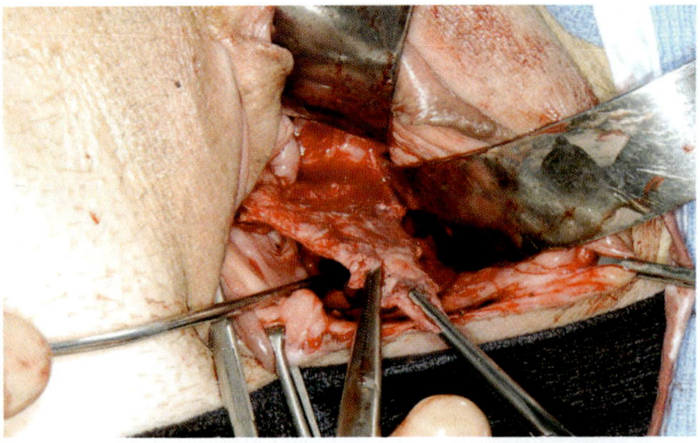

Fig. 25.6 Technique for transvaginal removal of mesh. Note the synthetic mesh is sharply dissected off the underlying viscera and overlying vaginal epithelium.

transection to decrease the risk of bleeding. After mesh removal, when possible, midline plication of underlying connective tissue is performed to help resupport the prolapsed tissue and possibly decrease the risk of recurrent prolapse. Also, if appropriate, a native tissue suture suspension of the vaginal apex to the uterosacral ligaments or sacrospinous ligaments can be performed (Video 25.2). If mobilization of the vaginal tissue does not allow for a tension-free closure of the vaginal epithelium, porcine small intestine submucosa graft (Surgisis Biodesign; Cook Surgical, Bloomington IN) or porcine bladder (Matristem; Acell Inc.; Columbia MD) can be secured in place over the vaginal defect (Khong & Lam, 2011) to act as a scaffold and encourage host response to mediate the healing process. In other words, porcine graft can be used as a patch to close a vaginal defect. Both of these tissues will ultimately convert to normal skin in the majority of cases, assuming a good blood supply is maintained (Video 25.3). Vulvar skin flaps may also be used in instances where large defects are present after mesh removal.

Two recent publications have reported good patient-reported outcomes after surgical management of transvaginal mesh complications (Crosby et al., 2014; Warembourg et al., 2017).

Dyspareunia and Pelvic/Vaginal Pain. Dyspareunia and/or pain may develop after transvaginal mesh placement for POP. In a systemic review, the overall incidence of new-onset dyspareunia after vaginal mesh placement was 9.1% (with a range of 0% to 67%) (Abed et al., 2011). Pelvic muscle spasm/pelvic floor tension myalgia can present as chronic pelvic pain and may be confused with mesh-related pain. Although they may be difficult to distinguish from each other, both may improve with nonsurgical treatments such as pelvic floor physical therapy (Rosenbaum & Owens, 2008). The authors recommend exhausting nonsurgical measures for the treatment of pelvic pain possibly related to mesh placement, because patients undergoing surgical excision often have persistent pain (El-Nashar & Trabuco, 2012). Of all mesh-related complications, pain remains the symptom most resistant to medical and surgical treatment. It is often improved after mesh excision but may never disappear completely (Skala et al., 2011). Thus, counseling patients before surgery about the risks associated with mesh removal is paramount. These include bleeding, infection, injury to adjacent organs, new/persistent pain, and recurrent prolapse.

El-Nashar and Trabuco (2012) performed an early excision of vaginal mesh 11 days after implantation. This was performed for severe vaginal pain and urinary urgency/frequency that began immediately after vaginal mesh placement. Complete excision, including mesh arms, was performed, and the patient had resolution of all symptoms. The implanting surgeon was not the referring provider in the case above, and this is consistent with findings by Blandon and colleagues. In their study, only 14% of patients with mesh-related complications were referred by the surgeon who placed the mesh; about half were referred by a different physician/health care provider, and the remainder were self-referred.

Visceral Injury. Albeit rare, injury to the bladder and bowel can occur during placement of vaginal mesh. Significant emphasis has been placed on the concept that mesh placement requires a deeper dissection plane, that is, through the full thickness of the vaginal epithelium, to avoid vaginal erosion. However, the surgeon must also go to great lengths to avoid an inadvertent proctotomy or cystotomy, as well as to avoid placing the mesh too deep (i.e., in the wall of the bladder or rectum).

In the rare situation where mesh is found postoperatively in the bladder or rectum, usually a major surgical procedure will be required to remove the mesh. If mesh is found in the rectum, a diverting colostomy may be necessary before attempting mesh removal. Videos 25.4 and 25.5 review techniques of removing synthetic mesh from the bladder and the rectum.

CONCLUSION

Complications and untoward sequelae from reconstructive pelvic surgery occur with both native-tissue and graft-augmented surgeries. Gauging the true incidence of these complications is difficult, because there is no good source for how many total procedures are being done and the frequency with which new materials are being used. As new procedures to correct pelvic floor disorders continue to evolve, open discussions among surgeons on how best to manage new and or unforeseen complications are important.

BIBLIOGRAPHY

Abed H, Rahn DD, Lowenstein L, et al. Incidence and management of graft erosion, wound granulation, and dyspareunia following vaginal prolapse repair with graft materials: a systematic review. *Int Urogynecol J*. 2011;22:789.

Abramov Y, Golden B, Sullivan M, et al. Histologic characterization of vaginal vs. abdominal surgical wound healing in a rabbit model. *Wound Repair Regen*. 2007;15:80.

Achtari C, Hiscock R, O'Reilly BA, et al. Risk factors for mesh erosion after transvaginal surgery using polypropylene (Atrium) or composite polypropylene/polyglactin 910 (Vypro II) mesh. *Int Urogynecol J Pelvic Floor Dysfunct.* 2005;16:389.

Amid P. Classification of biomaterials and their relative complications in abdominal wall hernia surgery. *Hernia.* 1997;1:15.

Araco F, Gravante G, Vita DDE, et al. Obturator abscess with spread to the thigh after three years from a transobturator procedure. *Aust N Z J Obstet Gynaecol.* 2009a;49:335.

Araco F, Gravante G, Piccione E. Bladder erosion after 2 years from cytocele repair with type I polypropylene mesh. *Int Urogynecol J Pelvic Floor Dysfunct.* 2009b;20:731.

AUGS. *Position Statement: Mesh Midurethral Slings for Stress Urinary Incontinence.* Available at: https://www.augs.org/assets/1/6/AUGS-SUFU_MUS_Position_Statement.pdf.

AUGS/ACOG Pelvic Organ Prolapse Practice Guidleine. *Female Pelvic Med Reconstr Surg.* 2019;25:387.

Babalola EO, Famuyide AO, McGuire LJ, et al. Vaginal erosion, sinus formation, and ischiorectal abscess following transobturator tape: ObTape implantation. *Int Urogynecol J Pelvic Floor Dysfunct.* 2006;17:418.

Baessler K, Hewson AD, Tunn R, et al. Severe mesh complications following intravaginal slingplasty. *Obstet Gynecol.* 2005;106:713.

Barendse-Hofmann MG, van Doorn LP, Oskam J, Steenvoorde P. Extracellular matrix prevents split-skin grafting in selected cases. *J Wound Care.* 2007;16:455.

Birnbaum SJ. Rational therapy for the prolapsed vagina. *Am J Obstet Gynecol.* 1973;115:411.

Blandon RE, Gebhart JB, Trabuco EC, Klingele CJ. Complications from vaginally placed mesh in pelvic reconstructive surgery. *Int Urogynecol J Pelvic Floor Dysfunct.* 2009;20:523.

Brizzolara S, Pillai-Allen A. Risk of mesh erosion with sacral colpopexy and concurrent hysterectomy. *Obstet Gynecol.* 2003;102:306.

Brubaker L, Cundiff G, Fine P, et al. A randomized trial of colpopexy and urinary reduction efforts (CARE): design and methods. *Control Clin Trials.* 2003;24:629.

Brubaker L, Cundiff GW, Fine P, et al. Abdominal sacrocolpopexy with Burch colposuspension to reduce urinary stress incontinence. *N Engl J Med.* 2006;354:1557.

Buechel M, Tarr ME, Walters MD. Vaginal apical pain after sacrocolpopexy in absence of vaginal mesh erosion; a case series. *Female Pelvic Med Reconstr Surg.* 2016;22:e8.

Carson SN, Travis E, Overall K, Lee-Jahshan S. Using becaplermin gel with collagen products to potentiate healing in chronic leg wounds. *Wounds.* 2003;15:339.

Chen HW, Guess MK, Connell KA, Bercik RS. Ischiorectal abscess and ischiorectal-vaginal fistula as delayed complications of posterior intravaginal slingplasty: a case report. *J Reprod Med.* 2009;54:645.

Chermansky CJ, Winters JC. Complications of vaginal mesh surgery. *Curr Opin Urol.* 2012;22:287.

Chien HW, Kumakura E, Koyama M. Iliosacral bacterial arthritis and retroperitoneal abscess after tension-free vaginal mesh reconstruction. *Int Urogynecol J.* 2010;21:753.

Clavé A, et al. Polypropylene as a reinforcement in pelvic surgery is not inert: comparative analysis of 100 explants. *Int Urogynecol J.* 2010;21:261.

Collinet P, Belot F, Debodinance P, et al. Transvaginal mesh technique for pelvic organ prolapse repair: mesh exposure management and risk factors. *Int Urogynecol J Pelvic Floor Dysfunct.* 2006;17:315.

Committee on Gynecologic Practice. Committee Opinion no. 513: vaginal placement of synthetic mesh for pelvic organ prolapse. *Obstet Gynecol.* 2011;118:1459.

Corona R, De Cicco C, Schonman R, et al. Tension-free vaginal tapes and pelvic nerve neuropathy. *J Minim Invasive Gynecol.* 2008;15:262.

Crosby EC, Abernethy M, Berger MB, et al. Symptom resolution after operative management of complications from transvaginal mesh. *Obstet Gynecol.* 2014;123:134.

Culligan PJ, Littman PM, Salamon CG, et al. Evaluation of a transvaginal mesh delivery system for the correction of pelvic organ prolapse: subjective and objective findings at least 1 year after surgery. *Am J Obstet Gynecol.* 2010;203:506.e1.

Culligan PJ, Murphy M, Blackwell L, et al. Long-term success of abdominal sacral colpopexy using synthetic mesh. *Am J Obstet Gynecol.* 2002;187:1473.

Cundiff GW, Varner E, Visco AG, et al. Risk factors for mesh/suture erosion following sacral colpopexy. *Am J Obstet Gynecol.* 2008;199:688.e1.

Davila GW. Optimizing safety and appropriateness of graft use in pelvic reconstructive surgery: introduction to the 2nd IUGA Grafts Roundtable. *Int Urogynecol J.* 2012;23:S3.

Davila GW, Baessler K, Cosson M, Cardozo L. Selection of patients in whom vaginal graft use may be appropriate. Consensus of the 2nd IUGA Grafts Roundtable: optimizing safety and appropriateness of graft use in transvaginal pelvic reconstructive surgery. *Int Urogynecol J.* 2012;23:S7.

Debodinance P, Berrocal J, Clavé H, et al. Changing attitudes on the surgical treatment of urogenital prolapse: birth of the tension-free vaginal mesh. *J Gynecol Obstet Biol Reprod (Paris).* 2004;33:577.

Dietz HP, Erdmann M, Shek KL. Mesh contraction: myth or reality? *Am J Obstet Gynecol.* 2011;204:173.e1.

Doumouchtsis SK, Lee FY, Bramwell D, et al. Evaluation of holmium laser for managing mesh/suture complications of continence surgery. *BJU Int.* 2011;108:1472.

Dwyer PL, O'Reilly BA. Transvaginal repair of anterior and posterior compartment prolapse with Atrium polypropylene mesh. *BJOG.* 2004;111:831.

El-Nashar SA, Trabuco EC. Is early excision the right answer for early onset pain related to vaginal mesh placement? A case report and a systematic review of the literature. *Female Pelvic Med Reconstr Surg.* 2012;18:185.

Fatton B, Amblard J, Debodinance P, et al. Transvaginal repair of genital prolapse: preliminary results of a new tension-free vaginal mesh (Prolift technique)—a case series multicentric study. *Int Urogynecol J Pelvic Floor Dysfunct.* 2007;18:743.

FDA Public Health Notification: Serious Complications Associated with Transvaginal Placement of Surgical Mesh in Repair of Pelvic Organ Prolapse and Stress Urinary Incontinence. Available at: http://www.fda.gov/MedicalDevices/Safety/AlertsandNotices/ucm262435.html.

FDA's Activities: Urogynecologic Surgical Mesh. Available at: https://www.fda.gov/medical-devices/urogynecologic-surgical-mesh-implants/fdas-activities-urogynecologic-surgical-mesh.

Feiner B, Jelovsek JE, Maher C. Efficacy and safety of transvaginal mesh kits in the treatment of prolapse of the vaginal apex: a systematic review. *BJOG.* 2009;116:15.

Feiner B, Maher C. Vaginal mesh contraction: definition, clinical presentation, and management. *Obstet Gynecol.* 2009;115:325.

Feldman GB, Birnbaum SJ. Sacral colpopexy for vaginal vault prolapse. *Obstet Gynecol.* 1979;53:399.

Finamore PS, Hunter K, Goldstein HB, et al. Does local injection with lidocaine plus epinephrine prior to vaginal reconstructive surgery with synthetic mesh affect exposure rates? A retrospective comparison. *Arch Gynecol Obstet.* 2011;284:659.

Firoozi F, Goldman HB. Transvaginal excision of mesh erosion involving the bladder after mesh placement using a prolapse kit: a novel technique. *Urology.* 2010;75:203.

Firoozi F, Ingber MS, Goldman HB. Pure transvagianl removal of eroded mesh and retained foreign body in the bladder. *Int Urogynecol J.* 2010;21:757.

FitzGerald MP, Payne CK, Lukacz ES, et al. Randomized multicenter clinical trial of myofascial physical therapy in women with interstitial cystitis/painful bladder syndrome and pelvic floor tenderness. *J Urol.* 2012;187:2113.

Foon R, Toozs-Hobson P, Latthe PM. Adjuvant materials in anterior vaginal wall prolapse surgery: a systematic review of effectiveness and complications. *Int Urogynecol J Pelvic Floor Dysfunct.* 2008;19:1697.

Gauruder-Burmester A, Koutouzidou P, Rohne J, et al. Follow-up after polypropylene mesh repair of anterior and posterior compartments in patients with recurrent prolapse. *Int Urogynecol J Pelvic Floor Dysfunct.* 2007;18:1059.

Ginath S, Garely AD, Condrea A, Vardy MD. Mesh erosion following abdominal sacral colpopexy in the absence and presence of the cervical stump. *Int Urogynecol J.* 2013;24:113.

Gold KP, Ward RM, Zimmerman CW, et al. Factors associated with exposure of transvaginally placed polypropylene mesh for pelvic organ prolapse. *Int Urogynecol J.* 2012;23:1461.

Guidelines for providing privileges and credentials to physicians for transvaginal placement of surgical mesh for pelvic organ prolapse. *Female Pelvic Med Reconstr Surg.* 2012;18:194.

Haylen BT, Freeman RM, Swift SE, et al. An International Urogynecological Association (IUGA)/International Continence Society (ICS) joint terminology and classification of the complications related directly to the insertion of prostheses (meshes, implants, tapes) and grafts in female pelvic floor surgery. *Int Urogynecol J.* 2011;22:3.

Helström L, Nilsson B. Impact of vaginal surgery on sexuality and quality of life in women with urinary incontinence or genital descensus. *Acta Obstet Gynecol Scand.* 2005;84:79.

Hinoul P, Ombelet WU, Burger MP, Roovers JP. A prospective study to evaluate the anatomic and functional outcome of a transobturator mesh kit (prolift anterior) for symptomatic cystocele repair. *J Minim Invasive Gynecol.* 2008;15:615.

Hodde J, Janis A, Ernst D, Zopf D, Sherman D, Johnson C. Effects of sterilization on an extracellular matrix scaffold: part I. Composition and matrix architecture. *J Mater Sci Mater Med.* 2007a;18:537.

Hodde J, Janis A, Hiles M. Effects of sterilization on an extracellular matrix scaffold: part II. Bioactivity and matrix interaction. *J Mater Sci Mater Med.* 2007b;18:545.

Hodde JP, Ernst DM, Hiles MC. An investigation of the long-term bioactivity of endogenous growth factor in OASIS Wound Matrix. *J Wound Care.* 2005;14:23.

Hurtado EA, Appell RA. Management of complications arising from transvaginal mesh kit procedures: a tertiary referral center's experience. *Int Urogynecol J Pelvic Floor Dysfunct.* 2009;20:11.

Information on Surgical Mesh for Pelvic Organ Prolapse and Stress Urinary Incontinence. US Food and Drug Administration; 2009. Available at: http://www.fda.gov/cdrh/consumer/surgicalmesh-popsui.html.

Jia X, Glazener C, Mowatt G, et al. Efficacy and safety of using mesh or grafts in surgery for anterior and/or posterior vaginal wall prolapse: systematic review and meta-analysis. *BJOG.* 2008;115:1350.

Joint Position Statement on the Management of Mesh-Related Complications for the FPMRS Specialist. *Female Pelvic Med Reconstr Surg.* 2020;26:219.

Joint Report on terminology for surgical procedures to treat stress urinary incontinence in women. *Female Pelvic Med Reconstr Surg.* 2020;26(3):162-172.

Joint Writing Group of the American Urogynecologic Society and the International Urogynecological Association. Joint Position Statement on the Management of Mesh-Related Complications for the FPMRS Specialist. *Female Pelvic Med Reconstr Surg.* 2020;26:219.

Karateke A, Akdemir Y, Kucukbas M, et al. Recurrent ischiorectal abscess secondary to transobturator tape erosion: an unusual chronic complication. *Eur J Obstet Gynecol Reprod Biol.* 2011;158:364.

Karlovsky ME, Thakre AA, Rastinehad A, et al. Biomaterials for pelvic floor reconstruction. *Urology.* 2005;66:469.

Kaufman Y, Singh SS, Alturki H, Lam A. Age and sexual activity are risk factors for mesh exposure following transvaginal mesh repair. *Int Urogynecol J.* 2011;22:307.

Khong SY, Lam A. Use of Surgisis mesh in the management of polypropylene mesh erosion into the vagina. *Int Urogynecol J.* 2011;22:41.

Kowalik CG, Cohn JA, Kakos A, et al. Road to recovery after transvaginal surgery for urethral mesh perforation: evaluation of outcomes and subsequent procedures. *Int Urogynecol J.* 2018;29:887.

Lee SY, Kim JY, Park SJ, et al. Bilateral recurrent thigh abscesses for five years after a transobturator tape implantation for stress urinary incontinence. *Korean J Urol.* 2010;51:657.

Letouzey V, Deffieux X, Levailolant J, et al. Ultrasound evaluation of polypropylene mesh contraction at long term after vaginal surgery for cystocele repair (abstract). *Int Urogynecol J Pelvic Floor Dysfunct.* 2009;20:S205.

Lin X, Du P, Chen L, et al. A case of mesh erosion to the sigmoid after laparoscopic sacrocolpopexy and a literature review of mesh related complications. *Female Pelvic Med Reconstr Surg.* 2018;24:e12.

Lo TS, Ashok K. Recurrent mesh erosion and retropubic abscess following anterior intravaginal slingplasty. *J Obstet Gynaecol Res.* 2011;37:363.

Luck AM, Steele AC, Leong FC, McLennan MT. Short-term efficacy and complications of posterior intravaginal slingplasty. *Int Urogynecol J Pelvic Floor Dysfunct.* 2008;19:795.

Madjar S, Frischer Z, Nieder AM, Waltzer WC. Bladder wall abscess following midurethral sling procedure. *Int Urogynecol J Pelvic Floor Dysfunct.* 2006;17:180.

Maher CM, Feiner B, Baessler K, Glazener CM. Surgical management of pelvic organ prolapse in women: the updated summary version Cochrane review. *Int Urogynecol J.* 2011;22:1445.

Management of mesh and graft complications in gynecologic surgery. *Female Pelvic Med Reconstr Surg.* 2017;23:171.

Margulies RU, Lewicky-Gaupp C, Fenner DE, et al. Complications requiring reoperation following vaginal mesh kit procedures for prolapse. *Am J Obstet Gynecol.* 2008;199:678.e1.

Marks BK, Goldman HB. Controversies in the management of mesh-based complications: a urology perspective. *Urol Clin North Am.* 2012;39:419.

Milani R, Salvatore S, Soligo M, et al. Functional and anatomical outcome of anterior and posterior vaginal prolapse repair with prolene mesh. *BJOG.* 2005;112:107.

Miller D, Milani AL, Sutherland SE, et al. Informed surgical consent for a mesh/graft-augmented vaginal repair of pelvic organ prolapse. Consensus of the 2nd IUGA Grafts Roundtable: optimizing safety and appropriateness of graft use in transvaginal pelvic reconstructive surgery. *Int Urogynecol J.* 2012;23:S33.

Moore RD, Miklos JR. Vaginal repair of cystocele with anterior wall mesh via transobturator route: efficacy and complications with up to 3-year followup. *Adv Urol.* 2009;2009:743831.

Muffly TM, Barber MD. Insertion and removal of vaginal mesh for pelvic organ prolapse. *Clin Obstet Gynecol.* 2010;53:99.

Murphy M, Society of Gynecologic Surgeons Systematic Review Group. Clinical practice guidelines on vaginal graft use from the Society of Gynecologic Surgeons. *Obstet Gynecol.* 2008;112:1123.

Ng CC, Chong CY. The effectiveness of transvaginal anterior colporrhaphy reinforced with polypropylene mesh in the treatment of severe cystoceles. *Ann Acad Med Singapore.* 2006;35:875.

Nygaard IE, Brubaker L, Zyczynski HM, et al. Long-term outcomes following abdominal sacrocolpopexy for pelvic organ prolapse. *JAMA.* 2013;39:2015.

Nygaard IE, McCreery R, Brubaker L, et al. Abdominal sacrocolpopexy: a comprehensive review. *Obstet Gynecol.* 2004;104:805.

Obstetrical and Gynecological Devices; Reclassification of Surgical Mesh for Transvaginal Pelvic Organ Prolapse Repair. 2016. Available at: https://www.federalregister.gov/documents/2016/01/05/2015-33165/obstetrical-and-gynecological-devices-reclassification-of-surgical-mesh-for-transvaginal-pelvic.

Occhino JA, Casiano ER, Trabuco EC, Klingele CJ. A three-incision approach to treat persistent vaginal exposure and sinus tract formation related to ObTape mesh insertion. *Int Urogynecol J.* 2012;23:1307.

Ogah J, Cody DJ, Rogerson L. Minimally invasive synthetic suburethral sling operations for stress urinary incontinence in women: a short version Cochrane review. *Neurourol Urodyn.* 2011;30:284.

Ogle CA, Linder BJ, Elliott DS. Holmium laser excision for urinary mesh erosion: a minimally invasive treatment with favorable long-term results. *Int Urogynecol J.* 2015;26:1645.

Ogle CA, Shepherd JP, Sutkin G. Posterior rectus abdominis sheath abscess after tension-free vaginal tape. *Int Urogynecol J.* 2012;23:1469.

Olsen AL, Smith VJ, Bergstrom JO, et al. Epidemiology of surgically managed pelvic organ prolapse and urinary incontinence. *Obstet Gynecol.* 1997;89:501.

Rafii A, Jacob D, Deval B. Obturator abscess after transobturator tape for stress urinary incontinence. *Obstet Gynecol.* 2006;108:720.

Richter HE, Albo ME, Zyczynski HM, et al. Retropubic versus transobturator midurethral slings for stress incontinence. *N Engl J Med.* 2010;362:2066.

Ridgeway B, Walters MD, Paraiso MF, et al. Early experience with mesh excision for adverse outcomes after transvaginal mesh placement using prolapse kits. *Am J Obstet Gynecol.* 2008;199:703.e1.

Rosenbaum TY, Owens A. The role of pelvic floor physical therapy in the treatment of pelvic and genital pain-related sexual dysfunction (CME). *J Sex Med.* 2008;5:513.

Sajid MS, Parampalli U, McFall MR. A meta-analysis comparing tacker mesh fixation with suture mesh fixation in laparoscopic incisional and ventral hernia repair. *Hernia.* 2013;17:159.

Sanders DL, Kingsnorth AN. Prosthetic mesh materials used in hernia surgery. *Expert Rev Med Devices.* 2012;9:159.

Scott NW, McCormack K, Graham P, et al. Open mesh versus non-mesh for repair of femoral and inguinal hernia. *Cochrane Database Syst Rev.* 2002;4:CD002197.

Skala CE, Renezeder K, Albrich S, et al. Mesh complications following prolapse surgery: management and outcome. *Eur J Obstet Gynecol Reprod Biol.* 2011;159:453.

Slack M, Ostergard D, Cervigni M, Deprest J. A standardized description of graft-containing meshes and recommended steps before the introduction of medical devices for prolapse surgery. Consensus of the 2nd IUGA Grafts Roundtable: optimizing safety and appropriateness of graft use in transvaginal pelvic reconstructive surgery. *Int Urogynecol J.* 2012;23:S15.

Smith FJ, Holman CD, Moorin RE, Tsokos N. Lifetime risk of undergoing surgery for pelvic organ prolapse. *Obstet Gynecol.* 2010;116:1096.

South MM, Foster RT, Webster GD, et al. Surgical excision of eroded mesh after prior abdominal sacrocolpopexy. *Am J Obstet Gynecol.* 2007;197:615.e1.

Svabík K, Martan A, Masata J, et al. Ultrasound appearances after mesh implantation—evidence of mesh contraction or folding? *Int Urogynecol J.* 2011;22:529.

Tijdink MM, Vierhout ME, Heesakkers JP, Withagen MI. Surgical management of mesh-related complications after prior pelvic floor reconstructive surgery with mesh. *Int Urogynecol J.* 2011;22:1395.

Trabuco EC, Klingele CJ, Gebhart JB. Xenograft use in reconstructive pelvic surgery: a review of the literature. *Int Urogynecol J Pelvic Floor Dysfunct.* 2007;18:555.

Urogynecologic Surgical Mesh Implants. 2019. Available at: https://www.fda.gov/medical-devices/implants-and-prosthetics/urogynecologic-surgical-mesh-implants.

Urogynecologic Surgical Mesh: Update on the safety and effectiveness of transvaginal placement for pelvic organ prolapse. Silver Spring, MD: Safety Communication, Food and Drug Administration; 2011.

Vassallo BJ, Karram MM. Management of iatrogenic vaginal constriction. *Obstet Gynecol.* 2003;102:512.

Velemir L, Amblard J, Fatton B, et al. Transvaginal mesh repair of anterior and posterior vaginal wall prolapse: a clinical and ultrasonographic study. *Ultrasound Obstet Gynecol.* 2010;35:474.

Warembourg S, Labaki M, de Tayrac R, et al. Reoperations for mesh-related complications after pelvic organ prolapse repair: 8-year experience at a tertiary referral center. *Int Urogynecol J.* 2017;28:1139.

Winters JC, Jacquetin B, Castro R. Credentialing for transvaginal mesh placement a case for "added qualification" in competency. Consensus of the 2nd IUGA Grafts Roundtable: optimizing safety and appropriateness of graft use in transvaginal pelvic reconstructive surgery. *Int Urogynecol J.* 2012;23:S27.

Withagen MI, Vierhout ME, Hendriks JC, et al. Risk factors for exposure, pain, and dyspareunia after tension-free vaginal mesh procedure. *Obstet Gynecol.* 2011;118:629.

Wolter CE, Starkman JS, Scarpero HM, Dmochowski RR. Removal of transobturator midurethral sling for refractory thigh pain. *Urology.* 2008;72:461.e1.

Yamada BS, Govier FE, Stefanovic KB, et al. Vesicovaginal fistula and mesh erosion after Perigee (transobturator polypropylene mesh anterior repair). *Urology.* 2006;68:1121.e5.

26

Complications of Pelvic Reconstructive Surgery

Ellen R. Solomon, Matthew D. Barber, Mickey M. Karram, and John B. Gebhart

CHAPTER OUTLINE

This chapter discusses the evaluation, prevention, and management of many complications commonly associated with pelvic reconstructive surgery. Of note, it does not include a discussion of the evaluation and management of lower urinary tract injuries, which can be found in Chapter 24, or management of mesh complications, which can be found in Chapter 25.

EVALUATING COMORBIDITIES AND PERIOPERATIVE RISK

Before a patient undergoes pelvic reconstructive surgery, the risk of potential complications should be carefully assessed and addressed with the patient. Complications may occur in the perioperative period, and it is necessary to recognize high-risk patients and minimize risk from surgery before their arrival to the operating room. The lifetime risk of a woman undergoing prolapse or incontinence surgery by the age of 80 years is 19% to 25% (Maher et al., 2013; Smith et al., 2010; Wu et al., 2014). The prevalence of perioperative complications among women undergoing reconstructive pelvic surgery has been reported to be as high as 33% (Lambrou et al., 2000). A large cross-sectional study including 366 women who had undergone prolapse surgery found an overall complication rate of 11.3% (Alshankiti et al., 2019). Risk factors for complications in the perioperative period are listed in Box 26.1.

Age is an important factor to consider when assessing perioperative risk. The median age of patients who undergo pelvic reconstructive surgery is 61.5 years (Luber et al., 2001). Increasing age corresponds with increasing medical comorbidities, including chronic illness, hypertension, coronary heart disease, diabetes, pulmonary disease, and central nervous system disease (Toglia & Nolan, 2003). A retrospective cohort study of 264,340 women undergoing pelvic surgery found that increasing age is associated with higher mortality risks and higher complication risks. Specifically, elderly women (>80 years of age) were found to have increased risk of perioperative complications compared with younger women (Sung et al., 2006). In this same study, elderly women who underwent obliterative procedures (e.g., colpocleisis) had a lower risk of complications compared with patients who underwent reconstructive procedures for prolapse. Furthermore, in a decision analysis by Jones et al. (2016), it was found that Le Fort colpocleisis is the preferred obliterative procedure, and that, as patients age, the difference between Le Fort alone and hysterectomy with colpocleisis widens, favoring Le Fort. In a retrospective review of patients 75 years and older, 25.8% of patients had significant perioperative complications including significant blood loss, pulmonary edema, and congestive heart failure. Independent risk factors that were predictive of perioperative complications in this patient population included length of surgery, coronary artery disease, and peripheral vascular disease (Stepp et al., 2005). In a retrospective cohort study including 508 women undergoing urogynecologic surgery, women who were older than age 65 years had an increased risk of postoperative complications on the Dindo–Clavien scale compared to women who were younger than age 65 years (Bretschneider et al., 2015). When surgeons are determining the best procedure for the patient, age should play a role in that decision.

BOX 26.1 General Risk Factors of Pelvic Reconstructive Surgery

Age	Hypertension
Central nervous system disease	Obesity
Coronary heart disease	Peripheral artery disease
Diabetes	Pulmonary disease

Cardiac risk factors also impact postoperative morbidity in pelvic surgery. In a retrospective cohort study by Heisler et al. (2010), perioperative complications were increased in patients with a history of myocardial infarction or congestive heart failure, perioperative hemoglobin decrease greater than 3.1 g/dL, preoperative hemoglobin less than 12.0 g/dL, or history of prior thrombosis. In a retrospective cohort study of 4315 patients undergoing elective major noncardiac surgery, predictors of major cardiac complications included high-risk types of surgeries, history of ischemic heart disease, history of congestive heart failure, history of cerebrovascular disease, preoperative treatment with insulin, and a serum creatinine of 2.0 mg/dL or greater (Lee et al., 1999). To decrease cardiac morbidity in patients undergoing surgery, it has been shown that continuing β blockers in the perioperative period in patients with chronic β blockade will decrease cardiovascular mortality (Shammash et al., 2001). In a very large retrospective cohort study by Sheyn et al. (2018), the rate of myocardial infarction or cardiac arrest was 0.11% among 46,367 women who underwent pelvic reconstructive surgery. In a retrospective chart review by Unger et al. (2015), 983 women who underwent transvaginal colpopexy were found to have a 0.8% rate of cardiac complications. These numbers are reassuring when considering pelvic floor surgery for many patients, even those who are elderly or with comorbidities. Consultation with the patient's primary care physician or cardiologist before surgery is often warranted in patients with cardiac disease.

Obesity is a significant risk factor for perioperative complications. With obesity, there is an increase in comorbid conditions, including cardiac disease, type 2 diabetes, hypertension, stroke, sleep apnea, and some cancers (Must et al., 1999). One study of obese and overweight women undergoing retropubic surgery for stress urinary incontinence found that obese women had significantly increased estimated blood loss and operative time (Rogers et al., 2006). In a retrospective cohort study, obese patients who underwent vaginal surgery were matched to patients who were of normal weight, and perioperative comorbidities and complications were analyzed. This study found that there was no difference in perioperative complications between obese and nonobese patients; however, there was a higher rate of surgical site infection in the obese population (Chen et al., 2007). In a large retrospective cohort study of 16,639 women who underwent pelvic floor reconstructive surgery, 10% of the patients were obese, and the overall perioperative complication rate during the surgical admission was 25%. On multivariable analysis, obesity increased the odds of perioperative complications by approximately 40% after adjusting for age, race, income, concomitant hysterectomy, and medical comorbidities (Pratt et al., 2018).

In obese women undergoing hysterectomy, the abdominal approach results in significantly higher rates of wound infection than vaginal hysterectomy (Pitkin, 1977). In a systematic review, compared with vaginal and laparoscopic hysterectomy, patients with body mass index (BMI) over 35 kg/m^2 who underwent abdominal hysterectomy had more postoperative complications and longer hospitalizations (Blikkendaal et al., 2015). Overall, vaginal surgery appears to be the safest approach for obese women. Despite this, in a large retrospective study of over 18,800 women undergoing hysterectomy for benign conditions, rates of abdominal hysterectomy increased from 46% in patients with ideal body weight to 62% in morbidly obese patients (Mikhail et al., 2015).

It is important to assess BMI when planning route of surgery and to consider the increased risks with obesity. In a large Swedish retrospective cohort study, women with a BMI of 25 kg/m^2 or greater were more likely to have increased blood loss and longer duration of surgery, and women with a BMI of 35 kg/m^2 or greater were more likely to have postoperative infections (Bohlin et al., 2016). Furthermore, in a large retrospective study of the American College of Surgeons National Surgical Quality Improvement Program (NSQIP) database, 55,409 women who underwent hysterectomy for benign conditions were studied, and patients with a BMI of 40 kg/m^2 or greater had five times the odds of wound dehiscence, five times the odds of wound infection, and 89% higher odds of sepsis compared to women with normal BMI (Shah et al., 2015).

In conclusion, when considering pelvic reconstructive surgery it is important to examine and evaluate the whole patient, including her medical comorbidities to appropriately assess her perioperative risk. Because of age and comorbidities, many patients should be evaluated by their primary care doctor or cardiologist before undergoing surgery. In high-risk patients, the vaginal route is often the lowest risk approach. In elderly patients no longer interested in sexual activity, obliterative procedures should be considered because of their shorter surgical times and low risk of complications relative to reconstructive procedures. Furthermore, when considering obliterative procedures, a LeFort colpocleisis tends to be the safest obliterative procedure to perform if feasible.

ENHANCED RECOVERY

Before bringing the patient to the operating room, careful planning and preoperative protocols may contribute to reduced complications and hospital stays through the use of Enhanced Recovery After Surgery (ERAS) pathways. Although not standardized specifically for pelvic floor surgeries, ERAS pathways were developed to decrease postoperative pain and recovery times, and, in many cases, promote shorter hospital stays. In general, ERAS consists of preoperative counseling about expectations after surgery; preoperative nutritional strategies; use of analgesic, neuropathic, and antiemetic medications in the preoperative environment; a perioperative focus on multimodal analgesia, fluid balance, and maintenance of normothermia; and promoting early mobilization after surgery.

In a prospective observational study of women undergoing minimally invasive hysterectomy via laparoscopy or robotic approaches in an ERAS pathway, rates of same-day discharge increased, with no increase in emergency room visits or readmissions compared with a non-ERAS historical control group. Factors that were more common in those admitted after surgery included a higher (worse) American Society of Anesthesiologists physical status score, Black race, urinary retention, and postoperative pain (Keil et al., 2019). In a retrospective study, women who underwent surgery for prolapse or incontinence before and after implementation of an ERAS pathway were compared (Carter-Brooks et al., 2018). The ERAS (vs. non-ERAS) group had a higher proportion of same-day discharge (91.7% vs. 25.9%, $P < .001$) and a 13.8-hour shorter duration of stay. Patients in the ERAS group were more likely to be discharged using a urethral catheter. There were no differences in total 30-day postoperative complications, but the ERAS group had a slightly increased rate of 30-day readmission (6.7% vs. 1.5%, $P = .048$). The ERAS group had high patient satisfaction scores. Their urogynecology tailored ERAS protocol is shown in Table 26.1.

The American College of Obstetricians and Gynecologists (ACOG) recommends using ERAS pathways "to promote more rapid surgical recovery, shorter length of stay, greater patient satisfaction, and decreased costs when compared with traditional approaches" (ACOG Committee Opinion No. 750, 2018).

PULMONARY COMPLICATIONS

Postoperative pulmonary complications are a frequent cause of morbidity and mortality in the urogynecology patient. Postoperative pneumonia, atelectasis, pneumothorax, and respiratory failure are postoperative complications that increase length of stay and are more common than postoperative cardiac complications (Lawrence et al., 1995). The incidence of postoperative pulmonary complications in gynecologic patients has been reported to be between 1.22% and 2.3% (Pappachen et al., 2006; Unger et al., 2015). Multiple risk factors may increase pulmonary complications in the postoperative surgical patient. In a randomized trial of patients who underwent nonthoracic surgery, multivariate analysis identified four risk factors for postoperative pulmonary complications, including age greater than 65 years, positive "cough test," perioperative nasogastric tube, and duration of anesthesia (procedures lasting >2.5 hours) (McAlister et al., 2005). A retrospective review of patients undergoing gynecologic laparoscopy found that operative time greater than 200 minutes and age greater than 65 years contributed to hypercarbia. Predictors of the development of pneumothorax included pneumoperitoneum pressure greater than 50 mm Hg and operative time greater than 200 minutes (Murdock et al., 2000). In a retrospective review of 3226 patients who underwent hysterectomy for benign conditions, the incidence of pulmonary complications was extremely low, at 0.3% (Solomon et al., 2013).

Surgical approach may also be a contributing factor to postoperative pulmonary complications. A study of patients undergoing abdominal surgery found that age greater than 60 years, smoking history within the past 8 weeks, BMI 27 kg/m^2 or more, history of cancer, and incision site in the upper abdomen were independent risk factors for postoperative pulmonary complications (Brooks-Brunn et al., 1997). In a clinical trial involving 994 patients performed by Xue et al. (1999), patients were divided into three groups: (1) elective superficial plastic surgery, (2) upper abdominal surgery, and (3) thoracoabdominal (TA) surgery. It was found that the incidence of hypoxemia in the postoperative period was closely related to the operative site, with the upper abdominal and TA sites associated with the greatest risk. When evaluating this study, patients undergoing pelvic reconstructive surgery would most likely fall into the low-risk category, similar to elective superficial plastic surgery, with a low risk of hypoxemia in the postoperative period.

Smoking is another risk factor associated with postoperative pulmonary complications. In a prospective cohort study of patients referred for nonthoracic surgery, the risk for postoperative pulmonary complications was increased with age greater than 65 years and smoking history of 40 pack-years or more (Pappachen et al., 2006). In a large retrospective review of 635,265 patients from the NSQIP database, current smokers had increased odds of postoperative pneumonia and unplanned intubation (Turan et al., 2011). Pulmonary complications significantly decrease after 8 weeks of smoking cessation (Warner et al., 1984).

Patients with chronic obstructive pulmonary disease are also at increased risk of having postoperative pulmonary complications, and preoperative pulmonary function tests may help to identify patients with increased pulmonary risk (Doyle, 1999). Patients with chronic obstructive pulmonary disease were 300 to 700 times more likely to have a postoperative pulmonary complication in a prospective cohort study (Pappachen et al., 2006). Of note, nasogastric intubation instead of orogastric intubation increases the risk of pneumonia in this patient population as well (Ephgrave et al., 1993).

Sleep apnea is an additional risk factor for postoperative pulmonary complications. Obstructive sleep apnea is defined as partial or complete obstruction of the upper airway during sleep. The prevalence of sleep apnea ranges from 1% to 24% (Medlin et al., 2018). For gynecologic patients, diagnosing and treating sleep apnea is very helpful for the postoperative course. Regional anesthesia should be used on these patients when possible and reducing the length of surgery is imperative for safety. In a retrospective cohort study of orthopedic and general surgery patients by Memtsoudis et al. (2011), 51,509 patients with sleep apnea who underwent general surgery procedures were assessed for postoperative pulmonary complications. Patients with sleep apnea developed pulmonary complications more frequently than their matched controls. Because of relaxation of the pharyngeal muscles from anesthetic agents, sedatives, and opioids, patients with obstructive sleep apnea may have increased airway collapse in the postoperative period (Bolden et al., 2009). Anesthesia may also blunt the hypercapnic and hypoxic respiratory drive, as well as the arousal response. In a

TABLE 26.1 Example of a Urogynecology Enhanced Recovery After Surgery (ERAS) Pathway

Preoperative Optimization	
Assessment	Pre-operative office visit or phone call Screen for chronic conditions and assess optimization for surgery Screen for tobacco & alcohol abuse Assess for weight loss & malnutrition Assess post-operative nausea and vomiting risk using simplified Apfel criteria
Education	Tobacco & alcohol cessation 4–6 weeks prior to surgery ERAS pathway Peri-operative expectations, reinforcing the patient's role in their own recovery Provide ERAS brochure and nutrition patient information
Exercise	30 minutes of walking daily until surgery
Diet	Protein and carbohydrate rich foods 1 week prior to surgery Regular diet until midnight the night before surgery Clear liquids until 3 hours prior to surgery • Clear liquids include: water, black coffee or clear tea, carbonated beverages, fruit juice without pulp, or Gatorade • Patients with diabetes – avoid sugar containing liquids
Verification	Preoperative phone call the day prior to surgery NPO instructions reviewed Medications reviewed Shower with soap the night before surgery
Day of Surgery	
Pre-operative	Multimodal pain management: • Celecoxib 400 mg PO (200 mg if age >65); omit if GFR <60 • Acetaminophen 1000 mg PO (omit if hepatic dysfunction) • Morphine sulfate ER 30 mg PO (15 mg if age >65) Postoperative nausea and vomiting prevention: • Perphenazine 8 mg PO • Anesthesia can add scopolamine patch if age <65 Antibiotic prophylaxis • Cefotetan 2 grams IV within 60 minutes of incision No routine fluid administration No IV opioid premedication
Intra-operative	Induction: • Propofol (1–2 mg/kg, or titrate to amnesia and anesthesia) • Ketamine 20 mg (20, 21) • Lidocaine 100–200 mg bolus • Muscle relaxant (no opioids) • Dexamethasone 4–5 mg IV (avoid if diabetes) Maintenance: • Ketamine 10mg q1 hour (avoid in final hour) • Lidocaine boluses q1 hour (1mg/kg) • Avoid opioids intra-op, unless patient c/o pain at emergence • Avoid routine use of NGT Fluid management: • Goal is euvolemia • Laparoscopic and vaginal cases: 2 mL/kg/hr • Boluses for MAP < 60 mmHg or 20% of baseline Emergence: • Propofol titration • Ondansetron 4 mg IV • No IV ketorolac (unless celecoxib not given pre-op) • No IV acetaminophen (unless not given pre-op)
Post-operative	Transition from IV to PO opioids for rescue pain management Avoid patient controlled anesthesia Ketorolac and acetaminophen scheduled Start ice chips/sips of clear liquids as tolerated IV fluids at 40ml/hour until tolerating po
Discharge checklist	Tolerating po w/o nausea and emesis Pain controlled (pain score < 5) Voiding trial complete Independent ambulation No signs of delirium (oriented to person, place, time, current events)
Post-Operative Follow-up	
Assessment POD 1	Phone call from office nurses Home Health if required (urinary retention, DVT prophylaxis)

DVT, Deep vein thrombosis; *ER*, extended release; *GFR*, glomerular filtration rate; *IV*, intravenous; *MAP*, mean arterial pressure; *NGT*, nasogastric tube; *PO*, per os; *POD*, postoperative day; *q*, every day.
Carter-Brooks et al. Urogynecology-specific ERAS outcomes. *Am J Obstet Gynecol 2018*

study performed by Bolden et al. (2007), the frequency of postoperative hypoxemia was measured in sleep apnea patients in the postoperative period, and 16% of the patients studied had postoperative sleep-related episodes of oxygen desaturation.

To avoid hypoxemia in obstructive sleep apnea patients, it is necessary to encourage patients to bring in their home continuous positive airway pressure (CPAP) machines or to order home CPAP settings for hospital machines. Careful evaluation of the patient is essential to prevent postoperative complications. If a patient is suspected to have sleep apnea but has not been diagnosed, it is useful to place the patient under continuous pulse oxygen saturation monitoring for the first 24 hours after surgery (Adesanya et al., 2010).

Atelectasis and hypoxemia are common after surgery, especially surgeries that involve the abdomen or thorax. Early on, atelectasis may result from soft tissue edema from the upper pharynx because of intubation and tongue manipulation. Later, especially in patients who have undergone abdominal surgery, there is decreased ability to take deep breaths or cough because of postoperative pain. Postoperative patients have decreased functional residual capacity (Wahba, 1996). These factors lead to hypoventilation. Diagnosis of atelectasis may be made clinically and/or via imaging tests. Atelectasis may present as postoperative fever or decreased breath sounds at the lung bases and can be found on chest x-ray or computed tomography (CT).

Pre- and postoperative incentive spirometry is the most common prevention and treatment intervention for atelectasis. Incentive spirometry used in the perioperative period enhances postoperative functional residual capacity and reminds patients to continue to take in large breaths. If a patient becomes hypoxic from atelectasis, bronchoscopy may be performed to remove secretions from the airway (Barrett, 1978). CPAP can be used in the postoperative period, and has also been shown to decrease the need for intubation in patients at high risk of hypoxemia from atelectasis after abdominal surgery (Squadrone et al., 2005).

Postoperative pneumonia is a common postoperative pulmonary complication. Hospital-acquired pneumonia refers to pneumonia that develops after 48 hours in the hospital. Diagnosing postoperative pneumonia can be difficult, as infiltrates from atelectasis, pulmonary edema, and acute lung injury can all look identical to pneumonia on chest x-ray. Diagnosis should be suspected if patient has new-onset fever, purulent sputum, leukocytosis, hypoxemia, and an infiltrate on chest x-ray. In a prospective case series of patients presenting with postoperative pneumonia within 14 days of surgery, 61% of patients developed pneumonia within the first 5 days postoperatively. The most common etiologic agents were *Staphylococcus aureus*, *Streptococci*, and *Enterobacter* (Montavers et al., 2002).

Treatment of postoperative pneumonia should begin with broad-spectrum antibiotics, given the polymicrobial nature of hospital-acquired pneumonia. Recommendations by the American Thoracic Society and the Infectious Disease Society of America (Kalil et al., 2016) include coverage for aerobic bacteria, as well as anaerobic bacteria. Most hospitals have guidelines for treating hospital-acquired pneumonia based on regional microbial patterns and antibiotic sensitivities.

VENOUS THROMBOEMBOLISM

Deep venous thrombosis (DVT) and pulmonary embolism (PE), jointly referred to as venous thromboembolism (VTE), are among the leading causes of preventable perioperative morbidity and mortality. In the perioperative period, the risk of death after VTE is approximately 3% to 4% (Colwell et al., 1999). The combination of epithelial damage, venous stasis, and hypercoagulability, collectively referred to as Virchow's triad, increases the risk of VTE for any patient undergoing surgery. Many pelvic reconstructive surgeries require the dorsal lithotomy and steep Trendelenburg positions; both exacerbate the risk of venous stasis. The postoperative risk of VTE may be elevated up to 1 year after the initial procedure has been performed but is highest in the immediate perioperative period (Sweetland et al., 2009).

The risk of VTE has been well studied in the general surgery, urology, and gynecologic oncology population. Recently there have been large studies that have addressed this issue in the population of patients who undergo pelvic reconstructive surgery. In a large cohort study by Montoya et al. (2014), the risk of VTE in this patient population that used intermittent pneumatic compression devices as the main form of postoperative thromboprophylaxis was 0.25%. Similarly, in an NSQIP registry study, the incidence of VTE was 0.3% among 20,687 women who underwent reconstructive pelvic surgery (Mueller et al., 2014). Overall, it seems that the risk is below 0.5% in the population undergoing these procedures.

A number of risk factors for VTE have been suggested for women in general and for those undergoing pelvic surgery. In a retrospective review of 1232 patients who underwent surgery for gynecologic conditions in Japan, it was found that malignancy, history of VTE, age greater than 50 years, and allergic-immunologic disease were all risk factors for VTE (Suzuki et al., 2010). However, this study only found three episodes of VTE in patients with benign disease, making it underpowered for this patient group. In a large prospective study by Lindqvist et al. (2008) that included 40,000 women, moderate drinkers of alcohol, women who engaged in strenuous exercise most days, and nonsmokers had the lowest risk of VTE.

In a retrospective review of 1862 gynecologic surgery patients given VTE prophylaxis with intermittent compression devices alone, the incidence of VTE was 1.3%. The risk factors associated with VTE in this study were diagnosis of cancer, age over 60 years, and anesthesia time over 3 hours. Patients with two or three of these variables had a 3.2% incidence of developing VTE, versus 0.6% in patients with zero or one risk factor (Clarke-Pearson et al., 2003). A large systematic review by Rahn et al. (2011) concluded that intermittent pneumatic compression devices provide sufficient prophylaxis for most patients undergoing pelvic reconstructive surgery. The authors determined that additional chemoprophylaxis should be added to the use of intermittent compression devices in patients with at least two out of three risk factors assessed: age over 60 years, history of cancer, or history of past VTE.

The question of which thromboprophylactic modality is best in the perioperative period for women undergoing pelvic reconstructive surgery is still uncertain. As mentioned previously, in the study by Montoya et al. (2014) the rate of VTE among patients who underwent pelvic reconstructive surgery was 0.25% where the only thromboprophylaxis used was sequential compression devices placed during the perioperative period. ACOG follows the recommendations provided by the American College of Chest Physicians from the Seventh ACCP Conference on Antithrombotic and Thrombolytic Therapy, published in 2004. The American College of Chest Physicians has since updated its recommendations for prophylaxis in all surgical patients (Table 26.2). Furthermore, they recommend chemothromboprophylaxis in patients who are at moderate and high risk. Most female pelvic reconstructive surgery patients fall into the "high" risk category, suggesting they should

TABLE 26.2 American College of Chest Physicians Assessment of Risk for Venous Thromboembolism in Patients Undergoing Surgery

Level of Risk	Definition	Recommended Prevention Strategy
Very low	A <0.5% risk of VTE (most outpatient or same-day surgery)	No specific recommendations
Low	Minor surgery (1.5% risk) (e.g., spinal surgery for nonmalignant disease)	Mechanical prophylaxis, preferably with SCDs
Moderate	Major surgery includes most general, open gynecologic and urologic cases (3% risk) (gynecologic noncancer surgery, cardiac surgery, thoracic surgery, spinal surgery for malignant disease)	LMWH, LDUH, plus mechanical thromboprophylaxis with ESs or SCDs
High	Major surgery, or patients with additional VTE risk factors (6% risk) (bariatric surgery, gynecologic cancer surgery, craniotomy, traumatic brain injury, spinal cord injury)	LMWH or LDUH, plus mechanical prophylaxis; use mechanical prophylaxis until bleeding risk diminishes
High-risk cancer surgery		LMWH or LDUH plus mechanical prophylaxis and extended-duration prophylaxis with LMWH postdischarge
High risk, LDUH and LMWH contraindicated or not available		Fondaparinux or low-dose aspirin (160 mg); mechanical prophylaxis with SCDs, ESs, or both

LDUH, Low-dose unfractionated heparin; *LMWH,* low-molecular-weight heparin; *VTE,* venous thromboembolic events; *SCDs,* sequential compression devices; *ESs,* elastic stockings.
(From Gould MK, Garcia DA, Wren SM, et al. Prevention of VTE in nonorthopedic surgical patients: Antithrombotic Therapy and Prevention of Thrombosis, 9th ed: American College of Chest Physicians Evidence-Based Clinical Practice Guidelines. *Chest.* 2012;141:e227S.)

receive chemothromboprophylaxis (Gould et al., 2012). However, as the rate of VTE appears to be below 0.5% in the urogynecologic population, it could be argued that our patients fall into the very low risk category, where no specific recommendations for prophylaxis are made.

It is essential to be able to recognize the symptoms of VTE in the postoperative patient. Although many patients who have VTE may be asymptomatic, the symptoms of dyspnea, orthopnea, hemoptysis, calf pain, calf swelling, chest pain, and tachypnea may signify a thrombotic event (Okadome et al., 2010). The physical signs that suggest VTE include hypotension, tachycardia, crackles, decreased breath sounds, lower extremity edema, tenderness in lower extremities, and hypoxia (Stein et al., 2007). Although the signs and symptoms of VTE are well known, it is difficult to rule out VTE by clinical diagnosis alone. A systematic review evaluating the D-dimer test used in combination with clinical probability to rule out VTE found that the D-dimer test is a safe and relatively reliable first-line test to use. After a 3-month follow-up, only 0.46% of patients were later diagnosed with PE (Cate-Hoek et al., 2005). However, the D-dimer test is not useful in pregnant patients, elderly patients, and hospitalized patients owing to decreased specificity (Agnelli et al., 2010).

Compression ultrasonography is a noninvasive, easy, and cost-effective procedure for the diagnosis of DVT in the lower extremities. The sensitivity and specificity for detecting DVT using compression ultrasonography in symptomatic patients is 89% to 96%, although the sensitivity is decreased in patients with calf DVT or in asymptomatic patients (Qaseem et al., 2007). Compression ultrasonography may also be used in conjunction with other diagnostic tests if PE is suspected (Moores et al., 2011). If compression ultrasound is negative but the patient remains symptomatic, venography may be used to further rule out DVT.

Indicated imaging for patients presenting with signs and symptoms of PE include ventilation perfusion (V/Q) scanning, CT, pulmonary angiography, and spiral CT of the chest. The V/Q scan was the imaging modality of choice for decades; however, owing to lack of ease of use and potential for indeterminate testing, CT has become the modality of choice (Desciak et al., 2011). CT angiography has a specificity of 96%, as well as 83% sensitivity, and has become the gold standard for PE diagnosis (Okadome et al., 2010).

It is important to start anticoagulation immediately once VTE has been diagnosed; furthermore, if there is high suspicion for PE, anticoagulation may be started even before the diagnosis is confirmed. Acute PE should be treated initially with a rapid-onset anticoagulant, which may be followed by treatment with an oral anticoagulant for at least 3 months (Cate-Hoek et al., 2005). For rapid-onset anticoagulation, patients may be started on intravenous unfractionated heparin, subcutaneous unfractionated heparin, subcutaneous low-molecular-weight heparin, and subcutaneous fondaparinux. The American College of Chest Physicians recommends using subcutaneous low molecular weight heparin for the initial treatment of acute, nonmassive PE. If the patient has decreased kidney function, is morbidly obese, or is pregnant, intravenous unfractionated heparin may be used, because of its shorter duration and titratability (Desciak et al., 2011). Once anticoagulation therapy has been established, the patient may continue on subcutaneous therapy or can be bridged to warfarin or other oral anticoagulant for at least 3 months. If the patient has contraindications to anticoagulation therapy, an inferior vena cava filter can be considered.

DELIRIUM

Delirium is an acute confusional state characterized by an alteration of consciousness with reduced ability to focus, sustain, or shift attention. Postoperative delirium is a common complication in elderly patients and can be life-threatening. Five percent of low-risk older adults having minor surgical procedures, and up to 50% of high-risk older adults having high-risk operations develop postoperative delirium. The sequelae include cognitive impairment, lack of functionality, and prolonged hospitalization with other associated morbidity. Symptoms of delirium can include hyperactive (e.g., agitation, heightened arousal, aggression) or hypoactive (e.g., withdrawn, decreased motor activity) behavior.

Delirium has been shown to be preventable in up to 40% of cases. Thus, prevention is the main management intervention, and commences by identifying high-risk patients who are aged 65 years or older, with past or present cognitive impairment, with current hip fracture, and with severe illness. Other risk factors include depression, alcohol or substance abuse, sleep deprivation, hypoxia, anemia, poor functional status, and polypharmacy, but preexisting cognitive impairment and dementia are the strongest predisposing factors. For any patient without known cognitive impairment, obtaining a detailed history and performing a cognitive assessment, such as the Mini-Cog, is strongly recommended. Trowbridge et al. (2016) found the following rates of cognitive impairment using the Mini-Cog in elderly urogynecology patients: 65 to 74 years, 5.3%; 75 to 85 years, 13.7%; and 85 years and older, 30%. Interviewing family members or other close contacts about the evolution of any cognitive or functional decline can be very helpful. Nonpharmacologic interventions to prevent postoperative delirium may include the following elements: cognitive reorientation, sleep enhancement (i.e., nonpharmacologic sleep protocol and sleep hygiene), early mobility and/or physical rehabilitation, adaptations for visual and hearing impairment, nutrition and fluid repletion, pain management, appropriate medication usage, adequate oxygenation, and prevention of constipation. Postoperative pain control should be optimized, preferably with nonopioid medications. Medications known to be associated with delirium, such as anticholinergic medications (particularly oxybutynin), benzodiazepines, diphenhydramine, sedative-hypnotics, and meperidine, should be avoided in at-risk patients.

Treatment of delirium should consist primarily of multidisciplinary nonpharmacologic interventions as described above for prevention. Supportive and restorative care to prevent further physical and cognitive decline should be implemented. Additionally, any underlying acute illness that may be contributing should be identified and treated. A focused history and physical should be performed, and medications reviewed. Basic laboratory studies that should be considered include blood count, metabolic panel, serum glucose, and urinalysis, as well as pulse oximetry and electrocardiogram. Focal neurologic findings should prompt a CT of the brain, and findings suggesting infection should prompt relevant intraabdominal or pelvic imaging. Alcohol or drug withdrawal should also be considered. Supportive care can include reorientation, mobilization, avoidance of restraints, reassurance, noise reduction, hydration, pain control, and bedside sitters. Where appropriate, low-dose, short-acting pharmacologic agents can be used to control dangerous and severely disruptive behaviors. Antipsychotic medications, such as low-dose haloperidol 0.5 to 1 mg as needed (maximum dose of 5 mg per day), can be used to treat moderate to severe hyperactive delirium that does not respond to behavioral and nonpharmacologic interventions. Benzodiazepines should not be used as first-line treatment for agitation associated with delirium. Importantly, antipsychotics and benzodiazepines should be avoided in the treatment of hypoactive delirium.

FEVER AND PERIOPERATIVE INFECTIONS

The most common postoperative complication of pelvic surgery is febrile morbidity, which occurs in 10% to 20% of women. Fevers after pelvic surgery can occur for the following reasons: (1) an operative site infection such as vaginal cuff cellulitis, pelvic abscess, or abdominal wound infection; (2) an infection remote from the operative site such as pneumonia or pyelonephritis; or (3) unexplained fever that resolves without consequence (up to 50% of cases). Recent evidence suggests that most unexplained postoperative fevers are not because of pulmonary atelectasis, but are the result of an increase in interleukins and cytokines. Regardless of the cause, a postoperative fever after pelvic surgery increases the hospital stay an average of 1 to 2 days. Fevers that persist and are associated with clinical signs, symptoms, and laboratory findings suggestive of a surgical site or other infection require appropriate treatment with antibiotics.

Urinary Tract Infection

Urinary tract infection (UTI) is one of the most common infections seen in the postoperative period. (See also Chapter 36.) The incidence of UTI rises with increasing age. Some 80% of UTIs are caused by bladder instrumentation, with catheter-associated UTI being most common (Lo et al., 2008). The rate of bacteriuria after undergoing an antiincontinence procedure has been estimated to be between 17% and 85% (Nygaard & Kreder, 1994). Reconstructive pelvic surgery almost always involves bladder instrumentation via cystoscopy and/or catheter placement, thereby increasing the risk of UTI in these patients. Additional risk factors for UTI include inefficient bladder emptying, pelvic relaxation, neurogenic bladder, asymptomatic bacteriuria, decreased ability to get to the toilet, nosocomial infections, physiologic changes, and sexual intercourse (Karram et al., 2007). Development of a fever in the postoperative period after female pelvic reconstruction should warrant a urinary tract evaluation; however, it is rare that lower UTI causes fever in itself. Fever may also warrant upper tract evaluation if urinalysis and/or urine culture is suspicious.

Multiple trials have evaluated the risk of UTI after urogynecological procedures. In a recent study by Thomas-White et al. (2018), female patients were more likely to develop UTI after pelvic surgery depending on their preoperative microbiome. In this study, UTI risk was associated with depletion of *Lactobacillus* and enrichment of a diverse mixture of uropathogens, and *Lactobacillus iners* appeared to be protective. In another recent study by El-Nashar et al. (2018), women who underwent hysterectomy for benign indications were evaluated for postoperative

UTI, and those who had hysterectomy without concomitant prolapse repair had a low rate of UTI (7.3%). Women who were postmenopausal, had anterior vaginal wall prolapse, and had high postvoid residuals (>150 mL) after surgery were at increased risk for postoperative UTI, with a range of 4.3% to 59.9% over an 8-week period.

In the Stress Incontinence Surgical Treatment Efficacy (SISTEr) trial, which compared Burch colposuspension to autologous fascial sling for treatment of stress urinary incontinence, the reported rate of UTI was 48% in the sling cohort and 32% in the Burch cohort during the first 24 months of follow-up (Albo et al., 2007). In the Trial of Midurethral Slings (TOMUS) study, retropubic midurethral slings were associated with significantly more UTIs than were transobturator slings in the first 6 weeks after surgery (13% vs. 8%, $P = .03$) and after 24 months' follow-up (21% vs. 13%, $P = .02$) (Brubaker et al., 2011).

Signs and symptoms of UTI in women are varied. Common cystitis symptoms include frequency, urgency, nocturia, dysuria, suprapubic discomfort, hematuria, and occasional mild incontinence. Fever, chills, general malaise, and costovertebral angle tenderness are associated with upper UTI (Nygaard & Kreder, 1994). There are multiple ways to diagnose UTI. Urine dipstick testing, often used as a rapid diagnostic test in the office, can detect the presence of leukocytes, bacteria, nitrites, and red blood cells. It also measures glucose, protein, ketones, blood, and bilirubin. In the setting of leukocytosis, and/or nitrites and hematuria, the sensitivity to detect UTI is 75%, but the specificity is 66% with a positive predictive value of 81% and a negative predictive value of 57% (Little et al., 2010). The most important predictor of UTI measured by microscopy is leukocytosis; however, leukocytosis alone is not sufficient to diagnose UTI (Komoroff et al., 1986). The gold standard to diagnosing UTI is a urine culture. The traditional diagnosis of UTI by culture is greater than 100,000 colony forming units (CFU)/mL; however, many women may have asymptomatic bacteriuria. In a study performed by Schiotz et al. (1994), 193 women who underwent gynecologic surgery and had a Foley catheter for 24 hours were assessed for bacteriuria; 40.9% of patients had asymptomatic bacteriuria, whereas only 8.3% of patients actually developed UTI. In contrast, those with fewer than 100,000 CFU/mL but symptoms of UTI can also be appropriately diagnosed as having a UTI.

The most common pathogen causing complicated and uncomplicated UTI is *Escherichia coli*. The definition of complicated UTI is UTI associated with a condition that increases the risk of acquiring infection or failing first-line treatment. Many patients with pelvic floor disorders with UTI may fit into the complicated category because they are currently catheterized or recently postcatheterization, as well as postprocedure (Hooten et al., 1997). Other uropathogens include *Klebsiella*, *Pseudomonas*, *Enterobacter*, *Enterococcus*, and *Candida*. The initial therapy for treatment of UTI traditionally has been trimethoprim-sulfamethoxazole (TMP-SMX) if the resistance in the population is less than 20%. However, owing to empiric treatment of UTI in the past, resistance to TMP-SMX and penicillins is high (up to 54% and 46%, respectively). Nitrofurantoin has been well-studied and is an additional agent used frequently to treat UTI. It is a cost-effective agent that may be used in the setting of fluroquinolone and TMP-SMX resistance (Mckinnell et al., 2011). Each hospital system should have an antimicrobiogram, which will indicate the most effective antibiotics for treatment of UTI in that region.

It is clear that patients who undergo female pelvic reconstructive procedures require antibiotic prophylaxis at the time of the procedure. The American Urologic Association Best Practice Guidelines recommend antibiotic prophylaxis for vaginal surgery to prevent both postoperative UTI and postoperative pelvic infection. A prospective randomized trial by Ingber et al. (2010) found that patients who were given single-dose antibiotic therapy for midurethral slings had a low rate of postoperative UTI (5.9%). Clinical trials have been mixed about whether multiple doses of antibiotics in the perioperative period decrease UTI rates beyond single-dose therapy. What is also unclear is the need for prophylactic antibiotics beyond the perioperative period in patients who will require prolonged catheterization. In a randomized, double-blind controlled trial conducted by Rogers et al. (2004), 449 patients who underwent pelvic organ prolapse and/or stress urinary incontinence surgery and had suprapubic catheters placed were given either placebo or nitrofurantoin monohydrate daily while the catheter was in place to assess rate of UTI. The study found a significant decrease in positive urine cultures, as well as symptomatic UTI, at suprapubic catheter removal with nitrofurantoin prophylaxis; however, there was no difference in symptomatic UTI at the 6- to 8-week postoperative visit. Two more recent randomized trials evaluating nitrofurantoin daily prophylaxis in patients with prolonged transurethral catheterization after pelvic reconstructive surgery found that daily nitrofurantoin during catheterization did not reduce risk of postoperative UTI (Dieter et al., 2014; Lavelle et al., 2019).

Surgical Site Infection

Infection complicating pelvic surgery can occur in multiple different settings. Mainly, infections are discovered as fever of unknown origin, operative site infection, and infections that are remote from surgery. The pathological source of most surgical site infections is from bacteria located on the skin or in the vagina. Skin flora are usually aerobic gram-positive cocci, but may include gram-negative, anaerobic, and/or fecal flora if incisions are made near the perineum and groin. Also, many pelvic reconstructive procedures may include implanted grafts or mesh, which can further complicate a postoperative infectious scenario (Bhatia et al., 1989).

Other patient comorbidities that may increase the risk of surgical site infections include advanced age, obesity, medical conditions, cancer, smoking, malnutrition, and immunosuppressant use (Walsh et al., 2009). Other risk factors for surgical site infection include poor hemostasis, length of stay, length of operative time, and tissue trauma. Specific risk factors for obese patients include increased bacterial growth on skin, decreased vascularity in the subcutaneous tissue, increased tension on wound closure because of increased intraabdominal pressure, decreased tissue concentrations of prophylactic antibiotics, a higher prevalence of diabetes with the potential of poor glucose control, and longer operating time (Boesch et al., 2009). In a retrospective review of patients who underwent midline abdominal incisions, patients with increased subcutaneous fat were 1.7 times more likely to develop a superficial incisional infection (Brummer et al., 2011). In a prospective study of 5279 patients who underwent hysterectomy, it was found that obese patients who underwent abdominal hysterectomy were five times more likely to have wound infection. Route of surgery was an additional risk factor for infection, with the highest risk in patients who underwent abdominal hysterectomy. Patients who underwent laparoscopic or vaginal hysterectomy were more likely to have remote pelvic infections compared with abdominal hysterectomy (Walsh et al., 2009). In a large retrospective study of over 22,000 patients undergoing hysterectomy, the rate of surgical site infection overall was 2.04%, and administration of β-lactam antibiotics before incision was associated with the lowest rate of surgical site infections (Uppal et al., 2016). It is therefore advised that patients with penicillin allergies should be questioned on their reaction thoroughly and undergo penicillin allergy testing before surgery to avoid alternate antibiotics if possible. In another large retrospective study of over 55,000 patients undergoing hysterectomy, it was found that, compared with those of normal BMI, women with BMI of 40 kg/m^2 or greater had five times the odds of wound dehiscence, five times the odds of wound infection, and 89% higher odds of sepsis (Shah et al., 2015).

Use of synthetic mesh may be an additional risk factor for surgical site infection, particularly when combined with concurrent hysterectomy. A retrospective analysis of over 200 patients who had vaginal hysterectomy at the time of sacrocolpopexy revealed a vaginal mesh exposure rate of 7.7%, and 1.9% of patients were treated for pelvic abscess (Jones et al., 2020). In randomized trials comparing native tissue vaginal repair to transvaginal mesh placement using wide-pore polypropylene, the risk of infection appears to be low in some trials (Hiltunen et al., 2007) and elevated in others (Vakili et al., 2005); however, many of these studies are small and are not adequately powered to detect differences in infectious morbidity.

Diagnosis of surgical site infection includes pain and tenderness at the operative site and fever. Postoperative fever is typically defined as a temperature of greater than 38°C on two or more occasions occurring at least 4 hours apart. Skin erythema, induration, and/or drainage of purulent or serosanguinous fluid may be visualized on examination. On pelvic exam, there may be pelvic, vaginal cuff, or parametrial tenderness. There may also be a leukocytosis on complete blood count. If pelvic abscess is suspected, ultrasound, CT scan, or magnetic resonance imaging (MRI) should be used for diagnosis. Ultrasound is a cost-effective way to image a patient with a suspected abscess. The sensitivity and specificity of pelvic ultrasound for detecting pelvic abscess are 81% and 91%, respectively (Moir et al., 1982) CT may be used to diagnose pelvic abscess when the diagnosis by ultrasound is equivocal. However, CT increases exposure to ionizing radiation, which may be problematic in younger patients.

Patients with superficial wound cellulitis may be treated with oral therapy. If there is evidence of a wound seroma or hematoma, a small portion of the wound may be opened and/or evacuated. It is important to probe the wound to ensure the fascia is intact. It may be necessary to remove staples and sutures in the infected area. Admission is recommended if a patient is febrile, has signs of peritonitis, has failed oral agents, has evidence of a pelvic or intraabdominal abscess, is unable to tolerate oral intake, or has laboratory evidence of sepsis (Vakili et al., 2005). Patients requiring admission should receive broad-spectrum parenteral antibiotics. Pelvic abscess may need drainage via opening of the vaginal cuff; CT- or ultrasound-guided drainage may also be used. A vaginal cuff abscess may necessitate opening part of or, in some cases, the entire cuff to allow for sufficient drainage. If mesh has been placed, it may need to be removed if directly involved with the infection to achieve adequate resolution.

Prevention of wound infection is paramount to the practice of reconstructive pelvic surgery. Good surgical technique, hemostasis, and gentle tissue handling may decrease risk of infection. There have been multiple studies that suggest perioperative cleansing of the vagina with saline (i.e., douching) increases infection rate (Kjolhede et al., 2009). Currently, there is no evidence to suggest that cleansing the vagina with any preparation reduces postoperative infection. However, in a retrospective cohort trial of 669 patients who underwent sacral nerve modulation therapy, it was found that chlorhexidine washing before the procedure may decrease rates of surgical site infections in this population (Brueseke et al., 2015).

The use of prophylactic antibiotics is an imperative strategy for lowering surgical site infection. Antibiotics should be given within 30 minutes of incision time to allow for the minimal inhibitory concentrations of the drug to be in the skin and tissues at time of incision. Recommendations for prophylactic antibiotic regimens from ACOG are listed in Table 26.3. Cephalosporins are commonly used in pelvic surgery because of their broad antimicrobial spectrum, with cefazolin the most

TABLE 26.3 American College of Obstetricians and Gynecologists Recommendations for Antibiotic Prophylaxis

Procedures	Antibiotic: Single Dose Intravenously Before Surgery
Hysterectomy, female pelvic reconstructive procedures, procedures involving mesh	Cefazolin 2 g; 3 g for patients weighing greater than 120 kg[a] If immediate hypersensitivity reactions to penicillin: Clindamycin 900 mg or Metronidazole 500 mg PLUS Gentamicin 5 mg/kg[b] or Aztreonam 2 gm

[a]Alternatives include cefotetan, cefoxitin, cefuroxime, or ampicillin-sulbactam.

[b] Dosage is based on the patient's actual body weight. If the patient's actual weight is more than 20% above ideal body weight (IBW), the "dosing weight" (DW) can be determined as follows: DW = IBW+0.4 (actual weight – IBW).

(Modified from ACOG Practice Bulletin, No. 195.)

BOX 26.2 American College of Obstetricians and Gynecologists Recommendations for Reducing Surgical Site Infections

Ensure preoperative glycemic control with target blood sugar levels of ≤200 mg/dL in diabetic and nondiabetic patients
Do not shave before surgery, use clippers for hair removal
Perform preoperative surgical site skin preparation with an alcohol-based or chlorhexidine alcohol–based agent

commonly used agent (ACOG Practice Bulletin, No. 195, 2018). Patients who are morbidly obese, with a BMI greater than 35 kg/m^2, should receive increased dosing of antibiotics (Walsh et al., 2009) Procedures lasting longer than 3 hours and involving blood loss greater than 1500 mL require redosing of antibiotics. Other considerations recommended by ACOG are shown in Box 26.2.

SMALL BOWEL OBSTRUCTION

Postoperative small bowel obstruction (SBO) is a relatively rare complication of female pelvic surgery; however, it can be debilitating and cause prolonged postoperative recovery. The incidence of SBO after hysterectomy can be as high as 1.1%, depending on route of surgery (Muffly et al., 2012). Most SBOs are considered to form because of intraabdominal adhesions, but when SBO occurs in the immediate postoperative period, it may be attributed to mechanical reasons related to the surgery (Pickleman et al., 1989). In a large retrospective study by Sheyn et al. (2019), 286 patients were diagnosed with SBO from among 47,937 women who underwent hysterectomy for benign indications, a rate of 5.9 per 1000 hysterectomies. Older patients and those who smoked were at higher risk. Surgical procedures that increased the risk of SBO included abdominal hysterectomy, lysis of adhesions, cystotomy, and cystotomy repair. Patients also were at increased risk of SBO if they had undergone blood transfusion during the surgery, lysis of adhesions, or concurrent appendectomy. A meta-analysis by Campbell et al. (2016) comparing abdominal versus laparoscopic sacrocolpopexy identified an increase in SBO in patients who underwent the abdominal approach versus the laparoscopic approach (odds ratio, 2.88; 95% confidence interval [CI], 1.3–6.33).

Although there are case reports of SBO occurring after vaginal prolapse procedures (Ridgeway et al., 2007), the rate is extremely low. In a retrospective review by Unger et al. (2015) describing 983 patients who underwent uterosacral vaginal vault suspension, it was found that the rates of postoperative ileus and SBO were 0.1% (95% CI, 0.02–0.6) and 0.8% (95% CI, 0.4–1.6), respectively. There have been numerous case reports describing SBO after using a thrombin-gelatin hemostatic matrix (Flo-seal; Baxter Healthcare, Deerfield, IL) (Clapp et al., 2011; Suzuki et al., 2010). These reports describe SBO detected early in the postoperative period, and these patients required additional surgery with removal of the material that caused inflammation around the small bowel. Overall, when feasible, vaginal or laparoscopic procedures have decreased rates of SBO relative to the open approach.

SMALL BOWEL INJURY

Bowel injury is a rare complication of pelvic reconstructive surgery but can occur with the abdominal, laparoscopic, or vaginal approaches. Intraoperative recognition and repair are essential to avoid the potentially devastating sequelae of peritonitis, abscess, and sepsis that can be associated with delayed recognition. Other potential sequelae of small bowel injury include fistula, prolonged ileus, and bowel obstruction. Potential mechanisms of intestinal injury include laceration, perforation, thermal or burn injury, crush with associated ischemic injury, and mensenteric/vascular injury. It is important to be cognizant of the mechanism of injury, as it will dictate the management approach. Tears that involve only the serosa can typically be managed with simple interrupted sutures or imbrication using a Lembert-style repair. Small serosal tears may require no treatment. Intramural hematomas will usually heal spontaneously and do not typically require intervention. Full-thickness defects will require either a primary repair or resection and primary anastomosis, depending on the nature and extent of the injury. A mesenteric vascular injury will require careful inspection of the bowel to assess for viability. All bowel with compromised vasculature will require wide resection with primary anastomosis of the viable bowel. When a bowel injury occurs because of trocar injury, whether laparoscopic or from a sling or prolapse mesh device, it is prudent to leave the trocar in position until the full nature of the injury is known, as it is much easier to identify the location of the injury with the trocar in place. Ileostomy is rarely, if ever, required to manage an intraoperative small bowel injury. If the surgeon is in doubt about the appropriate approach or does not feel comfortable repairing a small bowel injury, then the next step is to obtain an intraoperative general surgical consult.

Enterotomy Repair

Small bowel lacerations of less than half of the circumference of the small bowel without associated vascular or thermal injury may be repaired primarily without bowel resection. The surgical steps are as follows:

1. Isolate and expose injury: Identify and adequately expose the bowel injury. The small bowel should be inspected in its entirety to ensure that all injuries are identified (e.g., "run the bowel"). Isolate the site of injury with noncrushing bowel clamps or Babcock clamps to prevent further spillage of bowel contents. The mesentery should be inspected for any vascular compromise. Any active mesenteric bleeding should be controlled by isolation and ligation of individual vessels, rather than by mass ligation of the mesentery, which can produce ischemia.
2. Repair enterotomy: Although single-layer closure has been described, we prefer a two-layered closure. It is essential that the edges of the repair be viable; any devascularized or nonviable tissue should be debrided. The first layer of closure can be performed with simple interrupted sutures or a

running suture of No. 3-0 or 4-0 absorbable suture material incorporating all layers. The closure should run perpendicular to the direction of the bowel (transverse closure), regardless of the direction of the tear (Fig. 26.1). This layer is then buried by an interrupted longitudinal mattress stitch through the seromuscular layer using No. 3-0 delayed absorbable suture or silk. The reason for the direction of closure is to prevent stricture at the site of the repair, as longitudinal closure can cause narrowing of the lumen. The integrity of the repair may be assessed by milking small bowel contents across the line of repair and observing for leakage.

3. Irrigate the area copiously.

Small Bowel Resection and Primary Anastomosis

Full-thickness small bowel injuries that are larger than 50% of the bowel circumference, or injuries that include significant thermal or vascular injury should be repaired with small bowel resection and primary anastomosis. Also, if multiple enterotomies occur within a localized segment of small bowel, it is often prudent to resect the entire damaged segment rather than perform multiple primary enterotomy repairs, regardless of their size. Similarly, if primary repair will result in significant narrowing of the small bowel lumen, resection and primary anastomosis should be performed. Small bowel resection can be repaired using either an end-to-end hand-sewn repair or a side-to-side (functional end-to-end) anastamosis with a linear stapler; here we focus on a stapled repair. Gastrointestinal anastomosis (GIA) and TA staplers are required for a stapled small bowel repair. Noncrushing bowel clamps and/or Babcock clamps are also useful.

1. Isolate and expose injury: Identify and adequately expose the bowel injury. The small bowel should be inspected in its entirety to ensure that all injuries are identified (e.g., "run the bowel"). Isolate the site of injury with noncrushing bowel clamps or Babcock clamps to prevent further spillage of bowel contents. Moist laparotomy sponges can be used to isolate the damaged bowel from the remaining peritoneal contents. The mesentery should be inspected for any vascular compromise. Any active mesenteric bleeding should be controlled by isolation and ligation of individual vessels, rather than by mass ligation of the mesentery, which can produce ischemia. Direct observation of the affected bowel, Doppler ultrasound, or intravenous fluorescein can be used to determine the adequacy of blood flow to the affected small bowel. After the margins of the resection have been determined, electrocautery is used to score the peritoneum on either side of the mesentery in a V shape to encompass only vessels related to the section to be removed (Fig. 26.2A).
2. Divide the small bowel segment: A window is made in an avascular section of the mesentery adjacent to the bowel at the site of the planned margins. Using this window, the GIA stapler is passed through on either side of the segment of bowel being divided and engaged, creating two staple lines and two ends (Fig. 26.2A). Typically, the 3.8-mm GIA stapler is adequate, although a larger size may be needed if the bowel is thickened. This is repeated on the other side to isolate the bowel segment to be resected.
3. Divide the mesentery: After the bowel is divided, the mesentery is divided using electrocautery. Lifting the small bowel, the vascular arcade of the mesentery can typically be seen by transillumination. The vascular pedicles are ligated with No. 3-0 absorbable suture, hemoclips, or a harmonic scalpel. The isolated segment of damaged bowel is removed.
4. Side-to-side anastomosis: The two segments of small bowel to be used for the anastomosis are positioned for the side-to-side anastomosis with their antimesenteric sides in contact.

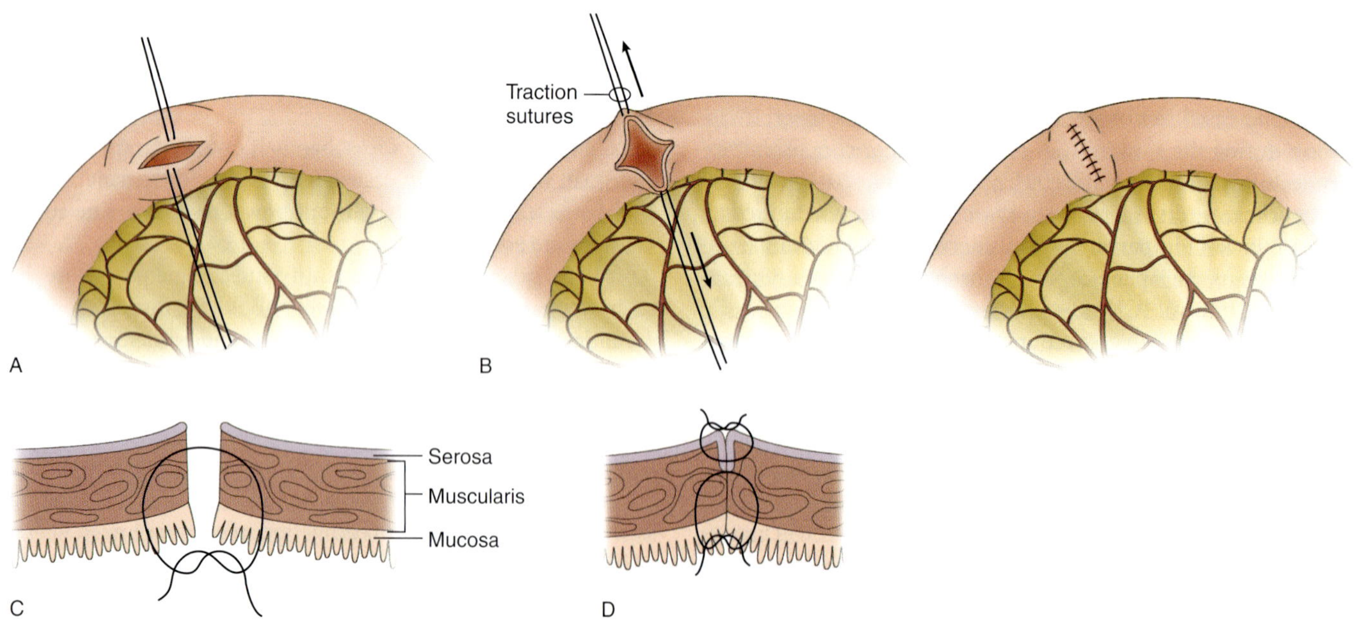

Fig. 26.1 Repair of enterotomy. **A** and **B**, The repair should be performed so that the closure is perpendicular to the axis of the small bowel. **C** and **D**, Two-layer closure incorporating the mucosa and muscularis in the inner layer and the serosa and muscularis on the outer layer. (From Nichols DH, Clarke-Pearson DL, eds. *Gynecologic, Obstetric and Related Surgery*, 2nd ed. St. Louis: Mosby; 2000.)

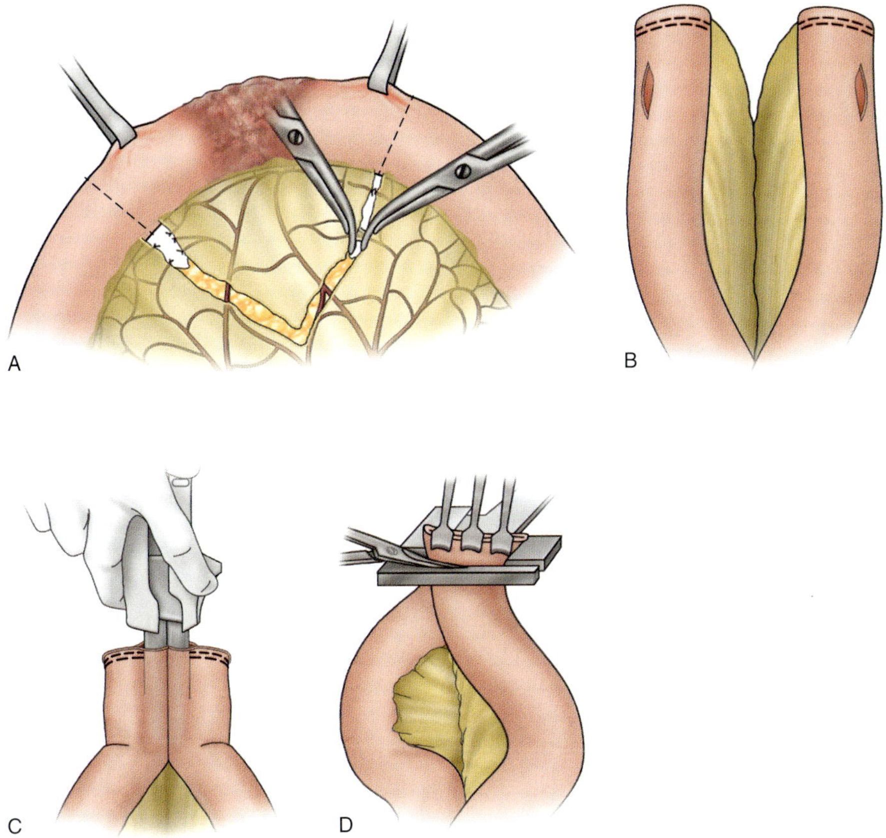

Fig. 26.2 Repair of small bowel injury with side-to-side intestinal anastomosis **A**, Electrocautery is used to score the peritoneum on either side of the mesentery in a V shape of resection margins. **B,** Enterotomy on the antimesenteric side. **C**, The opposing limbs of a gastrointestinal anastomosis stapler are then placed within the lumens, and the stapler is closed and fired along the antimesenteric border. **D**, Stapling below the clamps. (Modified from Smith JA, Howards SS, Preminger GM, Dmochowski RR, eds. *Hinman's Atlas of Urologic Surgery*, 4th ed. Philadelphia, 2018, Elsevier.)

Stay sutures of No. 3-0 suture can be used to assist with orientation if needed. Adjacent corners of the staple lines are cut off, and a GIA cutting stapler (60 mm or 80 mm) is inserted, with one arm of the stapler in the distal small bowel and the other in the proximal small bowel (Fig. 26.2C). The stapler is engaged, creating a connection with the length of the stapler between the two ends of the bowel that establishes the functional side-to-side anastomosis. This internal staple line should be inspected to identify any sites of bleeding. Interrupted No. 4-0 sutures can be placed for hemostasis in any bleeding areas.

5. Close the end of the anastomosis: The open end of the anastomosis is closed by firing a TA stapler across the free ends of the joined bowel loops (Fig. 26.2D). The staple line can be inverted using a row of No. 3-0 or 4-0 interrupted Lembert sutures to ensure closure. A simple suture can also be placed at the "crotch" of the anastomosis for additional support. The integrity of the repair may be assessed by milking small bowel contents across the line of repair and observing for leakage.
6. Close the mesenteric defect: Large mesenteric defects should be closed with continuous or interrupted No. 3-0 absorbable suture.
7. Irrigate the area copiously.

Although once common practice, the literature does not support routine nasogastric suction after repair of a small bowel injury. Multiple randomized trials have demonstrated that routine nasogastric decompression is associated with an increased rate of pneumonia, atelectasis, and fever in the postoperative period compared with no decompression. Moreover, nasogastric suction increases patient discomfort, sinus infection, and epistaxis. As such, nasogastric suction should not be performed routinely after small bowel resection. Patients should be monitored closely, and, if they develop signs and symptoms of a postoperative ileus, selective use of nasogastric suction is warranted. As with nasogastric suction, delayed postoperative feeding after bowel resection was once common practice. Current data support early postoperative feeding even after small bowel resection. Randomized trials demonstrate similar rates of ileus, anastomotic leak, and time required for return to normal bowel function between patients receiving early feeding compared with those receiving delayed feeding after surgery. There is no need to continue antibiotics into the postoperative period after an isolated small bowel injury.

RECTAL INJURY

As with small bowel injuries, intraoperative recognition and repair of rectal injury are also essential to avoid the significant complications that can be associated with delayed recognition, including abscess, sepsis, and rectovaginal fistula. Because of the high bacterial count of the colon and rectum, rectal injury imparts a significantly higher risk of infection than small bowel injury. Intraoperative detection of rectal injury is aided by liberal use of digital rectal examinations during and after surgery, particularly vaginal surgery. The use of a rigid protoscope or flexible sigmoidoscope should also be considered when a rectal injury is suspected. A "bubble test," where air is insufflated into the rectum via proctoscope while sterile water or saline is in the operative field, is also a useful technique for intraoperative detection of rectal injuries.

Also similar to small bowel injury, the location and mechanism of injury dictate the appropriate management of rectal injuries. Serosal tears can typically be managed with simple single-layer closure using No. 2-0 or 3-0 absorbable suture. Full-thickness extraperitoneal rectal lacerations can typically be repaired with primary closure. Injuries that occur during vaginal surgery can often be satisfactorily repaired transvaginally. Intraperitoneal injuries that involve less than 50% of the bowel wall and are not devascularized or that involve thermal injury or significant peritonitis can also be managed with primary closure. Large tears that involve more than 50% of the bowel wall, particularly when intraperitoneal or when associated with devascularization or significant thermal injury, will require rectosigmoid resection and primary anastomosis. Diverting colostomy should be considered in the presence of shock or sepsis, previous radiation, delayed recognition, and/or significant fecal contamination. Historically, mechanical bowel preparation has often been recommended before laparoscopic or open pelvic reconstructive procedures. However, the currently available data do not support this practice. A metaanalysis evaluating the value of preoperative mechanical bowel preparation before elective colorectal surgery suggests an increased rate of anastomotic leak after bowel preparation, with no benefit in postoperative infectious morbidity compared with no preoperative bowel preparation. If the surgeon is in doubt about the appropriate approach or does not feel comfortable repairing a rectal injury, then an intraoperative general surgery or colorectal surgery consult should be obtained.

Primary Repair of Proctotomy

Most extraperitoneal injuries and intraperitoneal injuries that involve less than 50% of the bowel wall and are not devascularized or involve thermal injury or significant peritonitis can be managed with primary closure. The surgical steps are as follows:

1. Isolate and expose the injury: Identify and adequately expose the bowel injury. Isolate the site of injury with atraumatic clamps to prevent further spillage of bowel contents. For intraperitoneal lesions, the mesentery should be inspected for any vascular compromise. Any active mesenteric bleeding should be controlled by isolation and ligation of individual vessels rather than by mass ligation of the mesentery, which can produce ischemia.
2. Repair proctotomy: Although single-layer closure has been described, we prefer a two-layered closure. It is essential that the edges of the repair be viable; any devascularized or nonviable tissue should be debrided. The first layer of closure can be performed with simple interrupted sutures or a running suture of No. 3-0 absorbable suture material incorporating all layers. With rectum or colon injuries, the direction of closure is less critical than with small bowel injuries, as narrowing of the rectal lumen is unlikely. A second layer consisting of interrupted longitudinal mattress stitches through the seromuscular layer using No. 2-0 or 3-0 delayed absorbable suture is performed. The integrity of the repair may be assessed via digital rectal exam, proctoscopy, or a "bubble test" as described earlier.
3. Irrigate the area copiously.

Rectosigmoid Resection With Primary Anastomosis

Large intraperitoneal rectal injuries that involve more than 50% of the bowel wall or a rectal injury associated with significant devascularization or thermal injury should be repaired with rectosigmoid resection and primary anastomosis. GIA and end-to-end anastomosis (EEA) staplers are required for a rectosigmoid resection and stapled EEA. Noncrushing bowel clamps and Babcock clamps are also useful. The surgical steps are as follows:

1. Isolate and expose the injury: Identify and adequately expose the bowel injury. Isolate the site of injury with atraumatic clamps to prevent further spillage of bowel contents. For intraperitoneal lesions, the mesentery should be inspected for any vascular compromise. Any active mesenteric bleeding should be controlled by isolation and ligation of individual vessels rather than by mass ligation of the mesentery, which can produce ischemia.
2. Rectosigmoid resection: Proximal to the area of injury, a small mesenteric window is made adjacent to the sigmoid colon. A GIA stapler is placed across the bowel and fired, transecting the sigmoid colon proximately and creating two staple lines isolating the proximal and distal ends. The sigmoid mesentery is transected parallel to the rectum to below the area of injury, ligating the vascular pedicles with sutures, hemoclips, and/or the harmonic scalpel. If possible, the left colonic branch of the inferior mesenteric artery should be preserved. The perirectal, rectovaginal and rectorectal spaces are developed, mobilizing the rectosigmoid until normal rectum is encountered distally. Care should be taken to avoid ureteral injury and injury to presacral vessels during this dissection. The TA stapler is placed distally across the rectum below the level of injury. The stapler is locked in the proper position and fired to place a staple line across the distal rectum. An atraumatic bowel clamp is placed just proximal to this staple line, and the rectum is transected between the clamp and the staple line. The rectal segment is removed from the operative field.
3. Mobilize the sigmoid colon: The remaining sigmoid and left colon should be mobilized to ensure a tension-free

anastomosis. The colon is retracted medially, and the lateral peritoneal attachments are incised with electrocautery, starting at the pelvic brim and extending cephalad parallel to the descending colon. If necessary, this can be carried up to the splenic flexure to transect the splenocolic ligament and mobilize the transverse colon to provide adequate mobilization.

4. Rectosigmoid anastomosis: An atraumatic bowel clamp is placed across the end of the descending colon, and the proximal staple line is excised with a scalpel. An appropriately-sized EEA stapler is selected by determining the largest EEA obturator that can be inserted without difficulty into the bowel lumen. The "anvil and spike" of the EEA sizer is inserted into the distal end of the descending colon and secured with a purse string suture placed circumferentially around the open lumen so that the anvil is within the lumen, and the "spike" protrudes out the end (Fig. 26.3). The EEA stapler is introduced into the anus and guided to the end of the rectal stump. The wing nut on the handle of the stapler is turned clockwise to advance a sharp trocar that pierces through the middle of the rectal stump. This sharp trocar is removed exposing a hollow shaft. The spike protruding from the end of the descending colon is placed into this hollow shaft and locked into place. Additional clockwise rotation of the wing nut brings the ends of the rectal stump and sigmoid colon in direct opposition, as indicated by the indicator line being visible in the indicator window on the stapler device. After assuring appropriate alignment of the sigmoid mesentery, the safety is released, and the handles are closed to fire the EEA stapler. The stapler tip is gently freed from the anastomosis and slowly withdrawn from the rectum.
5. Assess integrity of anastomosis: The integrity of the anastomosis is assessed in three ways: direct inspection of the surgical site, verification of an intact "O" ring from the stapler (two complete 360-degree tissue rings from the rectal and colonic ends should be present), and performance of a "bubble test." Finally, proctoscopy should be performed to inspect the staple line. If there is any concern for an incomplete anastomosis, reinforcement with interrupted No. 3-0 sutures should be performed and the integrity of the anastomosis retested.
6. Irrigate the area copiously.

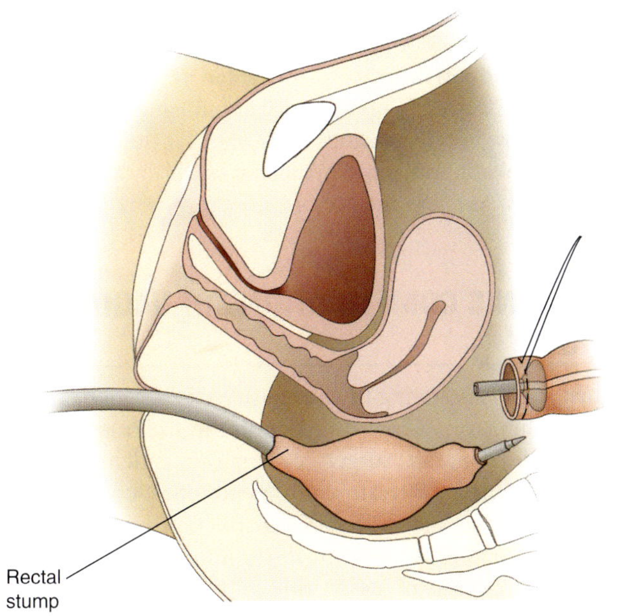

Fig. 26.3 Rectosigmoid anastomosis using end-to-end anastomosis stapler. (Modified from Smith JA, Howards SS, Preminger GM, Dmochowski RR, eds. *Hinman's Atlas of Urologic Surgery*, 4th ed. Philadelphia, 2018, Elsevier.)

As with small bowel injury, there is no need for routine nasogastric suction after large bowel injury and repair. Patients should be monitored closely, and in those who develop signs and symptoms of an ileus, selective nasogastric decompression may be warranted. Recent trends also support early postoperative feeding after large bowel injury or resection. There is no need to delay feeding in most cases. Broad-spectrum antibiotics should be continued for 24 hours into the postoperative period after large bowel injury without significant intraperitoneal fecal spillage. When there is gross contamination of the peritoneal cavity, antibiotics should be continued for 48 to 72 hours after surgery.

NERVE INJURY

Intraoperative nerve injury is a preventable iatrogenic complication. Injury to nerves in the upper and lower extremities, although uncommon, may occur during laparotomy, robotic, laparoscopic, and vaginal procedures. In a prospective cohort study of women who underwent elective gynecologic surgery, the overall incidence of postoperative neuropathy was 1.8% (Bohrer et al., 2009). Brachial plexus injury has a reported incidence of 0.16% (Romanowski et al., 1993). Risk factors for developing nerve injury during surgery include increased operating room time, patient positioning, and history of smoking (Warner et al., 2000). Stretching or direct compression of the nerve results in ischemia, and, when prolonged, necrosis can develop (Britt & Gordon, 1964). With muscle relaxants given during anesthesia, patients are unable to reposition themselves from nonphysiologic positions, and risk of nerve damage increases. With nerve compression, blood flow to the nerve is decreased, therefore operating room time is a critical factor for nerve injury. The longer a patient is incorrectly positioned, the worse the nerve injury. With the development of robotic surgery, it has been theorized that brachial plexus injuries may become more common (Shveiky et al., 2010). Most robotic procedures require steep Trendelenburg positioning and, depending on the operator, may require longer operating room times. Other risk factors include history of diabetes, alcoholism, and history of herpes zoster (Parks, 1973).

Nerve injuries to the upper extremity mostly occur from overstretching or compression of the brachial plexus or the ulnar nerve. Brachial plexus injury may result in both sensory and/or motor injury. Risk factors for brachial plexus injury include Trendelenburg positioning, longer operating room time, use of shoulder braces, abduction of the arm at 90 degrees or greater, and unequal shoulder support. Patients with brachial plexus injury may present with numbness of the first, second, and third digits and the radial side of the fourth digit. Patients may experience motor deficits that involve the shoulder, wrist, arm, and hand. In severe cases, patients may experience Erb palsy or Klumpke paralysis. Patients with ulnar nerve injury may present with the sensory loss of the lateral hand, with loss of sensation in the fourth and fifth digits.

Management of brachial plexus injury includes physical therapy, analgesics, nonsteroidal antiinflammatory medications, physical therapy, and neuropathic pain medications such as gabapentin. Prevention of brachial plexus injury includes utilizing the minimum amount of Trendelenburg positioning, decreasing operating room time as much as possible, avoiding abduction or extension of the upper extremities, and avoiding shoulder braces (Britt et al., 1964). For robotic and laparoscopic surgeries, we recommend padding and tucking the patient's arms to her sides, using a "thumbs-up" hand position with the patient's palms facing her thighs to avoid overabduction. Egg crate foam or "sticky mats" may be placed under the patient to decrease movement or sliding down the operating table.

Common lower extremity nerve injuries associated with female pelvic reconstructive surgery include femoral, lateral femoral cutaneous, obturator, sciatic, and common peroneal nerve injuries. Risk factors for lower extremity nerve injuries include ill positioning of the lower extremities using stirrups, lithotomy position, underweight, smoking, Trendelenburg position, and operating room time greater than 4 hours (Barnett et al., 2007). In laparoscopic and vaginal surgeries, the femoral nerve may be injured because of stretch encountered from the lithotomy position. The lateral cutaneous femoral nerve is one of the nerves most commonly injured from lithotomy position, and injury is caused from compression and stretching under the inguinal ligament, most likely from prolonged flexion of the lower extremities. The obturator nerve may be injured from prolonged flexion of the legs in the lithotomy position. Sciatic nerve injury is less common in the dorsal lithotomy position; however, it may be caused by overflexion of the hip with abduction and external rotation. The common peroneal nerve can be injured via direct pressure on the nerve when the lateral calf is touching the pole of the candy cane stirrups—boot stirrups may aid in decreasing risk of injury to this nerve (Parks, 1973).

To prevent lower extremity neuropathies caused by female pelvic reconstructive surgery, it is necessary to use correct positioning of the lower extremities. When positioning the lower extremities in boot stirrups, make sure the heel of the patient's foot fits directly into the boot. Padding the lateral aspect of the knee avoids injury to the peroneal nerve. When placing a patient in high lithotomy, the knee should be flexed 90 to 120 degrees, hip flexion should be less than 60 degrees, and abduction of the thighs should be no greater than 90 degrees. Nerve injuries from reconstructive pelvic surgery are minimized when the patient's extremities are positioned correctly.

Injury to the pudendal and other pelvic nerves may occur during specific pelvic reconstructive procedures. In the Operations and Pelvic Muscle Training in the Management of Apical Support Loss (OPTIMAL) trial, 374 women with apical vaginal prolapse were randomized to either sacrospinous ligament fixation or uterosacral vault suspension, and neurologic pain requiring intervention (medications, trigger point injections, or suture release) occurred more frequently after sacrospinous ligament fixation (6.9% vs. 12.4%) and persisted to 4 to 6 weeks after surgery more often (0.5% vs. 4.3%) (Barber et al., 2015). In the TOMUS study, neurologic complications were noted more frequently in sling procedures performed via the transobturator than the retropubic approach (9.7% vs. 5.0%, $P = .04$); however, most of these were minor and represented transient inner thigh numbness and weakness that resolved by 6 weeks (Brubaker et al., 2011). Of note, four patients (0.7%) had persistent postoperative neurologic symptoms at 24 months after surgery, without any difference between the transobturator and retropubic approaches.

TABLE 26.4 Motor and Sensory Defects Associated With Lower Extremity Neuropathy

Nerve	Motor Function	Sensory Loss
Femoral	Hip flexion and knee extension	Anterior and medial thigh, medial calf
Lateral femoral cutaneous	N/A	Anterior and lateral thigh
Sciatic	Foot dorsiflexion and eversion	Foot, toes
Obturator	Thigh adduction and internal rotation	Medial aspect of the thigh
Common peroneal	Foot dorsiflexion and eversion	N/A

N/A, Not applicable.

Diagnosis of postoperative neuropathy should include a thorough musculoskeletal and neurological examination (Table 26.4). Patients may experience pain, numbness, and tingling in dermatomes of the nerve routes. Electromyography and MRI are procedures that may further aid in diagnosis. Treatment includes oral analgesics, nonsteroidal antiinflammatory medications, low-dose antidepressants, medications including gabapentin and pregabalin, and physical therapy, especially for prolonged neuropathies. Surgery and steroid injections may be used for severe cases.

IATROGENIC COMPLICATIONS OF VAGINAL SURGERY

Vaginal surgery resulting in vaginal stenosis, severe pain, vaginal shortening, or vaginal constriction can occur after vaginal native tissue (nongraft) surgery, especially in patients who have received radiation for treatment of gynecologic malignancy or who have undergone overzealous correction of pelvic organ prolapse, such as excessive vaginal trimming or aggressive levatorplasty at the time of a posterior colporrhaphy. This section of the chapter will discuss how best to avoid and manage a foreshortened vagina, vaginal constriction, and loss of denuded vaginal and/or perineal skin after traditional suture repairs for pelvic organ prolapse.

Foreshortened Vagina

Before undertaking an operation for pelvic organ prolapse, the surgeon should determine the anticipated length of the vagina. Although there are little data to support how long a vagina needs to be to facilitate normal sexual function, we believe that the vagina should be suspended or supported to between 7 and 9 cm cephalad to the hymenal ring. This reference point is the approximate location of the ischial spine, which is a good anatomic marker to use in whatever procedure is being performed to support or suspend the vaginal apex. Suspension of the apex should be done in such a way that it does not greatly alter the axis of the vagina. The surgeon should always keep in mind that anatomy varies, and that patient expectations differ. Some patients' anatomy allows for greater depth; conversely, some patients do not desire a functional vagina, and the surgeon can intentionally reduce the depth and diameter.

A foreshortened vagina presents a difficult surgical dilemma. The majority of affected patients have considerable scarring. In such situations, we prefer to use a unipolar cautery device to cut through this scar tissue and to open the apex of the vagina. To keep the upper part of the vagina open, local estrogen and daily dilation should be initiated in the immediate postoperative period to keep scar from reforming. If the vagina can be kept open, it often heals well by secondary intention. Another approach is to cover these raw areas with a free skin graft or a biologic material, such as porcine-derived small intestinal submucosa or urinary bladder extracellular matrix. It is important in the postoperative period to see the patient frequently, to apply transvaginal estrogen cream, and to keep the vagina open by means of frequent examinations, an intravaginal mold, and early initiation of a vaginal dilator. See Video 26.1 for the correction of a foreshortened vagina and Video 26.2 for the use of biologic grafts in the correction of apical vaginal banding.

When less aggressive approaches are not successful, other, more advanced surgical options can be used. One approach is to manage the situation as we would for a patient with vaginal agenesis, by opening the top of the vagina and placing a skin graft with a mold. If using a transvaginal approach, every effort should be made to avoid entering the peritoneal cavity. The peritoneum provides the blood supply to the skin graft and confines the skin graft and mold within the vagina. If the peritoneum is entered, the skin graft or other material used to replace the vagina then requires fixation and a compensatory blood supply. Often an abdominal approach to mobilize an omental J-flap to provide a blood supply and support for the skin graft is then used. Finally, a colon interposition graft (sigmoid) can be used to create a neovagina or to augment a severely foreshortened vagina.

Vaginal Constriction

Vaginal constriction can occur after any vaginal procedure, including prolapse and episiotomy repair. Avoiding vaginal constriction is of paramount importance, and thus the surgeon should always ensure the ability to place two or three fingers into the vaginal canal during the repair and at the completion of the procedure. If repair has been too extensive and a constriction band is noted intraoperatively, immediate takedown of the offending suture is indicated. If, however, the vagina was not examined during the repair, and the epithelium has already been trimmed and closed, a relaxing incision can be made through the constriction band at 4 o'clock, 8 o'clock, or bilaterally (Fig. 26.4A–F). After hemostasis is ensured, this area usually heals well by secondary intention, thus maintaining appropriate caliber of the vagina. All patients who undergo vaginal surgery for pelvic organ prolapse should have a vaginal examination within 2 to 3 weeks after surgery to identify and prevent fusion or scarification that can occur when raw surfaces from the anterior and posterior vaginal walls come into contact with each other. If the patient is not examined in the postoperative period, the vaginal canal may fuse or severely constrict. If the early development of a tight or constricted vagina is detected in the postoperative period, application of local estrogen and use of a vaginal dilator may help prevent the process from continuing.

When a patient presents with postoperative vaginal constriction, we have not had much success with vaginal dilators. Usually, the dilator cannot be advanced beyond the point of constriction because of patient discomfort; thus, the majority of these patients are treated surgically. Surgical management depends on the severity of the constriction and, more importantly, the location of the constriction. Distal vaginal constrictions can be treated by introitoplasty procedures, where the constriction is cut longitudinally and then closed horizontally by mobilizing and advancing the vagina (Fig. 26.5 and Videos 26.3 and 26.4). Alternatively, various Z-plasty procedures can be used (Fig. 26.6). Both of these approaches require sufficient vaginal length, as they address only the constriction band.

For midvaginal constrictions, cutting through the constriction band sharply with a scalpel or electrosurgical instrument has been successful. The area is then either allowed to heal by secondary intention, or a skin graft or other biologic material is placed to patch the defect in the vaginal canal (Figs. 26.7 and 26.8 and Video 26.5). Usually packing is left in place after ensuring hemostasis in the operating room. The packing is removed within 24 hours (sometimes it is left longer, with more extensive dissections), and the area is inspected on a regular basis, with vaginal examinations recommended at least twice weekly for the first 2 weeks. If the midvaginal constriction is not amenable to simple incision, a vertical Z-plasty or a unilateral or bilateral perineal flap may be required to address severe constrictions. These procedures require a large incision through the constriction band, extending outward like a mediolateral episiotomy. The perineal flap is created and rotated into the vaginal incision, where it is secured in place.

Denuded or Lost Vaginal or Perineal Skin

The vagina and perineum are well-vascularized and reepithelialize well. Small, denuded areas heal by secondary intention, with no long-term sequelae. However, excision of a larger area, for example, after removal of mesh or release of large constriction rings, leaves large, deep denuded areas that require coverage. Historically, the only option was use of a skin graft. This has traditionally been reserved for use in patients with congenital anomalies of the vagina (e.g., thick transverse vaginal septum and vaginal agenesis) or for vaginal constrictions or

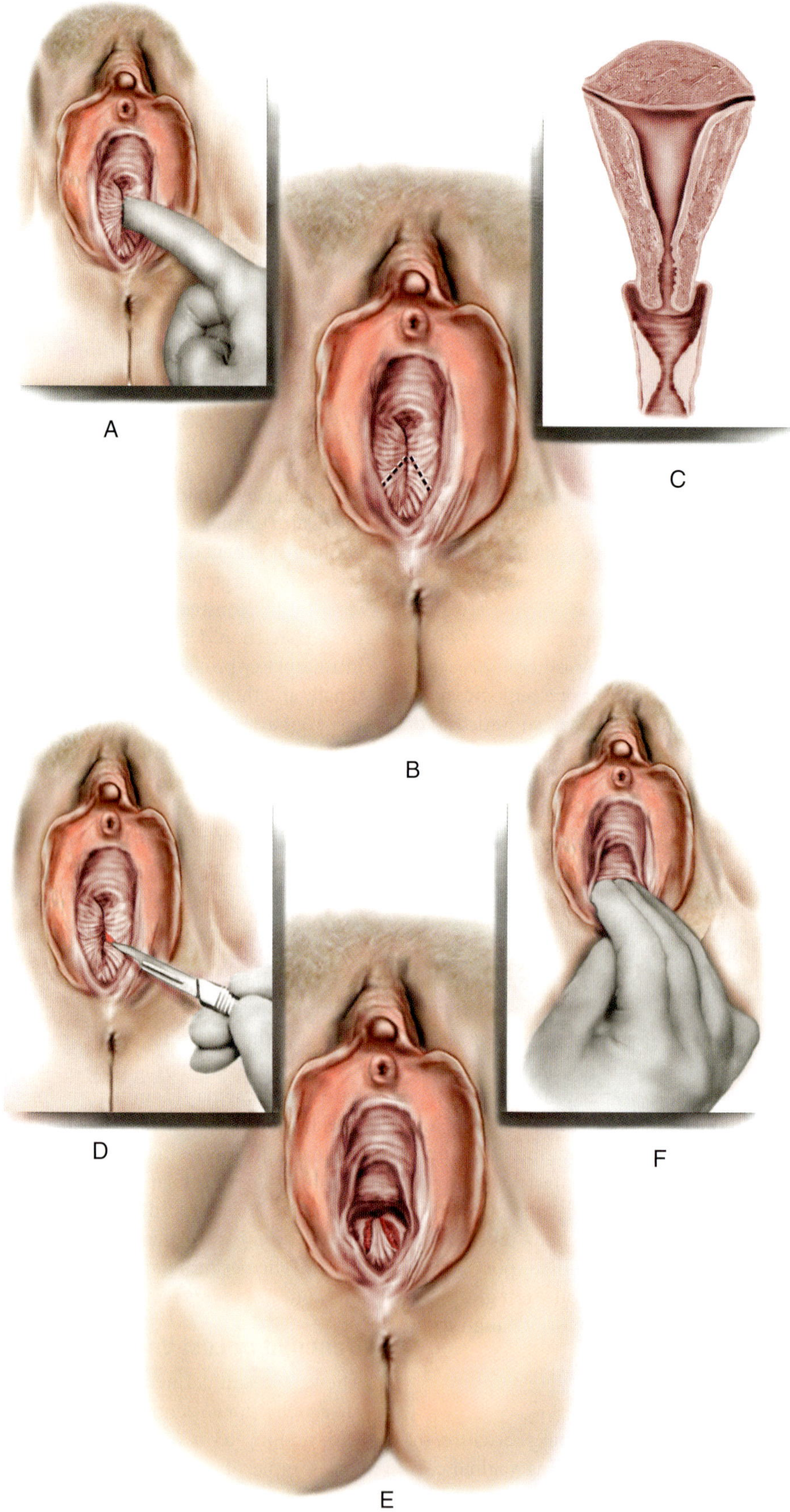

Fig. 26.4 Bilateral relaxing incisions for mid- to distal vaginal constriction. **A**, Midvaginal constriction allows penetration of only one finger. **B**, Sites of relaxing incisions are marked at 4 o'clock and 8 o'clock. **C**, Cross-section showing midvaginal constriction. **D**, Relaxing incisions are made with scalpel or monopolar cautery. Incision should extend through the complete thickness of the constriction band. **E**, Bilateral vaginal defects with complete release of constriction band. **F**, Examination allows penetration of two fingers.

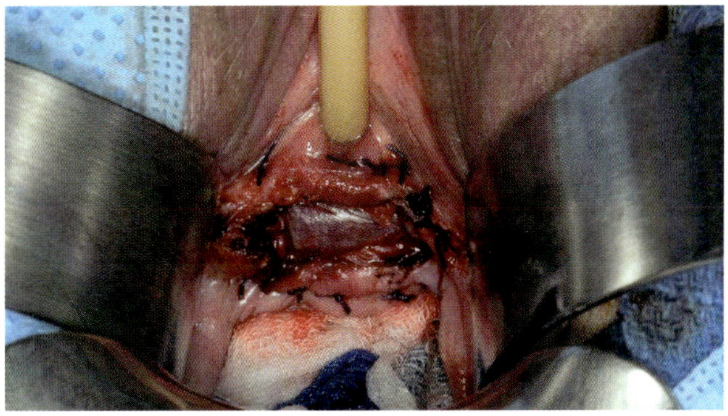

Fig. 26.5 Use of biologic graft (acellular, extracellular matrix derived from porcine small intestinal submucosa) to patch anterior vaginal wall defect.

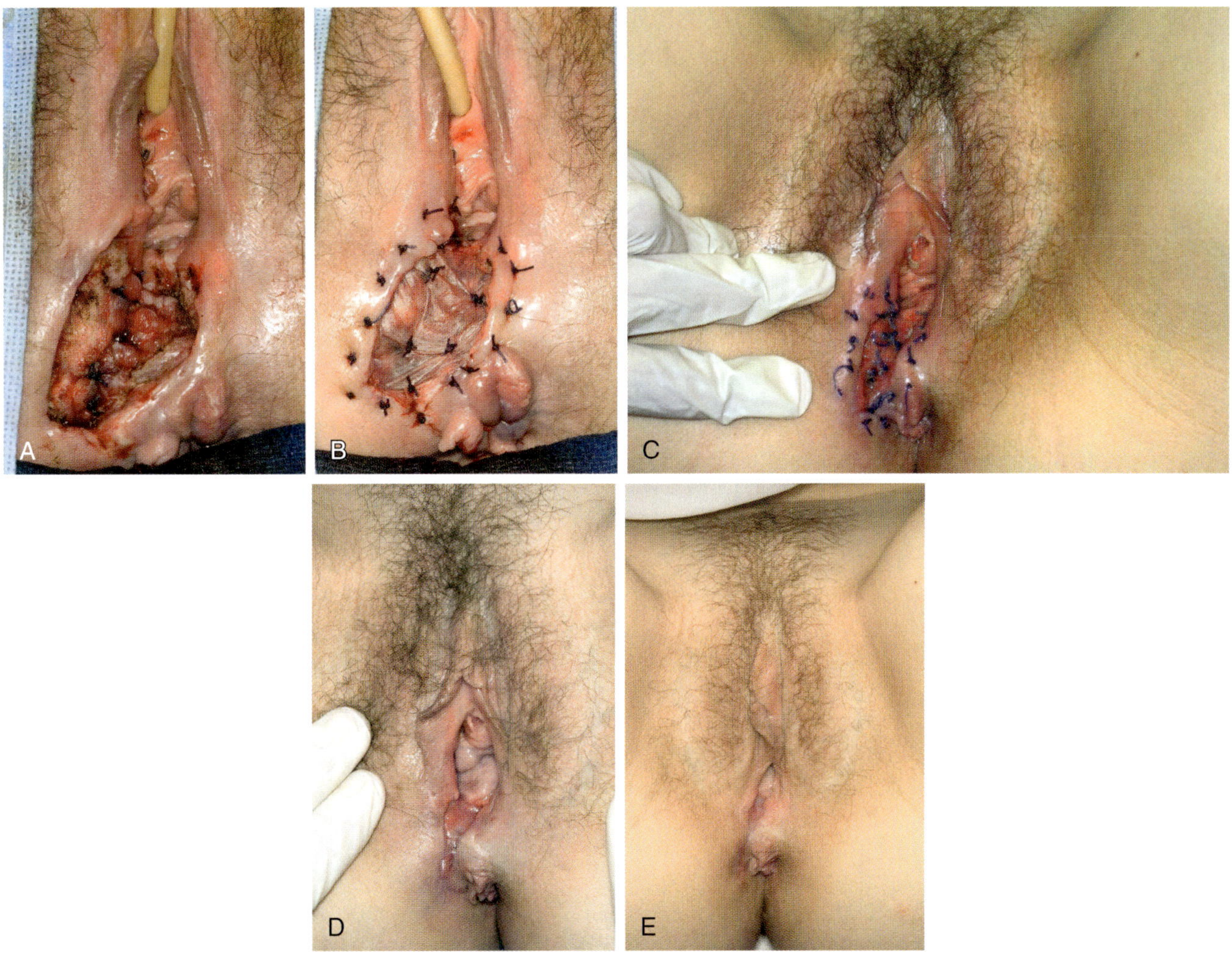

Fig. 26.6 Use of biologic graft (acellular, extracellular matrix derived from porcine small intestinal submucosa) to patch a large perineal breakdown. **A**, Photograph of perineal breakdown. **B**, Placement of graft to replace perineal and vaginal skin. **C**, Healing process at 2 weeks postoperatively. **D**, Healing process at 6 weeks postoperatively. **E**, Healing process at 3 months postoperatively.

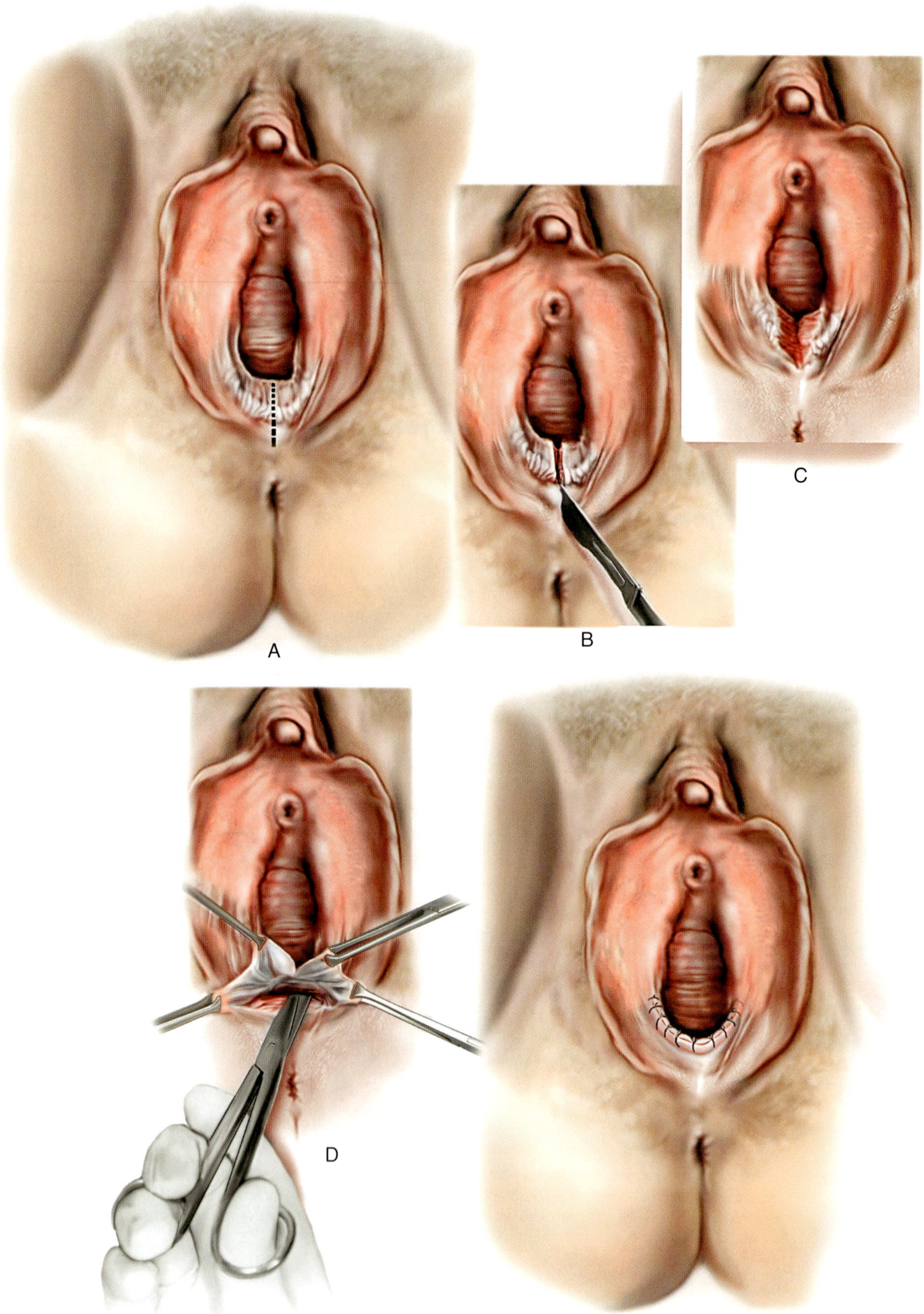

Fig. 26.7 Technique for vaginal introitoplasty. **A**, Longitudinal skin incision is marked. **B**, Constriction band is taken down in the midline. **C**, Incision should continue through the full thickness of the constriction band. **D**, Mobilization of posterior vaginal wall to allow for vaginal advancement. **E**, Vaginal wall is advanced and sutured in a horizontal direction to the perineal skin.

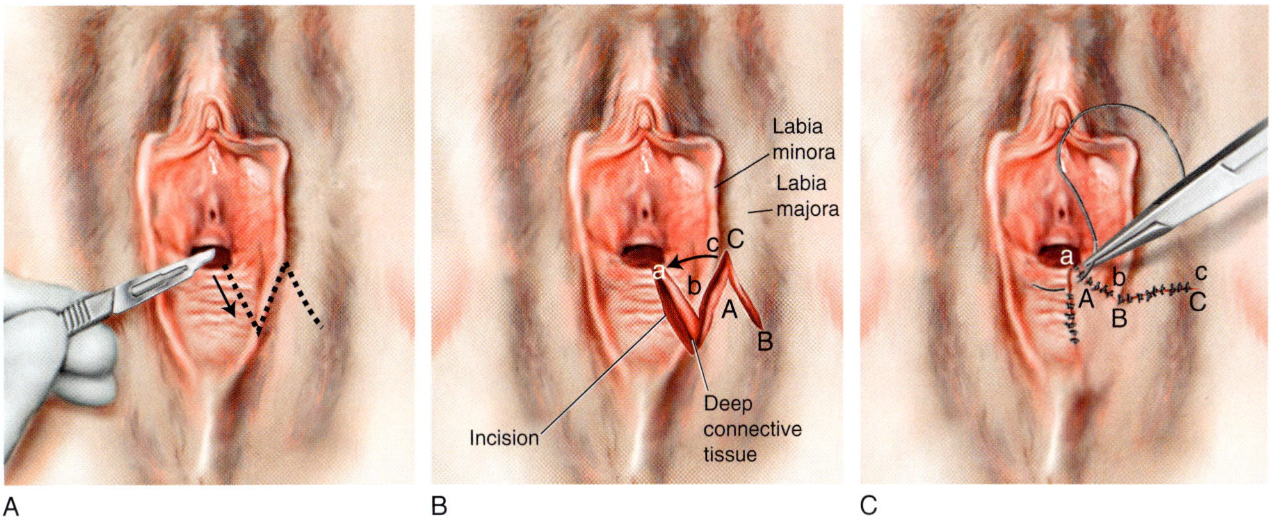

Fig. 26.8 Z-plasty for distal vaginal constriction. **A**, Z-plasty incisions are marked. **B**, Vaginal and perineal incisions are made cutting through full thickness of constriction band. **C**, Flaps are created and sutured in place.

obliterations. Free skin grafts work well to cover a denuded area, where it is impossible to reapproximate the epithelium. The disadvantages are morbidity and cosmesis of the graft harvest site. Cutaneous grafts have the added benefit of bringing to an area of need a more vascular, bulkier graft, which is often necessary when dealing with recurrent conditions or irradiated tissue. The disadvantage of cutaneous grafts is that they generally need to lie close to the defect, and they often do not cover as large an area as a skin graft. Harvest site morbidity and cosmesis are also considerations with these grafts.

We have had some preliminary experience with the use of biologic grafts, including an acellular, extracellular matrix derived from porcine small intestinal submucosa (Biodesign, Cook Medical, Bloomington, IN) and urinary bladder extracellular matrix (Matristem, Acell, Columbia, MD). Porcine small intestinal submucosa has been extensively evaluated in preclinical models and clinical studies, and recently has been used to facilitate wound closure in patients with diabetic ulcers, burns, and various other skin conditions (Barendse-Hofmann et al., 2007; Carson et al., 2003). Data suggest that healing of vaginal or vulvar epithelium is analogous to healing of epidermal skin (Abramov H et al., 2007). Unlike purified collagen wound-care products, other components of the extracellular matrix are retained in intact, active forms (Hodde et al., 2007). These include glycosaminoglycans, such as hyaluronic acid, proteoglycans, fibronectin, and other matrix-associated factors such as fibroblast growth factor and transforming growth factor-β. Similarly, porcine urinary bladder derived extracellular matrix has been shown to improve wound healing, including chronic wounds, nonhealing diabetic foot ulcers, and burns (Kimmel et al, 2010; Frykberg et al, 2016). Numerous patients in our practices have had perineal and vaginal epithelial defects replaced with a piece of these graft materials (Figs. 26.9 and 26.10). Our early results with these materials appear promising, thus offering an alternative to skin graft in women with extensive perineal or vaginal scarring (see Videos 26.2 and 26.6).

CONCLUSION

Complications and untoward sequelae from reconstructive pelvic surgery occur with both native-tissue and graft-augmented surgeries. Gauging the true incidence of these complications is difficult. As new procedures to correct pelvic floor disorders continue to evolve, open discussions among surgeons on how best to manage new and or unforeseen complications are important.

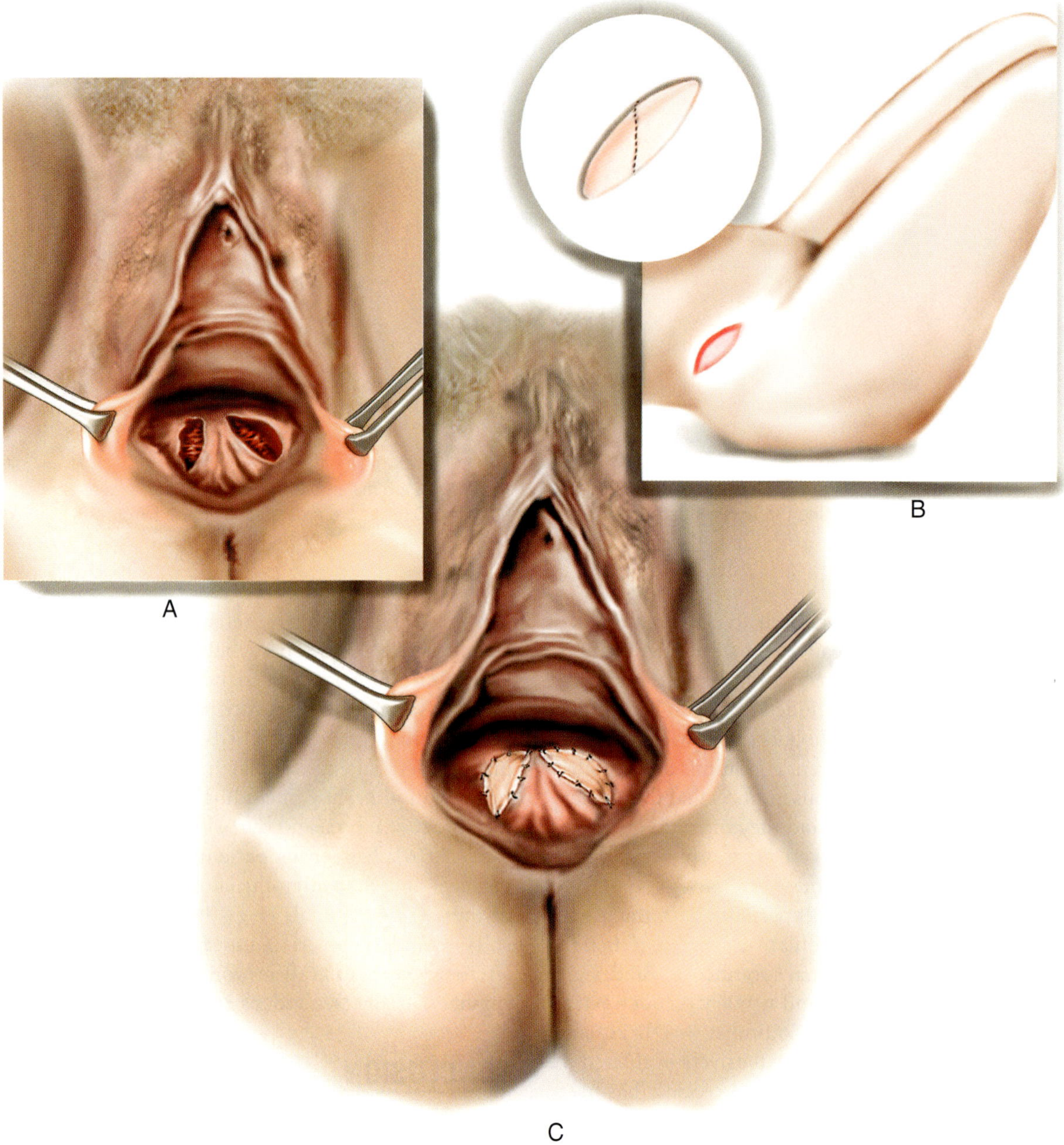

Fig. 26.9 Relaxing incisions for management of a midvaginal constriction band. Defects closed with either a skin graft or biologic graft. **A**, Constriction band cut at 4 o'clock and 8 o'clock. **B**, Skin graft harvested. **C**, Skin graft sutured into defect.

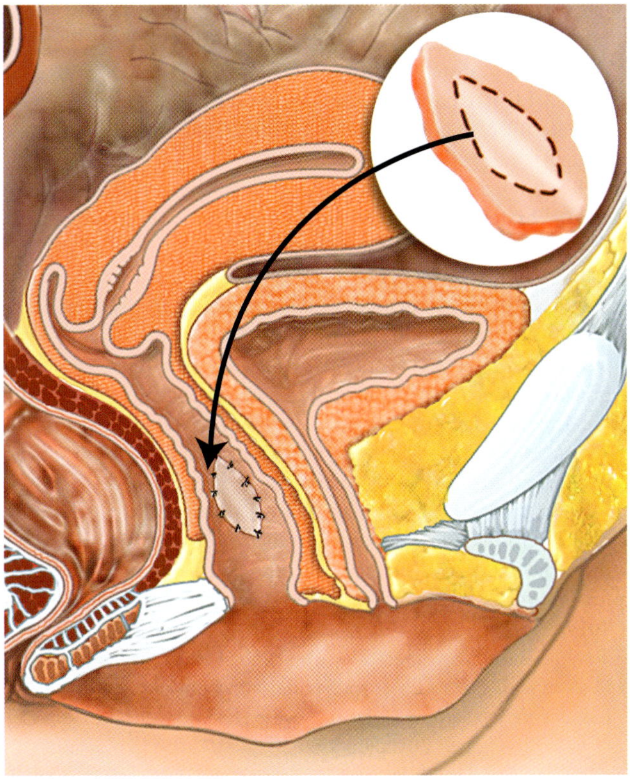

Fig. 26.10 Lateral view of pelvis after placement of skin graft for vaginal constriction.

BIBLIOGRAPHY

Abramov Y, Golden B, Sullivan M, et al. Histologic characterization of vaginal vs. abdominal surgical wound healing in a rabbit model. *Wound Repair Regen.* 2007;15:80.

Committee on Practice Bulletins—Gynecology, American College of Obstetricians and Gynecologists. ACOG Practice Bulletin No. 84: Prevention of deep vein thrombosis and pulmonary embolism. *Obstet Gynecol.* 2007;110:429.

ACOG Committee Opinion No. 750 Summary: perioperative pathways: enhanced recovery after surgery. *Obstet Gynecol.* 2018;132:801.

ACOG Practice Bulletins No. 195: prevention of infection after gynecologic procedures. *Obstet Gynecol.* 2018;131:e172.

Adesanya AO, Lee W, Greilich NB, Joshi GP. Perioperative management of obstructive sleep apnea. *Chest.* 2010;138:1489.

Agnelli G, Becattini C. Acute pulmonary embolism. *N Engl J Med.* 2010;363:266.

Albo ME, Richter HE, Brubaker L, et al. Burch colposuspension versus fascial sling to reduce urinary stress incontinence. *N Engl J Med.* 2007;356:2143.

Alshankiti H, Houlihan S, Robert M, Calgary Women's Pelvic Health Research Group. Incidence and contributing factors of perioperative complications in surgical procedures for pelvic organ prolapse. *Int Urogynecol J.* 2019;30:1945.

Al-Sunaidi M, Tulandi T. Adhesion-related bowel obstruction after hysterectomy for benign conditions. *Obstet Gynecol.* 2006;108:1162.

Andy UU, Harvie HS, Ackenbom MF, Arya LA. Single versus multi-dose antibiotic prophylaxis for pelvic organ prolapse surgery with mesh/graft. *Eur J Obstet Gynecol.* 2014;181:37.

Ansell J, Hirsch J, Hylek E, Jacobson A, et al. Pharmacology and management of the vitamin K antagonists: American College of Chest Physicians Evidence-Based Clinical Practice Guidelines (8th edition). *Chest.* 2008;133:160S.

Baessler K, Hewson AD, Tunn R, et al. Severe mesh complications following intravaginal slingplasty. *Obstet Gynecol.* 2005;106:713.

Barber MD, Brubaker L, Burgio KL, et al. Comparison of 2 transvaginal surgical approaches and perioperative behavior therapy for apical vaginal prolapse: the OPTIMAL randomized trial. *JAMA.* 2014;311:1023. Erratum *JAMA* 2015;313:2287.

Barendse-Hofmann MG, van Doorn LP, Oskam J, Steenvoorde P. Extracellular matrix prevents split-skin grafting in selected cases. *J Wound Care.* 2007;16:455.

Barnett JC, Hurd WW, Rogers RM, et al. Laparoscopic positioning and nerve injuries. *J Minim Invasive Gynecol.* 2007;14:664.

Barrett CR. Flexible fiberoptic bronchoscopy in the critically ill patient, methodology and indications. *Chest.* 1978;73:746.

Bent AE. Postoperative delirium in older adults. *Female Pelvic Med Reconstr Surg.* 2015;21:181.

Bhatia NN, Karram MM, Bergman A. Role of antibiotic prophylaxis in retropubic surgery for stress urinary incontinence. *Obstet Gynecol.* 1989;74:637.

Blikkendaal MD, Schepers EM, van Zwet EW, et al. Hysterectomy in very obese and morbidly obese patients: a systematic review with cumulative analysis of comparative studies. *Arch Gynecol Obstet.* 2015;292:723.

Boesch CE, Umek W. Effects of wound closure on wound healing in gynecologic surgery. *J Reprod Med.* 2009;54:139.

Bohlin KS, Ankardal M, Stjerndahl JH, et al. Influence of the modifiable life-style factors body mass index and smoking on the outcome of hysterectomy. *Acta Obstet Gynecol Scand.* 2016;95:65.

Bolden N, Smith CE, Auckley D. Avoiding adverse outcomes in patients with obstructive sleep apnea (OSA): development and implementation of a perioperative OSA protocol. *J Clin Anesth.* 2009;21:286.

Bolden N, Smith CE, Auckley D, et al. Perioperative complications during use of an obstructive sleep apnea protocol following surgery and anesthesia. *Anesth Analg.* 2007;105:1869.

Bohrer JC, Walters M, Park A, et al. Pelvic nerve injury following gynecologic surgery: a prospective cohort study. *Am J Obstet Gynecol.* 2009;201:531.

Bretschneider CE, Robinson B, Geller EJ, Wu JM. The effect of age on postoperative morbidity in women undergoing urogynecologic surgery. *Female Pelvic Med Reconstr Surg.* 2015;21:236.

Britt BA, Gordon RA. Peripheral nerve injuries associated with anesthesia. *Can Anaesth Soc J.* 1964;11:514.

Brooks-Brunn JA. Predictors of postoperative pulmonary complications following abdominal surgery. *Chest.* 1997;111:564.

Brubaker L, Norton PA, Albo ME, et al. Adverse events over two years after retropubic or transobturator midurethral sling surgery: findings from the Trial of Midurethral Slings (TOMUS) study. *Am J Obstet Gynecol.* 2011;205:498.

Brueseke T, Livingston B, Warda H, et al. Risk factors for surgical site infection in patients undergoing sacral nerve modulation therapy. *Female Pelvic Med Reconstr Surg.* 2015;21:198.

Brummer THI, Jalkanen J, Fraser J, et al. Prevention and management of surgical site infections in morbidly obese women. *Hum Reprod.* 2011;26:1741.

Campbell P, Cloney L, Jha S. Abdominal versus laparoscopic sacrocolpopexy: a systematic review and meta-analysis. *Obstet Gynecol Surv.* 2016;71:435.

Carson SN, Travis E, Overall K, Lee-Jahshan S. Using becaplermin gel with collagen products to potentiate healing in chronic leg wounds. *Wounds*. 2003;15:339.

Carter-Brooks CM, Du AL, Ruppert KM, et al. Implementation of a urogynecology-specific enhanced recovery after surgery (ERAS) pathway. *Am J Obstet Gynecol*. 2018;219:495.e1.

Cate-Hoek AJT, Prins MH. Management studies using a combination of D-dimer test results and clinical probability to rule out venous thromboembolism: a systematic review. *J Thromb Haemost*. 2005;3:2465.

Chen CCG, Collins SA, Rodgers AK, et al. Perioperative complications in obese women vs normal-weight women who undergo vaginal surgery. *Am J Obstet Gynecol*. 2007;197:98.

Clapp B, Santillan A. Small bowel obstruction after FloSeal use. *JSLS*. 2011;15:361.

Clarke-Pearson DL, Dodge RK, Synan I, et al. Venous thromboembolism prophylaxis: patients at high risk to fail intermittent pneumatic compression. *Obstet Gynecol*. 2003;101:157.

Colwell CW, Collis DK, Paulson R, et al. Comparison of enoxaparin and warfarin for the prevention of venous thromboembolic disease after total hip arthroplasty. *J Bone Joint Surg Am*. 1999;81:932.

Dieter AA, Amundsen CL, Edenfield AL, et al. Oral antibiotics to prevent postoperative urinary tract infection: a randomized controlled trial. *Obstet Gynecol*. 2014;123:103.

Desciak MC, Martin DE. Perioperative pulmonary embolism: diagnosis and anesthetic management. *J Clin Anesth*. 2011; 23:153.

Doyle RL. Assessing and modifying the risk of postoperative pulmonary complications. *Chest*. 1999;115:77S.

El-Nashar SA, Singh R, Schmitt JJ, et al. Urinary tract infection after hysterectomy for benign gynecologic conditions or pelvic reconstructive surgery. *Obstet Gynecol*. 2018;132:1347.

Ephgrave KS, Kleiman-Wexler R, Pfaller M, et al. Postoperative pneumonia: a prospective study of risk factors and morbidity. *Surgery*. 1993;114:815.

Frykberg RG, Cazzell SM, Arroyo-Rivera J, et al. Evaluation of tissue engineering products for management of neuropathic diabetic foot ulcers: an interim analysis. *J Wound Care*. 2016;25:S18.

Gebhart JB, Schmitt JJ. Surgical management of the constricted or obliterated vagina. *Obstet Gynecol*. 2016;128:284.

Gould MK, Garcia DA, Wren SM, et al. Prevention of VTE in nonorthopedic surgical patients: Antithrombotic Therapy and Prevention of Thrombosis, 9th ed: American College of Chest Physicians Evidence-Based Clinical Practice Guidelines. *Chest*. 2012;141:e227S.

Heisler CA, Aletti GD, Weaver AL, et al. Improving quality of care: development of a risk-adjusted perioperative morbidity model for vaginal hysterectomy. *Am J Obstet Gynecol*. 2010;202:137.

Hiltunen R, Nieminen K, Takula T, et al. Low-weight polypropylene mesh for anterior vaginal wall prolapse. *Obstet Gynecol*. 2007;110:455.

Hodde J, Janis A, Ernst D, et al. Effects of sterilization on an extracellular matrix scaffold: part I. Composition and matrix architecture. *J Mater Sci Mater Med*. 2007;18:537.

Hodde J, Janis A, Hiles M. Effects of sterilization on an extracellular matrix scaffold: part II. Bioactivity and matrix interaction. *J Mater Sci Mater Med*. 2007;18:545.

Hooten TM, Stamm WE. Diagnosis and treatment of uncomplicated urinary tract infection. *Infect Dis Clin North Am*. 1997;11:551.

Ingber MS, Vasavada SP, Firoozi F, Goldman HB. Incidence of perioperative urinary tract infection after single-dose antibiotic therapy for midurethral slings. *Urology*. 2010;76:830.

Isik-Akbay EF, Harmanli OH, Panganamamula UR, et al. Hysterectomy in obese women: a comparison of abdominal and vaginal routes. *Obstet Gynecol*. 2004;104:710.

Jones K, Thompson N, Imamoglu G, et al. Short-term outcomes of vaginal hysterectomy at the time of robotic sacrocolpopexy. *Female Pelvic Med Reconstr Surg*. 2021;27:e223.

Jones KA, Zhuo Y, Solak S, Harmanli O. Hysterectomy at the time of colpocleisis: a decision analysis. *Int Urogynecol J*. 2016;27:805.

Kalil AC, Metersky ML, Klompas M, et al. Management of adults with hospital-acquired and ventilator-associated pneumonia: 2016 clinical practice guidelines by the Infectious Diseases Society of America and the American Thoracic Society. *Clin Infect Dis*. 2016;63:e61.

Karram MM, Kleeman SD. Lower urinary tract infection. In: Walters M, Karram MM, eds. *Urogynecology and Reconstructive Pelvic Surgery*. 3rd ed. Philadelphia: Mosby Elsevier; 2007:413.

Keil DS, Schiff LD, Carey ET, et al. Predictors of admission after the implementation of an enhanced recovery after surgery pathway for minimally invasive gynecologic surgery. *Anesth Analg*. 2019;129:776.

Kimmel H, Rahn M, Gilbert TW. The clinical effectiveness in wound healing with extracellular matrix derived from porcine urinary bladder matrix: a case series on severe chronic wounds. *J Am Col Certif Wound Spec*. 2010;30:55.

Kjolhede P, Shefquet H, Lofgren M. Vaginal cleansing and postoperative infectious morbidity in vaginal hysterectomy. A register study from the Swedish National Register for Gynecological Surgery. *Acta Obstet Gynecol Scand*. 2011;90:63.

Kjolhede P, Shefqet H, Lofgren M. The influence of preoperative vaginal cleansing on postoperative infectious morbidity in abdominal total hysterectomy for benign indications. *Acta Obstet Gynecol*. 2009;88:408.

Komoroff AL. Urinalysis and urine culture in women with dysuria. *Ann Intern Med*. 1986;104:212-218.

Krivak TC, Zorn KK. Venous thromboembolism in obstetrics and gynecology. *Obstet Gynecol*. 2007;109:761.

Lambrou NC, Buller JL, Thompson JR, et al. Prevalence of perioperative complications among women undergoing reconstructive pelvic surgery. *Am J Obstet Gynecol*. 2000;183:1355.

Lawrence VA, Hilsenbeck SG, Mulrow CD, et al. Incidence and hospital stay for cardiac and pulmonary complications after abdominal surgery. *J Gen Intern Med*. 1995;10:671.

Lavelle ES, Alam P, Meister M, et al. Antibiotic prophylaxis during catheter-managed postoperative urinary retention after pelvic reconstructive surgery: a randomized controlled trial. *Obstet Gynecol*. 2019;134:727.

Lazenby GB, Soper DE. Prevention, diagnosis, and treatment of gynecologic surgical site infections. *Obstet Gynecol Clin North Am*. 2010;37:379.

Lee TH, Marcantonio ER, Mangione CM, et al. Derivation and prospective validation of a simple index for prediction of cardiac risk of major non cardiac surgery. *Circulation*. 1999;100:1043.

Levenson RB, Pearson KM, Saokar A, et al. Image-guided drainage of tuboovarian abscesses of gastrointestinal or genitourinary origin: a retrospective analysis. *J Vasc Interv Radiol*. 2011;22:678.

Lightner DJ, Wymer K, Sanchez J, Kavoussi L. Best practice statement on urologic procedures and antimicrobial prophylaxis. *J Urol*. 2020;203:351.

Lindqvist PG, Epstein E, Olsson H. The relationship between lifestyle factors and venous thromboembolism among women: a report from the MISS study. *Br J Haematol.* 2008;114:234.

Little P, Moore MV, Turner S, et al. Effectiveness of five different approaches in management of urinary tract infection: radomised controlled trial. *BMJ.* 2010;340:c199.

Lo E, Nocolle L, Classen D, et al. Strategies to prevent catheter-associated urinary tract infections in acute care hospitals. *Infect Control Hosp Epidemiol.* 2008;29:S41.

Luber KM, Boero S, Choe JY. The demographics of pelvic floor disorders: current observations and future projections. *Am J Obstet Gynecol.* 2001;184:1496.

Maher C, Feiner B, Baessler K, Schmid C. Surgical management of pelvic organ prolapse in women. *Cochrane Database Syst Rev.* 2013;4:CD004014.

Mattox TF, Sanford EJ, Varner E. Infected abdominal sacrocolpopexies: diagnosis and treatment. *Int Urogynecol J Pelvic Floor Dysfunct.* 2004;15:319.

McAlister FA, Bertsch K, Man J, et al. Incidence of and risk factors for pulmonary complications after nonthoracic surgery. *Am J Respir Crit Care Med.* 2005;171:514.

Mckinnell JA, Stollenwerk NS, Jung CW, Miller LG. Nitrofurantoin compares favorably to recommended agents as empirical treatment of uncomplicated urinary tract infections in a decision and cost analysis. *Mayo Clin Proc.* 2011;86:480.

Medlin EE, Rice LW, Al-Niaimi A. Obstructive sleep apnea and the impact on surgical outcomes in gynecology. *Obstet Gynecol Surv.* 2018;73:242.

Memtsoudis S, Liu SS, Ma Y, et al. Perioperative pulmonary outcomes in patients with sleep apnea after noncardiac surgery. *Anesth Analg.* 2011;112:113.

Mikhail E, Miladinovic B, Velanovich V, et al. Association between obesity and the trends of routes of hysterectomy performed for benign indications. *Obstet Gynecol.* 2015;125:912.

Moir C, Robins ER. Role of ultrasonography, gallium scanning, and computed tomography in the diagnosis of intraabdominal abscess. *Am J Surg.* 1982;143:582.

Montavers P, Veber B, Auboyer C, et al. Diagnostic and therapeutic management of nosocomial pneumonia in surgical patients: results of the Eole study. *Crit Care Med.* 2002;30:368.

Montoya TI, Leclaire EL, Oakley SH, et al., Fellows' Pelvic Research Network of the Society of Gynecologic Surgeons. Venous thromboembolism in women undergoing pelvic reconstructive surgery with mechanical prophylaxis alone. *Int Urogynecol J.* 2014;25:921.

Moores LK, King CS, Holley AB. Current approach to the diagnosis of acute nonmassive pulmonary embolism. *Chest.* 2011;140:509.

Mueller MG, Pilecki MA, Catanzarite T, et al. Venous thromboembolism in reconstructive pelvic surgery. *Am J Obstet Gynecol.* 2014;211:552.e1.

Muffly TM, Ridgeway B, Abbott S, et al. Small bowel obstruction after hysterectomy to treat benign disease. *J Minim Invasive Gynecol.* 2012;19:615.

Murdock CM, Wolff AJ, Van Geem T. Risk factors for hypercarbia, subcutaneous emphysema, pneumothorax and pneumomediastinum during laparoscopy. *Obstet Gynecol.* 2000;95:704.

Must A, Spandano J, Coakley EH, et al. The disease burden associated with overweight and obesity. *JAMA.* 1999;282:1523.

Nichols DH, Clarke-Pearson DL, eds. *Gynecologic, Obstetric and Related Surgery*, 2nd ed. St. Louis: Mosby; 2000.

Nygaard I, Brubaker L, Zyczynski HM, et al. Long-term outcomes following abdominal sacrocolpopexy for pelvic organ prolapse. *JAMA.* 2013;309:2016. Erratum *JAMA.* 2013;310:1076.

Nygaard IE, Kreder KJ. Complications of incontinence surgery. *Int Urogynecol J.* 1994;5:353.

Okadome M, Saito T, Miyahara D, et al. Postoperative pulmonary embolism including asymptomatic cases in gynecologic oncology. *Int J Gynecol Cancer.* 2010;20:655.

Pappachen S, Smith PR, Shah S, et al. Postoperative pulmonary complications after gynecologic surgery. *Int J Gynaecol Obstet.* 2006;93:74.

Parks BJ. Postoperative peripheral neuropathies. *Surgery.* 1973; 74:348.

Pickleman JA, Lee RM. The Management of patients with suspected early postoperative small bowel obstruction. *Ann Surg.* 1989;210:216.

Pitkin RM. Vaginal hysterectomy in obese women. *Obstet Gynecol.* 1977;49:567.

Pratt TS, Hudson CO, Northington GM, Greene KA. Obesity and perioperative complications in pelvic reconstructive surgery in 2013: analysis of the national inpatient sample. *Female Pelvic Med Reconstr Surg.* 2018;24:51.

Qaseem A, Snow V, Barry P, et al. Current diagnosis of venous thromboembolism in primary care: a clinical practice guideline from the American Academy of Family Physicians and the American College of Physicians. *Ann Intern Med.* 2007;146:454.

Rahn DD, Mamik MM, Sanses TV, et al. Venous thromboembolism prophylaxis in gynecologic surgery: a systematic review. *Obstet Gynecol.* 2011;118:1111.

Ridgeway B, Barber MD, Walters MD, Paraiso MF. Small bowel obstruction after vaginal vault suspension: a series of three cases. *Int Urogynecol J Pelvic Floor Dysfunct.* 2007;18:1237.

Rogers RG, Lebkuchner U, Kammerer-Doak DN, et al. Obesity and retropubic surgery for stress incontinence: is there really an increased risk of intraoperative complications? *Am J Obstet Gynecol.* 2006;195:1794.

Rogers RG, Kammerer-Doak D, Olsen A, et al. A randomized, double-blind, placebo-controlled comparison of the effect of nitrofurantoin monohydrate macrocrystals on the development of urinary tract infections after surgery for pelvic organ prolapse and/or stress urinary incontinence with suprapubic catheterization. *Am J Obstet Gynecol.* 2004;191:182.

Romanowski L, Reich H, McGlynn F, et al. Brachial plexus neuropathies after advances laparoscopic surgery. *Fertil Steril.* 1993;60:729.

Schiotz HA. Urinary tract infections and bacteriuria after gynecological surgery: experience with 24-hour Foley catheterization. *Int Urogynecol J.* 1994;5:345.

Shah DK, Vitonis AF, Missmer SA. Association of body mass index and morbidity after abdominal, vaginal, and laparoscopic hysterectomy. *Obstet Gynecol.* 2015;125:589.

Shammash JB, Trost JC, Gold JM, et al. Perioperative beta-blocker withdrawal and mortality in vascular surgical patients. *Am Heart J.* 2001;141:148.

Sheyn D, Mahajan S, El-Nashar S, et al. Prevalence and risk factors for cardiac arrest and myocardial infarction after pelvic reconstructive surgery: a national, multi-institutional, surgical database study. *Int Urogynecol J.* 2018;29:229.

Sheyn D, Bretschneider CE, Mahajan ST, et al. Incidence and risk factors of early postoperative small bowel obstruction in patients undergoing hysterectomy for benign indications. *Am J Obstet Gynecol.* 2019;220:251.

Shveiky D, Aseff JN, Iglesia CB. Brachial plexus injury after laparoscopic and robotic surgery. *J Minim Invasive Gynecol.* 2010;17:414.

Smith JA, Howards SS, Preminger GM, Dmochowski RR, eds. *Hinman's Atlas of Urologic Surgery*, 4th ed. Philadelphia, 2018, Elsevier.

Smith FJ, Holman CD, Moorin RE, Tsokos N. Lifetime risk of undergoing surgery for pelvic organ prolapse. *Obstet Gynecol.* 2010;116:1096.

Solomon ER, Muffly TM, Barber MD. Common postoperative pulmonary complications after hysterectomy for benign indications. *Am J Obstet Gynecol.* 2013;208:54.

Squadrone V, Coha M, Cerutti E, et al. Continuous positive airway pressure for treatment of postoperative hypoxemia. *JAMA.* 2005;293:589.

Stein PD, Beemath A, Matta F, et al. Clinical characteristics of patients with acute pulmonary embolism: data from PIOPED II. *Am J Med.* 2007;120:871.

Stepp KJ, Barber MD, Yoo EH, et al. Incidence of perioperative complications of urogynecologic surgery in elderly women. *Am J Obstet Gynecol.* 2005;192:1630.

Sung VW, Weitzen S, Sokol ER, et al. Effect of patient age on increasing morbidity and mortality following urogynecologic surgery. *Am J Obstet Gynecol.* 2006;194:1411.

Suzuki N, Yoshioka N, Ohara T, et al. Risk factors for perioperative venous thromboembolism: a retrospective study in Japanese women with gynecologic diseases. *Thromb J.* 2010;8:1.

Suzuki Y, Vellinga TT, Istre O, Einarsson JI. Small bowel obstruction associated with use of a gelatin-thrombin matrix sealant (FloSeal) after laparoscopic gynecologic surgery. *J Minim Invasive Gynecol.* 2010;17:641.

Sweetland S, Green J, Liu B, et al. Duration and magnitude of the postoperative risk of venous thromboembolism in middle aged women: prospective cohort study. *BMJ.* 2009;339:1.

Thomas-White KJ, Gao X, Lin H, et al. Urinary microbes and postoperative urinary tract infection risk in urogynecologic surgical patients. *Int Urogynecol J.* 2018;29:1797.

Toglia MR, Nolan TE. Morbidity and mortality rates of elective gynecologic surgery in the elderly woman. *Am J Obstet Gynecol.* 2003;189:1584.

Turan A, Mascha EJ, Roberman D, et al. Smoking and perioperative outcomes. *Anesthesiology.* 2011;114:837.

Trowbridge ER, Kim D, Barletta K, et al. Prevalence of positive screening test for cognitive impairment among elderly urogynecologic patients. *Am J Obstet Gynecol.* 2016;215:e1.

Unger CA, Walters MD, Ridgeway B, et al. Incidence of adverse events after uterosacral colpopexy for uterovaginal and posthysterectomy vault prolapse. *Am J Obstet Gynecol.* 2015;212:603.

Uppal S, Harris J, Al-Niaimi A, et al. Prophylactic antibiotic choice and risk of surgical site infection after hysterectomy. *Obstet Gynecol.* 2016;127:321.

Vakili B, Huynh T, Loesch H, et al. Outcomes of vaginal reconstructive surgery with and without graft material. *Am J Obstet Gynecol.* 2005;193:2126.

Wahba RM. Airway closure and intraoperative hypoxaemia: twenty-five years later. *Can J Anaesth.* 1996;43:1144.

Walsh C, Scaife C, Hopf H. Prevention and management of surgical site infections in morbidly obese women. *Obstet Gynecol.* 2009;113:411.

Walters MD, Barber MD. Complications of hysterectomy. In: Karram M, ed. *Hysterectomy for Benign Disease.* Philadelphia: Saunders Elsevier; 2010:195.

Warner MA, Divertie MB, Tinker JH. Preoperative cessation of smoking and pulmonary complications in coronary artery bypass patients. *Anesthesiology.* 1984;60:380.

Warner MA, Warner DO, Harper CM, et al. Lower extremity neuropathies associated with lithotomy positions. *Anesthesiology.* 2000;93:938.

Wu JM, Vaughan CP, Goode PS, et al. Prevalence and trends of symptomatic pelvic floor disorders in U.S. women. *Obstet Gynecol.* 2014;123:141.

Xue FS, Li BW, Zhang GS, et al. The influence of surgical sites on early postoperative hypoxemia in adults undergoing elective surgery. *Anesth Analg.* 1999;88:213.

PART 5

Fecal Incontinence and Defecation Disorders

27

Fecal Incontinence

Catherine S. Bradley and Yehudith Assouline Dayan

CHAPTER OUTLINE

EPIDEMIOLOGY

Fecal incontinence, the involuntary leakage of liquid or solid stool, and anal incontinence, including the involuntary leakage of gas, are devastating problems. Many people find these conditions socially incapacitating and stay home, minimizing social contact to avoid embarrassing situations. Estimates of the number of people afflicted with fecal incontinence likely underrepresent the prevalence, because many do not mention the problem to their caregivers, and health care providers do not routinely screen for these symptoms (Boreham et al., 2005). Definitions of fecal incontinence also vary from report to report, making comparisons difficult. A 2013 review performed as part of a National Institutes of Health State of the Science Workshop reported that fecal incontinence occurred in 7% to 15% of community-dwelling people (Bharucha et al., 2015). In a large systematic review, the median prevalence of fecal incontinence in women in the community was 8.9% (range 2.0%–20.7%), and the median prevalence of anal incontinence was 15.9% (range 2.2%–47.0%) (Ng et al., 2015).

The economic burden of fecal incontinence is high, including direct medical and surgical costs, as well as costs for pads, diapers, and other personal hygiene products. Fecal incontinence is one of the most common reasons for nursing home placement. Fecal incontinence increases progressively with age, although it can affect all ages. Although obstetric trauma is a known risk factor for fecal incontinence in women, fecal incontinence impacts both genders with similar prevalence rates. Other risk factors for fecal incontinence include diarrhea, chronic illness, smoking, and obesity. More information about the epidemiology and significant psychosocial impact of fecal incontinence can be found in Chapter 6.

ETIOLOGY

Defecation is a complex process that involves the interaction between anal function and sensation, rectal compliance, stool consistency, stool volume, colonic transit, and cognitive control. An alteration in any of these can lead to incontinence. Box 27.1 lists some common causes of fecal incontinence.

A large component of continence is the function of the anal sphincter complex, consisting of the internal anal sphincter muscle, the external anal sphincter muscle, and the puborectalis muscle (Fig. 27.1). The smooth muscle of the internal sphincter is innervated by the autonomic nervous system, whereas the external sphincter striated muscle is innervated by the inferior rectal branch of the pudendal nerve. Traditionally, the internal anal sphincter has been thought to be largely responsible for sphincter resting tone, with a smaller contribution by the external sphincter muscle. However, others suggest that the external sphincter may play a greater role in baseline sphincter pressure (Wong et al., 1998). The external anal sphincter is voluntarily recruited during rectal filling, aiding with increased sphincter pressure and maintenance of continence. Defecation is a result of voluntary relaxation of the external sphincter and puborectalis muscles, innervated by the S3–S4 nerves, in response to

BOX 27.1 Causes of Fecal Incontinence

Anal
Injury
Obstetric (vaginal delivery/trauma)
Surgical (fistulotomy, hemorrhoidectomy, sphincterotomy, stretch)
Irradiation
Trauma
Congenital (e.g., imperforate anus)

Intestinal
Colitis or proctitis
Colon, rectum, or small bowel resection
Tumors
Fecal impaction
Decreased rectal compliance
Rectal prolapse

Neurologic
Central nervous system
Dementia
Neoplasm
Stroke
Trauma
Multiple sclerosis
Peripheral (e.g., diabetes)

Other
Diarrhea
Combinations of anal and rectal causes
Myopathy (e.g., scleroderma)
Functional
Obesity

rectal distension that is dictated by receptors in the pelvic floor and the anal transition zone. Chapter 4 includes a detailed description of the anatomy, innervation, and function of the anorectum.

Anatomic disruption of the sphincter complex and dysfunction because of neurologic reasons are frequent causes of fecal incontinence. Vaginal birth, and particularly forceps-assisted operative vaginal delivery, commonly injures the mother's sphincter complex. In seminal research, Sultan et al. (1993) studied women before and after childbirth, with interviews, anal physiology testing, and anal endosonography, and found that 35% of primiparous women and 44% of multiparous women had sphincter defects as seen on endoanal ultrasound after delivery. The internal anal sphincter was injured more often than the external sphincter—sometimes even when no breach occurred in the perineal skin. A strong correlation was found between sphincter defects and the development of bowel symptoms, although only about a third of women with sphincter defects developed bowel symptoms. Studies have reported worsening fecal continence status in women with prior anal sphincter injury and subsequent vaginal delivery, particularly those with an anal sphincter defect seen on ultrasound after first delivery (Faltin et al., 2001). However, subsequent vaginal delivery appears safe in some women with prior sphincter injury. Vaginal delivery was not associated with significant worsening of anorectal symptoms or function in 99 women with prior obstetric anal sphincter injury who did not have significant fecal incontinence symptoms or anal sphincter defect on ultrasound after the birth injury (Jordan et al., 2018).

This and other research have demonstrated a clear association between obstetric injury and early-onset fecal incontinence. In some women, fecal incontinence symptoms may develop decades after an obstetric injury, possibly because other mechanisms maintain continence during that interval. The long-term risk of incontinence in women with a prior sphincter injury is still unclear. An epidemiological study including over 7000 Swedish women 40 to 60 years of age demonstrated that the risk of new fecal incontinence increased after age 52 years to a significantly greater extent in women with a history of obstetric anal sphincter injury compared with women without a sphincter injury, suggesting that a persistent risk extends at least into early menopause (Nillson et al., 2021). However, similar to urinary incontinence, obstetric injury appears to be a less important risk factor for fecal incontinence that occurs in elderly women, when other contributing factors are common (see Box 27.1).

EVALUATION

History

A comprehensive history is critical to the evaluation of a patient with fecal incontinence, focusing on bowel habits and incontinence symptoms (see also Chapter 9). Important questions to ask include duration of the problem, frequency of incontinence, time of day of incontinence, type of stool lost, ability to control flatus, use of pads, frequency of bowel movements, typical stool consistency, and effects of incontinence on daily life. The presence of fecal urgency is important. Urgency may reflect inability of the rectal reservoir to store stool (as with diarrhea or proctitis) rather than a sphincter problem. The consistency of incontinent stool may be related to the severity of the incontinence. Flatus is more difficult to control than liquid stool, and solid stool is the most easily controlled. Patients with incontinence of solid stool without knowledge of the loss of stool may be more distressed than those with incontinence of flatus only.

The obstetric history may also be relevant, including number of vaginal deliveries, use of vacuum or forceps, episiotomy, perineal tears or infections, and neonatal weight. A sexual history, including the practice of anal intercourse and the effect of incontinence on sexual behavior, should be obtained. Other medical and surgical conditions must be ascertained, particularly gastrointestinal and neurological disorders, as well as back injuries, previous anorectal or abdominal surgeries, irradiation history, and diabetes. Medications, food intolerance, and activity restrictions may add information.

The Bristol Stool Form Scale and bowel diaries may be used to complement the history (Lewis & Heaton, 1997). The well-validated Bristol Stool Form Scale provides descriptions of stool consistency ranging from 1 (separate hard lumps of stool) to 7 (watery diarrhea), which can aid patients in characterizing stool consistency. This is often used with a bowel diary to provide an

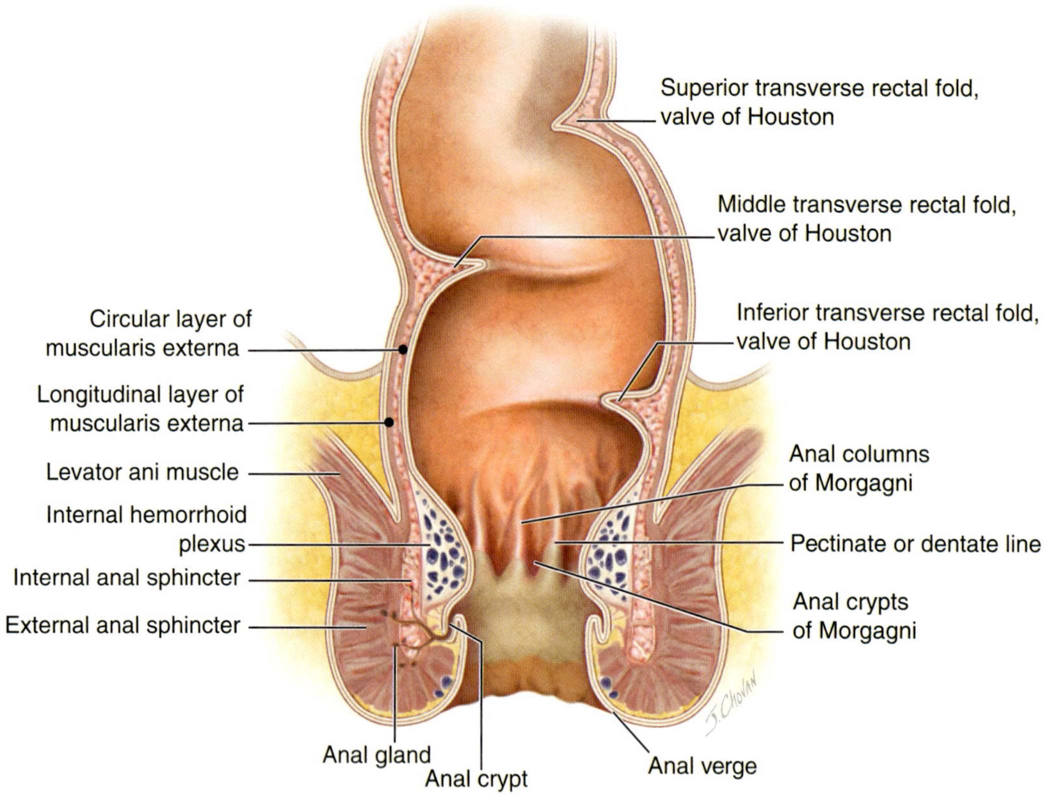

Fig. 27.1 Anatomy of the distal anal region. (Reprinted with permission from Baggish M, Karram M. *Atlas of Pelvic Anatomy and Gynecologic Surgery.* 5th ed. Philadelphia: Elsevier; 2020.)

objective record of stool frequency, consistency, and incontinence episodes.

Physical Examination

Physical examination should include abdominal, pelvic, and rectal examinations. Abdominal evaluation may help identify stool burden or other masses. Pelvic examination is used to assess for pelvic organ prolapse, including rectocele, and fistula.

The anorectal physical examination starts with inspection of the anal area, looking for soilage of stool on the skin and evidence of skin irritation. The anus is inspected, looking for gaping of the muscles and any scarring. A "dovetail" sign, where the anterior perianal folds are absent, and a shortened or thin perineal body are suggestive of an external anal sphincter defect. The patient is asked to squeeze and to simulate holding in a bowel movement to look for uniform circular contraction of muscle. Patients with a weak sphincter may contract the gluteal muscles instead of the anal sphincter. Next, asking the patient to strain may show exaggerated perineal descent or prolapse of hemorrhoids or even the rectum. The anocutaneous reflex can be checked by rubbing the perianal skin gently (a Q-tip works well) and looking for the reflex contraction of the anal sphincter mechanism, also referred to as "anal wink." Sensation to pinprick can also be assessed. Both of these give a crude assessment of sphincter innervation.

Palpation of the sphincter is next done with digital examination. The initial tone should be noted, as it reflects the internal sphincter. Then the patient is asked to squeeze on the index finger in the anus as if she were holding in a bowel movement. Strength, defects in the circle of muscle, and early fatigability are assessed. Scars or masses are appreciated. The digital rectal examination is also used to evaluate for rectal or anal masses, occult or gross blood, fistula, and the presence of a rectocele. Anoscopy and proctoscopy may be added to the examination to help diagnose anal lesions (such as hemorrhoids or neoplasms) or proctitis (also see Colonoscopy section later).

Questionnaires for Fecal Incontinence

The use of validated questionnaires may be helpful clinically to assess fecal incontinence severity and functional impact (quality of life) before and after treatment. One commonly used severity scale for fecal incontinence is the American Society of Colon and Rectum Fecal Incontinence Severity Index (FISI). The FISI consists of questions that rate continence to gas, mucus, solid, and liquid stool. Other popular tools also rate lifestyle alterations and wearing of a pad, in addition to incontinence to solid and liquid stool and gas, including the Wexner Score and St. Marks (Vaizey) Score. Recently, Rogers et al. (2020) developed and validated a new measure, the Accidental Bowel Leakage Evaluation questionnaire, based on a more comprehensive conceptual framework that includes patient-important domains of predictability, awareness, control, emptying, and discomfort. Initial reliability and validity testing in a care-seeking population of women with fecal incontinence is promising.

A validated questionnaire for measuring quality of life, the Fecal Incontinence Quality of Life (FIQL), was reported in 2000 by Rockwood et al. and has 29 items that relate to four scales: lifestyle, coping/behavior, depression/self-perception, and embarrassment. The FIQL is currently used routinely to assess quality of life during the patient's follow-up after any mode of treatment.

Treatment success is frequently defined as at least 50% reduction in fecal incontinence episodes, although patients would prefer this number to be greater than 75%. See Chapter 41 for further discussion of these and other patient-reported outcome measures.

Diagnostic Testing

Diagnostic testing for fecal incontinence may include the use of colonoscopy, endoanal ultrasound, magnetic resonance imaging (MRI), anorectal physiologic testing, and defecography. Additional testing is not required to begin treatment of fecal incontinence but is most often used if patients do not respond to conservative treatments and in more complex cases. (See Chapter 9 for further discussion.)

Colonoscopy. Colonoscopy is indicated with new-onset fecal incontinence, mainly in the context of new onset of diarrhea and loose stool, to evaluate for cancer and inflammation seen with inflammatory bowel disease and microscopic colitis. Additionally, red flags identified during evaluation, such as weight loss, anemia, and family history of colorectal cancer or inflammatory bowel disease, will also warrant a colonoscopy. In other patients, providers should ensure that colorectal cancer screening is up to date. American Cancer Society guidelines now recommend colorectal cancer screening, which may include colonoscopy, in adults with average risk of colorectal cancer beginning at age 45 years (Wolf et al., 2018).

Endoanal Ultrasonography. Endoanal ultrasonography is a valuable tool in the assessment of fecal incontinence, particularly in patients with a history of birth trauma or anorectal surgery or when examination suggests a sphincter defect is present. A probe inserted into the rectum and withdrawn through the anal canal allows for a 360-degree visualization of the internal and external anal sphincter muscles. Imaging of the anal sphincter is most useful when anal sphincter injury is suspected and when planning anal sphincter repair, allowing visualization of the extent and location of muscular defects (Fig. 27.2). Clinical guidelines support this practice and recommend considering endoanal ultrasound or other imaging in patients with reduced anal pressures who have failed conservative therapy, particularly if surgery is being considered (Wald et al., 2014). Findings on endoanal ultrasound do not predict clinical outcomes following conservative treatment or sacral neuromodulation (SNM). Chapter 13 includes a more detailed discussion of endoanal and transperineal ultrasonography to evaluate anal sphincter defects.

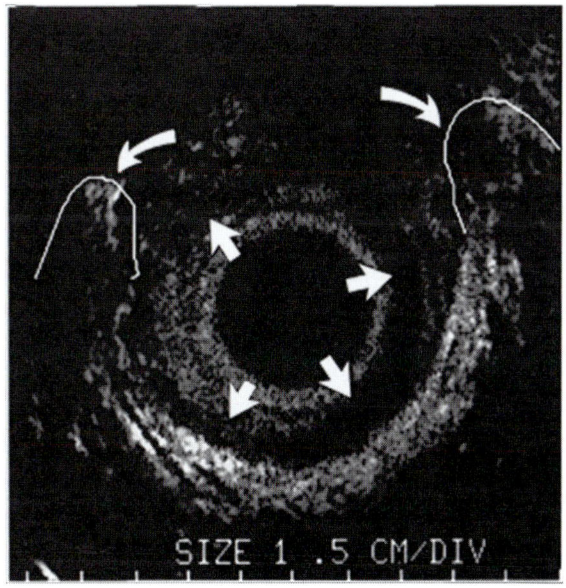

Fig. 27.2 Endoanal ultrasonography at the midanal canal in a woman with fecal incontinence and prior vaginal delivery. The internal anal sphincter is intact (*straight arrows*). The external anal sphincter has an anterior defect (*curved arrows*).

Magnetic Resonance Imaging. Magnetic resonance imaging (MRI) can also be used to identify sphincter anatomy and defects, as it identifies external anal sphincter atrophy and can differentiate a scar from a tear. Because of high cost and high interobserver variability in pelvic MRI interpretation, endoanal ultrasound is preferable in most cases (Lockhart et al., 2008).

Anorectal Physiology Testing. Anorectal physiology testing may include manometry, rectal sensation testing, and pudendal nerve studies. Anorectal function is most often assessed by anorectal manometry (ARM), which provides quantitative measurement of the resting anal pressure generated mainly by the internal anal sphincter and the squeeze pressure generated by the external anal sphincter. ARM also provides information about the length of the anal canal, rectal sensitivity, rectal compliance, and the integrity of the rectoanal inhibitory reflex. A short anal canal and/or decreased resting and squeeze pressures are found in the majority of patients with fecal incontinence.

Rectal sensation can be studied by inserting a balloon and determining the minimal volume that the rectum can sense, then sequentially inflating the balloon to a volume that cannot be tolerated. Increased rectal sensitivity signals a rectal reservoir that does not appropriately store stool and may push the fecal bolus past sphincter muscles, even if the sphincter muscle pressures are adequate. Pudendal nerve terminal motor latency can be determined using an electrode attached to a glove inserted into the anal canal. A prolonged conduction in the pudendal nerve may signal damage to the innervation of the external sphincter and puborectalis muscle.

Anorectal physiology tests can provide information about specific elements of anorectal dysfunction, and thus contribute to treatment planning, particularly in more complex patients. However, the clinical utility of ARM is questionable, as its results do not consistently correlate with fecal incontinence severity or predict treatment outcomes. Most current practice guidelines do not recommend routine use of ARM in patients with fecal incontinence (Paquette et al., 2015; American College of Obstetricians and Gynecologists, 2019). Based on moderate-quality evidence, an American College of Gastroenterology Clinical Practice Guideline (Wald et al., 2014) recommended the use of ARM and balloon expulsion and rectal sensation tests in patients who do not respond to conservative treatments. Pudendal nerve latency results also do not predict treatment success, and this test is not recommended for most patients.

Defecography. Defecography is indicated if rectal prolapse or internal intussusception (occult prolapse) is suspected. Of note: if fecal incontinence is severe, the rectal contrast may leak before initiation of the test, and results will be of limited value. See Chapter 13 for a more thorough discussion of defecography.

NONSURGICAL TREATMENT

Fig. 27.3 presents a stepwise algorithm for clinical management of patients with fecal incontinence recently proposed by Brown et al. (2020). Treatment should begin with patient education, the identification of possible food triggers to loose stools and fecal urgency (e.g., fructose, lactose, caffeine), and conservative approaches, initially focusing on dietary changes and supplements to manage stool consistency, antidiarrheal medications, and pelvic floor strengthening (physical therapy/biofeedback). The cause of fecal incontinence is often multifactorial, so no single therapy will benefit all patients. Expert opinion suggests at least 3 months of conservative therapy including stool bulking and pelvic floor strengthening should be pursued prior to offering more invasive treatment options (Ivatury et al., 2021).

Dietary and Medical Treatments

Dietary and medical treatments of fecal incontinence primarily focus on fiber supplementation to increase stool bulk and reduce watery stools, anticonstipation efforts (increased fluid and fiber, and/or laxatives) in patients with hard consistency stools, and antidiarrheal medications in those with loose stools. Because of their low risk, such conservative measures are recommended as initial treatments; however, the evidence base supporting their use is relatively sparse (Paquette et al., 2015; Wald et al., 2014).

The use of fiber bulking agents, such as psyllium husk (Metamucil; Procter & Gamble, Cincinnati, OH) and methylcellulose (Citrucel; GSK, Philadelphia, PA), can change stool consistency, making it firmer and more easily controlled. One small trial found psyllium to be superior to other fibers (methylcellulose and gum arabic) and to placebo in terms of reducing the frequency of fecal incontinence. Participants reported a 51% reduction in fecal incontinence episodes per week after treatment with psyllium, compared with a 32% increase, 20% reduction, and 11% reduction in the methylcellulose, gum arabic, and placebo groups, respectively (Bliss et al., 2014). Gradually increasing fiber intake may help reduce side effects such as abdominal distension and bloating. For example, we recommend starting with a teaspoon of psyllium daily and working up to a tablespoon up to two times daily as tolerated. If one fiber causes side effects, sometimes another will be better tolerated.

Agents designed to slow down the intestinal tract may also help with stool control. Even in patients without diarrhea, these agents may cause slight constipation, improving continence. Loperamide hydrochloride (Imodium; Johnson & Johnson, New Brunswick, NJ) is most often prescribed in this category. Loperamide prolongs intestinal transit time, allowing fecal volume to be reduced (secondary to the increased time allowed for removal of fluid from stool) and bulk density to be increased. It also increases rectal compliance, which decreases urgency. The dosage can be individualized for each patient, and it can be taken regularly or as needed. If patients have particular trouble after meals, 2 to 4 mg may be given before a meal to decrease the chance of stooling. The maximum daily dosage is 16 mg. A double-blind, randomized crossover trial compared the efficacy of psyllium and loperamide and found both to be similarly efficacious in reducing fecal incontinence episodes, but side effects were more common during loperamide treatment (29% of participants reported constipation) (Markland et al., 2015).

Diphenoxylate hydrochloride with atropine sulfate (Lomotil; Pfizer, New York, NY) can also be used to treat fecal incontinence, especially if diarrhea is a primary contributor to the incontinence. It is dosed similar to loperamide, with one or two 2.5-mg tablets taken up to four times daily. As with loperamide, the dosing must be individualized, and the most common side effect is constipation. Other less commonly used agents that focus on control of diarrhea may include cholestyramine, anticholinergic agents, and codeine. The anticholinergic agent darifenacin showed preliminary but encouraging results in an open-label, prospective study of 32 women with double urinary and fecal incontinence. Following 8 weeks of 15 mg darifenacin daily, 19 subjects reported reduced frequency of fecal incontinence and urinary symptoms and improved quality of life (Kissane et al., 2020).

Pelvic Floor Muscle Exercises and Biofeedback

Pelvic floor muscle rehabilitative treatments are another mainstay of conservative treatment for fecal incontinence. Despite conflicting evidence in support of their effectiveness, these treatments are safe and low cost. Treatments in this category are variable and may include patients performing unsupervised pelvic floor exercises ("Kegels") or engaging in supervised pelvic floor muscle training/exercise programs, often with a physical therapist. Electrical stimulation therapy can be used with either approach. These treatments typically focus on strengthening the external anal sphincter and pelvic floor muscles. Pelvic floor muscle training can also be augmented with manometric or electromyography (EMG)-assisted biofeedback, a type of neuromuscular retraining. In addition to strengthening the anal sphincter and pelvic floor muscles, biofeedback programs also aim to improve coordination of rectal distension and anal sphincter contraction and to improve sensation of stool in the rectum.

For biofeedback-assisted training, a balloon is placed in the rectum to simulate stool. Anal sphincter contraction is measured with a different balloon in the anal canal, by an anal plug, or by perianal surface electrodes. When contraction of the

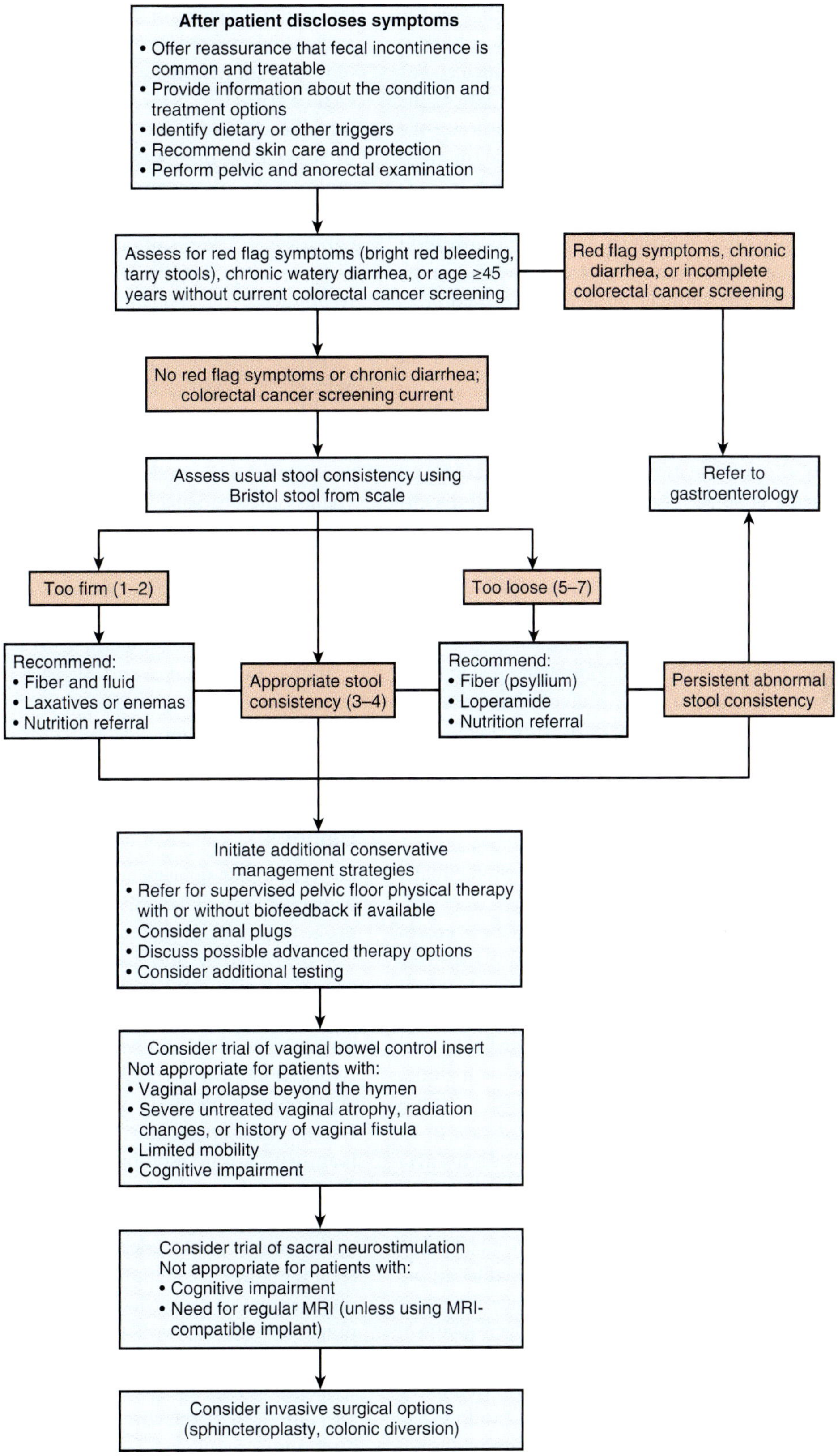

Fig. 27.3 Algorithm for management of fecal incontinence. *MRI*, Magnetic resonance imaging. (Reprinted with permission from Brown HW, Kyer KY, Rogers RG. Management of fecal incontinence, *Obstet Gynecol.* 2020;136:811.)

sphincter muscles is initiated, the patient observes this on the monitor. Visual (and, in some systems, auditory) feedback is given regarding contraction of the external sphincter. For sphincter strengthening, patients are encouraged when the proper sphincter response is made. They can then exercise the muscle by replicating this type of contraction outside the therapy session to increase the strength of the striated muscle.

Rectoanal coordination uses the same equipment. The goal is to train patients to achieve maximum voluntary squeeze in less than 1 second after the balloon is inflated in the rectum by consciously contracting the sphincter muscles. This method is customized for each patient, and patients may need one or more sessions to be able to perform the maneuver correctly at home. Rectal sensory perception is used to teach patients to sense smaller volumes of stool. The patients are urged to defecate with the balloon in the rectum, and observe this on the monitor. Gradually, the volume in the balloon is decreased, and patients learn to sense smaller volumes with less rectal distension. In one study, Rao et al. (1996) found that anal squeeze pressures, duration of squeeze, and capacity to retain liquid increased after biofeedback, and these findings correlated with a decrease in the number of episodes of fecal incontinence. However, these results have not been replicated.

Clinical trials for fecal incontinence comparing pelvic floor exercises, electrical stimulation, and biofeedback methods have reported conflicting results, possibly because of a lack of standardization in treatments and outcomes (Norton & Cody, 2012). One well-performed trial demonstrated superior outcomes for biofeedback compared with pelvic floor exercises alone in patients with at least weekly fecal incontinence unresponsive to other conservative measures (76% of biofeedback patients vs. 41% of pelvic floor exercise patients were improved at 3-month follow-up, $P < .001$) (Heymen et al., 2009). Norton et al. (2003) randomized 171 patients to four treatment groups: (1) standard care (dietary and behavioral education, medications); (2) standard care plus instruction on pelvic floor exercises; (3) standard care plus biofeedback; and (4) standard care plus biofeedback and the use of a home EMG biofeedback device. In contrast to the previous study's findings, biofeedback was not superior to standard care or to standard care with pelvic floor exercises, with equal numbers (54% vs. 53%) in the biofeedback and nonbiofeedback groups reporting improvement at 3 months. A systematic review of biofeedback and electrical stimulation by Vonthein et al. (2013) found sufficient evidence for the efficacy of biofeedback plus electrical stimulation in treating fecal incontinence. In addition, amplitude-modulated medium-frequency stimulation, also termed premodulated interferential stimulations, combined with biofeedback was superior to both low-frequency electrical stimulation and biofeedback alone. A randomized trial testing four different pelvic floor strengthening with biofeedback protocols that varied the number of in-person visits (from one to four) found that all were similarly effective, but that patient satisfaction was higher with more face-to-face contact (Young et al., 2018).

A recent multicenter, randomized factorial trial compared four different nonsurgical interventions in 300 women with fecal incontinence: oral placebo plus education only, placebo and ARM-assisted biofeedback, loperamide plus education only, and loperamide and ARM-assisted biofeedback (Jelovsek et al., 2019). After 24 weeks, all groups showed improvement in fecal incontinence severity score and bowel diary outcomes, but there were no differences between treatments (loperamide vs. oral placebo, biofeedback vs. education, loperamide and biofeedback vs. oral placebo, and biofeedback vs. loperamide plus education). The results can be partially explained by the fact that the control group, which received placebo plus education, responded better than anticipated, emphasizing the importance of patient education.

Pelvic floor muscle exercises are often grouped together with other conservative treatments. A recent randomized trial tested a group behavioral intervention ("Mind Over Matter: Healthy Bowels, Healthy Bladder") led by a trained community member (Brown et al., 2019). Older women with fecal and/or urinary incontinence were randomized to the intervention or a waitlist control group. The program provided education and promoted evidence-based self-management strategies and behaviors, including pelvic floor muscle exercises, dietary changes for optimization of stool consistency with gradual fiber supplementation, fluid adjustment to avoid bladder irritants and optimize fluid intake, and bladder training techniques. Both urinary incontinence and fecal incontinence improved for the intervention compared to control (71% vs. 23%, $P < 0.001$ and 55% vs. 27%, $P < .005$, respectively), offering a feasible community-based treatment.

Devices

Passive barrier devices include anal plugs and a vaginal bowel control device. These devices offer another conservative approach for managing fecal incontinence, although their use has not been widely adopted as yet. Evidence supporting these treatments remains limited, but risks appear to be low.

Anal plugs are simple devices that act as barriers to stool leakage. The plugs can be inserted after a bowel movement and removed manually or expelled during defecation. The Peristeen anal plug (Coloplast, Humlebaek, Denmark), available in Europe and Canada only, comes in two sizes and is made of soft foam with a water-soluble film that dissolves in the anal canal. The plug expands to three to four times its size and can be retained for 8 hours. Limited evidence suggests that long-term use is successful and tolerated in select patients and may reduce fecal incontinence symptoms (Bond et al., 2007). Another anal plug (Renew; Renew Medical, Foster City, CA) is a soft silicone plug, self-inserted with the use of a fingertip applicator and available in two sizes. In a prospective multicenter study (n = 91), 80% of enrolled participants completed 12 weeks of device use, and 78% of the completers reported more than a 50% reduction in frequency of fecal incontinence episodes (Lukacz et al., 2015). Adverse effects were generally mild, and limited to anal irritation and rectal pressure or discomfort.

A vaginal bowel control system (Eclipse System; Pelvalon, Sunnyvale, CA) was introduced recently. The vaginal silicone-coated device contains a dynamic balloon oriented posteriorly that reversibly compresses the rectum to aid in continence. In a prospective multicenter study, 62% of women enrolled achieved a successful fit. Some 53 of 73 (73%) women who entered the treatment phase had success at 3 months (>50% reduction in fecal incontinence episodes), and 74% continued therapy through 12 months with greater than 90% satisfaction (Richter et al., 2019). Adverse effects occurred in 38% of women during the treatment period, were generally mild, and most often included pelvic or vaginal discomfort or irritation and vaginal wall injury.

Bowel Management

Some patients find that daily enemas with approximately two pints of tap water, usually at the same time each morning just after eating, induce a bowel movement and empty the rectum. A cone-tipped catheter (the same type used for colostomy irrigation) may be helpful for incontinent patients to instill an enema so that it does not run out with instillation. Some advocate inserting a glycerin or bisacodyl suppository 20 to 30 minutes after eating, along with abdominal massage, to induce a bowel movement daily. With either method, bulking agents can be used, in addition to medications, to stop stooling in between desired defecation.

For patients with fecal incontinence associated with more severe dysfunction, such as neurogenic bowel, there is also a designated colonic irrigation system that combines tap water irrigation with a rectal balloon (Peristeen System; Coloplast, Humlebaek, Denmark). Inflation of the balloon prevents the water from leaking, and deflation results in irrigation of the rectosigmoid.

PROCEDURES AND SURGERY

Perianal Bulking Injections

Anal canal bulking injections have been performed using a wide variety of substances (including autologous fat, synthetic bovine dermal collagen, Teflon, silicone, and carbon beads) and techniques. In 2011 the US Food and Drug Administration (FDA) approved the use of dextranomer microspheres in non–animal-stabilized hyaluronic acid (NASHA Dx) (Solesta; Salix Pharmaceuticals, Raleigh, NC) injected into the anal canal as a treatment for fecal incontinence. In a multicenter randomized study, 52% of patients injected with NASHA Dx had a greater than 50% reduction in fecal incontinence episodes compared with 31% of those receiving a sham injection, and complications were rare (Graf et al., 2011). About 80% of the patients in both treatment arms had a second injection because of inadequate response. A Cochrane review concluded that NAHSA Dx may confer short-term benefits to just over half of patients treated (Maeda et al., 2013). Longer-term results subsequently published suggested that reductions in fecal incontinence episodes, as well as quality-of-life improvements, were sustained at 24 and 36 months in those patients with initial success (Mellgren et al., 2014). This and other smaller and uncontrolled studies support modest improvements in symptoms after perianal bulking injections with some sustained effects.

NASHA Dx is currently the only FDA-approved bulking product for fecal incontinence. Perianal bulking agents are administered in an outpatient setting and do not require anesthesia. The injection kit comes as four preloaded syringes holding 1 cc of the NASHA Dx gel. The gel is injected into the submucosal space in four areas 5 mm above the dentate line. The procedure is carried out in the office using a large beveled anoscope. This is a safe procedure, with minor bleeding being the most common complication, although rarely patients have developed a postprocedure abscess.

Although the assumption is that bulking agents improve closure of the anal canal, posttreatment anal manometry failed to show improvement of resting and squeeze pressures (Dehli et al., 2013). The original NASHA Dx trial included patients with severe fecal incontinence and with no sphincter defect, and it is unknown if patients with sphincter defects or with mild to moderate fecal incontinence will benefit. Clinical practice guidelines from the American College of Gastroenterology provide a weak recommendation that injectable anal bulking agents may have a role in treatment of fecal incontinence in patients who do not respond to conservative treatments, including biofeedback therapy (Bharucha et al., 2017; Wald et al., 2014).

Sacral Neuromodulation

SNM was approved by the FDA for treatment of fecal incontinence in 2011. The sacral nerve stimulation procedure, involving implantation of a wire electrode near the third sacral nerve root attached to a subcutaneous implantable pulse generator, is essentially the same as when used for treatment of urgency urinary incontinence. Chapter 32 includes a detailed discussion of procedure steps, reviewed briefly here.

As in treatment of urgency urinary incontinence, the procedure consists of two parts. Initially, a test phase is completed with placement of a sacral stimulation lead through the S3 sacral foramen. This can be performed using a less-invasive office-based percutaneous nerve evaluation (PNE) procedure, placing a temporary electrode wire with or without fluoroscopic guidance, or as an outpatient stage I procedure with placement of a permanent, self-anchoring lead (Fig. 27.4), which is confirmed radiologically (Fig. 27.5). During the 1- to 2-week test phase, the lead is connected to a temporary stimulation device, and the patient reports episodes of fecal incontinence and stool consistency in a diary. If the patient reports a greater than 50% improvement in frequency of fecal incontinence episodes compared with a preprocedure diary, the permanent neurostimulator is implanted in the upper buttock region. If the improvement seen is not sufficient, or if no improvement occurs, the lead is removed. When the staged approach is used, stage II is typically performed about 2 weeks after stage I to lessen the chance of infectious complications.

The option of performing the test phase using the PNE approach rather than a stage I procedure has been less widely used by surgeons performing SNM for fecal incontinence in the United States, but evidence suggests similar success rates for both approaches. A drawback of PNE is that the wire is not as secure as the tined lead and may migrate, giving a false negative result. For this reason, if the test is negative, formal operating room placement of the tined lead (a staged approach) may still

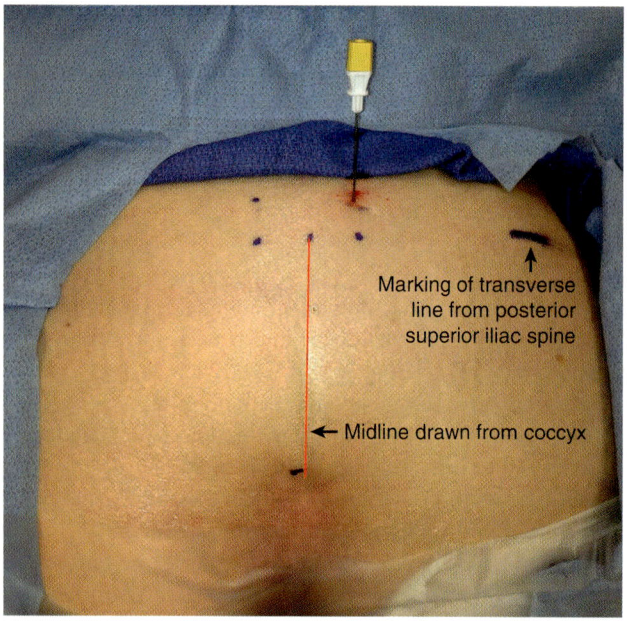

Fig. 27.4 Insertion of the needle and electrodes at the region of the S3 foramen.

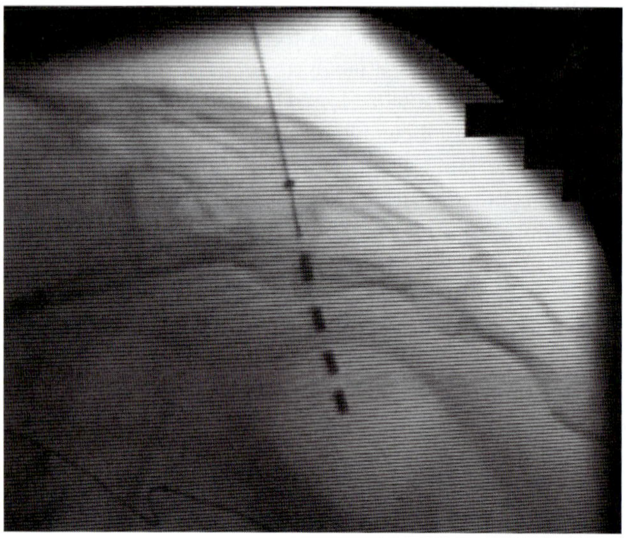

Fig. 27.5 Radiological confirmation of the electrode placement at the S3 foramen.

be considered. The popularity of PNE is owed in part to its low cost and commitment because it can be placed in the office and removed easily if there is not a benefit. If it is successful, the permanent device can be placed in the future with no mandatory time for implantation, as with stage II.

Results have been encouraging for SNM. In the uncontrolled FDA-monitored trial, 133 participants were eligible for stage I. Of those, 120 were implanted with the permanent device during stage II. The results over 1, 3, and 5 years of follow-up remained consistent, with approximately 85% maintaining the treatment goal of a greater than 50% reduction in fecal incontinence episodes (Hull et al., 2013; Mellgren et al., 2011; Wexner et al., 2010a), and 40% remaining totally continent. Devroede et al. (2012) documented sustained long-term improvement in quality of life in this group. Wexner et al. (2010b) showed that this appears to be a safe procedure, with an acceptable complication profile and infection rate of about 11%.

Despite significant evidence of the efficacy for SNM for fecal incontinence in uncontrolled trials, few randomized controlled trials have been performed comparing SNM to other medical or surgical treatments. Thaha et al. (2015) performed a Cochrane systematic review of SNM for fecal incontinence that included two small, parallel-group randomized trials (SNM vs. optimal medical therapy and vs. percutaneous tibial nerve stimulation), as well as several crossover trials. The parallel-group randomized trials both found greater reductions in fecal incontinence episodes in the SNM groups. The Cochrane authors concluded that limited evidence showed that SNM can improve continence in a proportion of patients with fecal incontinence. A more recent trial included 58 women with fecal incontinence after obstetric anal sphincter injury randomized to SNM versus submucosal anal bulking injection with cross-linked porcine dermal collagen. Similar to the previous trials, at 6 months incontinence and condition-specific quality of life scores all improved to a greater extent in the SNM group (Rydningen et al., 2017). SNM efficacy appears long-lasting. In a 10-year postprocedure follow-up of 360 patients, 45% of patients were still satisfied with their procedure, 39.1% were dissatisfied, and 23.1% were lost to follow-up. Of note, 64.7% of the patients needed a revision of their implant, and 26.1% had their device explanted (Desprez et al., 2020).

SNM was initially studied and FDA approved for patients with fecal incontinence and anal sphincter defects of less than 120 degrees. Ratto et al. (2012) systematically reviewed ten smaller studies of SNM for fecal incontinence in women with sphincter defects and found high success rates and improved quality-of-life outcomes, but study quality was generally low. More high-quality research is needed to better understand outcomes in patients with larger sphincter defects. To date no studies have directly compared SNM with anal sphincteroplasty for patients with fecal incontinence associated with anal sphincter defects.

The mechanism by which SNM improves fecal incontinence is not clear. SNM may activate pudendal nerve afferents, and afferent pudendal somatic fibers are believed to inhibit colonic motility and activate the internal anal sphincter (Gourcerol et al., 2011). Limited research to date (human- and animal-based) also suggests that SNM may function via the central nervous system, impacting brain activities and corticoanal pathways relevant to the continence mechanism (Janssen et al., 2017). Future research in these areas may help identify patient groups most likely to respond to SNM therapy.

Current practice guidelines for fecal incontinence give a strong recommendation for the use of SNM as an initial surgical option for patients who have failed medical measures because it has demonstrated good long-term efficacy in patients with or without anal sphincter defects, and low morbidity (American College of Obstetricians and Gynecologists, 2019; Bharucha et al., 2017; Paquette et al., 2015).

Anal Sphincteroplasty

For many years, anal sphincteroplasty was the primary surgical procedure performed for fecal incontinence in women who had

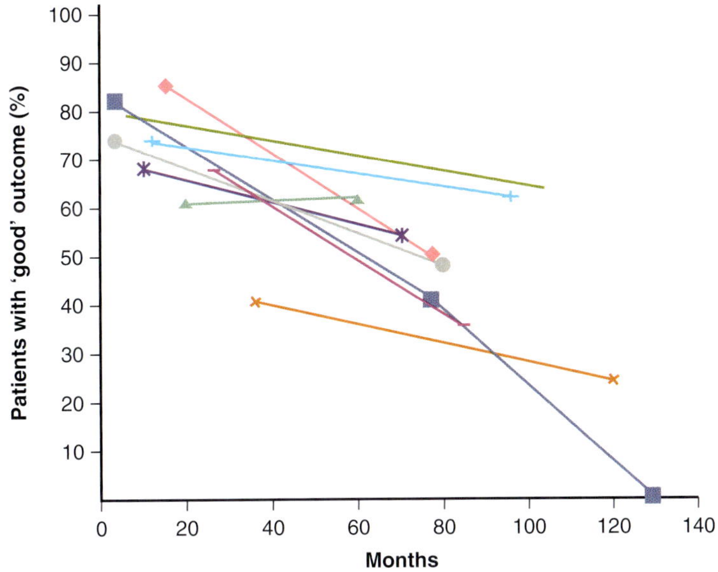

Fig. 27.6 Results from nine published studies examining long-term outcomes after anal sphincter repair. "Good" outcome was determined using varied definitions provided by the authors of each article, and included patients with improved incontinence, improved global score, and reduced impact on lifestyle. (Reprinted with permission from Glasgow SC, Lowry AC. Long-term outcomes of anal sphincter repair for fecal incontinence: a systematic review. *Dis Colon Rectum.* 2012;55:482.)

evidence of an anal sphincter defect. However, over the past decade, evidence has accumulated that favors improved results for SNM compared with sphincteroplasty, especially when long-term outcomes are considered (Fig. 27.6). Given this, most surgeons currently favor SNM before sphincteroplasty in the majority of patients. Still, sphincteroplasty remains an important treatment option for women with fecal incontinence who decline device implantation, those with a symptomatic cloacal perineal defect (in whom sphincteroplasty is performed as part of perineal reconstruction), and those who do not respond to SNM.

Anal sphincteroplasty is performed using the steps described below. See Figs. 27.7, 27.8, and 27.9 and Videos 27.1 and 27.2 for illustrations, surgical photographs, and videos of this procedure.

1. Preparation

   Many surgeons perform mechanical bowel preparation before sphincteroplasty, but we reserve this for more complex repairs or for patients with significant constipation. For most sphincter repairs, we feel bowel preparation is unnecessary. Some surgeons prefer to have patients use an enema before surgery to empty the rectum, or to perform an enema in the operating room just before surgery. Based on antibiotic prophylaxis recommendations developed for primary repair of obstetric anal sphincter injury, we administer a single dose of intravenous antibiotics just before incision (American College of Obstetricians and Gynecologists, 2018). General anesthesia is commonly used, although the procedure can be performed under epidural or spinal anesthesia. We perform anal sphincteroplasty in the lithotomy position using candy cane or boot stirrups, but this can also be performed in the prone, jackknife position (preferred by many colorectal surgeons). A Foley catheter is placed.

2. Incision (Fig. 27.7A, inset)

   An inverted-U incision is made close to the anal skin edge, typically extending from the 3 o'clock to the 9 o'clock position around the anus. We inject the area first with dilute lidocaine and epinephrine. Allis clamps may be placed at the lateral edges of this incision to provide countertraction while making the incision and during dissection.

3. Dissection and identification of the external anal sphincter muscle (Fig. 27.8C and D)

   The surgeon's finger is placed in the rectum during dissection to aid in identifying the correct plane of dissection and in avoiding rectal injury. Sharp dissection is used to separate the perineal and posterior vaginal skin away from the anterior rectal wall and sphincter complex. The skin incision may be extended vertically into the posterior vagina if needed. Any tears in the anal mucosa that occur during dissection can be repaired with No. 4-0 polyglactin suture.

   The external anal sphincter edges are typically retracted laterally and posteriorly. The extent and location of the external and/or internal anal sphincter defect(s) may be known in advance from a preoperative endoanal ultrasound. This may be helpful in locating the muscle edges in some cases. A nerve stimulator or electrocautery may aid in identifying viable muscle, as the muscle can be seen to contract when stimulated (if the patient is not paralyzed). The ends of the external sphincter muscles can be grasped with Allis clamps and elevated while being mobilized sharply from surrounding skin and anal mucosa. Any scar tissue and the sphincter capsule (if present) should be left attached to the muscles.

   It is important to remember that the branches of the pudendal nerves that innervate the external sphincter approach

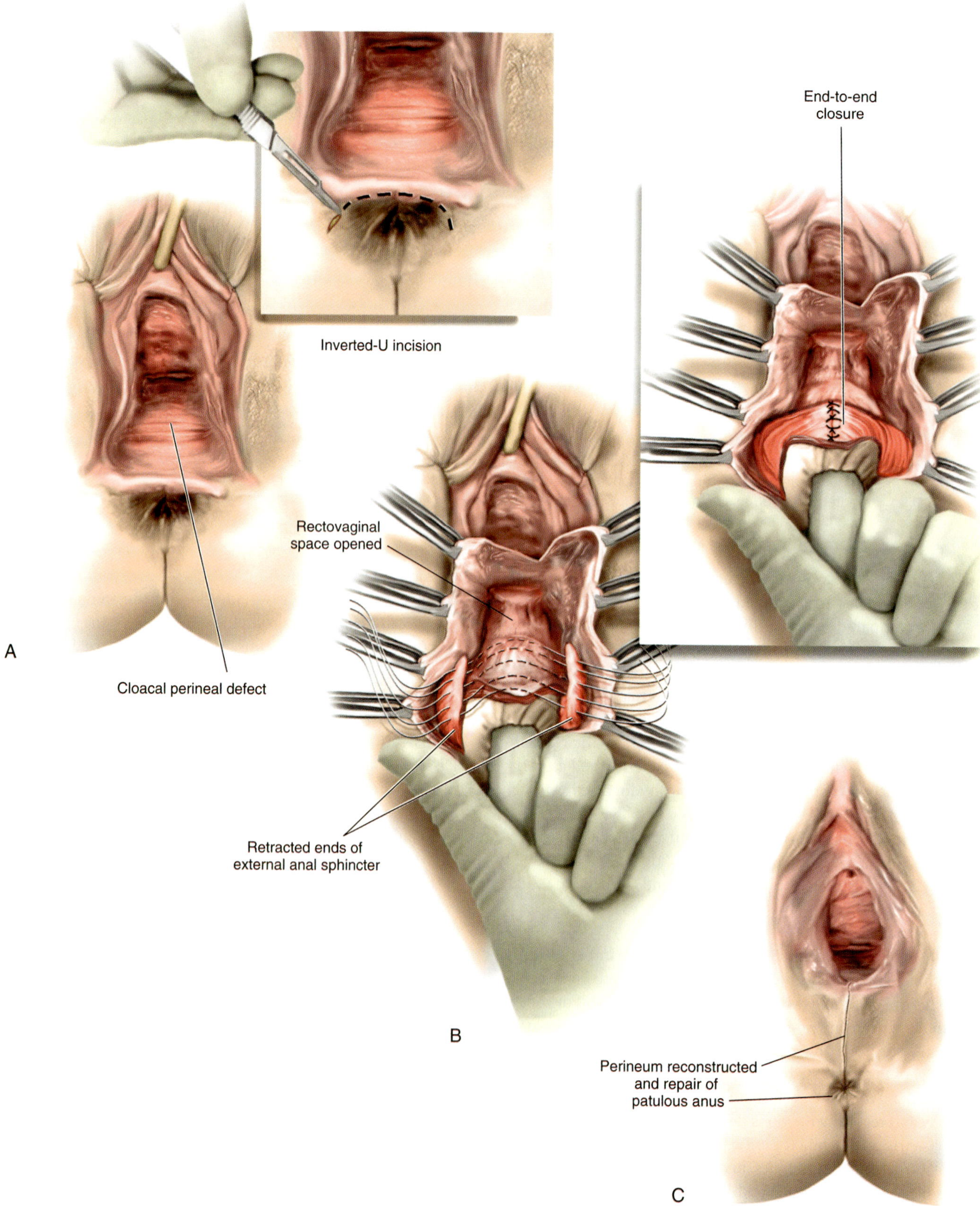

Fig. 27.7 Technique of end-to-end sphincteroplasty with perineal reconstruction. **A**, A cloacal perineal defect is noted, with the posterior vaginal and anterior rectal walls scarred together. An inverted-U incision is made (*inset*). **B**, The rectovaginal space has been opened, and the anterior rectal wall exposed. The retracted ends of the external anal sphincter have been identified. Sutures incorporate the external anal sphincter muscle on each side and include small bites through the internal anal sphincter. The completed end-to-end sphincteroplasty is shown (*inset*). **C**, The perineum has been completely reconstructed, an the patulous anal opening has been narrowed. (Reprinted with permission from Baggish M, Karram M. *Atlas of Pelvic Anatomy and Gynecologic Surgery*. 5th ed. Philadelphia: Elsevier; 2020.)

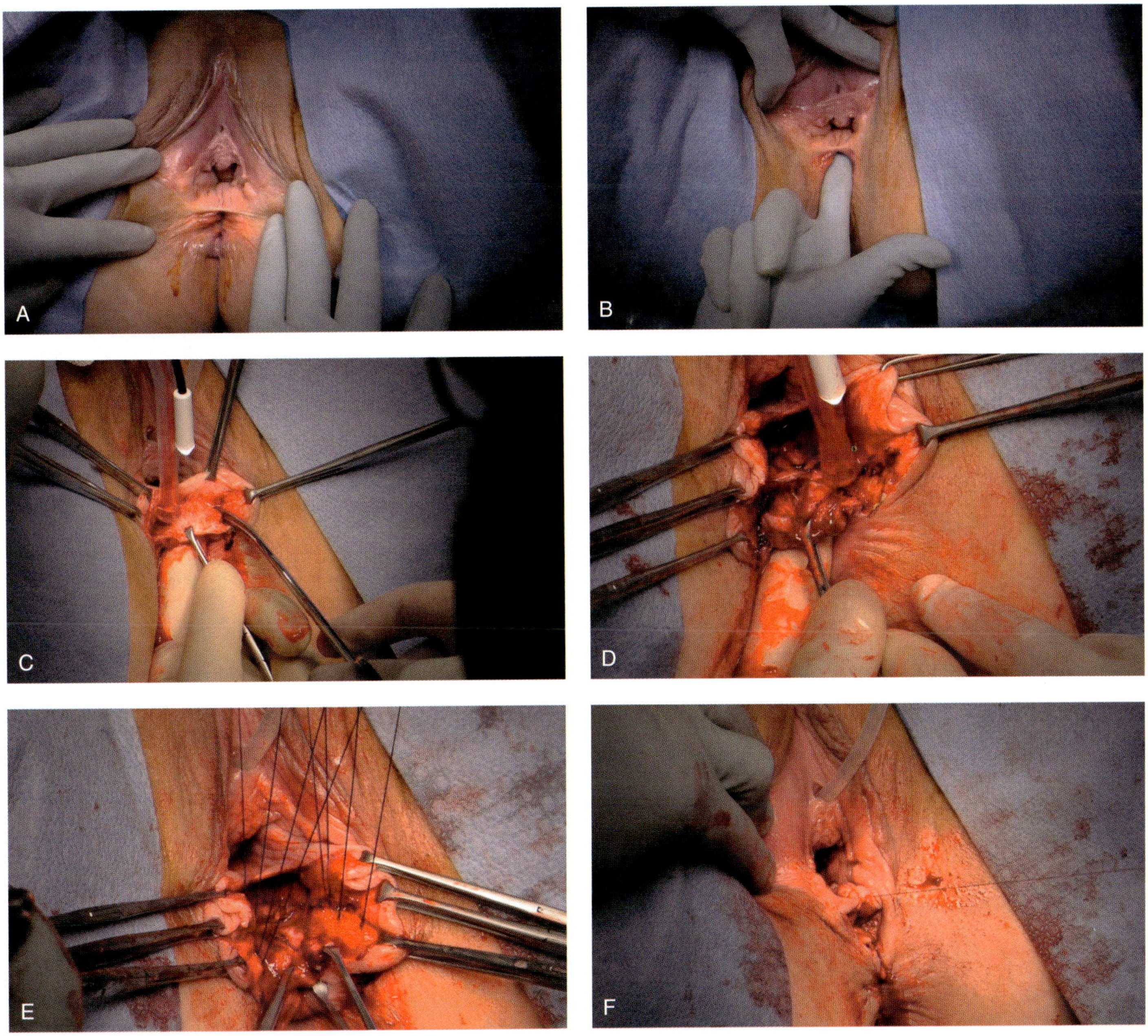

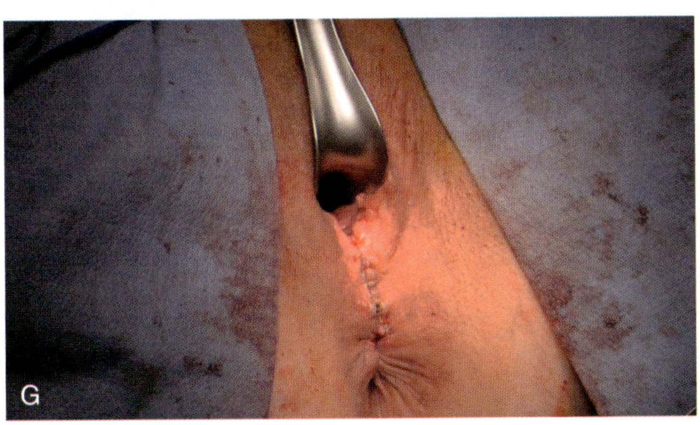

Fig. 27.8 Anal sphincteroplasty and perineal reconstruction in a patient with prior third-degree perineal laceration who presents with fecal incontinence and a cloacal perineal defect. **A** and **B**, Note retracted edges of the external anal sphincter, patulous anal opening, widened genital hiatus, and absent perineum. **C**, Sharp dissection is used to separate the posterior vaginal wall from the anterior wall of the rectum. **D**, Dissection is extended laterally to identify retracted edges of the external anal sphincter. **E**, Delayed absorbable sutures have been passed through the edges of the external anal sphincter, with the same sutures also incorporating bites of the internal anal sphincter. **F**, Anal sphincter sutures have been tied (in end-to-end fashion), and the posterior vaginal wall closed. **G**, The perineum has been reconstructed, and the perineal skin has been reapproximated. (Reprinted with permission from Baggish M, Karram M. *Atlas of Pelvic Anatomy and Gynecologic Surgery*. 5th ed. Philadelphia: Elsevier; 2020.)

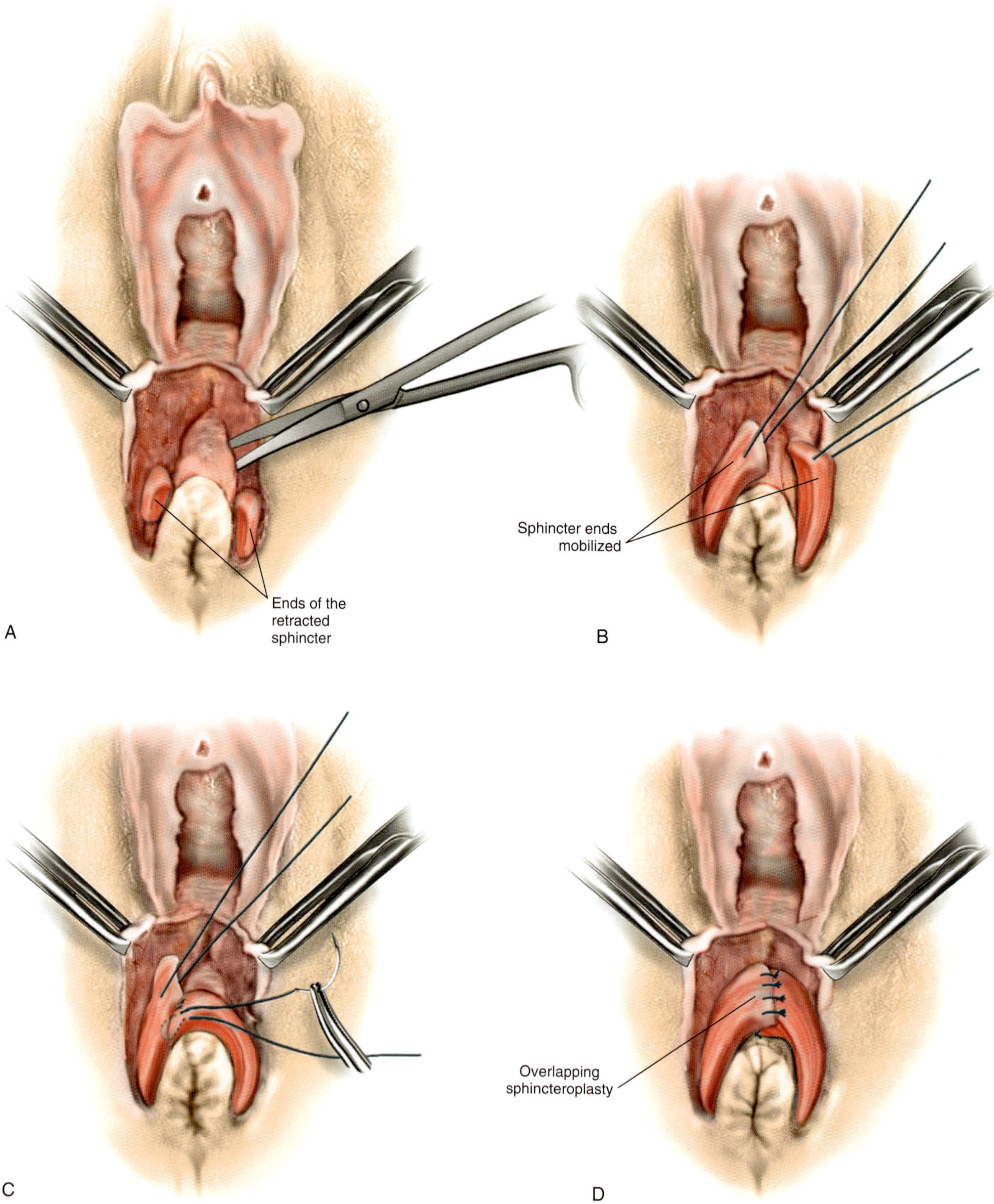

Fig. 27.9 Overlapping sphincteroplasty technique is illustrated. **A**, Dissection has been completed, exposing the anterior rectal wall and ends of the retracted external anal sphincter. **B** and **C**, Delayed absorbable sutures are placed through the mobilized ends of the external anal sphincter and tied (**D**) in an overlapping fashion. (Reprinted with permission from Baggish M, Karram M. *Atlas of Pelvic Anatomy and Gynecologic Surgery.* 5th ed. Philadelphia: Elsevier; 2020.)

the muscle from the posterolateral position at approximately the 5 o'clock and 7 o'clock positions. To avoid nerve injury, the arc of the incision should not extend to the extreme posterolateral position, and excessive mobilization of the sphincter muscle ends in this area should be avoided.

4. Sphincter muscle suture placement and reapproximation

The internal anal sphincter muscle, if identified, may be reapproximated to the midline over the anal mucosa using interrupted or continuous No. 3-0 polyglactin sutures. However, dissection of this layer is difficult, and if both internal and external muscles are injured, we prefer to leave them intact and repair them as one unit. If the internal sphincter is not disrupted, we identify and repair the external sphincter (but may incorporate the internal anal sphincter muscle in the sutures, as described later).

The external anal sphincter can be repaired using an end-to-end or overlapping technique. Whereas evidence does not clearly support improved outcomes for either approach (Fernando et al., 2013; Glasgow & Lowry, 2012), if adequate length of the sphincter ends can be mobilized, we prefer an overlapping technique. If the sphincter defect is large, dissection and mobilization of adequate lengths of the sphincter muscle to perform an overlapping repair may be challenging and potentially more morbid, and in this case end-to-end repair is typically performed.

For end-to-end repair, a series of No. 2-0 polyglactin or polydioxanone sutures are used, extending for the length of the sphincter complex (Figs. 27.7B and 27.8E). Each suture is placed through the exposed end of the left sphincter muscle, including scar or capsule tissue if present, and then similarly through the end of the right sphincter muscle. Small "bites" through the internal anal sphincter muscle (if intact) can be taken between the two sides. We place these sutures starting near the perineal skin and extending proximally, holding them without tying until all are placed. Typically, four or more sutures are used, which will reapproximate the sphincter complex for a length of at least 4 cm.

If using an overlapping technique, we place mattress sutures for the sphincteroplasty, using No. 2-0 polyglactin or polydioxanone sutures, in two columns of three to four sutures on each side (Fig. 27.9). Sutures from the underlying layer are all placed and then tied, before placing and tying sutures in the overlapping layer. The sphincter repair (whether end-to-end or overlapping) is performed to tighten the anal canal so that just an index finger is admitted.

5. Perineal reconstruction and skin closure

The perineal skin incision is usually closed in a vertical orientation, which helps lengthen the perineum. We often begin the inferior portion of the skin closure before tying the sphincter sutures, as the skin edges in this area may retract into the anal canal when the sutures are tied. The vaginal incision (if present) is closed, and perineal reconstruction is performed, using interrupted No. 2-0 polyglactin sutures. The perineal skin can be closed using a continuous subcuticular suture, but we prefer to use interrupted No. 2-0 or 3-0 absorbable sutures. In some cases, the skin incision may be closed in an inverted-Y configuration, if a simple vertical closure would place too much tension on the lateral skin edges.

6. Postoperative care

Patients are most often admitted overnight for observation and discharged home the next day, but healthy patients can be discharged home the same day per patient or provider preference. We advance the patient's diet and activity as tolerated and remove the Foley catheter as soon as the patient is able to void spontaneously. A postoperative bowel regimen is important. We recommend daily psyllium, with additional laxatives in patients who have preoperative constipation, with a goal of avoiding both liquid and very hard stool consistency. Superficial skin separation and wound drainage from the perineal incision are common, and we counsel patients not to be concerned if this occurs. We recommend Sitz baths once or twice daily starting on postoperative day two, keeping the perineum clean and dry at other times, and using a skin protectant and moisture barrier (Vaseline or zinc oxide ointment) on the perineal skin as healing occurs to avoid irritation.

In higher risk patients, a diverting stoma may be considered at time of sphincteroplasty—for example, in patients with complex anatomic defects, previous failed repairs, or concomitant inflammatory bowel disease. A stoma does not ensure success but may aid a successful outcome in such complex patients.

When sphincteroplasty is performed after breakdown of an obstetric anal sphincter injury repair, traditional recommendations are to allow time (typically 2–3 months) for tissue inflammation to resolve before attempting the secondary repair. However, small studies suggest that early secondary repair may be successful. In one recent case series, 17 women underwent overlapping external anal sphincteroplasty with perineorrhaphy a median of 30 days after their delivery (median 19.5 days [interquartile range 12–26.8 days]) after diagnosis of wound breakdown (Lewicky-Gaup et al., 2021). Surgery was performed after treatment of wound infection (if present). Postoperative superficial wound separation occurred in two women and deeper wound breakdown in one, but at 3 months all women had healed completely, and none reported fecal incontinence.

The literature, although generally limited to retrospective case series and uncontrolled prospective studies, suggests that initial improvement in fecal incontinence symptoms can be anticipated in 85% of patients after sphincteroplasty, although complete continence is rare. Continence of gas is least likely to improve, and patients should be counseled of this carefully before surgery. Long-term sphincteroplasty outcomes demonstrate gradual deterioration in function. In a systematic review of 16 studies with at least 5 years' follow-up, all but one study reported a decline over time in the percentage of patients reporting at least a "good" outcome (defined as any improvement in incontinence symptoms, improvement based on a global rating, or improved quality of life) (Fig. 27.6; Glasgow & Lowry,

2012). In more than half of the studies included, 50% or more patients had only fair (minimal improvement) or poor (worsened) outcomes 5 to 10 years after surgery. Predictors of success versus failure after sphincteroplasty have not been clearly defined. Pudendal nerve damage was associated with suboptimal results in one early study, but several later studies did not confirm this finding. Advanced age has also been reported to be associated with poorer outcomes in a few studies, but not in others.

Wound infection, the most common adverse event after sphincteroplasty, occurs in 6% to 35% of patients, and deep wound infection is associated with poorer long-term outcomes (Oom et al., 2009). Superficial skin separation is common and usually heals by secondary intention with adequate wound care. Other complications include hematoma, dyspareunia, and new defecatory dysfunction.

Based on available evidence, clinical practice guidelines from the American College of Obstetricians and Gynecologists (2019) and the American Society of Colon and Rectal Surgeons (Paquette et al., 2015) recommend that sphincteroplasty be considered in women with fecal incontinence and anal sphincter disruption who have failed conservative treatments. A 2017 American Gastroenterology Association Clinical Practice Update more narrowly defined the use of sphincteroplasty and recommended it as an option for postpartum women with fecal incontinence and in women with recent sphincter injuries. Additionally, the publication advised that sphincteroplasty be considered in women who present remote from likely sphincter injury with fecal incontinence and evidence of sphincter damage if they are unresponsive to conservative and biofeedback therapy, and if perianal bulking injections and SNM are not available or unsuccessful (Bharucha et al., 2017). Others have recommended that sphincteroplasty be reserved for women with sphincter defect present and less than 120 degrees or in younger women with recent sphincter injury, for example within the past year (Ivatury et al., 2021; Katuwal & Bhullar, 2021).

Very limited evidence is available regarding outcomes of patients who undergo repeat anal sphincteroplasty surgery. Given this and the availability of other treatments (in particular SNM), the American Society of Colon and Rectal Surgeons recommends that repeat anal sphincter reconstruction after a failed anal sphincteroplasty generally be avoided (Paquette et al., 2015).

Colostomy or Ileostomy

Fecal diversion, in the form of an end colostomy or, occasionally, an ileostomy, can be considered for patients with incapacitating fecal incontinence who have failed other treatments. In a UK survey of patients who had permanent colostomy for fecal incontinence, over 80% were positive about the stoma and its impact on their lifestyle and would undergo this treatment again (Norton et al., 2005).

ADDITIONAL TREATMENT CONSIDERATIONS

Percutaneous Tibial Nerve Stimulation

Percutaneous tibial nerve stimulation (PTNS) is currently not FDA approved for fecal incontinence, but is available to clinicians for the treatment of overactive bladder (Urgent PC; Cogentix Medical, Minnetonka, MN; and NURO; Medtronic, Minneapolis, MN). The procedure is done on an outpatient basis and involves stimulation of the posterior tibial nerve at the medial ankle, either by needle or surface electrode. See Chapter 32 for a detailed description of this procedure. Uncontrolled studies showed variable results; however, one randomized, multicenter, blinded, sham-controlled study enrolling 144 patients did not show any benefit of posterior tibial stimulation versus sham for the treatment of fecal incontinence (Leroi et al., 2012). Another large, multicenter, double-blind study from the United Kingdom enrolled 227 patients to receive either PTNS or sham and found no benefit of the active treatment: 39 (38%) of patients in the PTNS group had a 50% or greater reduction in episodes of fecal incontinence per week compared with 32 (31%) in the sham group ($P = .40$) (Knowles et al., 2015). A *post hoc* analysis of this trial showed that PTNS had better results compared with sham treatment in the small group of participants who did not report obstructive defecatory symptoms (Horrocks et al., 2017). More research is needed to confirm these results, but the best current evidence does not support the use of PTNS for the treatment of fecal incontinence.

Radiofrequency Energy Delivery

Radiofrequency energy delivery is an outpatient procedure done under conscious sedation and local anesthesia. The device used (Secca; Restech, Houston, TX) employs radiofrequency energy delivered to the anal sphincter and is proposed to improve sphincter function via collagen contraction and tissue remodeling. Although initial small studies suggested some benefits for this treatment and few risks, later prospective studies demonstrated low response rates and lack of a durable response (Lam et al., 2014). A single randomized, sham-controlled trial was performed in 40 participants with relatively severe fecal incontinence symptoms who had failed conservative treatments (Visscher et al., 2017). The study demonstrated statistically significant, small improvements in fecal incontinence symptom scores following radiofrequency energy treatment compared with sham, but these were thought to be clinically negligible. Quality-of-life scores and ARM outcomes did not differ between the groups. Given these findings, radiofrequency energy delivery treatment cannot be recommended in most patients with fecal incontinence and is rarely used. The American Society of Colon and Rectal Surgeons' Clinical Practice Guideline agreed that alternative treatments should be pursued before considering this option (Paquette et al., 2015).

Surgical Treatments Rarely Used or No Longer Available

In patients with severe fecal incontinence refractory to other surgical treatments, other surgeries have been offered in the past at specialized centers. In the graciloplasty (gracilis muscle transposition) procedure, the gracilis muscle was mobilized, wrapped around the anus, and stimulated with an implanted generator. Although successful outcomes were reported, the operation had a high risk of morbidity and a significant learning curve (Baeten et al., 2000). This procedure is rarely performed, and the generator used in the procedure is no longer available in the United States.

An artificial bowel sphincter was cleared by the FDA in 1999 through a humanitarian exemption (Acticon Neosphincter; American Medical Systems, Minnetonka, MN; no longer available). The device incorporated a balloon that, when fully inflated, occluded the anus, as well as a reservoir placed in the space of Retzius and a labial pump. The device was indicated for patients with severe symptoms in whom conventional management of fecal incontinence had failed. A similar artificial sphincter (Soft Anal Band System; A.M.I., Austria) is available in Europe, but evidence supporting use of this device is sparse. Few centers in the world perform artificial bowel sphincter procedures, and many technical challenges are associated with their implantation. Evidence supporting these devices is limited to one small randomized trial (n = 14) and uncontrolled case series (O'Brien et al., 2004). A systematic review of long-term outcomes of artificial bowel sphincter procedures (most using the Acticon Neosphincter) reported that 59% of devices were still functional at 5-year follow-up. However, complication and revision rates were high. Clinical practice guidelines recommend that the artificial bowel sphincter should be reserved for patients in whom all other treatments have failed, or those with extensive sphincter destruction, congenital malformations, neurogenic incontinence, or postsurgical significant bowel dysfunction with intact anal canal anatomy (Paquette et al., 2015).

Anal sphincter augmentation with a magnetic bead device was available that involved surgical implantation of magnetic beads threaded over a titanium wire around the anus (Fenix; Torax Medical, Inc., St. Paul, MN; no longer available). Defecation was achieved by mechanical separation of the beads induced by increased anal pressures. FDA approval for use as a humanitarian device was granted in 2015 following a report of 35 patients who failed conservative management, including SNM. In this report, 57% of patients had a greater than 50% reduction of their symptoms. One of five patients had to have the device explanted because of adverse events or lack of efficacy (Sugrue et al., 2017). Limited longer-term outcomes in this and additional studies demonstrated higher explantation and complication rates (17%–50%), and the device was voluntarily withdrawn from the market in 2017. It is unclear if future comparative trials will be completed, given the concern for adverse events with this implant.

Based on the success of the synthetic mesh midurethral sling as surgical treatment for stress urinary incontinence, the transobturator posterior anal sling procedure was developed as a surgical treatment for anal incontinence. In this procedure, a self-fixating polypropylene tape is inserted from a transgluteal approach through the obturator foramen bilaterally to create a U shape posterior to the anorectum with the arms extending in sling-like fashion. The mechanism of action is unknown, but the sling may help recreate the anorectal angle and aid the normal closure mechanism of the puborectalis muscle. The sling was implanted in 152 women in a multicenter study, with 69% of patients reporting at least a 50% reduction in fecal incontinence episodes after 1 year (Mellgren et al., 2016). Pelvic pain (31%) and infection (17%) were reported, but most adverse events were mild and were treated medically or required no treatment. Although early research results were promising, the company manufacturing the sling withdrew it from the FDA approval process in 2016. It is unclear if this device may become available to surgeons and patients in the future.

Stem Cell Therapy

Injection of stem cells into the anal sphincter has the potential of inducing muscle growth and improving muscle function. The first pilot study of autologous skeletal muscle–derived cell injection for treatment of fecal incontinence because of obstetric trauma showed promising results that were sustained at 5 years (Frudinger et al., 2015). A second, small, uncontrolled study reported that 78% of women at 12 months had a greater than 50% reduction in weekly incontinence episodes (Frudinger et al., 2018). Larger, controlled studies are needed before further recommendations can be made.

CONCLUSION

Fecal incontinence is a complex problem with many causes. Although it is not life-threatening, fecal incontinence may have a devastating impact on quality of life. Treatment can be initiated in most patients after a thorough history and physical examination. Additional diagnostic testing, such as endoanal ultrasound and ARM, may be helpful in patients with complex conditions and in those who fail conservative treatments. The majority of patients can be treated with dietary and medical management and/or pelvic floor muscle therapies. Anal and vaginal devices may help manage symptoms in some patients but are not yet commonly used. Patients whose symptoms do not respond after attempts at conservative treatments should be offered SNM or, in some cases, sphincteroplasty. More high-quality evidence from randomized controlled trials is needed to improve the strength of current fecal incontinence treatment recommendations.

BIBLIOGRAPHY

ACOG Practice Bulletin No. 198: Prevention and Management of Obstetric Lacerations at Vaginal Delivery. *Obstet Gynecol.* 2018;132:e87.

ACOG Practice Bulletin No. 210 Summary: Fecal Incontinence, *Obstet Gynecol.* 2019;133:837.

Baeten CG, Bailey HR, Bakka A, et al. Safety and efficacy of dynamic graciloplasty for fecal incontinence: report of a prospective, multicenter trial. *Dis Colon Rectum.* 2000;l43:743.

Baggish M, Karram M. *Atlas of Pelvic Anatomy and Gynecologic Surgery.* 5th ed. Philadelphia: Elsevier; 2020.

Bharucha AE, Dunivan G, Goode PS, et al. Epidemiology, pathophysiology, and classification of fecal incontinence: state of the science summary for the National Institute of Diabetes and Digestive and Kidney Diseases (NIDDK) workshop. *Am J Gastroenterol.* 2015;110:127.

Bharucha AE, Rao SSC, Shin AS. Surgical interventions and the use of device-aided therapy for the treatment of fecal incontinence and defecatory disorders. *Clin Gastroenterol Hepatol.* 2017;15:1844.

Bliss DZ, Savik K, Jung HG, et al. Dietary fiber supplementation for fecal incontinence: a randomized clinical trial. *Res Nurs Health.* 2014;37:367.

Bond C, Youngson G, MacPherson I, et al. Anal plugs for the management of fecal incontinence in children and adults: a randomized control trial. *J Clin Gastroenterol.* 2007;41:45.

Boreham MK, Richter HE, Kenton KS, et al. Anal incontinence in women presenting for gynecologic care: prevalence, risk factors, and impact upon quality of life. *Am J Obstet Gynecol.* 2005;192:1637.

Brown HW, Braun EJ, Wise ME, et al. Small-group, community-member intervention for urinary and bowel incontinence: a randomized controlled trial. *Obstet Gynecol.* 2019;134:600.

Brown HW, Kyer KY, Rogers RG. Management of fecal incontinence. *Obstet Gynecol.* 2020;136:811.

Brown SR, Wadhawan H, Nelson RL. Surgery for faecal incontinence in adults. *Cochrane Database Syst Rev.* 2013;7:CD001757.

Casal E, San Ildefonso A, Carracedo R, et al. Artificial bowel sphincter in severe anal incontinence. *Colorectal Dis.* 2004;6:180.

Deen KI, Kumar D, Williams JG, et al. The prevalence of anal sphincter defects in faecal incontinence: a prospective endosonic study. *Gut.* 1993;34:685.

Dehli T, Stordahl A, Vatten LJ, et al. Sphincter training or anal injections of dextranomer for treatment of anal incontinence: a randomized trial. *Scand J Gastroenterol.* 2013;48:302.

Desprez C, Damon H, Meurette G, et al. Ten-year evaluation of a large retrospective cohort treated by sacral nerve modulation for fecal incontinence: results of a French multicenter study. *Ann Surg.* July 24, 2020. Epub ahead of print.

Deutekom M, Dobben AC. Plugs for containing faecal incontinence. *Cochrane Database Syst Rev.* 2012;4:CD005086.

Devroede G, Giese C, Wexner SD, et al. Quality of life is markedly improved in patients with fecal incontinence after sacral nerve stimulation. *Female Pelvic Med Reconstr Surg.* 2012;18:103.

Efron JE, Corman ML, Fleshman J, et al. Safety and effectiveness of temperature-controlled radio frequency energy delivery to the anal canal (secca procedure) for the treatment of fecal incontinence. *Dis Colon Rectum.* 2003;46:1606.

Faltin DL, Sangalli MR, Roche B, et al. Does a second delivery increase the risk of anal incontinence? *BJOG.* 2001;10:684.

Faucheron JL, Sage PY, Trilling B. Erosion rate of the magnetic sphincter augmentation device is much higher for anal incontinence than for antireflux, *J Gastrointest Surg.* 2019;23:389.

Fernando RJ, Sultan AH, Kettle C, Thakar R. Methods of repair for obstetric anal sphincter injury. *Cochrane Database Syst Rev.* 2013;8:CD002866.

Frudinger A, Pfeifer J, Paede J, et al. Autologous skeletal-muscle-derived cell injection for anal incontinence due to obstetric trauma: a 5-year follow-up of an initial study of 10 patients. *Colorectal Dis.* 2015;17:794.

Frudinger A, Marksteiner R, Pfeifer J, et al. Skeletal muscle-derived cell implantation for the treatment of sphincter-related faecal incontinence. *Stem Cell Res Ther.* 2018;13:233.

George AT, Kalmar K, Panarese A, et al. Long-term outcomes of sacral nerve stimulation for fecal incontinence. *Dis Colon Rectum.* 2012;55:302.

Glasgow SC, Lowry AC. Long-term outcomes of anal sphincter repair for fecal incontinence: a systematic review. *Dis Colon Rectum.* 2012;55:482.

Goldman HB, Lloyd JC, Noblett KL, et al. International Continence Society best practice statement for use of sacral neuromodulation. *Neurourol Urodyn.* 2018;37:1823.

Gourcerol G, Vitton V, Leroi AM, et al. How sacral nerve stimulation works in patients with faecal incontinence. *Colorectal Dis.* 2011; 13:e203.

Graf W, Mellgren A, Matzel KE, et al. Efficacy of dextranomer in stabilised hyaluronic acid for treatment of faecal incontinence: a randomised, sham-controlled trial. *Lancet.* 2011;377:997.

Heymen S, Scarlett Y, Jones K, et al. Randomized controlled trial shows biofeedback to be superior to pelvic floor exercises for fecal incontinence. *Dis Colon Rectum.* 2009;52:1730.

Hong KD, Dasilva G, Kalaskar SN, et al. Long-term outcomes of artificial bowel sphincter for fecal incontinence: a systematic review and meta-analysis. *J Am Coll Surg.* 2013;217:718.

Hotouras A, Thaha MA, Allison ME, et al. Percutaneous tibial nerve stimulation (PTNS) in females with faecal incontinence: the impact of sphincter morphology and rectal sensation on the clinical outcome. *Int J Colorectal Dis.* 2012;27:927.

Horrocks EJ, Chadi SA, Stevens NJ, et al. Factors associated with efficacy of percutaneous tibial nerve stimulation for fecal incontinence, based on post-hoc analysis of data from a randomized trial. *Clin Gastroenterol Hepatol.* 2017;15:1915.

How P, Trivedi PM, Bearn PE, Thomas GP. Insert devices for faecal incontinence. *Tech Coloproctol.* 2021;25:255.

Hull T, Giese C, Wexner SD, et al. Long-term durability of SNS therapy for chronic fecal incontinence. *Dis Colon Rectum.* 2013;56:234.

Hull TL, Zutshi M. Chapter 31: Fecal incontinence. In: Karram MM, Walters MD, eds. *Urogynecology and Reconstructive Pelvic Surgery.* Philadelphia: Elsevier/Saunders; 2015:463.

Ivatury SJ, Wilson LR, Paquette IM. Surgical treatment alternatives to sacral neuromodulation for fecal incontinence: injectables, sphincter repair, and colostomy. *Clin Colon Rectal Surg.* 2021;34:40.

Janssen PTJ, Komen N, Melenhorst J, et al. Sacral neuromodulation for fecal incontinence: a review of the central mechanisms of action. *J Clin Gastroenterol.* 2017;51:669.

Jelovsek JE, Markland AD, Whitehead WE, et al. Controlling faecal incontinence in women by performing anal exercises with biofeedback or loperamide: a randomized clinical trial. *Lancet Gastroenterol Hepatol.* 2019;4:698.

Jordan PA, Naidu M, Thakar R, Sultan AH. Effect of subsequent vaginal delivery on bowel symptoms and anorectal function in women who sustained a previous obstetric anal sphincter injury. *Int Urogynecol J.* 2018;29:1579.

Katuwal B, Bhullar J. Current position of sacral neuromodulation in treatment of fecal incontinence. *Clin Colon Rectal Surg.* 2021;34:22.

Kissane LM, Martin KD, Meyer I, Richter HE. Effect of darifenacin on fecal incontinence in women with double incontinence. *Int Urogynecol J.* 2020;15:10.

Knowles CH, Horrocks EJ, Bremner SA, et al. Percutaneous tibial nerve stimulation versus sham electrical stimulation for the treatment of faecal incontinence in adults (CONFIDeNT): a double-blind, multicentre, pragmatic, parallel-group, randomised controlled trial. *Lancet.* 2015;386:1640.

La Torre F, de la Portilla F. Long-term efficacy of dextranomer in stabilized hyaluronic acid (NASHA/Dx) for treatment of faecal incontinence. *Colorectal Dis.* 2013;15:569.

Lam TJ, Visscher AP, Meurs-Szojda MM, Felt-Bersma RJ. Clinical response and sustainability of treatment with temperature-controlled radiofrequency energy (Secca) in patients with faecal incontinence: 3 years follow-up. *Int J Colorectal Dis.* 2014; 29:755.

Leroi AM, Siproudhis L, Etienney I, et al. Transcutaneous electrical tibial nerve stimulation in the treatment of fecal incontinence: a randomized trial (CONSORT 1a). *Am J Gastroenterol.* 2012; 107:1888.

Lewicky-Gaupp C, Mueller MG, Collins SA, et al. Early secondary repair of obstetric anal sphincter injury breakdown: contemporary surgical techniques and experiences from a peripartum subspecialty clinic. *Female Pelvic Med Reconstr Surg.* 2021;27:e333.

Lewis SJ, Heaton KW. Stool form scale as a useful guide to intestinal transit time. *Scand J Gastroenterol.* 1997;32:920.

Lockhart ME, Fielding JR, Richter HE, et al. Reproducibility of dynamic MR imaging pelvic measurements: a multi-institutional study. *Radiology.* 2008;249:534.

Lukacz ES, Segall MM, Wexner SD. Evaluation of an anal insert device for the conservative management of fecal incontinence. *Dis Colon Rectum.* 2015;58:892.

Maeda Y, Laurberg S, Norton C. Perianal injectable bulking agents as treatment for faecal incontinence in adults. *Cochrane Database Syst Rev.* 2013;2:CD007959.

Malouf AJ, Norton CS, Engel AF, et al. Long-term results of overlapping anterior anal-sphincter repair for obstetric trauma. *Lancet.* 2000;355:260.

Markland AD, Burgio KL, Whitehead WE, et al. Loperamide versus Psyllium fiber for treatment of fecal incontinence: The Fecal Incontinence Prescription (Rx) Management (FIRM) Randomized Clinical Trial. *Dis Colon Rectum.* 2015;58:983.

Matzel KE, Lux P, Heuer S, et al. Sacral nerve stimulation for faecal incontinence: long-term outcome. *Colorectal Dis.* 2009;11:636.

Mellgren A, Wexner SD, Coller JA, et al. Long-term efficacy and safety of sacral nerve stimulation for fecal incontinence. *Dis Colon Rectum.* 2011;54:1065.

Mellgren A, Matzel KE, Pollack J, et al. Long-term efficacy of NASHA Dx injection therapy for treatment of fecal incontinence. *Neurogastroenterol Motil.* 2014;26:1087.

Mellgren A, Zutshi M, Lucente VR, et al. for the TOPAS Study Group. A posterior anal sling for fecal incontinence: results of a 152-patient prospective multicenter study. *Am J Obstet Gynecol.* 2016;214:349.

Ng KS, Sivakumaran Y, Nassar N, Gladman MA. Fecal incontinence: Community prevalence and associated factors—a systematic review. *Dis Colon Rectum.* 2015; 58:1194.

Nilsson IEK, Åkervall S, Molin M, et al. Symptoms of fecal incontinence two decades after no, one, or two obstetrical anal sphincter injuries. *Am J Obstet Gynecol.* 2021;224:276.e1.

Norton C, Chelvanayagam S, Wilson-Barnett J, et al. Randomized controlled trial of biofeedback for fecal incontinence. *Gastroenterology.* 2003;125:1320.

Norton C, Burch J, Kamm MA. Patients' views of a colostomy for fecal incontinence. *Dis Colon Rectum.* 2005;48:1062.

Norton C, Cody JD. Biofeedback and/or sphincter exercises for the treatment of faecal incontinence in adults. *Cochrane Database Syst Rev.* 2012;7:CD002111.

O'Brien PE, Dixon JB, Skinner S, et al. A prospective, randomized, controlled clinical trial of placement of the artificial bowel sphincter (Acticon Neosphincter) for the control of fecal incontinence. *Dis Colon Rectum.* 2004;47:1852.

Oliveira L, Pfeifer J, Wexner SD. Physiological and clinical outcome of anterior sphincteroplasty. *Br J Surg.* 1996;83:502.

Omar MI, Alexander CE. Drug treatment for faecal incontinence in adults. *Cochrane Database Syst Rev.* 2013;6:CD002116.

Oom DM, Gosselink MP, Schouten WR. Anterior sphincteroplasty for fecal incontinence: a single center experience in the era of sacral neuromodulation. *Dis Colon Rectum.* 2009;52:1681.

Parker SC, Spencer MP, Madoff RD, et al. Artificial bowel sphincter: long-term experience at a single institution. *Dis Colon Rectum.* 2003;46:722.

Paquette IM, Varma MG, Kaiser AM, et al. The American Society of Colon and Rectal Surgeons' clinical practice guideline for the treatment of fecal incontinence. *Dis Colon Rectum.* 2015;58:623.

Rao SS, Welcher KD, Happel J. Can biofeedback therapy improve anorectal function in fecal incontinence? *Am J Gastroenterol.* 1996;91:2360.

Ratto C, Litta F, Parello A, et al. Sacral nerve stimulation in faecal incontinence associated with an anal sphincter lesion: a systematic review. *Colorectal Dis.* 2012;14:e297.

Reilly WT, Talley NJ, Pemberton JH, Zinsmeister AR. Validation of a questionnaire to assess fecal incontinence and associated risk factors. *Dis Colon Rectum.* 2000;43:146.

Rice TC, Quezada Y, Rafferty JF, Paquette IM. Dynamic article: percutaneous nerve evaluation versus staged sacral nerve stimulation for fecal incontinence. *Dis Colon Rectum.* 2016;59:962.

Richter HE, Dunivan G, Brown HW, et al. A 12-month clinical durability of effectiveness and safety evaluation of a vaginal bowel control system for the nonsurgical treatment of fecal incontinence. *Female Pelvic Med Reconstr Surg.* 2019;25:113.

Rockwood TH. Incontinence severity and QOL scales for fecal incontinence. *Gastroenterology.* 2004;126;S106.

Rockwood TH, Church JM, Fleshman JW, et al. Fecal incontinence quality of life scale: quality of life instrument for patients with fecal incontinence. *Dis Colon Rectum.* 2000;43:9.

Rogers RG, Sung VW, Lukacz ES, et al. Accidental bowel leakage evaluation: a new patient-centered validatd measure of accidental bowel leakage symptoms in women. *Dis Colon Rectum.* 2020;63:668.

Rosenblatt P, Schumacher J, Lucente V, et al. A preliminary evaluation of the TOPAS system for the treatment of fecal incontinence in women. *Female Pelvic Med Reconstr Surg.* 2014;20:155.

Ruiz D, Pinto RA, Hull TL, et al. Does the radiofrequency procedure for fecal incontinence improve quality of life and incontinence at 1-year follow-up? *Dis Colon Rectum.* 2010;53:1041.

Rydningen M, Dehli T, Wilsgaard T, et al. Sacral neuromodulation compared with injection of bulking agents for faecal incontinence following obstetric anal sphincter injury - a randomized controlled trial. *Colorectal Dis.* 2017;19:O134.

Schwandner O, Brunner M, Dietl O. Quality of life and functional results of submucosal injection therapy using dextranomer hyaluronic acid for fecal incontinence. *Surg Innov.* 2011;18:130.

Sultan AH, Kamm MA, Hudson CN, et al. Anal-sphincter disruption during vaginal delivery. *N Engl J Med.* 1993;329:1905.

Sugrue J, Lehur PA, Madoff RD, et al. Long-term experience of magnetic anal sphincter augmentation in patients with fecal incontinence. *Dis Colon Rectum.* 2017;60:87.

Takahashi-Monroy T, Morales M, Garcia-Osogobio S, et al. Secca procedure for the treatment of fecal incontinence: results of five-year follow-up. *Dis Colon Rectum.* 2008;51:355.

Thaha MA, Abukar AA, Thin NN, et al. Sacral nerve stimulation for faecal incontinence and constipation in adults. *Cochrane Database Syst Rev.* 2015;8:CD004464.

Vaizey CJ, Carapeti E, Cahill JA, Kamm MA. Prospective comparison of fecal incontinence grading systems. *Gut.* 1999;4:477.

Vaizey CJ, Norton C, Thornton MJ, et al. Long-term results of repeat anterior anal sphincter repair. *Dis Colon Rectum.* 2004;47:858.

Visscher AP, Lam TJ, Meurs-Szojda MM, Felt-Bersma RJF. Temperature-controlled delivery of radiofrequency energy in fecal incontinence: a randomized sham-controlled clinical trial. *Dis Colon Rectum.* 2017;60:860.

Vonthein R, Heimerl T, Schwandner T, Ziegler A. Electrical stimulation and biofeedback for the treatment of fecal incontinence: a systematic review. *Int J Colorectal Dis.* 2013;28:1567.

Wald A, Bharucha AE, Cosman BC, Whitehead WE. ACG clinical guideline: management of benign anorectal disorders. *Am J Gastroenterol.* 2014;109:1141.

Wexner SD, Gonzalez-Padron A, Rius J, et al. Stimulated gracilis neosphincter operation: initial experience, pitfalls, and complications. *Dis Colon Rectum.* 1996;39:957.

Wexner SD, Coller JA, Devroede G, et al. Sacral nerve stimulation for fecal incontinence: results of a 120-patient prospective multicenter study. *Ann Surg.* 2010a;251:441.

Wexner SD, Hull T, Edden Y, et al. Infection rates in a large investigational trial of sacral nerve stimulation for fecal incontinence. *J Gastrointest Surg.* 2010b;14:1081.

Whitehead WE, Rao SS, Lowry A, et al. Treatment of fecal incontinence: state of the science summary for the National Institute of Diabetes and Digestive and Kidney Diseases workshop. *Am J Gastroenterol.* 2015;110:138.

Wolf AMD, Fontham ETH, Church TR, et al. Colorectal cancer screening for average-risk adults: 2018 guideline update from the American Cancer Society. *CA Cancer J Clin.* 2018;68:250.

Wong RF, Bonapace Jr ES, Chung CY, et al. Simultaneous endoluminal sonography and manometry to assess anal sphincter complex in normal subjects. *Dig Dis Sci.* 1998;43:2363.

Wong WD, Jensen LL, Bartolo DC, et al. Artificial anal sphincter. *Dis Colon Rectum.* 1996;39:1345.

Young CJ, Zahid A, Koh CE, et al. A randomized controlled trial of four different regimes of biofeedback programme in the treatment of faecal incontinence. *Colorectal Dis.* 2018;20:312.

Zutshi M, Hull T, Gurland B. Biological implants in sphincter augmentation offer good short-term outcomes after a sphincter repair. *Colorectal Dis.* 2011;14:866.

Constipation

John Eric Jelovsek

CHAPTER OUTLINE

DEFINITION AND ETIOLOGY

Constipation is a broad term that is defined as difficult evacuation of feces, infrequent defecation, or inadequate defecation. Our understanding of the etiology of constipation has improved, resulting in an evolving definition. One commonly used definition is based upon bowel frequency of fewer than three stools per week. This definition is based on interviews of factory workers in the United Kingdom that found that 99% of the working population reported a frequency of bowel movements between three per day and three per week. The problem with this definition is that it ignores the symptoms reported by most patients who consider themselves constipated (i.e., straining, hard stools); it does not assist in separating out those patients with disorders of slowed intestinal transit and those with disorders of defecation, and it may not apply to patients who are taking laxatives.

Although physicians and patients often refer to constipation as a single disorder, it should be viewed as a symptom that means different things to different people. In 1987, Sandler and Drossman reported on the bowel habits of more than 1000 adults. The patients were asked how they define the term constipation. Some 52% said "straining at stool," 44% reported "hard stools," 34% reported "a sense of wanting to defecate but cannot," 32% reported "infrequent stools," 20% reported "abdominal discomfort," 19% reported "a sense of incomplete evacuation," and 11% said "spending too much time on the toilet." Therefore, simply asking a patient whether he or she has constipation is neither sensitive nor specific. However, there appears to be a large percentage of individuals who feel that they have constipation yet do not complain of any symptoms that physicians typically use to define constipation. This difference in definition between patient-centered self-report of constipation and objective criteria indicates that reliance on stringent symptom-based criteria may miss a large population who believe that they have constipation, whether they do or do not, based on those criteria.

Because constipation becomes a problem only when the patient complains of it, and because symptoms of constipation may occur in the absence of any physiologic abnormalities (i.e., stool frequency does not necessarily correlate with transit time), a symptom-based definition still holds some value and has become the standard. This led to the development of the Rome criteria (Drossman et al., 2000) for functional gastrointestinal disorders, with the most recent version summarized in the Rome IV criteria (Mearin et al., 2016). These symptom-based criteria are expert consensus guidelines for making the clinical diagnosis of the various types of functional bowel disorders, including constipation. The criteria have become the standard for the definition of constipation.

The Rome IV criteria divide patients complaining of symptoms of constipation into two major groups: those with functional bowel disorders and those with functional anorectal disorders. Functional bowel disorders include (1) functional constipation, (2) irritable bowel syndrome (IBS) with constipation (IBS-C), and (3) opioid-induced constipation. Experts continue to consider the first two disorders as part of a single continuum. Abdominal pain and bloating may be present in subjects with constipation but not be predominant symptoms (i.e., the patient does not meet criteria for IBS). Subjects with functional constipation often complain of fewer than three bowel movements per week, hard or lumpy stools, straining, feeling of incomplete emptying after a bowel movement, a sensation that stool cannot be passed, or a need to press on or around their bottom or vagina to complete a bowel movement.

Functional constipation may include patients who demonstrate slowed transit times on colonic transit studies or patients with normal transit or idiopathic constipation, because it is a symptom-based diagnosis. In fact, the latest American Gastroenterological Association (AGA) technical review does not use the term "functional constipation," because of this subset of patients who have slow transit constipation (Bharucha et al., 2013). Instead, the AGA criteria rely on assessments of colon transit and anorectal function to classify patients with constipation into one of three groups: normal-transit constipation, slow-transit constipation, and pelvic floor dysfunction or defecatory disorders.

The diagnostic criteria for functional constipation are shown in Box 28.1. Patients with IBS-C have the same symptoms, except that they often have a predominance of abdominal pain. This pain is related to (improved or worsened with) defecation, change in the number of bowel movements, or change in consistency of stools. Some experts have believed that constipation could be broken down into further subtypes based on the reported predominant evacuation symptoms, including IBS-outlet and outlet-type constipation. A subcategory of patients who fulfil criteria for either IBS-C or functional constipation also report one of the following evacuation symptoms: a sensation that stool cannot be passed when having a bowel movement, a need to press on or around their bottom or vagina to try to remove stool to complete a bowel movement, or difficulty relaxing or letting go to allow the stool to come out at least one-fourth of the time. These subtypes are now referred to as functional defecation disorders. The diagnostic criteria for functional defecation disorders are seen in Box 28.2.

Normal-transit constipation is probably the most common form of constipation, although this has not been formally studied. In these patients, stool frequency may be normal, but patients feel constipated and may report difficulty with defecation, bloating, abdominal pain, and hard stools. On testing, patients in this group may have increased rectal compliance, reduced rectal sensation, or both (Ashraf et al., 1996). Patients with slow-transit constipation typically have a decreased number of high-amplitude propagated contractions of the bowel. This may result from abnormalities of the myenteric plexus, decreased interstitial cells of Cajal that are required to generate smooth muscle electrical slow wave, diminished excitatory extrinsic nervous input, or extrinsic inhibitory activity (He et al., 2000). Those with defecation disorders may have normal or slightly slowed transit studies but have preferential storage of stool in the rectum. They also have higher defecatory sensation thresholds and may tolerate higher volumes in the rectum. Based on the Cleveland Clinic experience, outlet-type symptoms of constipation seem to be the predominate subtype seen in patients with other pelvic floor disorders such as pelvic organ prolapse and incontinence. Patients with dyssynergic defecation have paradoxical contraction or failure to relax the pelvic floor muscles during attempts to defecate. Physical examination may reveal a failure to relax the puborectalis or paradoxical contraction during an attempted defecation, and laboratory testing shows evidence of inappropriate contraction or failure of relaxation of the pelvic floor during attempts to defecate. Structural abnormalities are less common but include rectal prolapse and/or intussusception, rectocele, and excessive perineal descent.

The pathophysiology of constipation continues to evolve. Investigators have attempted to examine the relationships between slow transit disorders and external neuropathy conditions, such as spinal cord injury, Parkinson disease, multiple sclerosis, medications, and diabetes. The premise behind these disorders is that the symptoms of constipation result from motor and sensory disturbances, ultimately leading to delayed transit or physiologic disorders of the colon and pelvic floor, and, in women with slow-transit constipation refractory to medical therapy, colonic manometry can identify underlying neuropathy that may warrant colectomy (Singh et al., 2013). The primary causes of constipation are disordered regulation of the neuromuscular components within

BOX 28.1 Rome IV Diagnostic Criteria for Functional Constipation

Must Fulfill Both[a] Criteria:

1. Must include two or more of the following:
   - Straining >25% of defecations
   - Lumpy or hard stools (Bristol Stool Form Scale 1–2) >25% of defecations
   - Sensation of incomplete evacuation >25% of defecations
   - Sensation of anorectal obstruction/blockage >25% of defecations
   - Manual maneuvers to facilitate >25% of defecations
   - Less than three spontaneous bowel movements per week
2. Loose stools are rarely present without the use of laxatives.
3. There are insufficient criteria for irritable bowel syndrome.

[a]Criteria are met for the last 3 months with symptom onset at least 6 months before diagnosis.
(From Mearin F, Lacy BE, Chang L, et al. Bowel disorders. *Gastroenterol.* 2016;150;1393.)

BOX 28.2 Rome IV Diagnostic Criteria for Functional Defecation Disorders

Diagnostic Criteria[a] for Functional Defecation Disorders:

1. The patient must satisfy diagnostic criteria for functional constipation and/or irritable bowel syndrome with constipation
2. During repeated attempts to defecate, there must be features of impaired evacuation, as demonstrated by two of the following three tests:
   a. Abnormal balloon expulsion test
   b. Abnormal anorectal evacuation pattern with manometry or anal surface electromyography
   c. Impaired rectal evacuation by imaging

Subcategories for functional defecation disorders apply to patients who satisfy the following criteria:

1. Inadequate defecatory propulsion: Inadequate propulsive forces as measured with manometry with or without inappropriate contraction of the anal sphincter and/or pelvic floor muscles
2. Dyssynergic defecation: Inappropriate contraction of the pelvic floor as measured with anal surface electromyography or manometry, with adequate propulsive forces during attempted defecation

[a]Criteria fulfilled for the last 3 months with symptom onset at least 6 months before diagnosis.
(From Rao SS, Bharucha AE, Chiarioni G, et al. Anorectal disorders. *Gastroenterol.* 2016;150;1430.)

the colon and anorectum, as well as disruption in their corresponding ascending and descending pathways in the brain-gut axis (Sharma & Rao, 2017). Patients with slow colonic transit have a resting colonic motility similar to normal controls but have little or no increase in motor activity after meals or stimulation with bisacodyl (Waldron et al., 1988; Ravi et al., 2010). Neuropathy of the enteric nervous system may also occur in patients with Chagas disease secondary to infection by *Trypanosoma cruzi*, those with Hirschsprung disease, or those who engage in chronic laxative abuse. Genetic mutations demonstrated in patients with Hirschsprung disease include a mutation in the endothelin B receptor (Puffenberger et al., 1994) and an inactivating mutation in the *RET* protooncogene (Edery et al., 1994).

Studies of the pathophysiology of disorders of defecation have examined altered anorectal motor and sensory function. Recently, three patterns of disordered defecation have been recognized that involve impaired anal relaxation at the puborectalis, external anal sphincter, or both (Rattanakovit et al., 2015). These patterns were identified by studies involving perceptual responses to controlled rectal distension, alterations to visceral sensation, and pudendal nerve terminal motor latencies. Most patients with disorders of defecation suffer from the inability to coordinate the abdominal, rectoanal, and pelvic floor muscles during attempted defecation (Rao et al., 2004). For example, there is evidence that dyssynergia of the puborectalis and external anal sphincter muscles during defecation leading to outlet dysfunction and constipation in patients with multiple sclerosis is caused by a spinal lesion. Mathers et al. (1989) showed that this functional abnormality also occurred in patients with Parkinson disease, and that, in Parkinson disease, it was responsive to dopaminergic medication. De Groat et al. (1990) showed that interruption of pathways in the spinal cord can result in detrusor-sphincter dyssynergia, and it is therefore likely that paradoxical puborectalis contraction in multiple sclerosis is caused by interruption of spinal pathways by demyelination. The data provide evidence that functional bowel disorders may be more intimately associated with the neurologic system than is commonly thought. Despite these advances, our knowledge of neuroanatomy and its relationship to functional disorders of the bowel remains in its infancy.

EPIDEMIOLOGY

Constipation is a commonly encountered problem in medical practice and is expected to increase dramatically. The US population is becoming older, and more individuals are likely to be living with chronic neurologic disease and to reside in nursing homes. Estimates of incidence and prevalence vary depending upon the definition used (i.e., self-reported constipation or Rome criteria) and the population studied. Few data are available on the incidence of constipation. Talley et al. (1992) reported a rate of constipation onset of 40 per 1000 person-years in White residents of a single county in Minnesota. The symptom remission rate was 309 per 1000 person-years. Stewart et al. (1999), in a large US epidemiologic study of more than 10,000 individuals, found an overall constipation prevalence of 14.7% in the general population. Worldwide estimates are similar, with 12% of people reporting self-defined constipation (Wald et al., 2008). More recently, a systematic review and meta-analysis estimated the global prevalence and risk factors for chronic idiopathic constipation in 41 separate studies across several continents and estimated that the pooled prevalence in all studies was 14% (95% confidence interval: 12%–17%) (Suares & Ford, 2011). The pooled prevalence was largely stable across geographical locations and was slightly lower in South East Asian studies and higher in South American studies.

The global pooled prevalence of chronic idiopathic constipation appears to be higher in women compared with men (17% vs. 9%), and the rates of constipation subtypes in men and women in the United States are as follows: functional constipation 4.6%, IBS-C 2.1%, outlet constipation 4.6%, and IBS-outlet constipation 3.6% (Suares & Ford, 2011; Stewart et al., 1999). Overall, women had higher rates of outlet disorders. However, when constipation subtypes were broken down by gender, the only statistical difference was in women being more likely to have the IBS-outlet subtype of constipation. Most of the studies that stratified by age found consistent trends of increasing prevalence of constipation with age, with significant increases after age 70 years. Interestingly, when Sandler and Drossman (1987) stratified constipation subtypes in women by age, the prevalence of constipation actually decreased with increased age.

Most data suggest similar racial differences in the prevalence of constipation, with the average prevalence being 1.17- to 2.89-fold higher in non-Whites than in Whites. Outlet-type constipation was also more prevalent among non-Whites according to data from Sandler and Drossman (1987). In one meta-analysis of six studies, pooled estimates demonstrated an increase in the prevalence of constipation in those of lower socioeconomic status compared with those of higher socioeconomic status (Suares & Ford, 2011).

Because of the high prevalence, constipation consumes substantial health care resources. Constipation is one the five most common physician diagnoses for gastrointestinal disorders. Data from the National Ambulatory Medical Care Survey and the National Hospital Ambulatory Medical Care Survey suggest that ambulatory visits for constipation increased from 4 million visits per year from 1993 to 1996 to almost 8 million visits per year from 2001 to 2004 (0.72% of all ambulatory visits) (Shah et al., 2008). The annual direct medical costs for constipation were recently estimated to exceed $230 million, and the costs incurred by women with constipation were double those of women without constipation (Martin et al., 2006; Choung et al., 2011).

Among 300 women presenting to a urogynecology clinic for either pelvic organ prolapse or incontinence, the overall prevalence of constipation was 36%, as defined by the Rome II criteria. When this sample was stratified by subtype, 5% had functional constipation, 19% outlet-type, 5% IBS-C, and 7% IBS-outlet type (Fig. 28.1). Given recent population shifts in North America, constipation and its associated outlet disorders make this a condition with which gynecologists and urologists should be familiar.

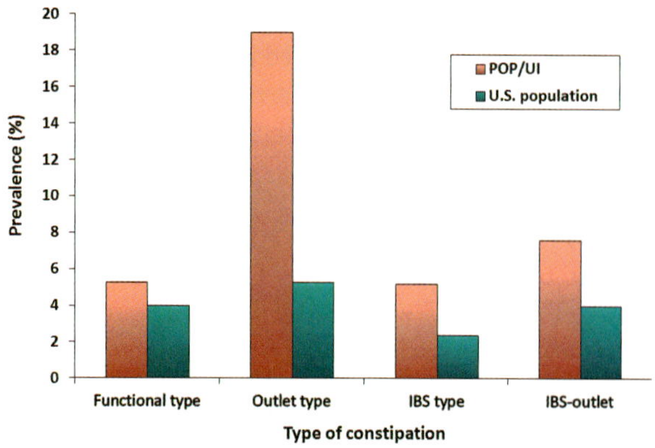

Fig. 28.1 Prevalence of constipation subtypes in 302 consecutive patients presenting to the Cleveland Clinic for pelvic organ prolapse (*POP*) and urinary incontinence (*UI*) versus the US population data. *IBS,* Irritable bowel syndrome. (From Stewart WF, Liberman JN, Sandler RS, et al. Epidemiology of constipation [EPOC] study in the United States: relation of clinical subtypes to sociodemographic features. *Am J Gastroenterol.* 1999;94:3530.)

EVALUATION

Patients who report constipation often have features of both slow-transit disorders and anorectal disorders. When attempting to evaluate constipation, it is convenient to try to separate out these two pathophysiologic mechanisms and tailor treatment accordingly. It is also helpful to distinguish between transient constipation that started at a time of change in dietary habits or lifestyle changes and those that are chronic. At the conclusion of the initial clinical evaluation, it should be possible to classify patients into the following categories (Bharucha et al., 2013; Rao et al., 2016):

1. Normal-transit constipation with normal colonic transit and defecation
2. Slow-transit constipation, when pelvic floor function is normal and there is evidence of slow transit
3. Defecatory disorders including failure of relaxing the pelvic floor during defecation or descending perineal syndrome
4. Combination of numbers 2 and 3
5. Organic constipation because of mechanical obstruction or side effects of medications
6. Secondary constipation owing to metabolic disorders

A thorough history and physical examination, minimal laboratory tests, colonoscopy, and other diagnostic tests are done as needed based on the history and physical examination.

History

The history begins with clarifying what the patient means when reporting constipation, such as number of stools per week, difficulty expelling stool or a feeling of incomplete defecation, pain with defecation, consistency of stool (including hard or lumpy stools), and duration of the problem. Some patients experience rectal pressure or fullness. Others may need to use their fingers to expel stool or stabilize the vagina or perineum, referred to as splinting, during defecation. They may be embarrassed to admit some of these practices and may need to be encouraged to tell this information. Features such as rectal bleeding in the absence of anal fissures or hemorrhoids, unintended weight loss, and family history of colon cancer should be elicited. Additionally, a dietary history, including questions about the amount of dietary fiber and fluid consumed daily, is necessary.

Objective measures of stool frequency, colonic transit, and anorectal function can also be performed when necessary. The Bristol Stool Form Scale is a useful tool that uses visual images of various forms of stool consistency on a 7-point scale. This scale has been compared against stool transit times and is easily understood by patients (Heaton & O'Donnell, 1994; Lewis & Heaton, 1997; Degen & Phillips, 1996). It may be particularly useful in patients who self-report constipation who have three or more bowel movements per week to establish whether hard or lumpy stools are present.

Ruling out associated medical problems that may lead to secondary constipation (Box 28.3) is important. Constipation is more common in people with neurologic disease, such as multiple sclerosis and spinal cord injury. Diabetes may also be associated with constipation. Recent changes in routine, such as levels of diet and exercise, may contribute to constipation. Sandler and Drossman (1987) found that decreased caloric

BOX 28.3 Possible Contributors to Constipation

Personal Habits
Low physical activity
Low calorie diet
Employment status

Obstructive
Colon
- Neoplasm
- Benign stricture (i.e., diverticula)
- Rectal prolapse

Anal outlet obstruction
- Pain (i.e., anal fissure)
- Stenosis
- Rectocele
- Pelvic floor dyssynergia

Medications
Narcotics
Antidepressants
Mineral supplements (i.e., iron, calcium)
Anticholinergics
β blockers, calcium channel blockers

Endocrine
Hypothyroidism
Hypercalcemia
Hypokalemia
Diabetes mellitus
Uremia

Neurologic
Aganglionosis (congenital: Hirschsprung disease; acquired: Chagas disease)
Central nervous system or spinal cord trauma or disease (Parkinson disease, multiple sclerosis)

Pregnancy
Psychiatric Causes
Other

intake favored constipation. Additionally, regular exercise is associated with a reduced risk of constipation (Nakaji et al 2002; Daley et al. 2008). In patients with severe constipation and no obvious cause, histories of physical and/or sexual abuse may be found.

Past surgeries may provide clues and should be elicited. Some debate exists as to whether hysterectomy causes constipation. In 1992, Prior et al. reported on 200 patients who underwent hysterectomy and found that 5% developed IBS-C. In 2004, Altman et al. reported on 120 consecutive patients who underwent either vaginal or abdominal hysterectomy. No statistical difference was present in preoperative and postoperative bowel emptying difficulties or incomplete bowel evacuation.

Physical Examination

The physical examination is tailored to the patient. The abdominal examination is usually normal, but masses, palpable stool in the colon, and surgical scars and hernias should be noted. The perineal examination starts with an inspection, looking for anal fissures or abnormalities. Asking the patient to strain may demonstrate perineal descent, widening of the perineal body, rectal prolapse, or a rectocele protruding into the vagina. Digital examination rules out fecal impaction, anal stenosis or stricture, external or internal rectal prolapse, pelvic or rectal masses, and rectocele. The examiner should note the consistency of stool in the rectum. The tone of the levator ani muscles on vaginal and rectal examination should be assessed at relaxation and with straining. Paradoxical contraction may be suspected if a failure to relax the puborectalis is noted when the patient is asked to simulate defecation. These patients often have a history of excessive straining before elimination. Even soft stools and enema fluid are difficult to pass. A carefully performed digital rectal examination has a high yield of detecting dyssynergia in patients with chronic constipation. The high specificity (87%) and positive predictive value (97%) make digital rectal examination an ideal test that can be used to diagnose dyssynergia in a patient with chronic constipation and symptoms of difficult defecation (Tantiphlachiva et al., 2010). Pain on the border of the puborectalis is a feature of some anorectal pain disorders with associated pelvic muscle spasm.

Few clinicians would dispute the association between vaginal prolapse and symptoms of constipation, although a direct relationship between the two is not clear. In 1998, Weber et al. described 143 women who completed a questionnaire assessment of bowel function and underwent standardized examination using the Pelvic Organ Prolapse Quantification method. In 26.6% it was rare to require straining to have a bowel movement, in 49.6% straining was sometimes required, in 14% straining was usually required, and in 9.8% straining was always required. Some 31% needed to help stool come out by pushing with a finger in the vagina or rectum. Severity of prolapse was not related to severity of bowel dysfunction. In a Swedish population of 491 women, when a rectocele was present 18% reported problems with emptying the bowel at defecation compared with 13% in the nonrectocele group (Samuelsson et al., 1999). However, constipation was not related to prolapse in this population.

Laboratory Evaluation

Blood work to assess a complete blood count, calcium, and thyroid-stimulating hormone should be carried out if a problem is suspected. Although these studies are often performed, their diagnostic utility and cost-effectiveness have not been evaluated and are likely low (Muller-Lissner et al., 2005).

Testing

Further testing depends on the severity of symptoms and findings on physical examination. At this stage in the management of constipation, the majority of patients require no further testing, and the physician can proceed to medical therapy. Patients older than age 50 years (≥45 years in Black people) should have a screening colonoscopy, based on national recommendations. This examination rules out neoplasms, a solitary rectal ulcer (erythema or ulceration on the lower anterior rectal wall thought to be from trauma secondary to internal rectal prolapse), or melanosis coli (brown-black discoloration of the mucosa from chronic use of certain laxatives).

A therapeutic trial of fiber is warranted if no cause has been found. Patients who do not respond may require further diagnostic evaluation to identify the subgroups of constipation. The tests chosen depends on patient characteristics and severity of symptoms. Testing is useful to distinguish between patients with defecatory dysfunction and slow transit. Three main physiologic tests can be used to assess defecatory dysfunction: balloon expulsion test, anorectal manometry, and colon transit studies. In patients with symptoms that are highly suggestive of pelvic floor dysfunction, anorectal testing with rectal balloon expulsion test and anorectal manometry are first considerations and may be considered even before trying laxatives (Bharucha et al. 2013).

Balloon Expulsion Test. The balloon expulsion test has been used to exclude patients with constipation suspected of having defecatory disorders. Normally, rectal distension is simulated with an air- or fluid-filled balloon, usually a lubricated latex condom, in the rectum. This is tied to a catheter that is introduced into the rectum. Fluid is instilled into the balloon, and total volume is measured when the patient has a sustained feeling of necessity to defecate. The time required to expel the rectal balloon in the seated position is measured. Patients should be able to expel the balloon in less than 1 minute to up to 5 minutes (Rao et al., 1999; Noelting et al., 2012). A 50-mL balloon filled with water can usually be expelled in 1 to 2 minutes. In 2004, Minguez et al. identified patients with functional constipation, both with and without pelvic floor dyssynergia. Balloon testing was performed, showing a specificity and negative predictive value of balloon testing for excluding defecation disorders of 89% and 97%, respectively. This may be a useful screening test in clinical practice because patients with a normal balloon expulsion test result, independent of the frequency of defecatory symptoms, do not need other functional studies that are more expensive and difficult to perform to rule out pelvic floor dyssynergia.

Anorectal Manometry Testing. In the evaluation of constipation, manometry is most helpful in excluding Hirschsprung disease by the presence of a normal rectoanal inhibitory reflex and a supporting clinical impression of defecatory disorders, as evidenced by high anal resting pressures, typically 90 mm Hg or more, with relatively little voluntary augmentation suggestive of a nonrelaxing pelvic floor (Bharucha et al., 2013). Brief distension of the manometry balloon normally leads to reflexive internal sphincter relaxation and external sphincter contraction. This is called the rectal anal inhibitory reflex. In patients with Hirschsprung disease, this does not occur. Compliance of the rectum can be calculated by measuring the sensitivity and maximal volume tolerated in a fluid-filled balloon. An increased compliance can be seen in patients with constipation and signals a megarectum or insensitive rectum (Bharucha et al., 2013). Manometry may also be therapeutically used for patients with constipation in anal manometry–assisted biofeedback, as discussed later.

Colon Transit Testing. The colonic transit study is an important test to evaluate the colon for slow transit but is not required nor justified in all patients for the evaluation of constipation (Mearin et al., 2016). Patients must stop all laxative use 48 hours before the study. They should also consume a high-fiber diet (30 g daily) and refrain from using enemas. Many variations of this study are known, but basically patients consume a commercially-prepared capsule that contains a certain number of radiopaque markers. The Hinton technique involves ingesting a capsule containing 24 radiopaque markers; normally, less than five markers should remain in the colon on an abdominal radiography 5 days later (Hinton et al., 1969). Another method involves ingesting a capsule containing 24 markers on days 1, 2, and 3 and then counting the markers remaining on a plain abdominal radiograph on days 4 and 7. Eight or fewer markers remaining in the colon is considered normal. Some clinicians divide the colon into right, left, and rectosigmoid to determine the transit time of each segment. This allows distinction between whole-gut dysmotility, as seen by evenly distributed markers throughout the colon to the rectum, versus anal outlet obstruction, in which the markers progress quickly through the colon and are held up in the rectal sigmoid region. In another pattern, markers proceed through the colon, accumulate in the left colon, and stop. This signals left colonic dysfunction.

Barium and Magnetic Resonance Defecography. The diagnostic role of defecography remains unclear, but this test is useful when anorectal testing results are inconsistent with the clinical impression and/or to identify anatomic abnormalities (Diamant et al., 1999; Rao et al., 2016). See Video 13.1 for a detailed demonstration of the indications, technique, and normal and abnormal findings of defecography. Defecography is performed by placing a paste of contrast material into the rectum to simulate stool. Radiographs are taken at rest and during straining. During the examination, the patient sits on a commode behind a curtain, and fluoroscopy is performed to obtain the pictures. The items examined include the angle between the anal canal and rectum at rest, strain, and squeeze. The ability to evacuate contrast material, presence of a rectocele, and evidence of intussusception should be noted. During normal defecation, the anal canal becomes straighter, which, in turn, increases the angle. If this does not occur, the puborectalis muscle may be inappropriately contracting and may prohibit the expulsion of the contrast (and stool). The amount of descent of the perineum is noted, because this may be associated with anal outlet obstruction and constipation. Additionally, enfolding of the walls of the rectum with defecation, as is seen with internal prolapse, is evaluated. Defecating proctogram may be useful in establishing the diagnosis of internal rectal prolapse or rectoceles. This study helps delineate the rectoceles that are displaced anteriorly, not fully emptying, and may require repair (Fig. 28.2). Also, enteroceles and sigmoidoceles can be seen. It should be noted that this test is embarrassing for the patient, and complicated and unstandardized for the radiologist to perform. Therefore, the results may not always demonstrate the abnormality or may not be totally accurate. Defecography is useful for assessing rectal evacuation. It provides functional or morphologic features of the defecatory maneuver. However, there is a poor correlation between defecography and electromyography or manometry for diagnosing pelvic floor dyssynergia.

A barium enema or colonoscopy will diagnose anatomic abnormalities, such as stricture or cancer. At times a barium enema is preferred because it defines the borders of the colon and may show a redundant or chronically dilated colon (megacolon) or rectum (megarectum). Colonoscopy should be performed in patients over 50 years of age to screen for colorectal cancer, or in those with alarming features such as unintentional weight loss, blood in the stool, anemia, sudden changes in bowel habits or abdominal pain, and a family history of colon malignancy. Magnetic resonance defecography avoids radiation exposure and is better for visualizing bony landmarks that are necessary for measuring pelvic floor motion. The main limitation is that most closed-configuration magnetic resonance

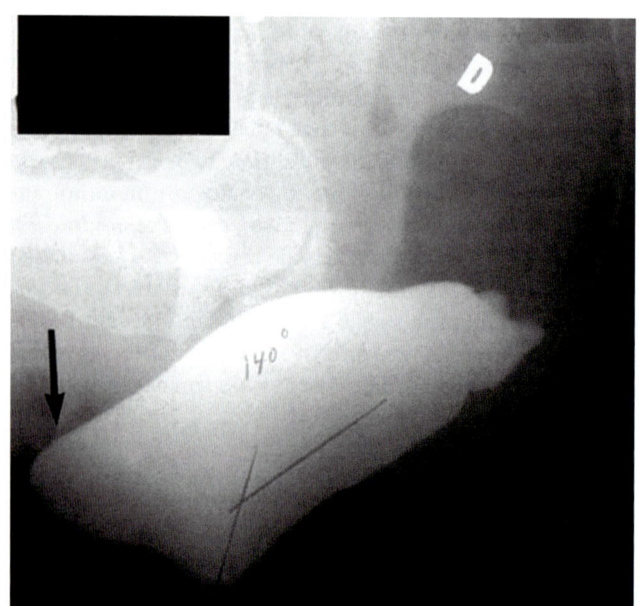

Fig. 28.2 Defecating proctogram demonstrating a rectocele (*arrow*) during defecation.

systems permit imaging in the supine position only, which limits the ability to identify intussception (Bertschinger et al., 2002).

NONSURGICAL TREATMENT

Most guidelines recommend that diet and lifestyle modifications be tried before pharmacological interventions. In general, recommended treatment pathways are to: (1) exclude other pathologies and secondary causes of constipation such as medications; (2) begin treatment with dietary and lifestyle adjustments such as routine bathroom times after meals; (3) suggest osmotic laxatives, stool softeners, and bulk laxatives, with no consensus on the order in which these are recommended; (4) suggest stimulant laxatives, suppositories, and/or enemas; and (5) consider surgery as a last resort or to treat identified disorders requiring surgical correction (Tack et al., 2011).

The majority of patients with constipation can be treated nonsurgically. If possible, it is important to correct associated medical or gastrointestinal abnormalities. These include problems such as hypothyroidism and hypokalemia. Hyperparathyroidism should be ruled out in patients with elevated calcium levels. Medications that are known to cause constipation sometimes can be modified to relieve the symptoms. Dispelling the myth that a daily bowel movement is "normal" can help avoid medical treatment. Many laxative manufacturers suggest that daily bowel movements are essential, in an effort to sell their products; however, this is not true. Next, a careful dietary history may provide clues to easily correctable problems that do not require specific drug treatment. However, there is no evidence that constipation can be treated by increasing fluid intake, unless there is evidence of dehydration (Muller-Lissner et al., 2005). Patients without these obvious or correctable problems should be started on medical management.

Medications

Bulk-Forming Laxatives and Fiber. Low dietary fiber is not the main determinant of constipation. A large British study by Connell et al. (1965) showed no relationship between dietary fiber intake and whole-gut transit time. Constipated patients on average do not eat less fiber than nonconstipated controls. Finally, patients who are constipated have lower stool weights and longer transit times than controls, whether or not they are treated with wheat bran. Despite this, fiber does work and is recommended if treatment is needed. Dietary fiber intake increases stool frequency in patients with constipation, but does not improve stool consistency, treatment success, laxative use, or painful defecation (Yang et al., 2012). Systematic reviews suggest that soluble (e.g., psyllium or ispaghula), but not insoluble, dietary fiber (e.g., wheat bran) supplements improve bowel symptoms in chronic constipation (Suares & Ford, 2011) and IBS (Bijkerk et al., 2004).

Fiber is the nondigestible segment of plants. Humans should consume 20 to 30 g of fiber daily for bowel health; however, the average American consumes only 11 g daily. Fiber promotes evacuation of the bowel by increasing the biomass volume and water content of feces. Fiber may improve constipation symptoms through four different mechanisms of action. First, stool is 30% to 50% bacteria; fiber provides substrate to increase the growth of bacteria and hence increase stool volume. Second, undigested hydrophilic components of fiber absorb fluid and can increase the fluidity of stool. Third, fermentation of fiber produces short-chain fatty acids that decrease transit time in the colon, which allows less time for the colonic mucosa to be in contact with the luminal contents to reabsorb water, thus increasing the fluidity of stool. Finally, the weight of the stool is increased simply by the nondigested components in fiber. The use of fiber is dose-dependent in its effect on stool weight. It requires a week to reach steady state, and patients who have slow transit require more fiber. Natural fiber is classified as soluble or insoluble fiber, and foods contain a mixture of these types. Stool size increases from the insoluble component of fiber. Foods high in insoluble fiber, as well as their fiber contents, are listed in Box 28.4.

Bulk-forming laxatives are thought to be among the safest laxatives. These include familiar products, such as Metamucil, Konsyl, Citrucel, and FiberCon. Dosage varies among products. Bulk-forming laxatives should be taken with sufficient fluids to avoid esophageal bolus obstruction and bowel obstruction from fecal impaction. The optimum quantity of "sufficient fluids" is unknown, but, in adults, drinking a full 8-ounce glass of fluid with each dose of bulk-forming laxative is recommended. For diabetic individuals, sugar-free varieties are manufactured. Side effects of bulk-forming laxatives include increased flatus, distension, poor taste, and bloating. Compliance with fiber supplementation regimens may be as low as 50%. More than 60% of patients randomized to psyllium report adverse effects such as constipation and diarrhea, and 40% of subjects drop out of clinical trials by 3 months (Suares & Ford, 2011). Generally, patients are instructed to start with one or two daily doses with fluids and/or meals and gradually adjust the dose after a 7- to 10-day period. This can be further increased, if needed, after several weeks. These agents take 12 to 72 hours to exert an effect, so patients should be encouraged to try the product for 1 to 2 weeks. Sometimes the problems of increased flatus and bloating decrease with continued use. If these symptoms are too distressing, the patient should switch to another

BOX 28.4 Insoluble Fiber Content of Selected Foods

Food (Total Fiber) (g)	Insoluble Fiber (g)
One pear (4.2)	2.9
One banana (3.9)	1.6
One cup strawberries (3.5)	3.0
One apple with skin (2.9)	2.8
Half cup frozen boiled peas (10.3)	3.2
Half cup cooked lima beans (5.5)	5.5
Half cup frozen broccoli (4.0)	2.1
Half cup cooked green beans (2.4)	1.2
Half cup raw tomatoes (1.9)	1.0
One cup chopped lettuce (0.9)	0.5

(Data from Dubuc MB, Lahaie LC. *Nutritive Value of Foods.* Ottawa: National Library; 1987.)

bulk-forming laxative, because the side effects may not be as distressing with another product.

Osmotic Laxatives. If more treatment is needed after bulk-forming laxatives, osmotic agents can be regularly used, supplemented by stimulant laxatives as needed. In general, there is more evidence of short-term and long-term efficacy for certain osmotic laxatives. A meta-analysis of seven controlled studies evaluating osmotic and stimulant laxatives reported a number needed to treat of 3 (Ford & Suares, 2011). Osmotic agents contain poorly absorbed substances that remain in the intestinal lumen, increasing the intraluminal osmotic pressure by drawing water into the lumen. The volume increases as the consistency decreases. The increased volume induces peristalsis.

There are four main types of osmotic agents: polyethylene glycol (PEG)-based solutions, magnesium citrate–based products, sodium phosphate–based products, and nonabsorbable carbohydrates. Patients with intractable constipation may benefit from daily administration of liquid PEG solutions, such as GoLYTELY or Colyte. A daily dosage of 8 to 16 ounces has been shown to improve stool frequency in chronically constipated patients. Another form of PEG (MiraLax) has been shown in placebo-controlled trials to increase bowel movement frequency. This medication is available in a powder form (17 g added to 8 oz of water) and may be useful for patients with slow-transit constipation. These compounds are not absorbed and do not cause a net ion gain or loss, and thus are safe for patients with concerns of fluid overload or renal insufficiency. In a Cochrane Database review of 10 randomized trials comparing PEG to lactulose, PEG was superior to placebo and lactulose for improving stool frequency, consistency, and abdominal pain (Lee-Robichaud et al., 2010).

Electrolyte-containing (magnesium- and sodium-based) laxatives are usually used to prepare patients for diagnostic bowel procedures and testing. They contain a magnesium cation or phosphate anion. Some believe that the nonabsorbed ion produces an osmotic effect, which increases the intraluminal fluid and thus increases the volume of stool. However, recent studies suggest that their method of action may be to stimulate the release of cholecystokinin, which stimulates small bowel motility and inhibits absorption of fluid and electrolytes from the small intestine. Saline laxatives can produce an evacuation within 2 to 6 hours if given orally or 15 minutes if given rectally. Oral administration should be accompanied by sufficient amounts of fluid to decrease holdover in the stomach and limit the possible effect of dehydration. Examples of these agents are magnesium citrate, milk of magnesia (magnesium hydroxide), magnesium sulfate, Phospho-soda (sodium phosphate and biphosphate), and Fleet enema (sodium biphosphate and phosphate). These agents should be used cautiously in patients with impaired renal function because magnesium and phosphate may cause electrolyte abnormalities. The sodium salts may cause congestive heart failure in susceptible patients. Electrolytes should be monitored in selected patients with use of these products. Additionally, enema preparations can cause rectal irritation.

Lactulose is a synthetic disaccharide that is not digested by gastrointestinal enzymes and is not significantly absorbed in the small intestine. Lactulose is metabolized by colonic bacteria to short-chain organic acids. The osmotic activity of the nonabsorbable short-chain organic acids draws water into the lumen. Lactulose is a syrup, and the dosage is 15 to 30 mL daily, increased to 60 mL daily if necessary. It may take up to 2 days to produce stool. Use as an enema in a 25% to 30% solution has been reported. Side effects include diarrhea, and the dosage must be titrated to each patient. Increased flatus and intestinal cramps can occur but usually subside with time. Lactulose contains galactose and lactose in small amounts and may alter serum glucose in diabetic persons.

Sorbitol, another poorly absorbed carbohydrate, can cause chronic diarrhea in persons who consume sugarless candy and gum that contain it. It works similarly to lactulose by reaching the colon as an active osmol. It can be administered orally or as an enema to treat constipation.

Glycerin suppositories promote fecal evacuation 15 to 30 minutes after administration by stimulating rectal evacuation as a hyperosmotic agent drawing fluid into the rectum. Possible side effects are abdominal cramping, rectal discomfort, and irritation of the rectal mucosa.

Stimulant Laxatives. Classes of stimulant laxatives include anthraquinones (cascara, senna [Senokot], and aloe), polyphenolic derivatives [phenolphthalein (Feen-a-Mint, Correctol, Ex-Lax], and bisacodyl [Dulcolax, Carter's Little Pills]), and castor oil. Oral, and some rectal, preparations are available for these medications. The anthraquinones and polyphenolic derivatives work in 6 to 8 hours. Short-term side effects include cramps, nausea, and abdominal pain. Castor oil works in 2 to 6 hours and is used mainly as a preparation for colonic procedures or radiologic studies. Stimulant laxatives produce their effect by inducing propagated colonic contractions and appear to be safe even with long-term use. These agents may be used as rescue agents if a patient has not had a bowel movement in 2 days or more regularly if needed. These agents may decrease water absorption and increase secretions, probably through prostaglandins. It was once believed that long-term use could lead to cathartic colon syndrome (a dilated and atonic colon following extensive and prolonged use of laxatives), melanosis coli (dark pigmentation of the colonic mucosa), or neuronal degeneration. However, studies suggest that stimulant laxatives (senna, bisacodyl) do not appear to damage the enteric nervous system (Dufour & Gendre, 1984; Kiernan & Heinicke, 1989).

Stool Softener Laxatives. Stool softeners exert a detergent-type effect through their hydrophilic and hydrophobic properties, which break down surface barriers, allowing water and lipids to enter the stool. This softens the stool and increases the fecal mass. Onset of action may take several days when administered orally, because it may take that long for the softened stool to reach the rectum. Rectal administration produces an effect in 2 to 15 minutes. Examples include docusate calcium (Surfak), docusate potassium (Dialose, Kasof), and docusate sodium (Colace, Comfolax, Modane Soft). Preparations of these in combination with stimulant laxatives include Feen-a-Mint, Correctol, Peri-Colace, and Doxidan. These agents have been suggested to decrease jejunal absorption and to damage villi, resulting in increased absorption of substances, such as mineral oil and phenolphthaleins. However, no serious adverse action is usually seen if these agents are taken alone. Side effects include diarrhea and mild abdominal cramping.

Lubricant Laxatives. Mineral oil is the most common lubricant laxative. A nondigested hydrocarbon with limited absorption, mineral oil decreases the absorption of water from stool and penetrates the stool to lubricate and soften. It can be used orally (15–45 mL daily in single or divided doses for adults) or in an enema (120 mL). Major concerns come with long-term use (>4 months) of this product. Oral use for more than 2 weeks coats the small intestine and may interfere with absorption of vitamins, especially vitamins A, D, E, and K (fat-soluble vitamins). For this reason, mineral oil should not be taken with meals. Additionally, many believe that it should not be administered at bedtime, to reduce the occurrence of aspiration of the mineral oil, which can produce lipoid pneumonia. Administration with docusate salts may enhance absorption of mineral oil, which can form lipoid granulomas in the reticuloendothelial system; therefore, administration of both together is usually avoided. Other side effects include pruritus ani, anal leakage, and diarrhea.

Intestinal Secretagogues. Patients who fail to respond to diet and laxatives are candidates for newer medications. Secretagogues (lubiprostone and linaclotide) accelerate transit and ease of defecation by stimulating a net efflux of ions and water into the intestinal lumen. Lubiprostone accelerates small-intestinal transit and colonic transit by activating prostaglandin E–type prostanoid receptors and the apical cystic fibrosis transmembrane regulator (CFTR), which mediates intestinal fluid secretion. It is approved by the FDA at a dosage of 24 μg twice daily for the treatment of chronic constipation. Linaclotide also acts to open the CFTR chloride channel and produce a net efflux of ions and water into the intestinal lumen. The FDA-approved dosages are 290 μg daily for IBS-C and 145 μg daily for chronic constipation. Plecanatide (3 mg once daily), a guanylate cyclase-C agonist, is also approved for constipation.

Serotonin 5-HT4 Receptor Agonists. Currently, prucalopride is a selective 5-HT4 receptor agonist approved by the FDA for chronic constipation. Trials have demonstrated that prucalopride (1–4 mg daily) improves stool frequency, consistency, and straining (Tack et al., 2009; Quigley et al., 2009).

Biofeedback

Patients with rectal evacuation problems manifested only by a hold-up of markers in the rectum during the colonic transit study, as well as those patients with defecation disorders diagnosed by balloon or anorectal manometry, testing should be managed with biofeedback-augmented pelvic floor therapy. Biofeedback strategies aim to instruct patients how to adequately contract the abdominal wall while relaxing the pelvic floor muscles during defecation. Visual or auditory signals are used to feedback physiologic activity to patients. In hyposensory patients, sensory training may be used by gradually reducing the volume of the rectal balloon, allowing patients to recognize earlier sensations of rectal filling. Controlled trials show that pelvic floor retraining with biofeedback is more effective in patients with defecatory disorders than in patients with slow colonic transit. One study demonstrated that 71% of patients with dyssynergic defecation, but only 8% of patients with isolated slow colonic transit, achieved adequate relief after biofeedback therapy (Chiarioni et al., 2005). Additionally, some patients with slow colonic transit appear to improve after pelvic floor therapy and biofeedback therapy, reinforcing the concept that delayed colonic transit may be secondary to pelvic floor dysfunction (Chiarioni et al., 2005). Moreover, three controlled studies showed that biofeedback therapy is more effective than polyethylene glycol (Chiarioni et al., 2006), sham feedback (Rao et al., 2007), or diazepam (Heymen et al., 2007) in defecatory disorders. These trials used five to six training sessions lasting 30 to 60 minutes at 2-weekly intervals. In summary, biofeedback therapy is essential in managing evacuation disorders because of pelvic floor dysfunction.

SURGICAL TREATMENT

A clinical decision-making tool has been developed by international consensus to assess whether a patient has had an adequate response to nonsurgical therapy for chronic constipation (Tack et al., 2017). When a patient is refractory to nonsurgical therapies, surgical treatments are warranted. Surgical treatment for patients with constipation can be divided into procedures for slow-transit constipation and for defecatory disorders.

Slow-Transit Constipation (Colonic Inertia)

Severely constipated patients with slow transit demonstrated on colonic transit studies who are medically refractory and who do not have pelvic floor dysfunction may benefit from subtotal colectomy. Colonic manometry with or without barostat testing should be performed to identify colonic inertia and upper gastrointestinal motility disorders. Operative choices include colectomy with ileosigmoid, ileorectal, or cecorectal anastomosis. Ileorectal anastomosis appears to be the procedure with the highest efficacy in properly selected patients (Hassan et al., 2006; You et al., 1998; Sunderland et al., 1992). Ileosigmoid anastomosis appears to result in persistence or recurrence of slow transit constipation, whereas anastomosis to the middle or lower rectum may result in abnormally high stool frequency, and sometimes fecal incontinence (Pemberton et al., 1991; Nyam et al., 1997). Symptoms of infrequent and difficult evacuation are most likely to improve after colectomy with ileorectal anastomosis. In up to 41% of patients, abdominal pain will persist after surgery, 14% of patients will develop diarrhea and/or fecal incontinence, and up to 18% will develop an adhesion-related small bowel obstruction.

Thus, patients who fail medical management are candidates for subtotal colectomy with ileorectal anastomosis. If a patient has slow-transit constipation and concomitant pelvic floor dysfunction, it is advisable to have treatment targeted at the pelvic floor dysfunction first and to offer colectomy if symptoms persist.

Sacral Nerve Stimulation

It has long been appreciated that patients undergoing sacral neuromodulation for urinary disorders also see improvement in bowel dysfunction. Because of this, sacral neuromodulation has been used for patients with constipation resistant to conservative treatment for over 10 years. Although the mechanism of action is unclear, there are findings indicating that neuromodulation alters the representation of the lower gastrointestinal tract in the sensory cortex. However, it remains unclear whether this affects bowel motility. A systematic review by Thomas et al. (2013) identified 13 studies (10 in adults and three in children) describing results of sacral neuromodulation for chronic constipation. Test stimulation was successful in 42% to 100% of patients, and of those who proceeded to permanent implant, up to 87% showed an improvement in bowel symptoms with a median follow-up of 28 months. Symptomatic improvement also correlated with improvement in quality of life and overall satisfaction. Most adverse events are similar to those seen in fecal incontinence and are related to reprogramming, pain, or infection. Sacral neuromodulation is not approved for treatment of constipation in the United States.

Defecatory Disorders

Dyssynergic Defecation. Surgical division of the pelvic floor or sphincter muscles has been tried for nonrelaxing or paradoxical puborectalis contraction. However, long-term improvement is seen in few patients, and biofeedback has become the mainstay of treatment for this problem.

Rectal Prolapse. Rectal prolapse or intussusception can be entirely internal (occult) or external and protrude through the anal sphincter complex. Patients with rectal prolapse and constipation should undergo a complete evaluation before surgery. If diffuse slow-transit constipation is found, a colectomy with ileorectal anastomosis and rectopexy may be the procedure of choice. Patients with normal transit and mild constipation may benefit from a sigmoid resection with a colorectal anastomosis and rectopexy. Chapter 30 more fully discusses this condition.

Rectocele. Defecatory dysfunction is commonly associated with rectoceles. This is a condition that results in the protrusion of the posterior vaginal wall and anterior rectal wall into the lumen of the vagina. Patients with a rectocele may complain of various symptoms during defecation, including straining, a feeling of incomplete emptying often necessitating the need for digitation or splinting to complete a bowel movement, rectal pain, a protrusion from the vagina, and vaginal and/or perineal bulge. Although clinical examination has demonstrated good sensitivity in the detection of rectoceles, there seems to be no correlation between bowel function and the size of the rectocele. Thus, indications for surgical repair of rectocele are variable and not well-defined. Because of this, investigators have attempted various tests to obtain insight into important dynamic information that may or may not improve with surgery.

Defecography is useful in determining size and position of rectoceles, perineal descent, rectal intussusception, and pelvic floor dyssynergia. However, data on whether size of a rectocele on defecography correlates with symptoms are conflicting. Although defecography is useful in evaluating how well a person evacuates the rectum, no correlation is found between women who retain contrast and symptoms of defecatory dysfunction or clinical outcome of surgical repair. Defecography may be useful in patients with pelvic floor dyssynergia, but the effects of this on the outcomes of rectocele repair are also contradictory. Other studies, such as anorectal manometry, pudendal nerve terminal motor latency, endoanal ultrasonography, and colonic transit studies, have not been helpful in clarifying which patients may benefit from surgery for rectocele in the presence of disorders of evacuation.

The approach to surgical repair of rectoceles is presented in Chapter 20. Outcomes of surgical intervention for rectocele are limited by a lack of standardized definitions in the literature. Gynecologists often operate on patients who suffer from the presence of a vaginal bulge or specific symptoms, such as splinting. A thorough history of symptoms of disordered defecation is often ignored, and classification of patients into standardized groups, such as those based on the Rome criteria, is lacking. Although most authors report that constipation improves after surgical repair, the symptoms reported are not specific and do not provide insight into the mechanism of improvement, because it appears that most symptoms do not necessarily correlate with anatomic severity. Table 28.1 illustrates the lack of standardized outcomes used for vaginal approaches to rectocele repair, resulting in a wide range of success rates. Investigators need to standardize subjective, anatomic, testing, and global satisfaction outcomes in this area.

CONCLUSION

Constipation is a common, complex constellation of symptoms with unclear pathophysiology that can produce mild or incapacitating symptoms. History and physical examination initiate therapy. Further laboratory, anatomic, and functional testing depend on the history and physical examination and the response to initial therapy. If the initial evaluation is normal or negative, an empiric trial of fiber (and/or dietary changes) can be followed by over-the-counter osmotic or stimulant laxatives. Most laxatives (and dietary fiber) are generally effective, inexpensive, and safe even for long-term use. For patients unresponsive to these measures, further investigation is warranted, using various imaging or physiologic tests. Behavioral therapy should be offered to patients with defecation disorders, as biofeedback is the mainstay of treatment for this group. For patients with continued constipation, newer agents such as secretagogues should be considered.

TABLE 28.1 **Transvaginal Rectocele Repair Symptoms**

Author (Year)	Number of Patients	Preoperative (%)	Postoperative (%)	Follow-Up (months)
Arnold et al. (1990)	29	Constipation (75)	Constipation (54) Anatomic cure (80)	
Mellegren et al. (1995)	25	Constipation (96) Rectal bleeding (16) Dyspareunia (4) Vaginal bulge (84)	Constipation (88) Vaginal bulge (4)	12
Kahn and Stanton (1997)	231	Constipation (22) Dyspareunia (18) Vaginal bulge (64)	Constipation (33) Dyspareunia (27) Vaginal bulge (24)	52
Kenton et al. (1999)	66	Constipation (41) Dyspareunia (28) Vaginal bulge (86)	Improved constipation (43) Dyspareunia (2) Vaginal bulge (9)	12
Porter et al. (1999)	125	Constipation (60) Vaginal bulge (38)	Constipation (50) Vaginal bulge (14) Anatomic cure (82)	6
Glavind and Madsen (2000)	67	Constipation (40) Dyspareunia (12) Vaginal bulge (100)	Improved constipation (88) Dyspareunia (6) Vaginal bulge (0)	3
Lopez et al. (2001)	25	Constipation (96) Dyspareunia (19) Vaginal bulge (84)	Improved constipation (91) Dyspareunia (33) Vaginal bulge (4)	60
Paraiso et al. (2001)	102	Straining (76) Manual evacuation (45) Fewer than two bowel movements/week (13)	Straining (45) Manual evacuation (8) Fewer than two bowel movements/week (6)	12
Sand et al. (2001)	70		Anatomic cure (90)	12
Singh et al. (2003)	42	Vaginal bulge (78)	Vaginal bulge (7) Anatomic cure (92)	18
Cundiff and Fenner (2004)	69	Constipation (46) Dyspareunia (29)	Constipation (13) Dysparenuia (19) Vaginal bulge (14)	12

Surgical intervention is mandated for patients with Hirschsprung disease and external rectal prolapse and for patients who are refractory to nonsurgical therapies. Women with a rectocele present with complex clinical pictures and often report mixed gynecologic and anorectal symptoms. Lack of standardized definitions and unclear data regarding testing modalities complicate the appropriate medical or surgical management in these patients.

BIBLIOGRAPHY

Altman D, Zetterstrom J, Lopez A, et al. Effect of hysterectomy on bowel function. *Dis Colon Rectum.* 2004;47:502.

Andorsky RI, Goldner F. Colonic lavage solution (polyethylene glycol electrolyte lavage solution) as a treatment for chronic constipation: a double-blind placebo-controlled study. *Am J Gastroenterol.* 1990;85:261.

Arnold MW, Stewart WR, Aguilar PS. Rectocele repair: four years' experience. *Dis Colon Rectum.* 1990;33:684.

Ashraf W, Park F, Lof J, Quigley EM. An examination of the reliability of reported stool frequency in the diagnosis of idiopathic constipation. *Am J Gastroenterol.* 1996;91:26.

Bassotti G, Chistolini F, Sietchiping-Nzepa F, et al. Biofeedback for pelvic floor dysfunction in constipation. *Br Med J.* 2004;328:393.

Bertschinger KM, Hetzer FH, Roos JE, et al. Dynamic MR imaging of the pelvic floor performed with patient sitting in an open-magnet unit versus with patient supine in a closed-magnet unit. *Radiology.* 2002;223:501.

Bharucha AE, Pemberton JH, Locke III GR. American Gastroenterological Association technical review on constipation. *Gastroenterology.* 2013;144:218.

Bharucha AE, Wald A, Enck P. Functional anorectal disorders. *Gastroenterology.* 2006;130:1510.

Bijkerk CJ, Muris JW, Knottnerus JA, et al. Systematic review: the role of different types of fibre in the treatment of irritable bowel syndrome. *Aliment Pharmacol Ther.* 2004;19:245.

Binder HJ. Use of laxatives in clinical medicine. *Pharmacology.* 1988;36:226.

Cerulli MA, Schuster MM. Medical treatment of constipation and fecal incontinence. In: Phillips SF, Pemberton JH, Shorter RG, eds: *The Large Intestine Physiology, Pathophysiology, and Disease.* New York: Raven; 1991.

Chiarioni G, Salandini L, Whitehead WE. Biofeedback benefits only patients with outlet dysfunction, not patients with isolated slow transit constipation. *Gastroenterology.* 2005;129:86.

Chiarioni G, Whitehead WE, Pezza V, et al. Biofeedback is superior to laxatives for normal transit constipation due to pelvic floor dyssynergia. *Gastroenterology.* 2006;130:657.

Choung RS, Branda ME, Chitkara D, et al. Longitudinal direct medical costs associated with constipation in women. *Aliment Pharmacol Ther.* 2011;33:251.

Connell AM, Hilton C, Irvine G, et al. Variation of bowel habit in two population samples. *Br Med J.* 1965;5470:1095.

Cundiff GW, Weidner AC, Visco AG, et al. An anatomic and functional assessment of the discrete defect rectocele repair. *Am J Obstet Gynecol.* 1998;179:1451.

Cundiff GW, Fenner D. Evaluation and treatment of women with rectocele: focus on associated defecatory and sexual dysfunction. *Obstet Gynecol.* 2004;104:1403.

Dahl J, Lindquist BL, Tysk C, et al. Behavioral medicine treatment in chronic constipation with paradoxical anal sphincter contraction. *Dis Colon Rectum.* 1991;34:769.

Daley AJ, Grimmett C, Roberts L, et al. The effects of exercise upon symptoms and quality of life in patients diagnosed with irritable bowel syndrome: a randomized controlled trial. *Int J Sports Med.* 2008;29:778.

Diamant NE, Kamm MA, Wald A, Whitehead WE. AGA technical review on anorectal testing techniques. *Gastroenterology.* 1999;116:735.

de Groat WC, Kawatani M, Hisamitsu T, et al. Mechanisms underlying the recovery of urinary bladder function following spinal cord injury. *J Auton Nerv Syst.* 1990;30:S71.

De Looze D, Van Laere M, De Muynck M, et al. Constipation and other chronic gastrointestinal problems in spinal cord injury. *Spinal Cord.* 1998;36:63.

Degen LP, Phillips SF. How well does stool form reflect colonic transit? *Gut.* 1996;39:109.

DiPalma JA, DeRidder PH, Orlando RC, et al. A randomized, placebo-controlled, multicenter study of the safety and efficacy of a new polyethylene glycol laxative. *Am J Gastroenterol.* 2000;95:445.

Drossman DA, Corazziari E, Talley NJ, et al. *Rome II. The Functional Gastrointestinal Disorders. Diagnosis, Pathophysiology and Treatment: A Multinational Consensus.* 2nd ed. McLean, VA: Degnon Associates; 2000.

Drossman DA, Sandler RS, McKee DC, Lovitz AJ. Bowel patterns among subjects not seeking health care. *Gastroenterology.* 1982;83:529.

Dubuc MB, Lahaie LC. *Nutritive Value of Foods.* Ottawa: National Library; 1987.

Dufour P, Gendre P. Ultrastructure of mouse intestinal mucosa and changes observed after long term anthraquinone administration. *Gut.* 1984;25:1358.

Edery P, Lyonnet S, Mulligan LM, et al. Mutations of the RET proto-oncogene in Hirschsprung's disease. *Nature.* 1994;367:378.

Ford AC, Suares NC. Effect of laxatives and pharmacological therapies in chronic idiopathic constipation: systematic review and meta-analysis. *Gut.* 2011;60:209.

Glavind K, Madsen H. A prospective study of the discrete fascial defect rectocele repair. *Acta Obstet Gynecol Scand.* 2000;79:145.

Goh JT, Tjandra JJ, Carey MP. How could management of rectoceles be optimized? *ANZ J Surg.* 2002;72:896.

Hassan I, Pemberton JH, Young-Fadok TM, et al. Ileorectal anastomosis for slow transit constipation: long-term functional and quality of life results. *J Gastrointest Surg.* 2006;10:1330.

He CL, Burgart L, Wang L, et al. Decreased interstitial cell of cajal volume in patients with slow-transit constipation. *Gastroenterology.* 2000;118:14.

Heaton KW, O'Donnell LJ. An office guide to whole-gut transit time. Patients' recollection of their stool form. *J Clin Gastroenterol.* 1994;19:28.

Heymen S, Scarlett Y, Jones K, et al. Randomized, controlled trial shows biofeedback to be superior to alternative treatments for patients with pelvic floor dyssynergia-type constipation. *Dis Colon Rectum.* 2007;50:428.

Hinds JP, Eidelman BH, Wald A. Prevalence of bowel dysfunction in multiple sclerosis: a population survey. *Gastroenterology.* 1990;98:1538.

Hinton JM, Lennard-Jones JE, Young AC. A new method for studying gut transit times using radioopaque markers. *Gut.* 1969;10:842.

Hull TL, Milsom JW. Constipation: results of surgical therapy. In: Brubaker LT, Saclarides TJ, eds. *The Female Pelvic Floor: Disorders of Function and Support.* Philadelphia: FA Davis; 1996.

Jorge JM, Wexner SD, Ger GC, et al. Cinedefecography and electromyography in the diagnosis of nonrelaxing puborectalis syndrome. *Dis Colon Rectum.* 1993;36:668.

Kahn MA, Stanton SL. Posterior colporrhaphy: its effects on bowel and sexual function. *BJOG.* 1997;104:82.

Kelvin FM, Maglinte DD, Benson JT. Evacuation proctography (defecography): an aid to the investigation of pelvic floor disorders. *Obstet Gynecol.* 1994;83:307.

Kenefick NJ, Vaizey CJ, Cohen CR, et al. Double blind placebo-controlled crossover study of sacral nerve stimulation for idiopathic constipation. *Br J Surg.* 2002;89:1570.

Kenny KA, Skelly JM. Dietary fiber for constipation in older adults: a systematic review. *Clin Effective Nurs.* 2001;5:120.

Kenton K, Shott S, Brubaker L. Outcome after rectovaginal fascia reattachment for rectocele repair. *Am J Obstet Gynecol.* 1999;191:1360.

Kiernan JA, Heinicke EA. Sennosides do not kill myenteric neurons in the colon of the rat or mouse. *Neuroscience.* 1989;30:837.

Lee-Robichaud H, Thomas K, Morgan J, Nelson RL. Lactulose versus polyethylene glycol for chronic constipation. *Cochrane Database Syst Rev.* 2010;7:CD007570.

Lewis SJ, Heaton KW. Stool form scale as a useful guide to intestinal transit time. *Scand J Gastroenterol.* 1997;32:920.

Longstreth GF, Thompson WG, Chey WD, et al. Functional bowel disorders. *Gastroenterology.* 2006;130:1480.

Lopez A, Anzen B, Bremmer S, et al. Durability of success after rectocele repair. *Int Urogynecol J.* 2001;12:97.

Martin BC, Barghout V, Cerulli A. Direct medical costs of constipation in the United States. *Manag Care Interface.* 2006;19:43.

Mathers SE, Kempster PA, Law PJ, et al. Anal sphincter dysfunction in Parkinson's disease, *Arch Neurol.* 1989;46:1061.

Mearin F, Lacy BE, Chang L, et al. Bowel disorders. *Gastroenterol.* 2016;150;1393.

Mellegren A, Anzén B, Nilsson BY, et al. Results of rectocele repair: a prospective study. *Dis Colon Rectum.* 1995;38:7.

Miller R, Duthie GS, Bartolo DC, et al. Anismus in patients with normal and slow transit constipation. *Br J Surg.* 1991;78:690.

Minguez M, Herreros B, Sanchiz V, et al. Predictive value of the balloon expulsion test for excluding the diagnosis of pelvic floor dyssynergia in constipation. *Gastroenterology.* 2004;126:57.

Muller-Lissner SA, Kamm MA, Scarpignato C, Wald A. Myths and misconceptions about chronic constipation. *Am J Gastroenterol.* 2005;100:232.

Nakaji S, Tokunaga S, Sakamoto J, et al. Relationship between lifestyle factors and defecation in a Japanese population. *Eur J Nutr.* 2002;41:244.

Nicholls RJ, Kamm MA. Proctocolectomy with restorative ileo-anal reservoir for severe idiopathic constipation. *Dis Colon Rectum.* 1988;31:968.

Noelting J, Ratuapli SK, Bharucha AE, et al. Normal values for high-resolution anorectal manometry in healthy women: effects of age and significance of rectoanal gradient. *Am J Gastroenterol.* 2012;107:1530.

Novick J, Miner P, Krause R, et al. A randomized, double blind, placebo controlled trial of tegaserod in female patients suffering from irritable bowel syndrome with constipation. *Aliment Pharmacol Ther.* 2002;16:1877.

Nyam DC, Pemberton JH, Ilstrup DM, Rath DM. Long-term results of surgery for chronic constipation. *Dis Colon Rectum.* 1997;40:273.

Paraiso MF, Weber AM, Walters MD, et al. Anatomic and functional outcome after posterior colporrhaphy. *J Pelvic Surg.* 2001;7:335.

Parkman HP, Rho SS, Reynolds JC, et al. Neurotrophin-3 improves functional constipation. *Am J Gastroenterol.* 2003;98:1338.

Pemberton JH, Rath DM, Ilstrup DM. Evaluation and surgical treatment of severe chronic constipation. *Ann Surg.* 1991;214:403.

Porter WE, Steele A, Walsh P, et al. The anatomic and functional outcomes of defect-specific rectocele repairs. *Am J Obstet Gynecol.* 1999;181:1353.

Prior A, Stanley KM, Smith AR, Read NW. Relation between hysterectomy and the irritable bowel: a prospective study. *Gut.* 1992;33:814.

Puffenberger EG, Hosoda K, Washington SS, et al. A missense mutation of the endothelin-B receptor gene in multigenic Hirschsprung's disease. *Cell.* 1994;79:1257.

Quigley EMM, Vandeplassche L, Kerstens R, Ausma J. Clinical trial: the efficacy, impact on quality of life, and safety and tolerability of prucalopride in severe chronic constipation—a 12-week, randomized, double-blind, placebo-controlled study. *Aliment Pharmacol Ther.* 2009;29:315.

Rao SS, Hatfield R, Soffer E, et al. Manometric tests of anorectal function in healthy adults. *Am J Gastroenterol.* 1999;94:773.

Rao SS, Mudipalli RS, Stessman M. Investigation of the utility of colorectal function tests and Rome II criteria in dyssynergic defecation (Anismus). *Neurogastroenterol Motil.* 2004;16:589.

Rao SS, Tuteja AK, Vellema T, et al. Dyssynergic defecation: demographics, symptoms, stool patterns, and quality of life. *J Clin Gastroenterol.* 2004;38:680.

Rao SS, Seaton K, Miller M, et al. Randomized controlled trial of biofeedback, sham feedback, and standard therapy for dyssynergic defecation. *Clin Gastroenterol Hepatol.* 2007;5:331.

Rao SS, Bharucha AE, Chiarioni G, et al. Anorectal disorders. *Gastroenterol.* 2016;150;1430.

Rattanakovit K, Rao SS, Amieva M, et al. Dyssynergia or no dyssynergia: phenotypic categorization of constipated patients with high-resolution anorectal manometry (HRAM). *Am J Gastroenterol.* 2015;110:S593.

Ravi K, Bharucha AE, Camilleri M, et al. Phenotypic variation of colonic motor functions in chronic constipation. *Gastroenterology.* 2010;138:89.

Samuelsson EC, Arne Victor FT, Tibblin G, Svärdsudd KF. Signs of genital prolapse in a Swedish population of women 20 to 59 years of age and possible related factors. *Am J Obstet Gynecol.* 1999;180:299.

Sand PK, Koduri A, Lobel RW, et al. Prospective randomized trial of polyglactin 910 mesh to prevent recurrence of cystoceles and rectoceles. *Am J Obstet Gynecol.* 2001;184:1357.

Sandler RS, Drossman DA. Bowel habits in young adults not seeking health care. *Dig Dis Sci.* 1987;32:841.

Schouten WR, Gordon PH. Constipation. In: Gordon PH, Nivatvongs S, eds. *Principles and Practice of Surgery for the Colon, Rectum, and Anus.* St. Louis: Quality Medical Publishing; 1992.

Shah ND, Chitkara DK, Locke GR, et al. Ambulatory care for constipation in the United States, 1993-2004. *Am J Gastroenterol.* 2008;103:1746.

Sharma A, Rao S. Constipation: pathophysiology and current therapeutic approaches. *Handb Exp Pharmacol.* 2017;239:59.

Singh K, Cortes E, Reid WM. Evaluation of the fascial technique for surgical repair of isolated posterior vaginal wall prolapse. *Obstet Gynecol.* 2003;101:320.

Singh S, Heady S, Coss-Adame E, Rao SS. Clinical utility of colonic manometry in slow-transit constipation. *Neurogastroenterol Motil.* 2013;25:487.

Siproudhis L, Ropert A, Vilotte J, et al. How accurate is clinical examination in diagnosing and quantifying pelvirectal disorders? *Dis Colon Rectum.* 1993;36:430.

Sloan S. Medical management of constipation. In: Brubaker LT, Saclarides TJ, eds. *The Female Pelvic Floor: Disorders of Function and Support.* Philadelphia: FA Davis; 1996.

Sonnenberg A, Koch TR. Epidemiology of constipation in the United States. *Dis Colon Rectum.* 1989;32:1.

Stewart WF, Liberman JN, Sandler RS, et al. Epidemiology of constipation (EPOC) study in the United States: relation of clinical subtypes to sociodemographic features. *Am J Gastroenterol.* 1999;94:3530.

Suares NC, Ford AC. Prevalence of, and risk factors for, chronic idiopathic constipation in the community: systematic review and meta-analysis. *Am J Gastroenterol.* 2011;106:1582.

Suares NC, Ford AC. Systematic review: the effects of fibre in the management of chronic idiopathic constipation. *Aliment Pharmacol Ther.* 2011;33:895.

Sunderland GT, Poon FW, Lauder J, Finlay IG. Videoproctography in selecting patients with constipation for colectomy. *Dis Colon Rectum.* 1992;35:235.

Tack J, van OM, Beyens G, Kerstens R, Vandeplassche L. Prucalopride (Resolor) in the treatment of severe chronic constipation in patients dissatisfied with laxatives. *Gut.* 2009;58:357.

Tack J, Muller-Lissner S, Stanghellini V, et al. Diagnosis and treatment of chronic constipation – a European perspective. *Neurogastroenterol Motil.* 2011;23:697.

Tack J, Boardman H, Layer P, et al. An expert consensus definition of failure of a treatment to provide adequate relief (F-PAR) for chronic constipation - an international Delphi survey. *Aliment Pharmacol Ther.* 2017;45:434.

Talley NJ, Weaver AL, Zinsmeister AR, Melton LJ. Onset and disappearance of gastrointestinal symptoms and functional gastrointestinal disorders. *Am J Epidemiol.* 1992;136:165.

Thomas GP, Dudding TC, Rahbour G, et al. Sacral nerve stimulation for constipation. *Br J Surg.* 2013;100:174.

Tantiphlachiva K, Rao P, Attaluri A, Rao SS. Digital rectal examination is a useful tool for identifying patients with dyssynergia. *Clin Gastroenterol Hepatol.* 2010;8:955.

Ting KH, Mangel E, Eibl-Eibesfeldt B. Is the volume retained after defecation a valuable parameter at defecography? *Dis Colon Rectum.* 1992;35:762.

Tjandra JJ, Ooi BS, Tang CL, et al. Transanal repair of rectocele corrects obstructed defecation if it is not associated with anismus. *Dis Colon Rectum.* 1999;42:1544.

Tramonte SM, Brand MB, Mulrow CD, et al. The treatment of chronic constipation in adults. A systematic review. *J Gen Intern Med.* 1997;12:15.

Van Dam JH, Ginai AZ, Gosseling MJ, et al. Role of defecography in predicting clinical outcome of rectocele repair. *Dis Colon Rectum.* 1997;40:201.

Van Dam JH, Schouten WR, Ginai AZ, et al. The impact of anismus on the clinical outcome of rectocele repair. *Int J Colorectal Dis.* 1996;11:238.

Van Laarhoven CJ, Kamm MA, Bartram CI, et al. Relationship between anatomic and symptomatic long-term results after rectocele repair for impaired defecation. *Dis Colon Rectum.* 1999;42:204.

Vickery G. Basics of constipation. *Gastroenterol Nurs.* 1997;20:125.

Wald A, Caruana BJ, Freimanis MG, et al. Contributions of evacuation proctography and anorectal manometry to evaluation of adults with constipation and defecatory difficulty. *Dig Dis Sci.* 1990;35:481.

Wald A, Scarpignato C, Mueller-Lissner S, et al. A multinational survey of prevalence and patterns of laxative use among adults with self-defined constipation. *Aliment Pharmacol Ther.* 2008;28:917.

Waldron D, Bowes KL, Kingma YJ, Cote KR. Colonic and anorectal motility in young women with severe idiopathic constipation. *Gastroenterology.* 1988;95:1388.

Weber AM, Walters MD, Ballard LA, et al. Posterior vaginal prolapse and bowel function. *Am J Obstet Gynecol.* 1998;179:1446.

Weber AM, Walters MD, Piedmonte MR. Sexual function and vaginal anatomy in women before and after surgery for pelvic organ prolapse and urinary incontinence. *Am J Obstet Gynecol.* 2000;182:1610.

Wexner SD, Cheape JD, Jorge JM, et al. Prospective assessment of biofeedback for the treatment of paradoxical puborectalis contraction. *Dis Colon Rectum.* 1992;35:145.

Wexner SD, Daniel N, Jagelman DG. Colectomy for constipation: physiologic investigation is the key to success. *Dis Colon Rectum.* 1991;34:851.

Yang J, Wang HP, Zhou L, Xu CF. Effect of dietary fiber on constipation: a meta analysis. *World J Gastroenterol.* 2012;18:7378.

You YT, Wang JY, Changchien CR, et al. Segmental colectomy in the management of colonic inertia. *Am Surg.* 1998;64:775.

Young FE, Heckler MM. Laxative drug products for over the counter human use: tentative final monograph. *Fed Regist.* 1985;50:2124.

29

Rectovaginal Fistula and Perineal Breakdown

Mickey M. Karram

CHAPTER OUTLINE

ANATOMY OF THE PERINEAL BODY, DISTAL VAGINA, RECTUM, AND ANUS

Perineal body defects and rectovaginal fistulas (RVFs) are part of a spectrum of conditions that impact the posterior pelvic floor. The surgical interventions used to address these defects must be based on a clear understanding of the anatomic structures involved. A postobstetric pinhole fistula may occur in isolation (i.e., the perineal body and anal sphincters [ASs] are completely intact) (Fig. 29.1); or maybe only the tip of an iceberg in which there is a significant defect of the entire perineal body and ASs (Fig. 29.2). Surgical management of these various defects requires a clear understanding of the anatomy of the distal portion of the posterior vaginal wall, the perineal body, the ASs, the rectum, and the anal canal.

The surgical anatomy of the posterior pelvic floor remains an area of controversy among surgeons and anatomists. In recent years, there has been a clearer understanding of the anatomy of the posterior vaginal wall and perineum; however, surgical studies in this area continue to use terms that are not anatomically based. Historically, the tissue that lies between the posterior vaginal wall and anterior wall of the rectum has been termed rectovaginal or Denonvilliers' fascia. Histologic studies have noted that what has previously been termed fascia is actually vaginal muscularis (Farrell et al., 2001). At the level of the midvagina, histological assessment of the posterior vaginal wall from the lumen of the vagina to the lumen of the rectum notes the following layers: the vaginal epithelium, the lamina propria of the vagina, the fibromuscular wall of the vagina (smooth muscle cells, elastin, and type II collagen), D the adventitia, the outer muscular wall of the rectum, the inner muscular wall of the rectum, the lamina propria of the rectum, and the rectal mucosa. Delancey (1999) discussed posterior vaginal wall anatomy in a review article and likened it to an open container. The front wall of the container is formed of the posterior vaginal wall, whereas the bottom of the container is made up of the perineal body and ASs. The levator ani muscles form the lateral sides of the container and the levator plate, where the muscles decussate behind the rectum to create the iliococcygeal raphe, which forms the back wall of the container. The uppermost portion of the container would then be created by the attachment of the posterior vaginal wall to the uterosacral ligaments, which extend below the peritoneum. All of these boundaries are subject to defects that can give rise to different structural failures.

The perineal body has been described as the central tendon between the urogenital and anal triangles (Fig. 29.3). It contains interlacing muscle fibers from the bulbospongiosus and superficial transverse perineal muscles, as well as the anterior portion of the external AS. There is also contribution from the longitudinal rectal muscle and medial portions of the puborectalis muscles.

Normally, the anus appears externally as a closed anterior/posterior lip, with its lateral walls closely opposed. Damage to

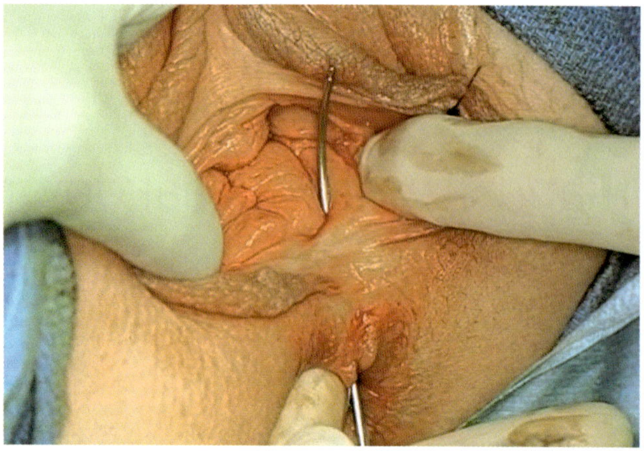

Fig. 29.1 Small rectovaginal fistula with intact perineum and anal sphincters.

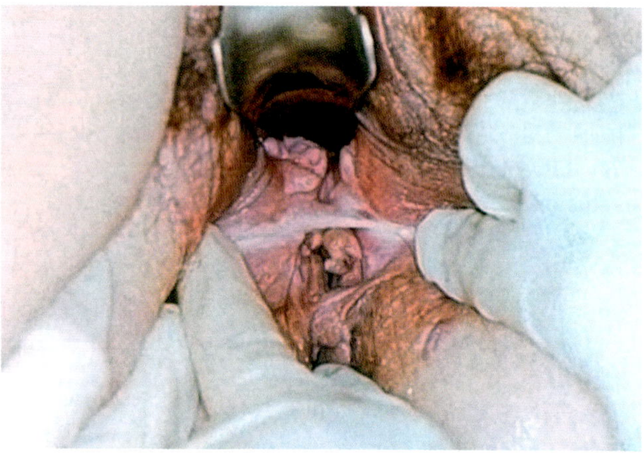

Fig. 29.2 Large rectovaginal fistula with complete perineal breakdown.

the surrounding sphincter mechanism may result in what has been termed a patulous anus (Fig. 29.2). The anus is anchored anteriorly by the perineal body and posteriorly by the anococcygeal ligament to the coccyx. The anal canal typifies the meeting of structures, with an endodermal and ectodermal derivation. The dentate line demarcates the boundary between the structures of the inferior hindgut and those of the proctodeum. The columns of Morgagni denote longitudinal folds of rectal mucosa that end as anal valves at the level of the dentate line. There are anal crypts present between the valves, most notably clustered in the posterior anus. Obstruction of these crypts can give rise to infection that may result in abscess or a fistula.

The AS apparatus involves the internal and external sphincters, as well as the conjoint longitudinal muscle that encircles the anus. These structures play a crucial role in fecal continence. The internal AS is a smooth muscle that is a dense continuation of the inner circular layer of the rectum and extends approximately 2.5 to 4 cm (Hauch et al., 2020). The internal AS arises at the junction of the anus and the rectum (anorectal ring) and ends approximately 1 to 1.5 cm distal to the dentate line. In contrast, the larger external AS is an elliptical band of skeletal muscle circumscribing the entire length of the anal canal. This structure makes up the majority of the perineal body from its anterior portion. Superiorly, the external AS continues as the puborectalis muscle. Many anatomists and surgeons believe it should be considered a component of the puborectalis muscle, even though the two muscles have separate embryologic derivations, and their muscle fibers do not intermingle (Fig. 29.3).

CLASSIFICATION AND PRESENTATION OF PERINEAL BREAKDOWN AND RECTOVAGINAL FISTULA

Obstetrical perineal tears are most commonly classified in the following fashion: first-degree is a laceration of the vaginal-epithelium or perineal skin only; second-degree is first-degree with involvement of the perineal muscles and fascia, but not the ASs; third-degree is disruption of the skin, mucous membrane, perineal body, and AS muscles; and fourth-degree is a third-degree tear with disruption of the anal mucosa. More recently, third-degree lacerations have been subdivided into three subcategories, with 3a lacerations involving less than 50% of the external AS, 3b involving more than 50% of external AS thickness, and 3c having both external and internal AS involvement (Practice Bulletin, 2016). Appropriate classification of lacerations is necessary, as incorrectly classified lacerations could result in inappropriate repair and suboptimal outcomes.

RVF is a congenital or acquired epithelialized tract between the rectum and the vagina. The communication may occur at any point along the vagina. Most fistulas actually arise in the anal canal distal to the pectinate line. RVFs are classified according to their location and size; careful attention to both features allows determination of the approach for surgical repair. In a low RVF, the rectal opening is located close to the dentate line, with the vaginal opening just inside the hymen. In a high RVF, the vaginal opening is near the cervix (or apex of the vagina in a posthysterectomy patient); the communication into the intestinal tract may be located in either the sigmoid colon or rectum. These fistulas usually require a laparotomy for repair. Such fistulas may not be readily apparent on physical examination or endoscopy and may require contrast studies for diagnosis. A mid-RVF is found somewhere between the hymen and the cervix. RVFs range in size from tiny (<1 mm in diameter) to large, where the rectovaginal defect encompasses the entire posterior vaginal wall. In using size as a criterion, fistulas less than 2.5 cm in diameter are considered small, and those greater than 2.5 cm are described as large. Simple RVFs consist of small, low fistulas secondary to infection or trauma. These fistulas generally have healthy, well-vascularized surrounding tissue that can be repaired with local techniques. RVFs are considered complex if they are large (>2.5 cm), high, or caused by inflammatory bowel disease (IBD). Recurrent fistulas are also considered complex because of their association with tissue scarring and decreased blood supply. Because healthy, well-vascularized tissue needs to be introduced after resection of diseased tissue, complex fistulas require more complicated surgical procedures for repair. A fistula-in-ano is an abnormal tract or cavity that is lined with granulation tissue and that connects a primary opening inside the anal canal to a secondary opening in the perianal skin or vulva; secondary tracts may be multiple

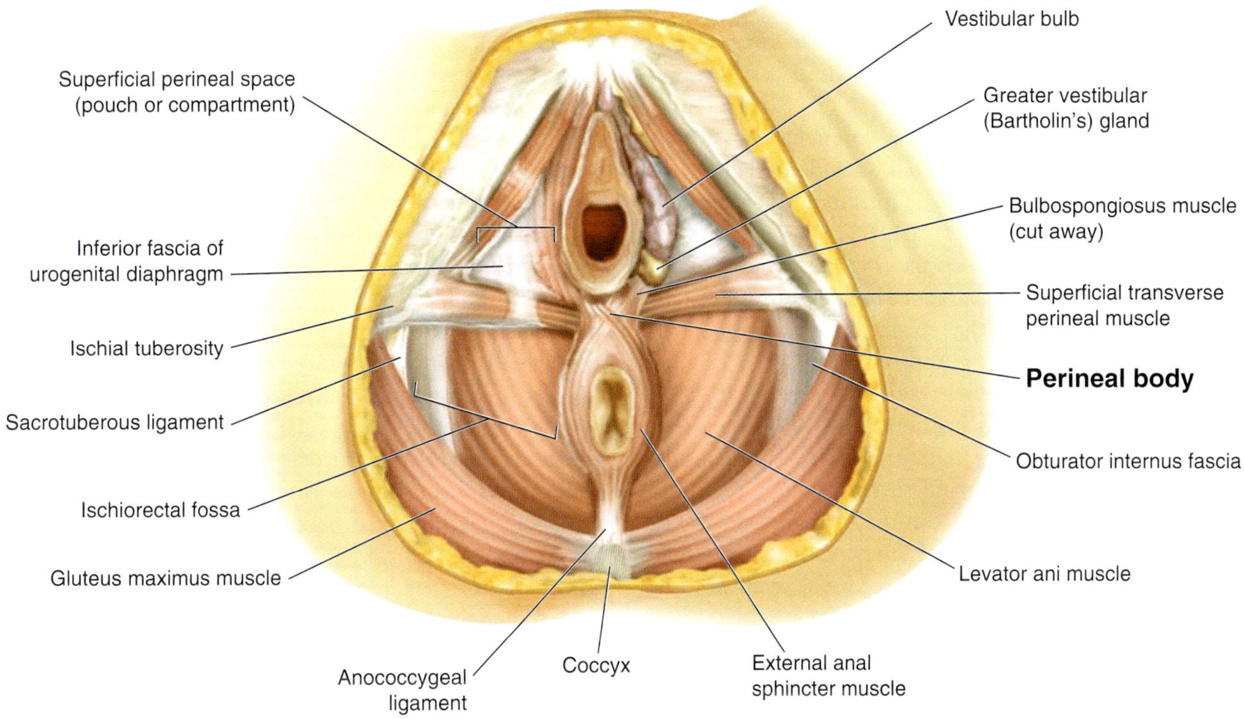

Fig. 29.3 The perineal body is the central point between the urogenital and anal triangles. It consists mainly of interlacing fibers from the bulbospongiosus muscle, the superficial transverse perineal muscle, and the external anal sphincter. There are also contributions from the longitudinal rectal muscle and the medial fibers of the puborectalis muscle.

and can extend from the same primary opening. Fistula-in-ano are only superficially discussed in this chapter; more detailed discussion of their diagnosis, evaluation, and treatment can be sought elsewhere.

Another method of classification is based on the underlying cause of the fistula, which will be a better predictor of the ultimate success of the repair, as it takes into consideration the integrity of the local tissue and the health of the patient. In 2017, a retrospective cohort study was conducted including 107 women who underwent surgical repair of RVF for various etiologies (cancer, IBD, infection, and other), and concluded that the rate of recurrence at 1 year was significantly different depending on surgical approach ($P < .001$), but not etiology ($P = .71$), and did not differ based on the surgical subspecialty performing the surgery (e.g., colorectal vs. female pelvic medicine and reconstructive surgery vs. combined/dual surgeon) (Byrnes et al., 2017).

A patient with a perineal breakdown may be asymptomatic or may present with an array of symptoms, including pain and dyspareunia, an enlarged introitus, and a variety of defecatory symptoms, including fecal incontinence if the sphincter mechanism is involved. A patient with an RVF is usually symptomatic. She most often complains of passage of flatus or stool through the vagina. Occasionally, the presenting complaint is a recurrent vaginal or bladder infection, which is the result of fecal soilage. A small fistula may be symptomatic only when gas or loose or liquid stool is passed. Determining the status of the AS mechanism is important when the patient's complaints are consistent with fecal seepage.

ETIOLOGIES OF RECTOVAGINAL FISTULA AND PERINEAL BREAKDOWN

Although the majority of cases of perineal breakdown are postobstetrical events, many different causes of RVFs have been identified (Box 29.1); the cause varies with the location of the fistula. Congenital RVFs are rare and are not discussed here.

Obstetric Injuries

Obstetric injuries are the most common cause of RVFs and perineal breakdown, causing up to 88% of fistulas in published series (Lowry et al., 1988). The incidence of perineal wound breakdown has been reported to be anywhere from 1% to nearly 25% of all lacerations (Gommesen et al., 2019; Jones et al., 2019). American College of Obstetricians and Gynecologists and World Health Organization guidelines recommend only one dose of antibiotics at the time of AS injury repair; however, a growing body of evidence (including a recent multicenter randomized controlled trial with 3400 women) suggests that a more liberal administration of antibiotic prophylaxis,

BOX 29.1 Causes of Rectovaginal Fistula

Congenital	Carcinoma
Obstetric	Radiation
Previous anorectal surgery	Lymphoproliferative malignancy
Inflammatory bowel disease	Endometriosis
Infection	

especially in obese women, after operative vaginal delivery may improve outcomes (Knight et al., 2019). A recent prospective cohort study with 24 months' follow-up of primiparous women after third- and fourth-degree laceration found that 9% and 24% of women suffered from fecal incontinence, respectively (Richter et al., 2015). Risk factors for development of an obstetric fistula (vesicovaginal or rectovaginal) include teenage status at delivery, primiparity, prolonged labor, home delivery, and short maternal height (Tebeu et al., 2012).

Historically, episiotomy was commonly performed during vaginal deliveries; however, this practice has decreased substantially with increasing evidence that episiotomies promote third- and fourth-degree perineal tears. Approximately 5% of vaginal deliveries or 20% of episiotomies result in a rectal tear or AS disruption. For women undergoing nonoperative vaginal deliveries, a policy of selective rather than routine episiotomy results in 30% fewer women experiencing severe (third- or fourth-degree) perineal tears or vaginal trauma (Jiang et al., 2017). Although the majority of perineal injuries are successfully repaired at the time of the delivery, dehiscence of an episiotomy repair can occur and is associated with infection, abscess, fistula, or sphincter disruption. Up to 1.5% of women who undergo an episioproctotomy develop an RVF. Such fistulas present either immediately postpartum from failed recognition of a fourth-degree injury or 7 to 10 days after an apparently normal repair. Midline episiotomy with resulting third-degree or fourth-degree laceration produces the greatest risk for development of an RVF. Mediolateral episiotomy, more common in British obstetric practice, causes fewer tears into the AS and rectum compared with midline incision. RVF after infection and dehiscence of an episiotomy most commonly occur low in the rectovaginal septum, but may extend much higher, especially in the case of a traumatic cloaca. Of paramount importance in these patients is an assessment of their degree of incontinence. Wise et al. (1991) noted that 27% of women with low RVFs had coexistent fecal incontinence, recommending a careful continence evaluation before embarking on a repair (see Chapter 27). A retrospective cohort spanning a 10-year period of women undergoing RVF repair compared the risk of failure of the repair in women with obstetric versus nonobstetric (IBD, iatrogenic, or traumatic) fistulas. The study concluded that women with nonobstetric fistula have a nearly four-fold increased risk of repair failure compared with obstetric fistula. This information is important in directing surgical outcome counseling and setting postoperative expectations (Karp et al., 2019).

Inflammatory Bowel Disease

IBD, specifically Crohn disease, is the second most common cause of RVFs and should be suspected in any instance when attempted repair has failed or in cases of spontaneous nonobstetric RVF. Because ulcerative colitis is not a transmural disease, it usually does not cause such problems. RVFs will occur in up to 10% of female patients with Crohn disease. These types of fistulas originate either from an inflamed anal gland (which is associated with a better prognosis) or from a rectal ulcer (which is associated with poorer prognosis). Low RVFs will usually follow a less aggressive disease course, especially in the absence of rectal inflammation. Symptoms tend to be worse in higher fistulas. Active small bowel Crohn disease and proctitis are usually associated with factors that result in a high risk of failure of fistula repair. Most commonly, RVFs from Crohn disease will occur in the mid portion of the rectovaginal septum; however, in patients with anorectal Crohn disease, a fistula can extend into the most distal aspect of the vagina or perineum. An anovaginal or RVF in Crohn disease is more likely to result in proctectomy or a dysfunctioning stoma than anal Crohn disease without a fistula.

Infection

The most common nonobstetric infectious cause of an RVF is formation of a cryptoglandular abscess in the anterior aspect of the anal canal. Extension of such an abscess into the vaginal wall can result in fistula formation. Other infectious processes that may fistulize into the vagina include lymphogranuloma venereum, tuberculosis, and formation of a Bartholin abscess. Acquired RVF may be an early manifestation of human immunodeficiency virus infection in women. Colovaginal fistula can result from diverticulitis, is usually located near the vaginal apex or cuff, and usually occurs in women who are postmenopausal and have previously undergone hysterectomy.

Prior Anorectal Surgery

RVF can occur after surgeries that involve the posterior vaginal wall or the anterior rectal wall. These include procedures such as vaginal hysterectomy, rectocele repair, hemorrhoidectomy, local excision of rectal tumors, and low anterior resection.

Cancer and Radiation Therapy

RVFs can result from invasive cervical or vaginal cancer or from anal or rectal cancer. They also develop in up to 6% of women after pelvic irradiation for endometrial, cervical, and vaginal cancer and are dependent on the radiation dosage. Fistulas that present early, during radiation therapy, are more likely to be caused by destruction of the carcinoma, whereas fistulas that occur later are caused by radiation injury to the tissue. Late fistulas are commonly associated with a rectal stricture. In a patient with a history of pelvic cancer, determining whether the RVF is caused by recurrent cancer is critical. This often requires examination with the patient under anesthesia, with tissue biopsies of the margins of the fistula. RVFs caused by radiation usually occur within 2 years of the completion of the radiation. They are usually located in the mid- or proximal vagina. Early warning signs of the development of a radiation-induced fistula include the passage of bright red blood per rectum, nonhealing rectal ulcerations, and anorectal pain.

DIAGNOSIS AND PREOPERATIVE EVALUATION

During the history-taking process, determining whether there is a previous history of anorectal surgery, complicated vaginal deliveries, radiation therapy, or IBD is important. Determining the patient's degree of continence is also important. The perineum and anus should be inspected and palpated (Fig. 29.4). A bidigital

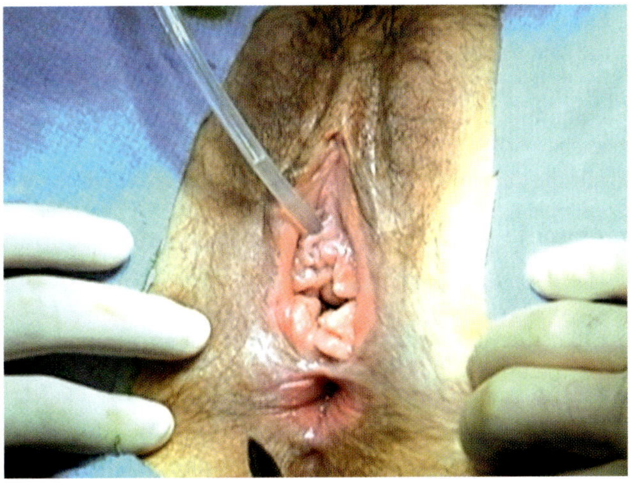

Fig. 29.4 Widened vaginal hiatus, patulous anal opening, and complete loss of perineal body with significant retraction of the ends of the anal sphincter.

examination is performed to palpate the thickness of the perineal body; the majority of RVFs will be appreciated during this maneuver. If a fistula is expected, and its location is not obvious with inspection and palpation, a careful vaginal speculum examination should be performed. A lacrimal duct probe is a useful adjunct to this examination. Rigid proctoscopy may give information regarding the compliance of the rectum and health of the surrounding tissue. If necessary, the vagina can be filled with water, and when the rectum is inflated via the proctoscope, the site of the fistula will show the escape of air bubbles. This "bubble test" can also be performed by inserting a lubricated red rubber catheter into the anus and introducing air into the rectum using an Asepto or similar syringe. Also, a vaginal tampon can be placed after instilling methylene blue in the rectum. The tampon is withdrawn and inspected for blue staining after 15 to 20 minutes. Another technique that can be helpful for low RVFs starts by mixing methylene blue into water-based lubricant. A rectal examination is then performed using this blue-colored lubricant. Palpating the anterior wall of the rectum and anus to "milk" the lubricant through any RVF present, while visualizing the posterior vaginal wall, will allow identification of even small distal RVFs. If the previously described maneuvers still do not demonstrate a fistula, the fistula may be located in the upper rectum, and contrast studies are needed to establish the diagnosis. Vaginography with a water-soluble contrast medium has a sensitivity of 79% to 100% (Bird et al., 1993; Giordano et al., 1996). A barium enema is not as sensitive in identifying the fistula but may provide general information as to the health of the colon. A computed tomography scan of the abdomen and pelvis, using gastrointestinal contrast, may be helpful, because it may show contrast in the vagina.

Magnetic resonance imaging (MRI) has been evaluated as a diagnostic tool for RVF. Dwarkasing et al. (2004), in a retrospective review, noted that MRI images correctly identified an RVF in 20 female patients with a known RVF. The MRI images also reclassified one patient as having a perianal fistula, a finding that was confirmed at the time of surgery. These authors concluded that MRI was superior to other radiologic tests in classifying RVF and identifying associated abscesses.

In most cases of perineal breakdown and/E or RVFs, especially postobstetric low fistulas, preoperative evaluation of the AS with transanal ultrasound should be considered. This allows clear visualization of the sphincter mechanism, which may be very useful in preoperative surgical planning. A prospective study published in 2017 evaluated the concordance between endoanal ultrasound detection of tract internal opening (IO), primary tract (PT), and AS defects and intraoperative findings (Emile et al., 2017). Overall accuracy of endoanal ultrasound was reported as 87%, 88.5%, and 89.5% in detection of IO, PT, and AS defects, respectively, and concordance between ultrasound and intraoperative findings was very good (Emile et al., 2017). An assessment of a patient's degree of fecal incontinence is critical, as one study noted that 48% of women with RVF have fecal incontinence (Tsang et al., 1998). Proctoscopy or even colonoscopy may also be necessary to evaluate for coexisting anorectal disease, particularly IBD.

SURGICAL TREATMENT OF RECTOVAGINAL FISTULA

Despite advances in medical therapy, surgery remains the mainstay of RVF treatment, and, like many surgical diseases, preoperative preparation and timing of repair are essential in planning an operation.

Preoperative bowel preparation should be done for all patients. This reduces the fecal and bacterial load, reducing the risk of postoperative infection and dehiscence of repair. Rectal irrigation as part of surgical prep can be performed in lieu of or in conjunction with a formal preoperative bowel preparation regimen. Perioperative antibiotics should be administered. Consideration should be given to the placement of intraoperative ureteral catheters when using a transabdominal approach to repair an RVF in a previously irradiated pelvis.

Several surgical techniques, alone or in combination, are used for the repair of RVFs. Approaches include transvaginal, transanal, perineal, and abdominal. Most postpartum RVFs are repaired transvaginally. The surgical procedure performed depends on the cause, location, and size of the fistula, as well as the condition of the involved tissues. RVFs after obstetric trauma may spontaneously heal; whereas those associated with Crohn disease, cancer, or radiation have little chance of healing without surgical intervention. The tissues involved in an RVF should be given adequate time to heal after the acute injury. This allows maximum resolution of inflammation, as well as a decrease in size of the fistula tract. Most authors recommend a waiting period of 8 to 12 weeks after the injury before attempting surgical repair, although immediate operative repair of a fourth-degree episiotomy dehiscence is recommended by some (Uygur et al., 2004). Fistulas associated with IBD are unlikely to heal if severe proctitis is present. Inflammation must be controlled by medical treatment, especially if the RVF is low because a reparative procedure is more likely to be successful if the proctitis has been controlled.

High Fistula Repair

Most surgeons use a transabdominal approach for the repair of a high rectovaginal or colovaginal fistula. The cause of high fistulas is usually inflammatory, including diverticulitis and Crohn disease. Radiation injury, traumatic injury, and carcinoma must also be considered. Bowel resection with primary reanastomosis, using nondiseased tissue, is the most successful approach. A prospective nonrandomized study found that 95% of women ($n = 40$) had resolution of high fistula after laparoscopic fistula excision, closure, and omental interposition (van der Hagen et al., 2011).

Midlevel Fistula Repair

A midlevel RVF caused by trauma can be repaired successfully transrectally or transvaginally once local tissue inflammation has resolved. For the patient with an intact perineum, an intact external AS, and a fistula in the lower third of the vagina, most gynecologists would perform a transvaginal fistula excision and layered closure, whereas most colorectal surgeons would perform an endorectal advancement flap repair (Champagne & McGee, 2010).

Most of these fistulas are secondary to obstetric trauma occurring in the mid to distal third of the vagina. The key to a successful repair is multilayered closure with a tension-free approximation of the edges of the defect. There should be excellent hemostasis, and perioperative antibiotics should be administered to decrease any potential for infection. The following are descriptions of both a vaginal repair and a rectal advancement flap for a primary, nonirradiated RVF with an intact perineum.

Transvaginal Repair of Rectovaginal Fistula (See Video 29.1)

1. The surgeon's nondominant index finger is placed in the rectum to aid in identification of the fistula and to assess the extent of scarification (Fig. 29.5A). A rectal finger will also facilitate dissection in the appropriate plane.
2. The initial incision depends on the anatomic location of the fistulous tract. A hemostatic solution of 0.5% lidocaine with 1:200,000 epinephrine may be injected submucosally. A midline incision in the posterior vagina can be used to the level of the fistulous tract, or an inverted-U perineal incision may also be beneficial in lower fistulas (Fig. 29.5B). This allows easy mobilization of the posterior vaginal wall from the anterior rectal wall, as well as a partial rebuilding of the perineal body if necessary. If the external AS is intact, there is no reason to disrupt it.
3. With traction on the vaginal wall, and with a finger in the rectum to provide support to the rectal wall, sharp dissection is used to mobilize the posterior vaginal wall from the anterior rectal wall (Fig. 29.5C).
4. After the vaginal walls are widely mobilized, the entire fistula tract can be excised (Fig. 29.5D). The rectal wall is cut back until fresh edges are encountered, as noted by fresh bleeding.
5. With the surgeon's index finger elevating the anterior rectal wall, an initial row of No. 3-0 or 4-0 delayed absorbable sutures is placed. These sutures are best placed extramucosally and should include a portion the muscularis and submucosa (Fig. 29.5E).
6. A second layer of inverted sutures is then placed; this inverts the first suture line into the rectum. Ideally, no sutures penetrate the rectal lumen (Fig. 29.5F).
7. If possible, a third layer of sutures is placed by plicating the fascia of the posterior vaginal wall over the rectal closure, and the vaginal epithelium is closed.

Transanal Endorectal Advancement Flap Procedure

1. The patient is placed in the prone position with the hips elevated (Fig. 29.6A).
2. The fistula is identified through the anus, and a small probe may be used to follow the tract into the vagina (Fig. 29.6B). A hemostatic solution of 0.5% lidocaine with 1:200,000 epinephrine may be injected submucosally. The rectal ostium is circumscribed by an incision placed 0.5 to 1 cm from the margins of the tract.
3. A broad-based flap of mucosa, submucosa, and circular muscle is developed and advanced distally. Before suturing the flap over the fistula site, the epithelium-lined tract is excised, and the muscular wall of the rectum is reapproximated with absorbable sutures (Fig. 29.6C).
4. The flap is then secured with interrupted absorbable sutures (Fig. 29.6D). The vaginal side is left open to provide drainage of the surgical site. Several authors report a high rate of success with this approach. Care must be taken to ensure that the rectal mucosa is not advanced too far, creating a mucosal ectropion and "wet anus."

Low Fistula Repair

Simple fistulotomy is the treatment of choice for low fistulas lying distal to the AS mechanism. Caution must be taken when considering a fistulotomy near the anterior AS mechanism, because even a normal sphincter mechanism is attenuated in this region.

For RVFs in the lower third of the vagina, especially those that have followed obstetric trauma and have resulted in a damaged perineal body and AS mechanism, some gynecologists favor conversion of the fistula to an episioproctotomy followed by layered closure. This is done with the patient in the supine position via a perineal approach, as described by Nichols (1993). Episioproctotomy permits excision of the entire fistulous tract followed by repair similar to that of a fresh fourth-degree perineal laceration. The technique requires transection and reunification of the external AS and the lower part of the internal sphincter. An overlapping or end-to-end external anal sphincteroplasty would be required to treat the anal incontinence. A risk of fistula recurrence, as well as anal incontinence, is present if the healing is imperfect.

For low fistulas above the external AS, as for lower midlevel fistulas, the approach favored by many colorectal surgeons is transanal repair using an endorectal advancement flap (Fig. 29.6A–D). Repair from the rectal side has the advantage of correction of the defect from the high-pressure side, perhaps resulting in less frequent failure of repair. The endorectal advancement flap also has the benefit of the interposition of healthy tissue, which is beneficial in the repair of both complex and recurrent fistulas. The benefit of a transvaginal or

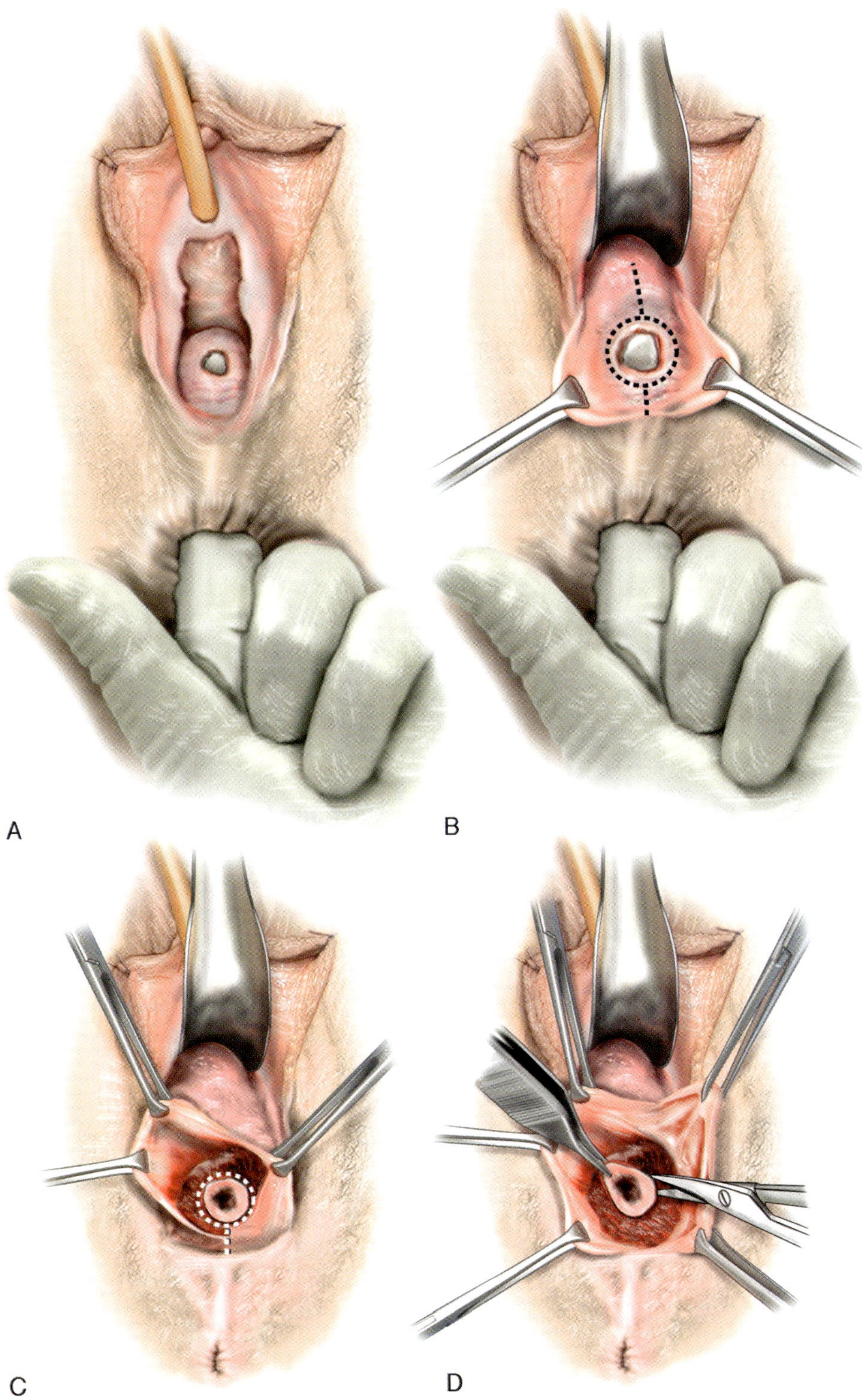

Fig. 29.5 Rectovaginal fistula repair in a patient with an intact perineum. **A**, A rectovaginal fistula present in the midportion of the posterior vaginal wall. **B**, The dashed line demonstrates the site of the posterior vaginal wall incision. **C**, The vaginal wall is mobilized off the anterior rectal wall. **D**, The fistulous tract is excised. The rectal wall is cut back until fresh edges are encountered. *Contined*

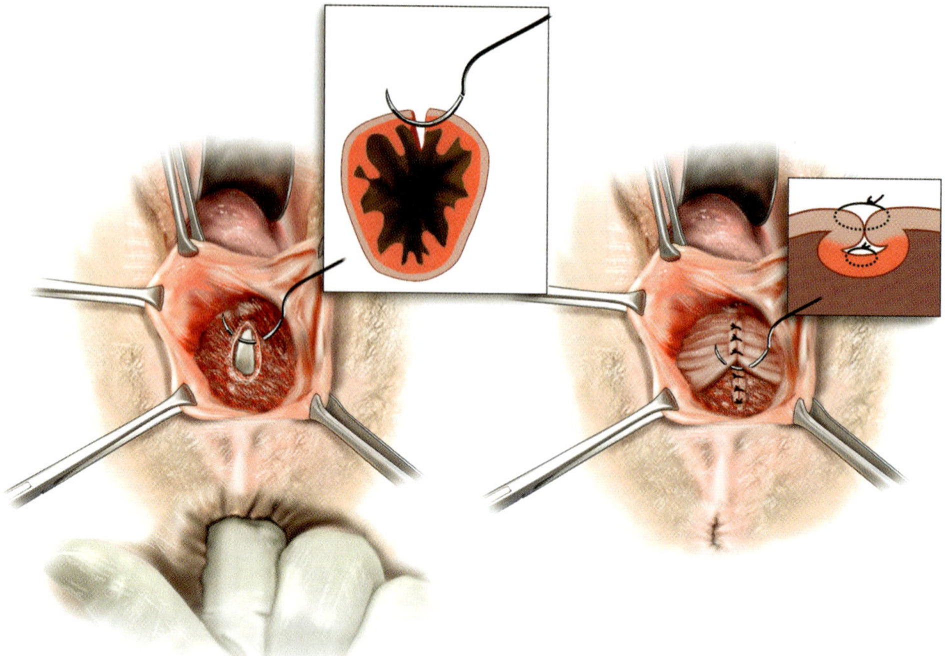

E F

Fig. 29.5, cont'd E, Extramucosal closure of the anterior rectal wall with interrupted, fine, delayed absorbable sutures. **F**, The second layer imbricates the muscular portion of the wall of the rectum over the initial layer. The repair is completed by plicating the rectovaginal fascia and closing the posterior vaginal wall.

transperineal approach, which would be performed by most gynecologists, is that the perineum can be more appropriately reconstructed.

Rectovaginal Fistula Secondary to Crohn Disease

At the present time, surgery is the only effective treatment for RVF secondary to Crohn disease. An extensive range of surgical options is available. A study comparing transrectal advancement flap techniques to transvaginal advancement flap techniques noted no significant differences in regard to outcomes (Ruffolo et al., 2009). Before this study, the rectal advancement flap route was generally considered to be the best treatment because repair was taken from a high-pressure side of a high–low pressure shunt, the primary source of the fistula was excised, and a layer of intact healthy tissue was interposed. The vaginal advancement flap technique instead consists of raising a vaginal flap, with the incision made in the posterior vaginal wall around the fistula opening. The vaginal and rectal orifices are identified and repaired with absorbable sutures. The vaginal advancement flap technique has been estimated to be less risky and easier to perform in the presence of anal rectal stenosis. In summary, there are no prospective randomized controlled trials for the surgical correction of Crohn disease–related RVF from which an evidence-based decision can be made. Until these data are available, the surgeon must use his or her clinical experience, personal knowledge, and assessment of the existing literature to formulate an optimal treatment plan for patients with RVF from Crohn disease. This topic is more extensively reviewed in an article by Hannaway and Hull (2008).

Rectovaginal Fistula Plug Repair

Biologic material placed through the RVF tract is one of the newer methods for repair and has been termed an anal fistula plug. The material used is a bioprosthetic made from porcine intestinal submucosa (Anal Fistula Plug, Cook Surgical Inc., Bloomington, IN). A tapered plug is placed through the rectovaginal tract. Excess plug length is excised at both the rectal and vaginal ends. The plug is then secured with an absorbable suture in a figure-eight fashion on the rectal side, and the vaginal side is left open for drainage. This way, the plug's bottom rests flatly against the anal opening. On the vaginal side, the surgeon should make sure it is not so tight at the exit site such that it prevents drainage. Postoperatively, patients are instructed to avoid strenuous activity or heavy lifting, as well as any sexual intercourse. Patients are given a 7-day course of oral antibiotics, as well as metronidazole cream to be placed at the external opening twice per day for 7 days. Experience with this technique in patients with RVF is limited. Smaller studies have noted that bioprosthetic plugs are more successful in the treatment of simple uncomplicated anorectal fistula (Ky et al., 2008). A study that used a Cook Surigis Anal Fistula Plug for complex anal fistulas noted only a 13.9% success rate (Safar et al., 2009). A systematic review of fistula plugs for fistula-in-ano from 2008 to 2015 reported success rates between 15.8% and 72.7%, with follow-up for between 2 and 19 months (Narang et al., 2016).

Complex or Recurrent Rectovaginal Fistulas

For complex or recurrent RVFs, more advanced procedures are considered. In certain situations, such as radiation-induced RVFs,

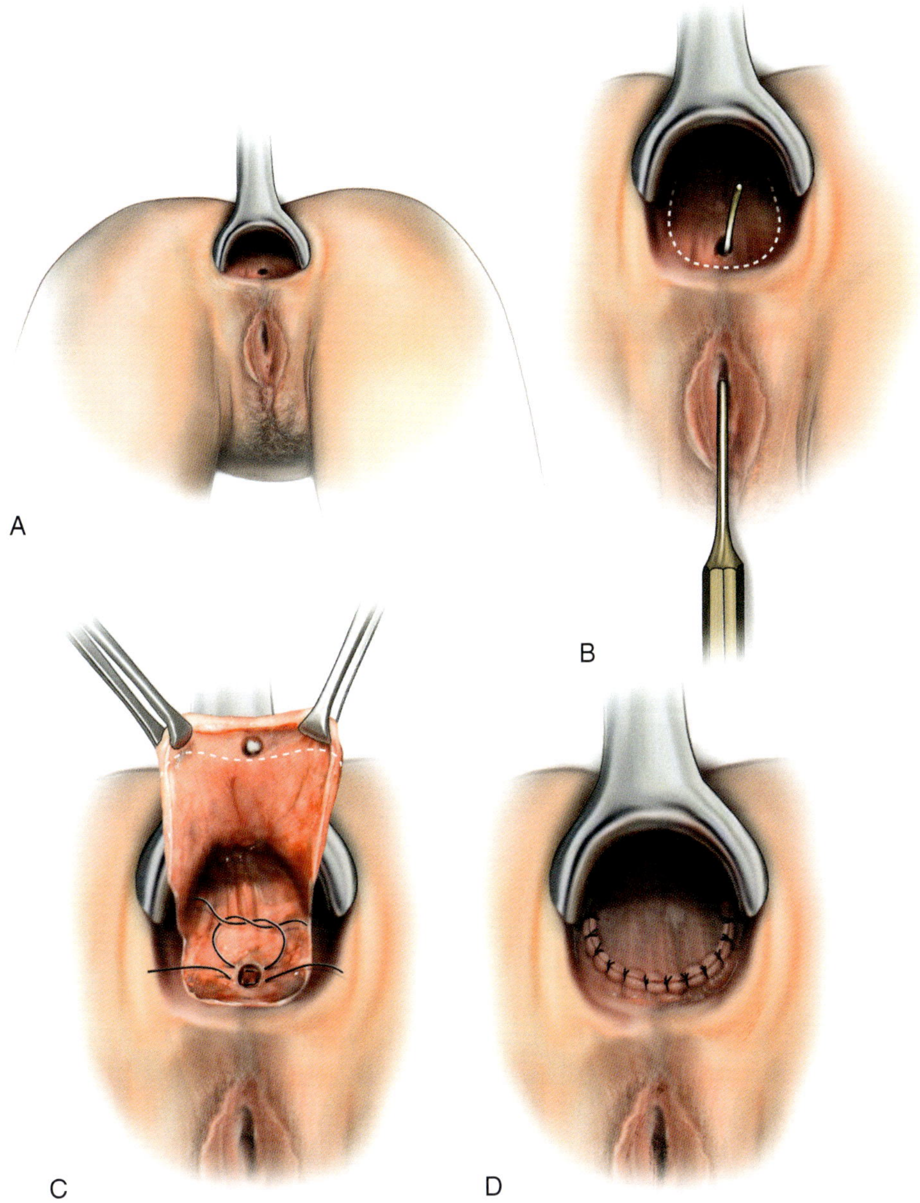

Fig. 29.6 Technique of endorectal advancement flap procedure. **A**, The patient is placed in the prone position with the hips elevated in preparation for a low or midlevel rectovaginal fistula repair. **B**, With the patient in the prone position, the anal speculum is placed posteriorly. The rectovaginal fistula is identified by placing a small probe from the anus into the vagina. The dotted line outlines the incision in the rectal mucosa used to develop the advancement flap. **C**, The epithelium-lined fistula tract is excised, and the muscular wall of the rectum is reapproximated with absorbable suture. The rectal advancement flap has been mobilized and is ready to be placed over the site of the fistula repair. **D**, The flap is secured with interrupted absorbable sutures.

healthy tissue must be brought into the rectovaginal space to allow appropriate healing and avoid any breakdown of the repair. Various materials have been interposed between the vaginal wall and rectal mucosa. These have included gracilis muscle, martius fat pad, and a variety of biologic materials (Fig. 29.7) (Video 29.2). Interposition of the gracilis muscles in the rectovaginal septum is usually performed in conjunction with a plastic surgeon, who will mobilize the distal insertion site of the muscle while preserving the neurovascular bundle that supplies the muscle and penetrates it more proximally. The plane between the rectum and vagina is developed, and both openings of the fistula are closed. The muscle is placed in the space between the rectum and vagina and then sutured into place to avoid dislodgment. The area is thoroughly drained, and, many times, a proximal stoma is used before this procedure. Martius graft has also been described as an interposition material for complicated urinary tract fistulas (Fig. 29.7). This involves mobilizing the bulbocavernous muscle and fat to be interposed in the rectovaginal space. Mobilization of a martius graft as an interposition material for urethrovaginal fistula is described in Chapter 38.

For complex fistulas that have failed multiple approaches, an abdominal approach with a full mucosectomy of the anal canal

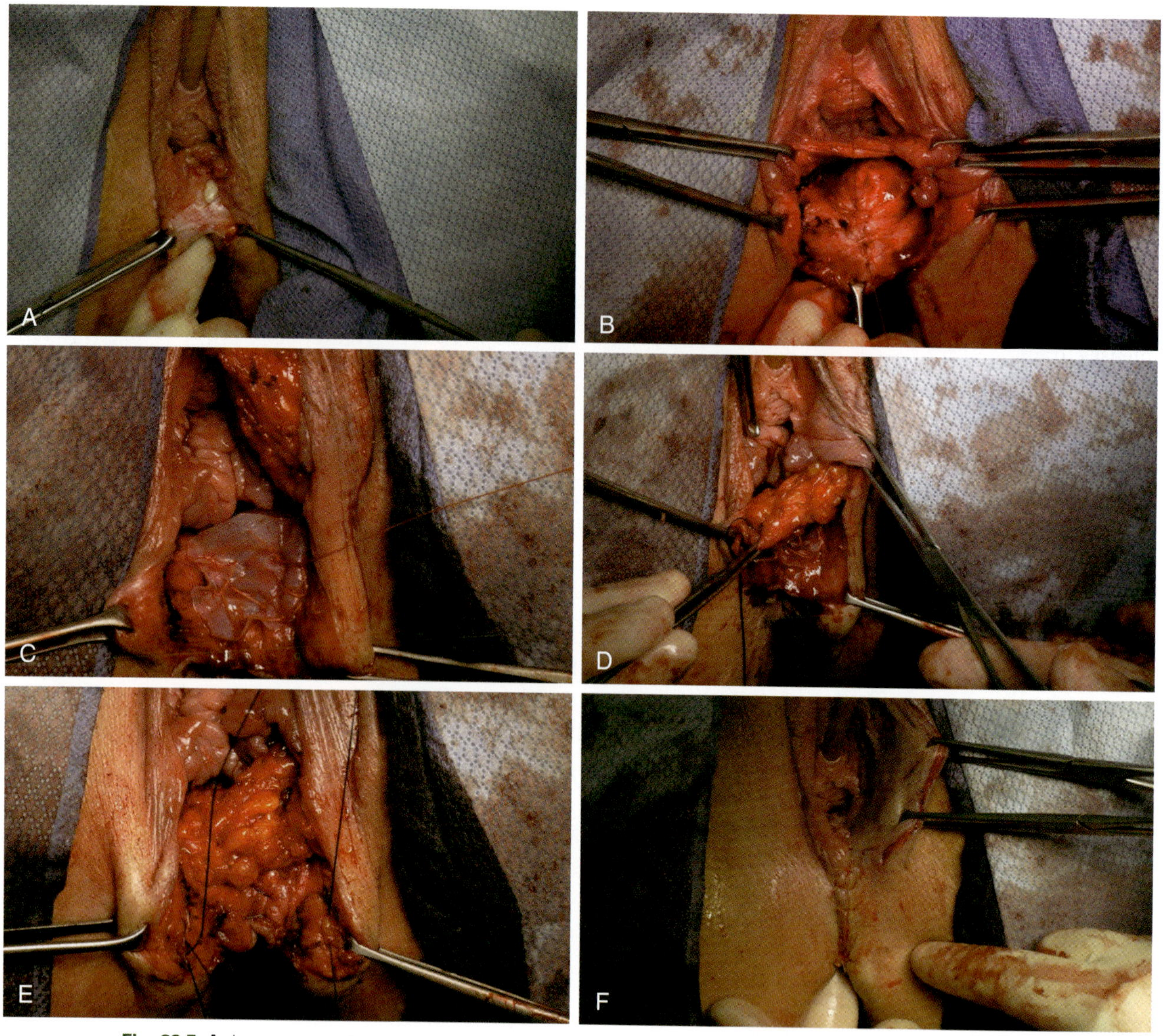

Fig. 29.7 **A**, Large, scarred, recurrent rectovaginal fistula; note that tissue appears devascularized, and that an obvious anal sphincter defect is present. **B**, Two-layered closure of the fistula, in a tension-free fashion, with a delayed absorbable suture has been performed. **C**, Interposition graft of matristem matrix or Acell has been placed over the layered fistula closure. **D**, Labial fat pad is mobilized and fixed to the posterior vaginal wall. **E**, External anal sphincter has been identified in preparation to performing an end-to-end sphinctero-plasty. **F**, Perineum has been reconstructed, and posterior vaginal wall and perineal skin have been closed.

and full rectal mobilization and formation of a coloanal anastomosis is done. This approach is always done using a covering stoma. Ileostomy is preferred over a colostomy to avoid compromising the reach of the rectum, which may occur with colostomy. Abdominal mobilization with a sleeve approach may be needed if there is insufficient bowel to reach the anus from the cut edge of the sleeve of rectal tissue. Abdominal mobilization of the rectum is usually carried out in the presacral plane. Occasionally, the splenic flexure must be mobilized, and/or the inferior mesenteric vessels divided, to allow for sufficient reach and to avoid tension. Great care must be taken, if either of these maneuvers is needed, to avoid injury to the marginal vessel that provides the blood supply to the distal cut bowel. Although this type of repair has typically been done as an open procedure, a laparoscopic or robotic approach in select women could be considered.

Fecal Diversion

Diversion of the fecal stream is sometimes required to allow adequate healing of the rectovaginal septum. Construction of a stoma is rarely necessary before attempt at primary repair. However, if perineal sepsis is severe, early diversion of the fecal stream may be necessary. Diversion of the fecal stream by construction of a proximal stoma should also be considered after a complex repair of RVF, such as a coloanal anastomosis, a Bricker onlay-type repair, or myofascial grafting. In addition, if previous attempts at repair of an RVF have failed, consideration should be given to construction of a stoma before an additional attempt at surgical reconstruction.

PERINEAL BREAKDOWN

Perineal tears most commonly occur at the time of delivery. Midline episiotomy is associated with an increased risk of extension of the laceration to the AS. To date, unfortunately, there is no consistent, mutually agreed-upon approach to reparative techniques for obstetric AS injury. Ultimately, more focused and intensive training of physicians and midwives in perineal anatomy and repair is imperative.

Breakdown of a perineal laceration may present weeks, months, or even years after delivery. Most cases of long-standing perineal laceration with disruption of the anterior AS complex lead to anal incontinence. The severity of symptoms varies with the degree of perineal laceration and sphincter loss. If the puborectalis portion of the levator muscle is well innervated and functional, it will provide some muscular contraction to permit control of feces. These patients often teach themselves a diet that will maintain their stools on the solid side.

The technique for appropriate episiotomy repair at the time of delivery should involve complete reconstruction of the perineal body with reapproximation of the external and internal ASs. Either an end-to-end or overlapping sphincteroplasty is appropriate. If the repair at the time of delivery breaks down, traditionally a second attempt should be deferred for a minimum of 8 weeks to provide sufficient time for resolution of the inflammatory response and return of adequate blood supply to the margins of the defect. Some surgeons have advocated an earlier repair so that the patient can avoid 2 months of uncomfortable symptoms (Uygur, 2004). If the entire perineal body is disrupted, including the internal and external ASs, and the posterior vaginal wall heals directly to the anterior rectal wall above the level of the hymenal ring, the patient is said to have a cloacal deformity (Fig. 29.8) (Video 29.3).

Several techniques have been described for reconstruction of a complete, chronic perineal laceration, including layered repair, the Warren's flap procedure, and the Noble–Mengert–Fish

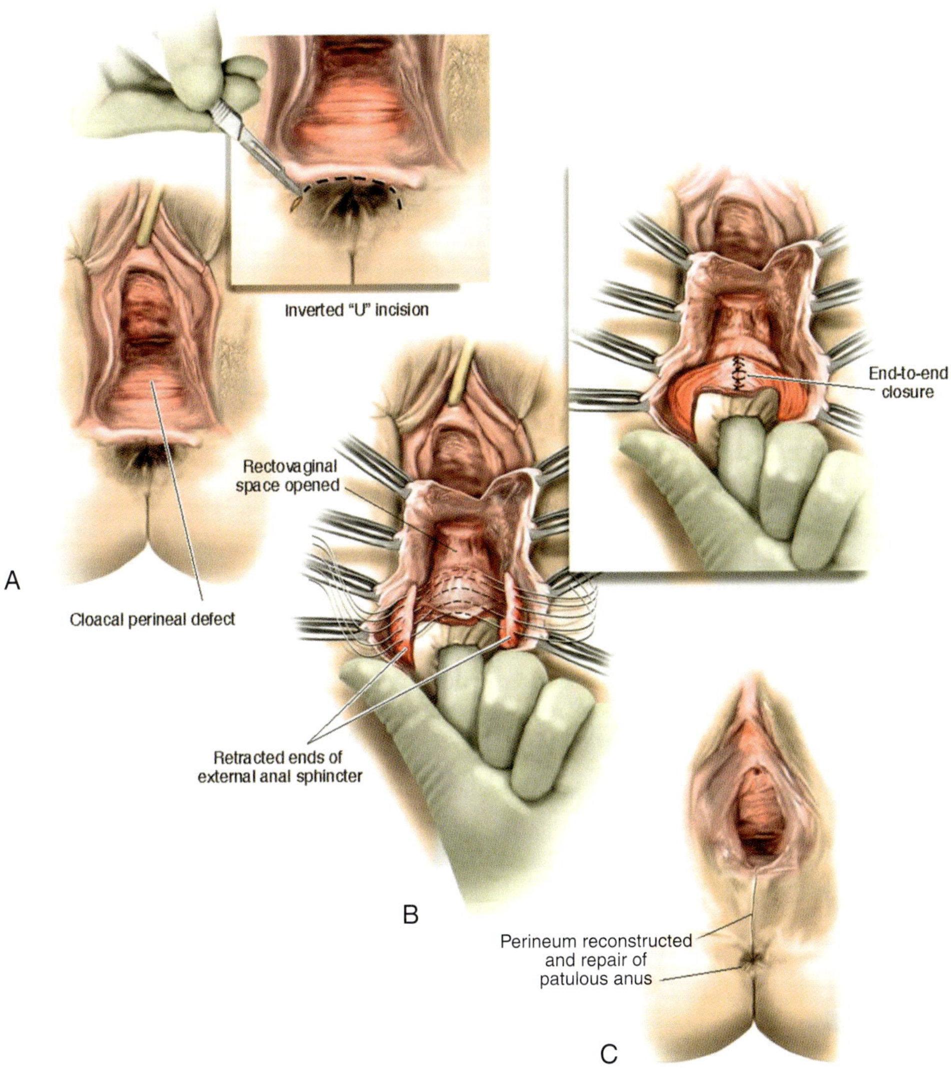

Fig. 29.8 Technique of repair of complete perineal breakdown. **A**, A cloacal defect is noted in which the posterior vaginal wall and the anterior wall of the rectum are fused. An inverted-U or transverse incision is made (*inset*). **B**, The rectovaginal space has been opened, and the posterior vaginal wall has been dissected away from the anterior wall of the rectum. The retracted ends of the external anal sphincter have been identified. Sutures incorporate small bites through the internal anal sphincter as they are passed to the opposite side. The completed end-to-end sphincteroplasty is shown (*inset*). **C**, The perineum has been completely reconstructed. The completed repair should show a perpendicular relationship between the posterior vaginal wall and the rebuilt perineum. Note that the anal opening becomes puckered and is no longer patulous.

operation. Most commonly, a layered repair is performed. The following is the technique for a layered closure of a complete perineal laceration that requires a sphincteroplasty:

1. A transverse or inverted-U perineal incision is made at the junction of the posterior vaginal wall and anal mucosa (Fig. 29.8A). The incision is extended far enough laterally to access the retracted external sphincter.
2. A midline incision is then made up along the posterior vaginal wall. Sharp dissection is used to completely mobilize the posterior vaginal wall from the anterior wall of the rectum. Any scar tissue is excised.
3. Any defect in the anal mucosa is closed with interrupted No. 3-0 delayed absorbable sutures.
4. The edges of viable external AS are at times identified with the help of a nerve stimulator and low-voltage cautery. The thickened, downward continuation of the circular, smooth muscle layer of the rectum, which is the internal AS, appears as a white, smooth layer of tissue between the anorectal mucosa and the external AS (Fig. 29.8B).
5. The external AS is brought together in an end-to-end fashion with interrupted No. 0 or 2-0 delayed absorbable sutures. We prefer to incorporate small bites of the internal AS in these sutures to reapproximate the internal AS well (Fig. 29.8B). Reapproximating this layer over a length of 3 to 5 cm is important, because the internal sphincter is responsible for most of the resting pressure, in what is normally a 4-cm high-pressure zone in the anal canal. Also, reapproximating the external sphincter in this fashion will close off dead space and decrease any tension on the mucosal layer if the repair involves closure of the anal mucosa. If the defect is small, or the external AS is easily mobilized, an overlapping sphincteroplasty can be considered as well.
6. Once the sphincter is reapproximated, the remainder of the perineal reconstruction should involve further support and elevation of the perineal body by bringing together the disrupted ends of the superficial transverse perineal muscles and bulbocavernous muscles. At times, because of a widened genital hiatus, a distal levatorplasty can be considered by bringing the puborectalis muscles closer together. One must remember that the arms of the puborectalis muscle do not normally come in contact with each other between the rectum and the vagina, so overzealous plication must be avoided, because it can create posterior tissue banding that will lead to dyspareunia. At completion of the repair, the posterior vaginal wall should be perpendicular to the perineal body (Fig. 29.8C).

CONCLUSION

RVF can be congenital or the result of trauma, IBD, carcinoma, radiation, or infection. Most RVFs seen by gynecologists follow traumatic obstetric delivery. The cause, location, and size of the fistula, as well as the competence of the AS mechanism, must be determined before repair. Repair of fistulas resulting from obstetric trauma has a high rate of success, but repair of those arising from other causes is more difficult and frequently requires consultation with a colorectal surgeon. Several different approaches to surgical repair have been described; the best approach is determined by the location, size, and cause of the fistula.

BIBLIOGRAPHY

Allen-Mersh TC, Wilson EJ, Hope-Stone HF. The management of late radiation-induced rectal injury after treatment of carcinoma of the uterus. *Surg Gynecol Obstet.* 1987;164:521.

American College of Obstetricians and Gynecologists' Committee on Practice Bulletins—Obstetrics. Practice Bulletin No. 165: Prevention and Management of Obstetric Lacerations at Vaginal Delivery. *Obstet Gynecol.* 2016;128:e1.

Bird D, Taylor D, Lee P. Vaginography—the investigation of choice for vaginal fistulae. *Aust N Z J Surg.* 1993;63:894.

Borgstein ES, Broadhead RL. Acquired rectovaginal fistula. *Arch Dis Child.* 1994;71:165.

Bricker EM, Kraybill WG, Lopez MJ. Functional results after postirradiation rectal reconstruction. *World J Surg.* 1986;10:249.

Byrnes JN, Schmitt JJ, Faustich BM, et al. Outcomes of rectovaginal fistula repair. *Female Pelvic Med Reconstr Surg.* 2017;23:124.

Champagne BJ, McGee MF. Rectovaginal fistula. *Surg Clin North Am.* 2010;90:69.

Chew SS, Rieger NA. Transperineal repair of obstetric-related anovaginal fistula. *Aust N Z J Obstet Gynaecol.* 2004;44:68.

Coats PM, Chan KK, Wilkins M, et al. A comparison between midline and mediolateral episiotomies. *Br J Obstet Gynaecol.* 1980;87:408.

Delancey JO. Structural atatomy of the posterior pelvic compartment as it relates to rectocele. *Am J Obstet Gynecol.* 1999;180:815.

Dwarkasing S, Hussain SH, Hop WC, et al. Anovaginal fistulas: evaluation with endoanal MR imaging. *Radiology.* 2004;231:123.

Emile SH, Magdy A, Youssef M, et al. Utility of endoanal ultrasonography in assessment of primary and recurrent anal fistulas and for detection of associated anal sphincter defects. *J Gastrointest Surg.* 2017;21:1879.

Farrell SA, Dempsey T, Geldenhuys L. Histologic examination of "fascia" used in colporraphy. *Obstet Gynecol.* 2001;98:794.

Froines EJ, Palmer DL. Surgical therapy for rectovaginal fistulas in ulcerative colitis. *Dis Colon Rectum.* 1991;34:925.

Fry RD, Kodner IJ. Rectovaginal fistula. *Surg Annu.* 1995;27:113.

Giordano P, Drew PJ, Taylor D, et al. Vaginography—investigation of choice for clinically suspected fistulas. *Dis Colon Rectum.* 1996;39:568.

Goligher JC. Rectovaginal fistula. In: Goligher JC, ed. *Surgery of the Anus, Rectum and Colon.* 4th ed. London: Spottiswoode Ballantyne; 1980.

Gommesen D, Nohr EA, Drue HC, et al. Obstetric perineal tears: risk factors, wound infection and dehiscence: a prospective cohort study. *Arch Gynecol Obstet.* 2019;300:67.

Greenberg JA, Lieberman E, Cohen AP, Ecker JL. Randomized comparison of chronic versus fast-absorbing polyglactin 910 for postpartum perineal repair. *Obstet Gynecol.* 2004;103:1308.

Hannaway CD, Hull TL. Current considerations in the management of rectovaginal fistula from Crohn's disease. *Colorectal Dis.* 2008;10:747.

Hauch A, Ramamoorthy S, Zelhart M, Dobke M. Refining approaches to surgical repair of rectovaginal fistulas. *Ann Plast Surg.* 2020;84:S250.

Homsi R, Daikoku NH, Littlejohn J, et al. Episiotomy: risks of dehiscence and rectovaginal fistula. *Obstet Gynecol Surv.* 1994;49:803.

Howard D, DeLancey JO, Burney RE. Fistula-in-ano after episiotomy. *Obstet Gynecol.* 1999;93:800.

Jiang H, Qian X, Carroli G, Garner P. Selective versus routine use of episiotomy for vaginal birth. *Cochrane Database Syst Rev.* 2017;2:CD000081.

Jones K, Webb S, Manresa M, et al. The incidence of wound infection and dehiscence following childbirth-related perineal trauma: a systematic review of the evidence. *Eur J Obstet Gynecol Reprod Biol.* 2019;240:1.

Karp NE, Kobernik EK, Berger MB, et al. Do the surgical outcomes of rectovaginal fistula repairs differ for obstetric and nonobstetric fistulas? A Retrospective Cohort Study. *Female Pelvic Med Reconstr Surg.* 2019;25:36.

Kimose H, Fischer L, Spjeldnaes N, et al. Late radiation injury of the colon and rectum: surgical management and outcome. *Dis Colon Rectum.* 1989;32:684.

Knight M, Chiocchia V, Partlett C, et al. Prophylactic antibiotics in the prevention of infection after operative vaginal delivery (ANODE): A multicentre randomised controlled trial. *Lancet.* 2019;393:2395.

Kodner IJ, Mazor A, Shemesh EI, et al. Endorectal advancement flap repair of rectal, vaginal, and other complicated anorectal fistulas. *Surgery.* 1993;114:682.

Kozok LJ. Surgical and non-surgical procedures associated with hospital delivery in the United States: 1980–1987. *Birth.* 1989;16:209.

Ky AJ, Sylla P, Steinhagen R, et al. Collagen fistula plug for the treatment of anal fistulas. *Dis Colon Rectum.* 2008;51:838.

Legino LJ, Woods MP, Rayburn WF, et al. Third- and fourth-degree perineal tears. 50 years' experience at a university hospital. *J Reprod Med.* 1988;29:423.

Lowry AC, Thorsen AG, Rothenberger DA. Repair of simple rectovaginal fistulas: influence of previous repairs. *Dis Colon Rectum.* 1988;31:676.

Narang SK, Jones C, Alam NN, et al. Delayed absorbable synthetic plug (GORE® BIO-A®) for the treatment of fistula-in-ano: a systematic review. *Color Dis.* 2016;18:37.

Nichols DH. Repair of rectal fistula and of old complete perineal laceration. In: Nichols DH, ed. *Gynecologic and Obstetric Surgery.* St. Louis: Mosby; 1993.

Nowacki MP. Ten years of experience with Park's coloanal sleeve anastomosis for the treatment of post-irradiation rectovaginal fistula. *Eur J Surg Oncol.* 1991;17:563.

Parker SL, Thorsen A. Fecal incontinence. *Surg Clin North Am.* 2002;82:1273.

Radcliffe AG, Ritchie JK, Hawley PR, et al. Anovaginal and rectovaginal fistulas in Crohn's disease. *Dis Colon Rectum.* 1988;31:94.

Rahman MS, Al-Sulerman SA, El-Yahia AR, Rahman J. Surgical treatment of rectovaginal fistula of obstetric origin: a review of 15 years' experience in a teaching hospital. *J Obstet Gynaecol.* 2003;6:607.

Richter HE, Nager CW, Burgio KL, et al. Incidence and predictors of anal incontinence after obstetric anal sphincter injury in primiparous women. *Female Pelvic Med Reconstr Surg.* 2015;21:182.

Ruffolo C, Penninckx F, Van Assche G, et al. Outcome of surgery for rectovaginal fistula due to Crohn's Disease. *Br J Surg.* 2009;96:1190.

Saclarides TJ. Rectovaginal fistula. *Surg Clin North Am.* 2002;82:1261.

Safar B, Jobanputra S, Sands D, et al. Anal fistula plug: initial experience and outcomes. *Dis Colon Rectum.* 2009;52:248.

Scott NA, Nair A, Hughes LF. Anovaginal and rectovaginal fistula in patients with Crohn's disease. *Br J Surg.* 1992;79:1379.

Snyder RR, Hammond TL, Hankins GD. Human papilloma virus associated with poor healing of episiotomy repairs. *Obstet Gynecol.* 1990;76:664.

Sultan AH, Thakar R. Lower genital tract and anal sphincter trauma. *Clin Obstet Gynecol.* 2002;16:99.

Tebeu PM, Fomulu JN, Khaddaj S, et al. Risk factors for obstetric fistula: a clinical review. *Int Urogynecol J.* 2012;23:387.

Thacker SB, Banta HD. Benefits and risks of episiotomy: an interpretive review of the English language literature, 1860–1980. *Obstet Gynecol Surv.* 1983;38:322.

Tsang CB, Mudoff RD, Wong RD, et al. Anal sphincter integrity and function influences outcome in rectovaginal fistula repair. *Dis Colon Rectum.* 1998;41:1141.

Uygur D, Yesildaglar N, Kis S, Sipahi T. Early repair of episiotomy dehiscence. *Aust N Z J Obstet Gynaecol.* 2004;44:244.

Van Der Hagen SJ, Soeters PB, Baeten CG, Van Gemert WG. Laparoscopic fistula excision and omentoplasty for high rectovaginal fistulas: a prospective study of 40 patients. *Int J Colorectal Dis.* 2011;26:1463.

Veronikis DK, Nichols DH, Spino C. The Noble-Mengert-Fish operation-revisited: a composite approach for persistent rectovaginal fistulas and complex perineal defects. *Am J Obstet Gynecol.* 1998;179:1411. Erratum *Am J Obstet Gynecol* 1999;180:257.

Wise WE, Aguilar PS, Padmanabtan A, et al. Surgical treatment of low rectovaginal fistulas. *Dis Colon Rectum.* 1991;34:271.

Yee LF, Birnbaum EH, Read TE, et al. Use of endoanal ultrasound in patients with rectovaginal fistulas. *Dis Colon Rectum.* 1999;42:1057.

30

Full-Thickness Rectal Prolapse

Ian M. Paquette and Liliana Bordeianou

CHAPTER OUTLINE

INTRODUCTION

Full-thickness rectal prolapse is a benign but debilitating condition involving full-thickness descent of the rectum through the anal canal (Fig. 30.1). It is important to distinguish full-thickness rectal prolapse from simple prolapse of the rectal mucosa on physical examination (Fig. 30.2). This chapter will focus on full-thickness rectal prolapse. The true cause of rectal prolapse is unknown, despite its long and extensive presence in medical history and literature. Numerous operations have been described in the literature since 1889, when Mikulicz described his series of six patients undergoing perineal excision for prolapse, and great variation in surgical management and approach still exists. In this chapter, we discuss the etiology, epidemiology, clinical features, evaluation, common surgical techniques, results, and our experience regarding rectal prolapse. This is an update from a previous chapter by Ashburn and Hull (2015), incorporating the latest clinical evidence and decision-making.

ETIOLOGY

A renowned English colorectal surgeon, Hugh Lockhart-Mummery of St. Marks' Hospital in London, wrote in 1972: "It is interesting to note that we still know so little about the cause of such a common condition." The most current and accepted theory was proposed by Broden and Snellman (1968) after they demonstrated with cinedefecography that full-thickness prolapse starts as an internal intussusception of the rectum with a lead point proximal to the anal verge. Years later, radiopaque markers were applied to the rectal mucosa in studies to demonstrate this phenomenon in real time and support the current theory that rectal prolapse is attributed to internal intussusception of the rectal wall.

There are many common anatomic features that may relate to rectal prolapse: a deep peritoneal cul-de-sac or pouch of Douglas, enterocele, loss of posterior rectal fixation, a patulous anal sphincter, diastasis of the levator ani, redundant rectum and sigmoid colon, and loss of the rectum's horizontal position may all contribute to the pathology. It is unclear whether these findings are a cause of the rectal prolapse, or if they are merely associated abnormalities. The goals of any operation to repair rectal prolapse should be to correct the prolapse of tissue, avoid worsening any concurrent issues such as incontinence or constipation, and avoid causing new problems, particularly new-onset constipation.

EPIDEMIOLOGY

Rectal prolapse is a relatively uncommon phenomenon, occurring in an estimated 0.5% of the population; however, the true incidence and prevalence are unknown, primarily because of underreporting, especially in the elderly population. The peak incidence is in the seventh decade of life, and it occurs more commonly in women, who are six times more likely to suffer from prolapse than are men (Kairaluoma & Kellokumpu, 2005). Although rectal prolapse is often associated with multiparity, nearly one-third of women with rectal prolapse are nulliparous. Male patients, although they represent a very small portion of this population, generally develop prolapse at a younger age than female patients (<40 years). There is also an association between younger presentation and psychiatric conditions requiring multiple medications, such as autism and developmental delay.

CLINICAL FEATURES

Patients with rectal prolapse generally present with fecal soilage, prolapse of tissue through the anal sphincter complex, mucoid discharge, and bleeding. Although the precise pathophysiology is unclear, Tjandra et al. (1993) found that 18% of patients with prolapse reported straining, and 42% had constipation as the most common associated symptom.

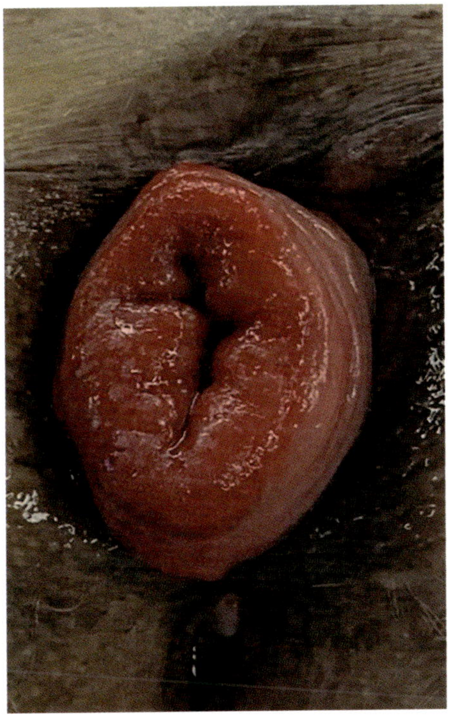

Fig. 30.1 Full-thickness rectal prolapse showing concentric folds of rectal mucosa indicating full–thickness protrusion of the rectum.

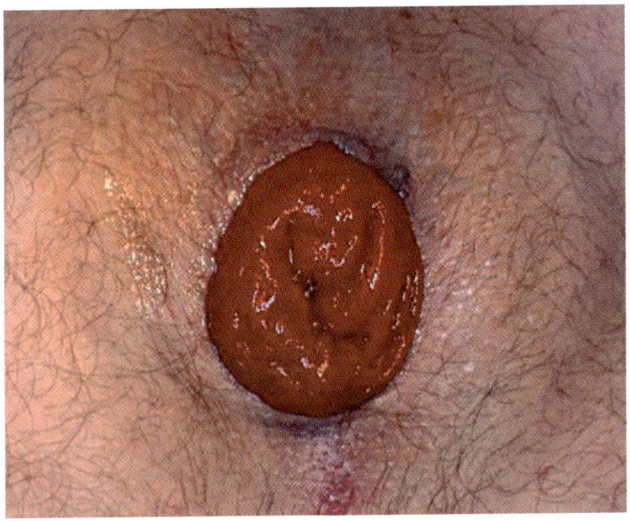

Fig. 30.2 Partial-thickness mucosal-only prolapse showing short segment protrusions and radial folding of the mucosa.

A complete assessment of female patients with rectal prolapse should include evaluation for constipation, urinary and fecal incontinence, and other pelvic floor disorders such as uterine prolapse, rectocele, cystocele, or enterocele. Staged or combined surgical correction of pelvic floor disorders, should they exist concurrently, is imperative for resolution of symptoms.

EVALUATION

Patients are often quite anxious when they present for evaluation for rectal prolapse. After a complete history of the type and duration of symptoms, a simple examination in the office is often sufficient. Symptoms related to fecal and urinary incontinence and constipation should be especially emphasized.

Physical examination entails visual inspection of the perineum, which often reveals a patulous anus. Additionally, mucous soiling of the perineum is often present because of the chronic external prolapse of the rectum. The examiner should be sure to rule out the presence of any palpable masses, and proctoscopy should be done to rule out a malignancy as a potential lead point. If the patient is overdue for a screening colonoscopy, or if symptoms suspicious for cancer are present, they should be referred for colonoscopy before surgical correction of the prolapse. Occasionally, rectal prolapse is not externally visible on initial examination. Examination of the patient in a squatting position or with Valsalva maneuver on a commode may be needed to reproduce the prolapse, but this is a necessary maneuver to distinguish between full-thickness and mucosal prolapse. During inspection, it is important to differentiate full-thickness rectal prolapse (concentric folds) from prolapsing internal hemorrhoids (radial invaginations) (see Figs. 30.1 and 30.2). Associated vaginal prolapse such as rectocele (posterior vaginal prolapse), cystocele (anterior vaginal prolapse), or enterocele (prolapse of small intestine, usually at the vaginal apex or posterior vagina) should be identified, if present.

When outlet obstruction or pelvic support disorders are suspected, defecography should be performed. (See Video 13.1 for a detailed description and demonstration of defecography.) This may provide important information like the presence of additional pathology, such as enterocele, rectocele, sigmoidocele, or concomitant vaginal vault prolapse. Additionally, looking at the anorectal angle at rest and straining can be used to assess for appropriate relaxation of the puborectalis muscle and whether or not conditions such as anismus need to be addressed before surgery. Although additional tests such as anal physiology testing can be done, they are typically not necessary in the work-up of an isolated rectal prolapse.

NONSURGICAL OPTIONS FOR PROLAPSE

No studies exist that compare operative repair with nonoperative therapy for rectal prolapse, nor are there definitive nonoperative alternatives to correct this condition. Aggressive treatment of constipation, if present, with medications may lessen symptoms. Applying table sugar to the prolapsed segment draws edema out of the segment and may facilitate reduction of the prolapse. Placing the patient in Trendelenburg position and administering intravenous benzodiazepines may ease reduction as well. However, none of these nonsurgical options will definitively repair prolapse, and surgery continues to be the preferred treatment.

COMMON SURGICAL REPAIRS FOR PROLAPSE

There are more than 300 procedures described to treat rectal prolapse, and new techniques are continually introduced in the literature. Despite this, there is no single operation that is preferred over the rest, and choosing the most appropriate procedure depends on individual patient factors. These factors include medical comorbid conditions, risk of recurrence, bowel function (fecal incontinence and constipation), degree of prolapse, and presence of associated pelvic disorders. Regardless of approach, the goals of any prolapse surgery are to treat the prolapse and to address associated constipation or incontinence.

Procedures for rectal prolapse can be classified into two main categories: perineal and transabdominal repairs. Perineal repairs are less invasive, cause less perioperative pain and morbidity, and are associated with reduced lengths of stay. They are often favored for frail, elderly patients, but at some institutions perineal repairs are recommended in healthy patients, too. The perineal approach includes a risk of infection and complications related to the suture line or wound. In addition, the perineal approach is known for recurrence rates that are four times higher than those of transabdominal operations; thus, the abdominal approach is often favored for medically-fit patients who can tolerate this operation.

A transabdominal repair requires general anesthesia and may have more devastating complications, such as anastomotic leak, abdominal sepsis, stricture, and adhesions. The introduction of minimally invasive approaches since the 1990s has added a new dimension to transabdominal prolapse surgery and has been shown to reduce postoperative convalescence, making this approach more appealing. Historical data have suggested a higher incidence of complications following an abdominal approach, and higher recurrence with a perineal approach. Senapati et al. (2013) randomized 293 patients with rectal prolapse to abdominal versus perineal surgery. Recurrence occurred in 20% of perineal procedures and 26% of abdominal procedures (P = .80). However, the recurrence from abdominal procedures in this study was much higher than that typically reported in the literature. In another small study, Emile et al. (2017) randomized 50 patients to ventral mesh rectopexy versus Delorme procedure. Clinical recurrence occurred in 8% of abdominal procedures versus 16% of perineal procedures (P = .66).

Perineal Repairs

Mucosal Sleeve Resection (Delorme Procedure). The choice between a mucosal sleeve resection such as Delorme or a full-thickness procedure such as an Altemeier is at the discretion of the surgeon, as most will choose the method they are most comfortable with. After positioning the patient, the perineum and vagina are prepared with an aseptic solution. The operation commences by injecting 1:100,000 epinephrine solution circumferentially into the submucosal plane just proximal to the dentate line. This allows delineation of the dissecting plane and diminishes blood loss. Using electrocoagulation, the dissection begins in circumferential manner 1 to 1.5 cm above the dentate line (Fig. 30.3), creating a plane between the submucosa and the internal anal sphincter. Once this plane is started, the free edge of the mucosa and submucosa is tagged with sutures for ease of handling and in creating traction for easier dissection. Continuing in a circumferential direction and using liberal amounts of injectable saline in the plane between the submucosa and the

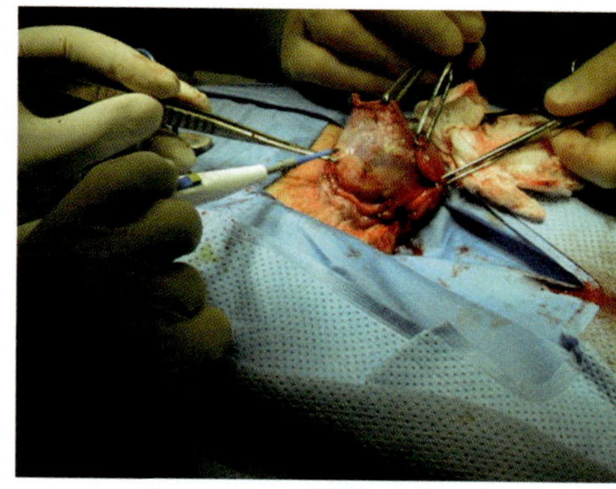

Fig. 30.3 Incision for a Delorme procedure 1 to 1.5 cm above the dentate line. The incision goes through the mucosa and submucosa initially, stripping this tube from the underlying internal anal sphincter and, more proximally, from the rectal muscular cuff.

muscular cuff, scissors are used to divide the attachments and to deliver the submucosa and mucosal cuff out of the rectum and anus (Fig. 30.4). Penetrating blood vessels encountered during the dissection can be treated with electrocoagulation. It is important to maintain strict hemostasis during the dissection to avoid hematomas after the procedure. The dissection continues until the rectal mucosa cannot be pulled down any farther; usually, 10 to 15 cm can be mobilized. During this phase of the operation, we use copious amounts of antibiotic solution such as tetracycline to irrigate the surgical field. After the dissection is completed, the rectal muscle is plicated with suture such as No. 2-0 Polyglactin 910 suture on a UR-6 needle (Vicryl; Ethicon, Inc., Somerville, NJ). A total of eight sutures are spaced circumferentially for this plication. The dissected mucosa is excised, and the proximal line of resection is approximated to the distal incision line. Interrupted sutures of No. 2-0 Vicryl on a UR-6 needle work well for this circumferential suture line (Fig. 30.5).

The reported rate of prolapse recurrence after the Delorme procedure varies from 10% to 15% in different series. The procedure is well tolerated in high-risk patients but still carries a risk for complications of bleeding, urinary retention, and fecal impaction in up to 12% of patients. In general, constipation and fecal incontinence tend to improve after surgery, the latter perhaps owing to the rectal muscular wall plication that creates

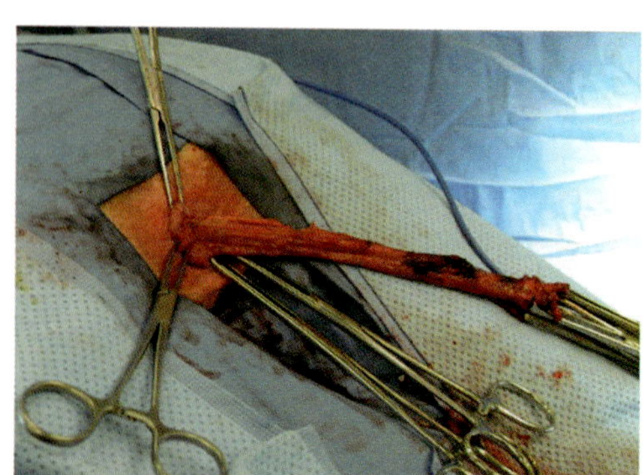

Fig. 30.4 Delorme procedure with stripping of the mucosa.

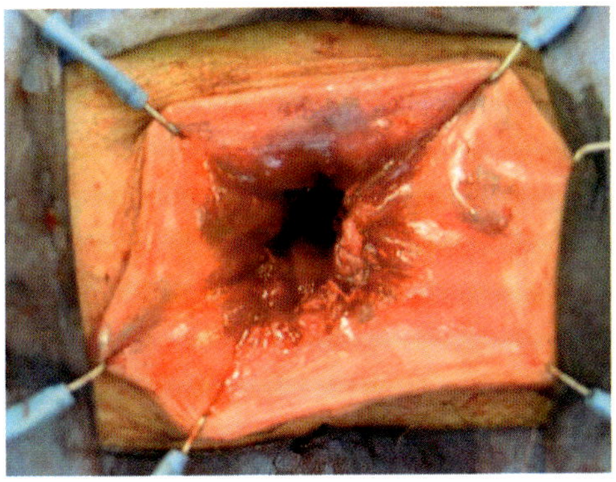

Fig. 30.5 Completed Delorme procedure. Notice that the rectal wall is plicated with sutures in an accordion-type fashion and is situated above the anal sphincters. The anastomosis is just above the dentate line.

a bulky, donut-like circumferential mass around the upper anal canal.

Perineal Rectosigmoidectomy (Altemeier Procedure). Perineal rectosigmoidectomy was first described in 1889 by Mikulicz; in 1952, Altemeier and coworkers described excellent results in elderly debilitated patients. This approach involves a full-thickness removal of the rectum and sigmoid colon via the perineum, with a coloanal anastomosis. This is a minimally invasive procedure, which is ideal for patients deemed too unhealthy for an abdominal procedure. However, in patients who have undergone previous rectal or sigmoid resections, care must be exercised in performing this operation, as the inferior mesenteric vessels may have been previously ligated, and the blood supply to this area may have been altered. Another application of this procedure is in the setting of incarcerated, irreducible prolapse.

First, the prolapse is established by gentle traction with the use of Allis or Babcock clamps. A circumferential incision is made 1.5 to 2.0 cm above the dentate line (Fig. 30.6) with electrocautery or a scalpel. The incision is deepened through the muscular layer until perirectal fat is encountered (Fig. 30.7). Mesorectal vessels are ligated (Fig. 30.8), proceeding in a circumferential manner. As the dissection continues in the cephalad direction, a hernia sac may be encountered anteriorly and opened, and the abdominal cavity may be entered (Fig. 30.9). When no additional bowel can be delivered without tension, the bowel is marked, as this will become the line of transection (Fig. 30.10). At this stage, particularly in incontinent patients, a levatorplasty can be performed by placing sutures such as No. 2-0 polypropylene suture (Prolene; Ethicon, Inc.) anteriorly to loosely approximate the levator muscles. The prolapsed rectal segment is transected (Fig. 30.11). An anastomosis is created with circumferential full-thickness interrupted No. 2-0 Vicryl sutures (Fig. 30.12).

Adding a levator repair to the perineal rectosigmoidectomy can dramatically improve continence postoperatively. Williams (1991), from the University of Minnesota, demonstrated improved incontinence in 91% of patients with the addition of levator repair versus 46% improvement without levatorplasty. This has been shown in more recent studies as

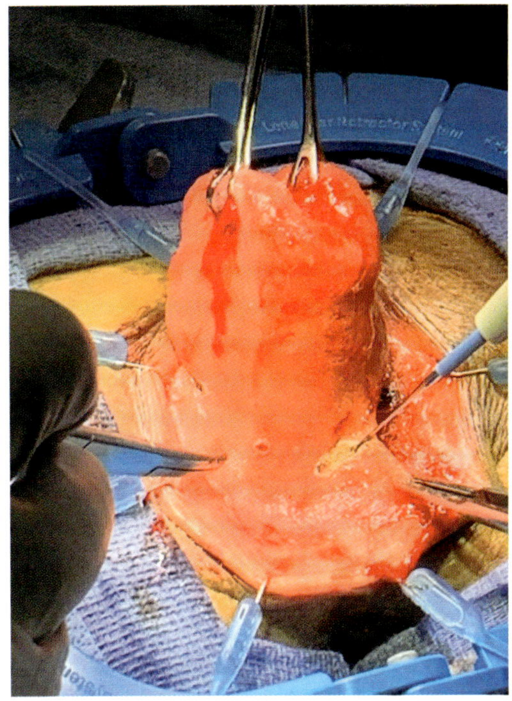

Fig. 30.6 Altemeier procedure (perineal proctosigmoidectomy). An incision is made with electrocautery (as shown here) or knife 1.5 to 2 cm above the dentate line. Note that the patient is in the prone jackknife position.

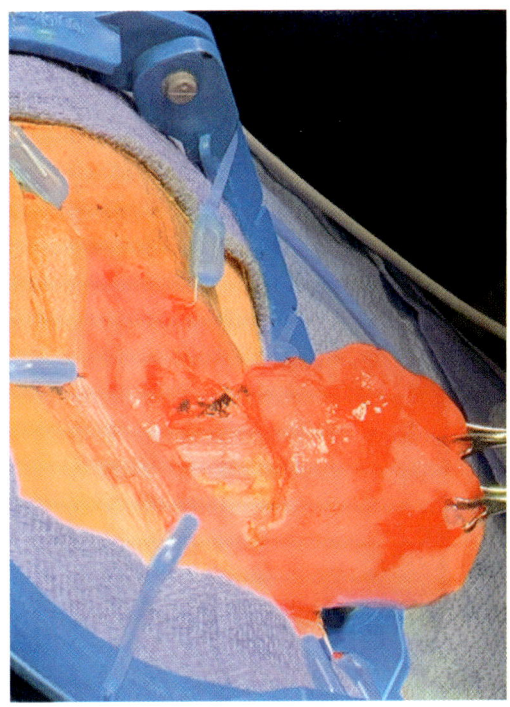

Fig. 30.7 The incision for the perineal proctosigmoidectomy divides all layers of the rectal wall until the extrarectal fat is encountered.

well (Glasgow et al., 2006). Of the three options for perineal repair (Delorme procedure, Altemeier procedure, and Altemeier procedure with levatorplasty), Altemeier with levatorplasty is associated with the lowest recurrence rate and best outcomes with respect to postoperative constipation and fecal incontinence.

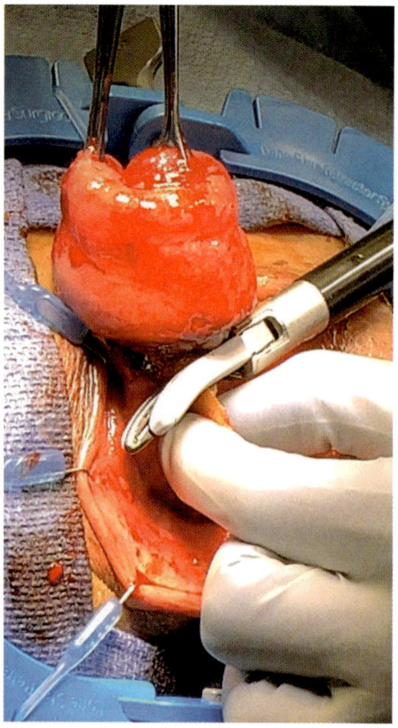

Fig. 30.8 The mesorectal vessels are divided and ligated.

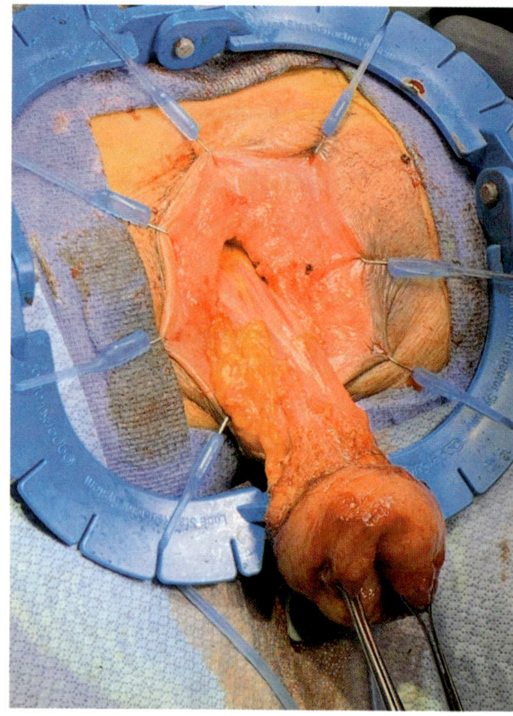

Fig. 30.10 Fully prolapsed segment.

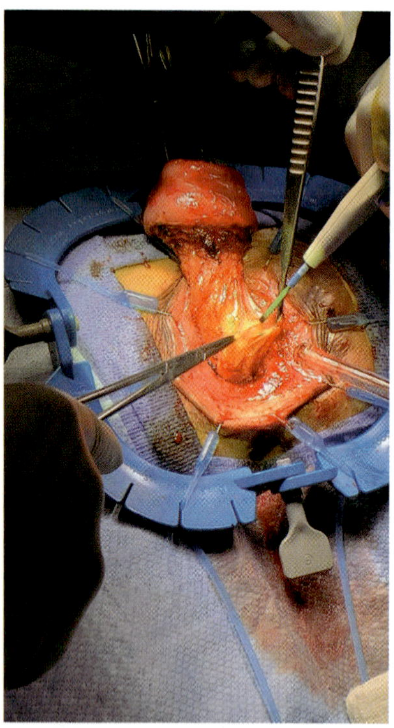

Fig. 30.9 The anterior peritoneal reflection is opened to enter the pelvis and allow more proximal dissection.

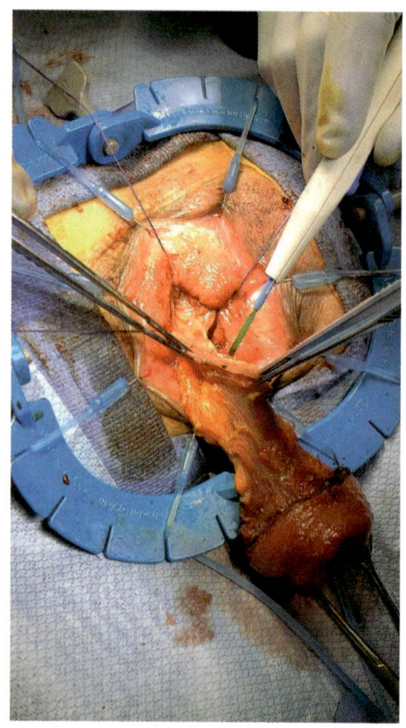

Fig. 30.11 The bowel is transected, preparing for full-thickness excision and hand-sewn coloanal anastomosis.

Anal Encirclement. With an abundance of successful abdominal and perineal operations, the anal encirclement procedure is not commonly done, and is essentially of historical interest. The concept of the procedure is to narrow the anal opening by external compressive means. This procedure should only be considered in patients who are at high enough risk that they cannot tolerate an Altemeier or Delorme procedure. It should be noted, however, that a typical perineal approach such as an Altemeier can commonly be done under a spinal anesthetic and with relative speed. If an anal encirclement is attempted, a foreign material, typically a biologic mesh, is encircled around the anal sphincter through a subcutaneous tunnel and tightened to

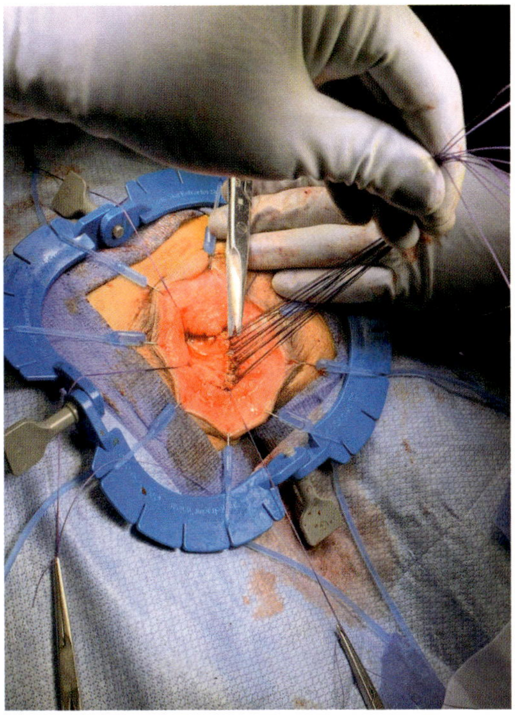

Fig. 30.12 Hand-sewn coloanal anastomosis.

narrow the anal opening. Recurrence is very high after this approach.

Transabdominal and Minimally Invasive Repairs

Transabdominal repairs provide the best outcomes and functional results for the treatment of rectal prolapse by restoring normal anatomy and repairing associated abnormalities. The American Society of Colon and Rectal Surgeons Practice Parameters for Rectal Prolapse (Bordeianou et al., 2017) recommend incorporating a transabdominal rectal fixation for patients with acceptable risk. Although it is often thought that older patients should have a perineal procedure, and younger patients should have an abdominal procedure, age is a relative consideration. If reasonably healthy, many elderly patients can still be treated by an abdominal approach with excellent results. Technical aspects of abdominal repairs for rectal prolapse include the type of rectal mobilization (posterior vs. ventral), the degree of rectal mobilization (with or without transection of lateral stalks), whether sigmoid resection is indicated, the method of rectal fixation, and which approach—either open or minimally invasive—is best. Since the 1990s, laparoscopy has been integrated into repairing prolapse and has brought a new dimension to the management of rectal prolapse in colorectal surgery.

All transabdominal operations involve a mode of rectopexy and can be classified into three groups: (1) posterior rectal mobilization with rectopexy alone, (2) ventral rectal mobilization with rectopexy alone, and (3) rectal mobilization with rectopexy and resection. The preferred type of transabdominal repair varies greatly from one country to another, from one institution to another, and even from one surgeon to another at the same institution.

Rectopexy. Although there are many variations of rectopexy, they all share the same basic principle, which is to suspend the rectum from the sacrum either with suture or with the assistance of material such as a synthetic or biologic mesh. The added benefit of sutured rectal fixation after rectal mobilization has been debated in prospective studies, which have claimed that rectal mobilization alone may be sufficient; however, one large randomized trial has examined the benefit of rectopexy versus no rectopexy after rectal mobilization in the treatment of prolapse (Karas et al., 2011) and definitively showed that addition of rectopexy to all abdominal rectal prolapse repairs is mandatory. This multicenter trial reported a higher recurrence rate in patients who did not undergo rectopexy after rectal mobilization (8.6% vs. 1.5%), despite no difference in complication rates.

Additional rectopexy-related considerations involve the mode of dissection before the rectopexy, the decision to add a concomitant bowel resection to the repair, and considerations in regard to use of mesh. Various rectopexy types will be individually discussed below.

Posterior Approaches. The extent and type of rectal mobilization determines the type of subsequent rectopexy offered. When aiming to perform a posterior suture rectopexy or a resection rectopexy procedure, rectal mobilization is performed posteriorly in the presacral space and carried to the coccyx or levators. Anteriorly, the rectum is mobilized to the perineal body. This circumferential mobilization is then tailored based on the decision concerning lateral mobilization. Division versus preservation of the lateral rectal stalks remains a controversial topic. Studies have shown that division of the lateral stalks may result in increased postoperative constipation, while preservation of these lateral stalks is associated with an increased rate of prolapse recurrence. Speakman et al. (1991), in a prospective randomized study of patients undergoing posterior mesh rectopexy, reported that constipation was increased by 50% if the lateral ligaments were divided, but that prolapse recurrence was increased by 33% if the lateral ligaments were not divided. Mollen et al. (2000) evaluated postoperative colonic transit in patients undergoing repair of rectal prolapse and found that transit was delayed in those patients undergoing division of the lateral stalks, supporting the theory that this is associated with postoperative constipation.

Suture Rectopexy. Cutait (1959) first described fixation of the rectum with suture as a component of treatment for rectal prolapse. Supporting surgeons argue that using foreign material to perform rectopexy is not only unnecessary but also may limit options in patients with constipation or extremely redundant sigmoid who would benefit from simultaneous colon resection. Whether artificial material should be used in the setting of bowel resection is controversial because the risk of infection may be increased. Because of these concerns, suture rectopexy has been advocated. Excellent results have been obtained in a number of series in which the lateral rectal stalks were sutured to the presacral fascia, with recurrence rates ranging from 3% to 9%. A drawback of this approach, however, is the development of new-onset constipation in 15% of patients or worsening constipation in patients (50%) with existing constipation symptoms.

Posterior Mesh Rectopexy (Ripstein Procedure). In 1963, Ripstein and Lanter described a posterior rectopexy involving the use of prosthetic material. After mobilization of the rectum in the mesorectal plane, the rectopexy is performed by placing a long strip of mesh (5 × 20 cm) around the anterior rectum and suturing the free ends of the mesh to the presacral fascia with nonabsorbable sutures. The mesh is also secured to the antimesenteric border of the rectum. The rectum is pulled straight out of the pelvis while the sutures are being placed. The mesh is wrapped loosely enough to allow a thumb or two fingers between the rectum and the sacrum. Alternatively, some surgeons secure the mesh to the presacral fascia at the midportion of the mesh and wrap each free end around the rectum, securing the ends to the antimesenteric border of the rectum. This modification attempts to decrease the rate of impaction or obstruction seen when the mesh completely encircles the rectum. Indeed, Ripstein now uses the posterior rectal sling rather than an anterior sling to decrease problems with constipation.

The Ripstein procedure has been praised for its low prolapse recurrence rate and criticized for postoperative obstructive complications. Gordon and Hoexter (1978) polled the members of the American Society of Colon and Rectal Surgeons, obtaining information on 1111 Ripstein procedures. This poll revealed a prolapse recurrence rate of 2.3%, sling-related complications in 16.5%, and a reoperation rate of 4.1%. Postoperative constipation should be interpreted carefully, as many patients who undergo prolapse surgery experience constipation preoperatively. Tjandra et al. (1993) reported that persistence of prior constipation occurred in 57% of patients after the Ripstein procedure (compared with 17% for resection rectopexy), and that 15% of patients developed new-onset constipation. The prolapse recurrence rate was 7%. However, 35% of patients were dissatisfied after the Ripstein procedure, based on personal interviews using a standard questionnaire, despite anatomic correction of the prolapse. Because of these results, we tend not to perform Ripstein procedures in patients with preoperative obstructive symptoms or significant bowel dysfunction.

Sigmoid Resection and Rectopexy. Resection rectopexy was initially described in 1955 by Frykman, with the appeal of treating prolapse with resection of redundant sigmoid colon and fixation without the use of mesh. The original concept was based on the idea of suspending the left colon from the splenic flexure to reduce prolapse recurrence. Subsequent studies have demonstrated that recurrence rates are similar with and without sigmoid resection, as low as 2% to 5% in some series. Resection does carry some additional risk of complication as a result of the presence of an anastomosis, and complication rates as high as 20% have been reported; they are generally related to anastomotic leak.

We perform rectopexy with resection by mobilizing the sigmoid colon and dividing the mesentery. The rectum is mobilized as previously described, circumferentially. We prefer to resect the sigmoid colon and next perform the anastomosis, either hand-sewn or with the circular stapler. The splenic flexure is usually not mobilized because the bowel by definition is very redundant. The rectopexy is performed by straightening the rectum (pulling it out of the pelvis) and placing two or three sutures from the lateral rectal stalks to the flat portion of the sacrum at the level of S2 or S3 (Fig. 30.13). We prefer to use No. 0 or No. 1 polypropylene suture.

Excellent results have been reported with rectopexy with resection. Patients with preoperative constipation reported lower constipation rates after resection rectopexy versus rectopexy alone. Patients with preoperative fecal incontinence may report an improvement in their symptoms after resection rectopexy, but resolution of fecal incontinence is much less common after sigmoid resection. Resection is indicated in patients who have preexisting constipation; however, care must be taken to identify patients with slow-transit constipation who may require subtotal colectomy combined with rectopexy. Resection in patients without preoperative constipation has not been advocated, as there is a lack of evidence in the literature to support resection in this population.

Anterior Approaches. When planning a ventral rectopexy, the rectal mobilization is only performed anteriorly. In these cases, a hockey-stick incision is made along the right side of the rectum and extending across the pouch of Douglas. The rectum is

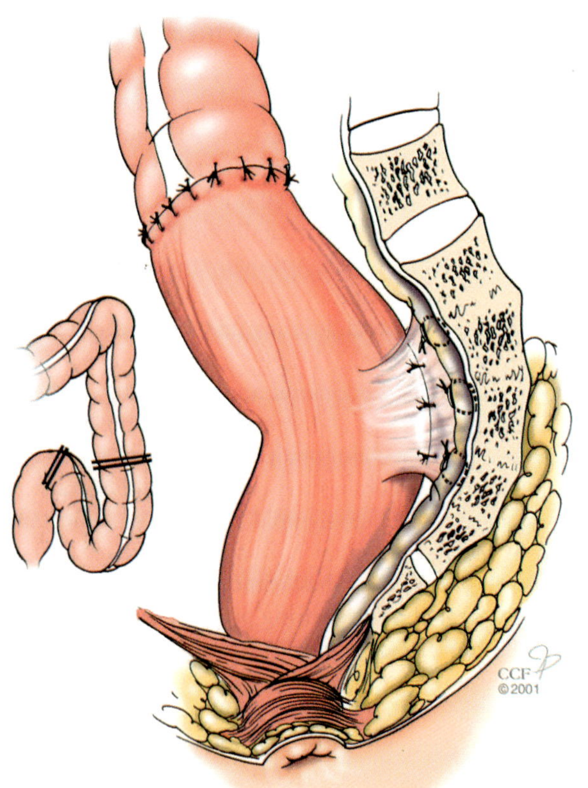

Fig. 30.13 Rectopexy with sigmoid resection. A sigmoid resection with a colorectal anastomosis has been performed. The rectum has been pulled out of the pelvis and straightened. The lateral rectal stalks have been sutured to the sacrum. (Reprinted with permission from The Cleveland Clinic Foundation.)

separated from the vagina until the perineal body is reached. Both lateral stalks are spared. No posterior rectal mobilization is performed. Avoidance of posterior mobilization appears to decrease risk of *de novo* constipation, while offering comparable recurrence rates in the short term. This dissection is followed by rectopexy with mesh.

In 2004, a ventral approach to rectopexy was described by D'Hoore et al., who advocated this approach because of its lower rates of postoperative constipation. This variation of mesh rectopexy involves isolated anterior mobilization of the rectum with mesh fixation of the anterior rectal wall and fixation of mesh to the sacrum (Fig. 30.14). It is thought that the mesh restores normal rectal anatomy without injuring the rectal innervation. Various centers have described the use of both permanent and biologic mesh, with reasonable short-term outcomes that are comparable to posterior rectopexy approaches from the standpoint of recurrence (3.4% in one series). These series also highlighted the possibility that the surgery offered lower rates of postoperative constipation. A recent randomized controlled trial supported these claims (Hidaka et al., 2019). Although there was no difference in short-term functional outcomes (fecal incontinence and constipation scores), ventral mesh repairs had more durable functional outcomes at 6 years, with suture rectopexy patients having greater deterioration in their constipation symptoms. Although not meeting statistical significance, there were lower rates of surgical recurrence at 6 years of follow-up for ventral rectopexy compared with suture rectopexy alone (9% vs. 23%; $P = .11$). This study and the numerous ventral rectopexy series may lead to a paradigm shift in rectal prolapse repairs, with many more colorectal surgeons considering this approach for their patients.

Minimally Invasive Approaches: Laparoscopy and Robotics

The difficulty in choosing between an abdominal approach and a perineal approach for the treatment of rectal prolapse is choosing between a lower recurrence rate (abdominal approach) and a lower surgical morbidity (perineal approach), as many patients with rectal prolapse are elderly and have significant comorbidity. A laparoscopic approach is conceptually attractive, as it combines the benefits of both approaches. Since laparoscopic rectopexy was first performed in 1992 by Berman, many studies have assessed and supported its feasibility and effectiveness in treating rectal prolapse.

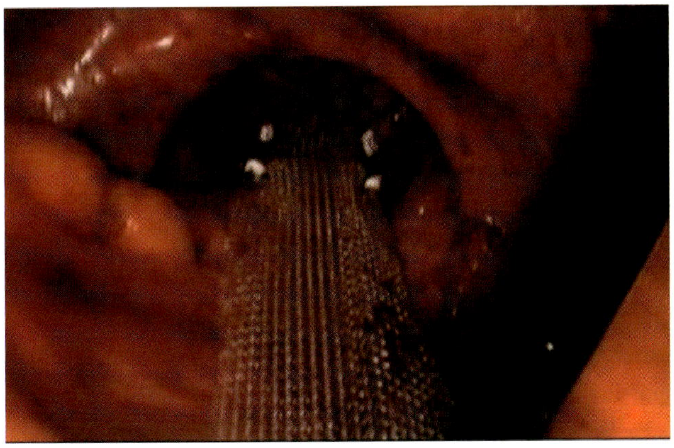

Fig. 30.14 Ventral mesh rectopexy. The mesh is sewn to the anterior rectal wall or the very distal rectum and secured to the sacral promontory.

There have been two prospective studies and several observational studies since that time that have shown consistently reduced postoperative pain, shortened hospital length of stay, and earlier return of bowel function in patients undergoing a laparoscopic approach compared with the open approach. Solomon et al. (2002) randomized 40 patients to either laparoscopic or open rectopexy. Operating time was significantly longer for the laparoscopic cases compared with the open cases (153 vs. 102 min), but the length of hospital stay was shorter (3.9 vs. 6.6 days), and more laparoscopic patients completed an established care pathway (75% vs. 35%). There was no difference in prolapse recurrence, but both major and minor morbidities were significantly lower for laparoscopic cases. Results were similar in a prospective study by Boccasanta et al. (1998), whose results showed low recurrence rates in both groups, with only one patient sustaining a recurrence after undergoing open repair. A subsequent Cochrane meta-analysis found both approaches to be comparable from the standpoint of recurrence, with improved morbidity with laparoscopic surgery.

Numerous observational studies have been conducted, and their findings support that laparoscopic rectopexy is a safe and cost-effective alternative to open rectopexy, with similar recurrence rates. Laparoscopy is associated with a longer operative time but results in less postoperative pain and a shorter hospital stay.

In terms of cost-effectiveness, Delaney et al. (2003) assessed the cost-effectiveness of both laparoscopic and abdominal approaches in a case-matched study of 150 colorectal operations. This study included a number of rectal prolapse cases, and the cost of laparoscopic cases was overall significantly lower.

With the inception of robotic surgery, surgeons have applied robotic techniques to colorectal surgery, with specific application to prolapse surgery. Robotic rectopexy allows for ideal visualization of the deep pelvis and a more facile arrangement for suturing. Compared with laparoscopy, outcomes are equivalent in terms of recurrence, but the robotic approach allows for an easier adoption of ventral mesh rectopexy, which requires higher-level laparoscopic skill.

OUTCOMES AND CHOICE OF PROCEDURE

In this chapter, different types of surgical procedures for the treatment of rectal prolapse have been discussed. There is no single "best" operation for patients with rectal prolapse. The choice of surgical procedure is tailored to each individual. Appropriate methods are considered to be those that provide optimal results with the lowest morbidity and mortality rates. To decide which operation is appropriate for each individual, all patient factors must be considered. Perineal repairs are associated with higher recurrence rates, but the morbidity is lower versus an abdominal approach. Therefore, the perineal approach may be the procedure of choice in frail patients with extensive comorbid conditions. If the prolapse is advanced, perineal proctosigmoidectomy should be considered. Levatorplasty (posterior and/or anterior) may be added, particularly if the patient is incontinent. In debilitated patients with previous left colon resections or minimal prolapse, the Delorme procedure may be optimal.

Overall, the abdominal laparoscopic or robotic approach is favored when considering recurrence rates and improved functional outcomes regarding fecal incontinence and constipation. However, the open abdominal approach is associated with higher morbidity and mortality rates. If the patient has no preoperative incontinence, and constipation is a contributing symptom, resection and rectopexy have been largely supplanted by ventral rectopexy, which is favored. Ventral rectopexy is especially beneficial for the patients with preoperative fecal incontinence, as resection may worsen their incontinence.

Many patients with rectal prolapse have functional defecatory problems. Correcting the prolapse may not change the abnormal defecatory patterns, and the patient must be counseled of this preoperatively. New advances in laparoscopic and robotic surgery have the potential to fundamentally alter the operative approach (although not the procedures) for abdominal repair of rectal prolapse, but long-term follow-up of outcomes is required.

BIBLIOGRAPHY

Aboul-Enein A. Prolapse of the rectum in young men: treatment with a modified Roscoe Graham operation. *Dis Colon Rectum.* 1979;22:117.

Agachan F, Pfeifer J, Wexner SD. Defecography and proctography. Results of 774 patients. *Dis Colon Rectum.* 1996;39:899.

Altemeier WA, Giuseffi J, Hoxworth P. Treatment of extensive prolapse of the rectum in aged or debilitated patients. *AMA Arch Surg.* 1952;65:72.

Ashburn JH, Hull TL. Rectal prolapse. In: Waters MD, Karram MM, eds. *Urogynecology and Reconstructive Pelvic Surgery,* 4th ed. Philadephia: Elsevier Saunders; 2015.

Berman IR. Sutureless laparoscopic rectopexy for procidentia: technique and implications. *Dis Colon Rectum.* 1992;35:689.

Blatchford GJ, Perry RE, Thorson AG, et al. Rectopexy without resection for rectal prolapse. *Am J Surg.* 1989;158:574.

Boccasanta P, Rosati R, Venturi M, et al. Comparison of laparoscopic rectopexy with open techniques in the treatment of complete rectal prolapse: clinical and functional results. *Surg Laparosc Endosc.* 1998;8:460.

Boccasanta P. Laparotomic vs. laparoscopic rectopexy in complete rectal prolapse. *Dig Surg.* 1999;16:415.

Bordeianou L, Paquette I, Johnson E, et al. ASCRS Clinical practice guideline for the management of rectal prolapse. *Dis Colon Rectum.* 2017;60:1121.

Broden B, Snellman B. Procidentia of the rectum studied with cine radiography: a contribution to the discussion of causative mechanism. *Dis Colon Rectum.* 1968;11:330.

Clark CE III, Jupiter DC, Thomas JS, Papaconstantinou HT. Rectal prolapse in the elderly: trends in surgical management and outcomes from the American College of Surgeons National Surgical Quality Improvement Program database. *J Am Coll Surg.* 2012;215:709.

Cutait DE. Sacro-promontory fixation of the rectum for complete rectal prolapse. *Proc R Soc Med.* 1959;52:105.

D'Hoore A, Cadoni R, Penninckx F. Long-term outcome of laparoscopic ventral rectopexy for total rectal prolapse. *Br J Surg.* 2004;91:1500.

Darzi A, Henry MM, Guillou PJ, et al. Stapled laparoscopic rectopexy for rectal prolapse. *Surg Endosc.* 1995;9:301.

Deen KI, Grant E, Billingham C, et al. Abdominal resection rectopexy with pelvic floor repair versus perineal rectosigmoidectomy and pelvic floor repair for full-thickness rectal prolapse. *Br J Surg.* 1999;81:302.

Delaney CP, Kiran RP, Senagore AJ, et al. Case-matched comparison of clinical and financial outcome after laparoscopic or open colorectal surgery. *Ann Surg.* 2003;238:67.

Delaney CP, Lynch AC, Senagore AJ, et al. Comparison of robotically performed and traditional laparoscopic colorectal surgery. *Dis Colon Rectum.* 2003;46:1633.

Delorme E. On the treatment of total prolapse of the rectum by excision of the rectal mucous membranes. *Bull Mem Soc Chir Paris.* 1900;26:499.

Duthie GS, Bartolo DC. Abdominal rectopexy for rectal prolapse: comparison of techniques. *Br J Surg.* 1992;79:107.

Emile SH, Elbanna H, Youssef M, et al. Laparoscopic ventral mesh rectopexy vs. Delorme's operation in management of complete rectal prolapse: a prospective randomized study. *Colorectal Dis.* 2017;19:50.

Fang SH, Cromwell JW, Wilkins KB, et al. Is the abdominal repair of rectal prolapse safer than perineal repair in the highest risk patients? An NSQIP analysis. *Dis Colon Rectum.* 2012;55:1167.

Finlay IG, Atchison M. Perineal excision of the rectum for the prolapse in the elderly. *Br J Surg.* 1991;78:687.

Frykman HM. Abdominal proctopexy and primary sigmoid resection for rectal procidentia. *Am J Surg.* 1955;90:780.

Glasgow SC, Birnbaum EH, Kodner IJ, et al. Preoperative anal manometry predicts continence after perineal proctectomy for rectal prolapse. *Dis Colon Rectum.* 2006;49:1052.

Gordon PH, Hoexter B. Complications of Ripstein procedure. *Dis Colon Rectum.* 1978;21:277.

Graf W, Karlbom U, Pahlman L, et al. Functional results after abdominal suture rectopexy for rectal prolapse or intussusception. *Eur J Surg.* 1996;162:905.

Halligan S, Sultan A, Rottenberg G, Bartram CI. Endosonography of the anal sphincters in solitary rectal ulcer syndrome. *Int J Colorectal Dis.* 1995;10:79.

Hidaka J, Efleki H, Dueland-Jakobsen J, et al. Functional outcome after laparoscopic posterior sutured rectopexy versus ventral mesh rectopexy for rectal prolapse: six-year follow-up of a double-blind, randomized single-center study. *EClinicalMedicine.* 2019;16:18.

Houry S, Lechaux JP, Huguier M, Moihou JM. Treatment of rectal prolapse by Delorme's operation. *Int J Colorectal Dis.* 1987;2:149.

Husa A, Salinio P, von Smitten K. Abdominal rectopexy and sigmoid resection for rectal prolapse. *Acta Chir Scand.* 1988;154:221.

Jacobs LK, Lin YJ, Orkin BA. The best operation for rectal prolapse. *Surg Clin North Am.* 1997;77:49.

Johansen OB, Wexner SD, Daniel N, et al. Perineal rectosigmoidectomy in the elderly. *Dis Colon Rectum.* 1993;36:767.

Kairaluoma MV, Kellokumpu IH. Epidemiologic aspects of complete rectal prolapse. *Scand J Surg.* 2005;94:207.

Karas JR, Uranues S, Altomare DF, et al. No rectopexy versus rectopexy following rectal mobilization for full-thickness rectal prolapse: a randomized controlled trial. *Dis Colon Rectum.* 2011;54:29.

Kling KM, Rongione AJ, Evans B, et al. The Delorme procedure: a useful operation for complicated rectal prolapse in the elderly. *Am Surg.* 1996;62:857.

Kupfer CA, Goligher JC. One hundred consecutive cases of complete rectal prolapse of the rectum treated by operation. *Br J Surg.* 1970;57:481.

Lechaux JP, Lechhaux D, Perez M. Results of Delorme's procedure for rectal prolapse: advantages of a modified technique. *Dis Colon Rectum.* 1995;38:301.

Lockhart-Mummery HE. Procidentia: recent experiences in the treatment of rectal prolapse. *Dis Colon Rectum.* 1972;15:347.

Lukkonen P, Mikkonen U, Jarvinen H. Abdominal rectopexy with sigmoidectomy vs rectopexy alone for rectal prolapse: a prospective, randomized study. *Int J Colorectal Dis.* 1992;7:219.

Madiba TE, Baig Mk, Wexner SD. Surgical management of rectal prolapse. *Arch Surg.* 2005;140:63.

Madoff RD, Mellgren A. One hundred years of rectal prolapse surgery. *Dis Colon Rectum.* 1999;42:441.

Madoff RD, Williams JG, Wong WD, et al. Long-term functional results of colon resection and rectopexy for overt rectal prolapse. *Am J Gastroenterol.* 1992;87:101.

Matheson DM, Keighley MRB. Manometric evaluation of rectal prolapse and fecal incontinence. *Gut.* 1981;22:126.

McKee RF, Lauder JC, Poon FW, et al. A prospective randomized study of abdominal rectopexy with and without sigmoidectomy in rectal prolapse. *Surg Gynecol Obstet.* 1992;174:145.

McMahan JD, Ripstein CB. Rectal prolapse. An update on the rectal sling procedure, *Am Surg.* 1987;53:37.

Mikulicz J. Zur operativen behandlung des prolapsus recti et coli invaginati. *Arch Klin Chir.* 1889;38:74.

Mollen RM, Kuijpers JH, van Hoek F. Effect of rectal mobilization and lateral ligaments division on colonic and anorectal function. *Dis Colon Rectum.* 2000;43:1283.

Monson JR, Jones NA, Vowden P, Brennan TG. Delorme's operation: the first choice in complete rectal prolapse? *Ann R Coll Surg Engl.* 1986;68:143.

Moschcowitz AV. The pathogenesis, anatomy and cure of prolapse of the rectum. *Surg Gynecol Obstet.* 1912;15:7.

Neill ME, Parks AG, Swash M. Physiological studies of the anal sphincter musculature in faecal incontinence and rectal prolapse. *Br J Surg.* 1981;68:531.

Novell JR, Osborne MJ, Winslet MC, et al. Prospective randomized trial of Ivalon sponge versus sutured rectopexy for full-thickness rectal prolapse. *Br J Surg.* 1994;81:904.

Oliver GC, Vachon D, Eisenstat TE, et al. Delorme's procedure for complete rectal prolapse in severely debilitated patients: an analysis of 41 cases. *Dis Colon Rectum.* 1994;37:461.

Parks AG, Swash M, Urich H. Sphincter denervation in anorectal incontinence and rectal prolapse. *Gut.* 1977;18:656.

Ramanjam PS, Venkatesh KS, Fietz MJ. Perineal excision of rectal procidentia in elderly high risk patients: a ten-year experience. *Dis Colon Rectum.* 1994;37:1027.

Riansuwan W, Hull TL, Bast J, et al. Comparison of perineal operations with abdominal operations for full-thickness rectal prolapse. *World J Surg.* 2006;34:1116.

Ripstein CB, Lanter B. Etiology and surgical therapy of massive prolapse of the rectum. *Ann Surg.* 1963;157:259.

Roberts PL, Schoetz DJ, Coller JA, Veidenheimer MC. Ripstein procedure. Lahey Clinic experience: 1963–1985. *Arch Surg.* 1988;123:554.

Sajid MS, Siddiqui MR, Baig MK. Open vs laparoscopic repair of full-thickness rectal prolapse: a re-meta-analysis. *Colorectal Dis.* 2010;12:515.

Sayfan J, Pinho M, Williams JA, et al. Sutured posterior abdominal rectopexy with sigmoidectomy compared with Marlex rectopexy for rectal prolapse. *Br J Surg.* 1990;77:143.

Scaglia M, Fasth S, Hallgren T, et al. Abdominal rectopexy for rectal prolapse. Influence of surgical technique on functional outcome. *Dis Colon Rectum.* 1994;37:805.

Schlinkert RT, Beart RW, Wolf BG, Pemberton JH. Anterior resection for complete rectal prolapse. *Dis Colon Rectum.* 1985;28:409.

Schultz I, Mellgren A, Johansson C, et al. Continence is improved after the Ripstein rectopexy. Different mechanisms in patients with rectal prolapse and rectal intussusception? *Dis Colon Rectum.* 1996;39:300.

Schultz I, Mellgren A, Nilsson BY, et al. Preoperative electrophysiologic assessment cannot predict continence after rectopexy. *Dis Colon Rectum.* 1998;41:1392.

Senagore AJ. Management of rectal prolapse: the role of laparoscopic approaches. *Semin Laparosc Surg.* 2003;10:197.

Senapati A, Gray R, Middleton L, et al. PROSPER: a randomized comparison of surgical treatments for rectal prolapse. *Colorectal Dis.* 2013;15:858.

Solomon MJ, Young CJ, Eyers AA, et al. Randomized clinical trial of laparoscopic versus open abdominal rectopexy for rectal prolapse. *Br J Surg.* 2002;89:35.

Speakman CT, Madden MV, Nicholls RJ, Kamm MA. Lateral ligament division during rectopexy causes constipation but prevents recurrence: results of a prospective randomized study. *Br J Surg.* 1991;78:1431.

Stern RC, Izant RJ, Boat TF, et al. Treatment and prognosis of rectal prolapse in cystic fibrosis. *Gastroenterology.* 1982;82:707.

Stevenson AR, Stitz RW, Lumley JW. Laparoscopic-assisted resection rectopexy for rectal prolapse. Early and medium follow up. *Dis Colon Rectum.* 1998;41:46.

Theuerkauf FJ, Beahrs OH, Hill JR. Rectal prolapse: causation and surgical treatment. *Ann Surg.* 1970;171:819.

Tjandra JJ, Fazio VW, Church JM, et al. Ripstein procedure is an effective treatment for rectal prolapse without constipation. *Dis Colon Rectum.* 1993;36:501.

Tobin SA, Scott IHK. Delorme operation for rectal prolapse. *Br J Surg.* 1994;81:1681.

Tou S, Brown SR, Malik AI, et al. Surgery for complete rectal prolapse in adults. *Cochrane Database Syst Rev.* 2015;11:CD001758.

Uhlig BE, Sullivan ES. The modified Delorme operation: its place in surgical treatment for massive rectal prolapse. *Dis Colon Rectum.* 1979;22:513.

Vongsangnak V, Varma JS, Watters D, Smith AN. Clinical, manometric and surgical aspects of complete prolapse of rectum. *J R Coll Surg Edinb.* 1985;30:251.

Watts JD, Rothenberger DA, Buls JG, et al. The management of procidentia: 30 years' experience. *Dis Colon Rectum.* 1985;28:96.

Wells C. New operation for rectal prolapse. *Proc R Soc Med.* 1959;52:602.

Williams JG. Perineal approaches to repair of rectal prolapse. *Semin Colon Rectal Surg.* 1991;2:198.

Williams JG, Wong WD, Jenson L, et al. Incontinence and rectal prolapse: a prospective manometric study. *Dis Colon Rectum.* 1991;34:209.

Yoshioka K, Hyland G, Keighley MR. Anorectal function after abdominal rectopexy: parameters of predictive value in identifying return of continence. *Br J Surg.* 1989;76:64.

PART 6

Lower Urinary Tract Disorders

31

Overactive Bladder Syndrome, Polyuria, and Nocturia

Siobhan M. Hartigan and Roger R. Dmochowski

CHAPTER OUTLINE

OVERACTIVE BLADDER SYNDROME

Overactive bladder (OAB) is a symptom syndrome defined as urinary urgency, with or without urgency incontinence, usually with urinary frequency and nocturia, and in the absence of urinary tract infection (UTI) or other obvious pathology (Haylen et al., 2010). Millions of Americans are affected by OAB at any given time, and the aging of the population ensures that the number of people who suffer from OAB will continue to increase over time. The symptoms of OAB can have a large negative impact on social and personal activities, which can cause significant psychological distress (Milsom et al., 2012). OAB continues to remain an underreported and undertreated condition, despite increased awareness, improved diagnosis, and increased treatment options in recent years. It is likely that the poorly understood etiology of OAB, the heterogeneity of symptom presentation and patient characteristics, and suboptimal patient-physician communication contribute to this problem.

Terminology, Prevalence, Epidemiology, and Economic Impact

The International Continence Society (ICS) is the governing body that has historically taken the lead in the standardization of terminology. The terminology used to describe OAB and associated symptoms has changed numerous times. The ICS recommends the use of symptoms, signs, and validated investigations to form workable diagnoses. In 2020, the ICS used the following terms:

- Increased daytime urinary frequency: Complaint that voiding occurs more frequently during waking hours than previously deemed normal by the individual (or caregivers) (D'Ancona et al., 2019).
- Nocturia:The number of times urine is passed during the main sleep period. Having woken to pass urine for the first time, each urination must be followed by sleep or the intention to sleep (D'Ancona et al., 2019).
- Urgency: Complaint of sudden, compelling desire to pass urine that is difficult to defer (D'Ancona et al., 2019).
- Overactive bladder (urgency) syndrome: Urinary urgency, usually accompanied by daytime frequency and/or nocturia, with or without urinary incontinence, in the absence of UTI or other obvious pathology (Haylen et al., 2010).
- Urgency urinary incontinence (UUI): Complaint of involuntary loss of urine associated with urgency (D'Ancona et al., 2019).
- Detrusor overactivity (DO): The occurrence of detrusor contraction(s) during filling cystometry. These contractions, which may be spontaneous or provoked, produce a waveform of variable duration and amplitude on the cystometrogram (CMG). The contractions may be phasic or terminal. They may be suppressed by the patient or be uncontrollable. Symptoms, for example, urgency and/or urgency incontinence or perception of the contraction, may or may not occur (D'Ancona et al., 2019). DO may be further qualified as neurogenic, when there is a relevant neurologic condition, or idiopathic, when the cause is unknown.

It is important to note that, although the current definition of OAB is based on symptoms, DO is a urodynamic observation. By definition, to diagnose a patient with DO, one must observe involuntary detrusor contractions during the filling phase of CMG during urodynamics testing. OAB and DO are thus not interchangeable terms, and it is important that the clinician use each term correctly.

The number of individuals affected by OAB is difficult to establish. The populations studied vary substantially from one publication to another, and the symptoms or signs used to define OAB may also vary between publications. Overall, however, the incidence of OAB is high, ranging between 7% and 27% in males and between 9% to 43% in females (Gormley et al., 2012; Haylen et al., 2016).

Based on data from the EPIC study, 10.7% of the world's population was found to be affected by OAB (i.e., almost 250 million women and over 200 million men) (Irwin et al., 2006). The Epidemiology of Lower Urinary Tract Symptoms (EpiLUTS) study, a cross-sectional, population-representative survey of men and women over 40 years old conducted via the internet in the United States, the United Kingdom, and Sweden, revealed the distribution of individual and the combination of various lower urinary tract symptoms (LUTS) within the OAB symptom complex by gender (Coyne et al., 2009; Coyne et al., 2011). In this large study that included 4562 women and 2559 men with OAB, 20.2% of women and 15.6% of men reported combined urgency, UUI, nocturia, and frequency.

In the United States alone, OAB has been estimated to affect up to 33 million people. However, it is estimated that only 15% of these patients with incontinence and OAB symptoms seek medical help. The National Overactive Bladder Evaluation program (Stewart et al., 2003) contacted more than 5000 households by telephone and, among those who responded, the overall prevalence of OAB was 16.6%. Men and women had a similar overall prevalence of OAB (16.0% and 16.9%, respectively) as defined by the ICS. The prevalence of symptoms increased sharply with age in both men and women (Fig. 31.1).

Men were shown to have a higher prevalence of "OAB dry," or OAB without UUI (13.4% vs. 7.6% in women), and women had a higher prevalence of "OAB wet," or OAB with UUI (9.3% vs. 2.6% in men) (Fig. 31.2). In women, the presence of "OAB wet" rose from 2% in the youngest group (ages 18–24 years) to 19.1% in those 65 to 74 years of age (Stewart et al., 2003).

In a secondary analysis of data from the EpiLUTS survey, Coyne et al. (2012) examined whether there were racial differences in the prevalence of OAB amongst men and women in the United States. Of the 20,000 US adults surveyed, OAB was found to be most prevalent in Black men and women. In this study, the prevalence of OAB in Black, Caucasian, Hispanic, and Asian women was 45.9%, 43.4%, 42.0%, and 26.6%, respectively.

Given that women between the ages of 60 and 80 are the most rapidly growing segment of the US population, and that up to 50% of women in this age group meet criteria for OAB syndrome, treatment of this condition clearly has a significant economic impact on our society. Using population prevalence estimates from the EpiLUTS study, Onukwugha et al. (2009)

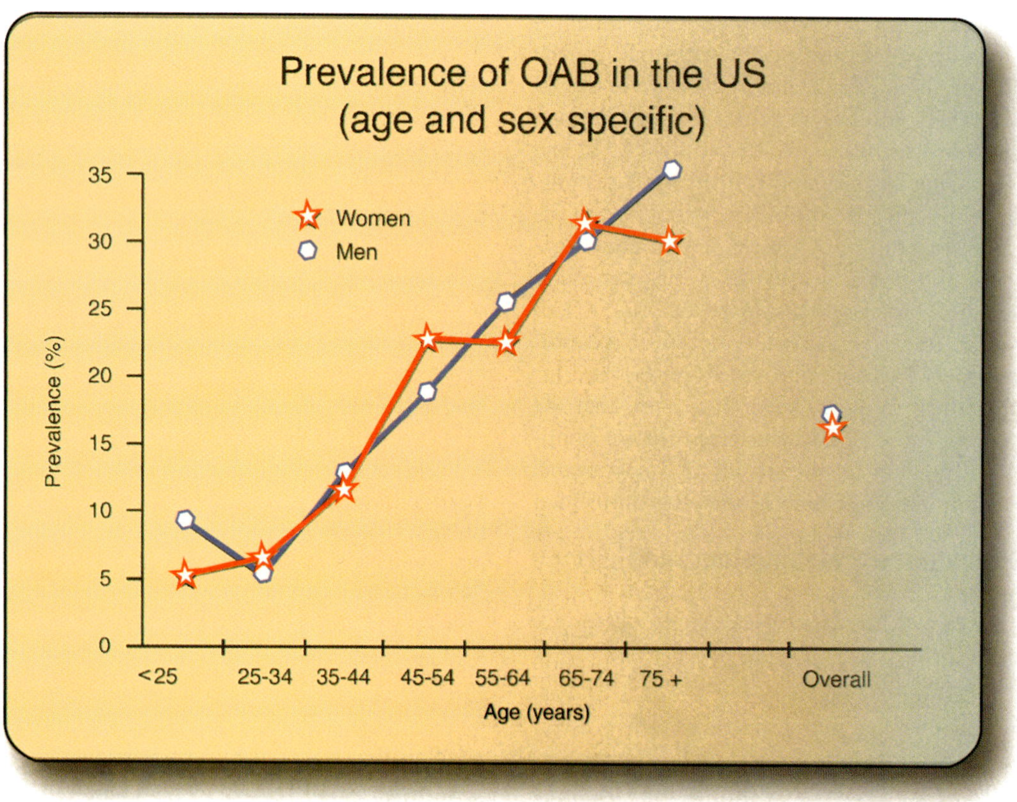

Fig. 31.1 Prevalence of overactive bladder (*OAB*) by age and sex in the United States. (Modified from Stewart WF, Van Rooyen JB, Cundiff GW, et al. Prevalence and burden of overactive bladder in the United States. *World J Urol.* 2003;20:327. With permission.)

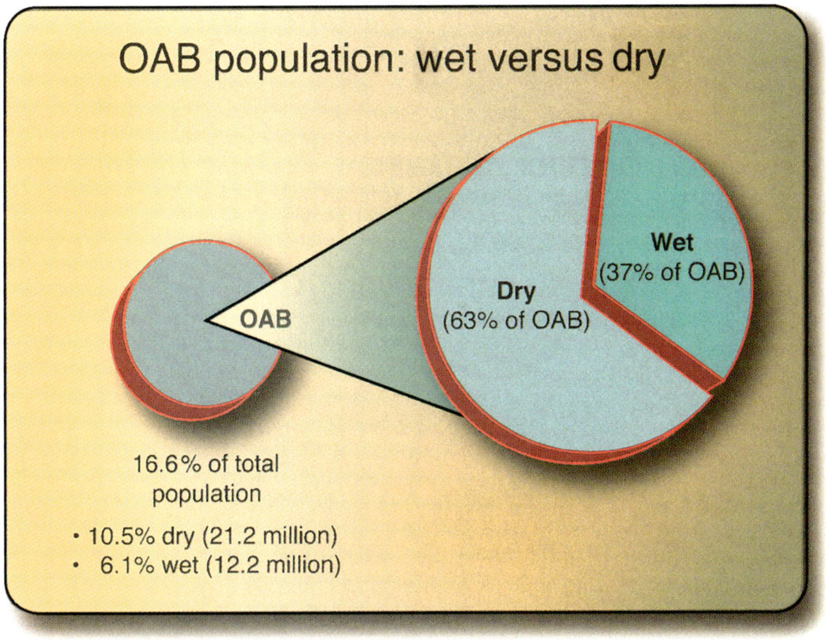

Fig. 31.2 Overall prevalence of overactive bladder (*OAB*) wet and OAB dry. (Modified from Stewart WF, Van Rooyen JB, Cundiff GW, et al. Prevalence and burden of overactive bladder in the United States. *World J Urol.* 2003;20:327. With permission.)

estimated the total cost at $24.9 billion annually. Another study estimated the current direct (medical and nonmedical) and indirect costs of OAB in the United States (Ganz et al., 2010). In 2007, average annual per capita costs of OAB were $1925 ($1433 in direct medical, $66 in direct nonmedical, and $426 in indirect costs). When applied to 34 million people in the United States with OAB, the total national costs were $65.9 billion ($49.1 billion direct medical, $2.3 billion direct nonmedical, and $14.6 billion indirect). This study, published in 2010, also predicted annual per capita costs to rise to $1944 in 2015 and $1969 in 2020, with total annual national costs rising to $76.2 billion in 2015 and $86.2 billion in 2020.

OAB can also have a significant impact on quality of life. Both men and women with bothersome OAB were more likely to report that their bladder condition caused them at least some problems (Milsom et al., 2012). These subjects reported worse scores on health-related quality of life questionnaires, anxiety assessments, and depression assessments. Men and women with bothersome OAB also had a greater number of health care visits annually compared to those with OAB without bother and those with minimal to no symptoms (Milsom et al., 2012).

Neurophysiology of the Lower Urinary Tract

To better understand the etiology and pharmacologic management of OAB, a brief review of the neurophysiology of the lower urinary tract is presented (see Chapter 3 for further details).

Autonomic Pathways. Sympathetic nerves, which help to control bladder relaxation, exit the spinal cord at levels T10 through L2 and synapse in paravertebral ganglions. Noradrenaline, the neurotransmitter of the sympathetic system, binds to α- and β-adrenergic receptors, and then postganglionic fibers travel to the bladder via the hypogastric nerve (Fig. 31.3). When norepinephrine binds to β-receptors on the bladder, it activates adenylate cyclase, which increases levels of cyclic adenosine monophosphate (AMP), thereby relaxing the detrusor muscle of the bladder (Fig. 31.4).

The parasympathetic nerves, which are important in the control of bladder contractility, exit the spinal cord at levels S2, S3, and S4. Preganglionic fibers travel to the bladder via the pelvic nerve, synapse close to the bladder, and then send short postganglionic fibers to the bladder (see Fig. 31.3). The parasympathetic system uses acetylcholine as its neurotransmitter and muscarinic receptors at target organs. Five subtypes of muscarinic receptors are known, with a predominance of M_2 and M_3 receptor subtypes in the bladder. Release of acetylcholine by postganglionic parasympathetic nerves activates both M_2 and M_3 receptor subtypes. M_2 receptors make up approximately 80% of the muscarinic receptors in the bladder. Activation of M_2 receptors negatively affects adenylate cyclase, thereby decreasing cyclic AMP, and ultimately inhibiting relaxation caused by the sympathetic system. M_3 subtypes, which make up the remaining 20% of muscarinic bladder receptors, activate phospholipase C, increase inositol triphosphate, and subsequently cause detrusor muscle contraction.

Somatic Pathways. The somatic pathway includes motor neurons that originate in Onuf's nucleus in the sacral spinal cord and exit the spinal cord at level S2, S3, and S4. Their axons travel via the pudendal nerve to the external urethral sphincter, where they innervate the striated smooth muscle. Acetylcholine is the neurotransmitter for the somatic nervous system, and binds to nicotinic receptors (see Fig. 31.3).

Central Regulation. The central regulation of micturition is controlled by several neurotransmitters, including acetylcholine, γ-aminobutyric acid (GABA), glycine, serotonin, dopamine, and noradrenaline. The pontine micturition center (Barrington nucleus or M region) is involved in regulating

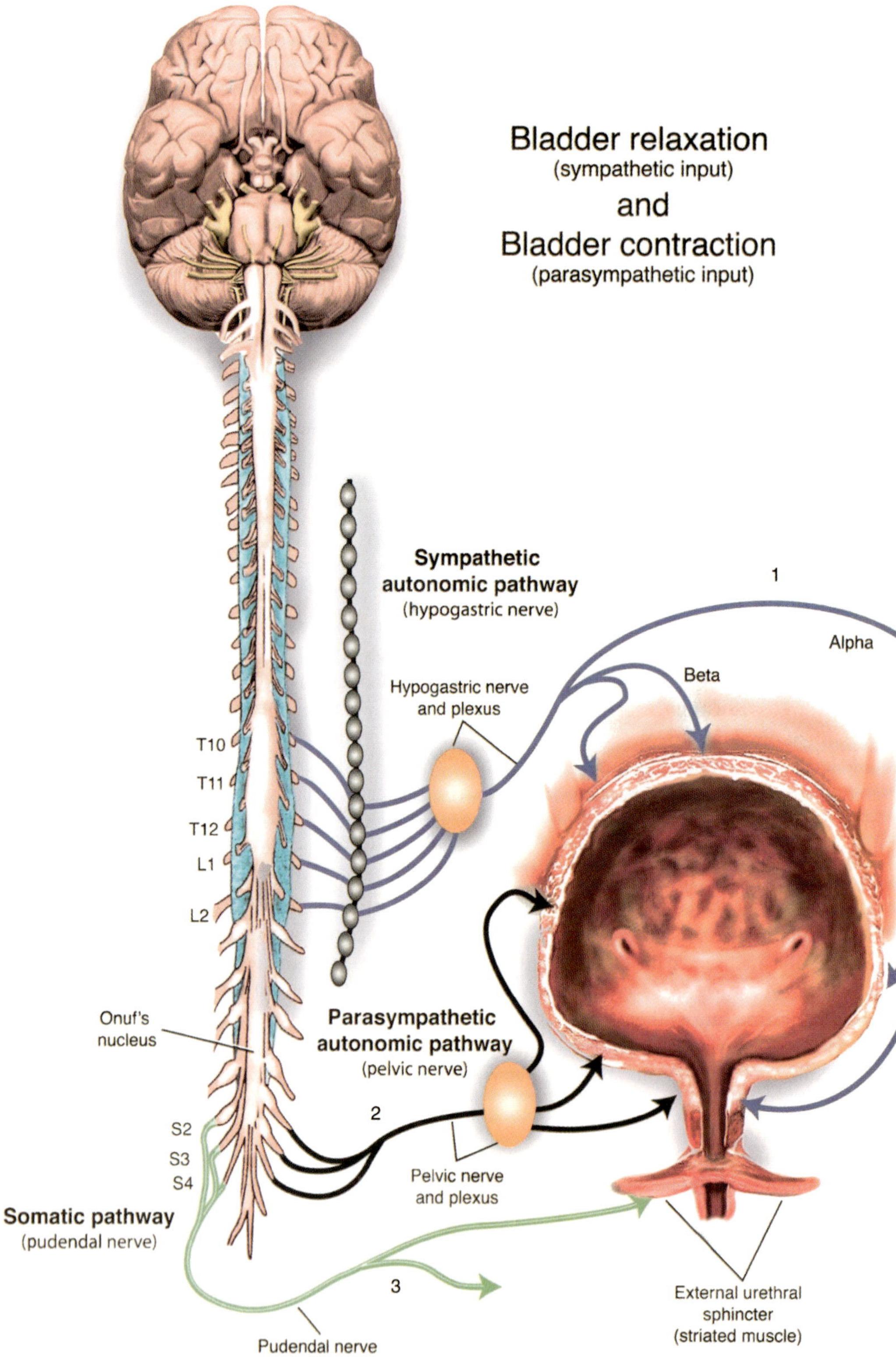

Fig. 31.3 Neurologic pathways for bladder storage and elimination. (1) Sympathetic nerves exit the spinal cord between T10 and L2 levels and synapse in the paravertebral ganglion. Postganglionic fibers then travel to the bladder via the hypogastric nerve. (2) Parasympathetic nerves exit the spinal cord via the sacral vertebral levels S2 through S4. Preganglionic fibers travel to the bladder via the pelvic nerve and synapse close to the bladder. Short postganglionic fibers are then sent to the bladder. (3) The external urethral sphincter is innervated by motor neurons that originate in Onuf's nucleus and travel via the pudendal nerve, part of the somatic pathway, to control this striated muscle.

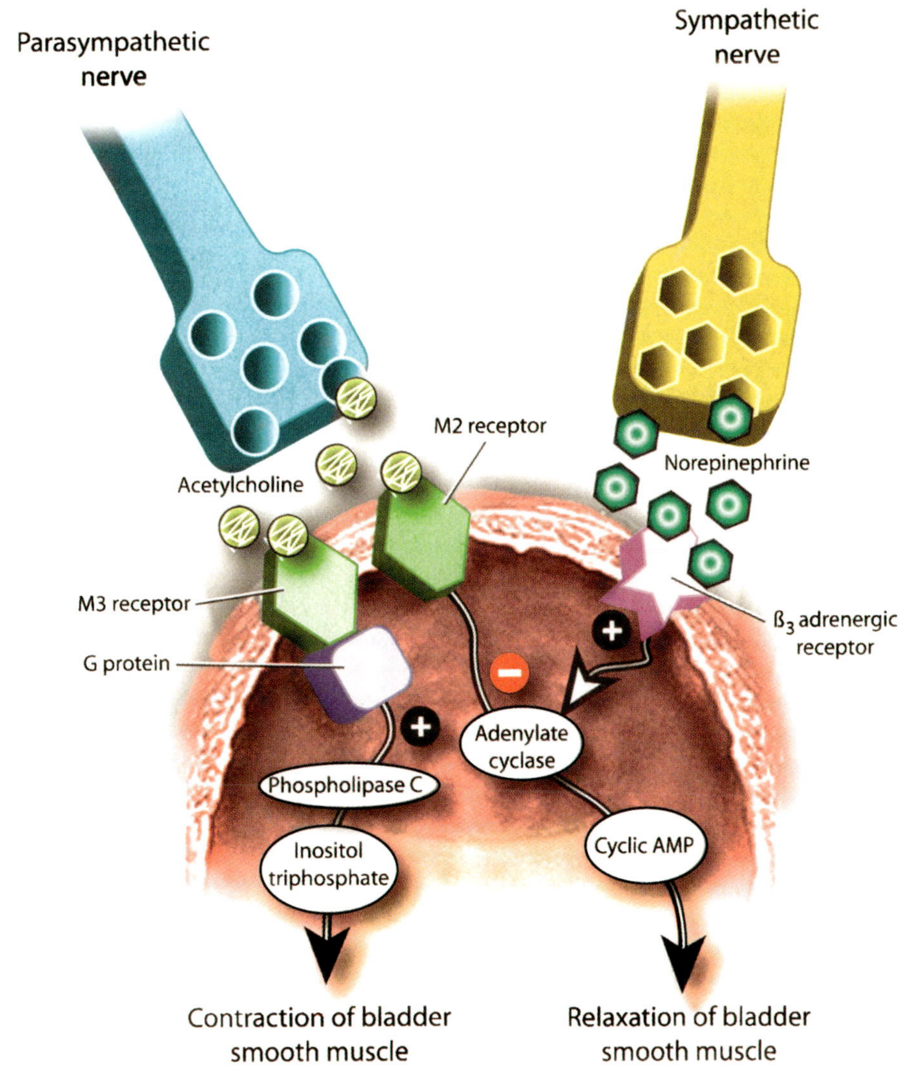

Fig. 31.4 A schematic representation of sympathetic and parasympathetic postjunctional receptors at the level of the bladder. *AMP*, Adenosine monophosphate.

voiding and incontinence by projecting directly to bladder motor neurons and indirectly to urethral motor neurons. The bladder motor neurons are preganglionic and parasympathetic (S2, S3, and S4) and located in the intramediolateral cell column of the sacral spinal cord. The urethral motor neurons are located in the sacral ventral horn (Onuf's nucleus). When the pontine micturition center is stimulated, the urethral motor neurons are inhibited, leading to a decrease in urethral pressure, and the bladder motor neurons are stimulated, leading to an increase in intravesical pressure, thus resulting in coordinated micturition between the bladder and the outlet (Fig. 31.5).

The pontine continence center projects to urethral sphincter motor neurons and, when stimulated, increases urethral sphincter tone. During the filling or storage phase, the pontine continence center sends continuous stimulation to urethral sphincter motor neurons to maintain urethral closure (see Fig. 31.5).

Afferent Information. Afferent sensory information is sent from the bladder via the pelvic nerve to the sacral dorsal root ganglia located within the spinal cord. These nerves are primarily made up of myelinated A and D fibers and unmyelinated C fibers. The A and D fibers respond to distension and active contraction, whereas C fibers respond to chemical irritation and pain (Fig. 31.6). There are several receptors that have been identified on these nerves, such as vanilloid, tachykinin, purinergic, and prostanoid receptors, which may have a role in the development of OAB syndrome and may be potential pharmacotherapy targets (Andersson, 2016).

Etiology of Overactive Bladder

Although there are numerous neurologic diseases associated with symptoms of OAB, the majority of women who present with this syndrome are neurologically intact. There are many conditions that are associated with OAB syndrome (Box 31.1) and the symptoms of this condition; however, the pathophysiology remains unknown for many patients, and the syndrome as a whole can have a heterogeneous presentation.

Neurologic Diseases. As discussed earlier, the process of bladder storage and emptying is controlled by the complex interplay

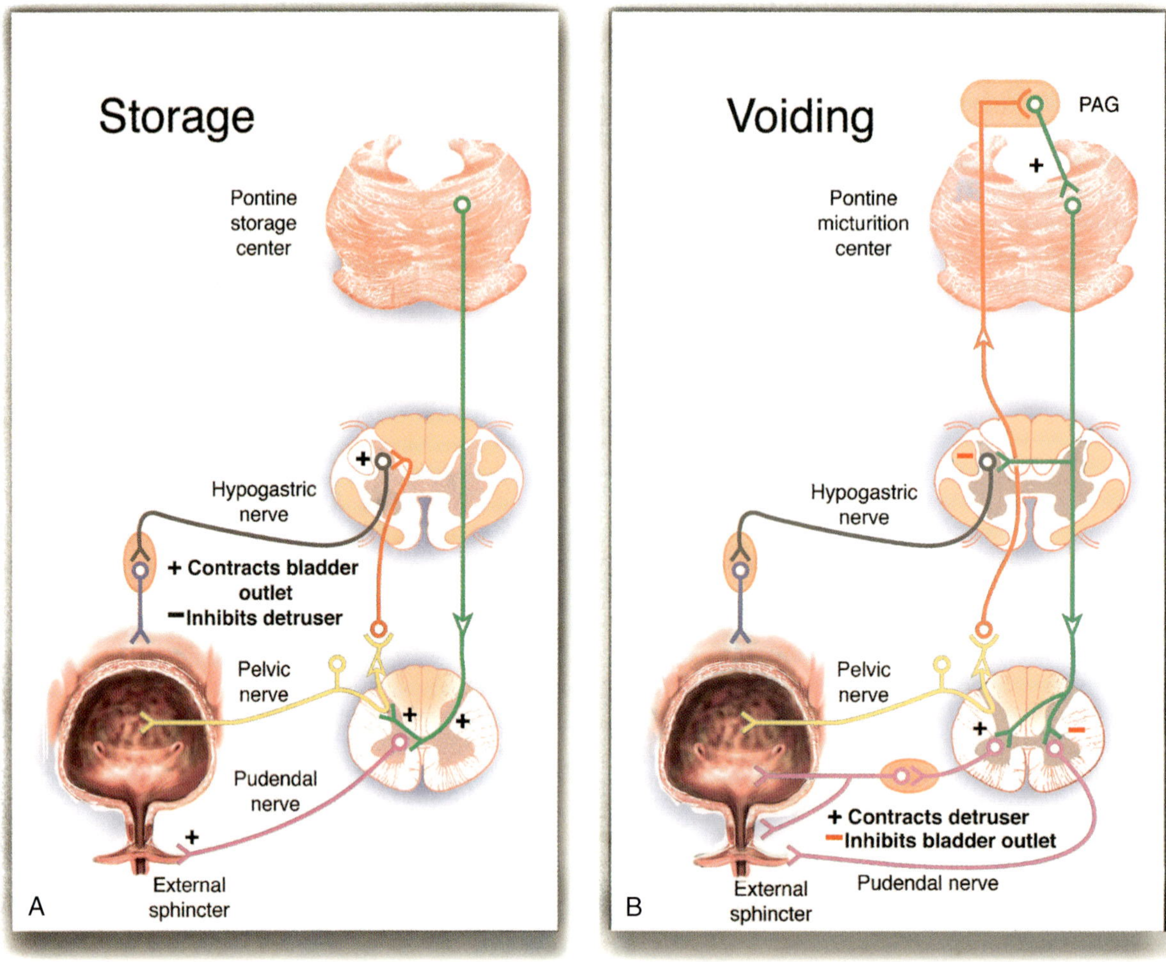

Fig. 31.5 A schematic representation of storage and voiding reflexes. **A**, During bladder storage, distension of the bladder causes afferent signals that, in turn, cause efferent signals via the hypogastric nerve (sympathetic system, relaxation) and the pudendal nerve (increased tone of the striated sphincter). **B**, During bladder elimination, increased afferent activity via the pudendal nerve travels through the periaqueductal gray matter through the pontine micturition center and, ultimately, sympathetic outflow (relaxation) and pudendal outflow (urethral tone), while increasing parasympathetic outflow (contraction). *PAG,* Periaqueductal gray.

of neurocircuits in the brain, spinal cord, and end-organ targets that coordinate the activity of smooth and striated muscle in the bladder and urethra. Neurologic lesions of the suprasacral spinal cord and higher centers are associated with DO because of their interruption of these circuits. Suprasacral lesions block the sacral reflex arc from the cerebral cortex and other higher centers that are crucial for both voluntary and involuntary inhibition of the bladder. Patients with suprasacral lesions typically have involuntary detrusor contractions that are usually associated with appropriate relaxation of the urethral sphincter due preservation of long tracts from the pontine region. Neurologic conditions that can result in DO include multiple sclerosis (MS), Parkinson disease (PD), dementia, and cerebrovascular disorders. (See Chapter 33 for more details.)

Multiple sclerosis. MS is a disease of unknown etiology characterized by demyelinated white matter plaque throughout the central nervous system (CNS), typically affecting patients between 20 and 40 years of age. The various locations of plaques within the CNS (cerebral cortex, cerebellum, brainstem, spinal cord, and optic nerve) produce varied neurologic dysfunction and symptoms. Plaques in the frontal lobe of the cerebral cortex or in the lateral columns of the spinal cord are associated with producing lower urinary tract dysfunction.

It is uncommon for patients with MS to report urological symptoms at initial presentation (only 3%–10%) (Aharony et al., 2017); however, because of the progressive nature of MS, close to 100% of patients report LUTS by 10 years following diagnosis (Panicker et al., 2015). Approximately two-thirds of MS patients with lower urinary tract dysfunction show DO on cystometry (de Seze et al., 2007; Litwiller et al., 1999), while approximately 20% to 25% of patients have an underactive or areflexic detrusor. About 25% of patients demonstrate detrusor sphincter dyssynergia (DSD) arising from the loss of coordination between the detrusor and sphincter muscles (Litwiller et al., 1999).

Cerebrovascular disease. Based on the 2018 National Health interview surveys, the prevalence of persons in the United States who report a medical history of stroke increases with age from 3.1% for those aged 45 to 64 years to 11.8% for those over age 75 years. Overall, there has been a trend toward

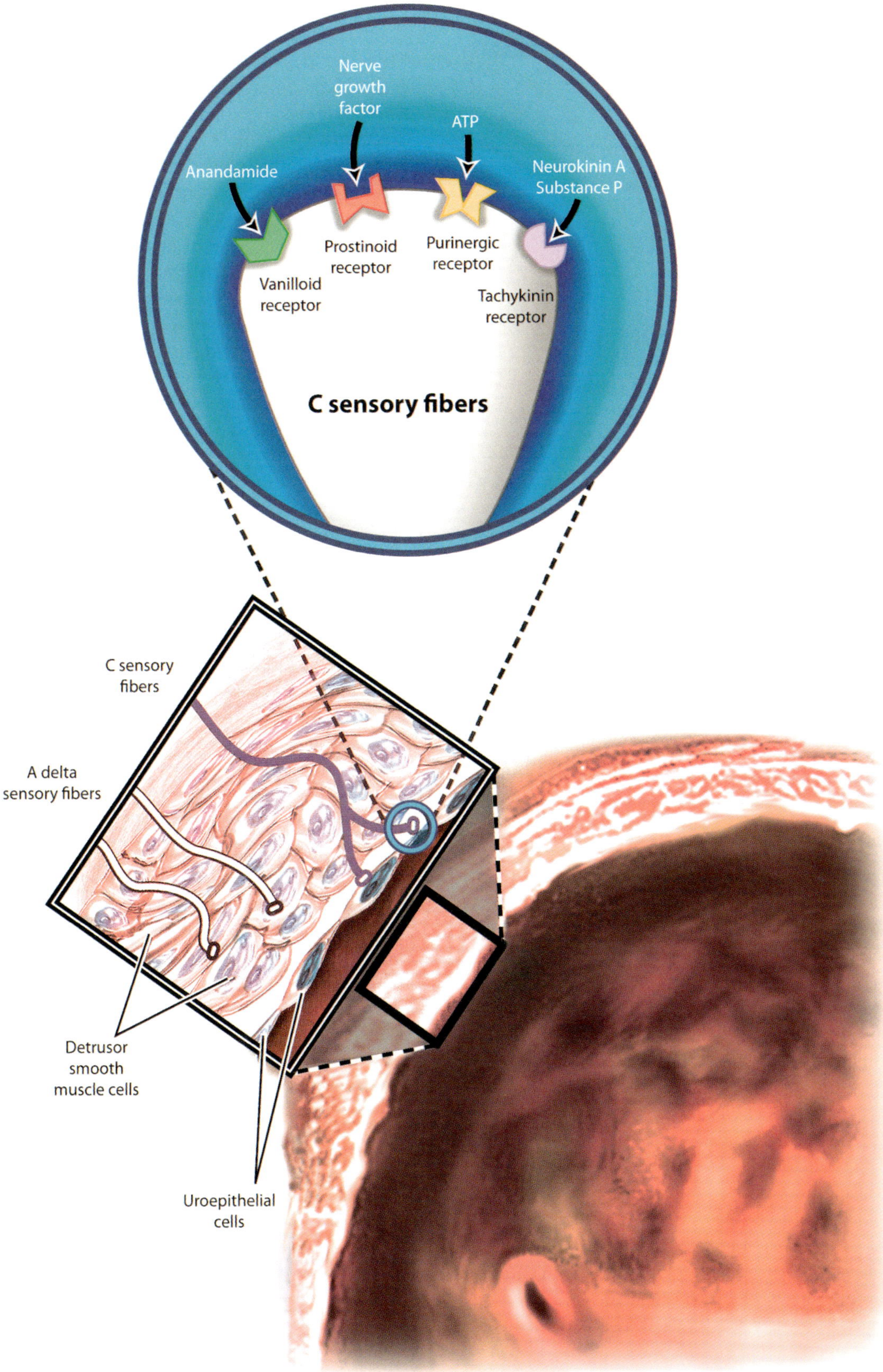

Fig. 31.6 Afferent signaling from the bladder. *ATP*, Adenosine triphosphate.

BOX 31.1 Conditions Associated with Overactive Bladder Syndrome

- Congenital
- Aging
- Neurogenic detrusor overactivity
  - Multiple sclerosis
  - Cerebrovascular disease
  - Parkinson disease
  - Dementia
  - Neoplasia
  - Spinal cord injury
- Bladder outlet obstruction and pelvic surgery
  - Antiincontinence surgery
  - Advanced pelvic organ prolapse
- Psychosomatic disease
- Urine in proximal urethra
- Detrusor overactivity
- Mixed incontinence

higher prevalence of stroke, which can result in varying degrees of chronic disability, including bladder dysfunction, over time in all age populations within the United States. Atherosclerosis, arteritis, intracranial hemorrhage, and arterial malformations may be etiologic factors. Infarction of discrete areas of the frontal lobe of the cerebral cortex, internal capsule (which sends axons between the thalamus and cerebral cortex), brainstem, or cerebellum can result in bladder dysfunction. During the initial phase following a cerebrovascular accident, urinary retention secondary to detrusor areflexia is common. However, during recovery, DO with an appropriate sphincteric response usually occurs. DSD can also rarely be seen in this patient population.

Parkinson disease. The prevalence of PD in industrialized countries is estimated at 0.3% of the entire population and approximately 1% in adults older than 60 years of age (de Lau & Breteler, 2006; Nussbaum & Ellis, 2003). The onset of disease usually occurs after 50 years of age, and the course of the disease is progressive. PD is associated with Lewy body formation and degeneration of cells within the substantia nigra of the midbrain that produce dopamine (Brucker & Kalra, 2017). Dopaminergic mechanisms have both inhibitory effects on micturition via D1 receptors and stimulatory effects via D2 receptors. When substantia nigra pars compacta cells are depleted in PD, there is a loss in D1-mediated inhibition, which leads to DO. The coordinated stimulation of the pontine micturition center at socially acceptable times to urinate is also prevented by the decreased integration of sensory input from the bladder to the periaqueductal gray and a defective ventral tegmental area (Brucker & Kalra, 2017). True DSD does not develop in patients with PD, because pontine micturition is spared.

The prevalence of LUTS in the presence of PD ranges from 27% to 85% (McDonald et al., 2017). A variety of storage symptoms are common, including nocturia (60% of patients), urgency (33%–54%), frequency (16%–36%), and urinary incontinence (26% of males and 28% of females) (Campos-Sousa et al., 2003). Voiding symptoms are less common than storage symptoms, but 44% to 70% of men report hesitancy and poor stream, and 28% of women report straining to void (Sakakibara et al., 2001). The relationship between motor symptoms in PD and bladder dysfunction is complex and nonlinear, and the effects of dopaminergic treatment on bladder control and urodynamic findings in patients with PD can be unpredictable.

Dementia. Dementia is a diffuse loss of cognitive functioning manifested by difficulty with thinking, remembering, and reasoning, as well as impairment of behavioral abilities to such an extent that it interferes with a person's daily life and activities. There are multiple causes of dementia, including aging, severe head injury, encephalitis, hydrocephalus, Pick disease, Alzheimer disease, Jakob–Creutzfeldt disease, and syphilis. Bladder dysfunction can occur in the presence of dementia either from direct involvement of cerebrocortical areas responsible for bladder control or from the loss or inability to control socially appropriate behavior. Depending on the cause or severity of dementia, DO or detrusor areflexia may also occur.

Neoplasia. Neoplasias within the CNS can interrupt normal micturition, resulting in bladder dysfunction. Brain tumors in the superior medial frontal lobe can result in irritative voiding symptoms and DO. Cervical spondylosis and spinal cord tumors above the level of the conus medullaris can also produce DO.

Spinal cord injury. Spinal cord injury is a common cause of DO. Any complete injury to the spinal cord that spares the S2, S3, and S4 segments eventually produces upper motor neuron lesions, resulting in DO. However, during the initial phase of spinal shock following a suprasacral spinal cord injury, the bladder can be areflexic, resulting in urinary retention and overflow incontinence.

Urogynecologic Conditions. Symptoms of urgency and frequency can be present with a variety of conditions, as listed in Box 31.2. Idiopathic DO describes symptoms of urgency and frequency, with or without incontinence, that cannot be explained by the presence of other conditions.

Cystitis. Inflammation of the bladder epithelium, with or without associated bacteriuria, has been suggested as a cause of bladder overactivity. A historic study by Bhatia and Bergman (1986) performed urodynamic studies in women before and

BOX 31.2 Conditions that Produce Symptoms of Urinary Frequency and Urgency

Urogynecologic
- Detrusor overactivity
- Urodynamic stress incontinence
- Mixed incontinence
- Interstitial cystitis
- Urinary tract infection
- Radiation cystitis
- Urogenital atrophy
- Urethral syndrome
- Pelvic organ prolapse
- Urethral diverticulum
- Pregnancy
- Pelvic mass
- Intravesical lesion

Medical
- Neurologic disease
- Congestive heart failure
- Diabetes mellitus
- Diabetes insipidus
- Diuretics

Psychological
- Habit
- Anxiety
- Excessive fluid intake

after treatment of acute UTI. These investigators found that half of patients with urodynamic evidence of DO before treatment for acute UTI had stable CMGs without DO following treatment. The symptoms of OAB syndrome and acute cystitis at onset are usually quite different because cystitis tends to cause an acute onset of dysuria, frequency, urgency, and often hematuria. It is important to distinguish the chronicity of symptoms and to obtain a urinalysis and, if indicated, urine culture to distinguish UTI as the etiology of symptoms and prevent overtreatment with antibiotics (Nik-Ahd et al., 2018).

Hypersensitive bladder disorders. Women with OAB do not usually have accompanying pain. The presence of persistent or recurrent chronic pelvic pain, pressure, or discomfort perceived to be related to the bladder in conjunction with at least one other urinary symptom, such as urgency or frequency, suggests a hypersensitive bladder condition, such as interstitial cystitis or bladder pain syndrome (Doggweiler et al., 2017) - see Chapter 35. Women who have had previous pelvic radiation and those with significant urogenital atrophy may also complain of OAB symptoms.

Urodynamic conditions. Detrusor activity can be triggered by a rise in intraabdominal pressure (seen as P_{abd} on CMG) if leakage of urine into the proximal urethra stimulates urethral afferents that induce involuntary voiding reflexes. If urinary incontinence occurs around the same time as an increase in intraabdominal pressure, this finding can be mistaken as stress incontinence, when in actuality the leakage occurs because of an involuntary detrusor contraction, not urethral sphincter weakness. This is called stress-induced DO and can be diagnosed on urodynamics. Stress urinary incontinence may also coexist with DO in many women, resulting in mixed urinary incontinence, and thus it is important to note if patients with stress-induced DO also have urodynamic stress urinary incontinence and/or DO independent of a stress event.

While studying urinary incontinence in the institutionalized elderly, Resnick and Yalla (1987) noted a subgroup of elderly women with DO resulting in incontinence who could not effectively empty their bladders when attempting to void. Urodynamic testing revealed that impaired voluntary detrusor contraction caused ineffective emptying, while the bladder also demonstrated involuntary overactivity. They named the condition DO with impaired contractility, now known as detrusor hyperactivity with impaired contractility (DHIC) and hypothesized that this may represent the last stage of DO, in which detrusor function deteriorates.

Structural or anatomic conditions. At the level of the urethra, urgency incontinence can occur with outlet obstruction. This is a well-known problem in men with benign prostatic hyperplasia and in younger men and women with spinal cord injuries or other neurologic impairments. In women, bladder outlet resistance from previous antiincontinence surgery can result in irritative voiding symptoms and urgency incontinence. Idiopathic bladder outlet obstruction is rare in women and requires video urodynamics to make a diagnosis of primary bladder neck obstruction (Nitti, 2005). Whereas abnormal voiding in women is often caused by poor detrusor function, rather than physical obstruction, obstructed voiding can be seen with advanced pelvic organ prolapse and after operations for stress incontinence.

Women who have undergone radical pelvic surgery may develop OAB postoperatively, likely because of partial denervation of the bladder during the operative process with subsequent development of detrusor dysfunction. Other conditions that can impact the lower urinary tract and result in OAB symptoms include pregnancy, pelvic mass, urethral diverticulum, and intravesical lesions including malignancy.

Orgasm. Urinary incontinence with orgasm has been found to be associated with DO (Mendez et al., 2018). The pathogenesis is unknown, but women sometimes experience urinary urgency or urgency incontinence, with a gush of urine during sexual climax. A prospective case-control study of 132 women found that 69% of women with climacturia also had DO on urodynamics, compared to only 39% of those with incontinence with vaginal penetration (Serati et al., 2008). Treatment is the same as for DO; sexual counseling and education are often helpful.

Mixed incontinence. The prevalence of mixed urinary incontinence in women ranges from 14% to 61% (Nitti, 2001). When surgery is performed for the correction of stress urinary incontinence in women, DO postoperatively may resolve, worsen, or remain unchanged. Women may condition themselves to have urgency and frequency by becoming habitual frequent voiders. This can be seen in women with long-standing stress incontinence, because they will consciously or subconsciously void more frequently to avoid or reduce leakage. Over time, it has been proposed that functional bladder capacity is reduced, and the bladder becomes more sensitive at lower volumes of urine, thus resulting in frequency and urgency (OAB dry). This same phenomenon can occur in women with urgency incontinence, resulting in more severe frequency. This can be viewed as a cycle in which symptoms continue to worsen unless intervention is undertaken (Fig. 31.7).

Idiopathic Detrusor Overactivity. Idiopathic DO is defined as involuntary detrusor contractions without an identifiable underlying cause (D'Ancona et al., 2019). Because of the difficulty

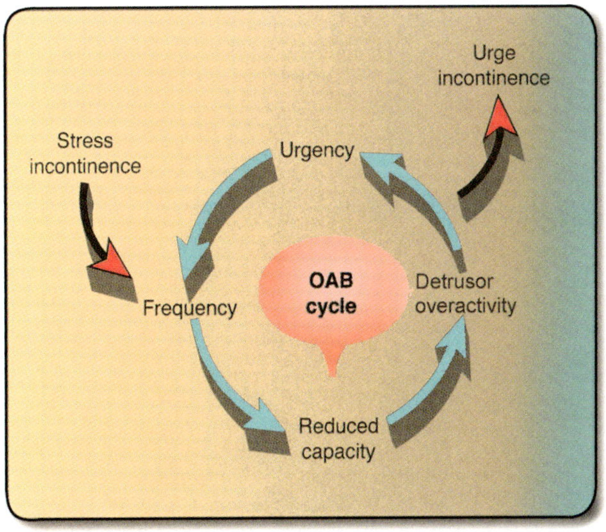

Fig. 31.7 Cycle of bladder dysfunction. *OAB,* Overactive bladder.

in identifying the underlying pathology for the development of OAB in most patients, their OAB is often labeled as "idiopathic." Prior hypotheses have thought of idiopathic DO as either being of neurogenic etiology (DO arising from generalized nerve mediated excitation of the detrusor muscle) or myogenic etiology (DO resulting from a combination of an increased likelihood of spontaneous excitation within smooth muscle of the bladder and enhanced propagation and subsequent spread of contractile signals via cell-to-cell coupling). However, more recently, OAB syndrome is thought to comprise several OAB phenotypes with different underlying mechanisms and pathophysiological causes (Peyronnet et al., 2019). Fig. 31.8 demonstrates a new diagnostic approach to seek the underlying pathophysiological phenotypes for OAB.

Evaluation

Per the joint guidelines on the Diagnosis and Treatment of Overactive Bladder (Non-Neurogenic) in Adults from the American Urological Association (AUA) and Society of Urodynamics, Female Pelvic Medicine, and Urogenital Reconstruction (SUFU), which were amended and endorsed by the American Urogynecologic Society in 2019, the minimum requirements in evaluation for OAB of an uncomplicated, non-neurogenic patient are careful history, physical exam, and urinalysis (Gormley et al., 2015; Lightner et al., 2019). One of the key elements in evaluating women with OAB is the impact of their symptoms on quality of life. Standardized quality-of-life questionnaires are available and can be administered to help with evaluation of quality of life and to track progression over time. In addition, it is important to assess concomitant pelvic organ prolapse, defecatory complaints, and sexual dysfunction. A thorough medical history should be taken, as well as a surgical history with emphasis on previous lower urinary tract or gynecologic surgery. A thorough review of all prescription medications that the patient is currently taking, and as well as previously tried OAB medications, is also vital.

Physical Examination. In the evaluation of OAB, a clinician should perform a general physical, neurologic, and pelvic examination (Gormley et al., 2015). Neurologic studies should include a brief mental status examination and evaluation of cranial nerves and deep tendon reflexes. Muscle strength can be assessed by having the patient actively move against resistance, such as shrugging her shoulders against downward pressure. Specifically testing the sacral spinal cord involves evaluating the patient's ability to extend and flex her hip, knee, and ankle, and invert and evert her foot. Deep tendon reflexes can be checked at the biceps (C5–C6), triceps (C7), knee (L3–L4), and Achilles tendon (L5–S2).

Spinal cord segments S2, S3, and S4 contain important neurons involved in micturition. The anal sphincter and pelvic reflexes are important indicators of sacral cord integrity. Voluntary contraction of the external anal sphincter indicates a minimum level of integrity of pelvic floor innervation. Stroking the skin lateral to the anus elicits a reflex anal sphincter contraction. The bulbocavernosus reflex involves tightening of the bulbocavernosus and ischiocavernosus muscles by tapping or squeezing the clitoris. The cerebellum should also be tested because it has major functions in the control of micturition. The cerebellum can be tested by evaluating finger/nose and heel/shin coordination and examining the patient's gait.

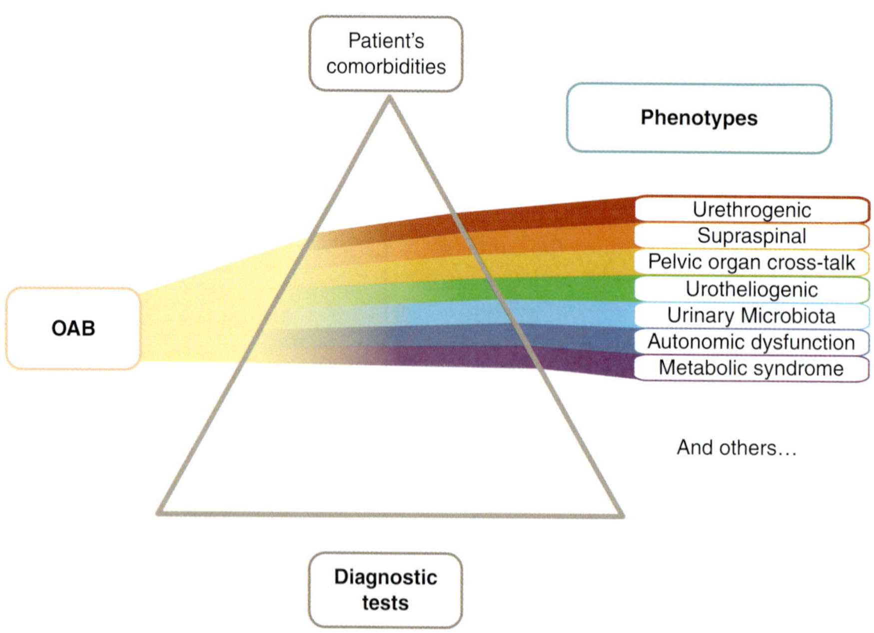

Fig. 31.8 Overactive bladder *(OAB)* syndrome with multiple possible underlying pathophysiological phenotypes. Identifying phenotypes could probably be achieved through a thorough clinical examination and may include urodynamic testing or other testing in selected cases. (From Peyronnet B, Mironska E, Chapple C, et al. A Comprehensive review of overactive bladder pathophysiology: on the way to tailored treatment. *Eur Urol.* 2019;75:988.)

A pelvic examination should include a thorough inspection of the perineal area and vulva, looking for excoriation, vaginal discharge, or atrophy, suggesting estrogen deficiency. Vaginal examination should include assessment for pelvic organ prolapse, pelvic muscle function, atrophy, and anatomic abnormalities. The urethra can be palpated through the anterior vagina, checking for a mass or purulent discharge from the urethral meatus consistent with a urethral diverticulum. Pelvic floor muscle function should be described by pelvic muscle tone at rest and by the strength of voluntary contraction (see Chapter 9). Determining the postvoid residual, either with ultrasound or by performing straight catheterization, can help rule out occult voiding dysfunction, as well as DHIC. However, postvoid residual measurement is not necessary for patients who are receiving first-line behavioral interventions or for uncomplicated patients (those without a history of or risk factors for urinary retention) receiving antimuscarinic medications (Gormley et al., 2015). Pelvic organ prolapse should be evaluated, specifically commenting on the support of the anterior, apical, and posterior vagina. Rectal examination should also be performed to rule out fecal impaction and rectal mass while assessing sphincter tone.

Diagnostic Studies

Urinalysis and urine culture. Because the symptoms of UTI and other irritative bladder conditions commonly mimic OAB, urinalysis should be performed before further investigations or treatments are initiated. As previously mentioned, bacteriuria may cause DO, which sometimes resolves after the infection has been treated. Urinalysis and, if indicated, microscopy, should also be used to screen for microhematuria, which would warrant further investigation for urothelial neoplasm.

Voiding diary. A voiding diary can be a useful tool for both patients and clinicians alike as a way to quantify and temporally map their urinary frequency and incontinence episodes. A completed voiding diary tracking up to 72 hours of a patient's fluid intake and voiding habits can help to corroborate their history and symptoms. A follow-up voiding diary can also be useful to provide evidence to both patient and clinician of treatment response.

Urodynamic testing

Cystometry. Cystometry is the critical portion of urodynamics testing for investigating bladder storage function, as it is the only method of objectively diagnosing detrusor contraction. Fig. 31.9 reviews the various cystometric patterns that may

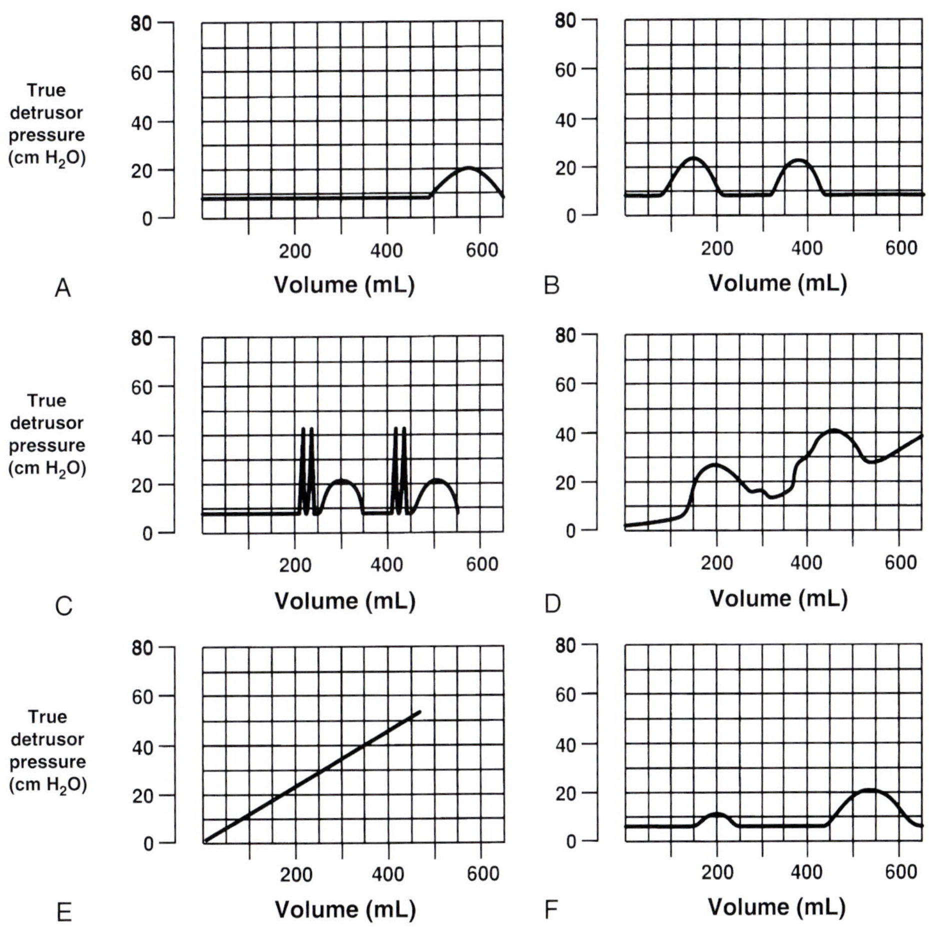

Fig. 31.9 Patients with detrusor overactivity can exhibit a variety of cystometric patterns. **A**, Normal filling cystometry with voluntary terminal detrusor contraction. **B**, Phasic involuntary detrusor contractions with detrusor pressure returning to baseline. **C**, Cough-provoked (or stress-induced) detrusor instability (intravesical instead of true detrusor pressure is depicted here). **D**, Phasic contractions with steady rise in detrusor pressure demonstrating poor compliance. **E**, Steady rise in detrusor pressure indicating a bladder with poor compliance. **F**, Subthreshold detrusor instability with voluntary terminal contraction.

be seen in patients with DO. (See Chapter 11 for more details.) Per the AUA/SUFU guidelines, "urodynamics are not recommended in the initial diagnostic workup of the uncomplicated OAB patient" (Lightner et al., 2019). However, for complicated patients or refractory patients who have failed multiple OAB treatments, urodynamics can be performed based on the clinician's judgment. Fig. 31.10 reviews the diagnosis and treatment algorithm from the AUA/SUFU guideline on Diagnosis and Treatment of Overactive Bladder (Non-Neurogenic) in Adults.

When performing urodynamic testing for a patient with OAB, it is important to try to replicate their bothersome symptoms during the study. Sometimes this requires clinicians to use provocative stimuli if detrusor contractions are not elicited during the filling phase. Testing should be performed with the patient in a sitting or erect position, because supine filling cystometry alone often fails to uncover a significant proportion of bladder overactivity. Other provoking factors that can be performed during the testing session include coughing, straining, heel-bouncing, jogging in place, listening to running water, and placing the patient's hands under running water. It is also useful to ask patients what typically prompts their symptoms and try to replicate those maneuvers during urodynamic testing.

It is important to remember that DO is a diagnosis made by findings on CMG, whereas OAB is a syndrome based on clinical symptoms; therefore, the absence of DO on urodynamics does not exclude a diagnosis of OAB. Al-Ghazo et al. (2011) found an overall incidence of DO in 76.1% of male patients and 58.7% of female patients with OAB. A higher percentage of patients (93% of men, 69.8% of women) were found to have DO when they had both symptoms of urgency and UUI. Overall, a combination of LUTS resulted in a higher likelihood of actually seeing DO on urodynamics.

Vecchioli-Scaldazza and Grinta (2010) explored the relationship between the presence of DO on urodynamics and the response to treatment with anticholinergics in patients with OAB. This study demonstrated that DO is not found in all subjects with OAB but that, when found, those patients respond more favorably to anticholinergic treatment. The authors suggested

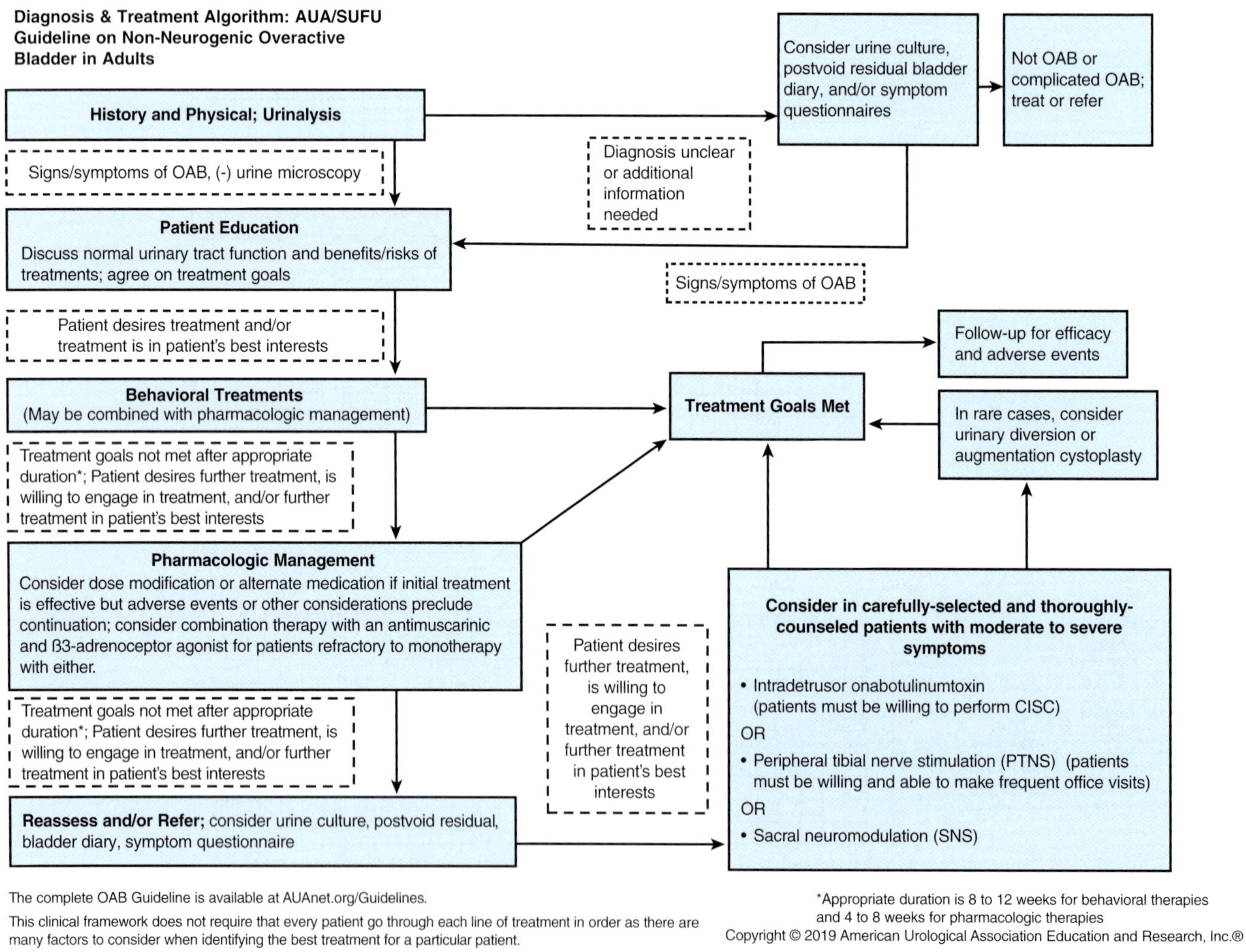

Fig. 31.10 Diagnosis and treatment algorithm from the American Urological Association (*AUA*) and Society of Urodynamics, Female Pelvic Medicine, and Urogenital Reconstruction (*SUFU*) guidelines on the Diagnosis and Treatment of Overactive Bladder (Non-Neurogenic) in Adults. *OAB*, Overactive bladder; *CISC*, clean intermittent self-catheterization. (From Lightner DJ, Gomelsky A, Souter L, Vasavada SP. Diagnosis and treatment of overactive bladder (non-neurogenic) in adults: AUA/SUFU guideline amendment 2019. *J Urol.* 2019;202:558.)

that anticholinergic therapy is most effective in patients with demonstrated DO and, thus, that urodynamics should be considered in all patients with OAB as a predictor for success of therapy. However, more importantly, this study sheds light on the point discussed above regarding a variety of different phenotypes of patients within the spectrum of OAB syndrome that may respond differently to various treatment options.

Overall, urodynamics testing is not necessary in a patient with uncomplicated (nonneurogenic) OAB before starting treatment and progressing through the treatment algorithm provided in the AUA/SUFU guideline (see Fig. 31.10). However, certain scenarios, such as refractory or complicated cases or concern for underlying neurogenic dysfunction, may warrant urodynamic testing based on the clinician's judgment.

Urethral pressure studies. Urethral pressure studies add little to the diagnosis of DO or to the differentiation of patients with stress incontinence from those with urgency incontinence. Detrusor contractions are almost always preceded by a drop in urethral pressure (Fig. 31.11). Bergman et al. (1989) studied urethral pressure tracings in 72 women with DO to learn whether urethral pressure changes may be the cause, rather than the effect, of bladder contractions. Patients who had urethral relaxation before detrusor contractions responded better to sympathomimetic drugs, whereas patients without urethral pressure changes responded more favorably to anticholinergic drugs.

Electromyography. Electromyography (EMG) gives information on the activity of the external striated urethral sphincter muscles. Its potential value in patients with DO is to document voluntary control of this sphincter, as well as to demonstrate that the external sphincter and detrusor muscle function in a coordinated fashion (Fig. 31.12). Mayo (1978) found that 48% of patients with idiopathic DO exhibited reflex relaxation of the sphincter at the time of a detrusor contraction. This observation is important because these patients are probably unable to voluntarily contract the external sphincter at the moment of the

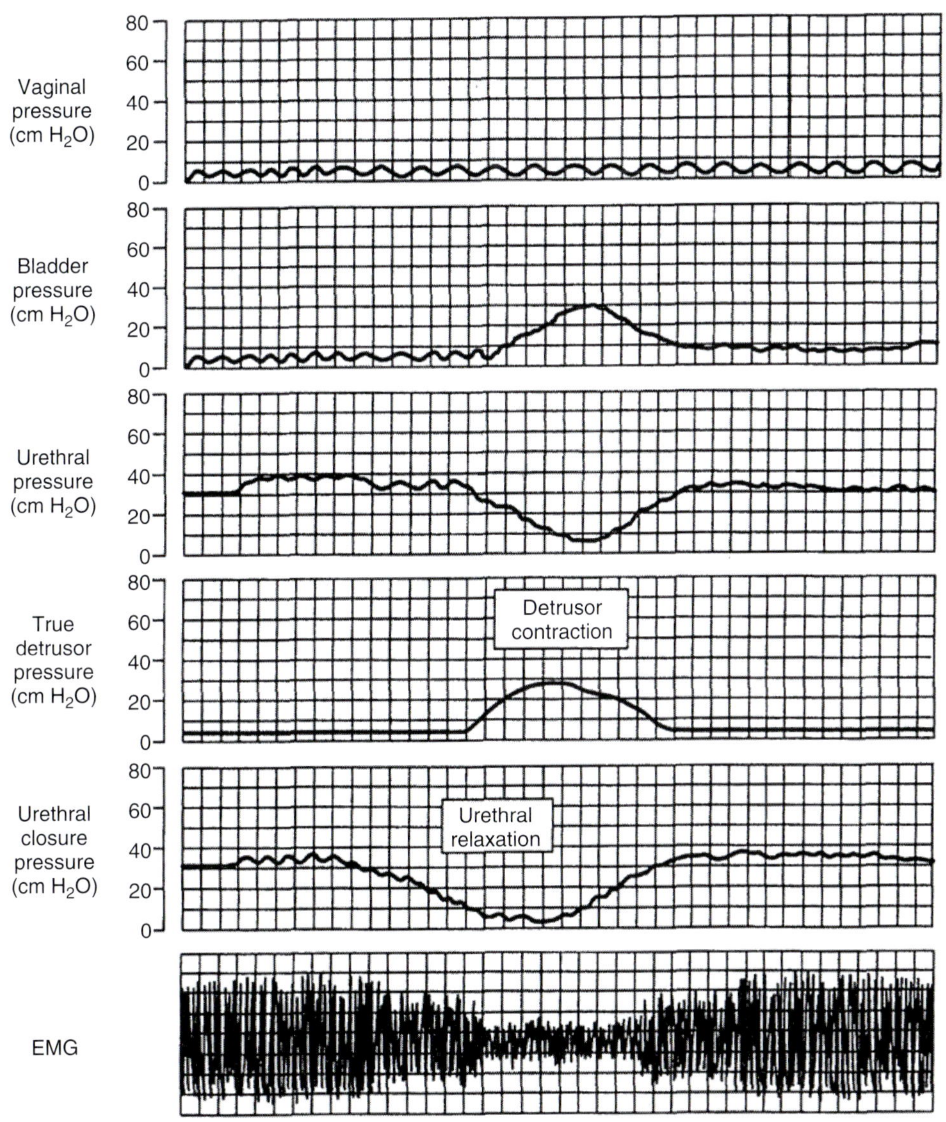

Fig. 31.11 Multichannel urethrocystometry showing detrusor contraction and concomitant urethral relaxation. In this example there is quieting of electromyography (*EMG*) activity; however, often with guarding, EMG activity will be increased with involuntary detrusor contraction.

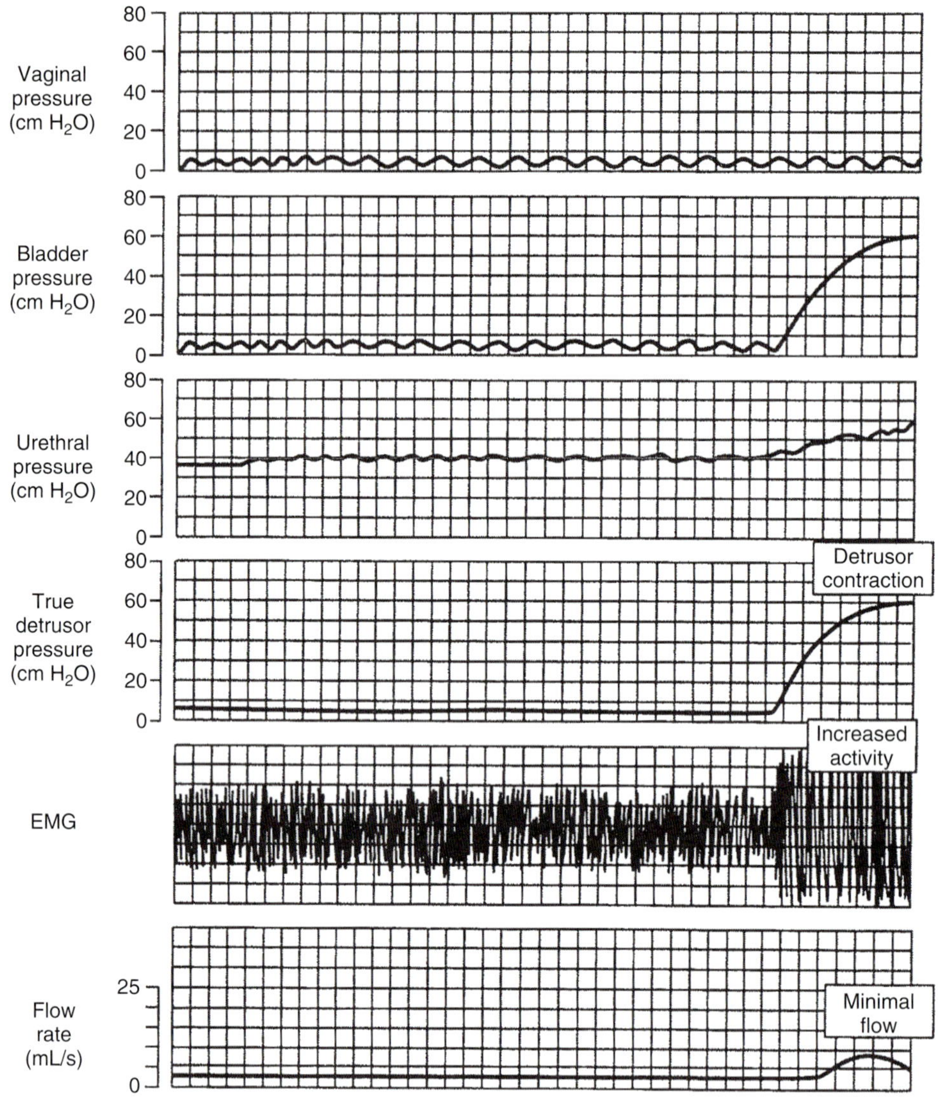

Fig. 31.12 Polypropylene mesh in the bladder of a patient who had previously undergone midurethral sling placement. *EMG*, Electromyography.

detrusor contraction; thus, their ability to inhibit urine loss is limited.

Endoscopy. Similar to urodynamics, the routine use of cystourethroscopy is not indicated in the evaluation of uncomplicated OAB (Lightner et al., 2019). However, certain findings during the evaluation of a patient with OAB may warrant cystourethroscopic examination. Box 31.3 lists clinical situations in which clinicians should consider cystourethroscopy in the setting of suspected OAB. For example, a history of a midurethral sling placement with polypropylene mesh and new onset of OAB symptoms might be indicative of mesh erosion into the urethra or bladder, which could be diagnosed with cystoscopy (see Chapter 25). Other indications for cystourethroscopy include physical examination findings of a mass below the urethra consistent with urethral diverticulum or concern for urethral malignancy. Nosti and Sokol (2012) reported an unusual case of an elderly woman with OAB and a history of lithium use for bipolar disorder. The patient was found to have suburothelial

BOX 31.3 Clinical Situations Where Cystourethroscopy Should Be Considered in the Setting of Overactive Bladder

- Hematuria
- History of recurrent UTIs
- Persistent or *de novo* OAB after an incontinence procedure
- *De novo* OAB after pelvic surgery
- Long-term indwelling catheter use
- Abnormal-appearing bladder on imaging
- Positive cytology
- Mixed symptoms with pain
- Prior mesh placement
- History of bladder cancer
- Occupational exposure

OAB, Overactive bladder; *UTIs*, urinary tract infections.

metal deposition that was felt to be related to her OAB by acting as a bladder irritant. The clinician should always pay attention to occupational exposures or medications that could potentially be bladder irritants.

Definitive indications for cystourethroscopy include gross or microscopic hematuria, see Chapter 40 (Lightner et al., 2019). Cystourethroscopy can also be considered if the diagnosis is in doubt or if the patient shows no response to appropriate behavioral and pharmacological therapy.

Management

There is a wide variety of treatment options available to the practitioner caring for patients with OAB. Treatments range from nonsurgical to surgical, with varying degrees of invasiveness and monetary and time investment. OAB can have a significant effect on a woman's quality of life, and, as already discussed, before discussing management option the specific patient's degree of bother should be assessed. The severity of the woman's symptoms, along with the degree of invasiveness of certain treatments and associated adverse events, most likely will contribute to a woman's perception of what will be the most reasonable therapeutic option for her to pursue. As there is no known "cure" for OAB, it is important that patients have a realistic expectation and aspiration for symptom management.

See Box 31.4 for a list of various treatment options for OAB. This chapter will specifically focus on first- and second-line treatments (see Fig. 31.10) for OAB. Third-line treatments are discussed in detail in Chapter 32.

Nonpharmacologic Management of Overactive Bladder. Behavioral modifications and lifestyle changes are an important first-line treatment for patients with OAB. Clinicians should have a conversation with patients to educate them about their symptoms and condition. There should be a thorough discussion of the nature and volume of fluid intake and dietary irritants. Fluid management remains an important method of self-management, as it requires a delicate balance between avoiding excess fluid consumption and preventing dehydration from too little fluid (Newman & Burgio, 2016).

Physicians should encourage patients to maintain adequate hydration by ingesting six 8-ounce glasses or 30 mL/kg body weight per day (minimum of 1500 mL/day) unless other medical comorbidities preclude this. And although overall fluid restriction should not be recommended, clinicians can help guide patients in restricting fluids at particular times to decrease the bother of OAB symptoms. Some possible times when fluid restriction could be helpful include when toilet access will be limited (e.g., sporting or social events) and in the hours leading up to bedtime, to decrease nocturia (Newman & Burgio, 2016). For patients who have increased overnight urine production owing to retained fluid during the day and fluid mobilization at night, behavioral modifications, such as wearing support stockings or elevating the lower extremities during the day, can be helpful to mobilize this fluid before bedtime.

Bladder retraining. Bladder retraining institutes a program of scheduled voiding with progressive increases in the interval between each void, based on the assumption that conscious efforts to suppress sensory stimuli will reestablish cortical control over an uninhibited bladder, thus reestablishing normal voiding patterns. This therapy has been studied by Frewen (1982), Fantyle et al. (1981), and others.

In several studies, Frewen reported success rates of approximately 80% using bladder retraining. However, his protocol included primarily in-hospital behavioral management, which is not realistic in a modern setting, and concurrent pharmacologic therapy. Fantl et al. reported on 92 patients with objective evidence of DO treated by bladder drill, with or without anticholinergic therapy. Cure rates were the same in both groups: 83% in patients treated with bladder drill and drugs, and 79% in patients treated with bladder drill alone. These high cure rates with bladder retraining drills have been substantiated by other authors.

The technique used for bladder retraining involves giving the patient insight into the nature of her dysfunction. The patient can be shown drawings demonstrating cerebral cortical inhibitory effects over bladder reflexes to assist in explaining lower urinary tract dysfunction. The patient's own cystometric tracing can be shown to her to illustrate the dysfunction. The patient is taught scheduled voiding at timed intervals, varying from 15 minutes to 1 hour, based on the patient's own frequency or incontinence intervals. One can typically start patients at voiding intervals of 30 to 60 minutes. Patients are given preprinted cards on which they record voiding (daily and nightly), involuntary leaking episodes, and occurrences that precipitate incontinence. Patients are instructed to make an earnest effort to follow the schedule during the day, attempting to suppress urgency and voiding only at the scheduled times regardless of the presence or absence of urinary urgency. Patients are instructed to contract their pelvic floor muscles when they feel urgency and impending urgency incontinence, to suppress involuntary bladder overactivity. Using this protocol, bladder training schedules are not followed during sleeping hours. Follow-up visits are scheduled every 1 to 2 weeks, at which time the cards are reviewed with the patient. Voiding intervals are increased periodically by 15 to 60 minutes, according to the patient's response in reducing urgency and urgency incontinence episodes. A 6- to 12-week treatment program is anticipated in most cases.

BOX 31.4 Nonsurgical Treatment Options for Overactive Bladder

- Treatment of associated conditions
  - Stress incontinence
  - Outlet obstruction
- Treatment of detrusor overactivity
  - Behavioral treatment
    - Bladder retraining
    - Biofeedback
  - Functional electrical stimulation
  - Acupuncture
- Pharmacologic treatment
  - Anticholinergic
  - Adrenergic agonists
  - Antispasmodic
  - β-3-adrenergic agonist
  - Afferent mechanisms
  - Central mechanisms
  - Tricyclic antidepressants

Enthusiastic patient contact, reassurance, good long-term support, and follow-up are important. Patients must be highly motivated to improve with this therapy, and the degree of patient compliance often coincides with success. Because the success rate is so good and the therapy involves low cost, bladder retraining drills should be offered as a first line of therapy in patients with DO. Modifications of the protocol listed above are clinician-dependent, but oftentimes include some form of patient education and timed voiding.

Biofeedback. Biofeedback is a form of patient reeducation, such that normally unconscious physiologic processes are made accessible by auditory, visual, or tactile signals, while attempts are made to modify the process by manipulating the signal presented to the patient. This method has been used with some success in the treatment of autonomic dysfunctions, hypertension, and cardiac dysrhythmias. Biofeedback appears to alter the faciliatory and inhibitory balance in the CNS to modify the complex events that result in the perception of the sensation of urinary urge (Dmochowski, 2002). This results in the urge to void being inhibited or not perceived as often.

As an example of how biofeedback can be used to treat DO, after cystometry is explained to the patient, bladder filling begins, and an audible signal is used to let the patient know that her bladder pressure is rising. The tone of the signal varies by the change in bladder pressure. The patient also visualizes the urodynamic tracing throughout the test. The bladder is repeatedly filled while the patient attempts to inhibit detrusor contractions. Individual treatment sessions are approximately one hour and are repeated weekly for up to 8 weeks.

Cardozo et al. (1978) found that biofeedback yielded 81% subjective and objective improvement for patients with DO. However, they did note that biofeedback was not as successful in patients with severe DO, particularly in women with high-amplitude detrusor contractions occurring at small bladder volumes. Another study by Burgio et al. (1985) combined biofeedback with behavioral treatments in patients with and without urodynamic evidence of DO and showed a large reduction in urge urinary incontinence. Patients with urodynamic evidence of DO had a mean 85% improvement, while patients without urodynamic evidence of DO had a mean 94% improvement.

Another study by Burgio et al. (2002) randomized 222 women to three different treatment arms, including a biofeedback-assisted behavior training, behavioral training without biofeedback (verbal feedback based on vaginal palpation), and self-administered behavioral treatment based on a self-help booklet. No significant differences were noted in symptom improvement between the three groups, but patient satisfaction was higher in the two groups receiving behavioral training. These findings are consistent with a systematic review published in 2005 that found no evidence that biofeedback in addition to pelvic floor muscle rehabilitation provided added benefit to pelvic floor muscle rehabilitation alone (Gray & David, 2005).

Many investigators use biofeedback techniques aimed at identifying and strengthening pelvic floor muscles. In addition, appropriate control of the external urethral sphincter mechanism may enhance the urethrovesical inhibitory reflex.

Functional electrical stimulation. Although less popular, because of the limitations that will be discussed, functional electrical stimulation (FES) is a nonsurgical option for treating OAB. FES stimulates the afferent limb of the pudendal reflex arc, increasing pelvic floor muscle and urethral striated muscle contractility and possibly stimulating reflex inhibition of detrusor contractility. Some patients who are refractory to behavioral and pharmacologic therapies respond to FES. The main difficulty with FES is patient acceptance of intravaginal or transrectal stimulation. Originally, patients were required to use the devices for several hours daily. The results reported in Leach and Bavendam (1989) clearly point out these limitations, showing a 94% dropout rate in a study of 36 patients using a transrectal stimulating device.

To overcome the requirement for long treatment sessions, investigators have studied the efficacy of intermittent maximal electrical stimulation in treating incontinence. With this therapy, the patient receives a short period of stimulation (e.g., 30 minutes) at maximum tolerable intensity. Treatment is continued over several weeks. Eriksen et al. (1989) reported short-term maximal pelvic floor electrical stimulation in 48 patients with idiopathic DO. Each patient received 20 minutes of simultaneous vaginal and anal electrical stimulation for an average of seven treatments. Initial clinical and urodynamic cures were observed in 50% of patients, with significant improvement in an additional 33%. At 1-year follow-up, persistent positive therapeutic effects were found in 77% of patients. In another study, Plevnik et al. (1986) treated 30 patients with DO with maximal electrical stimulation at home for 20 minutes per day for 30 days. Cure was noted in 29%; an additional 22% reported improvement. Bent et al. (1989) noted significant subjective improvement in 69% of patients with DO, using a regimen of 15 minutes of maximal stimulation twice daily for 6 weeks. Spruijt et al. (2003) randomized 24 postmenopausal women with urinary incontinence to intravaginal electrical stimulation or a daily Kegel exercise program. The effectiveness of FES was similar to Kegel exercises (29.2% vs. 36.4% for objective improvement, and 29.2% vs. 27.3% for subjective improvement). Wang et al. (2004) evaluated pelvic floor muscle training with and without biofeedback assistance and FES for 103 women with OAB. These authors found that OAB symptoms were reduced in about half of women treated with FES and biofeedback-assisted pelvic muscle training, compared with 38% treated with pelvic muscle training alone (although this difference was not statistically significant).

The role of FES as therapy for OAB is still evolving. Although currently not a first-line therapy, FES may be a beneficial option to certain groups of patients who have failed multiple treatments.

Pharmacologic Management of Overactive Bladder. Antimuscarinic pharmacotherapy has historically been a mainstay in the treatment for OAB. Over the past decade, β-3-adrenergic agonists have become a much-needed alternative for the pharmacologic treatment of OAB, either alone or in combination with anticholinergics. Other medications that work on different aspects of the neurophysiology of micturition will also be reviewed in this section (Table 31.1).

TABLE 31.1 Drug Classification and Mechanism of Action

Classification	Mechanism of Action/Comments	Drugs	Dosage
Anticholinergic	Inhibits muscarinic receptors	Oxybutynin	2.5–5 mg tid IR 5–15 mg qd ER 3.9 mg/4 days TD
		Tolterodine	1–2 mg bid IR 4 mg qd ER
		Propantheline	15 mg bid to 30 mg qid
		Trospium	20 mg bid
		Solifenacin	5–10 mg qd
		Darifenacin	7.5–15 mg qd
α-Adrenergic agonist	Increases urethral closure pressure	Ephedrine	25 mg PO qid
		Pseudoephedrine	Non-ER: 60 mg PO qid ER: 120 mg PO bid
Antispasmodic	Unknown	Baclofen	Initial dose: 5 mg orally three times a day for 3 days Then 10 mg orally three times a day for 3 days Then 15 mg orally three times a day for 3 days Then 20 mg orally three times a day Maintenance dose: 40–80 mg/day 80-mg/day doses should be administered in four divided doses
β-3-adrenergic agonist	Detrusor muscle relaxation	Mirabegron	25–50 mg qd ER
Afferent nerve inhibitor	Blocks sensory input to bladder	Capsaicin	Investigational
		Resiniferatoxin	Investigational
Tricyclic antidepressant	Some anticholinergic properties, smooth muscle relaxation, and norepinephrine reuptake inhibition	Imipramine	25 mg qd to 75 mg bid
		Amitriptyline	10 mg/d PO; titrate by 10 mg/week until maximum dose of 50 mg is reached, urinary symptoms disappear, or adverse effects become intolerable
Botulinum toxin	Inhibits release of acetylcholine	Toxins A and B	200–300 U injected cystoscopically
Central-acting	Serotonin and norepinephrine reuptake inhibitor	Duloxetine	Investigational

IR, Immediate release; *ER*, extended release; *TD*, transdermal; *PO*, per os.

There is no pharmacologic cure for OAB. Therefore, the goals of pharmacologic treatment are to reduce symptoms as much as possible and improve quality of life. It is always important to consider the side effect profile and possible polypharmacy interactions when prescribing medications for OAB. Per the AUA/SUFU guidelines (see Fig. 31.10), patients should be offered pharmacologic management for their OAB symptoms for an appropriate duration of 4 to 8 weeks. Following this, if their treatment goals are not met, dose modification or alternative pharmacologic treatment, such as switching to a different antimuscarinic medication or considering combination therapy with an antimuscarinic and a β-3-adrenoreceptor agonist, can be considered. Dose titration can be used in the hope of delivering the highest tolerable dose while limiting adverse side effects from medications.

Antimuscarinic agents. As previously mentioned, all five pharmacologically defined muscarinic receptors, M1 to M5, have been demonstrated to exist within the human bladder; however, the most prevalent types are the M2 and M3 receptors (Giglio & Tobin, 2009). Antimuscarinic drugs act by blocking the muscarinic receptors on the detrusor muscle from binding neurotransmitters released from activated cholinergic (parasympathetic) nerves, thereby inhibiting bladder contractility, decreasing sensory input, and increasing bladder capacity. In addition to muscarinic receptors within the lower urinary tract, muscarinic receptors are found in other regions of the body, such as the salivary glands, parotid gland, gastrointestinal tract, brain, eyes, and heart. Because the same subtypes of muscarinic receptors are found in these other organs and organ systems, antimuscarinic use in the treatment of lower urinary tract dysfunction is hindered by "uroselectivity" (Andersson, 1998) and the side effects caused by muscarinic blockade outside of the lower urinary tract.

Oxybutynin has some selectivity for M3 receptors to inhibit bladder contractions, but, because of muscarinic blockade in other parts of the body, it can have bothersome side effects. Oxybutynin has a higher affinity for muscarinic receptors in the parotid gland compared with the bladder, leading to the common side effect of dry mouth. Additionally, after first-pass hepatic metabolism, the concentration of the active metabolite of oxybutynin, *N*-desethyl-oxybutynin, can be six-fold higher than that of the parent compound after oral administration. Other side effects include constipation, gastrointestinal upset, blurred vision, dizziness, and impaired cognition. Alternative approaches have been developed to improve tolerability, including extended-release (ER) oral formulations, rectal or intravesical administration, and transdermal administration. In trials that compare ER with immediate-release (IR) formulations, ER oxybutynin had similar efficacy but reduced side effects. Absorption of ER oxybutynin may occur more in the large intestine, rather than the stomach and proximal small intestine, thereby decreasing conversion to *N*-desethyl-oxybutynin.

Transdermal oxybutynin affords the added benefit of bypassing hepatic metabolism, thereby providing more stable plasma concentrations and decreased levels of the primary active metabolite, *N*-desethyl-oxybutynin (Cohn et al., 2016). In a study of transdermal oxybutynin 3.9 mg per day and ER oxybutynin 10 mg once a day, the transdermal drug showed greater systemic availability, with less metabolism to *N*-desethyl-oxybutynin and greater salivary output. Dmochowski et al. (2002) studied 361 adults with OAB symptoms who were randomly assigned to transdermal oxybutynin, ER tolterodine 4 mg, or placebo. Transdermal oxybutynin and ER tolterodine were superior to placebo in reducing daily incontinent episodes and improving quality of life. Localized pruritus occurred in 14% of patients using transdermal oxybutynin. Despite an improved side effect profile, patients may still choose to discontinue transdermal oxybutynin use because of other anticholinergic side effects and application site reactions.

Under certain circumstances, it may be beneficial to increase oxybutynin above the recommended dose. In a study by Bennett et al. (2004), patients with neurogenic DO were treated with ER oxybutynin up to 30 mg per day. They found that oxybutynin dose escalation to 30 mg daily resulted in a statistically significant decrease in number of voids per day, episodes of nocturia, and incontinence episodes, without any serious adverse events or any patients dropping out of the study.

Tolterodine is a potent muscarinic receptor antagonist without selectivity for particular receptor subtypes. The major active metabolite shows a similar pharmacologic profile to its parent compound. Tolterodine is available in both IR and ER formulations. A large, multicenter, double-blind, randomized controlled study compared ER to IR tolterodine and placebo in 1529 adults with OAB symptoms (Van Kerrebroeck et al., 2001). The primary outcome was change in weekly number of incontinent episodes. Compared with placebo, both the IR and ER tolterodine showed a significantly better response compared with placebo; however, dry mouth was significantly lower with ER tolterodine compared with IR tolterodine and placebo.

The Overactive Bladder: Judging Effective Control and Treatment (OBJECT) trial (Appell et al., 2001), sponsored by the manufacturer of ER oxybutynin, was a prospective, randomized, double-blind parallel group study in which 378 patients were randomized to receive ER oxybutynin 10 mg per day or IR tolterodine 2 mg twice daily. Although both medications were found to decrease DO, ER oxybutynin had better efficacy and a small but statistically significant advantage for mixed incontinence and urinary frequency compared with IR tolterodine. Dry mouth and CNS side effects were similar for both treatment groups.

The Overactive Bladder: Performance of Extended Release Agents (OPERA) study (Diokno et al., 2003), also sponsored by the manufacturer of oxybutynin, was a randomized, double-blind, parallel group study of 790 women comparing ER formulations of oxybutynin 10 mg once per day with tolterodine 4 mg once per day. Inclusion criteria included DO of 21 to 60 episodes per week and frequency greater than 10 episodes per 24 hours. Both medications were similar in decreasing DO episodes and total incontinence episodes. However, 23% of women taking oxybutynin reported no episodes of incontinence, compared with 16.8% of women taking tolterodine, a statistically significant difference. Oxybutynin was significantly more effective in reducing frequency, although it was also more likely to cause dry mouth.

The Antimuscarinic Clinical Effectiveness Trial (ACET), which was sponsored by the manufacturer of tolterodine, involved two separate trials conducted in parallel, with individual centers evaluating one study drug only (Sussman & Garely, 2002). Patients in one trial were randomly assigned to open-label treatment with either 2 or 4 mg ER tolterodine. In the other trial, patients were randomized to 5 or 10 mg ER oxybutynin. Investigators were blinded to the existence of the other trial. A total of 1289 patients with symptoms of urinary frequency and urgency with or without incontinence (OAB wet and OAB dry) were enrolled. Although not designed to make direct comparisons between the two study populations, the authors reported that, after 8 weeks, ER tolterodine 4 mg was significantly more effective than ER oxybutynin 5 and 10 mg. ER tolterodine 2 mg once daily was similar to ER oxybutynin 5 and 10 mg once daily. Using a visual analog scale, patients taking ER tolterodine 4 mg had significantly less dry mouth than ER oxybutynin 10 mg. Interpretation of this study's results was limited by the lack of data supplied on the number of patients with isolated frequency and urgency versus those with DO and urgency incontinence. It is also important to note that no objective parameters, such as a voiding diary, were used for outcome measures.

Darifenacin, another antimuscarinic medication, shows high selectivity for M3 receptor subtypes, with an 11-fold higher affinity for M3 than M2 receptors. Haab et al. (2004) conducted a multicenter, double-blind, placebo-controlled, parallel-group study that enrolled 561 patients with OAB symptoms for more than 6 months. Subjects were randomized to receive once-daily ER oral darifenacin tablets of 3.75, 7.5, or 15 mg or matching placebo for 12 weeks. The authors found that doses of darifenacin at 7.5 and 15 mg were superior to placebo for reducing incontinent episodes, micturition frequency, bladder capacity, and urgency. The most common adverse events were mild to moderate dry mouth and constipation. Notably, the CNS and cardiac safety profile of darifenacin was found to be similar to placebo, which may be attributed to the M_3-selective receptor profile of darifenacin.

Solifenacin is another M_3-selective antagonist with selectivity for the bladder over salivary glands. Chapple et al. (2004) published results of a phase III trial that compared solifenacin and tolterodine with placebo. With tolterodine 2 mg twice daily, patients experienced a statistically significant decrease in the number of voids per 24 hours, but the decrease in incontinence and urgency episodes per 24-hour period was not statistically significant. In contrast, solifenacin showed statistically significant decreases for the number of voids, incontinent episodes, and urgency episodes per 24 hours. Dry mouth was seen in 18.6% of patients using IR tolterodine and in 14% and 21.3% using solifenacin 5 mg and 10 mg, respectively.

Trospium is a quaternary amine with some antimuscarinic activity. Because of its structure, trospium has limited passage across the blood–brain barrier into the CNS, and therefore has a low incidence of CNS side effects (Guay, 2003). This biochemical characteristic can justify the use of trospium in elderly patients or those with cognitive deficits (Coupland et al., 2019; Maggiore et al., 2012). With regard to its effectiveness in treating OAB, Zinner (2005) performed a multicenter, parallel, double-blind, placebo-controlled trial with 523 patients and found trospium 20 mg twice daily to be superior to placebo in decreasing the number of voids and incontinence episodes.

An updated Cochrane review of the literature published in 2012 sought to answer the common question in caring for patients with OAB of "which anticholinergic drug should be used?" (Madhuvrata et al., 2012). This review included trials that made four types of comparison, including comparisons of different anticholinergic drugs, different doses of the same drug, IR versus ER preparations, and comparisons of ER preparations. The analysis included 86 trials (70 parallel and 16 cross-over study designs) involving a total of 31,249 adults. Oxybutynin and tolterodine are the two most studied drugs, as they have been on the market longer than the others. Both have similar effects on OAB; however, on average, patients taking oxybutynin were more likely to withdraw from the studies because of adverse effects of the medication, mostly dry mouth. Regardless, both oxybutynin and tolterodine can cause dry mouth, more so in the IR formulations compared with the ER formulations. Overall, the authors concluded that tolterodine is preferred over oxybutynin if an oral IR formulation must be prescribed. ER formulations of either, however, are preferred because of their decreased side effect profile. Based on this meta-analysis, both solifenacin and fesoterodine were more effective than tolterodine. However, dry mouth was more likely in patients treated with fesoterodine and less likely in those treated with solifenacin.

The cognitive side effects associated with anticholinergic medications, including commonly used antimuscarinic medications for OAB, have long been a concern, especially when used in elderly populations. In a recent study by Coupland et al. (2019), increasing total cumulative use of bladder antimuscarinic in the 1 to 11 years before index date of dementia diagnosis was associated with a significantly increased risk of dementia (adjusted odds ratio 1.65; 95% confidence interval 1.56–1.75). Because antimuscarinics in the treatment of OAB are intended to be used continuously, caution should be used when prescribing these medications to middle-aged and older people, because of the cumulative total anticholinergic exposure risk.

Adrenergic medications. In addition to antimuscarinic medications, adrenergic agonists and antagonists have also been used to treat OAB. Because the bladder and urethra contain α- and β-adrenergic receptors, stimulation of these receptors can influence bladder and urethral function.

Mirabegron, a β-3-adrenergic agonist, was approved by the US Food and Drug Administration for the treatment of OAB in 2012 and for combination use with solifenacin in 2018. Mirabegron acts on the β-3-adrenoreceptors in the wall of the bladder. These receptors are involved in bladder wall relaxation during the filling and storage phase of micturition. Mirabegron was found in three separate randomized controlled clinical trials to significantly decrease the number of incontinence episodes and micturitions, while significantly increasing bladder capacity. Although the incidence of side effects with this medication is low, the most commonly reported adverse reactions are hypertension, nasopharyngitis, UTI, and headache. Mirabegron is not recommended in patients with uncontrolled hypertension, and blood pressure should be monitored in patients with a diagnosis of hypertension. Mirabegron is a CYP2D6 inhibitor, so in patients taking medications metabolized by this enzyme (e.g., metoprolol and desipramine), dosing may need to be adjusted. Patients on digoxin and warfarin should also be monitored closely, as mirabegron has been shown to increase the systemic effects of these medications.

A recently published systematic review by Kelleher et al. (2018) aimed to assess the efficacy and tolerability of mirabegron 50 mg versus antimuscarinic monotherapies and combination treatments. Some 64 studies including 46,666 subjects were included in the meta-analysis. Compared with placebo, mirabegron 50 mg was found to be more efficacious in improving micturition frequency, urgency incontinence, dry rate, and 50% reduction in incontinence. Mirabegron 50 mg was found to have comparable efficacy compared with most antimuscarinic monotherapies, but solifenacin 10 mg monotherapy and solifenacin 5 mg plus mirabegron 25 or 50 mg combination therapy were found to be more efficacious. Overall, mirabegron was found to be significantly better tolerated, with fewer common side effects such as dry mouth, constipation, and urinary retention. Mirabegron has also been found to have better persistence and compliance during long-term treatments compared with antimuscarinics alone (Chapple et al., 2017). When comparing mirabegron to tolterodine ER, Chapple et al. found a median time to discontinuation of 169 and 56 days, respectively, and 12-month persistence rates of 38% and 20%, respectively.

Ephedrine, phenylpropanolamine, and pseudoephedrine act via direct stimulation of α-adrenergic receptors to increase urethral tone and closure pressure. β-adrenergic agonists, including isoproterenol and terbutaline, induce bladder relaxation and decrease intravesical pressure. The Cochrane Database reviewed the efficacy of adrenergic drugs for urinary incontinence in adults (Alhasso et al., 2003). In 15 randomized trials, weak evidence suggested that adrenergic agonists were better than placebo for urinary incontinence.

Drugs that act on afferent mechanisms. Two medications that affect receptors on afferent nerves have been identified for potential use as therapeutic interventions: capsaicin and resiniferatoxin (RTX). Both medications are dissolved in ethanol and instilled into the bladder. Capsaicin may produce some discomfort when initially instilled, whereas RTX does not. RTX is 1000 times more potent than capsaicin, such that the nerve may be "burned out" before it can cause excitation. Kim et al. (2003) treated 36 patients with refractory neurogenic DO with intravesical RTX. Improvements were seen in mean cystometric capacity and incontinence episodes. Some patients had an increase in cystometric capacity of 500%. These agents are currently not commercially available and are thus only used under a research protocol.

Antidepressants. Potential neurotransmitter targets in the central mechanisms include serotonin, GABA, glycine, dopamine, and noradrenaline. Both sympathetic and parasympathetic autonomic nuclei, as well as urethral sphincter motor nuclei, receive serotonergic input from the raphe nuclei in the caudal brainstem. Serotonergic pathways promote urine storage by activating sympathetic pathways and inhibiting parasympathetic pathways. Duloxetine is a selective serotonin and norepinephrine reuptake inhibitor that has been shown to increase bladder capacity in animal models and shows promise for the treatment of both urge and stress incontinence. Phase III studies have shown duloxetine to be superior to placebo in the treatment of stress incontinence. Bump et al. (2003) also analyzed a subset of women with mixed incontinence and found that duloxetine showed equal efficacy in women with either mixed incontinence or pure stress urinary incontinence. In a study by Steers et al. (2007), 306 women were randomized to placebo or increasing doses of duloxetine (80–120 mg/day). The patients in the duloxetine group had significant improvements over the placebo group in terms of decreased number of voids and incontinence episodes, increased daytime voiding intervals, and overall improvement in quality-of-life scores on validated questionnaires. Adverse events included dry mouth, dizziness, constipation, insomnia, and fatigue. A slight increase in postvoid residual bladder volume was noted in the duloxetine group, but no patients reported hesitancy, and no evidence of urinary retention was noted. Until more data are available, duloxetine is not recommended for routine use in patients with OAB and is not included in current guidelines.

Tricyclic antidepressants, including amitriptyline and imipramine, produce smooth muscle relaxation, inhibit norepinephrine reuptake, and have anticholinergic properties. Woodman et al. (2001) reported that imipramine was an effective treatment in 25 patients with DO. Incontinent episodes were reduced, and quality of life was improved; however, 41% of patients experienced side effects and 14% ultimately withdrew from the study. Imipramine is also not currently recommended for use in treating OAB.

Conclusion. OAB affects millions of people, and the prevalence is likely to continue to increase as our population ages. As a syndrome of several symptoms that includes urinary urgency, frequency, urgency incontinence, and nocturia, an individual's presentation, degree of bother, and response to treatment can be quite heterogeneous. There are well-developed guidelines for clinicians to follow when treating patients with nonneurogenic OAB. For many years, the mainstay of pharmacologic treatment has been antimuscarinic therapy along with behavioral modifications; however, β-3-adrenergic agonists are also an excellent pharmacologic option, either as monotherapy or in combination with antimuscarinic medication. Third-line treatment options for OAB include sacral neuromodulation, intradetrusor onabotulinum toxin injection, and percutaneous tibial nerve stimulation, which are discussed in detail in Chapter 32. Further research must continue to investigate the various pathophysiologic phenotypes that likely contribute to the development of OAB.

POLYURIA

Definition

Polyuria is defined by the ICS as the excessive production of urine, defined by a voided volume of greater than 2.8 L in a 70-kg individual (or >40 mL of urine/kg of body weight) during a 24-hour period (D'Ancona et al., 2019). To accurately diagnosis polyuria, a thorough history is required, and a frequency-volume chart is critical to quantify the amount of urine produced within 24 hours. Patients may present with similar symptoms to OAB; however, if they meet criteria for polyuria, further investigation is warranted, and clinicians should have a heightened concern for diabetes mellitus (DM), diabetes insipidus (DI), and other medical conditions as an underlying etiology for polyuria. The exact prevalence of polyuria is unknown and is largely related to the underlying pathophysiology of the condition.

Pathophysiology

Polyuria may be caused by a solute or osmotic diuresis or by water diuresis (Box 31.5). Solute diuresis is typically associated with a urine osmolality greater than 600 mOsmol/kg and a total daily osmolar output greater than 1000 mOsmol (calculated as the urine osmolality multiplied by the 24-hour urine output), while water diuresis is typically associated with a urine osmolality less than 600 mOsmol/kg and often less than 300 mOsmol/kg and a total daily osmolar output less than 900 mOsmol (Rose & Post, 2001).

The maintenance of water homeostasis within the body is mainly determined by the hormone arginine vasopressin (AVP), also known as antidiuretic hormone, and thirst (Nigro et al., 2018). AVP, a nine–amino-acid peptide, is released from the posterior pituitary in response to an increase in serum osmolality. Healthy subjects have been found to have an osmotic threshold for AVP release of approximately 280 mOsmol/kg (Baylis & Robertson, 1980; Verbalis, 2003). Other triggers for AVP release are hypotension, sepsis, hypoglycemia, exercise, and nausea and emesis (Ball, 2007). AVP works in the kidney by binding to vasopressin-2 receptors on the basal membrane of the renal collecting tubular cell, which leads to an increase in the tubular fluid permeability by installing aquaporin-2 water channels, which allows for water retention and urinary concentration

BOX 31.5 Differential Diagnosis of Polyuria

- Solute Diuresis
  - Glucosuria
  - Mannitol (i.e., given to patients with increased intracranial pressure)
  - Sodium (e.g., because of intravenous volume expansion)
  - Urea
    - Tissue catabolism (e.g., because of glucocorticoid therapy)
    - Resolution from azotemia (e.g., following acute kidney injury)
    - Exogenous use of urea (e.g., in the use of patients with hyponatremia)
- Water Diuresis
  - Central diabetes insipidus
  - Nephrogenic diabetes insipidus
  - Primary polydipsia

(Juul et al., 2014). A rise in serum osmolality also leads to an increase in thirst sensation, prompting oral intake of water and maintenance of serum osmolality within the physiological range (Verbalis, 2003).

Osmotic Diuresis. An osmotic diuresis is most commonly caused by glucose-induced diuresis in patients with uncontrolled DM. Under normal physiologic conditions the urine contains no glucose because the kidneys are able to reabsorb all of the filtered glucose from the tubular fluid back into the bloodstream. However, in patients with uncontrolled DM and elevated blood glucose levels (typically exceeding 160–180 mg/dL), the proximal tubule becomes overwhelmed and begins to excrete glucose in the urine. Decreased glucose reabsorption from the proximal tubule leads to increased concentration of the filtrate, which pulls water into the urine to create an increased urine volume and can result in polyuria.

A simple urinalysis can be performed to reveal glucosuria in patients both with and without a known diagnosis of DM. Before treating a patient for any LUTs such as frequency or nocturia, it is important to investigate for glucosuria as a potential cause for underlying polyuria. If glucose is found to be present in the urine, the patient can be worked up for possible DM and can be treated with appropriate diet and medication.

Glucosuria can also develop in diabetic patients treated with sodium-glucose cotransporter 2 (SGLT2) inhibitors, which work by inhibiting renal glucose absorption, thereby leading to glucose excretion in the urine and an osmotic diuresis (Weir et al., 2014). Examples of SGLT2 inhibitors include canagliflozin, dapagliflozin, and empagliflozin. By thoroughly reviewing a patient's medication list as part of their history, clinicians can easily identify if one of these medications may be contributing to any urinary symptom complaints.

Urea diuresis is another type of solute diuresis in which urea acts as an osmotic agent. This can occur in several settings, such as the resolution of azotemia, with the use of urea therapy in patients being treated for hyponatremia, in tissue catabolism owing to glucocorticoid therapy, and with the administration of large amounts of protein, either orally, enterally via feeding tube, or intravenously, which will then be catabolized to urea.

In the setting of large-volume administration of intravenous saline or after the resolution of bilateral upper urinary tract obstruction (postobstructive diuresis syndrome), a sodium diuresis may occur leading to polyuria. Mannitol can also cause an osmotic diuresis and polyuria, which is commonly seen when it is used to treat increased intracranial pressure.

Water Diuresis. The three major causes of polyuria in water diuresis are primary polydipsia, central DI, and nephrogenic DI, which all result in relatively dilute urine (Nigro et al., 2018).

Primary polydipsia is caused by excessive water intake leading to a decrease in serum osmolality, and therefore a physiological suppression of AVP and hypotonic polyuria. Several psychiatric disorders have been linked to primary polydipsia, including schizophrenia, anxiety, depression, and addictive disorders (Dundas et al., 2007). Another form of primary polydipsia is dipsogenic polydipsia, in which there may be a disturbed thirst sensation, possibly caused by a lower osmotic limit of thirst sensitivity below the osmotic threshold for AVP secretion (Dundas et al., 2007; Nigro et al., 2018; Thompson et al., 1991). Healthy people can also have primary polydipsia.

Central DI results from the insufficient secretion of AVP, which may be attributed to several underlying etiologies, including pituitary surgery, some CNS tumors, trauma, hemorrhage, and autoimmune and granulomatous disease (Nigro et al., 2018). Neuroimaging can be used to investigate the underlying cause of central DI; however, in about 25% of patients with central DI, no abnormality is found on neuroimaging, and no clinical evidence of a related disease can be linked (classified as idiopathic central DI) (Maghnie et al., 2000).

Patients with nephrogenic DI have resistance to AVP action in the kidneys because of an acquired or genetic defect. Laboratory evaluation will reveal an elevated basal plasma AVP level. The majority of patients with nephrogenic DI (up to 95%) have the acquired form, which is most commonly caused by lithium treatment but can also be attributed to other drugs including antifungal agents (amphotericin B), antibiotics (ofloxacin, demeclocycline), dexamethasone, dopamine, ifosfamide, orlistat, and cisplatin (Moeller et al., 2013). In the genetic form of nephrogenic DI, 90% of patients have a mutation in the gene encoding the AVP-receptor 2, which is mostly inherited in an X-linked recessive manner. Therefore, most of these patients are male and will present with hypernatremia, dehydration, dilute urine, and failure to thrive (Bichet & Bockenhauer, 2016).

Evaluation

When polyuria is suspected, aside from a detailed history including medical, surgical, family, and medication history, and physical exam, clinicians can perform various tests to help decipher the underlying etiology and pathophysiology. A urinalysis should also be performed, with careful attention to any glucose being present in the urine and the specific gravity, and blood work can be checked for glucose and sodium levels.

Urine and serum osmolality can be measured to differentiate between a solute and a water diuresis. When urine osmolality is greater than serum osmolality, water conservation is present. A low plasma sodium concentration with a low urine osmolality is suggestive of water overload because of primary polydipsia. A high plasma sodium concentration is indicative of either an osmotic diuresis or, especially in the presence of a urine osmolality lower than the plasma osmolality, DI. If plasma sodium concentration is found to be normal, and there is a urine osmolality more than 600 mOsmol/kg in a patient with polyuria, DI can be excluded because the evidence points more toward a solute diuresis as the cause for polyuria.

To confirm the presence of polyuria, a 24-hour urine study can be done in which total solute excretion, urine osmolality, sodium, potassium, chloride, creatinine, urea nitrogen, and glucose can be measured. In addition to polyuria being present, total solute excretion will be normal in the presence of a water diuresis but will be elevated in osmotic diuresis.

The classic water deprivation test followed by injection of desmopressin (DDAVP) is a method that is commonly used to differentiate between the various causes of water diuresis polyuria.

AVP activity, either deficiency or resistance, can be indirectly evaluated through urine osmolality following prolonged fluid deprivation and then renal response to the administration of DDAVP (Dashe et al., 1963; Miller et al., 1970).

Management

The management of patients with polyuria will largely depend on the underlying etiology and the appropriate treatment for the identified pathophysiology. Clinicians should not hesitate to refer patients to the appropriate consultants for further workup of any suspected causes.

NOCTURIA

Definition

Nocturia is a well-recognized, highly prevalent symptom in both men and women, and is defined as "the number of times urine is passed during the main sleep period," that is the number of times a person wakes up to void after initially falling asleep (D'Ancona et al., 2019). To count as a nocturia event, each urination must be followed by sleep or the intention to sleep. Nocturia may be one of the symptoms experienced by a patient with OAB syndrome (Haylen et al., 2010). Nocturnal enuresis, the complaint of involuntary voiding that occurs at night during the main sleep period (i.e., bedwetting), does not count as nocturia because the patient fails to wake up when passing urine (Hashim et al., 2019). However, this must be clearly factored into any evaluation of LUTS and nocturnal urine production. Nocturia as a symptom may be the key to revealing significant underlying medical problems unrelated to the lower urinary tract, such as sleep disorders, heart failure, or DI.

Nocturnal urine volume, which should be quantified by a frequency-volume chart, is the total urine produced during the individual's main sleep period, including the first void after the main sleep period (Hashim et al., 2019). Nocturnal polyuria, defined as "passing large volumes of urine during the main sleep period" (Hashim et al., 2019) can be diagnosed using a frequency-volume chart to calculate the nocturnal polyuria index (NPi) (nighttime urine volume/24-hour urine volume). A patient has nocturnal polyuria if his or her NPi is greater than 20% in younger individuals, 20% to 33% in "middle age," or greater than 33% in the elderly (>65 years) (D'Ancona et al., 2019). If a patient is found to have polyuria (voided volume of >2.8 L in a 70-kg individual or >40 mL of urine/kg of body weight during a 24-hour period) based on the frequency-volume chart, the underlying etiology for his or her polyuria should be addressed before treatment of nocturia (D'Ancona et al., 2019).

Studies have shown that patients with more frequent episodes of nocturia have an increased degree of bother. Some consider a low number of nocturia episodes per night to be within a range of "normal" and not a reason for patients to seek treatment. However, like most LUTs, patients' subjective degree of bother will dictate the degree to which they seek and pursue treatment options. Tikkinen et al. (2010) found that patients who had two or more voids/night were found to be "bothered," whereas those with three or more voids/night reported "moderate-to-severe" bother. Frequent nocturia can also lead to daytime fatigue, decreased productivity, depression, and disruption to daily activities; therefore, it is important to identify and treat nocturia when it is a bothersome symptom.

Prevalence

The prevalence of nocturia increases with age in both men and women; however, gender does have a significant impact. The prevalence of nocturia among young adults is higher in women, whereas men have a greater prevalence in the elderly population with nocturia (Bosch & Weiss, 2010). A meta-analysis and systemic review by Cornu et al. (2012) found the prevalence of nocturia (≥2 voids/night) in men was 3.4% at ages 20 to 29 years, 17% at ages 50 to 59 years, and 53% at ages 80 to 90 years, with all intervening age ranges also increasing. In women, nocturia involving two or more voids/night also increased with age (9% at ages 20–29 years, 20% at ages 50–59 years, and 57% at ages 80–90 years). The prevalence of nocturia involving three or more voids/night was 17% of men aged 70 to 79 years and 24% of men aged 80 to 90 years, whereas in women nocturia involving three or more voids/night was found in 15% of those aged 70 to 79 years and 21% of those aged 80 to 90 years.

Ethnicity is also an important risk factor for nocturia, with African-Americans being more prone to nocturia than other ethnicities (Cornu et al., 2012). Burgio et al. (2010) looked at the prevalence of nocturia in 1000 older community-dwelling adults and found a significant association between nocturia and Black race. The higher prevalence of nocturia in Black individuals may be associated with a higher incidence of associated comorbidities (diabetes, hypertension, obesity, and cardiovascular disease) in this population.

Overall, nocturia has been found to be associated with a variety of other factors, including obesity, hypertension, metabolic syndrome, the winter season, increased C-reactive protein levels, lower educational achievement, lifestyle (alcohol consumption, smoking, and drug use), low testosterone levels in men, reproductive history in women, and/or low vitamin D levels (Cornu et al., 2012). A clear genetic predisposition for nocturia has not been identified. Nocturia is therefore a highly prevalent symptom that increases in prevalence with age in both sexes and has multiple contributory factors.

Pathophysiology

Although the definition of nocturia as a symptom is clear, it does not provide any indication of the underlying etiology. Fig. 31.13 details the potential causes or associated risk factors for nocturia, which can be quite varied. When a patient presents with a complaint of nocturia, the clinician must thoroughly evaluate the patient's complaints, signs, and symptoms so that they may categorize the patient as having polyuria, nocturnal polyuria, a bladder storage disorder, or possibly a primary sleep disorder. This may require ordering labs, performing additional workup, and/or consulting other physicians when indicated, and is critically important to avoid missing a serious underlying diagnosis.

Bing and colleagues (2007) compared 75 patients with nocturia to 75 controls. Bladder diaries revealed that 55% of

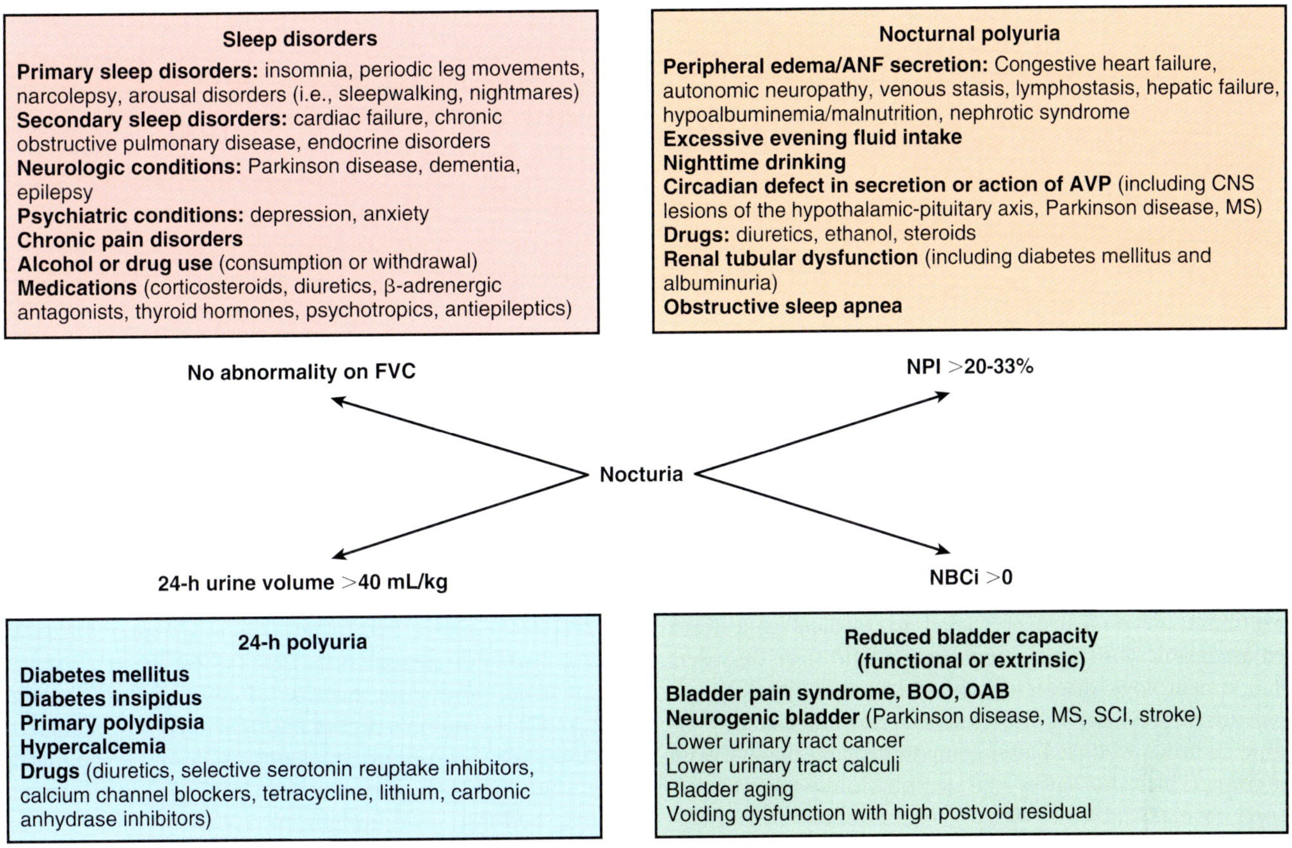

Etiologies of nocturia, classified according to the four definitions based on the frequency volume chart (FVC). Sleep disorders have been classified as a cause of nocturia, given the considerations exposed in the International Continence Society document [2].

Fig. 31.13 Potential underlying medical conditions associated with nocturia. *ANF*, Atrial natriuretic factor; *AVP*, arginine vasopressin; *BOO*, bladder outlet obstruction; *CNS*, central nervous system; *MS*, multiple sclerosis; *NBCi*, nocturnal bladder capacity index; *NPI*, nocturnal polyuria index; *OAB*, overactive bladder; *SCI*, spinal cord injury. (From Cornu JN, Abrams P, Chapple CR, et al. A contemporary assessment of nocturia: definition, epidemiology, pathophysiology, and management—a systematic review and meta-analysis. *Eur Urol*. 2012;62:877.)

patients had nocturnal polyuria, which was defined as a urine volume greater than 33% of the total voided 24-hour urine volume. In addition, patients were able to be categorized into an underlying pathophysiologic cause using bladder diaries 84% of the time. The percentage of patients who were able to be categorized based on the underlying pathophysiology increased to 96% when patient symptoms and urodynamic examination results were added in. These authors found nocturnal polyuria to be the most common cause of nocturia, occurring in 32% of patients, followed by a combination of nocturnal polyuria and OAB (25%) and OAB alone (17%). Some 21% of patients had polyuria alone or in combination with OAB or nocturnal polyuria. Overall, the authors suggest that an effective treatment approach may be tailored specifically for patients based on the underlying pathophysiology.

Identifying the underlying pathophysiology of nocturia requires a careful history and physical examination, as well as possible consultation with the patient's primary care provider to uncover other significant medical problems. Physical examination findings such as short neck and obesity might be suggestive of obstructive sleep apnea (OSA). OSA has been found to be associated with nocturnal polyuria, because of increased levels of atrial natriuretic peptide secretion resulting in nighttime diuresis (Lowenstein et al., 2008). Appropriate evaluation and treatment for OSA in these patients may resolve their nocturia without any intervention focused on the lower urinary tract (Fitzgerald et al., 2006; Guilleminault et al., 2004).

Vaughan et al. (2010) found that three or more episodes of nocturia were associated with a 28% increased risk of falling in an elderly population. A recent systematic review and meta-analysis by Pesonen et al. (2020) evaluated the association between nocturia and falls and fractures as a prognostic and as a causal risk factor. They found that nocturia is "probably associated with an approximated 1.2-fold increased risks of falls and possibly an approximately 1.3-fold increased risk of fractures." Given the significant consequences of falls in the elderly (i.e., loss of independence, injury, and injury-associated death), decreasing a patient's nocturia episodes may be one intervention that could help decrease this risk.

Evaluation

The initial evaluation of a patient with nocturia should start with a detailed history, including questions about voiding behavior, fluid intake, alcohol consumption, degree of bother from urinary symptoms, and previous UTIs, as well as a comprehensive review of medications (Cornu et al., 2012). A detailed medical and surgical history should be taken, and questions regarding possible sleep disturbances should also be asked. A physical examination should be performed, and a urinalysis should be done to rule out UTI.

A 24- to 72-hour frequency-volume chart, or bladder diary, is a key instrument in assessing a patient's complaint of nocturia to characterize the mechanism of nocturia and underlying etiology. The bladder diary should include a record of the volume and type of fluid ingested, as well as the volume and time of each void. It should also include the time the patient retires to bed, when she wakes up, and a subjective assessment of whether the patient felt that the night was good or bad in terms of her sleeping pattern. Review of the sleep pattern may reveal a concern for a sleep disorder, and, if so, the patient should be referred for further evaluation. Sleep disorders potentially related to nocturia include insomnia, obstructive and central apnea syndrome, restless legs syndrome, periodic legs syndrome, parasomnias, sleep disorders related to medical conditions (such as chronic obstructive lung disease), and sleep disorders related to neurologic diseases (such as Alzheimer disease).

Nocturnal polyuria, as discussed above, is measured by including all urine produced after going to bed and the first void after rising. This value varies considerably from person to person and normally increases with age. Causes of nocturnal polyuria include congestive heart failure, autonomic dysfunction, sleep apnea, renal insufficiency, estrogen deficiency, and circadian defect in secretion or action of antidiuretic hormones.

Patients with nocturia without polyuria or nocturnal polyuria on a frequency-volume chart will likely have reduced voided volume, potentially indicating a reduced bladder capacity or a sleep disorder. Bladder storage problems can be suspected from the bladder diary by comparing each nighttime voided volume with the patient's maximum bladder capacity. However, there is no definitive range of normal or abnormal volumes, and clinical judgment is required in reviewing the patient's bladder diary. Reduced bladder capacity may be caused by extrinsic compression of the bladder, as is common in pregnancy, or functional problems leading to reduced bladder storage, which can include bladder pain syndrome, neurogenic bladder, lower urinary tract cancer, bladder calculi, and incomplete bladder emptying. Some patients who might be suspected of having a bladder storage problem based on the bladder diary may in reality have a sleep disturbance. It is not uncommon for patients who wake frequently at night for other reasons to feel the need (or habit) to void each time they wake, voiding a small volume, as a "convenience void."

If there is a clear causative disease or a suspicion of one, consider referral for treatment of this underlying problem and then reassess nocturia after the patient has undergone the necessary workup and/or treatment. If there is no clear causative disease, then further treatment options for nocturia should be offered.

Management

An algorithm for initial evaluation and treatment of nocturia is provided in Fig. 31.14. When assessing a patient who has nocturia, one must first establish the degree of bother that the patient feels her nocturia causes her. So long as nocturia symptoms are not caused by an underlying comorbidity that should be addressed, such as OSA or congestive heart failure, the management of nocturia and treatment options pursued should match the patient's degree of bother in an attempt to improve quality of life. The initial treatment of nocturia should begin with education about the normal physiology of the bladder and behavioral modifications including voiding before bed, restricting fluids (particularly caffeinated beverages and alcohol) in the evening, elevating the legs and using compression stockings during the day to avoid lower extremity edema, and using protective undergarments (Cornu et al., 2012). Treating sleep disturbances, obesity, and hypertension in patients with nocturia may also decrease the number of nightly voids and improve quality of life (Saglam et al., 2013). Additionally, it is important to consider environmental conditions that may prevent complications related to nocturia, such as use of a bedside urinal or commode and a clear, lighted path to the bathroom to reduce the risk of falls (Kowalik et al., 2018).

As already discussed, for patients who have increased overnight urine production because of retained fluid during the day and fluid mobilization at night, behavioral modifications, such as wearing support stockings or elevating the lower extremities during the day, can be helpful to mobilize this fluid before bedtime. Additionally, if a patient takes a diuretic medication, the timing of dosing should be addressed. An ideal time to take a diuretic may be around noon, such that the patient has time to accumulate fluid throughout the morning, then diurese through the afternoon and early evening before sleeping, thus reducing third-space fluid that would be resorbed overnight. However, this should be considered for each patient's individual medication regimen and in coordination with her primary care physician.

Many of the studies evaluating different treatment methods for nocturia have focused on nocturia associated with benign prostatic hypertrophy (BPH) in men. α-Blocker therapy has been shown to have a modest benefit in decreasing the number of nightly voids. In a pooled analysis of three double-blind placebo-controlled studies, Roehrborn et al. (2003) found that alfuzosin 10 mg significantly improved the nocturia component of International Prostate Symptom Score questionnaire. Given that the underlying pathophysiology of nocturia in the setting of BPH is different than the underlying cause of nocturia in women, the ability to generalize the results of this study to both genders is limited.

Approximately 30% of patients with nocturia also report OAB symptoms (Tikkinen et al., 2007). When compared with placebo, several antimuscarinics (Dmochowski et al., 2010; Rackley et al., 2006; Toglia et al., 2010) and mirabegron (Chapple et al., 2014) demonstrate only about a 30% reduction in nighttime voids, despite improvement in LUTS. Brubaker and FitzGerald (2007) evaluated the use of solifenacin in both male and female patients with OAB and nocturia with and without nocturnal polyuria. In this study, no difference was seen in those patients with OAB and nocturnal polyuria. However, subjects with OAB and nocturia (without nocturnal polyuria) were found more likely to have one

Initial assessment and management of nocturia

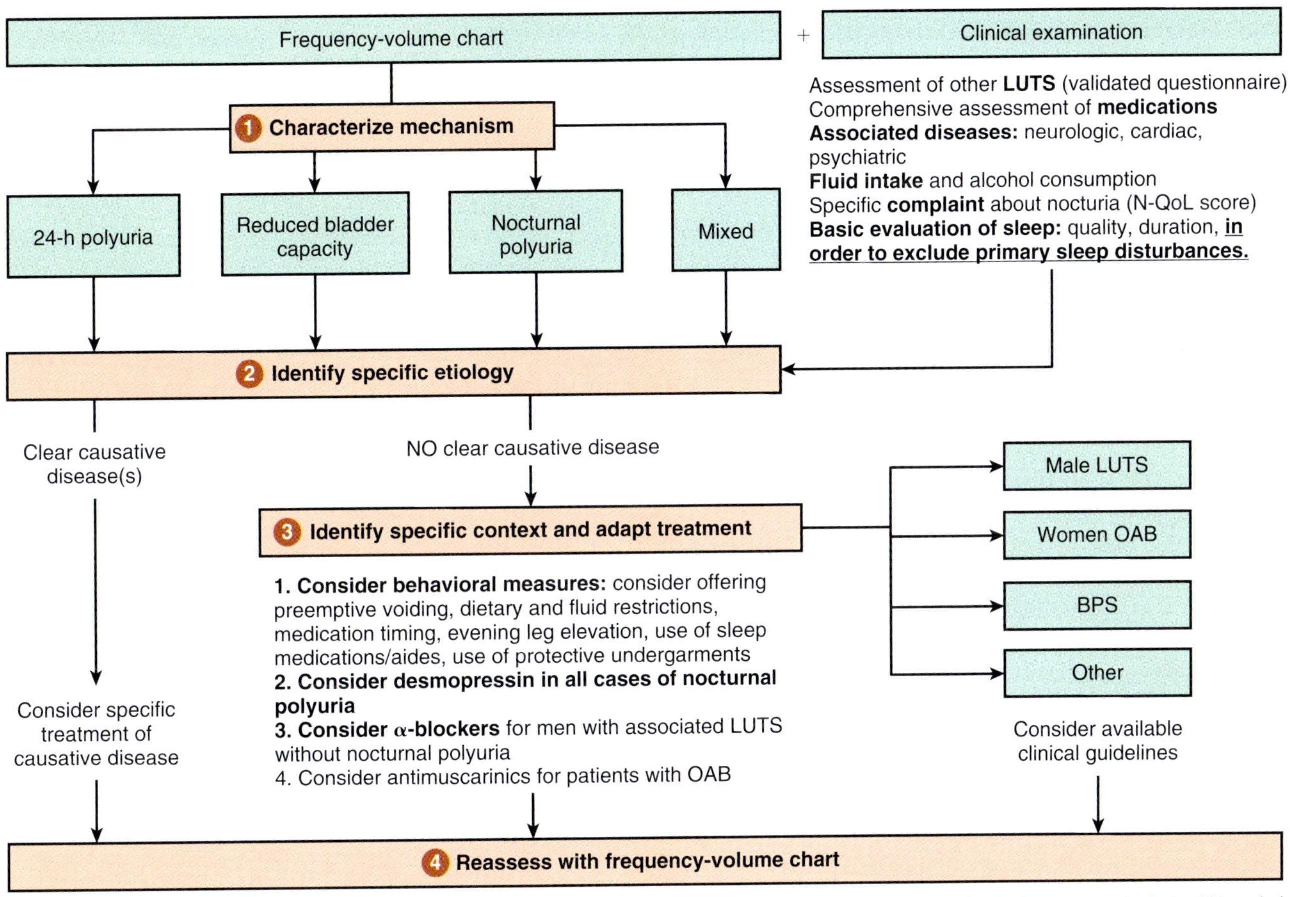

Algorithm for evaluation and treatment of nocturia. Primary sleep disorders (responsible for patient's awakening before the desire to pass urine) should be ruled out at clinical examination to avoid in-depth exploration.

Fig. 31.14 Algorithm for the initial assessment and management of nocturia. *BPS*, Bladder pain syndrome; *LUTS*, lower urinary tract symptoms; *N-QoL*, nocturia quality of life; *OAB*, overactive bladder. (From Cornu JN, Abrams P, Chapple CR, et al. A contemporary assessment of nocturia: definition, epidemiology, pathophysiology, and management—a systematic review and meta-analysis. *Eur Urol.* 2012;62:877.)

or fewer voids per night compared with placebo. In this study the nocturia episode reduction was not significant, but this was thought to be because of an unexpectedly high performance of placebo. Although a couple of other studies using trospium chloride showed similarly encouraging results, not all studies show similarly efficacious results with anticholinergics, and it may be that the patients who benefit the most are those with significant urgency associated with their nocturia episodes (Rackley et al., 2006).

Melatonin, a hormone produced by the brain that helps to regulate the sleep-wake cycle, is commonly used for the short-term treatment of difficulty sleeping. Melatonin, when used in men with nocturia and bladder outlet obstruction, was not found to significantly reduce nocturia (Drake et al., 2004). Drake et al. (2018) recently conducted a randomized, double-blind, placebo-controlled, crossover trial of melatonin in the treatment of nocturia in patients with MS. These authors found that melatonin did not significantly decrease nocturia episodes compared with placebo, nor was there a significant difference in LUTS, quality of life, or sleep quality while taking melatonin. Melatonin is likely not an adequate treatment option for most patients with nocturia.

The use of desmopressin for the treatment of nocturia has also been studied. Desmopressin is a synthetic analog of vasopressin, which is secreted by the posterior pituitary to increase water permeability within the renal parenchyma by acting on renal collecting ducts via V2 receptors. This leads to water reabsorption and decreased urine volume. Several formulations of desmopressin (oral tablets, orally disintegrating tablets, and intranasal spray) have been studied in patients with nocturnal polyuria. Two randomized studies found desmopressin to be effective in reducing nocturnal voids by more than 50% in 34% to 46% of subjects, compared with a reduction of just 3% to 7% in placebo groups (Lose et al., 2003; Mattiasson et al., 2002). A more recent study found that desmopressin oral disintegrating tablet in increasing doses was associated with a greater proportion of patients with a more than 33% reduction in nocturnal voids (Weiss et al., 2012). In another study, women who were prescribed 25 μg desmopressin oral disintegrating tablet had significantly increased odds of having a period of first interrupted sleep greater than 4 hours compared with placebo (Sand et al., 2013).

When using desmopressin for the treatment of nocturia, it is important to carefully review potential adverse effects and ensure the patient understands the need for continued monitoring. The most frequent adverse events include hyponatremia, headache, hypertension, edema, nausea, and abdominal pain. Although most cases of hyponatremia are asymptomatic, it is critical to monitor serum sodium levels after initiation of desmopressin therapy and with any dose adjustment. Overall, desmopressin can be a safe and effective treatment for nocturia in the properly selected patient, as long as there is careful attention paid to contraindications, and serum sodium levels are appropriately monitored.

Onabotulinum toxin injection into the bladder, a common treatment for OAB, has shown limited improvement in nocturia, with a decrease in nocturia episodes of 0.5 versus 0.25 with placebo (Chapple et al., 2013; Nitti et al., 2017). This may be a better option for patients with significant OAB in addition to nocturia that is not well controlled with oral medications. Similarly, sacral neuromodulation has been shown to decrease the number of nocturnal voids across all age groups, but this surgical option may be most beneficial in improving nocturia in patients with more severe OAB symptoms (Peters et al., 2013).

Conclusion

Nocturia is a highly prevalent symptom that can have a significant impact on quality of life. It is prudent to thoroughly evaluate patients with nocturia to identify the underlying etiology of their condition. The use of frequency-volume charts can greatly help to elucidate the cause of nocturia, identify polyuria and nocturnal polyuria, and guide treatment strategies. Comorbid conditions associated with nocturia should be identified, treated, and optimized. First-line therapy for nocturia includes behavioral and lifestyle modifications. Desmopressin is an effective treatment for nocturia that is attributed to nocturnal polyuria.

SUMMARY

Diagnosing OAB syndrome, polyuria, and nocturia can easily be accomplished with a careful medical history, physical examination, frequency-volume chart, and appropriate workup for any suspected underlying medical conditions. One must seek to understand the underlying pathophysiology and contributing factors to discover the etiology of each individual patient's symptoms. This, in turn, will help the clinician design an appropriate treatment plan that is tailored to and effective for the patient suffering from these conditions.

BIBLIOGRAPHY

Aharony SM, Lam O, Corcos J. Evaluation of lower urinary tract symptoms in multiple sclerosis patients: review of the literature and current guidelines. *Can Urol Assoc J.* 2017;11:61.

Al-Ghazo MA, Ghalayini IF, Al-Azab R, et al. Urodynamic detrusor overactivity in patients with overactive bladder symptoms. *Int Neurourol J.* 2011;15:48.

Alhasso A, Glazener CM, Pickard R, N'Dow J. Adrenergic drugs for urinary incontinence in adults. *Cochrane Database Syst Rev.* 2003;2:CD001842.

Andersson KE. The concept of uroselectivity. *Eur Urol.* 1998;33:7.

Andersson KE. Potential future pharmacological treatment of bladder dysfunction. *Basic Clin Pharmacol Toxicol.* 2016;119:75.

Appell RA, Sand P, Dmochowski R, et al. Prospective randomized controlled trial of extended-release oxybutynin chloride and tolterodine tartrate in the treatment of overactive bladder: results of the OBJECT Study. *Mayo Clin Proc.* 2001;76:358.

Ball SG. Vasopressin and disorders of water balance: the physiology and pathophysiology of vasopressin. *Ann Clin Biochem.* 2007;44:417.

Baylis PH, Robertson GL. Plasma vasopressin response to hypertonic saline infusion to assess posterior pituitary function. *J R Soc Med.* 1980;73:255.

Bennett N, O'Leary M, Patel AS, et al. Can higher doses of oxybutynin improve efficacy in neurogenic bladder? *J Urol.* 2004;171:749.

Bent AE, Sand PK, Ostergard DR. Transvaginal electrical stimulation in the treatment of genuine stress incontinence and detrusor instability. *Int Urogynecol J.* 1993;4:9.

Bergman A, Koonings PP, Ballard CA. Detrusor instability. Is the bladder the cause or the effect? *J Reprod Med.* 1989;34:834.

Bhatia NN, Bergman A. Cystometry: unstable bladder and urinary tract infection. *Br J Urol.* 1986;58:134.

Bichet DG, Bockenhauer D. Genetic forms of nephrogenic diabetes insipidus (NDI): Vasopressin receptor defect (X-linked) and aquaporin defect (autosomal recessive and dominant). *Best Pract Res Clin Endocrinol Metab.* 2016;30:263.

Bing MH, Moller LA, Jennum P, et al. Pathophysiological aspects of nocturia in a Danish population of men and women age 60 to 80 years. *J Urol.* 2007;178:552.

Bosch JL, Weiss JP. The prevalence and causes of nocturia. *J Urol.* 2010;184:440.

Brubaker L, FitzGerald MP. Nocturnal polyuria and nocturia relief in patients treated with solifenacin for overactive bladder symptoms. *Int Urogynecol J Pelvic Floor Dysfunct.* 2007;18:737.

Brucker BM, Kalra S. Parkinson's disease and its effect on the lower urinary tract: evaluation of complications and treatment strategies. *Urol Clin North Am.* 2017;44:415.

Bump RC, Norton PA, Zinner NR, et al. Mixed urinary incontinence symptoms: urodynamic findings, incontinence severity, and treatment response. *Obstet Gynecol.* 2003;102:76.

Burgio KL, Goode PS, Locher JL, et al. Behavioral training with and without biofeedback in the treatment of urge incontinence in older women: a randomized controlled trial. *JAMA.* 2002;288:2293.

Burgio KL, Johnson II TM, Goode PS, et al. Prevalence and correlates of nocturia in community-dwelling older adults. *J Am Geriatr Soc.* 2010;58:861.

Burgio KL, Whitehead WE, Engel BT. Urinary incontinence in the elderly. Bladder-sphincter biofeedback and toileting skills training. *Ann Intern Med.* 1985;103:507.

Campos-Sousa RN, Quagliato E, da Silva BB, et al. Urinary symptoms in Parkinson's disease: prevalence and associated factors. *Arq Neuropsiquiatr.* 2003;61:359.

Cardozo L, Stanton SL, Hafner J, Allan V. Biofeedback in the treatment of detrusor instability. *Br J Urol.* 1978;50:250.

Chapple C, Sievert KD, MacDiarmid S, et al. OnabotulinumtoxinA 100 U significantly improves all idiopathic overactive bladder symptoms and quality of life in patients with overactive bladder and urinary incontinence: a randomised, double-blind, placebo-controlled trial. *Eur Urol.* 2013;64:249.

Chapple CR, Cardozo L, Nitti VW, et al. Mirabegron in overactive bladder: a review of efficacy, safety, and tolerability. *Neurourol Urodyn.* 2014;33:17.

Chapple CR, Nazir J, Hakimi Z, et al. Persistence and adherence with mirabegron versus antimuscarinic agents in patients with overactive bladder: a retrospective observational study in UK clinical practice. *Eur Urol.* 2017;72:389.

Chapple CR, Rechberger T, Al-Shukri S, et al. Randomized, double-blind placebo- and tolterodine-controlled trial of the once-daily antimuscarinic agent solifenacin in patients with symptomatic overactive bladder. *BJU Int.* 2004;93:303.

Cohn JA, Brown ET, Reynolds WS, et al. An update on the use of transdermal oxybutynin in the management of overactive bladder disorder. *Ther Adv Urol.* 2016;8:83.

Cornu JN, Abrams P, Chapple CR, et al. A contemporary assessment of nocturia: definition, epidemiology, pathophysiology, and management—a systematic review and meta-analysis. *Eur Urol.* 2012;62:877.

Coupland CAC, Hill T, Dening T, et al. Anticholinergic drug exposure and the risk of dementia: a nested case-control study. *JAMA Intern Med.* 2019;179:1084.

Coyne KS, Margolis MK, Kopp ZS, Kaplan SA. Racial differences in the prevalence of overactive bladder in the United States from the epidemiology of LUTS (EpiLUTS) study. *Urology.* 2012;79:95.

Coyne KS, Sexton CC, Thompson CL, et al. The prevalence of lower urinary tract symptoms (LUTS) in the USA, the UK and Sweden: results from the Epidemiology of LUTS (EpiLUTS) study. *BJU Int.* 2009;104:352.

Coyne KS, Sexton CC, Vats V, et al. National community prevalence of overactive bladder in the United States stratified by sex and age. *Urology.* 2011;77:1081.

Crude percentages of stroke for adults aged 18 and over, United States, 2015-2018. *National Health Interview Survey.* 2011. Available at: https://www.cdc.gov/nchs/nhis/ADULTS/www/index.htm.

D'Ancona C, Haylen B, Oelke M, et al. The International Continence Society (ICS) report on the terminology for adult male lower urinary tract and pelvic floor symptoms and dysfunction. *Neurourol Urodyn.* 2019;38:433.

Dashe AM, Cramm RE, Crist CA, et al. A water deprivation test for the differential diagnosis of polyuria. *JAMA.* 1963;185:699.

de Lau LM, Breteler MM. Epidemiology of Parkinson's disease. *Lancet Neurol.* 2006;5:525.

de Seze M, Ruffion A, Denys P, et al. The neurogenic bladder in multiple sclerosis: review of the literature and proposal of management guidelines. *Mult Scler.* 2007;13:915.

Diokno AC, Appell RA, Sand PK, et al. Prospective, randomized, double-blind study of the efficacy and tolerability of the extended-release formulations of oxybutynin and tolterodine for overactive bladder: results of the OPERA trial. *Mayo Clin Proc.* 2003;78:687.

Dmochowski R. Interventions for detrusor overactivity: the case for multimodal therapy. *Rev Urol.* 2002;4:S19.

Dmochowski RR, Davila GW, Zinner NR, et al. Efficacy and safety of transdermal oxybutynin in patients with urge and mixed urinary incontinence. *J Urol.* 2002;168:580.

Dmochowski RR, Peters KM, Morrow JD, et al. Randomized, double-blind, placebo-controlled trial of flexible-dose fesoterodine in subjects with overactive bladder. *Urology.* 2010;75:62.

Doggweiler R, Whitmore KE, Meijlink JM, et al. A standard for terminology in chronic pelvic pain syndromes: A report from the chronic pelvic pain working group of the international continence society. *Neurourol Urodyn.* 2017;36:984.

Drake MJ, Canham L, Cotterill N, et al. Results of a randomized, double blind, placebo controlled, crossover trial of melatonin for treatment of nocturia in adults with multiple sclerosis (MeNiMS). *BMC Neurol.* 2018;18:107.

Drake MJ, Mills IW, Noble JG. Melatonin pharmacotherapy for nocturia in men with benign prostatic enlargement. *J Urol.* 2004;171:1199.

Dundas B, Harris M, Narasimhan M. Psychogenic polydipsia review: etiology, differential, and treatment. *Curr Psychiatry Rep.* 2007;9:236.

Eriksen BC, Bergmann S, Eik-Nes SH. Maximal electrostimulation of the pelvic floor in female idiopathic detrusor instability and urge incontinence. *Neurourol Urodyn.* 1989;8:219.

Fantl JA, Hurt WG, Dunn LJ. Detrusor instability syndrome: the use of bladder retraining drills with and without anticholinergics. *Am J Obstet Gynecol.* 1981;140:885.

Fitzgerald MP, Mulligan M, Parthasarathy S. Nocturic frequency is related to severity of obstructive sleep apnea, improves with continuous positive airways treatment. *Am J Obstet Gynecol.* 2006;194:1399.

Frewen WK. A reassessment of bladder training in detrusor dysfunction in the female. *Br J Urol.* 1982;54:372.

Ganz ML, Smalarz AM, Krupski TL, et al. Economic costs of overactive bladder in the United States. *Urology.* 2010;75:526.

Giglio D, Tobin G. Muscarinic receptor subtypes in the lower urinary tract. *Pharmacology.* 2009;83:259.

Gormley EA, Lightner DJ, Burgio KL, et al. Diagnosis and treatment of overactive bladder (non-neurogenic) in adults: AUA/SUFU guideline. *J Urol.* 2012;188:2455.

Gormley EA, Lightner DJ, Faraday M, et al. Diagnosis and treatment of overactive bladder (non-neurogenic) in adults: AUA/SUFU guideline amendment. *J Urol.* 2015;193:1572.

Gray M, David DJ. Does biofeedback improve the efficacy of pelvic floor muscle rehabilitation for urinary incontinence or overactive bladder dysfunction in women? *J Wound Ostomy Continence Nurs.* 2005;32:222.

Guay DR. Clinical pharmacokinetics of drugs used to treat urge incontinence. *Clin Pharmacokinet.* 2003;42:1243.

Guilleminault C, Lin CM, Goncalves MA, Ramos E. A prospective study of nocturia and the quality of life of elderly patients with obstructive sleep apnea or sleep onset insomnia. *J Psychosom Res.* 2004;56:511.

Haab F, Stewart L, Dwyer P. Darifenacin, an M3 selective receptor antagonist, is an effective and well-tolerated once-daily treatment for overactive bladder. *Eur Urol.* 2004;45:420.

Hashim H, Blanker MH, Drake MJ, et al. International Continence Society (ICS) report on the terminology for nocturia and nocturnal lower urinary tract function. *Neurourol Urodyn.* 2019;38:499.

Haylen BT, de Ridder D, Freeman RM, et al. An International Urogynecological Association (IUGA)/International Continence Society (ICS) joint report on the terminology for female pelvic floor dysfunction. *Int Urogynecol J.* 2010;21:5.

Haylen BT, de Ridder D, Freeman RM, et al. An International Urogynecological Association (IUGA)/International Continence Society (ICS) joint report on the terminology for female pelvic floor dysfunction. *Neurourol Urodyn.* 2010;29:4.

Haylen BT, Maher CF, Barber MD, et al. An International Urogynecological Association (IUGA) / International Continence

Society (ICS) Joint Report on the Terminology for Female Pelvic Organ Prolapse (POP). *Neurourol Urodyn.* 2016;35:137.

Irwin DE, Milsom I, Hunskaar S, et al. Population-based survey of urinary incontinence, overactive bladder, and other lower urinary tract symptoms in five countries: results of the EPIC study. *Eur Urol.* 2006;50:1306.

Juul KV, Bichet DG, Nielsen S, Norgaard JP. The physiological and pathophysiological functions of renal and extrarenal vasopressin V2 receptors. *Am J Physiol Renal Physiol.* 2014;306:F931.

Kelleher C, Hakimi Z, Zur R, et al. Efficacy and tolerability of mirabegron compared with antimuscarinic monotherapy or combination therapies for overactive bladder: a systematic review and network meta-analysis. *Eur Urol.* 2018;74:324.

Kim JH, Rivas DA, Shenot PJ, et al. Intravesical resiniferatoxin for refractory detrusor hyperreflexia: a multicenter, blinded, randomized, placebo-controlled trial. *J Spinal Cord Med.* 2003;26:358.

Kowalik CG, Cohn JA, Delpe S, et al. Nocturia: evaluation and current management strategies. *Rev Urol.* 2018;20:1.

Leach GE, Bavendam TG. Prospective evaluation of the incontan transrectal stimulator in women with urinary incontinence. *Neurourol Urodyn.* 1989;8:231.

Leone Roberti Maggiore U, Salvatore S, Alessandri F, et al. Pharmacokinetics and toxicity of antimuscarinic drugs for overactive bladder treatment in females. *Expert Opin Drug Metab Toxicol.* 2012;8:1387.

Lightner DJ, Gomelsky A, Souter L, Vasavada SP. Diagnosis and treatment of overactive bladder (non-neurogenic) in adults: AUA/SUFU guideline amendment 2019. *J Urol.* 2019;202:558.

Litwiller SE, Frohman EM, Zimmern PE. Multiple sclerosis and the urologist. *J Urol.* 1999;161:743.

Lose G, Lalos O, Freeman RM, et al. Efficacy of desmopressin (Minirin) in the treatment of nocturia: a double-blind placebo-controlled study in women. *Am J Obstet Gynecol.* 2003;189:1106.

Lowenstein L, Kenton K, Brubaker L, et al. The relationship between obstructive sleep apnea, nocturia, and daytime overactive bladder syndrome in women. *Am J Obstet Gynecol.* 2008;198:598.

Madhuvrata P, Cody JD, Ellis G, et al. Which anticholinergic drug for overactive bladder symptoms in adults. *Cochrane Database Syst Rev.* 2012;1:CD005429.

Maghnie M, Cosi G, Genovese E, et al. Central diabetes insipidus in children and young adults. *N Engl J Med.* 2000;343:998.

Mattiasson A, Abrams P, Van Kerrebroeck P, et al. Efficacy of desmopressin in the treatment of nocturia: a double-blind placebo-controlled study in men. *BJU Int.* 2002;89:855.

Mayo ME. Detrusor hyperreflexia: the effect of posture and pelvic floor activity. *J Urol.* 1978;119:635.

McDonald C, Winge K, Burn DJ. Lower urinary tract symptoms in Parkinson's disease: Prevalence, aetiology and management. *Parkinsonism Relat Disord.* 2017;35:8.

Mendez MH, Sexton SJ, Lentz AC. Contemporary review of male and female climacturia and urinary leakage during sexual activities. *Sex Med Rev.* 2018:6:16.

Miller M, Dalakos T, Moses AM, et al. Recognition of partial defects in antidiuretic hormone secretion. *Ann Intern Med.* 1970:73:721.

Milsom I, Kaplan SA, Coyne KS, et al. Effect of bothersome overactive bladder symptoms on health-related quality of life, anxiety, depression, and treatment seeking in the United States: results from EpiLUTS. *Urology.* 2012;80:90.

Moeller HB, Rittig S, Fenton RA. Nephrogenic diabetes insipidus: essential insights into the molecular background and potential therapies for treatment. *Endocr Rev.* 2013;34:278.

Newman D, Burgio K. Conservative management of urinary incontinence: behavioral and pelvic floor therapy and urethral and pelvic devices. In: Wein AJ, Kavoussi LR, Partin AW, Peters CA, eds. *Campbell-Walsh Urology.* 11th ed. Philadelphia: Elsevier; 2016:1876.

Nigro N, Grossmann M, Chiang C, Inder WJ. Polyuria-polydipsia syndrome: a diagnostic challenge. *Intern Med J.* 2018;48:244.

Nik-Ahd F, Lenore Ackerman A, Anger J. Recurrent urinary tract infections in females and the overlap with overactive bladder. *Curr Urol Rep.* 2018;19:94.

Nitti VW. The prevalence of urinary incontinence. *Rev Urol.* 2001;3:S2.

Nitti VW. Primary bladder neck obstruction in men and women. *Rev Urol.* 2005;7:S12.

Nitti VW, Dmochowski R, Herschorn S, et al. OnabotulinumtoxinA for the treatment of patients with overactive bladder and urinary incontinence: results of a phase 3, randomized, placebo controlled trial. *J Urol.* 2017:197:S216.

Nosti PA, Sokol AI. Unusual findings on cystoscopy in a patient with detrusor overactivity. *Female Pelvic Med Reconstr Surg.* 2012;18:186.

Nussbaum RL, Ellis CE. Alzheimer's disease and Parkinson's disease. *N Engl J Med.* 2003;348:1356.

Onukwugha E, Zuckerman IH, McNally D, et al. The total economic burden of overactive bladder in the United States: a disease-specific approach. *Am J Manag Care.* 2009;15:S90.

Panicker JN, Fowler CJ, Kessler TM. Lower urinary tract dysfunction in the neurological patient: clinical assessment and management. *Lancet Neurol.* 2015;14:720.

Pesonen JS, Cartwright R, Vernooij RWM, et al. The impact of nocturia on mortality: a systematic review and meta-analysis. *J Urol.* 2020;203:486.

Peters KM, Killinger KA, Gilleran J, Boura JA. Does patient age impact outcomes of neuromodulation? *Neurourol Urodyn.* 2013;32:30.

Peyronnet B, Mironska E, Chapple C, et al. A Comprehensive review of overactive bladder pathophysiology: on the way to tailored treatment. *Eur Urol.* 2019;75:988.

Plevnik S, Janez J, Vrtacnik P, et al. Short-term electrical stimulation: home treatment for urinary incontinence. *World J Urol.* 1986;4:24.

Rackley R, Weiss JP, Rovner ES, et al. Nighttime dosing with tolterodine reduces overactive bladder-related nocturnal micturitions in patients with overactive bladder and nocturia. *Urology.* 2006;67:731.

Resnick NM, Yalla SV. Detrusor hyperactivity with impaired contractile function. An unrecognized but common cause of incontinence in elderly patients. *JAMA.* 1987;257:3076.

Roehrborn CG, Van Kerrebroeck P, Nordling J. Safety and efficacy of alfuzosin 10 mg once-daily in the treatment of lower urinary tract symptoms and clinical benign prostatic hyperplasia: a pooled analysis of three double-blind, placebo-controlled studies. *BJU Int.* 2003;92:257.

Rose B, Post T. *Clinical Physiology of Acid-Base and Electrolyte Disorders.* 5th ed. New York: McGraw-Hill; 2001.

Saglam HS, Gokkaya CS, Salar R, et al. The effects of age, metabolic syndrome, nocturnal polyuria and sleep disorders on nocturia. *Adv Clin Exp Med.* 2013;22:489.

Sakakibara R, Hattori T, Uchiyama T, Yamanishi T. Videourodynamic and sphincter motor unit potential analyses in Parkinson's disease and multiple system atrophy. *J Neurol Neurosurg Psychiatry.* 2001;71:600.

Sand PK, Dmochowski RR, Reddy J, van der Meulen EA. Efficacy and safety of low dose desmopressin orally disintegrating tablet in women with nocturia: results of a multicenter, randomized, double-blind, placebo controlled, parallel group study. *J Urol.* 2013;190:958.

Serati M, Salvatore S, Uccella S, et al. Urinary incontinence at orgasm: relation to detrusor overactivity and treatment efficacy. *Eur Urol.* 2008;54:911.

Spruijt J, Vierhout M, Verstraeten R, et al. Vaginal electrical stimulation of the pelvic floor: a randomized feasibility study in urinary incontinent elderly women. *Acta Obstet Gynecol Scand.* 2003;82:1043.

Steers WD, Herschorn S, Kreder KJ, et al. Duloxetine compared with placebo for treating women with symptoms of overactive bladder. *BJU Int.* 2007;100:337.

Stewart WF, Van Rooyen JB, Cundiff GW, et al. Prevalence and burden of overactive bladder in the United States. *World J Urol.* 2003;20:327.

Sussman D, Garely A. Treatment of overactive bladder with once-daily extended-release tolterodine or oxybutynin: the antimuscarinic clinical effectiveness trial (ACET). *Curr Med Res Opin.* 2002;18:177.

Thompson CJ, Edwards CR, Baylis PH. Osmotic and non-osmotic regulation of thirst and vasopressin secretion in patients with compulsive water drinking. *Clin Endocrinol (Oxf).* 1991;35:221.

Tikkinen KA, Johnson TM, II, Tammela TL, et al. Nocturia frequency, bother, and quality of life: how often is too often? A population-based study in Finland. *Eur Urol.* 2010;57:488.

Tikkinen KA, Tammela TL, Rissanen AM, et al. Is the prevalence of overactive bladder overestimated? A population-based study in Finland. *PLoS One.* 2007;2:e195.

Toglia MR, Ostergard DR, Appell RA, et al. Solifenacin for overactive bladder: secondary analysis of data from VENUS based on baseline continence status. *Int Urogynecol J.* 2010;21:847.

Van Kerrebroeck P, Kreder K, Jonas U, et al. Tolterodine once-daily: superior efficacy and tolerability in the treatment of the overactive bladder. *Urology.* 2001;57:414.

Vaughan CP, Brown CJ, Goode PS, et al. The association of nocturia with incident falls in an elderly community-dwelling cohort. *Int J Clin Pract.* 2010;64:577.

Vecchioli-Scaldazza C, Grinta R. Overactive bladder syndrome: what is the role of evidence of detrusor overactivity in the cystometric study? *Minerva Urol Nefrol.* 2010;62:355.

Verbalis JG. Disorders of body water homeostasis. *Best Pract Res Clin Endocrinol Metab.* 2003;17:471.

Wang AC, Wang YY, Chen MC. Single-blind, randomized trial of pelvic floor muscle training, biofeedback-assisted pelvic floor muscle training, and electrical stimulation in the management of overactive bladder. *Urology.* 2004;63:61.

Weir MR, Januszewicz A, Gilbert RE, et al. Effect of canagliflozin on blood pressure and adverse events related to osmotic diuresis and reduced intravascular volume in patients with type 2 diabetes mellitus. *J Clin Hypertens (Greenwich).* 2014;16:875.

Weiss JP, Zinner NR, Klein BM, Norgaard JP. Desmopressin orally disintegrating tablet effectively reduces nocturia: results of a randomized, double-blind, placebo-controlled trial. *Neurourol Urodyn.* 2012;31:441.

Woodman PJ, Misko CA, Fischer JR. The use of short-form quality of life questionnaires to measure the impact of imipramine on women with urge incontinence. *Int Urogynecol J Pelvic Floor Dysfunct.* 2001;12:312.

Zinner NR. Trospium chloride: an anticholinergic quaternary ammonium compound for the treatment of overactive bladder. *Expert Opin Pharmacother.* 2005;6:1409.

32

Refractory Overactive Bladder

Megan S. Bradley and Cindy L. Amundsen

CHAPTER OUTLINE

INTRODUCTION

Overactive bladder (OAB) is characterized by urinary urgency, with or without urgency urinary incontinence (UUI), usually with increased daytime frequency and nocturia, if there is no proven infection or other obvious pathology. The American Urologic Association (AUA) defines the refractory patient as the patient who has failed a sufficient trial of behavioral therapy and at least one medication (antimuscarinic or β-3 agonist) for 4 to 8 weeks. This may be because of lack of efficacy and/or intolerable side effects (Gormley et al., 2012). Currently accepted options for third-line therapy for refractory OAB include: (1) percutaneous tibial nerve stimulation (PTNS), (2) intradetrusor onabotulinumtoxinA (BTX-A), and (3) sacral neuromodulation (SNM). Emerging therapies may include selective bladder denervation, newer, smaller, magnetic resonance imaging (MRI)-compatible and rechargeable SNM devices, and chronic peripheral neuromodulation. This chapter will focus on the three common options for refractory OAB, with a brief discussion of emerging therapies.

BOTULINUM TOXIN

Background

The US Food and Drug Administration (FDA) approved BTX-A for cosmetic use in 1991. It has since been FDA approved for many indications including blepharospasm, cervical neck dystonia, hyperhidrosis, chronic migraine, and upper limb spasticity. In August 2011, BTX-A was approved for the treatment of neurogenic bladder; in January 2013, it was approved for treatment of OAB. BTX-A is a potent neurotoxin derived from the anaerobic bacterium, *Clostridium botulinum.* Initially, the proposed method of action was based on data extrapolated from skeletal muscle, where BTX-A acts primarily as a muscle paralytic, inhibiting the presynaptic release of acetylcholine from motor neurons at the neuromuscular junction. As a result, a flaccid paralysis ensues. By cleaving protein receptors within the nerve terminals, BTX-A prevents the normal vesicular transport and release of acetylcholine from the motor nerve terminals into the neuromuscular junction. Since these initial theories were formulated, BTX-A has been found to also affect the afferent side of the nervous system by inducing changes like decreasing the sensory response of C-fibers (de Groat & Yoshimura, 2009). It is likely that BTX-A has a complex inhibitory effect on vesicular release of excitatory neurotransmitters and on the axonal expression of other important mediators. Based on histologic evidence, recovery of chemodenervation occurs after 3 to 6 months. This is thought to be the result of turnover of the presynaptic molecules and nerve sprouting from the nerve terminal, forming a new functional synapse.

There are seven immunologically distinct subtypes of botulinum toxin, but only types A and B are available for use in clinical practice. BTX-A, which is approved for OAB treatment, is available as Botox (Allergan Inc., Irvine, CA) in the United States and as Dysport (Medicis Aesthetics) in the United Kingdom. Type B is less potent and is commercially available as MyoBloc in the United States and as NeuroBloc in Europe (Solstice Neurosciences, Louisville, KY). BTX-A is administered by cystoscopic injection of multiple aliquots into the detrusor muscle. The FDA-approved dosage for the treatment of neurogenic bladder is 200 U; the FDA-approved dose for OAB is 100 U.

Efficacy

An extensive Cochrane review, and AUA systematic review summarize the literature surrounding the use of BTX-A for OAB (Duthie et al., 2011; Gormley et al., 2015). The results summarized in these reviews and newer, relevant randomized controlled trials (RCTs) are presented here and in Table 32.1. Four early randomized trials with placebo control groups evaluated intradetrusor injections of 50 to 300 U (Brubaker et al., 2008; Dmochowski et al., 2010; Flynn et al., 2009; Rovner et al., 2011). Overall, significant reductions in incontinence episodes and in urgency were reported in the active treatment groups. Voiding frequency results are less clear, with studies reporting a large range of reductions (e.g., from a nonsignificant 1.3 episodes per day to up to 14.2 episodes per day). This is likely because of the inclusion of patients with different baseline voiding frequency levels in these studies.

TABLE 32.1 Selected Randomized Controlled Trials of Botulinum Toxin a for Refractory Overactive Bladder (Listed by Dose Tested)

Author	N	Baseline UUIE/Day	Outcome Definition	Outcome	Urinary Retention or Postvoid Residual
200 U					
Brubaker et al. (2008)	43	5.17	Failure = PGI-I score ≥4;	60% response BTX group; median duration response: 373 days (BTX) vs. 62 (placebo)	12/28 (43%) BTX vs. 0 Placebo (PVR >200 mL)
Sahai et al. (2007)	34	4.98 (BTX); 3.91 (placebo)	UUIE on diary, QOL	Sig changes in freq and UUIE/day	6/18 (33%) BTX with PVR >150 mL
Flynn et al. (2009)	22	8 (BTX) 7.9 (placebo)	UUIE/day, QOL	QOL sig change; decreased UUIE/day in BTX (3.4/day) at 6 weeks	26.6% PVR >200 mL at 6 weeks, 1 symptomatic requiring ISC
Amundsen et al. (2016)	264	5.4 (BTX); 5.2 (SNM)	UUIE/day (average over 6 months)	Change 3.9 UUIE/day (BTX) vs. 3.3 (SNM)	8% ISC at 1 month, 2% at 6 months
Tincello et al. (2012)	240	6.2 both groups	Voiding frequency/24hours at 6 months	Voiding frequency (8.3/24 hours [BTX] vs. 9.67/24 hours [placebo])	16% ISC (BTX), 4% ISC (placebo)
Altaweel et al. (2011)	39	4.2 (100 U), 3.8 (200 U)	Improvement in urodynamic parameters at 3 months	Improved urodynamic both groups, no difference between groups	10% (100 U), 20% (200 U)
100–150 U					
Cohen et al. (2009)	44	9.8 (BTX) 9.3 (placebo)	>50% reduction of UUIE at 3 months	100 U: 8/12 (67%), 150 U 9/12 (75%)	2 pts, 1 in each group, ISC (PVR >350 mL)
Kuo (2007)	45	6.8 (suburo), 11.3 (detrusor), 11.1 (bladder base)	Satisfaction based on symptom improvement	Satisfied (order of detrusor, suburo, bladder base): 3 months: 93%, 80%, 67%; 9 months: 20%, 20%, 6.7%	Acute retention: 2 detrusor, 2 suburo, 0 bladder base; PVR >150 mL: 33%, 47%, and 13%
Dmochowski et al. (2010)	313	Not reported	Change from baseline in UUIE/week at 12 weeks	-17.4 (placebo), −20.7 (50 U), −18.4 (100 U), −23 (150 U), −19.6 (200 U), −19.4 (300 U)	PVR >200 mL at any visit; 2.3% (placebo), 8.9%–25.5% (BTX)
Kuo (2006)	75	Not reported	Self-reported UI (0 = none to 3 = severe), VD (0 = none to 3 = severe); Excellent (UI = 0 and VD increase <2), Improved (UI improved and VD increase <2)	Excellent or improved: 100 U 73.3%; 150 U 77.7%; 200 U 81.8%	PVR >150 mL: 100 U 30%, 150 U 72%, 200 U 52%
Visco et al. (2012)	241	5.2 (medication), 4.8 (BTX)	Mean UUIE/day at 6 months	3.4 (medication) and 3.3 (BTX)	5% in the BTX group ISC
Chapple et al. (2013)	548	5.2	Change from baseline UUIE/day	−2.95 (BTX) vs. −1.03 (placebo)	6.9% of BTX performed ISC
Denys et al. (2012)	99	5.9 (placebo), 3.9 (50 U), 5.9 (100 U), 3.9 (150 U)	>50% improvement in baseline urgency and UUI at 3 months	65% (100 U), 56% (150 U)	8 pts performed ISC
Jabs and Carleton (2013)	21	5.0 (placebo), 6.1 (BTX)	Maximum bladder capacity at cystoscopy	Mean max bladder capacity 161 mL higher in BTX vs. placebo	No ISC

BTX, Botulinum toxin; *ISC*, intermittent self-catheterization; *PGI-I*, patient global impression of improvement; *pts*, participants; *PVR*, postvoid residual; *QOL*, quality of life; *SNM*, sacral neuromodulation; *U*, Units; *UI*, urinary incontinence; *UUIE*, urgency urinary incontinence episodes; *VD*, voiding difficulty.

The 2015 AUA literature review retrieved four additional RCTs with placebo control groups (Chapple et al., 2013; Denys et al., 2012; Jabs & Carleton, 2013; Tincello et al., 2012) and two with nonplacebo comparator groups (Altaweel et al., 2011; Kuo, 2011). In general, most trials reported statistically significant improvements in measured voiding outcomes (UUI, urinary frequency, urgency, nocturia, pad use) and in quality-of-life (QOL) outcomes compared with placebo groups. Not included in these literature reviews was the Anticholinergic versus Botox Comparison (ABC) study, a multicenter RCT that compared the effectiveness of 6 months of daily anticholinergic therapy to a single intradetrusor injection of 100 U of BTX-A in patients with OAB symptoms (Visco et al., 2012). This study included women who were either drug-naïve or who had tried two or fewer prior anticholinergic medications. The results demonstrated that anticholinergic medication had similar rates of improvement in daily UUI episodes compared with BTX-A injections (3.4 anticholinergic vs. 3.3 BTX-A; $P = .81$). However, patients who underwent BTX-A injections had significantly higher cure rates compared with patients who received anticholinergic medication (13% anticholinergic vs. 27% BTX-A; $P < .01$).

Finally, in the 2016 Refractory Overactive Bladder: Sacral Neuromodulation Versus Botulinum Toxin Assessment (ROSETTA) study, 364 women were randomized to cystoscopic intradetrusor injection of 200 U of BTX-A or to SNM (Amundsen et al., 2016). The women in the BTX-A group had a greater reduction in 6-month mean number of episodes of UUI per day than did those in the SNM group (–3.9 vs. –3.3 episodes per day; $P = .01$).

Dosing Considerations

Although the current FDA-approved dose of BTX-A for idiopathic OAB is 100 U, there is significant variation in reported dose and comparator arms in the literature. RCTs with different doses are reported in Table 32.1. The studies reporting on active BTX-A (doses from 50–200 U) generally demonstrate improved efficacy of BTX-A compared with placebo, but there is not a clear relationship between dose and efficacy across these trials. One of the largest trials, performed by Chapple et al. (2013), randomized patients with idiopathic OAB (≥3 UUI episodes/3 days and ≥8 micturitions per day) to BTX-A at a dose of 100 U ($n = 277$) or placebo ($n = 271$). They found that, at 12 weeks, BTX-A significantly decreased UUI episodes/day compared with the control group (–2.95 BTX-A vs. –1.03 placebo; $P < .001$). As previously discussed, Visco et al. (2012) noted similar improvement in patients treated with BTX-A 100 U or anticholinergic medications, but an improved cure rate with BTX-A. Dmochowski et al. (2010) compared responses across a wide range of BTX-A doses (50–300 U) and reported that doses of 100 U or greater were sufficient to reduce UUI episodes and improve QOL measures, but without clear dose-response effects above 150 U. This study was limited by lack of statistical comparison between groups.

Tincello et al. (2012) randomized a total of 240 women with refractory OAB to receive either 200 U of BTX-A or placebo injection. The primary outcome was voiding frequency at 6 months. The median voiding frequency was lower after treatment with BTX-A compared with placebo (8.3 vs. 9.67, $P < .01$). Episodes of UUI also decreased (1.67 vs. 6.0, $P < .01$). Cure rates were higher in the BTX-A group compared with the placebo group (31% vs. 11%; $P = .002$). Given the available literature, our expert opinion is that patients should be counseled regarding the option for 100 U versus 200 U for refractory OAB.

Duration of Effect and Repeat Injections

Most studies suffer from lack of long-term follow-up, but longer-term efficacy has been demonstrated in some studies. Amundsen et al. (2018) investigated clinical responders in the ROSETTA trial to determine efficacy up to 2 years. Clinical responders were defined as those experiencing at least a 50% reduction in UUI episodes 1 month after administration of BTX-A. Over the course of 2 years, up to two additional BTX-A injections were allowed after the initial 6-month study. No difference in decreased mean UUI episodes per day was found between the BTX-A and SNM groups over 24 months (–3.88 vs. –3.50, $P = .15$). The BTX-A group maintained high satisfaction and treatment endorsement throughout the 24-month period. Importantly, of the 115 participants who requested a second BTX-A injection, the median interval between first and second injection was 350 days (interquartile range 242–465 days).

Other prospective and retrospective studies have helped illustrate the duration of efficacy of BTX-A, especially after the first injection., Granese et al. (2012) reported on 68 women (baseline 5.7 UUI episodes/day) who underwent an intradetrusor injection of 100 U BTX-A and were followed for 12 months. Patients were allowed repeat injection at 12 months if they experienced symptom relapse. On average, patients had sustained improvement in UUI episodes/day up to 9 months (5.7 at baseline vs. 1.9 at 9 months). Twenty-five of the 54 patients with 12-month data requested a second injection, with similar improvements. Veeratterapillay et al. (2014) reported on 125 patients who had two or more 200 U BTX-A injections (667 injections total). The median interval between injections was 14.4 months. There was sustained efficacy after repeat injections, with statistically similar times to repeat injections after the first four injections. Finally, Dowson et al. (2012) reported similar significant reductions in frequency, urgency, and UUI after BTX-A injections in 100 patients, 63 of whom had two or more injections (mostly of 200 U). Again, the average time between injections ranged between 300 and 450 days.

Rates of BTX-A discontinuation are difficult to estimate because of differences in reporting and poor patient follow-up in many studies. Reasons for BTX-A discontinuation are more consistently reported and include failure of therapy (either subjective or objective) and low tolerability (e.g., having to perform intermittent self-catheterization [ISC], urinary retention, and recurrent urinary tract infections [UTIs]). Given the wide range of times until return of symptoms reported in the literature, it is likely prudent to avoid scheduled repeat injections and to proceed only with return of bothersome symptoms.

Location and Depth of Botulinum Toxin Injection

The location and depth of intradetrusor BTX-A injections vary across studies. Two systematic reviews evaluated adverse events and short-term efficacy associated with trigonal and extratrigonal BTX-A (Davis et al., 2014; Jo et al., 2018). Importantly, both included studies that involved patients with neurogenic bladder. The earlier review by Davis et al. (2014) evaluated six studies (258 patients) that were carried out between 2006 and 2011. This meta-analysis did not show significant differences between trigonal and extratrigonal BTX-A for acute urinary retention (4.2% vs. 3.7%, $P = .93$), UTI, or short-term cure rates. In 2018, Jo et al. evaluated eight studies published from 2007 to 2016, only one of which was included in the previous systematic review. They found overall improved outcomes in the trigone inclusion arms based on higher complete dryness rates (odds ratio [OR] = 2.19, 95% confidence interval [CI] 1.32–3.63, $P = .002$) and fewer incontinence episodes (−0.85 per day, 95% CI −1.55 to −0.16, $P = .02$). No differences in safety or adverse events, including bladder discomfort, were seen between groups. A limitation of this meta-analysis was an overall small number of patients per study. In terms of depth of injection, the more recent systematic review evaluated an intradetrusor versus suburothelial approach and did not find a difference in reduction in UUI between groups (−1.32 episodes per day, 95% CI −5.69 to −3.06, $P = .56$; Jo et al., 2018).

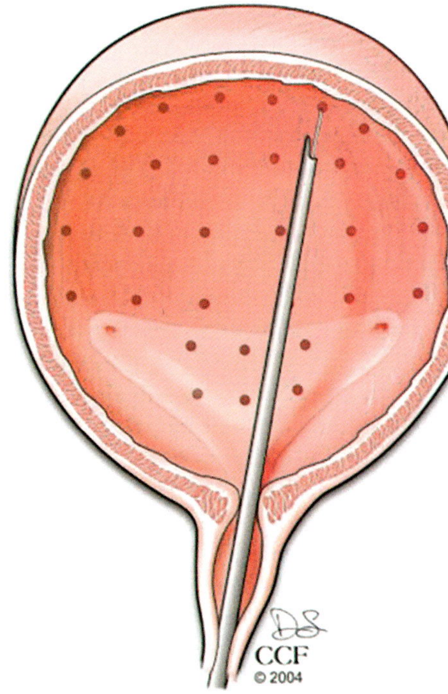

Fig. 32.1 Injection pattern for onabotulinum toxin A.

Technique for Botulinum Toxin Injection

The technique of mixing the BTX-A and how to inject it is described on the package insert and is standard (http://www.allergan.com/assets/pdf/botox_pi.pdf). The procedure is described here and demonstrated in Video 32.1.

BTX-A is a vacuum-dried protein available in 50-, 100-, and 200-U vials that must be refrigerated. Before injection, the vials of toxin must be reconstituted with preservative-free saline, and the mixture can be stored at 2° to 8° C for up to 24 hours. This outpatient procedure is easily performed in a clinical setting or, in rare circumstances, in an operating room. One trial reported similar pain scores of approximately 4/10 on a visual analog scale for subjects who had either local or general anesthetic (Denys et al., 2012). Experts agree that intravesical premedication can be given in the office, with approximately 30 to 40 mL of 2% lidocaine instilled via catheter into the bladder for about 20 minutes before injection. There is little evidence regarding other management options or the impact of this strategy, and future research would help standardize recommendations.

Cystoscopy may be performed using a 30-degree, 12-degree, or even 0-degree lens with a rigid cystoscope plus working element with channel for injection needle or disposable injection needle. A flexible cystoscope with injection needle may also be used. The bladder is filled with approximately 100 mL of 0.9% normal saline to achieve some tautness to the bladder wall. Injections are spread over different rows to equally cover the bladder dome and posterior base, sparing the ureteral orifices (Fig. 32.1). Some studies included a tiny amount of indigo carmine or methylene blue in the injection solution to facilitate visualization of the injection pattern. Again, depth of injection may not significantly impact efficacy, but visualization of injection may improve the ability to avoid extravasation of the injection through the bladder wall (Szczypior et al., 2017). The concentration of toxin and volume of fluid that is injected are not consistent across studies. Although one study showed that a single BTX-A injection can spread the neurotoxin activity to the opposite side of the bladder (Coelho et al., 2012), the standard technique uses between 10 and 20 injections. Liao et al. (2016) prospectively compared the therapeutic effects and safety of different numbers of BTX-A injections for patients with OAB and found that injection of 1 mL of BTX-A (10 U) at 10 sites was adequate for an optimal therapeutic effect. The BTX-A package insert recommends administering 100 U as 0.5-mL (5 U) injections across 20 sites into the detrusor, for a total volume of 10 cc, but, given the literature, a total of 10 to 20 sites is likely similarly efficacious.

Complications and Their Management

Urinary Retention and Self-Catheterization Recommendations. One of the most common complications after BTX-A injection is urinary retention. Rates of urinary retention range from 0% to 43% (Gormley et al., 2015). The definition of elevated postvoid residual (PVR) varies across studies, from 100 mL to 400 mL, with most studies defining an elevated PVR as 100 to 150 mL. Meta-analysis of data from RCTs comparing BTX-A to placebo showed a significant difference between BTX-A and placebo in terms of PVR-related catheterization (relative risk [RR]: 5.25; 95% CI 2.47–11.16; $P < .01$; Cui et al., 2013). The onset of urinary retention typically coincides with the clinical efficacy, beginning within the first week after injection. The duration of retention is variable, with some patients only requiring clean ISC for a few days, whereas for others the condition persists for the duration of the effects of the drug. Importantly, Kessler et al. (2009) examined QOL outcomes in women who had to perform ISC post–BTX-A treatment compared with those who did not and found no differences between groups.

We tend to recommend teaching patients ISC before injection, because if patients report minimal voiding or dribbling they are then able to perform ISC at home. Patients can be seen in the office for an assessment of PVR urine volume by catheterization or bladder ultrasonography either at a standard interval (1–2 weeks) or with symptoms of urinary retention. Multiple previous randomized trials chose to require self-catheterization at residual volumes greater than 300 mL (without symptoms) or greater than 150 to 200 mL in the presence of bothersome retention symptoms (Amundsen et al., 2016; Visco et al., 2012). In light of recent AUA guidelines regarding management of patients with nonneurogenic urinary retention (Stoffel et al., 2017), we continue to recommend ISC only for PVRs greater than 300 mL in the asymptomatic patient or greater than 200 mL in the presence of bothersome retention symptoms. For those patients sent home who require ISC, a clear follow-up plan should be outlined, including how often to use the catheter and at what volumes catheterization should be continued or discontinued.

Urinary Tract Infection and Antibiotic Prophylaxis. The other most common complication after BTX-A injection is UTI. Rates of UTI range from 3.6% to 54.5%, with four RCTs reporting rates of greater than 40%. In the aforementioned meta-analysis, there was a higher risk of UTI in the BTX-A group compared with the placebo group (RR: 2.36; 95% CI 1.58–3.53; $P < .0001$; Cui et al., 2013).

In terms of post–BTX-A UTI prevention, we adhere to AUA guideline recommendations for the use of prophylactic antibiotics for cystoscopy with manipulation for all patients (Lightner et al., 2020). These guidelines suggest administering antibiotics at the time of BTX-A, but specific recommendations are lacking. Antibiotic regimens can range from a single dose to use for 3 days before and 3 days after injection. A recent retrospective review of different prophylactic protocols found that starting antibiotics 1 day before BTX-A injection decreased the odds of postinjection UTI compared with postprocedure antibiotic prophylaxis only (OR, = 0.23; 95% CI 0.07–0.73; $P = .01$; Bickhaus et al., 2020). Based on these results, the authors recommended beginning antibiotic prophylaxis before the procedure and continuing it for 4 total days to decrease the risk of UTI. Similarly, the largest RCT to date used ciprofloxacin 500 mg on the day of procedure and for 3 days postprocedure (Amundsen et al., 2016). The aforementioned AUA guidelines recommend fluoroquinolones, trimethoprim/sulfamethoxazole, or even a second-generation cephalosporin. Considering patient antibiotic allergies or intolerances, any of the options are reasonable to give on at least day of procedure and may be continued for 1 to 3 days, per provider preference.

Additionally, the FDA-provided safety instructions for BTX-A state that it should not be administered to a patient suffering from a UTI, owing to concerns over adverse events (Allergan 2020). Although this recommendation seems prudent, given the discrepancy in UTI diagnostic criteria across studies and the high rates of asymptomatic bacteriuria in the elderly, we feel that current or recent bacteriuria is not an absolute contraindication to injection. In a cohort of patients undergoing BTX-A injection for either idiopathic or neurogenic detrusor overactivity, 38.8% of patients had asymptomatic bacteriuria (Aharony et al., 2019). Whereas postprocedure symptomatic UTI was more frequent in the asymptomatic bacteriuria group, there was no difference in serious adverse events like urosepsis, and there was similar efficacy between groups. Furthermore, performing BTX-A injection within 30 days of a recent UTI does not increase the odds of postprocedure UTI (Bickhaus et al., 2019). Our practice is to inquire about clinical symptoms and perform a urine dip on the day of injection. If patients are mildly symptomatic with a negative dipstick, we generally proceed with injection and send a urine culture to guide additional therapy in case they develop an increasingly symptomatic UTI. If patients have UTI symptoms and a positive dipstick, we tend to delay injection until a later date.

Conclusion

In conclusion, symptoms of OAB have been shown to significantly improve after BTX-A injections. Patients who are candidates for cystoscopic BTX-A injections should be counseled about the need for reinjections and possible postprocedure adverse events, including the risk of urinary retention requiring clean ISC and UTIs. Health care providers who perform BTX-A injections must have appropriate training and experience in treating women with pelvic floor disorders, operative cystoscopy privileges, and the ability to diagnose and manage any adverse outcomes after BTX-A injections into the bladder.

SACRAL NEUROMODULATION

Background and Possible Method of Action

SNM for treatment of refractory OAB has undergone modifications since the initial FDA approval of InterStim (Medtronic Inc., Minneapolis, MN) for urinary urgency/frequency in 1999. The initial one-step process was altered in 2003 to create a two-step algorithm for permanent implantation. Afferent neural activity from the pelvic and pudendal nerves is thought to be primarily responsible for the effects of neuromodulation at the sacral level of the spinal cord (S2–S4) (de Groat et al., 2014; Fowler et al., 2008). Normal voiding relies on intact neural pathways in the central nervous system. Pelvic parasympathetic nerves that arise at the sacral level of the spinal cord (S2–S4) are responsible for exciting the bladder and relaxing the urethra. The somatic nervous system acts on the external urethral sphincter via the pudendal nerve. The lumbar, pelvic, and pudendal nerves each contain both afferent and efferent axons that participate in feedback loops to manage voiding responses, which, if uninhibited, can result in urgency, frequency, and incontinence. Studies have evaluated multiple sites for neuromodulation, such as the sacral, tibial, pudendal, and genital nerves. However, the most commonly described site of neuromodulation for treatment of OAB is the third sacral nerve root (S3).

Efficacy

A variety of single-group observational studies were initially included in the evidence for SNM. The InSite Trial was a randomized, multicenter study evaluating the success rate of SNM compared with standard medical therapy in 147 patients with OAB (Siegel et al., 2015). Standard medical therapy was defined as antimuscarinic therapy, and inclusion criteria included failure of at least one medication. The primary objective was to compare the therapeutic success rate at 6 months, defined as 50% or greater improvement from baseline symptoms. For patients who were incontinent at baseline, 71% of those treated with SNM responded, compared with 47% of patients treated with standard medical therapy. Rates of complete continence were higher in those treated with SNM (39% vs. 21%), and this group showed statistically significant improvement over the standard medical therapy group in all measures of QOL. Follow-up studies continued to evaluate safety and efficacy of SNM over 5 years (Siegel et al., 2018). During the study period, 340 patients received test stimulation, and of those 272 (80%) had the SNM implanted. The overall therapeutic success rate at 5 years was 82% with sustained improvements in quality-of-life measurements. The 5-year cumulative rate of adverse events that required surgical intervention after the full SNM was implanted was 22%. The most common adverse event was an undesirable change in stimulation. Of note, the InSite trial does differ from many BTX-A trials in that patients had less severe symptoms at baseline. Again, in the ROSETTA trial, patients were randomized to receive either BTX-A 200 U or SNM. These patients had significant UUI, with an average of 5.2 UUI episodes per day in the SNM group. At 6 months, there were significant improvements in frequency of UUI episodes with a reduction to 3.3/day (Amundsen et al., 2016). Two-year outcomes confirmed that improvements in UUI episodes/day (−3.5) and QOL were sustained (Amundsen et al., 2018).

Progression from the advanced evaluation to pulse generator implantation ranges from approximately 70% to 80% (Amundsen et al., 2016; Davis et al., 2012; Siegel et al., 2018). One of the largest evaluations of SNM (n = 2765) found that 69% of patients undergoing an advanced evaluation via staged approach progressed to pulse generator implantation (Dobberfuhl et al., 2018). This study found that a diagnosis of UUI was associated with the highest success with advanced evaluation (72%).

Surgical Technique

The procedure is performed in one of two ways: an initial advanced evaluation (stage I, test stimulation) or basic evaluation (percutaneous nerve evaluation [PNE]). In some circumstances the procedure may involve a combined insertion of the lead and neurostimulator. The advanced evaluation (commonly referred to as test stimulation or stage I) is a clinical trial of a permanent tined lead with four electrodes using external stimulation. If the patient has appropriate symptom improvement with the test stimulation, a subcutaneous implantable pulse generator (IPG) is implanted. The basic evaluation (PNE) is placement of a temporary wire containing one electrode using external stimulation. Monitored anesthesia supplemented with local anesthesia is used for advanced evaluation, and local anesthesia alone is used for basic evaluation.

Advanced Evaluation (Test Stimulation or Stage I). The current commercially available electrode lead incorporates four equally spaced electrode contact points on a flexible lead that is inserted percutaneously under image guidance and anchored in place by several plastic tines. After the patient receives sedation and local anesthesia, the S3 foramina are identified. The location of the S3 foramina is identified via fluoroscopy and should correspond to approximately 9 cm cephalad to the drop-off of the sacrum and 1 to 2 cm lateral to the midline on either side. Important anatomic landmarks are shown in Fig. 32.2. The foramen needle is then inserted into the S3 foramen, ideally at a 45-degree angle. The position of the needle is confirmed using fluoroscopy. The nerve is test-stimulated for the appropriate motor and sensory responses, as listed in Table 32.2 (Matzel et al., 2017).

After appropriate motor/sensory responses are noted with the foramen needle, the incision is slightly extended, the needle

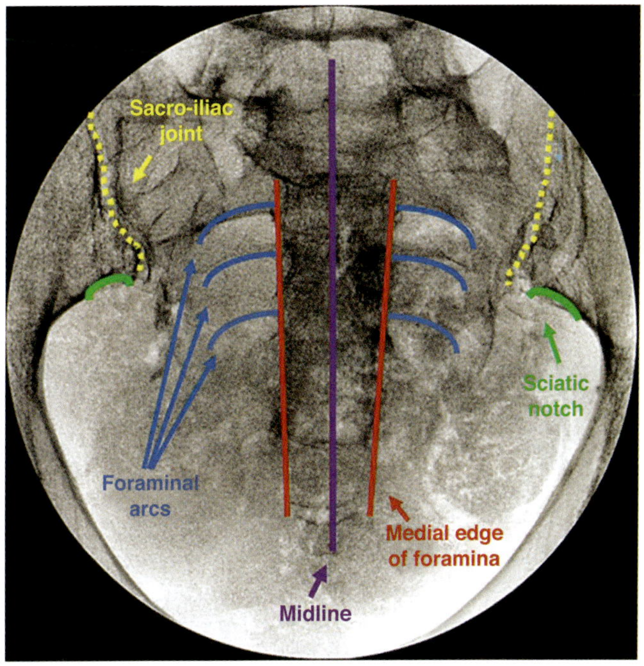

Fig. 32.2 Anatomic landmarks for sacral neuromodulation.

TABLE 32.2 Sacral Nerve Responses to Test Stimulation

Sacral Nerve	Response
S2	Plantar flexion of the entire foot with lateral rotation Clamp movement of the anal sphincter
S3	Dorsiflexion of the great toe Bellows reflex (anal wink) Parasthesias or sensation of pulling in the rectum or vagina
S4	Bellows only Sensation of pulling in the rectum only

stylet is removed, and the directional guide is inserted to a depth not significantly past the tip of the needle. The dilator is placed over the guidewire utilizing radiopaque marker to show progression just past the ventral portion of the sacrum. The lead is placed into the introducer sheath as directed to expose the electrodes. At this junction, it has been suggested that a curved stylet may allow for more accurate placement of the lead by allowing a more parallel association with the S3 nerve (Jacobs et al., 2014). Usually, electrodes are positioned such that electrodes 2 and 3 straddle the ventral surface of the sacrum, as shown in Fig. 32.3. Test stimulation is repeated on each electrode, and the responses are observed. Ideally, there are appropriate motor and sensory responses at all four electrodes, with amplitude of 3.0 mA or less (or even ≤2.0 mA; Matzel et al., 2017). If responses are not acceptable, the lead can be removed and replaced to try to follow the nerve. A lateral sacral view can be helpful at this timepoint to see if the lead placement is too lateral. If this is the case, it may be prudent to start again with the foramen needle on either side to attempt insertion closer to the sacral foramina. An appropriately placed lead is noted in Fig. 32.4. See also Video 32.2.

If appropriate responses are obtained, the tines are deployed. A 3- to 4-cm incision is made into the subcutaneous tissues in the upper lateral buttock and below the beltline or below the level of the ischial wings for connecting the permanent lead to the percutaneous extension lead wire. With the tunneling device, a tunnel is made to allow for passage of lead to the subcutaneous pocket. The lead is then cleaned and connected to the extension wire with a torque-limiting screwdriver. The percutaneous extension is tunneled subcutaneously to the contralateral side of the patient. The incision is closed in two layers after the wound is copiously irrigated. The extension wire is connected to the external pulse generator. Additional information is presented in Video 32.3, and Fig. 32.5 presents a summary of key points for optimal lead placement.

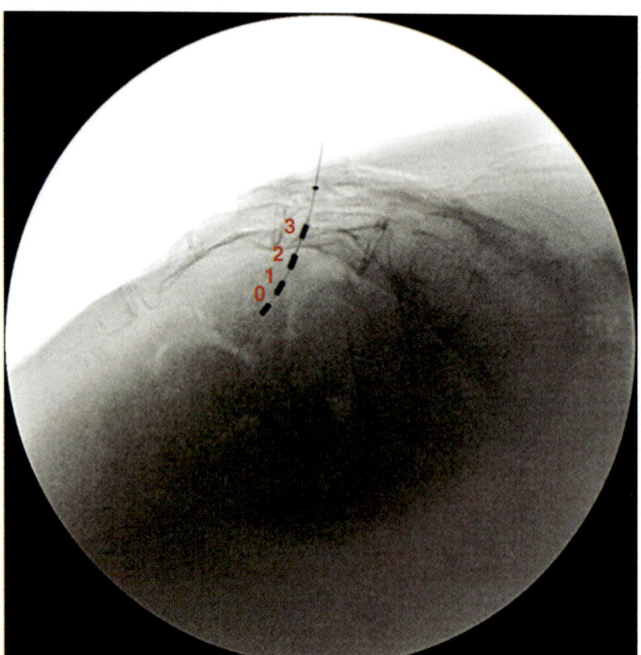

Fig. 32.3 Lateral fluoroscopic image of appropriately placed sacral neuromodulation lead. Usually, electrodes are positioned such that electrodes 2 and 3 straddle the ventral surface of the sacrum.

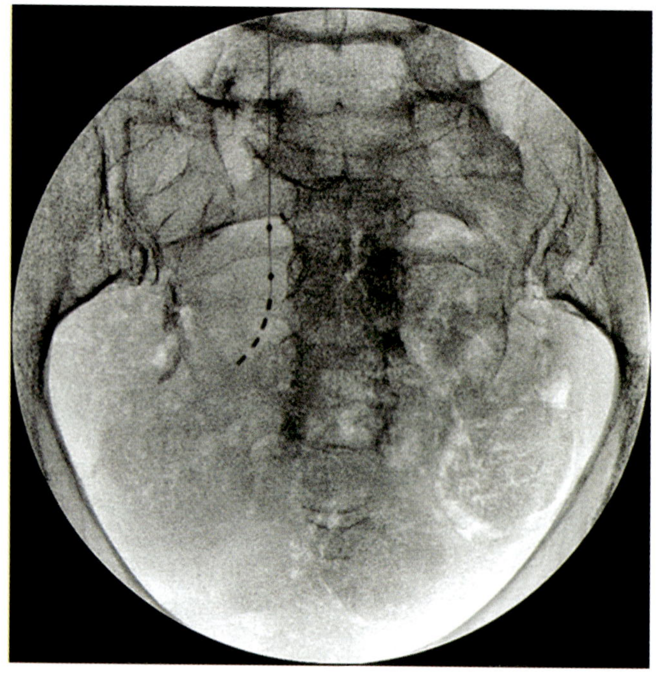

Fig. 32.4 Anteroposterior fluoroscopic image of appropriately placed sacral neuromodulation lead.

There is no consensus regarding the benefit of antibiotic-impregnated sheet use, wound irrigation with antibiotic solution, or postoperative antibiotics, although many will give 5 to 7 days of oral antibiotics postoperatively (Lee et al., 2017). During the test stimulation phase, patients are instructed to complete a daily bladder diary, and a stage II implant is planned for patients with greater than 50% improvement in symptoms.

Insertion of Pulse Generator (Stage II). The patient is placed in the prone position, and the previous buttock incision is opened with care to avoid damaging the permanent lead, which may be superficial. Once the connection between the lead and the extension wire is located, the temporary lead extension is cut. At the end of the case, the portion exiting the skin on the contralateral side is pulled and removed. The plastic protection sheath is removed, and the remaining portion of the temporary extension wire is unscrewed and completely removed. The electrodes of the permanent lead are cleaned and confirmed to be blood-free, and then secured to the IPG with the torque-limiting screwdriver. A pocket is created in the subcutaneous tissue that is large enough to avoid tension during closure and to provide a covering layer of subcutaneous tissue anterior to the pulse generator to prevent erosion. The implant area is copiously irrigated and closed in two layers.

Basic Evaluation (Percutaneous Nerve Evaluation). A basic evaluation is performed by placing bilateral percutaneous wires with one electrode in the S3 foramen (with or without fluoroscopic guidance) using local injectable anesthesia. The wires are then connected to an external pulse generator and

1. AP view	Identify **medial edge** of foramina	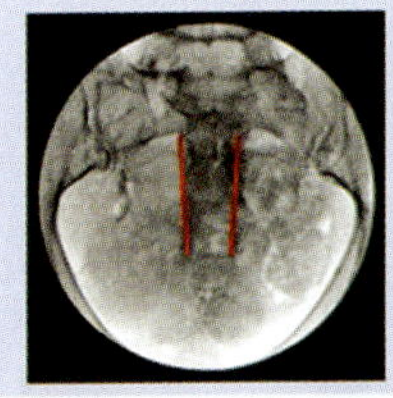
2. Lateral view	Identify **S3 bone seam** Mark skin needle entry point **parallel and cephalad** to bone seam	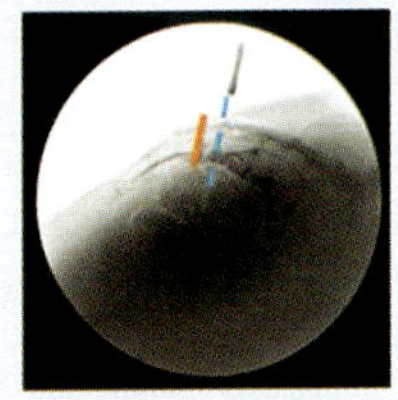
3. Needle placement	Parallel and cephalad to bone seam Parallel to **sagittal plane** **Small adjustments** based on fluoroscopy	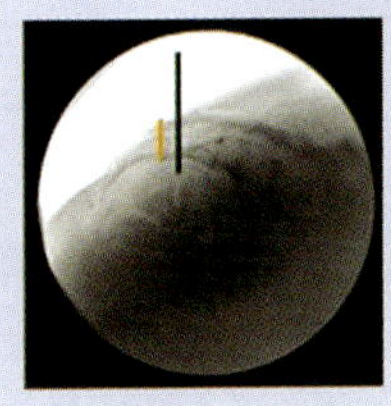 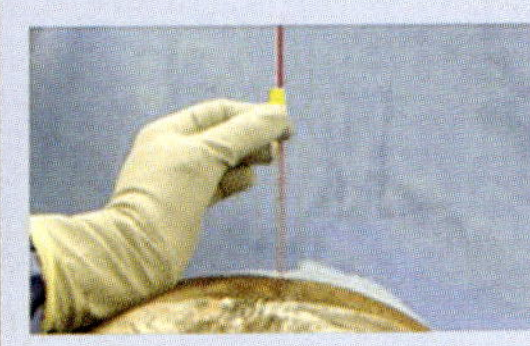

Fig. 32.5 Key points for optimal lead placement. *AP,* Anteroposterior.

worn by the patient for several days. Although PNE can be done in the office, it has a lower success rate, and therefore a lower implantation rate, compared with an advanced evaluation, which may be attributed to migration of the nonfixed wire, as well as an inability to trial multiple electrodes. Whereas upwards of 80% of patients progress to IPG placement after an advanced evaluation, only 40% to 50% progress to a full implant after a basic evaluation (Borawski et al., 2007; Marcelissen et al., 2011). If there is not a significant improvement in symptoms after a basic evaluation, an advanced evaluation is planned. The PNE procedure is demonstrated in Video 32.4.

Troubleshooting Sacral Neuromodulation in Follow-Up

In the InSite trial 5-year follow-up study, after initial successful implantation 22% of patients reported an undesirable change in stimulation, 15% reported implant site pain, and 13% reported ineffective stimulation. Two-year outcomes from a large, multicenter RCT comparing SNM with BTX-A found that 58% (81/139) of patients with SNM required reprogramming, with 17% (14/81) requiring three or more attempts at reprogramming. The most common reason for reprogramming was decreased efficacy. Device revisions occurred in only 3% (4/139) because of the inability to reprogram.

As reprogramming may be a common requirement for clinicians who perform SNM for OAB, we feel that an algorithmic approach is warranted. There are not a lot of data available to inform an evidence-based approach to programming, and most information is based on expert opinion or retrospective reviews. Some studies suggest performing a sacral radiograph as a part of the approach to help address the decreased efficacy of SNM. However, this suggestion was made before the evolution to a tined anchoring system, which involves less lead migration, and studies since then have failed to show a correlation between the long-term response to SNM and the electrode position on sacral x-rays (Gahzi et al., 2017). As such, we do not routinely recommend this in our evaluation.

Below we present our algorithms for either IPG site pain (Fig. 32.6) or change in perceived stimulation/efficacy of SNM device (Fig. 32.7). These are based on similar protocols used in the ROSETTA trial (Amundsen et al., 2016). For IPG site pain, the first step is to have the patient turn off her device. If discomfort resolves, then her discomfort is likely energy-related and may be improved by programming efforts. In general, unipolar stimulation is when at least one electrode is configured as negative, and the generator, or neurostimulator case, is configured as positive. This not only can deplete the battery at a higher rate but may also lead to uncomfortable buttock stimulation. If it is noted that the current stimulation is in a unipolar format, then a change to bipolar may alleviate discomfort. If reprogramming does not relieve discomfort, then replacement of the IPG and consideration of lead revision should occur.

For a change in perceived stimulation, especially a lack of stimulation, first confirm the device is on and that battery life remains. If the IPG is off, then turn on the device, confirm appropriate sensory sensations (i.e., vaginal), and monitor symptoms. If there has been a stimulation shift to an alternate location (i.e., down leg, up into sacral area), then reprogramming can often lead to a solution. In general, more superficial/proximal electrodes (i.e., 2 and 3) may cause sacral pain, whereas stimulation of distal electrodes (i.e., 0 and 1), depending on the track of the lead, may stimulate S2 (cause leg pain) or S4 (cause rectal discomfort). This can be taken into consideration for reprogramming. Finally, if stimulation is appropriately located but is uncomfortable to the patient, there are other parameters such as pulse width, frequency, and soft start/stop

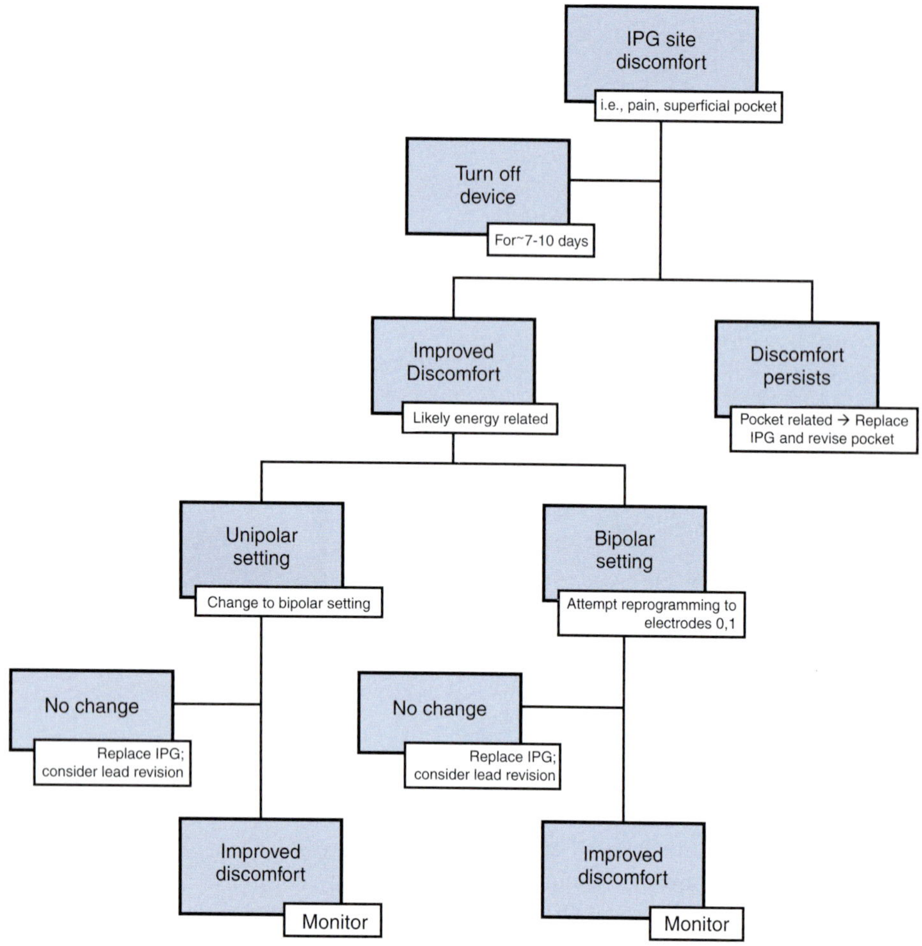

Fig. 32.6 Algorithm for approach to implantable pulse generator site pain. *IPG*, Internal pulse generator.

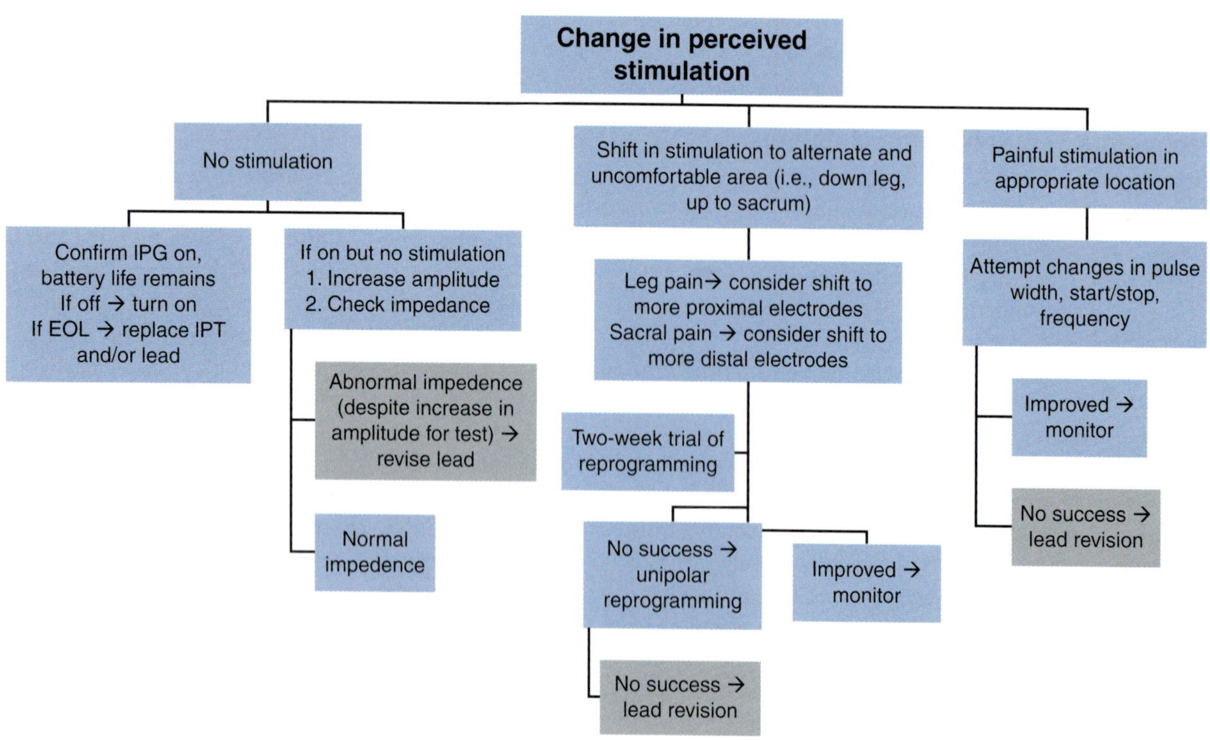

Fig. 32.7 Algorithm for approach to a change in perceived stimulation of sacral neuromodulation. *IPG*, Implantable pulse generator; *EOL*, end of life.

that may be modified to improve discomfort. After each reprogramming session, we allow at least 2 weeks to monitor symptoms before deciding on next steps. If a patient does not have success after two reprogramming sessions, then either lead revision or alternative options should be discussed. An "end-of-life" battery requires replacement of the IPG and/or lead revision based on previous symptom improvement.

Complications

Since the introduction of the tined lead, the frequency and profile of complications have changed dramatically (Sutherland et al., 2007). Reported complications of SNM are relatively minor and include lead migration with loss of efficacy (1.1%–8.6%), pain at the implant or lead site (3.3%–19.8%), superficial wound infection or implant (lead and/or IPG) infection (2.2%–14.3%), and need for surgical revision (6.25%–39.5%) (Gormley et al., 2012). The ROSETTA trial reported a rate of device revision and/or removal of only 3% in the first 6-month period (Amundsen et al., 2016). At 2-year follow-up, surgical revision was offered if reprogramming proved ineffective, and device removal was performed if symptoms continued. Device revisions occurred in 4/139 (3%) because of decreased efficacy. Device removal occurred in 12/139 (8.6%) (for infection [$n = 4$], decreased efficacy [$n = 4$], subject desire [$n = 2$], and pain [$n = 2$]). Optimization of lead placement with low amplitude response at all electrodes is the best way to avoid device revision for inefficacy.

Risk factors associated with complication after SNM are variably reported in the literature. A recent, large multicenter retrospective study did not determine any specific demographic or health characteristics that predicted risk of explant for infection, but, overall, the rate of device explant was low (1.97%; Myer et al., 2018). This study did find that having a postoperative hematoma or a deep pocket ($\geq$3 cm) significantly increased the risk of explant because of infection. These findings highlight the importance of meticulous hemostasis, as well as ensuring the pocket depth is less than 3 cm at the time of device implant.

Antibiotic choice may impact the risk of infection (Haraway et al., 2013). Placement of an antibiotic-impregnated collagen sheet in the wound has been investigated to determine if it may decrease risk of infection. One small study in patients undergoing SNM suggested benefit, but in larger trials there were no differences in infection with this approach (Bennett-Guerrero et al., 2010; Simpson et al., 2012). Currently, there is no guidance regarding skin preparation, but multiple studies in other disciplines have shown the benefit of chlorhexidine-alcohol. There are also no data regarding postprocedure antibiotics, but administration of oral antibiotics after cardiac pacemaker implantation has been shown to decrease infection.

Our general recommendations are supported by the literature (Lee et al., 2017):

1. Antibiotics: Before both test stimulation and implantation of pulse generator, we administer intravenous (IV) cefazolin (weight-based dosing) or 600 mg clindamycin IV if the patient is allergic to penicillin. The patient is managed postoperatively with trimethoprim-sulfamethoxazole twice daily for 5 days during test stimulation and after implantation of pulse generator. Alternative antibiotics such as amoxicillin/clavulanic acid, clindamycin, or ciprofloxacin are reasonable alternatives for patients with sulfa allergies.
2. Intraoperative: We use ChloraPrep (Becton, Dickinson and Company; Franklin Lakes, NJ) as our perioperative skin preparation. During the surgery, physicians may use iodine-impregnated adhesive drapes (such as Ioban 2 Antimicrobial Incise Drapes; 3M, St. Paul, MN) to cover the incision to provide an additional barrier for reduced contamination risk.
3. Test stimulation bandage: We use a large, transparent adhesive dressing to cover the entirety of all incisions to decrease infection.
4. Duration between stages: The duration between the two procedures is usually 1 to 2 weeks to reduce the risk of infection while allowing ample time to trial the device.

Considerations for Lead Removal

Explantation of the SNM device is occasionally necessary. Removing the tined lead can put strain on the lead, resulting in a possible break and retained fragments. The FDA released a notification regarding health consequences related to retained lead fragments. We support the techniques recommended by Sterling et al. (2016), in which an incision is made over the previous lead insertion site, and the lead is isolated and externalized. The fibrous encapsulation is dissected off the lead to expose the tines and ensure the lead is free from adhesions. The lead is removed by wrapping it around a curved hemostat and turning it under tension. If the lead breaks, the incision is extended, and dissection is carried down to the sacral body to remove all fragments. If the lead and/or IPG are removed because of infection a patient may undergo a reimplantation after an approximately 3-month interval and after any comorbidities like diarrhea, poorly controlled diabetes, and possibly smoking have been addressed.

Contraindications

In July 2012, the FDA approved that patients with InterStim II and specific InterStim I systems can undergo head MRI under specific conditions. Contraindications to implantation of the InterStim II device include the need for repeat back or body MRI. More recently, a new SNM system, Axonics (Axonics Modulation Technologies, Irvine, CA), has acquired FDA approval for OAB (see also Emerging Therapies section below). This device is full-body MRI 1.5T conditionally safe and Head Coil MRI 1.5T and 3T conditionally safe. Patients who have not demonstrated an appropriate response to test stimulation or who are unable to operate the neurostimulator should not be implanted with any SNM device.

Conclusions

In summary, SNM is a minimally invasive technique to treat refractory OAB. More recent high-quality RCTs have shown sustained efficacy with low complications for current SNM devices. Current and future derivations of SNM will allow for improved MRI compatibility, smaller devices, and longer battery life.

FACTORS ASSOCIATED WITH SUCCESS OF BOTULINUM TOXIN AND SACRAL NEUROMODULATION

Conclusions regarding factors predicting the success of either BTX-A or SNM have been mixed. However, two secondary analyses of the ROSETTA trial found that increasing age was associated with a lower treatment response. When split into groups by age, both groups experienced improvement in mean UUI episodes per day following each treatment. In the BTX-A group, women younger than 65 years had 3.3-fold greater odds of at least 75% resolution than women 65 years or older (Komesu et al., 2018). Older women had more UTI following BTX-A and SNM (OR = 1.9, 95% CI 1.2–3.3). There was no evidence of age differences in SNM revision/removal or catheterization following BTX-A. More severe symptoms (increased UUI episodes/day) at baseline seemed to improve treatment response, and higher body mass index was associated with reduced treatment response (Richter et al., 2017).

PERCUTANEOUS TIBIAL NERVE STIMULATION

Background and Proposed Method of Action

Percutaneous tibial nerve stimulation is a neuromodulation technique performed by percutaneous electrical stimulation of the posterior tibial nerve. McGuire et al. were the first to describe PTNS, in 1983. Subsequently, Stoller et al. (1999) further developed PTNS, initially referred to as the Stoller afferent nerve system, as a treatment for OAB. In July 2005, the Urgent PC Neuromodulation System (formerly Uroplasty, Inc, Minnetonka, MN; now Cogentix Medical, Holland) was introduced for patients suffering from urinary urgency, frequency, and urgency incontinence. In 2010, the cleared indication was changed to OAB. A second device, the NURO Neuromodulation system (formerly Advanced UroSolutions, Elizabethton, TN; now Medtronic Inc., Minneapolis, MN) was cleared by the FDA in November 2013.

The innervation of the lower urinary tract comes from the lumbar, sacral, and coccygeal segmental nerves originating from L2–S4. The sciatic nerve is composed of fibers from L4 to S3 and descends toward the lower extremities. One of its distal branches is the posterior tibial nerve. The exact mechanism of action of peripheral neuromodulation has not been clearly elucidated, but there is likely effect on the cross-signaling between nerve signals involved in the voiding reflex (de Groat et al., 2014). The pudendal nerve, the dorsal genital nerve, and the posterior tibial nerve are examples of such peripheral nerves that can affect bladder behavior.

Efficacy

A variety of observational trials initially reported on the efficacy of PTNS, showing decreased incontinence (reduction range 1–3 episodes/day), frequency (reduction range 2–5 episodes/day), nocturia (reduction range 1–2 episodes/night), and improved QOL (MacDiarmid et al., 2010; Vandoninck et al., 2003). Systematic reviews have identified two RCTs comparing PTNS to sham therapy (Gormley et al., 2015; Moossdorff-Steinhauser et al., 2013). The largest trial is "The Sham Effectiveness in Treatment of Overactive Bladder Symptoms (SUmiT) trial" (Peters et al., 2010). This trial randomized 220 adults with OAB symptoms (fewer mean UUI episodes/day as compared with trials on BTX-A or SNM) to 12 weeks' treatment with weekly PTNS or sham therapy. Finazzi-Agrò et al. (2010) reported on 35 female subjects randomized to PTNS or control (needle placed in gastrocnemius muscle). The voiding diary parameters showed a statistically significant improvement in frequency and incontinence episodes for the PTNS groups compared with sham. One study showed a statistically significant improvement in nocturia (P = .04) and urgency (P < .001) in the PTNS group compared with the sham group (Peters et al., 2010). One RCT compared PTNS with tolterodine ER, with no statistically significant difference between the groups regarding urinary urgency (P = .44) (Peters et al., 2009).

Regarding longer-term efficacy, 50 participants from the SUmiT trial who met the primary effectiveness endpoint after 12 weekly sessions were enrolled in a prospective study to assess long-term outcomes with PTNS. The Sustained Therapeutic Effects of Percutaneous Tibial Nerve Stimulation study patients were treated with a 14-week tapering protocol followed by a personal treatment plan (Peters et al., 2013). Although 97% of patients maintained moderate or marked improvement in OAB symptoms at 3 years, these promising results are limited by the small study size. Maintenance therapy with monthly sessions after the initial 12-week course is a common protocol for patients receiving this modality, but there is a paucity of information regarding the necessary length of maintenance therapy and the average interval until symptom recurrence after cessation of therapy.

Technique

Percutaneous tibial nerve stimulation is a nonsurgical, ambulatory treatment. Although this treatment requires weekly 30-minute treatment sessions for 12 consecutive weeks, the treatment has very few associated adverse events and is not painful. The procedure involves placing a small (34-gauge) needle electrode into the lower inner aspect of either leg cephalad to the medial malleolus (Fig. 32.8). A surface electrode is placed using sticker adhesive, and the needle electrode is then connected to a stimulator. The generated electrical pulse (current level of 0.5–9 mA at 20 Hz) then travels to the sacral nerve plexus via the tibial nerve. The initial 12-week course is followed by occasional treatments (usually monthly) as needed based on patient symptoms. A short video demonstrating the PTNS procedure is presented here (Video 32.5).

Side Effects and Cost

Adverse events associated with PTNS are reported as mild, transient, and relatively uncommon at 1% to 2% of cases, including bruising or bleeding at the needle site, tingling, and mild pain (Peters et al., 2009; Peterson et al., 2010). The cost effectiveness of PTNS is difficult to assess, owing to a wide range of coverage and patient copays for the procedure. A decision analysis using cost from a societal perspective did not find PTNS to be more cost effective than treatment with anticholinergic therapy

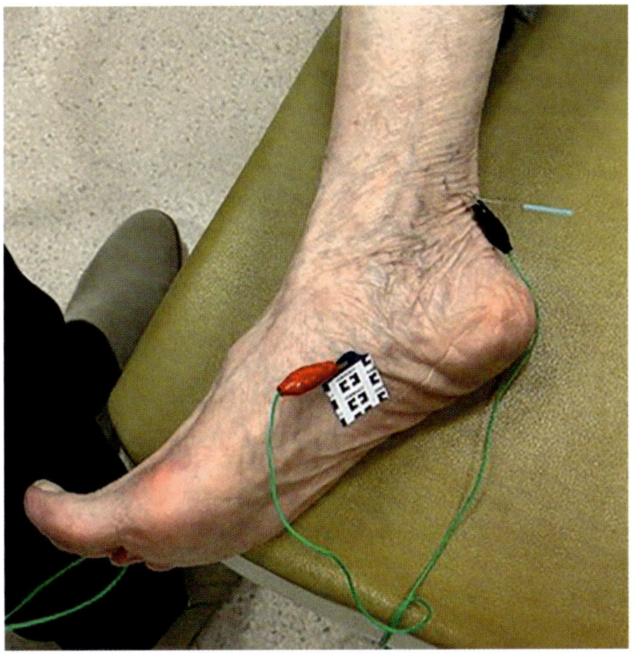

Fig. 32.8 Percutaneous tibial nerve stimulation needle placement.

(Chen et al., 2012). Given the ease of performing the procedure and the minimal adverse events, PTNS is a reasonable treatment option for patients with OAB. However, travel for weekly visits, prolonged monthly maintenance, and the burden of copayments/lack of insurance coverage does limit the wider dissemination of this therapy. There does not seem to be a difference in efficacy when medications are used with PTNS, but this body of literature is overall small (Sancaktar et al., 2010).

COST EFFECTIVENESS OF THERAPIES

It may be that, if medical management is effective, the lowest cost is associated with continued medical therapy (Chen et al., 2012). However, when medications are ineffective or not tolerable, it is important to consider comparative cost between the available third-line options. When considering third-line options for refractory OAB, accurate costs to patient and to society are important because the relative cost per improvement in health-related QOL may help patients, clinicians, and payers make informed decisions about therapy. Owing to the many variables that may affect cost and reported efficacy outcomes, evaluating these more advanced therapies in terms of cost can be challenging.

There is a dearth of literature examining the cost-effectiveness of PTNS. One study suggested that PTNS entail a substantially lower cost than SNM (Martinson et al., 2013). However, this study did not account for more recent, low SNM explantation rates. Furthermore, PTNS is variably covered by insurance plans and requires clinic visits for treatment, possibly over the course of a patients' lifetime. These are all variables that must be considered when recommending PTNS.

There is more cost evidence regarding BTX-A and SNM, but this body of literature mostly uses models with older data. A retrospective cost-effectiveness analysis of BTX-A compared with SNM for OAB suggested that SNM may become cost effective after 5 years compared with BTX-A, but many variables, including use of local anesthesia with BTX-A and PNE with SNM, may affect these results (Leong et al., 2011). A recent secondary analysis from a large, multicenter RCT found that, at 2 years, BTX-A had lower overall costs, and modeling out to 5 years showed that SNM remained more expensive, considering similar outcomes (Harvie et al., 2019). Sensitivity analyses from this study indicated how reduction of SNM device and implantation costs, limited need for SNM pulse generator replacement with rechargeable technology, increased BTX-A injection frequency, or higher UTI treatment costs would most directly impact cost-effectiveness.

EMERGING THERAPIES

Previously, only one SNM device was FDA-approved (Interstim; Medtronic, Minneapolis, MN). Limitations of this technology include the need for neurostimulator replacement after an expected 7-year life in the body, and the recommendation against performing nonhead MRI, although small case series have suggested safety of even body MRI with an implanted Interstim device (Chermansky et al., 2011). As discussed previously, Axonics Modulation Technologies (Irvine, CA) has developed a smaller, rechargeable, implantable pulse generator (neurostimulator) SNM device with an expected 15-year life in the body. The Axonics system is full-body MRI 1.5T conditionally safe and head coil MRI 1.5T and 3T conditionally safe, and it obtained FDA approval for OAB in 2019 (Elterman 2018). One limitation to the Axonics system is that the IPG only stores a single program. Although patients can turn the device off and change the amplitude, they are unable to trial different programs, which potentially means more frequent clinic visits for reprogramming. Medtronic received FDA approval in 2020 for a rechargeable neurostimulator (InterStim Micro) with accompanying MRI-safe lead (InterStim SureScan MRI lead) that will also allow patients with the implanted system to safely receive MRI scans, given certain precautions.

The Relax OAB trial described outcomes of the rechargeable Axonics sacral nerve stimulation device (Blok et al., 2018). Initially, this was a prospective, single-stage implant of the lead (opposed to advanced evaluation first) and IPG in 51 patients with refractory OAB. Three-month results demonstrated that 71% of patients were test responders (>50% improvement in UUI episodes/day), and the infection rate was less than 2%. Some 98% of patients were able to recharge the device within the first month. The same population was followed for 12 months, and, of those with follow-up (84%), UUI episodes/day were reduced from a baseline of 8.3 ($\pm$ 0.8) to 1.8 ($\pm$ 0.5) (Blok et al., 2019). The most common device-related adverse event was an undesirable or uncomfortable stimulation (13 events in 10 subjects), which resolved with reprogramming. Another study evaluated 129 patients with the Axonics SNM system and found that, at 6 months, 90% of participants were therapy responders (urinary UUI episodes/day reduced from 5.6 $\pm$ 0.3 at baseline to 1.3 $\pm$ 0.2) (McCrery et al., 2020). A total of three patients (2.3%) had

TABLE 32.3 Emerging Therapies for Refractory Overactive Bladder

Therapy	Company	Information	Data
StimRouter	Bioness Inc. (Valencia, CA)	• Implanted lead, integrated receiver, anchor and three electrode contacts close to the posterior tibial nerve • Transmitter and patch are worn only during periods of stimulation • Patient uses a programmer to track usage and change programs	Currently recruiting for US IDE trial
RENOVA	BlueWind Medical (Israel)	• Surgically implanted close to posterior tibial nerve • External control unit is worn around the ankle 30 minutes daily • Stimulation parameters can be altered to optimize	20 participants with 3-year follow-up; 75% with ≥50% improvement in OAB symptoms (Dorsthorst et al., 2020)
Radiofrequency ablation	Hologic Inc. (Marlborough, MA)	• Radiofrequency energy is used to ablate areas near the bladder trigone (selective bladder denervation)	29 women with 12-month follow-up; 69% had ≥50% reduction in UUI, 10% dry/cure rate (Rovner et al., 2019)

IDE, Investigational Device Exemption; *OAB*, overactive bladder; *UUI*, urgency urinary incontinence.

device removal owing to either infection or pain, and there were no serious device-related adverse events.

Additional emerging therapies for refractory OAB are discussed in Table 32.3. Because peripheral nerves such as the tibial nerve are more accessible, stimulation of other peripheral nerves have been investigated (i.e., pudendal nerve and dorsal genital nerve; Bartley et al., 2013). The pudendal nerve is composed mainly of afferent sensory fibers that originate from sacral nerve roots S1–S3 and innervate the pelvic floor muscles, the external urethral and anal sphincters, and the pelvic organs (Groen et al., 2005). To stimulate the pudendal nerve, both the transvaginal and posterior approach have been described (Fugett et al., 2018; Peters et al., 2010). Similarly, the dorsal genital nerve, a branch of the pudendal nerve, can be stimulated via needle placement in the midline of the midpubis and advanced to between the crura of the clitoris and the pubic bone. Feasibility studies for both these peripheral nerve stimulation techniques have looked promising for OAB treatment. However, neither have been extensively evaluated in larger studies.

FINAL CONCLUSIONS

In conclusion, PTNS, BTX-A, and SNM are all approved options for refractory OAB. Each modality has some risks and benefits, considering individual patient preferences, comorbidities, and previous therapies. Future research investigating improved prediction models surrounding optimal individual treatment plans is important to improve the care for women with refractory OAB.

BIBLIOGRAPHY

Aharony S, Przydacz M, Van Ba OL, Corcos J. Does asymptomatic bacteriuria increase the risk of adverse events or modify the efficacy of intradetrusor onabotulinumtoxinA injections? *Neurourol Urodyn*. 2019;39:203.

Allergan I. Botox: highlights of prescribing information. http://www.allergan.com/assets/pdf/botox_pi.pdf. Accessed March 1, 2020.

Altaweel W, Mokhtar A, Rabah D. Prospective randomized trial of 100u vs 200u botox in the treatment of idiopathic overactive bladder. *Urol Ann*. 2011;3:66.

Amundsen CL, Richter HE, Menefee SA, et al. OnabotulinumtoxinA vs sacral neuromodulation on refractory urgency urinary incontinence in women: a randomized clinical trial. *JAMA*. 2016;316:1366.

Amundsen CL, Komesu YM, Chermansky C, et al. Two-year outcomes of sacral neuromodulation versus onabotulinumtoxinA for refractory urgency urinary incontinence: a randomized trial. *Eur Urol*. 2018;74:66.

Apostolidis A, Dasgupta P, Fowler CJ. Proposed mechanism for the efficacy of injected Botulinum toxin in the treatment of human detrusor overactivity. *Eur Urol*. 2006;49:644.

Bartley J, Gilleran J, Peters K. Neuromodulation for overactive bladder. *Nat Rev Urol*. 2013;10:513.

Bennett-Guerrero E, Pappas TN, Koltun WA, et al. Gentamicin–collagen sponge for infection prophylaxis in colorectal surgery. *N Engl J Med*. 2010;363:1038.

Bickhaus JA, Bradley MS, Amundsen CL, et al. Does a recent urinary tract infection increase the risk of postprocedure urinary tract infection after onabotulinum toxin A? *Female Pelvic Med Reconstr Surg*. 2018;27:121.

Bickhaus JA, Vaughan M, Truong T, Li Y-J, Siddiqui NY. A comparison of antibiotic prophylaxis regimens to decrease the risk of post-procedure urinary tract infection after onabotulinum toxin A injection. *Int Urogynecol J*. 2020;31:1907.

Blok B, Van Kerrebroeck P, de Wachter S, et al. Three month clinical results with a rechargeable sacral neuromodulation system for the treatment of overactive bladder. *Neurourol Urodyn*. 2018;37:S9.

Blok B, Van Kerrebroeck P, de Wachter S, et al. A prospective, multicenter study of a novel, miniaturized rechargeable sacral neuromodulation system: 12-month results from the RELAX-OAB study. *Neurourol Urodyn*. 2019;38:689.

Borawski KM, Foster RT, Webster GD, Amundsen CL. Predicting implantation with a neuromodulator using two different test stimulation techniques: a prospective randomized study in urge incontinent women. *Neurourol Urodyn*. 2007;26:14.

Brubaker L, Richter HE, Visco A, et al. Refractory idiopathic urge urinary incontinence and botulinum A injection. *J Urol*. 2008;180:217.

Chen HW, Bercik RS, Werner EF, Thung SF. Cost-effectiveness of percutaneous tibial nerve stimulation versus extended release tolterodine for overactive bladder. *J Urol*. 2012;187:178.

Chapple C, Sievert KD, MacDiarmid S, et al. OnabotulinumtoxinA 100 U significantly improves all idiopathic overactive bladder symptoms and quality of life in patients with overactive bladder and urinary incontinence: a randomised, double-blind, placebo-controlled trial. *Eur Urol*. 2013;64:249.

Chermansky CJ, Krlin RM, Holley TD, et al. Magnetic resonance imaging following interstim®: An institutional experience with imaging safety and patient satisfaction. *Neurourol Urodyn.* 2011;30:1486.

Coelho A, Cruz F, Cruz CD, Avelino A. Spread of onabotulinumtoxinA after bladder injection. Experimental study using the distribution of cleaved SNAP-25 as the marker of the toxin action. *Eur Urol.* 2012;61:1178.

Cohen BL, Barboglio P, Rodriguez D, Gousse AE. Preliminary results of a dose-finding study for botulinum toxin-a in patients with idiopathic overactive bladder: 100 versus 150 units. *Neurourol Urodyn.* 2009;28:205.

Cui Y, Wang L, Liu L, et al. Botulinum toxin-A injections for idiopathic overactive bladder: a systematic review and meta-analysis. *Urol Int.* 2013;91:429.

Davis T, Makovey I, Guralnick ML, O'Connor RC. Sacral neuromodulation outcomes for the treatment of refractory idiopathic detrusor overactivity stratified by indication: Lack of anticholinergic efficacy versus intolerability. *Can Urol Assoc J.* 2012;7:176.

Davis NF, Burke JP, Redmond EJ, et al. Trigonal versus extratrigonal botulinum toxin-A: a systematic review and meta-analysis of efficacy and adverse events. *Int Urogynecol J Pelvic Floor Dysfunct.* 2014;26:313.

De Wachter S, Benson KD, Dmochowski RR, et al. Six-month results of selective bladder denervation in women with refractory overactive bladder. *J Urol.* 2019;201:573.

de Groat WC, Yoshimura N. Afferent nerve regulation of bladder function in health and disease. *Handb Exp Pharmacol.* 2009;194:91.

de Groat WC, Griffiths D, Yoshimura N. Neural control of the lower urinary tract. In: *Comprehensive Physiology*. Vol 5. Hoboken, NJ: John Wiley & Sons, Inc.; 2014:327.

Denys P, Le Normand L, Ghout I, et al. Efficacy and safety of low doses of onabotulinumtoxinA for the treatment of refractory idiopathic overactive bladder: a multicentre, double-blind, randomised, placebo-controlled dose-ranging study. *Eur Urol.* 2012;61:520.

Deveneau NE, Greenstein M, Mahalingashetty A, et al. Surface and boney landmarks for sacral neuromodulation: a cadaveric study. *Int Urogynecol J.* 2015;26:263.

Dmochowski R, Chapple C, Nitti VW, et al. Efficacy and safety of onabotulinumtoxinA for idiopathic overactive bladder: a double-blind, placebo controlled, randomized, dose ranging trial. *J Urol.* 2010;184:2416.

Dobberfuhl AD, Mahal A, Dallas KB, et al. Statewide success of staged sacral neuromodulation for the treatment of urinary complaints in California (2005-2011). *Female Pelvic Med Reconstr Surg.* 2020;26:437

Dorsthorst MJT, Digesu GA, Tailor V, et al. 3-year followup of a new implantable tibial nerve stimulator for the treatment of overactive bladder syndrome. *J Urol.* 2020;204:545.

Dowson C, Watkins J, Khan MS, et al. Repeated botulinum toxin type A injections for refractory overactive bladder: medium-term outcomes, safety profile, and discontinuation rates. *Eur Urol.* 2012;61:834.

Duthie JB, Vincent M, Herbison GP, et al. Botulinum toxin injections for adults with overactive bladder syndrome. *Cochrane Database Syst Rev.* 2011;12:CD005493.

Elterman DS. The novel Axonics® rechargeable sacral neuromodulation system: Procedural and technical impressions from an initial North American experience. *Neurourol Urodyn.* 2018;37:S1. Available at: https://www.axonics.com/hcp/axonics-system/mri-safety-compatibility.

Flynn MK, Amundsen CL, Perevich M, et al. Outcome of a randomized, double-blind, placebo controlled trial of botulinum A toxin for refractory overactive bladder. *J Urol.* 2009;181:2608.

Finazzi-Agrò E, Petta F, Sciobica F, et al. Percutaneous tibial nerve stimulation effects on detrusor overactivity incontinence are not due to a placebo effect: a randomized, double-blind, placebo controlled trial. *J Urol.* 2010;184:2001.

Fowler CJ, Griffiths D, De Groat WC. The neural control of micturition. *Nat Rev Neurosci.* 2008;9:453.

Fugett J, Phillips L, Tobin E, et al. Selective bladder denervation for overactive bladder (OAB) syndrome: From concept to healing outcomes using the ovine model. *Neurourol Urodyn.* 2018;37:2097.

Gahzi AA, Banakhar MA, Elterman DS, Hassouna M. Radiographic position of the electrode as a predictor of the outcome of InterStim therapy. *Int Neurourol J.* 2017;21:289.

Gamé X, Khan S, Panicker JN, et al. Comparison of the impact on health-related quality of life of repeated detrusor injections of botulinum toxin in patients with idiopathic or neurogenic detrusor overactivity. *BJU Int.* 2011;107:1786.

Goldman HB, Amundsen CL, Mangel J, et al. Dorsal genital nerve stimulation for the treatment of overactive bladder symptoms. *Neurourol Urodyn.* 2008;27:499.

Gormley EA, Lightner DJ, Burgio KL, et al. Diagnosis and treatment of overactive bladder (non-neurogenic) in adults: AUA/SUFU guideline. *J Urol.* 2012;188:2455.

Gormley EA, Lightner DJ, Faraday M, Vasavada SP. American Urological Association; Society of Urodynamics, Female Pelvic Medicine. Diagnosis and treatment of overactive bladder (non-neurogenic) in adults: AUA/SUFU guideline amendment. *J Urol.* 2015;193:1572.

Granese R, Adile G, Gugliotta G, et al. Botox® for idiopathic overactive bladder: Efficacy, duration and safety. Effectiveness of subsequent injection. *Arch Gynecol Obstet.* 2012;286:923.

Groen J, Amiel C, Bosch JLHR. Chronic pudendal nerve neuromodulation in women with idiopathic refractory detrusor overactivity incontinence: Results of a pilot study with a novel minimally invasive implantable mini-stimulator. *Neurourol Urodyn.* 2005;24:226.

Haraway AM, Clemens JQ, He C, Stroup C, Atiemo HO, Cameron AP. Differences in sacral neuromodulation device infection rates based on preoperative antibiotic selection. *Int Urogynecol J.* 2013;24:2081.

Harvie HS, Amundsen CL, Neuwahl SJ, et al. Cost-effectiveness of sacral neuromodulation versus onabotulinumtoxinA for refractory urgency urinary incontinence: results of the ROSETTA Randomized Trial. *J Urol.* 2020;203:969.

Hijaz A, Vasavada S. Complications and troubleshooting of sacral neuromodulation therapy. *Urol Clin North Am.* 2005;32:65.

Hijaz A, Vasavada SP, Daneshgari F, et al. Complications and troubleshooting of two-stage sacral neuromodulation therapy: a single-institution experience. *Urology.* 2006;68:533.

Jabs C, Carleton E. Efficacy of botulinum toxin a intradetrusor injections for non-neurogenic urinary urge incontinence: a randomized double-blind controlled trial. *J Obstet Gynaecol Can.* 2013;35:53.

Jacobs SA, Lane FL, Osann KE, Noblett KL. Randomized prospective crossover study of interstim lead wire placement with curved versus straight stylet. *Neurourol Urodyn.* 2014;33:488.

Jo JK, Kim KN, Kim DW, et al. The effect of onabotulinumtoxinA according to site of injection in patients with overactive bladder: a systematic review and meta-analysis. *World J Urol.* 2018;36:305.

Kessler TM, Khan S, Panicker J, et al. Clean intermittent self-catheterization after botulinum neurotoxin type A injections: short-term effect on quality of life. *Obstet Gynecol.* 2009;113:1046.

Ko CP. Do nerve terminal sprouts contribute to functional recovery from botulinum neurotoxin A? *J Physiol.* 2008;586:3021.

Komesu YM, Amundsen CL, Richter HE, et al. Refractory urgency urinary incontinence treatment in women: impact of age on outcomes and complications. *Am J Obstet Gynecol.* 2018;218:111.e1.

Kuo HC. Will suburothelial injection of small dose of botulinum A toxin have similar therapeutic effects and less adverse events for refractory detrusor overactivity? *Urology.* 2006;68:993; discussion 997.

Kuo HC. Comparison of effectiveness of detrusor, suburothelial and bladder base injections of botulinum toxin A for idiopathic detrusor overactivity. *J Urol.* 2007;178:1359.

Kuo HC. Bladder base/trigone injection is safe and as effective as bladder body injection of onabotulinumtoxinA for idiopathic detrusor overactivity refractory to antimuscarinics. *Neurourol Urodyn.* 2011;30:1242.

Leong RK, de Wachter SGG, Joore MA, van Kerrebroeck PEV. Cost-effectiveness analysis of sacral neuromodulation and botulinum toxin A treatment for patients with idiopathic overactive bladder. *BJU Int.* 2011;108:558.

Lee C, Pizarro-Berdichevsky J, Clifton MM, Vasavada SP. Sacral neuromodulation implant infection: risk factors and prevention. *Curr Urol Rep.* 2017;18:16.

Liao C-H, Chen S-F, Kuo H-C. Different number of intravesical onabotulinumtoxinA injections for patients with refractory detrusor overactivity do not affect treatment outcome: a prospective randomized comparative study. *Neurourol Urodyn.* 2016;35:717.

Lightner DJ, Wymer K, Sanchez J, Kavoussi L. Best practice statement on urologic procedures and antimicrobial prophylaxis. *J Urol.* 2020;203:351.

MacDiarmid SA, Peters KM, Shobeiri SA, et al. Long-term durability of percutaneous tibial nerve stimulation for the treatment of overactive bladder. *J Urol.* 2010;183:234.

Marcelissen T, Leong R, Serroyen J, et al. Is the screening method of sacral neuromodulation a prognostic factor for long-term success? *J Urol.* 2011;185:583.

Martinson M, MacDiarmid S, Black E. Cost of neuromodulation therapies for overactive bladder: Percutaneous tibial nerve stimulation versus sacral nerve stimulation. *J Urol.* 2013;189:210.

Matzel KE, Chartier-Kastler E, Knowles CH, et al. Sacral neuromodulation: standardized electrode placement technique. *Neuromodulation.* 2017;20:816.

McCrery R, Lane F, Benson K, et al. Treatment of urinary urgency incontinence using a rechargeable SNM system: 6-month results of the ARTISAN-SNM Study. *J Urol.* 2020;203:185.

McGuire EJ, Zhang SC, Horwinski ER, Lytton B. Treatment of motor and sensory detrusor instability by electrical stimulation. *J Urol.* 1983;129:78.

Moore DC, Cohn JA, Dmochowski RR. Use of botulinum toxin A in the treatment of lower urinary tract disorders: a review of the literature. *Toxins (Basel).* 2016;8:88.

Moossdorff-Steinhauser HFA, Berghmans B. Effects of percutaneous tibial nerve stimulation on adult patients with overactive bladder syndrome: a systematic review. *Neurourol Urodyn.* 2013;32:206.

Myer ENB, Petrikovets A, Slocum PD, et al. Risk factors for explantation due to infection after sacral neuromodulation: a multicenter retrospective case-control study. *Am J Obstet Gynecol.* 2018;219:78.e1.

Nigam PK, Nigam A. Botulinum toxin. *Indian J Dermatol.* 2010;55:8.

Nitti VW. Botulinum toxin for the treatment of idiopathic and neurogenic overactive bladder: state of the art. *Rev Urol.* 2006;8:198.

Noblett KL, Buono K. Sacral nerve stimulation as a therapy for patients with refractory voiding and bowel dysfunction. *Obstet Gynecol.* 2018;132:1337.

Peters KM, Macdiarmid SA, Wooldridge LS, et al. Randomized trial of percutaneous tibial nerve stimulation versus extended-release tolterodine: results from the overactive bladder innovative therapy trial. *J Urol.* 2009;182:1055.

Peters KM, Carrico DJ, Perez-Marrero RA, et al. Randomized trial of percutaneous tibial nerve stimulation versus sham efficacy in the treatment of overactive bladder syndrome: results from the SUmiT Trial. *J Urol.* 2010;183:1438.

Peters KM, Killinger KA, Boguslawski BM, Boura JA. Chronic pudendal neuromodulation: expanding available treatment options for refractory urologic symptoms. *Neurourol Urodyn.* 2010;29:1267.

Peters KM, Carrico DJ, Wooldridge LS, et al. Percutaneous tibial nerve stimulation for the long-term treatment of overactive bladder: 3-year results of the STEP study. *J Urol.* 2013;189:2194.

Powell LC, Szabo SM, Walker D, Gooch K. The economic burden of overactive bladder in the United States: a systematic literature review. *Neurourol Urodyn.* 2018;37:1241.

Richter HE, Amundsen CL, Erickson SW, et al. Characteristics associated with treatment response and satisfaction in women undergoing onabotulinumtoxinA and sacral neuromodulation for refractory urgency urinary incontinence. *J Urol.* 2017;198:890.

Rovner E, Kennelly M, Schulte-Baukloh H, et al. Urodynamic results and clinical outcomes with intradetrusor injections of onabotulinumtoxinA in a randomized, placebo-controlled dose-finding study in idiopathic overactive bladder. *Neurourol Urodyn.* 2011;30:556.

Rovner ES, Versi E, Le Mai T, et al. One-year results with selective bladder denervation in women with refractory overactive bladder. *Neurourol Urodyn.* 2019;38:2178.

Sahai A, Khan MS, Dasgupta P. Efficacy of botulinum toxin-A for treating idiopathic detrusor overactivity: results from a single center, randomized, double-blind, placebo controlled trial. *J Urol.* 2007;177:2231.

Sancaktar M, Ceyhan ST, Akyol I, et al. The outcome of adding peripheral neuromodulation (Stoller afferent neuro-stimulation) to anti-muscarinic therapy in women with severe overactive bladder. *Gynecol Endocrinol.* 2010;26:729.

Senaratne JM, Jayasuriya A, Irwin M, et al. A 19-year study on pacemaker-related infections: a claim for using postoperative antibiotics. *Pacing Clin Electrophysiol.* 2014;37:947.

Siegel S, Noblett K, Mangel J, et al. Results of a prospective, randomized, multicenter study evaluating sacral neuromodulation with InterStim therapy compared to standard medical therapy at 6-months in subjects with mild symptoms of overactive bladder. *Neurourol Urodyn.* 2015;34:224.

Siegel S, Noblett K, Mangel J, et al. Five-year followup results of a prospective, multicenter study of patients with overactive bladder treated with sacral neuromodulation. *J Urol.* 2018;199:229.

Simpson JA, Peacock J, Maxwell-Armstrong C. Use of a gentamicin-impregnated collagen sheet (Collatamp®) following implantation of a sacral nerve stimulator for faecal incontinence. *Colorectal Dis.* 2012;14:e200.

Sterling ME, Hartigan SM, Wein AJ, Smith AL. A standardized surgical technique for removal of the Interstim tined lead. *Can J Urol.* 2016;23:8471.

Stoffel JT, Peterson AC, Sandhu JS, et al. AUA white paper on nonneurogenic chronic urinary retention: consensus definition, treatment algorithm, and outcome end points. *J Urol.* 2017;198:153.

Sutherland SE, Lavers A, Carlson A, et al. Sacral nerve stimulation for voiding dysfunction: one institution's 11-year experience. *Neurourol Urodyn*. 2007;26:19; discussion 36.

Szczypior M, Połom W, Markuszewski M, et al. Overactive bladder treatment: application of methylene blue to improve the injection technique of onabotulinum toxin A. *Scand J Urol*. 2017;51:474.

Tincello DG, Kenyon S, Abrams KR, et al. Botulinum toxin a versus placebo for refractory detrusor overactivity in women: a randomised blinded placebo-controlled trial of 240 women (the RELAX study). *Eur Urol*. 2012;62:507.

Tuuli MG, Liu J, Stout MJ, et al. A Randomized trial comparing skin antiseptic agents at cesarean delivery. *N Engl J Med*. 2016;374:647.

Vandoninck V, van Balken MR, Agró EF, et al. Posterior tibial nerve stimulation in the treatment of urge incontinence. *Neurourol Urodyn*. 2003;22:17.

Veeratterapillay R, Harding C, Teo L, et al. Discontinuation rates and inter-injection interval for repeated intravesical botulinum toxin type A injections for detrusor overactivity. *Int J Urol*. 2014;21:175.

Visco AG, Brubaker L, Richter HE, et al. Anticholinergic versus botulinum toxin A comparison trial for the treatment of bothersome urge urinary incontinence: ABC trial. *Contemp Clin Trials*. 2012;33:184.

Visco AG, Brubaker L, Richter HE, et al. Anticholinergic therapy vs. onabotulinumtoxina for urgency urinary incontinence. *N Engl J Med*. 2012;367:1803.

Walker TJ, Dayan SH. Comparison and overview of currently available neurotoxins. *J Clin Aesthet Dermatol*. 2014;7:31.

33

Neurourology and Compliance Abnormalities

Elizabeth Rourke, Roger R. Dmochowski, and Stephen R. Kraus

CHAPTER OUTLINE

INTRODUCTION

The primary functions of the urinary bladder are storage and emptying, which are mediated by a combination of parasympathetic, sympathetic, and autonomic signaling (see Chapter 3). Bladder compliance is the ability of the bladder to accommodate changes in urinary volume during the storage phase, without a significant change in bladder pressure. Changes in compliance can result in a loss of bladder distensibility during bladder filling, as well as increases in intravesical pressures and/or decreased capacity during this phase.

Bladder compliance is a urodynamic measurement that is calculated by the change in detrusor pressure (P_{det}) during the change in bladder volume, and is expressed as ΔV (in mL)/Δ P_{det} (in cm H_2O) (Abrams et al., 2003). This can be calculated using a volume/cystometric pressure curve during urodynamic evaluation. Ultrastructural changes within the detrusor muscle, defects in the nervous system, and compromise or changes in bladder anatomy can all contribute to impaired bladder compliance through a loss of viscoelastic properties, replacement of bladder wall constituents by fibrosis, and/or changes in bladder muscle tone. Specifically, studies have demonstrated loss of bladder compliance with deposition of collagen within the extracellular matrix of the bladder as a result of chronic outlet obstruction, as well as radiation, pelvic/bladder injury, and so on (Madersbacher et al., 1999). This incites damage on the cellular level, including hypoxia, hypertrophy of myocytes causing thickening of the bladder wall, and decreases in neural density (Bellucci et al., 2017; Brierly et al., 2003). Pathologic conditions associated with impaired bladder compliance include radiation, chronic infection/inflammation including tuberculosis and schistosomiasis, outlet obstruction (urethral stricture, pelvic organ prolapse, benign prostatic hyperplasia, etc.), neurologic conditions (multiple sclerosis [MS], Shy–Drager syndrome, spinal cord injury [SCI], cauda equina), and surgical denervation (abdominoperineal resection, radical hysterectomy) (Liao et al., 2015).

COMPLIANCE AND CHANGES IN BLADDER NEUROPHYSIOLOGY

Normal bladder storage and emptying occur via a coordinated reflex arc involving the somatic and autonomic nervous systems. The sympathetic nervous system, through stimulation of efferent nerve fibers originating from T10 to L2 via the hypogastric nerve, allows for bladder storage (relaxation of the detrusor muscle and contraction of bladder neck/proximal urethra), while the parasympathetic nerves (S2–S4 efferents) are suppressed. In addition, the somatic efferents stimulate the contraction of the external urethral sphincter via the pudendal nerve, allowing for distensibility of the bladder at low pressures without urinary incontinence/leakage. This system, coupled with the ultrastructure of the bladder (the layers of the bladder wall, including urothelium, lamina propria, smooth muscle, and serosa), allows for bladder filling with low intraluminal pressures. See Chapter 3 for more details.

Disruption of the nervous system and/or bladder structure can result in impaired compliance (Uvelius & Gabella, 1980). SCIs, congenital disorders (i.e., spina bifida, myelomeningocele), vascular disease, diabetes, and demyelinating disorders (i.e., MS) can cause varying levels of neurologic injury, and ultimately neurogenic bladder. Injury to the various nervous systems can cause a disruption in signaling patterns between the bladder and the brain via the pontine micturition center (PMC), which plays a role in inhibition of bladder contractility. A disruption of the PMC can impair the bladder's ability to fill at low pressures, ultimately decreasing elasticity and bladder compliance. In addition, damage to the sympathetic nerves above the level of T10 results in bladder and sphincter spasticity, increased detrusor tone, and muscle hypertrophy, and contributes to loss of bladder compliance (Dorsher & McIntosh, 2012; Nseyo et al., 2017).

TYPES OF NEUROGENIC BLADDER

Several neurologic diseases, including SCIs, spina bifida, MS, Parkinson disease, stroke, and dementia, can result in neurogenic bladder with a variety of characteristic changes in bladder physiology and urodynamic parameters, which are summarized in Table 33.1.

Detrusor Overactivity

Neurogenic detrusor overactivity (DO), sometimes called detrusor hyperreflexia, results in the inability of the bladder to store urine secondary to unsolicited bladder contractions and, over time, can lead to impaired compliance. DO has been attributed to bladder denervation supersensitivity and hypertrophy, which in turn increase the collagen content of the bladder wall, ultimately leading to decreased viscoelasticity and impaired compliance (Cho et al., 2009). This is commonly seen in patients with MS, SCI, Parkinson disease, or stroke.

Detrusor Areflexia

A bladder pattern seen in SCI, MS, peripheral nerve injury, and occasionally stroke is detrusor areflexia/acontractile and hypocontractility. During the storage/filling phase, this is often associated with a decrease in or lack of sensation/urge to void, in addition to increased storage capacity. Over time this can contribute to impaired bladder compliance, especially when associated with elevated detrusor leak point pressures (DLPPs) and/or storage pressures greater than 40 cm H_2O.

Detrusor Sphincter Dyssynergia

Detrusor sphincter dyssynergia (DSD) in SCI and MS is a loss of coordination between the bladder and sphincter during the voiding phase. Normal physiology dictates sphincter relaxation before bladder contraction and micturition; DSD results in an involuntary contraction of the sphincter (periurethral striated external sphincter, and possibly smooth muscle of the internal sphincter) during an involuntary detrusor contraction. This discoordinated contraction should raise concern for risk of increased intravesical pressures causing reflux, urinary tract infection, hydronephrosis, renal failure, etc. (Abrams et al., 2003).

Intrinsic Sphincter Deficiency

Intrinsic sphincter deficiency (ISD) results from deinnervation of the external/internal sphincters as the result of a lower motor neuron disorder such as a low-level SCI, spina bifida/myelomeningocele, cauda equina, or peripheral injury (Myers et al., 2016). ISD often coexists with an areflexic bladder with impaired compliance, and is best studied with the use of video urodynamics (VUDs) to demonstrate incompetent/open sphincter during filling phases.

TABLE 33.1 Summary of Neuropathologies and Corresponding Bladder Patterns

Location of Disease	Neurologic Pathology	Bladder Pattern/Dysfunction
Brain (pons, cortex, etc.)	Stroke[a] Parkinson disease Dementia Closed head injury/traumatic brain injury[a] Frontal lobe lesion Normal pressure hydrocephalus[b] Multiple sclerosis	Detrusor overactivity ± Pseudodyssynergia ± Impaired contractility
Suprasacral (C1–L2)	Spinal cord injury[c] Tumors, infarction, infection of spinal cord Disc disease Spinal stenosis Tethered cord syndrome	Detrusor overactivity ± Detrusor sphincter dyssynergia
Lower lumbar and sacral	Peripheral nerve injury Pelvic plexus injury/trauma[d] Cauda equina syndrome Myelomeningocele[e]	Areflexic bladder Impaired contractility

[a]Initial insult results in urinary retention with temporary detrusor areflexia, which is replaced with detrusor overactivity with possible impaired contractility in the stable phase.
[b]Triad of gait disturbances, dementia, and urinary incontinence (additionally urinary frequency, urgency, and nocturnal enuresis). Treatment with neurosurgery consultation for shunt placement.
[c]Initial phase/spinal shock: detrusor areflexia, flaccid paralysis. Recovery of detrusor activity often coincides with return of reflexes below the level of the lesion.
[d]Hypogastric nerve injury resulting in incomplete bladder neck closure, pelvic nerve injury causing impaired detrusor contractility, and pudendal nerve injury rendering external sphincter incompetent.
[e]Areflexic, poorly compliant bladder with high storage pressures because of external sphincter hypertonicity (failure to relax during voiding) and incompetent/open bladder neck.

URODYNAMICS AND BLADDER COMPLIANCE

A standardized definition of bladder compliance has been established by the International Continence Society, which states that "compliance is calculated by dividing the change in volume by the change in detrusor pressure, reported in mL/cm H_2O" (Abrams et al., 2003). This value can be calculated through the use of urodynamics, specifically during filling cystometry, and it is recommended that bladder volume and P_{det} be measured at the start of filling and at capacity. Normal bladder compliance is typically defined as greater than 40 mL/cm H_2O, with the lower limit of normal being 20 to 30 mL/cm H_2O, and impaired compliance ranging from 1 to 20 mL/cm H_2O (Abrams et al., 1997). The criteria for defining impaired compliance are not well established, and have varied widely (Table 33.2). However, studies have demonstrated loss of compliance with transmission to the upper urinary tract at ranges of 5 to 12.5 mL/cm H_2O (Toppercer & Tetreault, 1979; Webster & Kreder, 1998).

During filling cystometry, early increases in P_{det} with increasing volume are seen in abnormal compliance instead of the normal bladder distensibility, yielding low storage pressures throughout the bladder filling phase (Fig. 33.1). Leakage of urine during the filling phase can also reflect a loss of compliance, and is known as the DLPP, which is the P_{det} at which leakage occurs in the absence of both a bladder contraction and an increase in intraabdominal pressure. A DLPP greater than 40 cm H_2O has been shown to transmit intravesical pressures to upper tracts as vesicoureteral reflux and ureteral dilation. (McGuire et al., 1981). Impaired compliance can also be seen with sustained bladder contractions, as storage of urine during these contractions occurs at high pressure, and risk of damage to upper urinary tracts should be considered.

URODYNAMIC FINDINGS IN NEUROGENIC BLADDER

The use of contrast urodynamics with fluoroscopy (VUDS) is recommended in patients with neurologic disorders that would place them at high risk for neurogenic bladder, to provide further insight into the anatomical function/dysfunction of the urinary system (Winters et al., 2012).

DO appears on the urodynamics study (UDS) tracing as a rise in P_{det} in conjunction with an increase in intravesical pressure and unchanged abdominal pressure. Phasic DO is seen throughout the study, and may or may not be associated with incontinence during this involuntary bladder contraction. Terminal DO is an involuntary detrusor contraction at capacity that results in bladder emptying/incontinence and cannot be suppressed by the patient. DO is typically associated with suprasacral causes of neurogenic bladder.

Detrusor external sphincter dyssynergia (DSD) can be diagnosed with the assistance of electromyography (EMG; via perineal surface electrodes) and fluoroscopy during contractions on VUDS. It is characteristically demonstrated as increased activity of the pelvic floor/sphincter complex via the EMG tracing in conjunction with bladder contractions. In addition, a voiding cystourethrogram can be helpful because in the setting of DSD, it may demonstrate concomitant urethral narrowing during the voiding phase with increased sphincter activity on EMG. DSD may also appear as a dilated proximal urethra and open bladder neck, secondary to an obstructing/contracting sphincter, during the voiding phase (Stoffel, 2016).

ISD can be difficult to diagnose on urodynamics because there is no standardized definition. However, ISD may be suspected in cases where maximal urethral closing pressure is less than 25 to 30 cm H_2O, and/or Valsalva leak point pressure is less than 60 cm H_2O (Krissi et al., 2005; Murphy et al., 2004). VUDS may demonstrate "funneling" of the bladder neck during voiding cystourethrogram (Macura et al., 2006).

Additionally, in the setting of a neurogenic bladder resulting in the loss of bladder compliance or increased storage pressures, VUDS can aid in the diagnosis of vesicoureteral reflux. If this is identified on VUDS, it is imperative to further evaluate the upper genitourinary tract with renal ultrasound and nuclear renal scan, as well as assess renal function with 24-hour creatinine clearance and serum creatinine.

Table 33.2 Summary of Studies Defining Bladder Compliance

Reference	Summary of Findings
Abrams et al., 2003	Normal compliance ratio >30.3 cc/cm H_2O at 100 cc bladder volume
Weld et al., 2000	Normal compliance ratio >12.5 cc/cm H_2O
Musco et al., 2018	Normal compliance in nonneurogenic >40 mL/cm H_2O and >30 mL/cm H_2O in neurogenic
	Low compliance (women) <30 mL/cm H_2O in nonneurogenic and <10 mL/cm H_2O in neurogenic
Webster and Kreder, 1998	Normal compliance 6–10 cm H_2O
Andersen, 1976	Low compliance 5 cm H_2O
	Normal compliance 50 cm H_2O
	High compliance 150 cm H_2O

PATIENT EVALUATION

The evaluation for compliance abnormalities and neurogenic bladder should begin with history and physical examination to ascertain the causes of the urinary tract dysfunction (Box 33.1). A careful history can provide insight into possible causes, including prior surgeries, chronic inflammation, anatomic abnormalities, neurologic symptoms, infectious etiology, prior urologic disease, and so on. Physical examination should not only include a complete genitourinary examination, but also focus on patient ambulatory status, manual dexterity, or other neurologic changes such as paresthesias or gait abnormalities. In addition, it is recommended that patients complete self-administered questionnaires that focus on bladder dysfunction and corresponding symptoms, such as the Urogenital Distress Inventory-Short Form and the Incontinence Impact Questionnaire-Short Form. Completion of these questionnaires can aid in establishing baseline symptoms and allow for monitoring of subjective improvement during the treatment period.

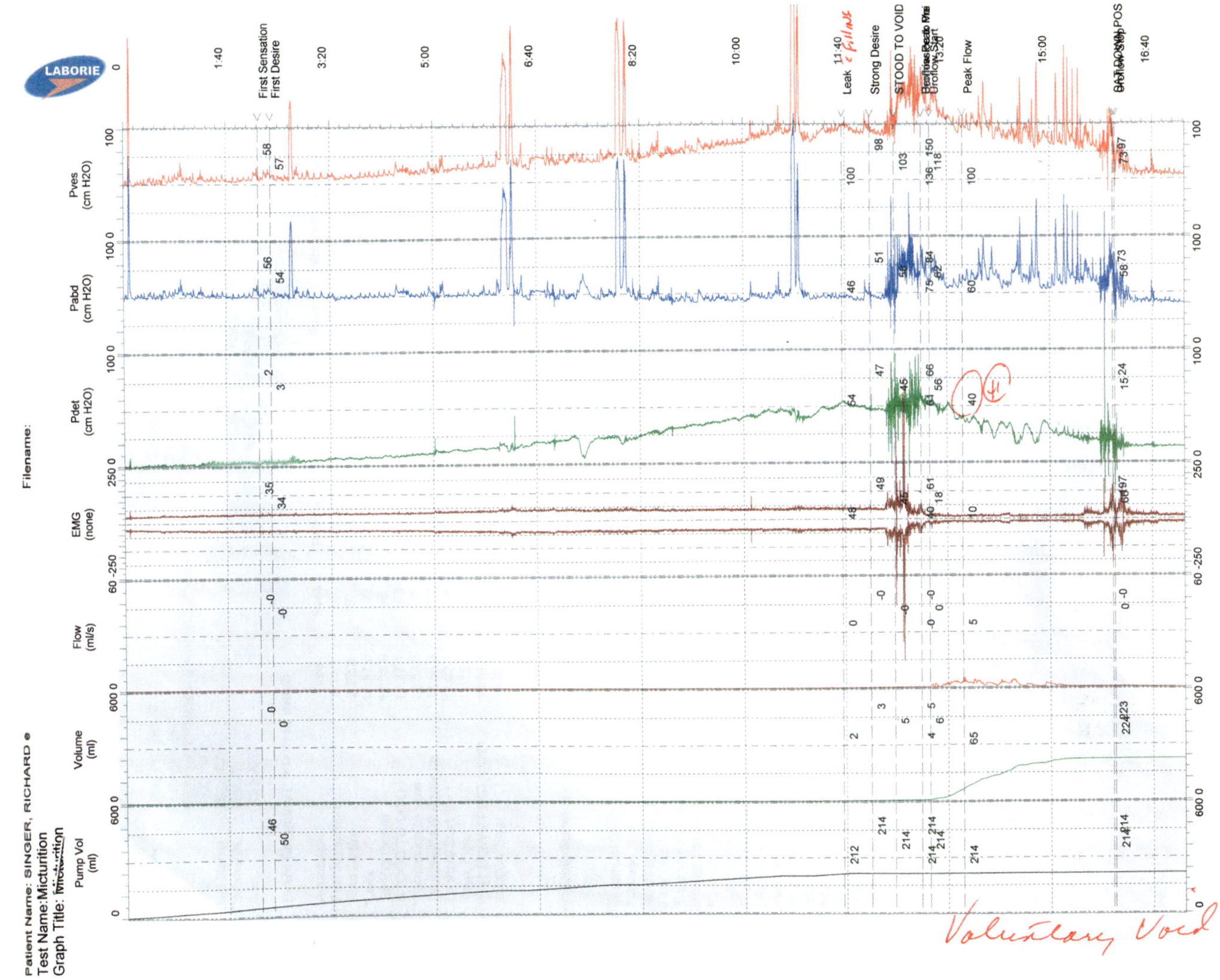

Fig. 33.1 Urodynamic tracing of impaired bladder compliance.

BOX 33.1 Salient Features of the Initial Evaluation of Patients with Suspected Neurogenic Bladder

History
- Sequential progression of urinary symptoms
- Neurologic symptoms (vision, gait, coordination, parasthesias, weakness, etc.)
- Bowel habits/constipation/fecal incontinence
- Sexual history
- Prior urologic disease
- Diabetes
- Thyroid disease
- Herpes simplex virus infection
- Back pain or disc disease
- Pelvic, anorectal, or spinal surgery
- Previous therapies, including medications

Physical Examination
- Ambulatory status
- Manual dexterity
- Back: skin or spinal cord anomalies
- Abdomen: scars, mass, tenderness
- Pelvic and vagina: pelvic organ prolapse, enlarged uterus, pelvic or vaginal mass
- Sacral neurologic examination: sensation, perineal reflexes, pelvic floor contraction
- Anal sphincter tone and squeeze
- Neurologic examination – sensation, motor, deep tendon reflexes

Urinalysis

Postvoid residual

Ultimately, assessment of bladder function is recommended in special cases where bladder dysfunction is suspected. A baseline postvoid residual (PVR) volume should be obtained to ensure complete bladder emptying. Urodynamics including cystometrogram, pressure-flow studies, and EMG can be performed, and in select cases can be completed with the addition of fluoroscopy/VUDS. VUDS in a noncompliant bladder may demonstrate a Christmas tree appearance with trabeculations, diverticula, and vesicoureteral reflux, and should be considered in patients with neurogenic causes of bladder dysfunction. Patients with compliance changes on UDS and sustained bladder pressures greater than 40 cm H_2O should undergo upper tract imaging (i.e., renal bladder ultrasound, voiding cystourethrogram, computed tomography urogram).

It is important to be aware of neurogenic patients who may experience autonomic dysreflexia during UDS. Autonomic dysreflexia is defined as an exaggerated response of the autonomic nervous system to noxious stimuli and is characteristically seen in SCI at the T6 level or higher. The response to the stimulus (often seen in overfilling of the bladder or urinary retention) is a reflex sympathetic vasoconstriction resulting in hypertension and a parasympathetic effect of diaphoresis, flushing, and reflex bradycardia (Linsenmeyer et al., 2006). The recommended initial treatment is to remove the noxious stimulus by terminating UDS and draining the bladder with either intermittent catheterization or indwelling urethral catheter placement. A patient with known autonomic dysreflexia should have continuous blood pressure/pulse monitoring during UDS. If draining the bladder is not sufficient to treat the patient's autonomic dysreflexia, pharmacologic agents such as nifedipine (immediate release/bite and swallow), morphine, and nitrate spray/paste/sublingual can be used. If a patient remains unstable, it is crucial to initiate a transfer to the emergency department or intensive care unit for continuous symptomatic treatment and monitoring.

MANAGEMENT OF IMPAIRED COMPLIANCE

Overall treatment goals for impaired compliance should be focused around lowering bladder storage pressures to minimize risk of damage to upper urinary tracts (via reflux, hydronephrosis, infection, etc.).

Pharmacologic Management

Oral Medications. The mainstay of medical management for bladder compliance has historically been anticholinergic medications. In cases of neurogenic bladder with incomplete emptying, these medications are often used in conjunction with intermittent catheterization. Studies have demonstrated optimized bladder compliance with a combination of anticholinergics, tricyclic antidepressants (imipramine), and α-adrenergic blockers. Muscarinic receptors in the bladder, which are responsible for bladder contraction, are targeted by anticholinergics; thus, blockade allows for bladder relaxation. The addition of an α-adrenergic blockade further allows for relaxation of the detrusor, bladder neck, and urethra. Imipramine causes a decrease in bladder contractility by inhibiting serotonin reuptake and blocking norepinephrine. A combination of two or three of these medications can ultimately help to improve bladder compliance by optimizing bladder relaxation during filling (Andersson, 2000; Cameron et al., 2009; McGuire et al., 1985).

A new addition to pharmacotherapy for bladder compliance is the β-3-adrenorecptor agonists such as mirabegron. Mirabegron has been demonstrated to improve bladder compliance and capacity and to lower grades of vesicoureteral reflux. It can be used alone or in conjunction with an anticholinergic medication. Mirabegron is often preferred over anticholinergics for patients who are unable to tolerate the side effects, such as dry mouth, constipation, and impaired cognition (Kamei et al., 2015; Wada et al., 2015).

Botulinum Toxin. Botulinum toxin is derived from *Clostridium botulinum*, a gram-negative, rod-shaped, anaerobic bacterium, and acts as a potent neurotoxin. There are seven immunologically different subtypes, including A, B, CI, D, E, F, and G; however, only types A and B are available for clinical use. BTX-A, known as Botox (Allergan Inc., Irvine, Ca), and type B, known as Myobloc (rimabotulinumtoxinB, US World, LLC, Louisville, KY), are the two subtypes available in the United States. Type A is more potent and has a longer duration of effect than type B.

Botulinum toxin binds to presynaptic cholinergic terminals and inhibits the release of acetylcholine from the neuromuscular junction, thus causing bladder smooth muscle relaxation and flaccid paralysis (Dolly, 1994). Each serotype of botulinum toxin contains a heavy and a light chain molecule linked by a disulfide bond, and the heavy chain is what gives the toxins specificity for cholinergic nerve endings. The heavy chain binds to the neuronal cell membrane and is internalized, after which the light and heavy chain are separated via a disulfide reaction. The cleaved light chain binds to acetylcholine vesicles and prevents acetylcholine exocytosis, resulting in blockade of the neuromuscular junction (Dolly et al., 1984; Mahajan & Brubaker, 2007). Muscle function returns over a period of 6 to 12 months as axons regenerate over the nerve endplates at the neuromuscular junction, allowing for new functional synapses to form (Sahai et al., 2010).

The US Food and Drug Administration (FDA) approved Botox in August 2011 for the treatment of medication-refractory urinary incontinence secondary to DO associated with neurological disease. Two phase III multicenter randomized controlled clinical trials were performed, and concluded the approved dose of 200 U. These trials also recommended that treatment with botulinum toxin could be repeated when the clinical effects diminished, with a minimum of 12 weeks in between injections. The maximum cumulative dose of botulinum toxin should not exceed 400 U in a 3-month period. Patients who are not performing intermittent catheterization should have their PVR assessed within 2 weeks of treatment, and use of botulinum toxin is contraindicated in patients with acute urinary tract infections.

Before proceeding with treatment, patients should be screened for urinary tract infection and have urinalysis performed. FDA recommendations state that prophylactic antibiotics, except for aminoglycosides, which are curare-like compounds that interfere with neuromuscular transmission, should be administered for 1 to 3 days. It is recommended to stop anticoagulation at least 3 days before the procedure, and patients on anticoagulation should be counseled appropriately on risk of bleeding.

Botulinum toxin injections can be performed in the office or in the operating room, and the choice is often dependent on the patient (i.e., neurogenic patients with spasticity, mobility issues that may not tolerate lithotomy). If the procedure is performed in the clinic, it is recommended to begin with intravesical instillation of diluted local anesthetic (100 mL of 2% lidocaine). The bladder should be drained and irrigated with sterile water after utilization of intravesical anesthetic before injection. A flexible cystoscope is recommended for male patients in the office setting; however, flexible or rigid cystoscopy can generally be used for female patients without additional discomfort. Per its prescribing information, a 200-U vial of Botox should be reconstituted with 6 mL of preservative-free 0.9% injectable sodium chloride. The endoscopic needle is inserted into the detrusor to a depth of approximately 2 mm, and 1 mL is injected into 30 total sites. Following injection, the bladder wall should be visualized to ensure appropriate hemostasis (electrocautery can be used if needed). The patient should be observed in the office or in the postoperative recovery unit for at least 30 minutes following the procedure. See Chapter 32 for more discussion on the use of botulinum toxin in refractory DO.

Before FDA approval, Schurch et al. (2005) published their prospective, randomized, placebo-controlled trial on the efficacy of botulinum toxin in SCI patients and demonstrated improvements in maximum cystometric capacity and a significant decrease in mean maximum detrusor voiding pressure in patients receiving 200 to 300 U of Botox (Schurch et al., 2005). Multiple studies/trials conducted from 2005 to 2011 have demonstrated improvements in urodynamic parameters, including mean maximum detrusor pressure and cystometric capacity for patients with neurogenic DO receiving Botox injections (typically 200–300 U) (Table 33.3). Reitz et al. (2004) published the largest study to date, with 200 patients treated with 300 U of Botox, demonstrating a complete resolution of symptoms in 73% of patients. They also noted improvements in posttreatment urodynamics, including improved mean cystometric capacity and decreased mean voiding pressures.

Botulinum toxin injection to the external urethral sphincter can be used in patients with DSD and resulting bladder outlet obstruction. Chemical alleviation of the outlet obstruction allows for voiding/incontinence via a low-pressure state. Typically performed in males (however, this procedure could be considered in certain female populations, with the understanding that the incontinence rate is high), the patient usually drains into an external collection device. Four randomized controlled trials have demonstrated improvement in urodynamic parameters, including voiding pressures and PVR. This can be performed cystoscopically or transperineally with ultrasound guidance, with two to four total injections of 100 U of Botox at the 9 o'clock and 3 o'clock positions (Mahfouz & Corcos, 2011; Utomo et al., 2014).

The side effects of botulinum toxin because of systemic absorption, albeit rare, include generalized weakness, optic changes (diplopia, blurred vision), and dysphagia. The most common adverse effects include urinary retention, postprocedural urinary tract infection, hematuria, and site injection pain. In patients who void, a preoperative history of elevated PVR volume greater than 100 mL may increase a patient's risk of postoperative acute urinary retention, and can be managed with intermittent catheterization or temporary indwelling urethral catheter (Bogdan & Sangeea, 2013; Leippold et al., 2003).

Surgical Management

Sacral Neuromodulation. Sacral neuromodulation (SNM) is an FDA-approved treatment modality for refractory urinary urgency/frequency, urge incontinence, nonobstructive urinary retention, and fecal incontinence. Currently, there are two approved SNM devices: InterStim (Medtronic, Inc., Minneapolis, MN) and Axonics (Axonics Modulation Technologies Inc., Irvine, CA). The overall mechanism of action for SNM has been theorized, but to date remains largely uncertain. Electrical impulses from the SNM are delivered to the S3 sacral nerve root, thus stimulating the pelvic plexus and pudendal nerve, which stimulate the bladder, pelvic floor (levator ani muscles), and rectum. It is believed that impulses from SNM activate bladder somatosensory afferent fibers that are responsible for regulation of the local hypogastric sympathetic nerves and central PMC, and function as a "pacemaker" for the bladder by downregulating contractile responses and decreasing detrusor muscle hyperactivity. See Chapter 32 for more details about SNM in the treatment of refractory overactive bladder. Currently, the data are limited on the use of SNM for impaired

Table 33.3 Summary of Evidence Detailing Effect of Botulinum Toxin on Compliance

Reference	Study Population	Summary of Outcomes
Schurch et al., 2005	Spinal cord injury (SCI) and multiple sclerosis (MS) $n = 59$	-Placebo vs. 200 U vs. 300 U -Mean change in detrusor pressure (P_{det}): decreased by 50% and 38% in response to 200 and 300 U, respectively -Mean change in maximum cystometric capacity (MCC): increased 67% and 32% in response to 200 and 300 U, respectively
Giannantoni et al., 2004	SCI $n = 75$	-Resiniferatoxin vs. Botox 300 U -Botox 44% decrease in baseline P_{det} -Botox 54% improvement in MCC
Popat et al., 2005	SCI, MS, and other $n = 44$	-Botox 300 U -42% decrease in baseline P_{det} -181% improvement in MCC
Reitz et al., 2004	SCI, MS, and other $n = 200$	-Botox 300 U at 12 and 36 weeks -58% and 21% decrease in baseline P_{det} at 12 and 36 weeks, respectively -54% and 29% improvement in MCC at 12 and 36 weeks, respectively

compliance; however, patients with neurogenic lower urinary tract dysfunction may be considered for SNM if previous therapies such as medications have failed, and if they are not at high risk for upper tract damage. SNM is a therapy modality that can be used before advancing to more invasive management such as augmentation cystoplasty or urinary diversion. Wöllner et al. (2016) demonstrated significant improvement in bladder compliance in patients with neurogenic DO who underwent SNM implantation (22.8 pretreatment vs. 53.6 posttreatment; $P < .046$).

This procedure is typically performed in two stages; however, the first stage can be performed as a percutaneous nerve evaluation (PNE) or as stage I placement of a permanent tined lead attached to an external stimulator. If PNE is performed, permanent implantation occurs in a combined stage I/II procedure. The stage II procedure includes implantation of an implantable pulse generator (IPG) to the tined lead. PNE is performed by placing percutaneous leads in the S3 foramen bilaterally, and can be done with or without the assistance of fluoroscopy. This can be performed in the office setting; however, studies have demonstrated high false-negative rates (50%) for PNE compared with stage I, with 46% of patients who undergo PNE advancing to stage II versus 69% to 88% of patients who undergo stage I advancing to stage II (Borawski et al., 2007; Marcelissen et al., 2011). The success of treatment is defined as greater than 50% improvement in average daily episodes of incontinence, number of voids, and/or return to normal voiding frequency (<8 voids a day), and can be ascertained by reviewing symptoms recorded in a daily bladder diary and by PVR assessment (especially in those who are undergoing placement for nonobstructive urinary retention). The length of the trial period for PNE/stage I is largely based on surgeon preference; however, 3 to 5 days is recommended for PNE, and 1 to 2 weeks for stage I.

The stage I procedure is typically performed in the operating room, and can be done under monitored anesthesia with local anesthetic or under general anesthesia, with care taken to avoid the use of long-acting paralytics. The patient is instructed to perform a chlorohexidine gluconate shower before surgery (typically the night before or the morning of the surgery) to reduce surgical site infection risk. Preoperative antibiotics are recommended, given that a foreign body implant is being used, and antibiotic selection is based on surgeon preference. In our experience, vancomycin and an aminoglycoside are preferred, as long as there are no patient contraindications (allergies, impaired renal function, etc.). The patient is placed in the prone position, allowing for 30-degree flexion at the hip (chest rolls and pillows to assist), with the buttock taped to allow for visualization of anus/bellows and foot exposed for movement during test stimulation. The patient's lower back and perineum should be prepped in the usual sterile fashion. The S3 foramina can be located 9 cm cephalad from the tip of the sacrum and 1 to 2 cm lateral of midline. A foramen needle should be inserted into the S3 foramina at a 45-degree angle. A larger needle is available for those patients whose habitus requires extra distance to reach the foramina. The position of the needle can be confirmed in both the anterior/posterior and lateral views. The nerve is then stimulated with the mini hook from the test stimulation cable. Stimulation of the S3 nerve should demonstrate bellows, flexing of the great toe, and an inward pull of the rectum and bellows (deepening and flattening of the buttock groove). S2 stimulation results in leg/hip rotation, heel rotation, plantar flexion, and calf contraction. S4 stimulation induces bellows and no foot movement. The amplitude of the external neurostimulator should be decreased to determine the intensity of response to the lowest level of stimulation. A contralateral test may be performed if the desired response or intensity of response is not seen. Once the needle has been placed in the appropriate position, and the desired response is obtained, the foramen needle stylet is removed and replaced with a directional guide to the appropriate depth (9 cm for a 3- to 5-inch needle and 12.5 cm for a 5-inch needle). The foramen needle is then removed over the directional guide, and a small skin incision is made alongside the directional guide to allow for placement of the lead. The dilator sheath is then placed over the guide and advanced into the foramen under fluoroscopic guidance to ensure the radiopaque marker is placed halfway through the foramen. The dilator and guide are removed from the sheath, and the lead is introduced into the sheath and advanced such that electrodes 2 and 3 are along the anterior edge of the sacrum. The lead is then stimulated to ensure proper positioning along the nerve; an S3 response should be obtained in at least two of the four electrodes (0, 1, 2, and 3). The recommended amplitude range for lead placement is 1 to 2 mA; an amplitude greater than 2 mA may result in compromise of battery longevity, so if this occurs one should consider repositioning the lead. The neurostimulator pocket is made by creating a 3- to 4-cm incision in the subcutaneous tissue of the upper lateral buttock (below the beltline). The lead is tunneled to the pocket incision with the tunneling device, with care taken to ensure that the lead is not tunneled too superficially. The lead is then connected to the extension lead and secured using the setscrew connector. The tunneling device is used again to transfer the extension wire from the pocket to an exit point just lateral to the incision, and then connected to an external pulse generator. The pocket is copiously irrigated and closed in multiple layers. It is recommended to continue a 5- to 7-day course of antibiotics during the test stimulation period. The test stimulator is programmed in the recovery unit.

The stage II implant occurs following a PNE or stage I demonstrating greater than 50% improvement in symptoms. The patient is again placed in the prone position; however, the buttocks do not need to be taped, as no additional test stimulation will occur, and fluoroscopy is not needed for this stage. This stage can be performed under monitored anesthesia with local anesthetic. The previously created generator pocket is reopened with a 15 blade, with care taken to avoid damage to the lead (minimize electrocautery, blunt dissection preferred). Once the lead is identified, the extension wire is cut and removed from the exiting portion of the skin. The boot is removed, and the torque wrench is used to unscrew the lead from the temporary extension wire. The lead is cleaned and dried and placed in the IPG and tightened (avoid overtightening). The pocket should be large enough to accommodate the

IPG without tension during closure of the wound, and should be closed in two layers with absorbable suture.

The adverse effects associated with SNM include pain at insertion site (most common), superficial wound infection, lead migration, seroma at IPG site, skin erosion, and sensation of electrical shock. Trauma to the lower lumbar/sacrum can result in device failures requiring lead and/or generator revision. Contraindications to SNM include less than 50% improvement in symptoms and urinary retention secondary to obstruction. Advances in SNM technology have addressed magnetic resonance imaging (MRI) compatibility, and currently both Medtronic and Axonics are MRI-compatible. MRI-compatible devices can be used in patients with neurogenic bladder secondary to MS, particularly those with urinary urgency, frequency, and urgency urinary incontinence.

Augmentation Cystoplasty and Urinary Diversion. Surgical management of impaired bladder compliance with augmentation cystoplasty or urinary diversion can be considered when a patient has failed all other interventions, including medications, botulinum toxin, and SNM. Bladder augmentation allows for an increase in bladder capacity and a reduction in detrusor storage pressures, especially for those who remain at high risk for upper tract damage despite all other interventions. Augmentation cystoplasty is indicated not only for patients with poor compliance, but also those with neurogenic and idiopathic DO who may have failed other therapies or who are not candidates for SNM or botulinum toxin. Patients who are candidates for augmentation cystoplasty must also demonstrate appropriate dexterity and willingness to perform clean intermittent catheterization (CIC) or have a caregiver willing to do so for them. Patients that are unwilling or unable to perform CIC are at risk for augment rupture that could result in death. For the patient with limited dexterity who cannot perform CIC via the urethra, an augmentation cystoplasty can be performed in conjunction with a continent catheterizable channel if the patient has enough dexterity to perform catheterization via a fixed abdominal wall stoma. Alternatively, a urinary diversion (i.e., ileal conduit) can be offered. Contraindications to augmentation cystoplasty include impaired renal function, bowel disease (inflammatory bowel disease, short gut syndrome as seen in cloacal exstrophy, congenital abnormalities), and malignancy.

The ileum is the preferred bowel segment for cystoplasty, and care must be taken to preserve the terminal ileum to prevent vitamin B12 and salt losses. Although other segments of bowel can be used for augmentation, including stomach, jejunum, and colon, the ileum is preferred because of a variety of factors, including proximity to bladder, metabolic issues (hyperchloremic metabolic acidosis), compliance, and production of mucus.

The procedure begins by placing the patient in the supine position and making an extended Pfannenstiel or midline abdominal incision. The bladder is bivalved in a transverse incision or in an inverted-U shape. A 20- to 25-cm segment of ileum is harvested at least 15 to 20 cm from the ileocecal valve. The harvested segment, with adequate mesenteric length to reach the bladder, is copiously irrigated and then detubularized along the antimesenteric border. The ileal segment is then folded into a U or cup shape, and the mucosal edges are anastomosed using a running absorbable suture to create the anterior and posterior walls of the augment. At this time, consideration should be given to the need for ureteral reimplantation, bladder neck closure, and/or placement of catheterizable channel. The posterior walls of the ileum and bladder are anastomosed, a suprapubic tube is placed through the augment and the lower abdominal wall, and then the anterior layer is closed (typically in two layers). It is recommended to place a drain in the pelvis before closure. The suprapubic catheter should be irrigated daily to prevent mucous accumulation, and the drain should be removed at the discretion of the surgeon (i.e., no concern for leak, minimal drainage). A cystogram is typically performed before catheter removal in 3 to 4 weeks.

Complications associated with augmentation cystoplasty include wound infection, postoperative ileus, small bowel obstructions, bleeding, metabolic derangements, acute renal failure, vitamin B12 deficiency, diarrhea, bladder stone formation, perforation, incontinence, and carcinoma (Husmann & Snodgrass, 2004). Postoperative irrigation of mucus is recommended to prevent stone formation and can be performed daily. It is recommended to evaluate for vitamin B12 deficiency 3 to 5 years following augmentation and to carry out cystoscopic surveillance for bladder tumors at 10 years. Overall, augmentation cystoplasty has demonstrated improvement in UDS parameters, including increase in maximum capacity (mean increase 400 mL) and decrease in mean maximal detrusor pressure (53–14 cm H_2O), and remains a viable surgical option for patients with impaired compliance who have failed other less invasive management strategies (Blaivas et al., 2005).

CONCLUSION

The management options available for neurogenic bladder and impaired bladder compliance have improved over time, and now less invasive interventions are available, including botulinum toxin (with or without CIC) and SNM. With the advent of these therapies, more invasive surgical options like augmentation cystoplasty have become less common. The overall benefits of SNM with regards to bladder compliance still require further investigation; however, it remains an option for neurogenic lower urinary tract dysfunction.

BIBLIOGRAPHY

Abrams P, Cardozo L, Fall M, et al. The standardization of terminology in lower urinary tract function: report from the standardization sub-committee of the International Continence Society. *Urology.* 2003;61:37.

Abrams P. Urodynamic techniques. In: *Urodynamics*. 2nd ed. London: Springer-Verlag; 1997.

Andersen JT. Detrusor hyperreflexia in benign intravesical obstruction. A cystometric study. *J Urol.* 1976;115:532.

Andersson KE. New roles for muscarinic receptors in the pathophysiology of lower urinary tract symptoms. *BJU Int.* 2000;86:36.

Bellucci C, Ribeiro W, Hemerly T, et al. Increased detrusor collagen is associated with detrusor overactivity and decreased bladder compliance in men with benign prostatic obstruction. *Prostate Int.* 2017;5:70.

Blaivas JG, Weiss JP, Desai P, et al. Long-term follow-up of augmentation enterocystoplasty and continent diversion in patients with benign disease. *J Urol.* 2005;173:1631.

Bogdan O, Sangeea M. The use of onabotulinum toxin for the treatment of overactive bladder syndrome. *Indian J Urol.* 2013;29:2.

Borawski KM, Foster RT, Webster GD, et al. Predicting implantation with neuromodulator using two different test stimulation techniques: a prospective randomized study in urge incontinent women. *Neurourol Urodyn.* 2007;26:14.

Brierly RD, Hindley RG, McLarty E, et al. A prospective evaluation of detrusor ultrastructural changes in bladder outlet obstruction. *BJU Int.* 2003;91:360.

Cameron A, Clemens Q, Latini J, et al. Combination drug therapy improves compliance of the neurogenic bladder. *J Urol.* 2009;182:1062.

Cho SY, Yi JS, Oh SJ. The clinical significance of poor bladder compliance. *Neurourol Urodyn.* 2009;28:1010.

Dolly J, Black J, Williams RS, Melling J. Acceptors for onabotulinum neurotoxin reside on motor nerve terminals and mediate its internalization. *Nature.* 1984;307:457.

Dolly J. General properties and cellular mechanisms of neurotoxins. In: Jankovic J, Hallet M, eds. *Therapy with Onabotulinum Toxin.* New York: Marcel Dekker; 1994.

Dorsher P, McIntosh P. Neurogenic bladder. *Adv Urol.* 2012;2012: 816274.

Giannantoni A, Mearini E, Di Stasi SM, et al. New therapeutic options for refractory neurogenic detrusor over- activity. *Minerva Urol Nefrol.* 2004;56:79.

Hassouna MM, Siegel SW, Nyeholt AA, et al. Sacral neuromodulation in the treatment of urgency-frequency symptoms: a multicenter study on efficacy and safety. *J Urol.* 2000;163:1849.

Husmann DA, Snodgrass WT. Augmentation cystoplasty: enteric and urothelial. *AUA Update Ser.* 2004; 23:282.

Kamei J, Furuta A, Akiyama Y, et al. Video-urodynamic effects of mirabegron, a β3-adrenoceptor agonist, in patients with low-compliance bladder. *Int J Urol.* 2015;22:956.

Karsenty G, Denys P, Amarenco G et al. Onabotulinum toxin A (Botox) intradetrusor injections in adults with neurogenic detrusor overactivity/neurogenic overactive bladder: a systematic literature review. *Eur Urol.* 2008;53:275.

Krissi H, Pansky M, Halperin R, Langer R. Maximum urethral closure pressure <20 cm H2O: Does it predict intrinsic sphincteric deficiency? *J Reprod Med.* 2005;50:824.

Leippold T, Reitz A, Schurch B. Onabotulinum toxin as a new therapy option for voiding disorders: current state of the art. *Eur Urol.* 2003;44:165.

Leng W, Morrisroe S. Sacral nerve stimulation for the overactive bladder. *Urol Clin North Am.* 2006;33:491.

Liao J, Lin Y, Liang C et al. Monitoring bladder compliance using end filling detrusor pressure: clinical results and related factors. *Taiwan J Obstet Gynecol.* 2015;54:709.

Linsenmeyer TA, Bodner DR, Creasey GH, et al. Bladder management for adults with spinal cord injury: a clinical practice guideline for health-care providers. *J Spinal Cord Med.* 2006;29:527.

Macura KJ, Genadry RR, Bluemke DA. MR Imaging of the female urethra and supporting ligaments in assessment of urinary incontinence: spectrum of abnormalities. *Radiographics.* 2006;26:1135.

Madersbacher S, Pycha A, Klingler C, et al. Interrelationships of bladder compliance with age, detrusor instability, and obstruction in elderly men with lower urinary tract symptoms. *Neurourol Urodyn.* 1999;18:3.

Mahajan ST, Brubaker L. Onabotulinum toxin: from life-threatening disease to novel medical therapy. *Am J Obstet Gynecol.* 2007;196:7.

Mahfouz W, Corcos J. Management of detrusor external sphincter dyssynergia in neurogenic bladder. *Eur J Phys Rehabil Med.* 2011;47:639.

Marcelissen T, Leong R, Serroyen J, et al. Is the screening method of sacral neuromodulation a prognostic factor for long-term success? *J Urol.* 2011;185:583.

McGuire EJ, Savastano JA. Effect of alpha- adrenergic blockade and anticholinergic agents on the decentralized primate bladder. *Neurourol Urodyn.* 1985;4:139.

McGuire EM, Woodside JR, Borden TA. Prognostic value of urodynamic testing in myelodysplastic children. *J Urol.* 1981;126:205.

Murphy M, Culligan PJ, Graham CA, et al. Is the leak point pressure alone an accurate indicator of intrinsic sphincteric deficiency? *Int Urogynecol J Pelvic Floor Dysfunct.* 2004;15:294.

Musco S, Padilla-Fernández B, Del Popolo G, et al. Value of urodynamic findings in predicting upper urinary tract damage in neuro-urological patients: a systematic review. *Neurourol Urodyn.* 2018;37:1522.

Myers JB, Mayer EN, Lenherr S. Neurogenic Bladder Research Group (NBRG.org): Management options for sphincteric deficiency in adults with neurogenic bladder. *Transl Androl Urol.* 2016;5:145.

Nseyo U, Santiago-Lastra Y. Long-term complications of the neurogenic bladder. *Urol Clin North Am.* 2017;44:355.

Popat R, Apostolidis A, Kalsi V, et al. A comparison between the response of patients with idiopathic detrusor overactivity and neurogenic detrusor overactivity to the first intradetrusor injection of botulinum-A toxin. *J Urol.* 2005;174:984.

Reitz A, Stöhrer M, Kramer G, et al. European experience of 200 cases treated with botulinum-A toxin injections into the detrusor muscle for urinary incontinence due to neurogenic detrusor overactivity. *Eur Urol.* 2004;45:510.

Sahai A, Dowson C, Khan MS, et al. Repeated injections of onabotulinum toxin-A for idiopathic detrusor overactivity. *Urology.* 2010;75:552.

Schmidt RA, Jonas U, Oleson KA, et al. Sacral nerve stimulation for treatment of refractory urinary urge incontinence. Sacral Nerve Stimulation Study Group. *J Urol.* 1999;162:352.

Schurch B, de Sèze M, Denys P, et al. Botulinum toxin type A is a safe and effective treatment for neurogenic urinary incontinence: results of a single treatment, randomized, placebo controlled 6-month study. *J Urol.* 2005;174:196.

Stoffel JT. Detrusor sphincter dyssynergia: a review of physiology, diagnosis, and treatment strategies. *Transl Androl Urol.* 2016;5:127.

Toppercer A, Tetreault J. Compliance of the bladder: an attempt to establish normal values. *Urology.* 1979;14:204.

Utomo E, Groen J, Blok BF. Surgical management of functional bladder outlet obstruction in adults with neurogenic bladder dysfunction. *Cochrane Database Syst Rev.* 2014;5:CD004927.

Uvelius B, Gabella G. Relation between cell length and force production in urinary bladder smooth muscle. *Acta Physiol Scand.* 1980;110:357.

Wada N, Okazaki S, Kobayashi S, et al. Efficacy of combination therapy with mirabegron for anticholinergic-resistant neurogenic bladder: videourodynamic evaluation. *Hinyokika Kiyo.* 2015;61:7.

Webster G, Kreder K. The neurourologic evaluation. In: Walsh PC, Retik AB, Vaughan Jr ED, et al. *Campbell's Urology*. 7th ed. Philadelphia: W.B. Saunders Co; 1998:935.

Weld K, Marshall J, Dmochowski R. Differences in bladder compliance with time and associations of bladder management with compliance in spinal cord injured patients. *J Urol.* 2000;163:1228.

Williams ER, Siegel SW. Procedural techniques in sacral nerve modulation. *Int Urogynecol J.* 2010;21(suppl 2):S453.

Winters JC, Dmochowski RR, Goldman HB, et al; American Urological Association; Society of Urodynamics, Female Pelvic Medicine & Urogenital Reconstruction. Urodynamic studies in adults: AUA/SUFU guideline. *J Urol.* 2012;188:2464.

Wöllner J, Krebs J, Pannek J. Sacral neuromodulation in patients with neurogenic lower urinary tract dysfunction. *Spinal Cord.* 2016;54:137.

34

Voiding Dysfunction in Women

Frank C. Lin and Victor W. Nitti

CHAPTER OUTLINE

INTRODUCTION

Lower urinary tract dysfunction describes various problems related to the bladder's ability to store or empty urine. Voiding dysfunction refers specifically to bladder emptying problems. Urinary retention is the inability to complete the voiding phase of the micturition cycle, and oftentimes represents the end stage of voiding dysfunction. Abnormal bladder emptying can occur as a result of dysfunction of the bladder or the outlet, and sometimes both. Voiding dysfunction manifests clinically in lower urinary tract symptoms (LUTS), which may be associated with voiding or emptying symptoms (decreased force of stream, incomplete emptying, hesitancy, straining to void, and urinary retention) or storage symptoms (frequency, urgency, nocturia, and urgency incontinence). Because symptoms do not always correlate with the underlying pathology, and numerous conditions may present similarly, it is a challenging task to determine the specific etiology involved. In many cases, voiding dysfunction can be explained by neurologic disease, learned behavioral patterns, or congenital, acquired, or iatrogenic bladder outlet obstruction. At other times the cause may not be readily apparent, such as in cases of idiopathic detrusor underactivity (DU). In this chapter, we discuss normal voiding and the pathophysiologic events that lead to abnormal lower urinary tract function, as well as the evaluation, management, and treatment of women with specific types of voiding problems.

NEUROPHYSIOLOGY OF MICTURITION

Normal voiding is accomplished by activation of the "micturition reflex" (Fig. 34.1). This is a coordinated event characterized by, in order: (1) relaxation of the striated urethral sphincter, (2) contraction of the detrusor, (3) opening of the vesical neck and urethra, and (4) onset of urine flow (Fig. 34.2). This reflex is normally controlled by the pontine micturition center (PMC) located in the rostral brainstem. A separate sacral micturition center is located at S2 to S4, through which the bladder can contract independent of cortical and pontine input. The PMC, through its neural pathways to the sacral micturition center, is responsible for coordinated and voluntary voiding. Both the autonomic and somatic nervous systems play a crucial role in lower urinary tract function. Normal voiding occurs when the bladder responds to threshold tension via its mechanoreceptors. To avoid a random occurrence, central nervous system inhibitory and facilitatory pathways are involved in coordination of urine storage and micturition.

Micturition depends on a spinobulbospinal reflex that is relayed through the PMC, which receives input from the cerebral cortex, cerebellum, basal ganglia, thalamus, and hypothalamus, and is the final common pathway to the bladder motor neurons. Much of the input from suprapontine centers is inhibitory, although some facilitatory influences are involved. The central facilitatory areas are the anterior pons and the posterior hypothalamus, and the inhibitory areas include the cerebral cortex, basal ganglia, and cerebellum. The cerebellum also is implicated in the maintenance of tone in the pelvic floor striated musculature and coordination between bladder contraction and periurethral striated muscle relaxation. Because the suprapontine input to the PMC is mostly inhibitory, interruption of this input (e.g., cerebrovascular accident, cerebral atrophy, Parkinson disease, brain tumor, or trauma) often results in uncontrolled detrusor activity, or involuntary contractions, but the "micturition reflex" is left intact. The typical presentation of a suprapontine lesion is loss of voluntary control of micturition. Uninhibited detrusor

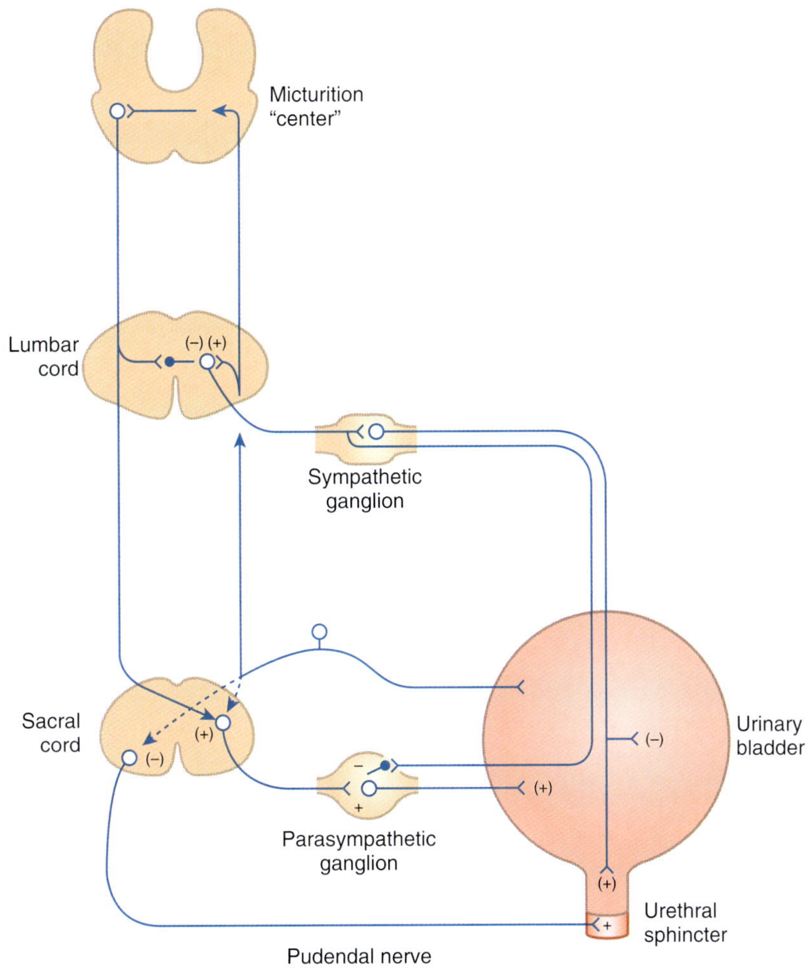

Fig. 34.1 Diagram of reflex pathways involved in micturition (according to deGroat). Plus and minus signs indicate, respectively, excitatory and inhibitory synaptic actions. The connection of the pontine micturition center to the cerebral cortex and other suprapontine areas is not pictured. (From deGroat WC, Booth AM. Physiology of the urinary bladder and urethra. *Ann Intern Med.* 1980;92:312.)

contractions may result in urinary frequency, urgency, and urgency incontinence. Little risk is present for developing renal deterioration because voiding is coordinated, even if not always voluntary.

Anatomically, the two areas of the spinal cord responsible for transmitting afferent input from the lower urinary tract are the lateral spinothalamic tracts and the posterior columns. The lateral spinothalamic tracts contain ascending routes responsible for transmitting bladder sensation and triggering voiding. Proprioceptive sensory impulses generated in bladder muscle and periurethral striated muscle travel in the posterior columns. The PMC controls efferent input to the bladder and external sphincter via two separate regions. The medial region is responsible for motor input to the bladder detrusor muscle via the reticulospinal tracts to the sacral intermediolateral cell groups, which contain preganglionic parasympathetic neurons that form the motor supply of the bladder detrusor muscle. Electrical stimulation of this region results in a prompt decrease in pelvic floor electromyography (EMG) and urethral pressure followed by an increase in intravesical pressure (normal voiding). The lateral region has specific projections via the corticospinal tracts to the nucleus of Onuf in the sacral cord that contains motor neurons innervating the pelvic floor, including the urethral and anal sphincters. Electrical stimulation of this region results in a rapid increase in urethral pressure and pelvic floor EMG but little increase in intravesical pressure (normal storage).

Storage and evacuation of urine depend on neural integration at the peripheral, spinal cord, and central levels. Normally, bladder distension will cause low-level firing of afferent nerves. This will cause a reflex inhibitory response to the bladder via the hypogastric nerve and a stimulatory response to the external sphincter from the pudendal nerve. With further distension, myelinated A delta fiber afferents are activated. Afferents travel up the spinal cord to the PMC. Here, central input, mostly inhibitory, is received from suprapontine centers. If voiding is not desired, the voiding reflex can be suppressed or interrupted. If voiding is desired, efferent output to the pelvic plexus at S2–S4 via the spinal cord is initiated. Ultimately, the stimulatory message is sent to the bladder via the pelvic nerve. At the same time, inhibitory messages are sent via the hypogastric and pudendal pathways to allow for relaxation of the urethral sphincter mechanisms and coordinated voiding.

Peripheral innervation to the bladder and to the internal and external sphincters is provided by the pelvic, hypogastric, and

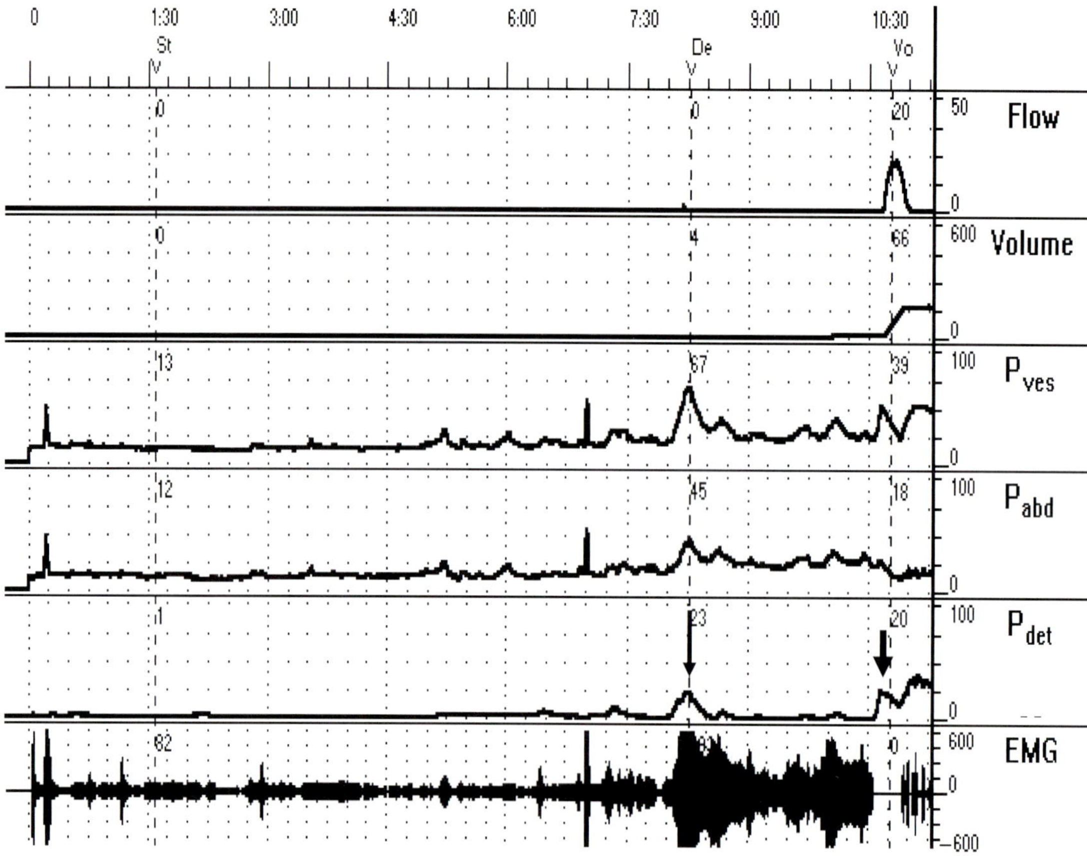

Fig. 34.2 Urodynamic representation of the micturition cycle. Note that during filling there is an involuntary detrusor contraction (*arrow*) accompanied by an increase in external sphincter activity, as portrayed by increased EMG activity (guarding reflex). The contraction abates, and then normal voiding ensues (*large arrow*). First there is relaxation of the external sphincter, followed by a voluntary detrusor contraction and initiation of flow. P_{ves}, Intravesical pressure; P_{abd}, intraabdominal pressure; P_{det}, detrusor pressure; *EMG*, electromyography.

pudendal nerves. Parasympathetic efferent input to the bladder arises from the intermediolateral cell column of S2–S4 and travels as preganglionic fibers via the pelvic nerve to the pelvic plexus located on both sides of the rectum, from which postganglionic fibers innervate the bladder. Efferent sympathetic nerves to the bladder and urethra arise from the intermediolateral cell column of T10 to L2 as preganglionic fibers that travel to ganglia located in the superior hypogastric plexus, from which arises the hypogastric nerve that contains the postganglionic sympathetic efferents to the bladder and urethra. The pudendal nerve carries the somatic input from S2–S4 to the external sphincter. Injury to any one of these nerves or their branches can result in a partial or complete denervation to the involved end organ.

In addition to the neurophysiologic pathways, other pharmacologic factors are responsible for normal voiding. The lower urinary tract is rich in both cholinergic and adrenergic receptors. Muscarinic receptors are located in the body of the bladder, and they are activated by parasympathetic release of acetylcholine to induce bladder contraction. Also, β-adrenergic receptors in the detrusor cause relaxation in response to increasing levels of cyclic adenosine monophosphate. In the bladder neck and urethra, α-adrenergic receptors are responsible for the increase in urethral tone and rise in intraurethral pressure during sympathetic stimulation via the hypogastric nerve. Each of these receptor types have been the basis for pharmacologic therapy of the lower urinary tract.

Anticholinergic medications can cause bladder relaxation by inhibiting parasympathetic pathways; β-adrenergics also treat bladder overactivity by stimulating adrenoreceptors and causing detrusor relaxation. α-Agonist medications have been used to treat stress incontinence, whereas α-blockers can facilitate emptying by relaxation of bladder neck smooth muscle.

CLASSIFICATION OF VOIDING DYSFUNCTION

Many complex classification systems for voiding dysfunction have been proposed; however, they failed to be diagnostically and therapeutically oriented. We have found the functional classification system proposed by Wein (1981) to be the most useful. This simple and practical classification system can be applied easily to our diagnostic criteria (e.g., urodynamics). Of equal importance is that treatment options can be chosen based on the classification.

The functional classification is based on a simple understanding of urine storage and micturition. For normal urine storage and voiding to occur, there must be proper and coordinated functioning of the bladder and the bladder outlet. Therefore, in simple anatomic terms, voiding dysfunction can be divided into the following categories:

1. Bladder dysfunction
2. Bladder outlet dysfunction (bladder neck, urethra, external sphincter)
3. Combined bladder and outlet dysfunction

Similarly, the effects of these problems can be classified as follows:

1. Failure to properly store urine
2. Failure to properly empty urine
3. Failure to store and empty urine

Voiding dysfunction can be characterized as neurogenic or nonneurogenic. Furthermore, nonneurogenic voiding dysfunction related to outlet obstruction can be classified as functional or anatomical. Bladder outlet obstruction is characterized by a reduced urine flow rate and/or a raised postvoid residual (PVR) associated with an elevated voiding detrusor pressure. It is usually diagnosed by studying the synchronous values of urine flow rate and detrusor pressure and any PVR measurements. Common anatomic causes of female bladder outlet obstruction include advanced pelvic organ prolapse, stress incontinence surgery, and urethral stricture (Haylen et al., 2010). Neurogenic obstruction is functional and the result of dyscoordination of the external and/or internal sphincter during voiding.

EVALUATION OF FEMALE VOIDING DYSFUNCTION

The evaluation of LUTS and potential voiding dysfunction in women begins with a thorough history focusing on the type and duration of symptoms and voiding habits over time. Historically, women have fewer reported classic voiding (obstructive) symptoms and have more commonly presented with storage symptoms and recurrent urinary tract infections. Two studies showed that, with a high index of suspicion and careful questioning, voiding symptoms were noted in 71% to 76% and storage symptoms were present in 79% to 92% of women with obstruction; therefore, voiding symptoms should not be overlooked when evaluating a woman who complains primarily of storage symptoms. A complete medical, surgical, obstetric-gynecologic, neurologic, and urologic history may uncover possible causes of voiding dysfunction. Any inciting events, such as surgeries to treat stress urinary incontinence (SUI) or any other procedures in the lower urinary tract or vagina, must be recorded. Other relevant information that may aid in the diagnosis of obstruction include history of urogenital trauma, history of falls, back injury, or surgery, and other medical conditions, such as diabetes, neurological disease, or psychiatric conditions.

A complete physical examination including a pelvic examination is required. An abdominal examination is performed to evaluate for abdominal masses or a palpable distended bladder. A pelvic examination then is performed, and one should first inspect the vagina and the epithelium for atrophic changes, signs of prior surgery, and possible foreign body. Attention should be paid to the positions of the urethra, bladder neck, and bladder at rest and with Valsalva by visualizing the amount of anterior, apical, and posterior compartment prolapse. One should inspect the anterior vaginal wall for existing scars or hypersuspension or urethral kinking caused by prior surgery. The posterior blade of a small vaginal speculum is helpful in visualizing the anterior vaginal wall. The cotton swab test can be used to quantify urethral hypermobility when needed. The patient also should be assessed for SUI. Vaginal apex support and position are important, as uterine or apical prolapse are potential causes of obstruction. After examination of the anterior vaginal wall is completed, the blade of the speculum is rotated, and the posterior wall and apex are inspected. Similar to other forms of prolapse, posterior vaginal wall prolapse, including rectocele and posterior enterocele, can cause obstruction and voiding dysfunction. Bimanual examination with palpation of the uterus and cervix should be done to determine uterine size and position, and to identify the presence of any pelvic masses, including fibroids, which may cause or contribute to voiding dysfunction.

In patients with LUTS, a focused neurologic examination should also be performed. Attention should be paid to the sensory and motor functions of the sacral nerves, including anal sphincter tone, perineal sensation, bulbocavernosus and anal wink reflexes, strength of lower extremities, and deep tendon reflexes (knee and ankle). A careful neurologic examination may help to confirm suspected disease or uncover an unknown lesion, and a formal neurologic consultation may be appropriate.

Simple office-based tests can give insight to the cause of LUTS. Urine analysis (and culture, if indicated) is done routinely. Intake and voiding diaries are helpful in quantifying fluid consumption, symptoms, voiding habits, and urine production. Diaries log the number of incontinence episodes and type (stress, urgency, insensible). Noninvasive uroflowmetry and PVR volume determination are good methods to screen for disorders of bladder emptying. A PVR assessment can be performed initially as a safety measure to rule out significant retention of urine, and later to monitor changes in bladder emptying ability, especially in neurologic conditions, as some patients may develop bladder dysfunction at any point in their disease process. There is no standard definition as to what constitutes a clinically significant PVR; however, recent studies have commonly used 100 or 150 mL as limits. No data suggest that higher residuals indicate pathological conditions. Absolute volumes, proportion of bladder capacity, or presence of relevant symptoms are all used in some contexts (Mevcha & Drake, 2010).

Acute urinary retention is defined as a relatively sudden inability to pass urine associated with bladder distension. Chronic retention is less specifically defined but usually presents as an elevated PVR of at least 250 mL without pain. Individuals with chronically elevated PVR may be at increased risk of ongoing voiding dysfunction, recurrent urinary tract infections, and stone disease, but often are asymptomatic or minimally symptomatic and may not require intervention. Although uroflowmetry and PVR cannot determine why voiding or emptying are abnormal (e.g., DU vs. obstruction), they may prompt more thorough evaluation with urodynamics. Thus, we consider uroflowmetry and PVR to be good screening tests for a woman with LUTS. A single elevated PVR should not be considered the sole assessment of bladder emptying ability and should be confirmed with a repeat measurement on a follow-up visit. PVR volume should be interpreted with respect to LUTS, urinary tract infections, and other symptoms.

Urodynamic testing can be an important part of the evaluation of female voiding dysfunction. It should be performed in patients for whom additional information is needed to make an accurate diagnosis and to guide therapy and/or counseling, and in those patients whose condition has the potential to have deleterious and irreversible effects on the upper urinary tract. Urodynamic findings inconsistent with patient symptoms or events occurring during testing that are uncharacteristic for patients during normal activity should be interpreted with caution. This is especially true for uroflowmetry, where it is very important to correlate catheterized uroflow with what is normal or characteristic for the patient. Multichannel urodynamics with simultaneous measurement of vesical and abdominal pressure and "subtracted" detrusor pressure during filling and voiding (see Fig. 34.2) is the standard. The filling phase (cystometry) evaluates the ability of the bladder to effectively store urine by assessing bladder stability, compliance, and capacity. Pressure-flow analysis during voiding assesses bladder contractility and bladder outlet resistance. EMG may be added to assess the pelvic floor musculature and external sphincter. Videourodynamics is the addition of simultaneous fluoroscopy during urodynamics, and is particularly helpful in confirming and localizing anatomic or functional obstruction. It can discover an obstruction that would not have been found on the basis of multichannel urodynamics alone. If videourodynamics are not available, then a separate voiding cystourethrogram that examines the bladder, bladder neck, and urethra during voiding can be helpful in localizing obstruction.

The final component of the evaluation is cystourethroscopy, when indicated. Scarring, kinking, or deviation of the urethra, especially after previous surgery, may be responsible for incomplete emptying. Rarely, a urethral lesion responsible for obstruction may be found. Examination of the bladder may uncover a lesion, such as a tumor or stone, and may identify some of the changes associated with obstruction or retention.

DIAGNOSIS AND MANAGEMENT

Treatment of voiding dysfunction is dictated by several factors. First is the potential danger to the upper urinary tract associated with high storage pressures or urinary retention, which can lead to renal deterioration. Although this is less common in nonneurogenic voiding dysfunction, any evidence of upper tract decompensation (hydronephrosis, renal insufficiency, recurrent pyelonephritis) should be given immediate attention. Second is the degree of bother of the patient's symptoms. In many cases, empiric therapy is an appropriate first step for patients with symptoms caused by voiding dysfunction. In patients without neurologic disease whose primary complaints are storage symptoms, that is, urgency incontinence without emptying disorder, behavioral modification with pelvic floor muscle exercises or oral pharmacotherapy is effective in relieving overactive bladder symptoms. In cases in which the diagnosis is not clear, or when abnormal emptying and storage coexist, a more comprehensive workup is necessary. When empiric therapy fails, or if voiding dysfunction is associated with neurologic disease, further investigation with urodynamic testing is usually indicated. In these instances, the specific cause for the voiding dysfunction will direct treatment. On the other hand, if a patient presents with an incidental finding of an elevated PVR, no further testing may be necessary. For example, if an asymptomatic woman presents after routine pelvic ultrasound that showed a PVR of 200 mL, there is no compromise of the upper urinary tract, and she remains asymptomatic, further diagnostic studies are usually unnecessary, and monitoring of PVR may be sufficient.

Distinguishing neurogenic from nonneurogenic voiding dysfunction is important. The distinguishing feature is a known neurological disease. In most cases, neurogenic voiding dysfunction is related to either neurogenic DU or acontractility, or functional obstruction from detrusor-sphincter dyssynergia (DSD). Nonneurogenic voiding dysfunction can also be caused by DU or obstruction, which can be functional, as in the case of dysfunctional voiding and primary bladder neck obstruction (PBNO), or anatomic, as in the case of pelvic organ prolapse, urethral stricture, postsurgical obstruction, etc. A complete list of causes for bladder outlet obstruction in women is shown in Table 34.1.

NEUROGENIC VOIDING DYSFUNCTION

Pathophysiology

A wide range of neurological diseases can affect the complex central and peripheral neural networks that regulate the function of the lower urinary tract, resulting in storage and voiding dysfunction. This can have a profound effect on the urinary system, and the pattern of voiding dysfunction depends on the extent, the evolution, and the site of the neurological dysfunction (Georgopoulos & Apostolidis, 2017). The term neurogenic bladder is often used loosely by clinicians to describe a bladder that is not functioning normally. It is critical to be more precise in assessment and classification for diagnostic and therapeutic purposes. Thus, the goals in assessing patients with neurogenic voiding dysfunction are to determine the effects of the neurologic disease on the entire urinary tract in such a way that treatment can be implemented to relieve symptoms and prevent damage to the upper and lower urinary tracts. For the patient with neurologic disease, global symptoms do not always indicate the magnitude to which the disease is affecting the urinary tract.

Pathologic processes at each level of innervation must be considered when evaluating neurogenic voiding dysfunction (Box 34.1). For example, suprapontine lesions (e.g., cerebral atrophy, cerebrovascular accident, brain tumor) cause a loss of inhibitory input to the PMC and subsequent uninhibited bladder contractions, a condition known as neurogenic detrusor overactivity (NDO) when evaluated urodynamically. Sphincter

TABLE 34.1 Anatomic and Functional Causes of Bladder Outlet Obstruction in Women

Anatomic Obstruction	Functional Obstruction
A. Inflammatory processes	A. Detrusor-sphincter dyssynergia
1. Bladder neck fibrosis	
2. Urethral stricture	
3. Atrophic vaginitis/urethritis	
4. Meatal stenosis	
5. Urethral caruncle	
6. Skene's gland cyst/abscess	
7. Urethral diverticulum	
B. Pelvic prolapse	B. Dysfunctional voiding
1. Anterior vaginal wall	
2. Posterior vaginal wall	
3. Apical (uterine prolapse/enterocele)	
C. Neoplastic	C. Primary bladder neck obstruction
1. Urethral carcinoma	
2. Bladder carcinoma	
D. Gynecologic (extrinsic compression)	
1. Retroverted uterus	
2. Lower segment uterine or vaginal leiomyoma	
3. Cervical carcinoma	
4. Vaginal carcinoma	
E. Iatrogenic obstruction	
1. Antiincontinence procedures	
2. Multiple urethral dilations	
3. Urethral excision/reconstruction	
F. Miscellaneous	
1. Urethral valves	
2. Ectopic ureterocele	
3. Bladder calculi	

BOX 34.1 Summary of Lesions Found in Common Neurogenic Voiding Dysfunctions

Suprapontine Lesions
Cerebrovascular disease
Parkinson disease
Multiple sclerosis
Concussion
Brain tumor
Shy–Drager syndrome
Normal pressure hydrocephalus

Pontine-Sacral Spinal Cord Lesions
Spinovascular disease
Spinal cord injury
Multiple sclerosis
Spinal dysraphism
Tabes dorsalis
Spinal stenosis
Disk herniation

Infrasacral/Peripheral Lesions
Sacral agenesis
Low spinal cord tumor
Spinal cord injury
Cauda equina syndrome
Diabetes
Herpes zoster
Tabes dorsalis
Radical pelvic surgery

reflexes are not affected and coordinated uninhibited voiding can result.

Clinically, interruption of the neural pathways connecting the PMC to the sacral micturition center (e.g., spinal cord injuries or lesions) usually results in NDO and a dyscoordination of the bladder and external sphincter (detrusor sphincter dyssynergia [DSD]). DSD is characterized by simultaneous contractions of the detrusor and external (and sometimes internal) urethral sphincter. The involuntary detrusor contractions cause incontinence, and the involuntary sphincter contractions cause bladder outlet obstruction and retention of urine. DSD is commonly seen in suprasacral spinal cord lesions and multiple sclerosis, and, less commonly, in myelodysplasia and lumbosacral lesions. Untreated DSD can result in high storage pressures (loss of bladder compliance) and resultant vesicoureteral reflux, hydronephrosis, urolithiasis, and urosepsis. Suprasacral spinal cord lesions also result in loss of supraspinal input; however, the complexity of the resulting voiding dysfunction depends on the level and completeness of the lesion. Also, input to the sphincters may be disrupted, resulting in DSD. A complete spinal cord lesion will result in the development of a spinal micturition reflex, in which unmyelinated C-fiber afferents excite sacral neurons and trigger a bladder contraction. In addition, incomplete relaxation of the external sphincter results in a contraction against a closed outlet, with subsequent incontinence, retention, and eventual loss of bladder compliance. When the lesion is above the lower thoracic spinal cord, internal sphincter dyssynergia can also develop as the autonomic neural input to the internal sphincter/bladder neck is disrupted. This can occur with spinal cord injury, lesions, or infarction, as well as with multiple sclerosis that affects the suprasacral spinal cord.

Infrasacral cord and peripheral nerve lesions generally result in loss of sensation and contractility, leading to a large, hypercompliant, areflexic bladder. The external sphincter also may be deficient of contractility and tone. Neurologic lesions that interfere with the sacral reflex arc most often are seen in patients with myelodysplasia, diabetic cystopathy, ruptured discs, or low spinal cord tumors. These diminish reflexive voiding and result in various degrees and combinations of detrusor areflexia, intrinsic urethral sphincter deficiency, and paralysis of the external urethral striated sphincter.

Neurologic lesions can be "complete" or "incomplete"; therefore, the exact manifestations of a particular disease or lesion are not absolutely predictable. A complete urologic evaluation for patients with neurogenic voiding dysfunction is always recommended. A single disease process such as multiple sclerosis can affect multiple areas of the central nervous system. Urologic presentations include detrusor overactivity, detrusor overactivity with DSD, and impaired or absent detrusor contractility. The latter two presentations can result in impaired bladder emptying.

Evaluation

The urodynamic evaluation often is integral to the evaluation of patients with suspected neurologic voiding dysfunction, especially when emptying is incomplete and elevated storage pressures are suspected (Fig. 34.3). Incontinence is a common complaint of these individuals and can be secondary to NDO or decreased compliance. Multichannel urodynamics is key to understanding the underlying pathology. The detrusor leak point pressure (DLPP) is the amount of detrusor pressure, in the absence of an increase in abdominal pressure, required to cause incontinence. It is a direct reflection of the amount of resistance provided by the external sphincter; the higher the resistance, as with DSD, the higher the DLPP. The higher the DLPP, the more likely pressure will be transferred to the upper tract. High storage pressures are potentially dangerous to the upper urinary tract. McGuire et al. (1981) showed that storage pressures of greater than 40 cm H_2O are associated with upper tract deterioration in myelomeningocele patients. Although this number should not be taken as a definitive cutoff (it was determined in a very specific population), storage pressures that approach or exceed 40 cm H_2O should prompt an evaluation of the kidneys for hydronephrosis.

The evaluation of upper urinary tract health and function is paramount in women with neurogenic voiding dysfunction. Several diagnostic tools can be helpful. Renal ultrasound can assess the absence, presence, and degree of hydronephrosis. Renal scintigraphy is best used to evaluate renal function and scarring and can determine the presence or absence of obstruction. When videourodynamic studies are not available, it may be necessary to perform a cystogram or voiding cystourethrogram to assess for vesicoureteral reflux.

Treatment of Neurogenic Storage Dysfunction

The main goal in the treatment of neurogenic lower urinary tract dysfunction, first and foremost, is to protect the upper urinary tracts from damage. This is accomplished by maintaining low storage pressures in the lower urinary tract and facilitating bladder emptying. A secondary and also important goal is to alleviate the patient's bothersome LUTS. Treatment should be directed at the specific problems uncovered during the evaluation, regardless of the neurologic disease associated with those problems.

For detrusor overactivity and impaired compliance, anticholinergic medications have traditionally been first-line therapy, and, in many cases, are sufficient to lower storage pressures and reduce or abolish involuntary detrusor contractions. Less is known about β-3-agonists in the neurogenic bladder. In cases of outlet dysfunction, like DSD, anticholinergic medication

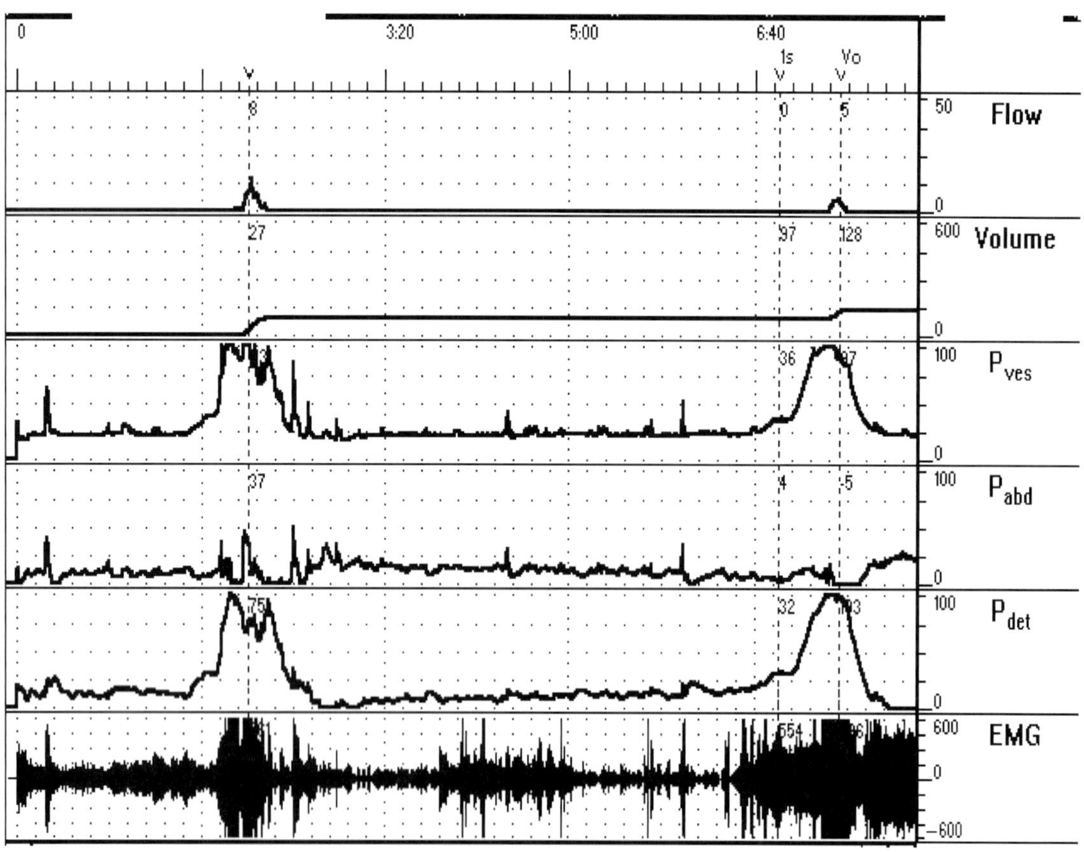

Fig. 34.3 Urodynamic tracing of a young woman with incontinence and a tethered cord. Note the first involuntary detrusor contraction (IDC) accompanied by increased EMG activity and incontinence, as registered on the flow curve. The second IDC is also accompanied by increased EMG activity that does not abate when the patient is asked to voluntarily void. Diagnosis: neurogenic detrusor overactivity with detrusor external sphincter dyssynergia. P_{ves}, Intravesical pressure; P_{abd}, intraabdominal pressure; P_{det}, detrusor pressure; *EMG*, electromyography.

may reduce storage pressures, but also will likely produce urinary retention, necessitating intermittent self-catheterization.

In 2011, the US Food and Drug Administration (FDA) approved intradetrusor onabotulinumtoxinA (Botox; Allergan Inc., Irvine, CA) for use in patients with NDO who are refractory to antimuscarinic medications. Although onabotulinumtoxinA does not treat the voiding dysfunction, it can successfully reduce bladder pressures. In cases of DSD, it is usually combined with clean intermittent catheterization (CIC). In such cases a 200-unit dose is recommended (Cruz et al., 2011; Ginsberg et al., 2012; Carlson et al., 2013).

Treatment of Neurogenic Voiding Dysfunction

The main goals of treating neurogenic voiding dysfunction are improving bladder emptying and decreasing elevated intravesical pressures during storage. Complete bladder emptying results in reduction of urinary tract infection, stone formation, and overflow incontinence. Low voiding bladder pressure is key to the prevention of upper tract deterioration (Georgopoulos & Apostolidis, 2017).

Active surveillance with or without manipulation techniques such as double voiding and Credé maneuver and/or Valsalva maneuver can be appropriate for patients with low intravesical pressures and good empting ability (Kim, 2017). No effective oral pharmacotherapy exists at this time for the treatment of neurogenic DU, although the use of bethanacol has been reported anecdotally, without proven success (also see Detrusor Underactivity section later).

In patients who have a problem with emptying, either secondary to DSD or impaired contractility, emptying must be facilitated. For DSD, CIC has been a mainstay of therapy and is most effective when detrusor overactivity is controlled by one of the means described previously. The same is true for retention secondary to DU, because no therapies are available that increase detrusor contractility. In some cases, a catheterizable stoma can facilitate independence when neurologic disease is advanced and urethral catheterization cannot be performed independently.

OnabotulinumtoxinA has been injected transurethrally into the external sphincter for the treatment of DSD, and both open-label and randomized controlled studies have shown mixed results. Chen et al. (2008) evaluated the effect of 100 U of onabotulinumtoxinA on the external urethral sphincter in treatment of DSD in 20 patients with suprasacral spinal cord injury. After 4 weeks of treatment, there were significant reductions in static and maximal urethral pressure, EMG activity, and PVR, but not in maximal detrusor pressure or DLPP. The largest randomized controlled trial to date assessed 86 multiple sclerosis patients and concluded that a single 100-U injection of onabotulinumtoxinA did not decrease PVR volume (Gallien et al., 2005).

Endoscopic sphincterotomy is an alternative that can be used to treat DSD in men; however, lack of an appropriate external collection device other than a diaper makes this option less desirable in women. Chronic indwelling catheters generally are not recommended as a first choice for treatment of chronic retention in the neurological patient but may be used as a last resort in select patients. In situations in which this form of management is desirable and necessary, appropriate catheter care, with frequent changing of the catheter, is recommended. We always recommend using the smallest size catheter, usually 14-French or 16-French, and a 5-mL balloon. Urinary leakage around the catheter becomes common, and there is a tendency for providers to continuously upsize the catheters, causing further trauma and complications related to erosions. A propensity also exists for chronic infections, stone formation, bladder neck erosions, and the development of squamous cell carcinoma. Calculi have been reported to occur in more than 30% of patients managed with an indwelling catheter. Urethral erosions are a well-known complication of long-term indwelling catheters, because of pressure and traction causing necrosis of the urethra. In women, especially those who are not fully sensate, the risk of urethral erosion is significant. When this occurs, oftentimes the bladder neck must be closed, and the catheter converted to a suprapubic tube. Consideration of an early suprapubic catheter placement can alleviate some of this risk.

In 2015, the FDA approved the inFlow Urinary Prosthesis in the United States (Vesiflo, Redmond, WA) for female patients with impaired detrusor contractility of neurologic origin. This is a magnetically-activated intraurethral valve-pump that drains the bladder. Chen et al. (2005) tested the inFlow device, recruiting 273 women who performed CIC for this prospective study. Although most women withdrew (most commonly because of discomfort or urinary leakage), 77 (28%) completed the trial. In this group, PVR volumes were comparable to those when using CIC, and quality-of-life outcomes improved during use of the prosthesis for bladder emptying. These results suggest this nonsurgical prosthesis may be a viable treatment alternative to CIC for a subgroup of women with a hypocontractile or acontractile bladder.

Skeletal muscle wraps have been used as surgical therapy for neurogenic underactive bladder (UAB), including latissimus dorsi (Gakis et al., 2011) and rectus abdominis (Agarwal et al., 2018). These investigations using skeletal muscle show promise for spinal cord injury patients who have no alternative to CIC. In the latissimus dorsi detrusor myoplasty study, 17 of 24 patients (71%) gained complete spontaneous voiding with a mean PVR volume of 25 mL (range 0–100 mL), and complete spontaneous voiding was achieved in all five patients who had rectus abdominis detrusor myoplasty. Additional, larger studies are needed.

Finally, in patients with high storage pressures and DSD or those with DU and incomplete emptying who cannot perform self-catheterization and have or are trying to avoid complications of indwelling catheters who do not respond to any of the aforementioned therapies for neurogenic voiding dysfunction, augmentation cystoplasty, with or without continent catheterizable stoma or urinary diversion, can be considered. These operations are indicated in patients with functionally decreased bladder capacities and refractory storage symptoms. Intermittent catheterization will be required for emptying. They are, however, major operations with obvious risks and, with the exception of an ileal conduit, require the use of upper extremities for self-catheterization.

Therapies exist on the horizon, including electrical neuromodulation techniques, bladder injection with stem cells, and novel receptor targets. While some have shown potential benefits, further research is needed.

Nonneurogenic Voiding Dysfunction

Dysfunctional Voiding. Dysfunctional voiding, or micturition that is obstructed because of failure of the external urethral sphincter-pelvic floor complex to relax appropriately (in the absence of any neuroanatomical abnormality), has high rates of urinary tract infection, incontinence, and vesicoureteric reflux. Complaints of urinary incontinence and recurrent urinary tract infection are oftentimes the presenting symptoms (Clothier & Wright, 2018).

The prevalence of dysfunctional voiding in the adult population is unknown. In 1999, Nitti et al. found dysfunctional voiding to be the most common abnormality of the voiding phase in women presenting with LUTS, and in a retrospective study Groutz et al. (2001) found that 2% of patients referred for urodynamic evaluation met the criteria. Dysfunctional voiding is a learned behavior, which differentiates it from true DSD, which was described earlier (Fig. 34.4). Thus, the terms learned voiding dysfunction and pseudodyssynergia also have been used to describe the condition. Dysfunctional voiding may result in various LUTS, including both storage and emptying symptoms. Carlson et al. (2001) investigated the presenting symptoms in patients with a urodynamic diagnosis of dysfunctional voiding and found that frequency and urgency were the most common symptoms in 82% of patients, urgency and stress incontinence were present in 23% and 15% of patients, respectively, and 42% of patients had a history of recurrent urinary tract infections. Dysfunctional voiding also may be responsible for episodes of acute or chronic urinary retention, and, in severe cases, upper and lower urinary tract decompensation.

In 1973, Hinman and Bauman popularized the concept of dyscoordination between the detrusor and the activity of the pelvic floor–external sphincter complex in neurologically normal individuals. Much of the literature describes this phenomenon, also known as the nonneurogenic neurogenic bladder, or Hinman syndrome, as occurring in children and adolescents who typically present with enuresis, recurrent urinary tract infections, and sometimes hydronephrosis. In 1978, Allen and Bright used the term dysfunctional voiding to describe failure to coordinate detrusor and sphincter activity in children. The literature is replete with reports of this condition in children; in adults, however, much less has been written, although it has been reported to cause various LUTS, incomplete emptying, incontinence, and recurrent urinary tract infections.

Dysfunctional voiding in children originally was thought to be a response to psychosocial problems. The condition is now recognized as a developmental abnormality, whereby there is persistence of the transitional phase between infantile

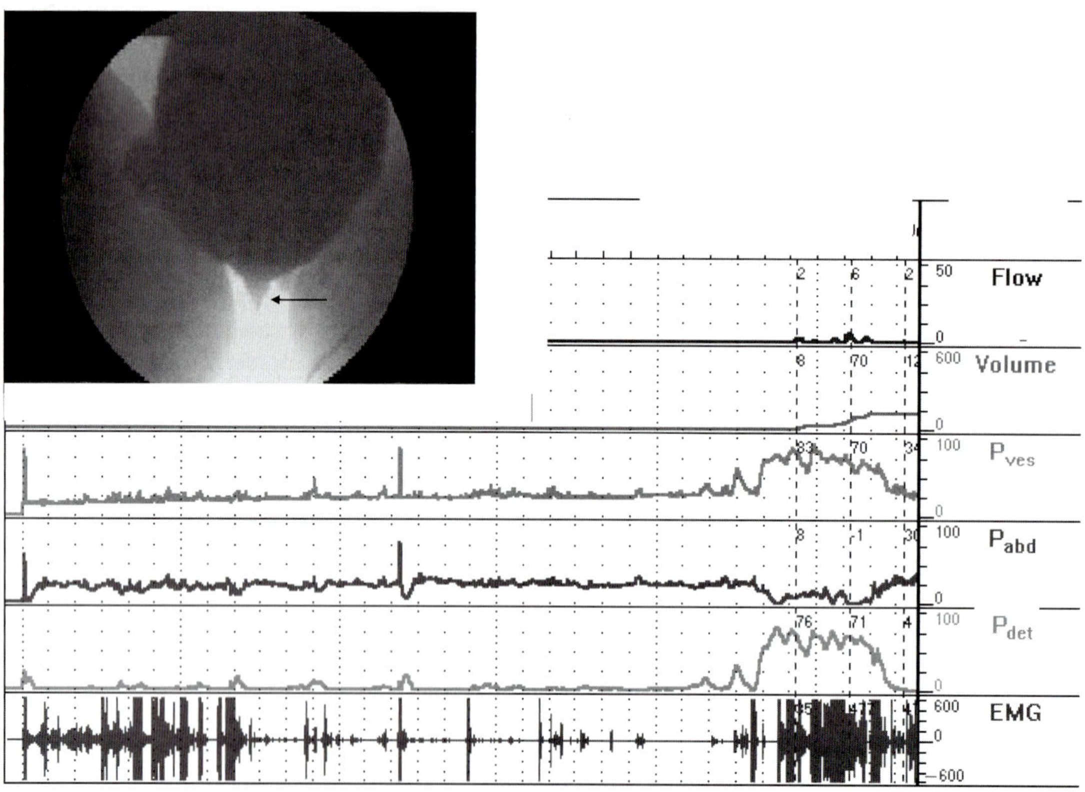

Fig. 34.4 Videourodynamic study of a 23-year-old woman with urgency incontinence and incomplete emptying. Note the high-pressure detrusor contraction that occurs before void, accompanied by decreased flow and increased EMG activity. *Arrow* indicates location of external sphincter. Fluoroscopic image taken during voiding shows a spinning top urethra with obstruction at the level of the external sphincter. Neurologic evaluation was negative. Diagnosis: dysfunctional voiding. P_{ves}, Intravesical pressure; P_{abd}, intraabdominal pressure; P_{det}, detrusor pressure; *EMG*, electromyography.

reflexogenic voiding and the normal volitional voiding of adulthood. There are several theories on why dysfunctional voiding occurs in adults. The most plausible is that it represents a learned behavior in response to an adverse event or condition, such as inflammation, irritation, infection (cystitis, urethritis, vaginitis), urethral diverticulum, pelvic inflammatory disease, anorectal disease, or trauma. Other authors have suggested that dysfunctional voiding may result from voluntary withholding of urination in individuals who work long hours. Kaplan et al. (1980) proposed that "the stress of modern society may manifest itself in this region of the body." McGuire and Savastano (1984) attributed the behavior to a primary abnormality of detrusor overactivity, with the dyssynergic sphincter response developing as a result of sudden unanticipated detrusor contractility. Contraction of the pelvic floor–external sphincter complex is a normal response to the need to control urgent urination, and results in a reflex inhibition of the detrusor. When this becomes habitual over time, the abnormal incoordination carries over to voluntary voiding, resulting in an intermittent urinary stream and residual urine.

The treatment of dysfunctional voiding has evolved over the years. The goal is to facilitate the patient's return to normal micturition. Usually a combination of behavioral, cognitive, and pharmacological therapies can be used to achieve this. Pelvic floor physical therapy has been shown to be effective and has become the first-line treatment. In 2010, Minardi et al. evaluated the efficacy of biofeedback and pelvic floor relaxation biofeedback on urodynamic and voiding parameters in 86 women with dysfunctional voiding and recurrent urinary tract infections for 1 year. There was significant decrease in storage and emptying symptoms, as well as improvement in urodynamic parameters including mean flow rate, flow time, and voided volume, and a decrease in PVR. There is an increased incidence of dysfunctional voiding in sexual abuse victims that has been linked to psychological stressors and elevated stress and anxiety scores; therefore, certain individuals may benefit from mental health therapy and support as well.

Some pharmacotheraputic options have been shown to be beneficial in patients with dysfunctional voiding. Xu et al. (2007) showed that oral baclofen, a γ-aminobutyric acid β receptor agonist, could be used to improve urinary symptoms in patients with dysfunctional voiding. They conducted a double-blind, placebo-controlled, crossover trial of baclofen 10 mg three times daily or placebo in 60 women with LUTS and urodynamic evidence of dysfunctional voiding. There were significantly fewer voids per 24-hour period (9.6 placebo vs. 6.7 baclofen, $P = .001$) in baclofen-treated patients, as well as an increase in maximal flow rate and a significant decrease in detrusor pressure at maximal flow rate. Baclofen was well-tolerated, and adverse events were similar between groups.

Some clinicians have had anecdotal success with amitriptyline. Vaginal benzodiazepine suppositories also have been used as an adjunct treatment in high-tone pelvic floor dysfunction associated with dyspareunia. In cases in which there is also detrusor overactivity or impaired compliance, anticholinergic medications can be used in addition to other therapies. Just as in the treatment of DSD, endoscopic and transperineal urethral injections of onabotulinum toxin A have been performed in women with dysfunctional voiding, although there are only limited and poor-quality data available.

Finally, sacral neuromodulation (SNM) has been shown to be beneficial in nonobstructive urinary retention. Tanagho and Schmidt (1988) first reported electrically stimulating sacral nerve roots for the treatment of nonobstructive urinary retention. Although the mechanism of action of SNM continues to remain unclear, FDA approval was granted in 1999 for its use in the treatment of nonobstructive urinary retention. A 5-year prospective, multicenter study conducted by van Kerrebroeck et al. (2007) included 152 patients treated with SNM (InterStim; Medtronic Inc., Minneapolis, MN), 31 of whom had an indication of urinary retention. On average, the number of catheterizations per day and the catheterized volume decreased (from 5.3 to 1.9, and from 379 to 109 mL, respectively). There was evidence of clinical success defined as a 50% or greater reduction in daily catheterizations and catheterized volumes in 58% and 71% of patients, respectively, 5 years after implantation.

Percutaneous tibial nerve stimulation performed for 30 minutes once a week for 12 weeks has been shown to benefit patients with dysfunctional voiding. Patients with dysfunctional voiding were significantly more likely to benefit than those with overactive bladder. However, storage symptoms were more likely to demonstrate an objective benefit than residual urine and flow rates (Capitanucci et al., 2009; Sinha, 2011). The exact mechanism of action by which neuromodulation may restore function in dysfunctional voiding is unknown, but it may work by reducing high-tone pelvic floor muscle dysfunction.

Fowler Syndrome. Fowler syndrome is a failure of the urethral sphincter to relax during voiding in patients in whom other types of urologic, gynecologic, or neurologic pathologies have been excluded. In 1985, Fowler et al. reported EMG abnormalities of the striated urethral sphincter in 15 women with voiding symptoms and urinary retention. It was hypothesized that these abnormal EMG patterns could be impairing relaxation of the urethral sphincter. Fowler syndrome usually is diagnosed in young women in their 20s or 30s who develop urinary retention. Many of these women have a history or findings consistent with polycystic ovary, which suggests that the abnormal sphincter may be under the influence of estrogen and could be attributed to a hormone-sensitive channelopathy confined to the urethral sphincter; however, the exact pathophysiology of the disease is still unknown. Many of these women have a trigger such as general anesthesia, urinary tract infection, gynecologic surgery, or childbirth. In an evaluation of 91 women with complete urinary retention conducted by Swinn et al. (2002), two-thirds presented after a gynecologic operation, and one-third developed retention spontaneously.

EMG is used to confirm the diagnosis and may show complex repetitive discharges and a decelerating component. Other useful diagnostic modalities include urethral pressure profile (UPP) and urodynamics, which may show a prolonged filling phase and reduced filling sensation, as well an increase in EMG activity, with no rise in the detrusor pressure during voiding, which differentiates Fowler syndrome from dysfunctional voiding. Other radiologic modalities that may be used are magnetic resonance imaging and ultrasound, which can show increased sphincteric volume. The goal of treatment is to ensure adequate bladder emptying.

SNM has been shown to be an efficient treatment that may restore normal voiding, and many feel it is the treatment of choice for Fowler syndrome. In 2000, Swinn et al. reported results of peripheral nerve stimulation in 38 women with urinary retention, 34 of whom had a diagnosis of Fowler syndrome. The overall success rate was 68%, with 12 patients undergoing permanent implantation; 10 patients were able to void normally, and two patients still needed to catheterize. In 2007, De Ridder et al. studied 62 women, 30 with Fowler syndrome and 32 with idiopathic retention. At 5 years after SNM, 72% of women with Fowler syndrome still had normal micturition, compared with 46% of women in the idiopathic retention group. Complications included lead migration, pain at the implantable pulse generator site, and possible infection. SNM is usually well-tolerated and safe and provides a useful therapeutic option to restore voiding in these patients.

Panicker et al. (2016) evaluated sphincteric onabotulinumtoxinA injections in 10 women with a primary disorder of urethral sphincter relaxation (elevated UPP, sphincter volume, and abnormal EMG). In this study, 100 U of onabotulinumtoxinA was injected into the striated urethral sphincter under EMG guidance. This pilot study showed an improvement in patient-reported LUTS and the objective parameters of maximum flow rate, PVR, and UPP, at 10 weeks posttreatment. No serious side effects were reported. Similarly, a retrospective study (Jiang et al., 2018) reported outcomes in 53 patients with voiding dysfunction attributed to nonneurogenic urethral sphincter hyperactivity who had sphincteric injections of 100 U of onabotulinum toxin A. Some 59% had a satisfactory improvement for an average duration of 9.6 months. Increased urinary incontinence or new urinary tract infections were noted in 10% to 20% of patients after treatment. This treatment could represent a safe outpatient treatment for young women with retention owing to a primary disorder of urethral sphincter relaxation. However, larger studies are required to confirm these findings.

Primary Bladder Neck Obstruction. PBNO is characterized by failure of the bladder neck to open properly in the presence of a detrusor contraction of normal or increased pressure and duration (Fig. 34.5). Marion (1933) originally described it in a male patient, and it was later described by Diokno et al. in 1984 in a group of women who underwent videourodynamic tests for nonneurogenic voiding dysfunction. Nitti et al. (1999) found the prevalence of PBNO to be 0.5% in women overall and 16% in obstructed women.

The exact etiology of PBNO is unknown. One theory is that it is caused by smooth muscle hypertrophy or an increase in collagen deposition at the bladder neck. Another is that a continual high tonus in the smooth muscle of the posterior urethra causes rigidity of the bladder neck. A theory that there is an increased number of α-adrenergic receptors, resulting in nonrelaxation

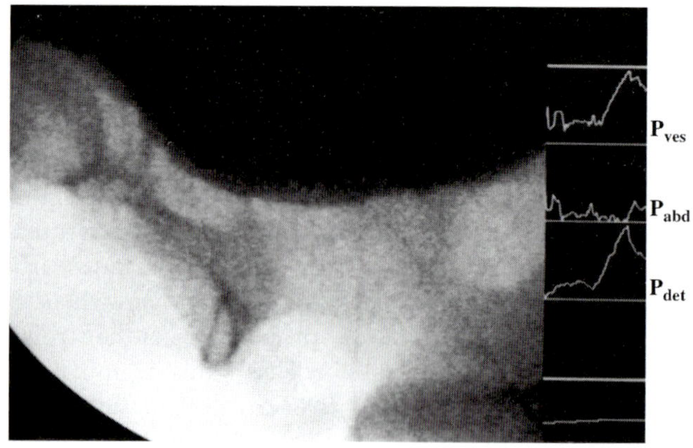

Fig. 34.5 Videourodynamic study of a 36-year-old woman with obstructive voiding symptoms and intermittent urinary retention. There is a sustained detrusor contraction of more than 50 cm H_2O with failure of the bladder neck to open. Diagnosis: primary bladder neck obstruction. P_{ves}, Intravesical pressure; P_{abd}, intraabdominal pressure; P_{det}, detrusor pressure.

during voiding, also has been suggested. Women with PBNO typically present initially with storage symptoms, and often are treated for bladder overactivity. Voiding symptoms then may become more prominent, and patients may even progress to periodic urinary retention and have high PVR volumes. Recurrent urinary tract infections commonly can result.

Diagnostic criteria for PBNO include high voiding pressure and low urine flow, along with fluoroscopic evidence of incomplete or nonopening of the bladder neck with voiding. Brucker et al. (2012) reported on urodynamic differences between dysfunctional voiding and PBNO in women. They showed that patients with dysfunctional voiding have greater mean maximum flow rate (12 vs. 7 mL/s, P = .027) and lower mean PVR (125 vs. 400 mL, P = .012). They also showed that EMG alone would have led to an erroneous diagnosis in 20% of patients with voiding dysfunction and 14% of patients with PBNO, supporting the use of fluoroscopy to differentiate between these two functional disorders.

The treatment options for PBNO in women include expectant management, pharmacotherapy, and surgical intervention. Expectant management is an option for patients whose symptoms are not bothersome and who do not have clinical or urodynamic evidence of upper or lower urinary tract decompensation. Unfortunately, little is known about the natural history of PBNO in women. The number of those who elect observation (watchful waiting) and have progressive symptoms, experience decompensation, or receive treatment is unknown.

In our practice, we follow watchful waiting patients periodically with a semiannual or annual uroflow, PVR, and assessment of symptoms. If there are any significant findings or a change in the patient's symptoms, we perform a renal ultrasound, and measure renal function as clinically indicated. The main focus of pharmacotherapy is α-adrenoreceptor blockade. One published study by Kumar et al. (1999) documented treatment of 24 women with PBNO. This was a highly symptomatic group: all had significantly elevated PVR volumes, and stringent urodynamic criteria were used to make the diagnosis. All women were treated initially with phenoxybenzamine, prazosin, or terazosin, and 50% responded to α-blockade with decreased symptoms, increased flow, and decreased residual volumes. Specifically, in responders maximum flow rates increased from 9.5 to 15.1 mL/s, and PVR decreased from 277 to 27 mL. No validated symptom assessment was used to assess symptom response. In 2006, Kessler et al. found significant improvement in symptoms and urodynamic parameters with the use of terazosin in 67% of women with PBNO. Although we have had success with α-blockers in cases of milder, nonretention PBNO, we have not been as successful in more severe cases or in women with urinary retention. We follow patients on medical therapy for PBNO similarly to those on watchful waiting.

PBNO can be treated surgically with transurethral incision of the bladder neck. This can be done either unilaterally or bilaterally, but the main concern of bladder neck incision is the development of postoperative SUI. The concept of bladder neck incision initially was described by Turner-Warwick et al. (1973) in men with voiding dysfunction. Jonas et al. (1979) applied the technique to women, showing a 71% improvement of symptoms in women with functional or mechanical outlet obstruction.

In the largest study of PBNO treatment published by Zhang et al. (2014), 84 women were diagnosed using video urodynamic criteria and treated with bladder neck incisions. Postoperative follow-up ranged from 6 to 78 months (average 27.4). Successful recovery after bladder neck incision without serious complications was achieved in 71 (84.5%) patients. The maximum uroflow rate increased from 9.8 to 18.8 mL/s ($P < .01$), and PVR decreased from 115.1 to 23.3 mL ($P < .01$). The maximal detrusor pressure at the maximum flow rate decreased from 69.6 to 20.5 cm H_2O ($P < .01$). Several complications were identified after surgery, including hemorrhage, need for reincision of the bladder neck, vesicovaginal fistula ($n = 3$), SUI ($n = 4$), and urethral stricture ($n = 3$).

Pelvic Organ Prolapse. Prolapse of pelvic organs can have a profound effect on lower urinary tract function. Urinary frequency, urgency, incontinence, and bladder outlet obstruction with varying degrees of urinary retention can occur. Patients may report the need to position themselves in a certain way to void (e.g., leaning backward or squatting) or may need to manually reduce the prolapse (splinting) to void.

Obstruction from prolapse can be caused by kinking of the urethra in cases of anterior vaginal wall prolapse (cystocele) or by direct compression of the prolapsing organ on the urethra. It can be demonstrated urodynamically by evaluating patients with the prolapse unreduced. The effect of the prolapse on voiding function can be seen further by then reducing the prolapse (with a pessary, speculum, or large swab) and repeating the study. Using this technique, Romanzi and Blaivas (1999) found urinary obstruction in 4% of patients with grade one or grade two cystocele and 58% of women with grade three or grade four cystocele. After pessary placement, 94% reverted to normal flow. Oftentimes simply inserting a pessary to facilitate bladder emptying is enough to make a diagnosis of obstruction related to prolapse, and urodynamic testing is not always necessary (Glass et al., 2020).

Iatrogenic Postsurgical Obstruction. Surgical procedures for the correction of SUI are designed to restore support to the urethrovesical junction or to improve coaptation of the urethra (in cases of intrinsic sphincter deficiency). This can be accomplished in various ways, including Burch retropubic colposuspension and pubovaginal and midurethral sling procedures. A potential complication of all these procedures is iatrogenic outlet obstruction leading to voiding dysfunction.

The incidence of iatrogenic urethral obstruction varies widely in the literature, from 2.5% to 24% (Tran & Rutman, 2017). Discrepancies in reported rates across studies may be explained by various factors, such as differences in definition, varying patient populations, and surgical differences. Obstruction after incontinence surgery is typically a result of technical factors, such as improper placement or excessive tensioning of sutures or slings. In 2007, Albo et al. found a surgical retention rate of 0% after Burch procedures versus 6.1% after pubovaginal sling procedures. Urinary retention is uncommon after midurethral sling surgery, but higher rates of retention have been reported after retropubic versus transobturator midurethral slings. Richter et al. (2010) performed a large, multicenter randomized trial of retropubic versus transobturator slings for SUI ($n = 597$). Postoperative voiding dysfunction that required surgery occurred in 2.7% of participants after retropubic and 0% after transoburator slings ($P = .004$).

Some additional factors may affect a patient's ability to empty after antiincontinence surgery. Obstruction may be caused indirectly by a cystocele or other prolapse that either was uncorrected at the time of surgery or had occurred postoperatively. Prolapse of sufficient size may kink the urethra. Impaired detrusor contractility, a condition that was likely present preoperatively, may cause obstruction in the face of the increased urethral resistance created by an antiincontinence procedure. Finally, the patient who habitually voids by abdominal straining may have difficulty emptying after pubovaginal sling surgery because the sling acts to increase urethral resistance with increases in abdominal pressure.

The evaluation of postsurgical voiding dysfunction should be thoughtful. Transient voiding dysfunction is frequent and expected after many types of antiincontinence surgery. Most women will begin voiding sufficiently on their own within a few days to weeks, whereas others may take longer to resume normal voiding and may need to perform intermittent catheterization as a bridge. Return to normal voiding may take longer in patients who have been obstructed chronically or have had an autologous pubovaginal sling procedure. Storage symptoms of urgency, frequency, and urgency incontinence are often more refractory than retention because they can be related to bladder changes. These symptoms may resolve as late as 6 months after surgery. For traditional procedures like Burch colposuspension and pubovaginal sling, it is not uncommon to delay evaluation of the patient with urinary retention or severe storage symptoms after incontinence surgery for 1 to 3 months postoperatively. Although this time frame is arbitrary, most data in the literature are based on a waiting period of at least 3 months, to ensure adequate time for retention from obstruction to resolve and to minimize the risk of recurrent stress incontinence. After

3 months, there is very low probability that any persistent retention will resolve without intervention.

We currently offer surgical revision beginning at about 1 month for patients requiring catheterization after a pubovaginal sling procedure, although continued watchful waiting is also an option. In the case of synthetic midurethral slings, some have advocated quicker intervention, within 7 to 10 days, when complete retention or severe obstructive symptoms are present. After retropubic and transobturator midurethral sling procedures, temporary voiding dysfunction resolved in 25% to 66% of patients in 1 to 2 weeks, and in 66% to 100% of patients by 6 weeks. Because of the immobility of the polypropylene mesh and the ingrowth of fibroblastic tissue at 1 to 2 weeks, patients with severe symptoms or urinary retention are less likely to improve after this period, and the traditional 3-month waiting period seems unwarranted. In our experience, symptoms persisting beyond 6 weeks likely will not respond and require surgical intervention. If there is no other explanation for the patient's voiding symptoms, intervention as early as 7 to 14 days may be reasonable, especially for those patients in complete retention. The decision to intervene early, however, should be discussed with the patient, as well as the risk of recurrent stress incontinence.

The diagnostic evaluation of the patient with voiding dysfunction after incontinence surgery begins with a focused history and physical examination. Key points in the history are the patient's preoperative voiding status and the temporal relationship of the LUTS to the surgery. The type of procedure performed and the number and type of other procedures done are also important. In cases of urinary retention and incomplete emptying, urodynamic studies are not necessary before intervention, particularly if preoperative contractility and emptying are known to be normal. It is well established that urodynamic tests may fail to diagnose obstruction in a significant number of women obstructed from antiincontinence procedures. Additionally, patients with nondiagnostic urodynamic studies, or those who fail to produce a detrusor contraction during urodynamics, have the same outcomes as those with urodynamic findings that are classic for obstruction. In cases of *de novo* or worsened storage symptoms, including urgency incontinence without a significantly elevated PVR or decreased flow rate, a formal urodynamic evaluation to assess for occult obstruction should be considered. The physical examination may reveal a hypersuspended urethra or significant prolapse that could point to the cause of obstruction, but often the examination is normal.

Treatment is dictated by the degree of bother of postoperative symptoms. In some cases, an obstructed patient, at least temporarily, will opt for conservative management with CIC. Occasionally, a woman who had severe SUI before surgery and is not very bothered by catheterization may prefer CIC to repeat surgery and a risk of recurrent stress incontinence. Most patients with significant symptoms from iatrogenic obstruction, however, choose definitive treatment. The role for urethral dilation in such cases is not known, but we feel it is of limited use and may be detrimental. Most commonly, obstructed slings are treated by sling excision, or by incision, which involves a vaginal incision and the use of a right-angle clamp to identify the sling, followed by incision of the sling with or without removal of the suburethral segment. Success rates vary, but they usually are reported in the 80% to 100% range, with recurrent stress incontinence rates between 0% and 36%.

Urethrolysis, whether by retropubic, transvaginal, or suprameatal approach, appears to have a similar success rate, ranging from 65% to 93%. The type of urethrolysis (or sling incision) chosen will depend on several factors, including patient presentation, type of incontinence procedure performed, whether she had a previously failed urethrolysis, and surgeon preference. It has been our practice to perform a transvaginal procedure for a sling incision, with suburethral sling excision for synthetic slings, a sling incision for an autologous or biological sling or urethrolysis when an autologous or biological sling cannot be identified, and urethrolysis for all nonsling revisions, as well as sling incisions that have failed. Typically, urethrolysis will involve mobilizing the urethra to varying degrees, depending on the extent of the obstruction. The procedure may be performed transvaginally, retropubically, or by a combination of the two. Reported success rates after urethrolysis vary from 66% to 93%, and recurrent rates of stress incontinence after the procedure vary from 3% to 20%. Our experience with sling incisions, including retropubic and transobturator midurethral slings, has shown results equivalent to formal urethrolysis. In the case of synthetic midurethral slings, we have also performed sling "adjustment" by pulling the sling down at 1 week, either as an in-office procedure or in the operating room with local anesthesia. If SUI recurs, it can be treated with a urethral bulking agent, or even repeat surgical procedure, in the future.

Detrusor Underactivity. DU can be a contributor to LUTS. DU is defined as a detrusor contraction of reduced strength and/or duration, resulting in prolonged bladder emptying and/or a failure to achieve complete bladder emptying within a normal time span (Chapple et al., 2018). Strictly speaking, DU is a urodynamic diagnosis without any strict pressure flow criteria being applied. The clinical findings of reduced urinary flow rate and/or an increased PVR have been used to describe UAB. The International Continence Society characterizes UAB by a slow urinary stream and hesitancy and straining to void, with or without a feeling of incomplete bladder emptying, sometimes with storage symptoms. An analogy can be drawn to the terms "overactive bladder" and "detrusor overactivity." Several conditions can result in DU of nonneurogenic origin, including radiation cystitis, tuberculosis, chronic outlet obstruction, diabetic cystopathy, and idiopathic processes.

UAB and DU have remained poorly researched and, therefore, poorly treated. DU can be diagnosed only on the basis of an urodynamic study to evaluate detrusor contractility, and can have idiopathic, neurogenic, myogenic, and iatrogenic causes. Gammie et al. in 2016 reviewed 1788 pressure-flow studies in an attempt to identify specific symptoms and signs in patients with DU versus normal findings. Patients with DU reported a higher occurrence of decreased and/or interrupted urinary stream, hesitancy, feeling of incomplete bladder emptying, palpable bladder, and absent and/or decreased sensation compared with patients with normal pressure-flow study results. Results from this and future studies may help in developing a specific symptom questionnaire to assess DU. This would have high utility for screening patients for DU without subjecting them to costly and invasive urodynamics studies.

Management goals for DU and UAB include improving LUTS and reducing urinary retention complications, such as recurrent urinary tract infection, stone formation, renal failure, and overflow incontinence. In general, the treatment for DU of nonneurogenic origin is similar to that described for neurogenic origin earlier in this chapter. Many patients ultimately become dependent on indwelling catheters (urethral vs. suprapubic). However, indwelling urinary catheters are known to have a high rate of adverse events, including infection, encrustation, leakage, discomfort, urethral erosion, and bladder spasm (Hartigan et al., 2019).

There are a number of other potential treatments, including CIC, pharmacotherapy, surgical treatments (SNM, deobstructing surgeries, reduction cystoplasty, and detrusor myoplasty), and stem cell and gene therapies. CIC is the only treatment shown to be uniformly reliable, and it is the mainstay for patients with significant retention. Pharmacotherapy with cholinergic agonists, such as bethanecol, has not proven to be successful in randomized controlled trials, although its use has been reported anecdotally by some (Gaitonde et al., 2019).

As described previously, SNM is an approved intervention for nonobstructive urinary retention (see the Treatment of Neurogenic Voiding Dysfunction section). In a multicenter randomized trial of 177 patients with nonneurogenic urinary retention, 68 were randomized to SNM versus a wait-list control group (Jonas et al., 2001). Those with SNM implants demonstrated 83% success (69% eliminated catheterization, and an additional 14% had a 50% or greater reduction in catheter volume per catheterization) compared with 9% success in the control group at 6 months ($P < .0001$). Implant efficacy was sustained 18 months after implantation. This treatment option may become more common, as magnetic resonance imaging–compatible SNM devices are now available.

Research related to novel therapies for UAB, including stem cells and gene therapy, is currently underway. Studies have demonstrated that autologous muscle-derived cells can be harvested, processed, and injected into the detrusor, but evidence for treatment outcomes (beyond case reports) is not yet available There remains a significant amount of research potential in this area, as the need for successful UAB treatment modalities is largely unmet. Future developments in the pharmaceutical industry, gene therapy, and biomedical applications are expected to eventually close this gap (Bayrak et al., 2019).

CONCLUSION

The evaluation, management, and treatment of women with voiding dysfunction and urinary retention is often complex and must take multiple factors into consideration, including symptoms, degree of bother, and whether there is a history or suspicion of neurologic disease. A patient-specific diagnostic approach is recommended and should prioritize preservation of renal function when appropriate, followed by treatment of symptoms. In many cases, empiric treatment is appropriate. When a formal diagnosis is indicated, specific therapy can be directed based on urodynamics (or video urodynamics) and other tests.

BIBLIOGRAPHY

Agarwal P, Husain S, Wankhede S, et al. Rectus abdominis detrusor myoplasty (RADM) for acontractile/hypocontractile bladder in spinal cord injury patients: Preliminary report. *J Plast Reconstr Aesthet Surg*. 2018;71:736.

Ahmed HU, Shergill IS, Arya M, Shah PJ. Management of detrusor-external sphincter dyssynergia. *Nat Clin Pract Urol*. 2006;3:368.

Albo ME, Richter HE, Brubaker L, et al. Burch colposuspension versus fascial sling to reduce urinary stress incontinence. *N Engl J Med*. 2007;356:2143.

Allen TD. The non-neurogenic neurogenic bladder. *J Urol*. 1977;117:232.

Allen TD, Bright TC III. Urodynamic patterns in children with dysfunctional voiding problems. *J Urol*. 1978;119:247.

Amundsen CL, Guralnick ML, Webster GD. Variations in strategy for the treatment of urethral obstruction after a pubovaginal sling procedure. *J Urol*. 2000;164:434.

Bayrak Ö, Dmochowski RR. Underactive bladder: a review of the current treatment concepts. *Turk J Urol*. 2019;45:401.

Bellina JH, Schenck D, Millet AH, et al. Outflow uropathy: occupational disorder? *J La State Med Soc*. 1999;151:414.

Blaivas JG. The neurophysiology of normal micturition: a clinical study of 550 patients. *J Urol*. 1982;127:958.

Blaivas JG, Singa HP, Zayed AA, Labib KB. Detrusor-external sphincter dyssynergia. *J Urol*. 1981;125:541.

Bosch JL, Groen J. Sacral nerve neuromodulation in the treatment of patients with refractory motor urge incontinence: long-term results of a prospective longitudinal study. *J Urol*. 2000;163:1219.

Bradley WE, Sundin T. The physiology and pharmacology of urinary tract dysfunction. *Clin Neuropharmacol*. 1982;5:131.

Bradley WE, Timm GW, Scott FB. Innervation of the detrusor muscle and urethra. *Urol Clin North Am*. 1974;1:3.

Brucker BM, Fong E, Shah S, Kelly C, Rosenblum N, Nitti VW. Urodynamic differences between dysfunctional voiding and primary bladder neck obstruction in women. *Urology*. 2012;80:55.

Capitanucci ML, Camanni D, Demelas F, et al. Long-term efficacy of percutaneous tibial nerve stimulation for different types of lower urinary tract dysfunction in children. *J Urol*. 2009;182:2056.

Carlson JJ, Hansen RN, Dmochowski RR, et al. Estimating the cost-effectiveness of onabotulinumtoxinA for neurogenic detrusor overactivity in the United States. *Clin Ther*. 2013;35:414.

Carlson KV, Rome S, Nitti VW. Dysfunctional voiding in women. *J Urol*. 2001;165:143.

Carlsson CA. The supraspinal control of the urinary bladder. *Acta Pharmacol Toxicol*. 1978;43:8.

Carr LK, Webster GD. Voiding dysfunction following incontinence surgery: diagnosis and treatment with retropubic or vaginal urethrolysis. *J Urol*. 1997;157:821.

Chaabane W, Guillotreau J, Castel-Lacanal E, et al. Sacral neuromodulation for treating neurogenic bladder dysfunction: clinical and urodynamic study. *Neurourol Urodyn*. 2011;30:547.

Chaikin DC, Rosenthal J, Blaivas JG. Pubovaginal fascial sling for all types of stress urinary incontinence: long-term analysis. *J Urol*. 1998;160:1312.

Chapple CR, Osman NI, Birder L, et al. Terminology report from the International Continence Society (ICS) Working Group on Underactive Bladder (UAB). *Neurourol Urodyn.* 2018;37:2928.

Chen SL, Bih LI, Huang YH, et al. Effect of single botulinum toxin A injection to the external urethral sphincter for treating detrusor external sphincter dyssynergia in spinal cord injury. *J Rehabil Med.* 2008;40:744.

Chen TY, Ponsot Y, Carmel M, et al. Multi-centre study of intraurethral valve-pump catheter in women with a hypocontractile or acontractile bladder. *Eur Urol.* 2005;48:628.

Clothier JC, Wright AJ. Dysfunctional voiding: the importance of non-invasive urodynamics in diagnosis and treatment. *Pediatr Nephrol.* 2018;33:381.

Cross CA, Cespedes RD, English SF, McGuire EJ. Transvaginal urethrolysis for urethral obstruction after anti-incontinence surgery. *J Urol.* 1998a;159:1199.

Cross CA, Cespedes RD, McGuire EJ. Our experience with pubovaginal slings in patients with stress urinary incontinence. *J Urol.* 1998b;159:1195.

Cruz F, Herschorn S, Aliotta P, et al. Efficacy and safety of onabotulinumtoxinA in patients with urinary incontinence due to neurogenic detrusor overactivity: a randomised, double-blind, placebo-controlled trial. *Eur Urol.* 2011;60:742.

Dasgupta R, Wiseman OJ, Kitchen N, Fowler CJ. Long-term results of sacral neuromodulation for women with urinary retention. *BJU Int.* 2004;94:335.

deGroat WC, Booth AM. Physiology of the urinary bladder and urethra. *Ann Intern Med.* 1980;92:312.

Deindl FM, Vodusek DB, Bischoff C, et al. Dysfunctional voiding in women: which muscles are responsible? *Br J Urol.* 1998;82:814.

De Ridder D, Ost D, Bruyninckx F. The presence of Fowler's syndrome predicts successful long-term outcome of sacral nerve stimulation in women with urinary retention. *Eur Urol.* 2007;51:229.

de Sèze M, Raibaut P, Gallien P, et al. Transcutaneous posterior tibial nerve stimulation for treatment of the overactive bladder syndrome in multiple sclerosis: results of a multicenter prospective study. *Neurourol Urodyn.* 2011;30:306.

Diokno AC, Hollander JB, Bennett CJ. Bladder neck obstruction in women: a real entity. *J Urol.* 1984;132:294.

Dunn JS Jr, Bent AE, Ellerkman RM, et al. Voiding dysfunction after surgery for stress incontinence: literature review and survey results. *Int Urogynecol J Pelvic Floor Dysfunct.* 2004;15:25.

El Badawi A. Neuromorphologic basis of vesicourethral function. I. Histochemistry, ultrastructure, and function of intrinsic nerves of the bladder and urethra. *Neurourol Urodyn.* 1982;1:3.

Fan YH, Lin AT, Wu HM, et al. Psychological profile of female patients with dysfunctional voiding. *Urology.* 2008;71:625.

Foster HE, McGuire EJ. Management of urethral obstruction with transvaginal urethrolysis. *J Urol.* 1993;150:1448.

Fowler CJ, Betts CD, Christmas TJ, et al. Botulinum toxin in the treatment of chronic urinary retention in women. *Br J Urol.* 1992;70:387.

Fowler CJ, Christmas TJ, Chapple CR, et al. Abnormal electromyographic activity of the urethral sphincter, voiding dysfunction, and polycystic ovaries: a new syndrome? *BMJ.* 1988;297:1436.

Fowler CJ, Kirby RS. Abnormal electromyographic activity (decelerating burst and complex repetitive discharges) in the striated muscle of the urethral sphincter in 5 women with persisting urinary retention. *Br J Urol.* 1985;57:67.

Gaitonde S, Malik RD, Christie AL, et al. Bethanechol: Is it still being prescribed for bladder dysfunction in women? *Int J Clin Pract.* 2019;73:e13248.

Gakis G, Ninkovic M, van Koeveringe GA, et al. Functional detrusor myoplasty for bladder acontractility: long-term results. *J Urol.* 2011;185:593.

Gallien P, Reymann J, Amarenco G, et al. Placebo controlled, randomised, double blind study of the effects of botulinum A toxin on detrusor sphincter dyssynergia in multiple sclerosis patients. *J Neurol Neurosurg Psychiatry.* 2005;76:1670.

Gammie A, Kaper M, Dorrepaal C, et al. Signs and symptoms of detrusor underactivity: an analysis of clinical presentation and urodynamic tests from a large group of patients undergoing pressure flow Studies. *Eur Urol.* 2016;69:361.

Georgopoulos P, Apostolidis A. Neurogenic voiding dysfunction. *Curr Opin Urol.* 2017;27:300.

Ginsberg D, Gousse A, Keppenne V, et al. Phase 3 efficacy and tolerability study of onabotulinumtoxinA for urinary incontinence from neurogenic detrusor overactivity. *J Urol.* 2012;187:2131.

Glass D, Lin FC, Khan AA, et al. Impact of preoperative urodynamics on women undergoing pelvic organ prolapse surgery. *Int Urogynecol J.* 2020;31:1663.

Goldman HB. Simple sling incision for the treatment of iatrogenic urethral obstruction. *Urology.* 2003;62:714.

Goldman HB, Rackley RR, Appell RA. The efficacy of urethrolysis without re-suspension for iatrogenic urethral obstruction. *J Urol.* 1999;161:196.

Groutz A, Blaivas JG, Pies C, Sassone AM. Learned voiding dysfunction (non-neurogenic, neurogenic bladder) among adults. *Neurourol Urodyn.* 2001;20:259.

Hartigan SM, Reynolds WS, Dmochowski RR. Detrusor underactivity in women: a current understanding. *Neurourol Urodyn.* 2019;38:2070.

Haylen BT, Law MG, Frazer M, Schulz S. Urine flow rates and residual urine volumes in urogynecology patients. *Int Urogynecol J Pelvic Floor Dysfunct.* 1999;10:378.

Haylen BT, Lee J, Logan V, et al. Immediate postvoid residual volumes in women with symptoms of pelvic floor dysfunction. *Obstet Gynecol.* 2008;111:1305.

Haylen BT, de Ridder D, Freeman RM, et al. International Urogynecological Association; International Continence Society. An International Urogynecological Association (IUGA)/International Continence Society (ICS) joint report on the terminology for female pelvic floor dysfunction. *Neurourol Urodyn.* 2010;29:4.

Hinman F Jr. Nonneurogenic neurogenic bladder (the Hinman syndrome)—15 years later. *J Urol.* 1986;136:769.

Hinman F, Bauman FW. Vesical and ureteral damage from voiding dysfunction in boys without neurologic or obstructive disease. *J Urol.* 1973;109:727.

Jiang YH, Chen SF, Jhang JF, et al. Therapeutic effect of urethral sphincter onabotulinumtoxinA injection for urethral sphincter hyperactivity. *Neurourol Urodyn.* 2018;37:2651.

Jin XB, Qu HW, Liu H, et al. Modified transurethral incision for primary bladder neck obstruction in women: a method to improve voiding function without urinary incontinence. *Urology.* 2012;79:310.

Jonas U, Petri E, Hohenfellner R. Indication and value of bladder neck incision. *Urol Int.* 1979;34:260.

Jonas U, Fowler CJ, Chancellor MB, et al. Efficacy of sacral nerve stimulation for urinary retention: results 18 months after implantation. *J Urol.* 2001;165:15.

Jorgensen TM, Djurhuus JC, Schroder HD. Idiopathic detrusor sphincter dyssynergia in neurologically normal patients with voiding abnormalities. *Eur Urol.* 1982;8:107.

Kaplan WE, Firlit CF, Schoenberg HW. The female urethral syndrome: external sphincter spasm as etiology. *J Urol.* 1980;124:48.

Kessler TM, La Framboise D, Trelle S, et al. Sacral neuromodulation for neurogenic lower urinary tract dysfunction: systematic review and meta-analysis. *Eur Urol.* 2010;58:865.

Kessler TM, Studer UE, Burkhard FC. The effect of terazosin on functional bladder outlet obstruction in women: a pilot study. *J Urol.* 2006;176:1487.

Kim DK. Current pharmacological and surgical treatment of underactive bladder. *Investig Clin Urol.* 2017;58:S90.

Kim YH, Kattan MW, Boone TB. Bladder leak point pressure: the measure for sphincterotomy success in spinal cord injured patients with external detrusor-sphincter dyssynergia. *J Urol.* 1998;159:493.

Klutke C, Siegle S, Carlin B, et al. Urinary retention after tension-free vaginal tape procedure: incidence and treatment. *Urology.* 2001;58:697.

Kumar A, Mandhani A, Gogoi S, Srivastava A. Management of functional bladder neck obstruction in women: use of a-blockers and pediatric resectoscope for bladder neck incision. *J Urol.* 1999;162:2061.

Kuo HC. Botulinum A toxin urethral injection for the treatment of lower urinary tract dysfunction. *J Urol.* 2003;170:1908.

Levanovich PE, Diokno A, Hasenau DL, et al. Intradetrusor injection of adult muscle-derived cells for the treatment of underactive bladder: pilot study. *Int Urol Nephrol.* 2015;47:465.

Lombardi G, Del Popolo G. Clinical outcome of sacral neuromodulation in incomplete spinal cord injured patients suffering from neurogenic lower urinary tract symptoms. *Spinal Cord.* 2009;47:486.

Lyon RP, Smith DR. Distal urethral stenosis. *J Urol.* 1963;89:414.

Marion G. Surgery of the neck of the bladder. *Br J Urol.* 1933;5:351.

Mayo ME. Primary bladder neck obstruction. *Surg Rounds.* 1982;5:66.

McGuire EJ, Savastano JA. Urodynamic studies in enuresis and the nonneurogenic neurogenic bladder. *J Urol.* 1984;132:299.

McGuire EJ, Woodside JR, Borden TA, Weiss RM. The prognostic significance of urodynamic testing in myelodysplastic patients. *J Urol.* 1981;126:205.

Mevcha A, Drake MJ. Etiology and management of urinary retention in women. *Indian J Urol.* 2010;26:230.

Minardi D, d'Anzeo G, Parri G, et al. The role of uroflowmetry biofeedback and biofeedback training of the pelvic floor muscles in the treatment of recurrent urinary tract infections in women with dysfunctional voiding: a randomized controlled prospective study. *Urology.* 2010;75:1299.

Mishra VC, Mishra N, Karim OM, Motiwala HG. Voiding dysfunction after tension-free vaginal tape: a conservative approach is often successful. *Int Urogynecol J Pelvic Floor Dysfunct.* 2005;16:210.

Morgan TO, Westney OL, McGuire EJ. Pubovaginal sling: 4-year outcome and quality-of-life assessment. *J Urol.* 2000;163:1845.

Nitti VW, Carlson KV, Blaivas JG, Dmochowski RR. Early results of pubovaginal sling lysis by midline sling incision. *Urology.* 2002;59:47.

Nitti VW, Fiske J. Cystometrogram versus cystometrogram plus voiding pressure—flow studies in women with lower urinary tract symptoms. *J Urol.* 1999;161:201.

Nitti VW, Raz S. Obstruction following anti-incontinence procedures: diagnosis and treatment with transvaginal urethrolysis. *J Urol.* 1994;152:93.

Nitti VW, Tu LM, Gitlin J. Diagnosing bladder outlet obstruction in women. *J Urol.* 1999;161:1535.

Norgaard JP, Swartz-Sorenson S, Djurhuus JC. Functional bladder neck obstruction in women. *Urol Int.* 1984;39:207.

Opisso E, Borau A, Rodríguez A, et al. Patient controlled versus automatic stimulation of pudendal nerve afferents to treat neurogenic detrusor overactivity. *J Urol.* 2008;180:1403.

Panicker JN, Seth JH, Khan S, et al. Open-label study evaluating outpatient urethral sphincter injections of onabotulinumtoxinA to treat women with urinary retention due to a primary disorder of sphincter relaxation (Fowler's syndrome). *BJU Int.* 2016;117:809.

Pannek J, Einig EM, Einig W. Clinical management of bladder dysfunction caused by sexual abuse. *Urol Int.* 2009;82:420.

Peters KM, Kandagatla P, Killinger KA, et al. Clinical outcomes of sacral neuromodulation in patients with neurologic conditions. *Urology.* 2013;81:738.

Petit H, Wiart L, Gaujard E, et al. Botulinum A toxin treatment for detrusor-sphincter dyssynergia in spinal cord disease. *Spinal Cord.* 1998;36:91.

Petrou SP, Brown JA, Blaivas JG. Suprameatal transvaginal urethrolysis. *J Urol.* 1999;161:1268.

Petrou SP, Young PR. Rate of recurrent stress urinary incontinence after retropubic urethrolysis. *J Urol.* 2002;167:613.

Reitz A, Schmid DM, Curt A, et al. Afferent fibers of the pudendal nerve modulate sympathetic neurons controlling the bladder neck. *Neurourol Urodyn.* 2003;22:597.

Reitz A, Stohrer M, Kramer G, et al. European experience of 200 cases treated with botulinum—a toxin injections into the detrusor muscle for urinary incontinence due to neurogenic detrusor overactivity. *Eur Urol.* 2004;45:510.

Richter HE, Albo ME, Zyczynski HM, et al. Retropubic versus transobturator midurethral slings for stress incontinence. *N Engl J Med.* 2010;362:2066.

Rogalski MJ, Kellogg-Spadt S, Hoffmann AR, et al. Retrospective chart review of vaginal diazepam suppository use in high-tone pelvic floor dysfunction. *Int Urogynecol J.* 2010;21:895.

Romanzi L, Blaivas JG. The effect of genital prolapse on voiding. *J Urol.* 1999;161:581.

Scarpero HM, Dmochowski RR, Nitti VW. Repeat urethrolysis after failed urethrolysis for iatrogenic obstruction. *J Urol.* 2003;169:1013.

Scheepens WA, Jongen MM, Nieman FH, et al. Predictive factors for sacral neuromodulation in chronic lower urinary tract dysfunction. *Urology.* 2002;60:598.

Schurch B, Schmid DM, Stohrer M. Treatment of neurogenic incontinence with botulinum toxin A. *N Engl J Med.* 2000;342:65.

Sinha S. Dysfunctional voiding: a review of the terminology, presentation, evaluation and management in children and adults. *Indian J Urol.* 2011;27:437.

Spinelli M, Malaguti S, Giardiello G, et al. A new minimally invasive procedure for pudendal nerve stimulation to treat neurogenic bladder: description of the method and preliminary data. *Neurourol Urodyn.* 2005;24:305.

Steers WD. Physiology of the urinary bladder. In: Walsh PC, Retik AB, Stamey TA, Vaughan ED Jr, eds. *Campbell's Urology.* 6th ed. Philadelphia: WB Saunders Co; 1992.

Swinn MJ, Kitchen ND, Goodwin RJ, Fowler CJ. Sacral neuromodulation for women with Fowler's syndrome. *Eur Urol.* 2000;38:439.

Swinn MJ, Wiseman OJ, Lowe E, Fowler CJ. The cause and natural history of isolated urinary retention in young women. *J Urol.* 2002;167:151.

Tanagho EA, Miller ER, Lyon RP, Fisher R. Spastic striated external sphincter and urinary tract infections in girls. *Br J Urol.* 1971;43:69.

Tanagho EA, Schmidt RA. Electrical stimulation in the clinical management of the neurogenic bladder. *J Urol.* 1988;140:1331.

Tang PC. Levels of the brainstem and diencephalon controlling micturition reflex. *J Neurophysiol.* 1955;18:583.

Tang PC, Ruch TC. Localization of brainstem and diencephalic areas controlling the micturition reflex. *J Comp Neurol.* 1956;106:213.

Thiel DD, Pettit PD, McClellan WT, Petrou SP. Long-term urinary continence rates after simple sling incision for relief of urinary retention following fascia lata pubovaginal slings. *J Urol.* 2005;174:1878.

Tran H, Rutman M. Female outlet obstruction after anti-incontinence surgery. *Urology*. 2017;112:1.

Turner-Warwick R, Whiteside CG, Worth PH, et al. A urodynamic view of the clinical problems associated with bladder neck dysfunction and its treatment by endoscopic incision and trans-trigonal posterior prostatectomy. *Br J Urol.* 1973;45:44.

van Kerrebroeck PE, van Voskuilen AC, Heesakkers JP, et al. Results of sacral neuromodulation therapy for urinary voiding dysfunction: outcomes of a prospective, worldwide clinical study. *J Urol.* 2007;178:2029.

Wein AJ. Classification of neurogenic voiding dysfunction. *J Urol.* 1981;125:605.

Wood SK, Baez MA, Bhatnagar S, Valentino RJ. Social stress-induced bladder dysfunction: potential role of corticotropin-releasing factor. *Am J Physiol Regul Integr Comp Physiol.* 2009;296:R1671.

Xu D, Qu C, Meng H, et al. Dysfunctional voiding confirmed by transdermal perineal electromyography, and its effective treatment with baclofen in women with lower urinary tract symptoms: a randomized double-blind placebo-controlled crossover trial. *BJU Int.* 2007;100:588.

Zhang P, Wu ZJ, Xu L, et al. Bladder neck incision for female bladder neck obstruction: long-term outcomes. *Urology*. 2014;83:762.

35

Interstitial Cystitis/Bladder Pain Syndrome

Elizabeth B. Takacs, Kimberly A. Kenne, Joseph T. Kowalski, and Catherine S. Bradley

CHAPTER OUTLINE

INTRODUCTION

Interstitial cystitis/bladder pain syndrome (IC/BPS) is a heterogeneous and symptom-based condition marked by bladder or urethral pain and associated lower urinary tract symptoms, especially urinary frequency and urgency, in the absence of infection and other demonstrated pathology. Tremendous efforts have been made to gain an understanding of this disease, but the etiology remains unclear. This chapter will present current understanding and controversies surrounding nomenclature and definition of the disorder, pathogenesis, and diagnostic approach. Finally, management options, from conservative to surgical, are presented incorporating the latest clinical evidence and consensus guideline recommendations.

NOMENCLATURE

Efforts to improve the clinical outcomes of women with IC/BPS have been complicated by a lack of international consensus on the definition of and diagnostic criteria for this challenging condition. In 1987, for research purposes, the National Institutes of Health (NIH) established standardized diagnostic criteria for IC (Gillenwater & Wein, 1988; Box 35.1). However, these expert consensus–based research criteria were quite restrictive and were found to be less useful for clinical purposes. In fact, among 269 women followed for 1 year as part of the National Interstitial Cystitis Database study, 60% of those thought very likely to have IC would not be diagnosed based on these criteria (Hanno et al., 1999).

Over the last 20 years, various professional organizations have proposed different nomenclature for painful bladder conditions, with differing diagnostic recommendations. In 2002, the International Continence Society focused on bladder pain and introduced the term painful bladder syndrome (PBS). PBS was defined as the complaint of suprapubic pain related to bladder filling accompanied by other symptoms, such as increased daytime and nighttime frequency, in the absence of proven urinary infection or other obvious pathology (Abrams et al., 2002).

In 2008, the European Society for the Study of Interstitial Cystitis (ESSIC) reached a consensus to rename IC and PBS to BPS (van de Merwe et al., 2008). BPS would be diagnosed on the basis of chronic pelvic pain, pressure, or discomfort perceived to be related to the urinary bladder accompanied by at least one other urinary symptom, such as persistent urge to void or urinary frequency for greater than 6 months. In a departure from other contemporaneous guidelines, ESSIC recommended that classification of BPS types might be performed according to findings at cystoscopy with hydrodistention, as well as histologic findings in bladder biopsies (Box 35.2). Confusable diseases as the cause of the symptoms must be excluded (Table 35.1). The presence of other organ symptoms, as well as cognitive, behavioral, emotional, and sexual symptoms, should be addressed.

The terminology most widely used clinically in the United States is IC/BPS, defined by the Society for Urodynamics and Female Urology as "[a]n unpleasant sensation (pain, pressure, discomfort) perceived to be related to the urinary bladder,

BOX 35.1 The 1987 National Institutes of Health/National Institute of Diabetes and Digestive and Kidney Diseases Diagnostic Criteria for Interstitial Cystitis

Category A: At Least one of the Following Findings on Cystoscopy:

- Diffuse glomerulations (≤10 per quadrant) in at least three quadrants of the bladder
- A classic Hunner ulcer

Category B: At Least one of the Following Symptoms:

- Pain associated with the bladder
- Urinary urgency

Exclusion Criteria:

- Age <18 years[a]
- Urinary frequency while awake <8 times per day
- Nocturia fewer than two times per night
- Maximal bladder capacity >350 mL while patient is awake
- Absence of an intense urge to void with bladder filled to 150 mL of water with medium filling rate (30–100 mL/min) during cystometry
- Involuntary bladder contractions on cystometry using medium filling rate
- Duration of symptoms <9 months[a]
- Symptoms relieved by antimicrobial agents (antibiotics, urinary antiseptics), anticholinergics, or antispasmodics[a]
- Urinary tract infection in the past 3 months[a]
- Active genital herpes
- Vaginitis[a]
- Uterine, cervical, vaginal, or urethral cancer within the past 5 years[a]
- Bladder or ureteral calculi[a]
- Urethral diverticulum[a]
- History of cyclophosphamide or chemical cystitis or tuberculosis or radiation cystitis
- Benign or malignant bladder tumors

[a]Relative exclusion criteria.
(From Gillenwater JY, Wein AJ. *Summary of the National Institute of Arthritis, Diabetes, Digestive and Kidney Diseases Workshop on Interstitial Cystitis*, Bethesda, MD, August 28–29, 1987, National Institutes of Health. *J Urol.* 1988;140:203.)

BOX 35.2 Schematic Representation of the ESSIC Approach for Diagnosis of Interstitial Cystitis/Bladder Pain Syndrome (2008)

PATIENT SELECTION
patient with chronic pelvic pain, pressure or discomfort perceived to be related to the urinary bladder accompanied by at least one other urinary symptom such as persistent urge to void or frequency

↓

EXCLUSION OF CONFUSABLE DISEASES
medical history, physical examination, urinalysis, urine cultures, PSA in males >40 yrs, uroflowmetry, post-void residual urine volume by ultrasound scanning, cystoscopy and biopsy

↓

CLASSIFICATION OF BPS
cystoscopy with hydrodistension[1] and biopsy if indicated

symbol 1: cystoscopy findings	symbol 2: biopsy findings
X: not done 1: normal 2: glomerulations grade II or III 3: Hunner's lesion (with or without glomerulations)	X: not done A: normal B: inconclusive C: inflammatory infiltrates, granulation tissue, detrusor mastocytosis or intra-fascicular fibrosis

[1] in the same session as the cystoscopy above if possible

BPS, Bladder pain syndrome; *ESSIC*, European Society for the Study of Interstitial Cystitis; *IC*, interstitial cystitis.
(From van de Merwe JP, Nordling J, Bouchelouche P, et al. Diagnostic criteria, classification, and nomenclature for painful bladder syndrome/interstitial cystitis: an ESSIC proposal. *Eur Urol.* 2008;53:60. With permission.)

associated with lower urinary tract symptoms of more than six weeks duration, in the absence of infection or other identifiable causes" (Hanno & Dmochowski, 2009). This definition allows treatment to begin after a relatively short symptomatic period (6 weeks rather than 6 months, as in the ESSIC definition) and was used by the American Urological Association (AUA) in their IC/BPS guidelines published in 2011 and amended in 2015 (Hanno et al., 2015).

Recently, international IC/BPS experts have called for the development of more consistent nomenclature and guidelines for IC/BPS (Hanno et al., 2020; Homma, 2019). It has long been recognized that some patients with IC/BPS have erosive bladder lesions ("Hunner lesions"), and increasing evidence supports different treatment outcomes in patients with such lesions. Given this, interest has grown in classifying and defining IC/BPS based on the presence or absence of these lesions, sometimes called Hunner lesion disease versus non–Hunner lesion disease, or ulcerative IC and nonulcerative IC (Whitmore et al.). We anticipate that future diagnostic classifications for IC/BPS are likely to include this categorization.

EPIDEMIOLOGY

First described over a century ago by Skene (1887), Nitze (1907), and Hunner (1915), IC/BPS was not studied from an epidemiologic standpoint until the last several decades. Likely related to changing definitions of IC, reported prevalence rates varied substantially among early population-based studies, ranging widely from 18 to 865 women per 100,000 (0.02%–0.9% prevalence; Jones & Nyberg, 1997). Use of more modern definitions and varying study methodology led to subsequent prevalence estimates ranging from 0.45% (Leppilahti et al., 2002) to as high as 12.6% (Rosenberg & Hazzard, 2005).

Given the lack of objective tests available to diagnose the condition, epidemiologic studies generally fall into three categories: self-report studies, symptom assessments, and review of billing data/diagnosis codes (Hanno et al., 2015). These varied methods likely contribute to the wide range of estimates regarding burden of disease. In a population-based, cross-sectional survey of individuals in the Boston area, Clemens

TABLE 35.1 Confusable Diseases for Bladder Pain Syndrome in Women

Confusable Disease	Excluded or Diagnosed by
Carcinoma and carcinoma *in situ*	Cystoscopy and biopsy
Infection with	
Common intestinal bacteria	Routine bacterial culture
Chlamydia trachomatis, Ureaplasma urealyticum, Mycoplasma hominis, Mycoplasma genitalium, Corynebacterium urealyticum, Candida species	Special cultures
Mycobacterium tuberculosis	Dipstick, if sterile pyuria, culture for *M. tuberculosis*
Herpes simplex virus or human papillomavirus	Physical examination, culture
Radiation	Medical history
Chemotherapy, including immunotherapy with cyclophosphamide	Medical history
Antiinflammatory therapy with tiaprofenic acid	Medical history
Bladder neck obstruction or neurogenic outlet obstruction	Uroflowmetry and ultrasound
Bladder stone	Imaging or cystoscopy
Lower ureteric stone	Medical history and/or hematuria: upper urinary tract imaging such as CT or IVP
Urethral diverticulum	Medical history, physical examination, MRI or ultrasound
Urogenital prolapse	Medical history, physical examination
Endometriosis	Medical history, physical examination
Vaginal candidiasis	Medical history, physical examination
Cervical, uterine, or ovarian cancer	Physical examination, biopsies
Incomplete bladder emptying (retention)	Postvoid residual urine volume measured by ultrasound scanning
Overactive bladder	Medical history
Pudendal nerve entrapment	Medical history, physical examination, nerve block may help confirm diagnosis
Pelvic floor muscle–related pain	Medical history, physical examination

The diagnosis of a confusable disease does not necessarily exclude a diagnosis of bladder pain syndrome.
CT, Computed tomography; *IVP*, intravenous pyelogram; *MRI*, magnetic resonance imaging.
(Modified from van de Merwe JP, Nordling J, Bouchelouche P, et al. Diagnostic criteria, classification, and nomenclature for painful bladder syndrome/interstitial cystitis: an ESSIC proposal. *Eur Urol.* 2008;53:60.)

et al. (2007) reported the prevalence of PBS as 0.83% to 2.71% of women, depending on the definition used. Perhaps the most rigorous large-scale estimate of disease prevalence is provided by the RAND Interstitial Cystitis Epidemiology (RICE) study, a US population-based telephone survey. RICE investigators estimated the prevalence of IC/BPS in women 18 years of age and older to range from 2.7% to 6.5%, which translated to 3.3 to 7.9 million adult US women (Berry et al., 2011). Prevalence estimates in female populations are consistently higher than in male populations, with investigations based on diagnosis in clinical practice suggesting a female-to-male ratio of 5:1 (Clemens et al., 2005), whereas population-based studies find a lower ratio (2–3:1; Clemens et al., 2007). In population-based studies, IC/BPS is not consistently associated with any racial/ethnic background but is most common in middle-aged groups (40–59 years range) and those with lower socioeconomic status (Clemens et al., 2007; Berry et al., 2011).

Regardless of the exact prevalence of IC/BPS, this condition has been shown to overlap with many other pain syndromes and has a significant impact on patients' quality of life. Many IC/BPS patients suffer from fibromyalgia, irritable bowel syndrome, anxiety, and depression (Lai et al., 2016; Naliboff et al., 2015; Krieger et al., 2015). As many as 85% of patients with IC/BPS will be diagnosed with high-tone pelvic floor dysfunction or levator ani pain, which often manifests as general pelvic pain, dyspareunia, urinary hesitancy, and difficulty with defecation (Peters et al., 2007). Epidemiologic studies confirm that women with IC/BPS symptoms have poorer self-reported physical and mental health than the general US population (Berry et al., 2011).

ETIOLOGY

The etiology of IC/BPS is currently unknown and likely to be multifactorial. A comprehensive review of this broad topic is beyond the scope of this chapter; therefore, we briefly review several potential IC/BPS etiologies, including both peripheral and central causes, with a focus on recent research results.

Epithelial Alterations

Increasing evidence suggests that alterations of the urothelium (specialized transitional epithelium lining the renal pelvis, ureters, and bladder) play an important role in IC/BPS. Both molecular and structural uroepithelial changes have been observed in patients with IC/BPS and in animal models of the disease (Birder, 2019). The urothelium forms an efficient barrier against potentially harmful urine components. Also, activation of urothelial cells by chemical, thermal, or mechanical stimuli can cause the release of various mediators or neurotransmitters, which may influence nerve activity, detrusor cell contraction, and ultimately bladder function (Birder & Andersson, 2013). Thus, a wide variety of epithelial dysfunctions, such as altered expression or sensitivity of molecular targets, channels, or receptors, might lead to abnormal sensation and function such as that seen in IC/BPS.

Histologic examination of the bladder in IC/BPS differs based on the presence or absence of Hunner lesions identified during cystoscopy (see Diagnostic Cystoscopy). The bladder mucosa of patients with Hunner lesion disease is characterized by chronic inflammatory changes, including lymphocytes, plasma cells, macrophages, neutrophils, and mast cells, particularly between the urothelium and lamina propria (suburothelium) (Logadottir et al., 2014). Similar inflammation is not seen in non–Hunner lesion IC/BPS. Others have reported that findings of pancystitis, clonal B-cell expansion, and epithelial denudation are unique to Hunner lesion disease (Maeda et al., 2015). These differences suggest that different disease mechanisms are involved in IC/BPS patients with and without Hunner lesions, supporting proponents of new IC/BPS diagnostic classifications that separate Hunner lesion disease from other types of IC/BPS (Hanno et al., 2020).

Other mucosal abnormalities do not clearly differ in IC/BPS patients with or without Hunner lesions. Immunohistological studies of bladder mucosa from bladder biopsies of IC/BPS patients with and without Hunner lesions have demonstrated differences in markers related to inflammation, angiogenesis, fibrosis, and denudation compared with controls. In some cases, the changes correlate with symptom outcomes. Furuta et al. (2019) reported increased TNF-α, VEGF, CD31, and TGF-β in IC/BPS patients with and without Hunner lesions compared with controls, whereas increased mast cell tryptase and collagen were observed in Hunner lesion patients only (compared with non–Hunner lesion patients and controls). The increased expression of CD31, a protein marker related to angiogenesis, in IC/BPS patients had the highest correlations with pain and urinary symptoms.

Gene expression studies in RNA taken from bladder biopsies also suggest that disease mechanisms may differ in IC/BPS patients with and without Hunner lesions. In one study, patients with Hunner lesions had a distinct gene expression profile, with upregulation of genes involved in biological pathways related to cell proliferation, the immune system, and infectious processes (Akiyama et al., 2019). The RNA sequence analysis from IC/BPS patients without Hunner lesions did not differ from controls.

An elevated mast cell count in the bladder muscularis was long promoted as a diagnostic histopathologic feature of IC/BPS, and different values for mast cell counts in the detrusor layer were proposed as a diagnostic marker. Akiyama et al. (2018) studied 69 patients with IC/PBS (diagnosed based on the 1987 NIH criteria and including both ESSIC types 2 and 3) and 37 controls (with and without non-IC/BPS chronic cystitis) and demonstrated that the presence of mast cells correlated with the level of background lymphoplasmacytic infiltrate, but not with the diagnosis of IC. This suggests that mast cell counts are not of value in diagnosing IC/BPS.

The urothelium's surface coat of glycosaminoglycans (GAG) has been proposed to be deficient in some patients with IC/BPS. When the GAG layer is damaged, the urothelium has increased permeability to urine components, which may result in local inflammation, neural sensitization, and subsequent pain, frequency, and urgency. Important components of the GAG layer include chondroitin sulfate, hyaluronic acid, heparin sulfate, dermatan sulfate, and keratin sulfate (Hurst & Zebrowski, 1994), and early research identified a lack of chondroitin sulfate in the GAG layer of IC/BPS patients (Hurst et al., 1996). Several agents with GAG-like properties, such as sodium hyaluronate, heparin, and pentosan polysulfate, are administered intravesically as treatment for IC/BPS, based on the hypothesis that replenishing the GAG layer might lead to urothelial layer recovery. Indeed, intravesical instillation of chondroitin sulphate into the rat bladder was shown to restore a damaged epithelial permeability barrier (Hauser et al., 2009).

Alternatively, dysfunction in other components of the urothelium may also be related to increased permeability. Jhang et al. (2018) considered electron microscopy characteristics of the urothelium and demonstrated defects in umbrella cells (denudation, increased pleomorphism, and decreased microplicae of the cell membrane) in patients with IC/BPS (diagnosed using ESSIC 2008 criteria) compared with controls. Importantly, the severity of these defects correlated with symptom severity and bladder capacity.

Neurogenic Inflammation

Neurogenic inflammation involves the enhanced release of proinflammatory neuropeptides (such as substance P) from sensory and/or sympathetic nerves, which can lead to persistent afferent nerve sensitization and local inflammatory changes. This process is mediated by mast cells, as the neurotransmitters released by peripheral neurons induce mast cell degranulation and the release of additional proinflammatory mediators. It is proposed that the inflammatory mediators' actions on afferent neurons create a positive feedback loop, resulting in altered neural plasticity and central nervous sensitization in the dorsal root ganglia and the upper spinal cord and contributing to symptom persistence in IC/BPS (Akiyama et al., 2020). This process, mediated by mast cells, has been proposed to be a nidus for induction, establishment, and chronicity of the various tissue changes seen in IC/BPS. Other conditions in which neurogenic inflammation may be implicated include irritable bowel syndrome, vulvodynia, migraines, and fibromyalgia, conditions that frequently overlap with IC/BPS.

Infectious Agents

Extensive efforts have been made, with limited success, to establish an infectious agent as the cause of IC. Hunner (1915) first suggested a hematogenously disseminated bacterial cystitis as the cause. Most patients with IC/BPS report a history of urinary tract infection and have received several courses of antibiotics based on their symptoms, not on positive urine cultures. To date, no single bacterium, virus, fungus, or fastidious microorganism has been isolated as an etiologic factor in IC/BPS.

More recently, molecular methods such as 16S rRNA rapid next-generation gene sequencing and expanded quantitative urine culture techniques have been employed to demonstrate that the lower urinary tract is not sterile, and alterations in the bladder microbiome ("dysbiosis") have been identified that are associated with other chronic urinary tract conditions, such as urgency urinary incontinence (Pearce et al., 2015). In the largest study to date focused on the bladder microbiome in women with IC/BPS, Nickel et al. (2019) compared microbiota in voided urine specimens obtained from 181 female IC/BPS and 182 female control participants. IC/BPS participants had a clinical diagnosis of IC/BPS, as well as current bladder pain or discomfort and associated urologic symptoms. A total of

92 bacterial species (41 genera) were identified, with similar mean species counts in IC/BPS and control participants (2.49 ± 1.48 vs. 2.30 ± 1.28). The species composition did not significantly differ between IC/BPS and control participants. Testing of individual genera showed a lower prevalence ($P = .002$) and relative abundance ($P = .001$) of *Corynebacterium* among IC/BPS participants compared with controls. Overall, this and smaller studies have reported differing and inconclusive results related to dysbiosis and IC/BPS, and more research is needed (Abernethy et al., 2017; Meriwether et al., 2019).

Centralized Pain Processing

Women with IC/BPS frequently have other concurrent functional pain syndromes, including fibromyalgia, irritable bowel syndrome, and vulvodynia. A key component of these conditions is diffuse hyperalgesia (increased pain to normally painful stimuli) and/or allodynia (pain to normally nonpainful stimuli), suggesting a fundamental problem with pain and/or sensory processing in the central nervous system (CNS), rather than a peripheral abnormality originating from the location of experienced pain (Clauw, 2015). Some studies suggest that patients with non–Hunner lesion IC/BPS are more likely to have such concurrent disorders, although results are conflicting (Braunstein et al., 2008; Peters et al., 2011). This potential difference has led experts to suggest that IC/BPS without Hunner lesions might share a neurophysiologic dysfunction affecting the CNS with the other functional pain syndromes. Regardless of the presence or absence of Hunner lesions, IC/BPS patients who have other concurrent pain syndromes are likely to have dysfunction in central pain pathways and increased pain perception. The mechanism(s) underlying central pain amplification and sensitization remains unclear. Increasing evidence suggests this may include altered processing of afferent signals in the brain (see below). Central visceral hypersensitivity/pain may also involve the persistent activation of dorsal horn neurons, resulting in changes within the spinal cord that can mediate pain long after resolution of inflammation or other pelvic insult.

Altered Brain Structure and Function

Neuroimaging research in chronic pain syndromes other than IC/BPS has demonstrated that brain structure and function are important factors related to chronic pain, creating the rationale for recent neuroimaging research in IC/BPS patients. The Multidisciplinary Approach to the Study of Chronic Pelvic Pain (MAPP) Research Network, an NIH program funded since 2008, developed a standardized protocol for functional magnetic resonance imaging (MRI) across sites (Alger et al., 2016). This protocol was implemented in a 1-year observational cohort study of IC/BPS patients and in healthy control participants. IC/BPS participants in this MAPP study had a clinical diagnosis of IC/BPS and reported current bladder pain or discomfort with associated urologic symptoms on enrollment.

Several studies from this MAPP cohort have demonstrated differences in the brains of women with IC/BPS compared with healthy, age-matched control participants (Fig. 35.1). Differences were particularly apparent in medial areas of the motor and sensory cortex, the right posterior insula, and the periaqueductal grey area of the brainstem, areas consistent with the sensorimotor representation of the pelvis (Bagarinao et al., 2014; Huang et al., 2016; Clemens et al., 2019), and previously implicated in viscerosensory bladder function, urinary continence, and descending modulation of nociceptive signals (Griffiths et al., 2007; Fowler et al., 2008; Tadic et al., 2012). Also, grey and white matter structure alterations and resting-state function were convergent in the supplementary motor area, a region with a role in providing corticospinal input to active pelvic floor muscles (Kuhtz-Buschbeck et al., 2005; Fowler et al., 2008; Tadic et al., 2012). These findings led to the investigators' conclusion that painful bladder conditions involve disturbances in brain-level sensorimotor systems that regulate urine storage and produce differences in brain structure and function (Clemens et al., 2019).

A subset of 52 MAPP participants with urologic chronic pelvic pain syndrome (including 34 women with IC/BPS) was imaged longitudinally. In these participants, brain functional connectivity (a measure of functional interaction among brain regions during rest) could predict short-term (3-month) pain reduction with 73.1% accuracy. Participants whose pain symptoms improved had stronger functional connectivity in the left frontoparietal brain network than those whose pain symptoms remained constant or worsened, possibly reflecting neural systems that regulate a patient's attention to her symptoms (Kutch et al., 2017). These findings suggest that differences in CNS pain processing may have a fundamental role in IC/BPS, in addition to dysfunction identified in the bladder and urinary tract.

CLINICAL PHENOTYPING

Most experts now agree that the IC/BPS diagnosis includes heterogeneous patients with varying pathologic etiologies. Given this, there are increasing efforts to phenotype or classify patients based on clinical factors to better target treatments to each patient (Khullar et al., 2019; Clemens et al., 2019). Many phenotyping approaches in IC/BPS have been proposed, and important clinical differences have been found between phenotypic groups. However, few data exist that demonstrate different treatment outcomes in phenotypically defined patients, with the exception of cystoscopic treatment of Hunner lesions (see Management of Interstitial Cystitis/Bladder Pain Syndrome).

The ESSIC guidelines emphasize use of cystoscopic findings and bladder biopsy results to classify IC/BPS patients (van de Merwe et al., 2008). Supporting this approach, IC/BPS patients with Hunner lesions have been found to differ from those without Hunner lesions, with more severe urinary frequency and smaller bladder capacity (Ahn et al., 2018). Logadottir et al. (2012) studied IC/BPS patients with Hunner lesions and abnormal bladder biopsy results (including histopathologic findings of inflammatory infiltrates, granulation tissue, overexpression of mast cells, and/or intrafascicular fibrotic changes), also called ESSIC type 3C disease (Box 35.2), and compared them to IC/BPS patients with normal cystoscopy and biopsy results. Those with type 3C disease had a lower

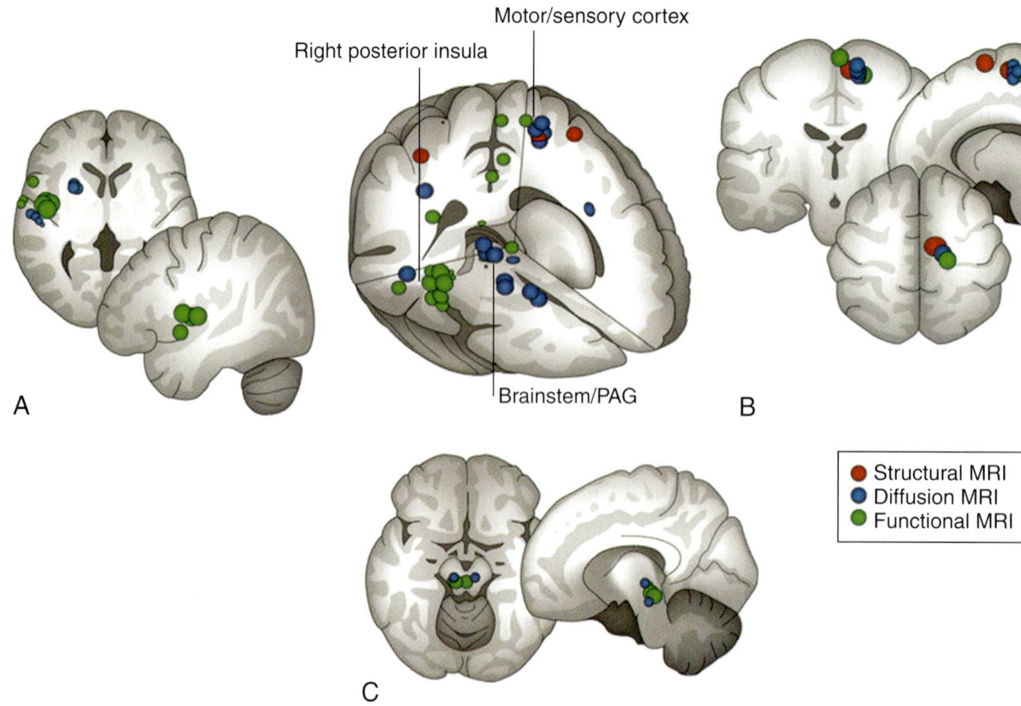

Fig. 35.1 Neuroimaging findings in urologic chronic pelvic pain syndrome. Locations in the brain of altered function (*green*; assessed using resting-state functional MRI), grey matter structure (*red*; assessed using T1-weighted MRI), and white matter structure (*blue*; assessed using diffusion tensor MRI) in participants with urologic chronic pelvic pain syndrome compared with matched healthy control individuals. There is overlap in the right posterior insula (A), the medial sensorimotor areas (B), and the brainstem and PAG (C). *MRI*, Magnetic resonance imaging; *PAG*, periaqueductal grey. (From Clemens JQ, Mullins C, Ackerman AL, et al. Urologic chronic pelvic pain syndrome: insights from the MAPP Research Network. *Nat Rev Urol*. 2019;16:187. With permission.)

average maximal voided volume and lower average bladder capacity under anesthesia. Others have reported that IC/BPS patients with Hunner lesions are older and more likely to have other comorbid pain syndromes, and that those patients without Hunner lesions more likely to have pelvic floor dysfunction and myofascial pain (Peters et al., 2011; Whitmore et al., 2019).

Nickel et al. (2009) used the U-POINT system to classify 100 IC/BPS patients into six clinically identifiable domains, including Urinary, Psychosocial, Organ-Specific, Infection, Neurological/Systemic, and Tenderness (muscle). Most female IC/BPS patients were categorized into multiple domains (87% into three or more), and the identification of impacted domains outside the bladder (e.g., psychosocial and muscle tenderness) was associated with more severe pain and urinary symptoms. Based on known mechanisms of action, treatments can be targeted to each U-POINT domain, as illustrated in Table 35.2 (Khullar et al., 2019).

Table 35.2 The U-POINT Classification and Proposed Treatment Options Based on the Predominant Clinical Phenotype of Interstitial Cystitis/Bladder Pain Syndrome Patients

Clinical Phenotype	Treatment Options
Urinary	Behavioral treatments, antimuscarinic drugs, intravesical treatment (heparin, DMSO, HA, CS, PPS), HD, onabotulinum toxin A, sacral neuromodulation, radical surgery
Psychosocial	Stress management and psychosocial support
Organ-specific	
Hunner lesion (−)	Amitriptyline, cimetidine, hydroxyzine, PPS, quercetin, intravesical treatment (DMSO, heparin, HA, CS, alkalinized lidocaine, PPS), HD, onabotulinum toxin A, radical surgery
Hunner lesion (+)	Cyclosporin A, endoscopic treatment (fulguration, laser ablation, resection, steroid injection), hyperbaric oxygen, radical surgery
Infectious	Antibiotics
Neurological/systemic	Gabapentanoids, cimetidine, hydroxyzine, sacral neuromodulation
Tenderness	Pelvic floor physiotherapy, massage therapy, acupuncture, trigger point injections

DMSO, Dimethylsulfoxide; *HA*, hyaluronic acid; *CS*, chondroitin sulfate; *PPS*, pentosan polysulfate; *HD*, hydrodistension.
(From Khullar V, Chermansky C, Tarcan T, et al. How can we improve the diagnosis and management of bladder pain syndrome? Part 1: ICI-RS 2018. *Neurourol Urodyn*. 2019;38:S66. With permission.)

Future research is needed to identify if treatment outcomes are improved using U-POINT or other phenotyping systems.

The clinical phenotyping of patients with urologic chronic pelvic pain disorders (including women with IC/BPS) is a major goal of the MAPP Research Network (Clemens et al., 2019). MAPP investigators performed a 1-year observational cohort study of over 200 women with IC/BPS and identified important clinical factors associated with quality-of-life outcomes and with symptom trajectories over time, including the presence of pain outside the pelvis, the presence of concurrent nonurological chronic pain conditions (such as fibromyalgia and irritable bowel syndrome), and the severity of bladder-focused symptoms (Lai et al., 2015; Naliboff et al., 2017; Clemens et al., 2019). Based on multiple MAPP studies, Clemens et al. (2019) suggest that IC/BPS patients who have concurrent nonurological chronic pain conditions or widespread pain have a more systemic condition and may be more likely to experience symptom progression and decreased quality of life than those with bladder-focused symptoms. Future MAPP research will validate such phenotypic profiles with longer-term outcomes in this patient population and will identify potential phenotypes based on both biological factors (for example urine biomarker, immune assay, and neuroimaging results) and clinical characteristics.

FLARES

Traditionally, the natural history of symptoms in IC/BPS has included periods of symptom exacerbation or "flares." The majority of IC/BPS patients report a history of symptom flares, and flare frequency is associated with symptom severity, bother, and disruption to normal activities (Sutcliffe et al., 2014). Although flares are an important part of the IC/BPS patient experience, little research has focused on flares. Sutcliffe et al. (2015) explored flares from the patient perspective by conducting focus groups of IC/BPS patients. In this study, the most commonly described flares were painful increases in symptoms lasting days, but the patient experience of flares varied widely, including in symptom type, severity, and duration (from minutes to weeks). Many factors have been reported to trigger symptom flares, including foods and drinks (e.g., citrus fruits, tomatoes, spicy food, alcoholic and caffeinated beverages), urinary tract infections, stress, and wearing tight clothing (Lai et al., 2019). One large case-crossover study conducted in the MAPP network found that, among many tested potential triggers, including dietary factors and stress, only recent sexual activity was associated with flare onset (Sutcliffe et al., 2018). However, in a subset of participants who identified dietary factors as causing flares, consumption of tomatoes, yogurt, spicy foods, alcohol, caffeinated beverages, and carbonated beverages was associated with flares. These results suggest that flare triggers may be specific to certain patients, and that implementing recommendations for prevention strategies in all patients may be too restrictive.

Almost no studies to date have tested treatments aimed specifically at flares, but many have reported patient self-management strategies, most commonly increased fluid intake, increased rest, dietary changes, heat or cold therapy, and relaxation techniques such as meditation and visualization (Lai et al, 2019). Research in this area is clearly needed.

EVALUATION

IC/BPS is a diagnosis of exclusion. The AUA established an evidence-based clinical framework for diagnosis and overall management of IC/BPS, last updated in 2015 (Fig. 35.2; Hanno et al., 2015). The guideline states that insufficient literature was identified to constitute an evidence base for diagnosis of IC/BPS in clinical practice. For this reason, diagnosis statements are largely based on clinical principles or expert opinion. The basic assessment should include a careful history, physical examination, and laboratory examination to document symptoms and signs that characterize IC/BPS and exclude other disorders commonly associated with IC/BPS in the differential diagnosis (Hanno et al., 2015). Cystoscopy and urodynamic testing may be considered but are not necessary for making the diagnosis in uncomplicated presentations. The following sections generally follow the AUA recommendations except where specifically noted.

History

The history should elucidate symptoms, their duration, and exacerbating and alleviating factors. Symptoms should be chronic in nature and present for at least 6 weeks. The number of voids per day, sensation of constant urge to void, and the location, character, and severity of pain, pressure, or discomfort should be documented. The patient should be queried regarding specific foods or drinks that worsen pain and whether pain worsens with bladder filling and/or improves with bladder emptying. Dyspareunia, dysuria and relationship of pain to menses should also be noted.

Confusable diagnoses must be excluded (see Table 35.1). Patients cannot have evidence of cystitis caused by infection, use of cyclophosphamide or other chemical agents, radiation, or tuberculosis. Other infections, such as vaginitis, urethritis, urethral ureaplasma, or genital herpes, cannot be present. Also, urethral diverticulum, bladder carcinoma, and carcinoma *in situ* must be excluded.

Although not mandatory for diagnosis, a voiding diary (an example is shown in Fig. 14.1) may be beneficial for documenting baseline symptoms and providing a benchmark for tracking changes in symptoms with treatment. Frequent low-volume voids are suggestive of IC/BPS. Validated symptom questionnaires, such as the Interstitial Cystitis (O'Leary–Sant) Symptom and Problem Indices (ICSI and ICPI), the Genitourinary Pain Index, and the Bladder Pain/Interstitial Cystitis Symptom Score may also be used to document baseline symptoms and their impact on quality of life (O'Leary et al., 1997; Clemens et al., 2009; Humphrey et al., 2012).

A comprehensive history should also include menstrual and sexual history, medical history with emphasis on other chronic pain disorders (i.e., fibromyalgia, irritable bowel syndrome, migraines, endometriosis, vulvodynia, etc.), surgical history, medication use and allergies, and use of tobacco, alcohol, and drugs. Given the known relationship between sexual abuse and/

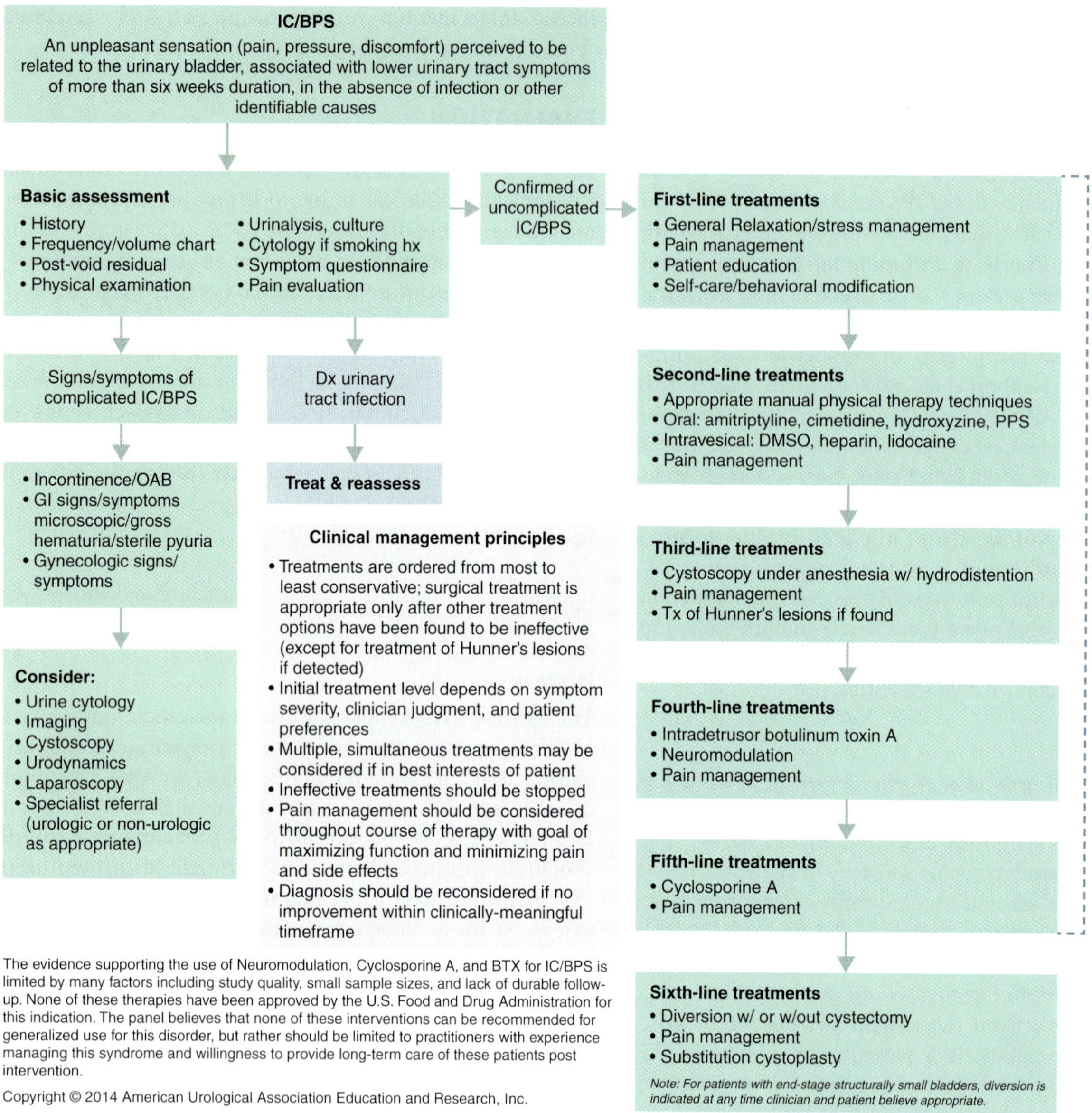

Fig. 35.2 American Urologic Association Guideline Amendment: Interstitial Cystitis/Bladder Pain Syndrome Diagnosis and Treatment Algorithm. *IC/BPS*, Interstitial cystitis/bladder pain syndrome; *hx*, history; *Dx*, diagnosis; *PPS*, pentosan polysulfate sodium; *DMSO*, dimethylsulfoxide; *OAB*, overactive bladder; *GI*, gastrointestinal; *Tx*, treatment; *BTX*, botulinum toxin A. (From Hanno PM, Erickson D, Moldwin R, Faraday MM, American Urological Association. Diagnosis and treatment of interstitial cystitis/bladder pain syndrome: AUA guideline amendment. *J Urol*. 2015;193:1545. With permission.)

or traumatic life events and pain syndromes including IC/BPS, it is also important to obtain this history as part of the evaluation (Mayson & Teichman, 2009; Link et al., 2008).

Physical Examination

A comprehensive physical examination should include an abdominal examination to detect tenderness, masses, hernias, and the presence of prior surgical incisions. A back examination to elicit costovertebral angle tenderness may be helpful if there is concern for infection. A focused neurologic examination to elicit the bulbocavernosus reflex and assess perineal sensation is recommended to help rule out an underlying neurologic condition.

The pelvic examination should begin with evaluation of the external genitalia for signs of infection, masses, dermatologic conditions, and vulvar pain disorders (i.e., vestibulitis or vulvodynia). The pelvic examination includes assessment for vaginitis with vaginal microscopy and/or cultures, if appropriate, and evaluation for signs of vulvovaginal atrophy, urethral caruncle, and cervical cancer screening if indicated. Evaluation for pelvic organ prolapse should be documented. Prolapse is not commonly associated with pain. However, anterior vaginal wall prolapse may be associated with frequency, urgency, incontinence, or obstructive urinary symptoms, and treatment of prolapse may be considered in select IC/BPS patients. The posterior bladder wall and urethra should be palpated to check for tenderness and masses. A bimanual examination should be performed to detect pelvic masses and uterine tenderness. A rectovaginal examination is performed to evaluate for tenderness and masses.

Lastly, the pelvic floor muscles should be palpated to determine tenderness, tone, strength, and ability to appropriately contract and relax. Meister et al. (2019) recently developed a standardized and reproducible pelvic floor muscle examination protocol intended to screen for the presence of pelvic floor myofascial pain. In addition to palpation of three external sites (bilateral sacroiliac joints, medial edge of the anterior superior iliac spine, and cephalad edge of the pubic symphysis) to screen for the presence or absence of self-reported pain, the examination includes internal vaginal palpation of the pelvic floor muscles. The internal examination calls for palpation of each muscle group in the center of the muscle belly, then along the length of the muscle, proceeding counter-clockwise: right obturator internus, right levator ani, left levator ani, and left obturator internus (with pain rated by the patient on a scale of 0–10 at each site; Fig. 35.3).

Laboratory and Radiographic Evaluation

The basic laboratory testing includes a urinalysis and urine culture. If the patient presents with unevaluated microscopic hematuria, then an appropriate evaluation should be completed (see Chapter 40). Urine cytology may also be considered in the presence of hematuria and persistent pain or lower urinary tract symptoms. Urine culture may be indicated even in patients with a negative urinalysis to detect lower levels of bacteria that are clinically significant but not readily identifiable with a dipstick or on microscopic examination. The potassium sensitivity test, although historically done, has neither the specificity nor sensitivity to change clinical decision-making and is not recommended. Additionally, the test is painful and may trigger a severe symptom flare.

Initial evaluation should also include measurement of postvoid residual urine volume (catheterized or with bladder ultrasound). A renal ultrasound, intravenous pyelogram, or computed tomography scan may be indicated in the presence of hematuria, history of recurrent urinary tract infection, or history of pelvic surgery. MRI or transperineal ultrasound may further delineate the urethra when evaluating for a urethral diverticulum (see Chapters 13 and 37).

MRI has also been used to attempt to differentiate IC/BPS from normal patients, as well as to phenotype IC/BPS with or without Hunner lesions (Ackerman et al., 2016; Charlanes et al., 2019; Tyagi et al., 2018). However, the findings required to make a relevant diagnosis based on MRI are not agreed upon. Additionally, studies that evaluate MRI have small sample sizes and/or demonstrate a lack of sensitivity and specificity. Thus, MRI should not be considered part of the routine evaluation of suspected IC/BPS at this time.

Diagnostic Cystoscopy

Cystoscopy should be considered when the diagnosis is in doubt or when the results may guide treatment; it is not necessary for making the diagnosis in uncomplicated presentations. Cystoscopy is also indicated in the presence of hematuria, persistent or recurrent urinary tract infection, prior urethral/bladder surgery, or suspected fistula or urethral diverticulum. There are no agreed-upon cystoscopic findings diagnostic for IC/BPS. The only specific cystoscopic finding that leads to a diagnosis of IC/BPS is one or more inflammatory-appearing lesions, initially described by Dr. Guy Hunner as patches of red mucosa and small vessels radiating to a central pale scar (Hunner, 1918). However, these Hunner lesions or ulcers are

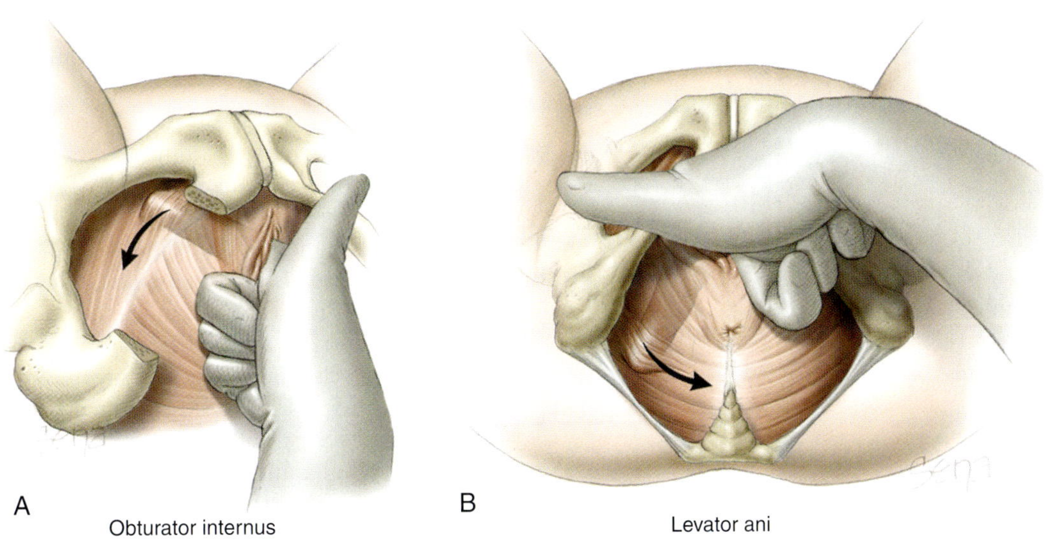

Fig. 35.3 Method of internal palpation of the pelvic floor muscles. Internal palpation is performed with the index finger of the dominant hand, once in the center of the muscle belly, then in a sweeping motion along the length of the muscle in the direction of the orientation of that muscle, and proceeds counter-clockwise: right obturator internus (**A**), right levator ani (**B**), left levator ani, and then left obturator internus. (From Meister MR, Sutcliffe S, Ghetti C, et al. Development of a standardized, reproducible screening examination for assessment of pelvic floor myofascial pain. *Am J Obstet Gynecol.* 2019;220:255.e1. With permission.)

only present in a subset of IC/BPS patients, with variable prevalence rates of 5% to 57% reported in different studies (Koziol, 1994; Peeker & Fall, 2002; Whitmore et al., 2019). Ronstrom and Lai (2020) recommend that evaluation for Hunner lesions first be performed without significant distention of the bladder, as their appearance may change with distention. Gentle distention to about half capacity can be considered if the initial appearance of the bladder does not confirm Hunner lesions but their presence is strongly suspected. Hunner lesions may be identified with several variations in appearance (Figs. 35.4 to 35.6). Bladder biopsy may be indicated to exclude other pathologies if a lesion of uncertain nature is present but is not part of the routine evaluation and presents a risk of bladder perforation.

Glomerulations (pinpoint petechial hemorrhages) may be detected on cystoscopy and can be consistent with IC/BPS, but these lesions are commonly seen in other conditions that may coexist with or be misdiagnosed as IC/BPS, such as chronic undifferentiated pelvic pain or endometriosis. Using hydrodistention to identify glomerulations does not improve diagnostic accuracy of cystoscopy and is not necessary for making a diagnosis of IC/BPS (Shear & Mayer, 2006). Determining bladder capacity during cystoscopy may be useful for guiding prognosis and treatment.

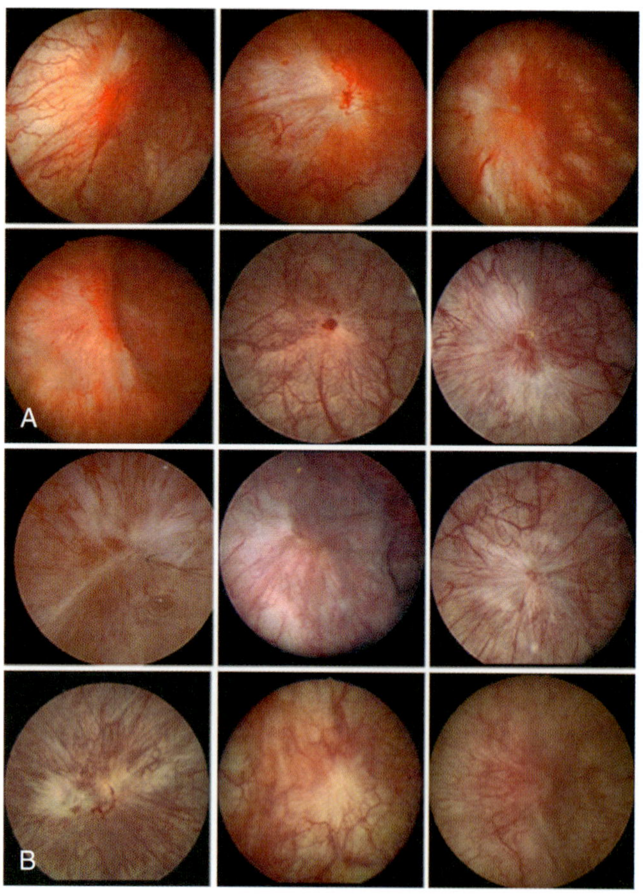

Fig. 35.4 Cystoscopic views of classic Hunner lesions. **A**, Classic Hunner lesions with coagulum: stellate appearance with neovascularity with central coagulum. **B**, Classic Hunner lesions without coagulum: stellate appearance with neovascularity without central coagulum. (From Ronstrom C, Lai HH. Presenting an atlas of Hunner lesions in interstitial cystitis which can be identified with office cystoscopy. *Neurourol Urodyn.* 2020;39:2394. With permission.)

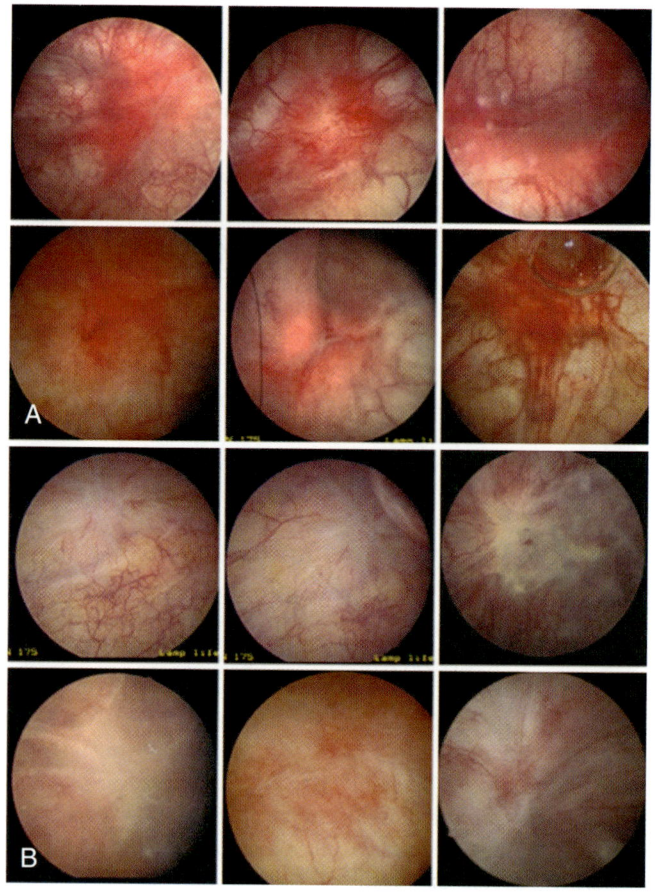

Fig. 35.5 Cystoscopic views of inflamed Hunner lesions. **A**, Inflamed Hunner lesions: inflamed lesion with neovascularity without stellate appearance. **B**, Noninflamed lesions: stellate, noninflamed, bland lesion (may represent a former, resolved Hunner lesion). (From Ronstrom C, Lai HH. Presenting an atlas of Hunner lesions in interstitial cystitis which can be identified with office cystoscopy. *Neurourol Urodyn.* 2020;39:2394. With permission.)

Notably, current European Association of Urology (EAU) recommendations on cystoscopy and bladder biopsy differ considerably from the AUA guidelines (Engeler et al., 2020). Despite admitting controversy over the value of cystoscopy in IC/BPS, the guideline authors believe that objective findings are important for diagnosis, prognosis, treatment, and ruling out other treatable diseases. The guidelines reference the ESSIC classification of IC/BPS subtypes (van de Merwe et al., 2008; Box 35.2). This classification scheme requires hydrodistention and bladder biopsy. Thus, cystoscopy under general anesthesia is recommended as part of the baseline diagnostic evaluation of suspected IC/BPS in the European guidelines. Other experts suggest that office cystoscopy to identify the presence or absence of Hunner lesions, without hydrodistention or biopsy, is preferred in the initial management of these patients (Ronstrom & Lai 2020). Our current practice, based on the AUA guideline, is to perform cystoscopy in patients who have unsatisfactory response to initial behavioral and pharmacologic treatment, more severe symptoms, or other indications for cystoscopic evaluation. Patients with high levels of anxiety or

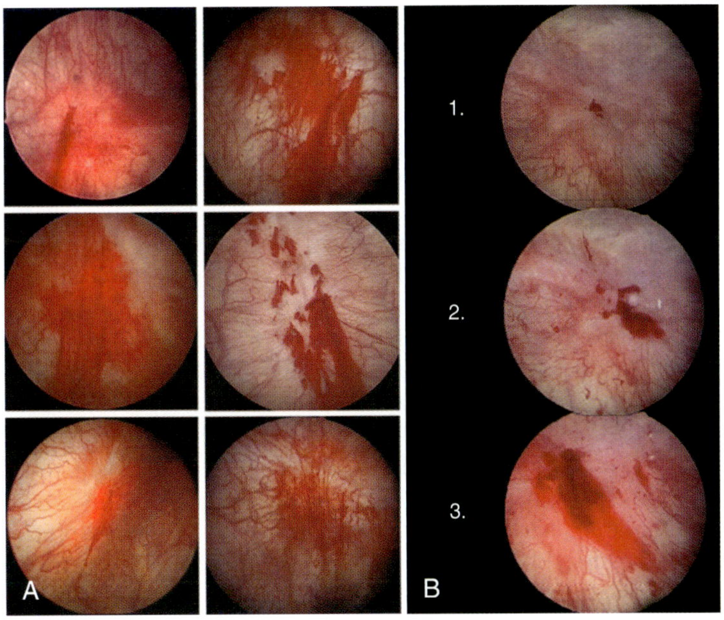

Fig. 35.6 Cystoscopic views of Hunner lesions with waterfall effect. **A**, Waterfall effect: Hunner lesion bleeds like a waterfall during bladder distention. **B**, Sequence of the development of a classic Hunner lesion (with coagulum) into a waterfall lesion with distension of the bladder during cystoscopy. (From Ronstrom C, Lai HH. Presenting an atlas of Hunner lesions in interstitial cystitis which can be identified with office cystoscopy. *Neurourol Urodyn*. 2020;39:2394. With permission.)

bladder pain may not tolerate office cystoscopy under local anesthesia. In such patients, or when hydrodistention is planned, we perform cystoscopy under anesthesia.

Urodynamic Tests

Similar to cystoscopy, urodynamics are not necessary for diagnosing IC/BPS. However, urodynamics may be helpful in ruling out alternative diagnoses or identifying factors that may inform prognosis and guide treatment. Common urodynamic findings in IC/BPS patients are increased bladder sensation and bladder outlet obstruction (Kuo & Kuo, 2018), presumably owing to pelvic floor dysfunction (Cameron & Gajewski, 2009). Mean bladder volume at first sensation and maximum bladder capacity have been demonstrated to be lower in patients with Hunner lesions compared with IC/BPS patients without Hunner lesions (Ahn et al., 2018). The presence of detrusor overactivity may be seen in IC/BPS, but the prevalence of this finding is similar to a severe overactive bladder population (Shim et al., 2016).

MANAGEMENT OF INTERSTITIAL CYSTITIS/ BLADDER PAIN SYNDROME

Numerous treatment modalities have been used in the treatment of IC/BPS. It is important to recognize that the approach to a patient with IC/BPS should epitomize the concept of patient-centered care. Treatments for IC/BPS must be tailored to the individual, with consideration of comorbid conditions, current medications, and goals of care. A key challenge of current management is a lack of consensus across organizations and researchers related to defined IC/BPS nomenclature, classification, and phenotypes, as well as the importance of these phenotypes in guiding management strategies. There is also a "disconnect" between patient-perceived effectiveness and the efficacy of treatments as reported in clinical trials and guidelines (Lusty et al., 2018). Recently, phenotypic-directed management has been recommended, distinguishing between bladder-centric (e.g., presence of Hunner lesions and small bladder capacity) and non–bladder-centric (e.g., absence of Hunner lesions, presence of pelvic floor dysfunction) disease and management. Contemporary publications on therapeutic algorithms for ulcerative or Hunner lesion IC have been published emphasizing rapid advancement to cystoscopy and bladder-specific approaches for patients identified as having ulcers (Crescenze et al., 2019; Han et al., 2018; Whitmore et al., 2019). Our approach in this chapter is to provide an overview of available strategies and to suggest a management algorithm based on published guidelines, systematic reviews, and recent research publications. We take into consideration that as patients progress through various levels of therapy there is increasing risk, and treatment is multimodal and often multidisciplinary. Frequent reassessment, patient education, and reassurance are recommended.

Conservative Therapies

Conservative treatment strategies should be considered first and are foundational for the management of patients with IC/BPS. These treatment modalities may require a motivated patient, as they often require changes to lifestyle, and a multidisciplinary approach (e.g., physical therapists and mental health providers). Evidence supporting conservative treatment strategies is limited, and treatment response may be variable across IC/BPS patients. However, conservative therapies have a low risk profile with potential benefit, so should be implemented early in the treatment course. The International Consultation on Incontinence–Research Society (ICI-RS) in

2018 identified the following as first-line conservative therapies: patient education, stress reduction, multimodal therapy, pelvic floor relaxation therapy, bladder retraining, fluid modification, timed voiding, dietary modifications, and environment factors (Khullar et al., 2019b). All major IC/BPS guidelines recommend dietary education and physical therapy as first-line interventions (Malde et al., 2018).

Dietary modifications are a key treatment strategy in the management of patients with IC/BPS. Many survey-based studies of patients with IC/BPS have demonstrated exacerbation of symptoms with ingestion of specific comestibles (Table 35.3) (Shorter et al., 2007; Bassaly et al., 2011). Both minor and major dietary changes can have a significant impact on symptoms and should be personalized to the patient (Rahnama'i et al., 2020). The elimination diet is a standard protocol used to identify dietary triggers (Friedlander et al., 2012). The general principle of dietary modification is to exclude or limit foods that create a more acidic urinary pH, increase potassium content in the urine, have an allergy-initiating component, or may stimulate sensitive pain receptors in the bladder (Rahnama'i et al., 2020).

The role of physical therapy has increased in many treatment algorithms, especially in patients with non–bladder-centric disease. Physical therapy may include the use of transcutaneous electrical nerve stimulation (TENS), the release of myofascial bands, and the relaxation of the pelvic floor muscle complex (Peters et al., 2007; FitzGerald et al., 2012). Pelvic floor muscle strengthening exercises are generally contraindicated for patients with IC/BPS (Rahnama'i et al., 2020). Trigger point injections may be used to aid in release of myofascial bands (Rahnama'i et al., 2020; Han et al., 2018). The various guidelines agree there is evidence to support the recommendation for physical therapy for IC/BPS; however, there is a lack of evidence to support recommendations for acupuncture, pelvic floor trigger point injections, or TENS, specifically (Malde et al., 2018).

In addition to the abovementioned conservative therapies, management of psychosocial comorbidities is recognized as being important. This often involves collaboration with mental health providers and/or the use of cognitive behavioral therapy (Rahnama'i et al., 2020). A systematic review determined that IC/BPS patients have high baseline assessment measures of anxiety, depression, and stress, as well as poor mental health–related quality of life; and furthermore, that anxiety or depressive disorders may present before and after diagnosis (McKernan et al., 2018). This review also suggested that early stages of illness are a particularly vulnerable time period, implying that early psychological intervention may interrupt development or worsening of these conditions and have implications for disease prognosis.

TABLE 35.3 Dietary Triggers of Worsened Symptoms in 598 Interstitial Cystitis/Bladder Pain Syndrome Survey Participants

Item	No. of Participants Consuming Item	% Reporting Worsening with Item
Oranges	417/597 (69.8%)	81.3
Grapefruits	297/596 (49.8%)	83.1
Lemons	404/593 (68.1%)	75.5
Chili peppers	314/593 (53.0%)	78.3
Orange juice	409/591 (69.2%)	84.1
Tomato juice	262/591 (44.3%)	80.2
Pineapple juice	279/590 (47.3%)	78.8
Cranberry juice	341/589 (57.9%)	78.6
Coffee	356/590 (60.3%)	79.2
Gin	177/591 (29.9%)	76.2
Beer	255/590 (43.2%)	77.2
Red wine	302/589 (51.3%)	83.7
White wine	319/589 (54.2%)	77.5
Champagne	237/590 (40.2%)	76.8
Coca-Cola	345/591 (58.4%)	83.2
Pepsi	322/591 (54.5%)	86.0
Dr Pepper	269/590 (45.6%)	83.6
Mountain Dew	243/591 (41.1%)	85.2
Monosodium glutamate	281/589 (47.7%)	75.4

Items listed scored at least 4 ("slightly" or "significantly" worsens symptoms) in more than 75% of those who responded and had an average score of 4 or greater.
(From Bassaly R, Downes K, Hart S. Dietary consumption triggers in interstitial cystitis/bladder pain syndrome patients. *Female Pelvic Med Reconstr Surg.* 2011;17:36. With permission.)

Pharmacologic Therapies

Both oral (with the exception of cyclosporine A) and intravesical medications are considered second-line therapies for patients with IC/BPS and are used in patients with and without Hunner lesions. Cyclosporine A is considered for patients with Hunner lesions who have failed fulguration (Crescenze et al., 2019; Han et al., 2018) and is classified as a fourth-line option (Malde et al., 2018).

Oral medications can be used as single agents or as combined medication therapy, and intravesical therapies are administered as a single agent or in a multidrug "cocktail." Oral and intravesical agents can be used in combination with each other and should be considered in patients who have failed to achieve adequate symptom control with conservative strategies alone. Here we focus on the most commonly used and recommended oral medications for IC/BPS, including amitriptyline, hydroxyzine, cimetidine, pentosan polysulfate sodium, and cyclosporine A.

Oral Agents. Amitriptyline is a tricyclic antidepressant that is commonly prescribed for IC/BPS, alone or in combination with other medications. Two randomized controlled trials (RCTs) demonstrate its effectiveness at symptom resolution at doses greater than 50 mg daily (Foster et al., 2010; van Ophoven & Hertle, 2005). The proposed mechanism of action is blockage of acetylcholine receptors, inhibition of serotonin and noradrenaline reuptake, and blockage of histamine (H1) receptors, which leads to improvement in urgency as well as pain (Giusto et al., 2018). Because of the side effect of somnolence, this medication is often dosed at bedtime (or 1–2 hours earlier) and may assist in improved sleep. Additional common side effects include fatigue, constipation, dry mouth, and dizziness. To improve tolerability, amitriptyline is usually started at a low dose, 10 to 25 mg before bedtime, and titrated up to 75 mg as tolerated. Across treatment guidelines, amitriptyline is given a grade A or B recommendation (Malde et al., 2018).

Antihistamines, including hydroxyzine and cimetidine, may be included in the management of IC/BPS. Given the increase in mast cells in the bladder mucosa of patients with IC/BPS, a hypersensitivity reaction may be the cause of urinary symptoms in some patients. Hydroxyzine is an H1 receptor antagonist that decreases mast cell activation and may also have some anticholinergic properties. It has been shown to significantly improve symptoms at doses ranging from 25 to 75 mg, with side effects including sedation and weakness (Sant et al., 2003; Theoharides et al., 1994; Theoharides et al. & Sant, 1997). Hydroxyzine appears equally effective in patients both with and without visible bladder lesions (Khullar et al., 2019b). Cimetidine is an H2 receptor antagonist with a similar mechanism of action to hydroxyzine but with a lower incidence of somnolence. With doses ranging from 200 mg three times daily to 300 to 400 mg twice daily, cimetidine has been shown to significantly improve suprapubic pain scores and nocturia symptoms (Giusto et al., 2018). Because of a weaker level of available evidence, both antihistamines are given lower grades of recommendation, are identified as having a limited value, or are not recommended, depending on the specific guideline (Malde et al., 2018).

Pentosan polysulfate sodium (PPS; Elmiron, Janssen Pharmaceuticals Inc., Belgium) is the only US Food and Drug Administration (FDA)-approved oral medication for the treatment of IC/BPS. Pentosan polysulfate sodium is a low molecular weight heparinoid with a proposed mechanism of action of correction of a GAG layer deficiency of the bladder epithelium improving protection from substances in the urine. Despite initial demonstration of efficacy, recent reports have raised questions regarding the overall benefit (Taneja et al., 2020). Review of the contemporary literature demonstrates that phenotype may be important, as four of five RCTs identified used cystoscopic findings as criteria for inclusion, and in those studies PPS demonstrated a beneficial role (Taneja et al., 2020). Large meta-analyses conclude that oral PPS has a positive impact on symptom management in patients with IC/BPS (Taneja et al., 2020). Although the recommended dosing is 100 mg three times per day, clinical improvement may be dependent more on duration of use than on dose (Khullar et al., 2019b). Across guidelines there is no consensus on the grade of recommendation of PPS (Malde et al., 2018).

Side effects of PPS include diarrhea, headache, nausea, and laboratory abnormalities, including increases in liver function tests and low platelets (Mogica & De, 2020). Recently, a specific form of pigmented maculopathy has been associated with PPS use (Pearce et al., 2018; Hanif et al., 2019). Development of this disorder appears to be related to cumulative dose, and the reported prevalence varies widely (Mogica & De, 2020). Recent studies suggest that the vision changes may be progressive after discontinuation of the medication (Huckfeldt & Vavvas, 2019; Shah et al., 2020). Symptoms include difficulty reading, difficulty seeing in dim or night light, and distorted vision. Both Canadian and US regulatory agencies have published postmarket warnings for PPS, recommending baseline and regular interval ophthalmic assessment during use (Mogica et al., 2020; Health Canada, 2020; U.S. Food and Drug Administration, 2020).

Cyclosporine A has shown promise for use in IC/BPS in several small studies, particularly in IC/BPS with Hunner lesions. The mechanism of action for this systemic immunosuppressant is suppression of T-cell activation through inhibition of calcineurin (Han et al., 2018). Several studies have shown a positive response to cyclosporine A (Forrest et al., 2012; Crescenze et al., 2017). Recommended dosing is 2 mg/kg divided into two daily doses (Hanno et al., 2015), although some authors have reported use of 3 mg/kg (Han et al., 2018). Dose adjustment is recommended to achieve cyclosporine A levels of less than 700 ng/mL and titration to the lowest necessary level or discontinuation based on symptom control (Crescenze et al., 2019; Crescenze et al., 2017; Forrest et al., 2012). Drug monitoring is required and includes 2-hour post-dose cyclosporine A serum levels, renal and hepatic function, complete blood count, uric acid levels, and magnesium levels, as well as blood pressure monitoring and assessment for clinical signs and symptoms of immunosuppression. Continued surveillance is recommended 1 month after initiation and then every 3 months for duration of drug use (Crescenze et al., 2019; Han et al., 2018). Consistent across studies was the risk of reversible nephrotoxicity (Crescenze et al., 2019; Han et al., 2018; Forrest et al.); other side effects include hypertension, infection, possible alopecia, somatic pains, and electrolyte changes (Forrest et al., 2012). There is no consistent recommendation for the use of cyclosporine A across IC/BPS treatment guidelines (Malde et al., 2018).

Intravesical Agents. The theory behind use of intravesical therapies is to replace components of the urothelium's damaged GAG layer and restore its impermeability (Giusto et al., 2018). Bladder instillations may include a single agent or multiple drugs (i.e., an "intravesical cocktail"). Importantly, intravesical therapies may be burdensome to patients because of the inconvenience of treatment and/or cost (Barua et al., 2016). During shared decision-making, it is important to consider the frequency of instillation (weekly vs. every 2 to 3 weeks), duration of treatment, use of in-office or at-home administration, cost of medication, and side effect/benefit profile. In addition, there is increased morbidity to the patient with initiation of catheterization. Similar to oral agents, numerous intravesical medications have been used, and our focus will be on those commonly used and consistently recommended across treatment guidelines (Table 35.4). Similar to many of the oral medications, the grade of recommendation for use is highly variable across guidelines (Malde et al., 2018).

Dimethyl sulfoxide (DMSO; Rimso-50, Mylan Laboratories Inc, Canonsburg, PA) is the only FDA-approved pharmacologic agent for intravesical use in IC/BPS and can be used as a single agent or administered as a "cocktail," often combined with heparin and lidocaine. DMSO has antiinflammatory effects, promotes smooth muscle relaxation through nerve blockade, and inhibits collagen (Giusto et al., 2018). Recommended dosing is 50 mL of 50% DMSO with variable administration

TABLE 35.4 Grade of Recommendation for Intravesical Therapy for Interstitial Cystitis/Bladder Pain Syndrome Based on Professional Organization Guidelines

Intravesical Agent	EAU (2020)	AUA[a] (2015)	RCOG (2016)	ICI (2017)
DMSO	NR	Option	C	B
Heparin	C	Option	D	C
Hyaluronic acid	B	—	B	D
Pentosan polysulphate	A	—	—	D
Lidocaine	A	Option	B	C

[a]AUA did not provide evidence grades but instead listed those they considered as options.
Grade explanation: (A) clinical studies of good quality and consistency that include at least one randomized trial; (B) well-conducted clinical studies without randomized trials; (C) absence of directly applicable clinical studies of good quality; (D) evidence level 3 or 4, or extrapolated evidence from studies rated as 2+, or formal consensus.
AUA, American Urologic Association; *DMSO*, dimethyl sulfoxide; *EAU*, European Association of Urology; *ICI*, International Consultation on Incontinence; *NR*, not recommended; *RCOG*, Royal College of Obstetricians and Gynaecologists.
(Modified from Malde S, Palmisani S, Al-Kaisy A, Sahai A. Guideline of guidelines: bladder pain syndrome. *BJU Int.* 2018;122:729. With permission.)

schedules, but typically weekly or every 2 weeks up to monthly, retention for 15 to 20 minutes, and a total of between four and six instillations (Hanno et al., 2015). Two randomized crossover studies have demonstrated its efficacy, and it is listed as a second-line therapy by the AUA (Giusto et al., 2018). A common side effect of DMSO is the taste of garlic or a garlic smell from the patient, which can last several hours.

Heparin is another option for intravesical administration in IC/BPS. Although there is a lack of strong evidence for use as monotherapy, when combined with alkalinized lidocaine there is reasonable evidence to support its use (Giusto et al., 2018). Heparin seems to mimic the GAG layer of the bladder, act as an antiinflammatory, and play a role in fibroblast proliferation, smooth muscle proliferation, and angiogenesis. Given little systemic absorption, side effects are limited. Dosage is generally between 10,000 and 25,000 units two to three times per week (Hanno et al., 2015).

Lidocaine works as a temporary local anesthetic to the bladder. Alkalization helps the drug penetrate through the epithelium. As an intravesical agent, it is most commonly combined with other medications or used intraoperatively at the time of hydrodistention or fulguration for postoperative pain control (Crescenze et al., 2019; Kirk et al., 2018). Lidocaine appears to be useful for providing acute relief but has minimal efficacy as a stand-alone monotherapy for repeated use (Giusto et al., 2018).

As mentioned previously, PPS is a heparin analog, and its use intravesically in IC/BPS is thought to restore the damaged GAG layer, with the goal of reducing permeability of the bladder mucosa (Giusto et al., 2018; Khullar et al., 2018). At a dose of 300 mg in 50 mL of normal saline instilled twice a week, several small studies (controlled and uncontrolled) demonstrated successful outcomes in IC/BPS patients, including increased bladder capacity, improvement in visual analog scale pain ratings, improved IC questionnaire scores, and better health-related quality of life (Bade et al., 1997; Daha et al., 2008; Davis et al., 2008). In contrast, a larger and more recent trial by Nickel et al. (2015) failed to demonstrate improvement with PPS intravesical instillation compared with placebo. The authors suggested that their negative findings may have resulted in part from the composition of the study population. The older trials enrolled patients using a more conservative definition of IC/BPS, whereas the recent trial included patients with milder IC/BPS symptoms and no required cystoscopic findings.

Both hyaluronic acid and chondroitin sulfate are components of the GAG layer of the bladder epithelium. Intravesical instillation is aimed at replenishing the potential defects through direct contact with these agents. The EAU identifies both agents as having significant value in the treatment of IC/BPS. Hyaluronic acid is generally dosed at 40 mg in 50 mL of saline. In observational studies, hyaluronic acid demonstrated efficacy as a monotherapy, but this was not maintained long-term (Pyo & Cho, 2016; Porru et al., 1997). As monotherapy or in combination with chondroitin sulfate, hyaluronic acid has been found to reduce pain ratings and increase voided volume and bladder capacity (Pyo & Cho, 2016). An RCT demonstrated a greater reduction in pain in patients receiving instillations with hyaluronic acid and chondroitin sulfate versus DMSO (Gafni-Kane et al., 2013; Cervigni et al., 2017).

Cystoscopic Procedures

Cystoscopy with hydrodistension is recommended as third-line treatment for IC/BPS by the AUA, but its level of recommendation is variable across other guidelines (Malde et al., 2018). The proposed mechanism of action for hydrodistension is relative ischemia induced through distention causing degeneration of the unmyelinated motor and sensory nerve fibers in the bladder wall (Olson et al., 2018). Although there is considerable variability in the technique used, per the AUA guideline hydrodistension should be performed under general anesthesia, to a pressure of 60 to 80 cm H_2O, and held for less than 10 minutes (Hanno et al., 2015). This procedure is performed using a rigid cystoscope. The recommended pressure is obtained by placing the fluid instillation bag 60 to 80 cm above the bladder. Digital compression in the vagina around the urethra may be needed to prevent leakage around the scope. The inflow of irrigation fluid is stopped when no further fluid enters the drip chamber, and a timer for the distention is started. In addition to variations in technique, many studies incorporate the use of hydrodistension with other therapeutic modalities, such as fulguration of Hunner lesions, bladder instillations, or onabotulinum toxin A injections, making determination of outcomes challenging.

Results of hydrodistention alone were reviewed in a 2018 systematic review of 17 studies. The evidence was overall weak: heterogenous patient populations and treatments were used, along with unvalidated, subjective outcome measures. Rates of improvement also varied widely (5%–100%), with a mode of 57% (Olson et al., 2018). A recent prospective study of IC/BPS patients with or without Hunner lesions undergoing hydrodistension reported a time to therapeutic failure of 28.5 months and 25.2 months, respectively (Niimi et al., 2016). In a second retrospective study, patients without Hunner lesions were treated with hydrodistension and intravesical lidocaine at the conclusion of the procedure. Thirty-six percent of patients required repeat hydrodistension at a mean of 253 days, and no change in mean bladder capacity was seen over time (Kirk et al., 2018).

For patients with cystoscopic findings of Hunner lesions, targeted treatment of the ulcerative lesion with or without hydrodistension is recommended in both the AUA and Royal College of Obstetricians and Gynaecologists guidelines; this treatment approach is given a grade B recommendation by the EAU and by the East Asian and Canadian Urologic Associations (Malde et al., 2018). Unlike studies of many other IC/BPS therapies, those that examined the effect of treatment of ulcerative lesions reflect a more uniform patient population. Procedural approaches to the management of IC/BPS with ulcerative lesions include fulguration with laser or electrocautery, resection of the ulcerative site, and injection with triamcinolone, all with or without simultaneous hydrodistension.

Cystoscopic fulguration, laser ablation, and resection of the ulcer aim to remove the inflammatory infiltrates and activated nerve endings (Niimi et al., 2016). Literature to date reveals that targeted treatment of ulcerative lesions results in approximately 78% to 94% of patients having initial symptom improvement; however, 14% to 67% will require repeat procedures at a mean of 11 to 16 months (Hillelsohn et al., 2012; Ryu et al., 2013; Chennamsetty et al., 2015; Payne et al., 2009; Neale et al., 2021).

Cystoscopy with triamcinolone injections is also performed for those IC/BPS patients with Hunner lesions. Injection of the lesions is performed centrally and peripherally in the submucosal layer, using 40 mg/mL triamcinolone in normal saline with a maximum dose of 400 mg triamcinolone administered in 0.5- to 1-mL aliquots (Crescenze et al., 2019; Cox et al., 2009). Using this technique, 70% to 85.7% of patients reported improvement. Because of lack of safety testing for the 400-mg dose, the AUA guideline recommends a maximum dose of 60 mg administered at a concentration of 10 mg/mL or 40 mg/mL (Hanno et al., 2015).

Onabotulinum toxin A (Botox; Allergan Inc, Irvine, CA) is considered a fourth-line therapy in the current AUA guideline (Hanno et al., 2015). Across guidelines there is sufficient evidence to provide this treatment modality with grade B, C, and D recommendations, although predominately grade C (Malde et al., 2018). It is suggested this may be offered after failed conservative strategies, oral medications and intravesical instillations, cystoscopy with hydrodistention, destruction of ulcerative lesions, or a combination of these treatments. Onabotulinum toxin A cleaves SNAP-25 proteins in motor neurons, preventing acetylcholine release at the motor endplate, and inhibits the vanilloid type 1 receptor (Giusto et al., 2018; Khullar et al., 2018). Onabotulinum toxin A is administered cystoscopically into the detrusor muscle at a dose of 100 to 200 units. At present, there are somewhat limited data to support the use of this procedure for IC/BPS because of the lack of well-conducted RCTs. The ICI-RS in 2017 concluded that a consistent positive effect was not demonstrated, as published studies were small and heterogeneous in design (Rahnama'i et al., 2018). Potential adverse outcomes from onabotulinum toxin A administration include dysuria, urinary tract infection, and incomplete bladder emptying requiring catheterization.

Sacral Neuromodulation

The ICI-RS reported consensus that sacral neuromodulation (SNM) should be tried before radical surgery for IC/BPS (Khullar et al., 2019b). The mechanism of action for SNM in improving IC/BPS is not clearly understood but is hypothesized to be related to the gate-control theory and/or reduction in pelvic floor hypertonicity. In the gate-control theory, nonpainful neuronal input from SNM acts to close the "gate" to the CNS, preventing the entrance of pain sensation from the bladder. SNM provides a nonnoxious stimulus, and thus increased signaling through pain fibers is suppressed (Rahnama'i et al., 2018).

Similar to many other therapies, the quality of research studies assessing the impact of SNM on IC/BPS is low, with few RCTs available. Several systematic reviews have been published on SNM for IC/BPS specifically or for treatment of chronic pelvic pain. In the systematic review performed by Mahran et al. (2019) examining SNM use in chronic pelvic pain, six included studies were in an IC/BPS-only population. Results from these studies demonstrated that 56% to 100% of patients progressed to full implant after either percutaneous nerve evaluation or advanced evaluation; in these patients, there was a 0% to 30% failure rate defined as no improvement, no satisfactory response after implantation, or device removal (Mahran et at., 2019). The results of the ICI-RS in 2017 determined that 38% to 72% of patients experience a reduction in symptom scores in the short term, with a long-term success of 72% to 77%. Overall, the explant rate ranged from 28% to 50% (Rahnama'i et al., 2018). Another systematic review with meta-analysis determined that, across subjective outcomes (visual analog scale pain rating, ICPI, and ICSI), there is a significant decrease in symptom scores, with a success rate across 10 studies (258 subjects) of 84% (Wang et al., 2017). The meta-analysis also demonstrated significant improvements in daytime frequency, nocturia, and voids per 24 hours. The pooled complication rate was 3% (0%–56%), and the explant rate 8%. All three studies concluded that SNM is an effective therapy for IC/BPS; however, individual study quality remains low (Mahran et al., 2019; Wang et al., 2017; Rahnama'i et al., 2018).

Surgical Interventions

Consensus across guidelines is that radical surgery should be considered a last-resort option in patients with IC/BPS; not because of lack of efficacy, but because of the permanent nature of the procedures and the risk for associated morbidity. It is recommended that, before proceeding with radical surgery, patients be reviewed and discussed by a full multidisciplinary team (Khullar et al., 2019b). Radical surgery options for this patient population include augmentation cystoplasty, supra- or subtrigonal cystectomy, and continent diversion or incontinent diversion, such as an ileal conduit. In addition to other associated procedural risks, it is important to counsel patients on the risk of persistent pain after surgery because the evidence related to pain outcomes after radical surgery for IC/BPS is unclear. Studies examining the risk of persistent pain after radical surgery have reported persistent pain in 10% to 20% of patients following supratrigonal cystectomy combined with substitution cystoplasty, augmentation cystoplasty, or ileocecal pouch (Linn et al., 1998; Kim et al., 2014; Mateu Arrom et al., 2018). Other studies demonstrated that removal of the entire bladder is not required to achieve pain resolution, so the role of cystectomy remains unclear (Norus et al., 2014; Redmond & Flood, 2017). Unfortunately, it is still unknown which patients might best benefit from radical surgery.

Pain Management

Just as the conservative first-line strategies are important in management of this patient population, having a plan for pain management with escalation through pharmacologic therapies is imperative. Given increasing concerns and risks related to use of opioid medications for chronic pain disorders, pain management should use nonsteroidal antiinflammatory drugs and weak opioids (if needed) like tramadol. Management of neuropathic pain with medications like gabapentin or pregabalin can be used in monotherapy or combination with other agents (Giusto et al., 2018). The Global IC/BPS Society also recommended consideration of pudendal or hypogastric plexus nerve blocks for patients refractory to other pain management strategies combined with multimodal therapies (Rahnama'i et al., 2020).

BIBLIOGRAPHY

Nomenclature and Epidemiology

Abrams P, Cardozo L, Fall M, et al. The standardization of terminology in lower urinary tract function. Report from the Standardization Sub-committee of the International Continence Society. *Neurourol Urodyn.* 2002;21:167.

Berry SH, Elliott MN, Suttorp M, et al. Prevalence of symptoms of bladder pain syndrome/interstitial cystitis among adult females in the United States. *J Urol.* 2011;186:540.

Bologna RA, Whitmore KE. Hypersensitivity disorders of the lower urinary tract. In: Karram MM, Walters MD, eds. *Urogynecology and Reconstructive Pelvic Surgery.* Philadelphia: Elsevier/Saunders; 2015:542.

Clemens JQ, Meenan RT, O'Keeffe Rosetti MC, et al. Prevalence of interstitial cystitis symptoms in a managed care population. *J Urol.* 2005;174:576.

Clemens JQ, Link CL, Eggers PW, et al. Prevalence of painful bladder symptoms and effect on quality of life in black, Hispanic and white men and women. *J Urol.* 2007;177:1390.

Curhan GC, Speizer FE, Hunter DJ, et al. Epidemiology of interstitial cystitis: a population based study. *J Urol.* 1999;161:549.

Doggweiler R, Whitmore KE, Meijlink JM, et al. A standard for terminology in chronic pelvic pain syndromes: a report from the chronic pelvic pain working group of the international continence society. *Neurourol Urodyn.* 2017;36:984.

Gillenwater JY, Wein AJ. *Summary of the National Institute of Arthritis, Diabetes, Digestive and Kidney Diseases Workshop on Interstitial Cystitis,* Bethesda, MD, August 28–29, 1987, National Institutes of Health. *J Urol.* 1988;140:203.

Hanno PM, Landis JR, Matthews-Cook Y, et al. The diagnosis of interstitial cystitis revisited: lessons learned from the National Institutes of Health Interstitial Cystitis Database study. *J Urol.* 1999;161:553.

Hanno PM, Erickson D, Moldwin R, Faraday MM, American Urological Association. Diagnosis and treatment of interstitial cystitis/bladder pain syndrome: AUA guideline amendment. *J Urol.* 2015;193:1545.

Hanno P, Fall M, Meijlink J, Nordling J. Towards a new paradigm in bladder pain syndrome and interstitial cystitis. *BJU Int.* 2020;126:549.

Homma Y. Interstitial cystitis, bladder pain syndrome, hypersensitive bladder, and interstitial cystitis/bladder pain syndrome - clarification of definitions and relationships. *Int J Urol.* 2019;26:20.

Hunner GL. A rare type of bladder ulcer in women: report of cases. *Boston Med Soc J.* 1915;172:660.

Jones CA, Nyberg L. Epidemiology of interstitial cystitis. *Urology.* 1997;49:2.

Krieger JN, Stephens AJ, Landis JR, et al. Relationship between chronic nonurological associated somatic syndromes and symptom severity in urological chronic pelvic pain syndromes: baseline evaluation of the MAPP study. *J Urol.* 2015;193:1254.

Lai HH, Jemielita T, Sutcliffe S, et al. Characterization of whole body pain in urological chronic pelvic pain syndrome at baseline: a MAPP Research Network study. *J Urol.* 2007;198:622.

Lai HH, Shen B, Rawal A, Vetter J. The relationship between depression and overactive bladder/urinary incontinence symptoms in the clinical OAB population. *BMC Urology* 2016;16:60

Leppilahti M, Tammela TL, Huhtala H, Auvinen A. Prevalence of symptoms related to interstitial cystitis in women: a population based study in Finland. *J Urol.* 2002;168:139.

Naliboff BD, Stephens AJ, Afari N, et al. Widespread psychosocial difficulties in men and women with urologic chronic pelvic pain syndromes: case-control findings from the Multidisciplinary Approach to the Study of Chronic Pelvic Pain Research Network. *Urology.* 2015;85:1319.

Nitze M. *Lehrbuch de cystoscopie: ihre technik und kinsche bedeutung.* Berlin: JE Bergman; 1907.

Peters KM, Carrico DJ, Kalinowski SE, et al. Prevalence of pelvic floor dysfunction in patients with interstitial cystitis. *Urology.* 2007;70:16.

Rosenberg MT, Hazzard M. Prevalence of interstitial cystitis symptoms in women: a population based study in the primary care office. *J Urol.* 2005;174:2231.

Skene AJ. *Diseases of Bladder and Urethra in Women.* New York: William Wood; 1887.

van de Merwe JP, Nordling J, Bouchelouche P, et al. Diagnostic criteria, classification, and nomenclature for painful bladder syndrome/interstitial cystitis: an ESSIC proposal. *Eur Urol.* 2008;53:60.

Whitmore KE, Fall M, Sengiku A, et al. Hunner lesion versus non-Hunner lesion interstitial cystitis/bladder pain syndrome. *Int J Urol.* 2019;26:26.

Etiology

Abernethy MG, Rosenfeld A, White JR, et al. Urinary microbiome and cytokine levels in women with interstitial cystitis. *Obstet Gynecol.* 2017;129:500.

Akiyama Y, Maeda D, Morikawa T, et al. Digital quantitative analysis of mast cell infiltration in interstitial cystitis. *Neurourol Urodyn.* 2018;37:650.

Akiyama Y, Maeda D, Katoh H, et al. Molecular taxonomy of interstitial cystitis/bladder pain syndrome based on whole transcriptome profiling by next-generation rna sequencing of bladder mucosal biopsies. *J Urol.* 2019;202:290.

Akiyama Y, Luo Y, Hanno PM, et al. Interstitial cystitis/bladder pain syndrome: The evolving landscape, animal models and future perspectives. *Int J Urol.* 2020;27:491.

Alger JR, Ellingson BM, Ashe-McNalley C, et al. Multisite, multimodal neuroimaging of chronic urological pelvic pain: methodology of the MAPP Research Network. *Neuroimage Clin.* 2016;12:65.

Apkarian AV, Baliki MN, Geha PY. Towards a theory of chronic pain. *Prog Neurobiol.* 2009;87:81.

Bagarinao E, Johnson KA, Martucci KT, et al. Preliminary structural MRI based brain classification of chronic pelvic pain: a MAPP network study. *Pain.* 2014;155:2502.

Birder L, Andersson KE. Urothelial signaling. *Physiol Rev.* 2013;93:653.

Birder LA. Pathophysiology of interstitial cystitis. *Int J Urol.* 2019;26:12.

Braunstein R, Shapiro E, Kaye J, Moldwin R. The role of cystoscopy in the diagnosis of Hunner's ulcer disease. *J Urol.* 2008;180:1383.

Clauw DJ. Fibromyalgia and related conditions. *Mayo Clin Proc.* 2015;90:680.

Clemens JQ, Mullins C, Ackerman AL, et al. Urologic chronic pelvic pain syndrome: insights from the MAPP Research Network. *Nat Rev Urol.* 2019;16:187.

Fowler CJ, Griffiths D, de Groat WC. The neural control of micturition. *Nat Rev Neurosci.* 2008;9:453.

Furuta A, Suzuki Y, Igarashi T, et al. Angiogenesis in bladder tissues is strongly correlated with urinary frequency and bladder pain in patients with interstitial cystitis/bladder pain syndrome. *Int J Urol.* 2019;26:35.

Geppetti P, Nassini R, Materazzi S, Benemei S. The concept of neurogenic inflammation. *BJU Int.* 2008;101:2.

Griffiths D, Tadic SD, Schaefer W, Resnick NM. Cerebral control of the bladder in normal and urge-incontinent women. *Neuroimage.* 2007;37:1.

Hanno P, Fall M, Meijlink J, Nordling J. Towards a new paradigm in bladder pain syndrome and interstitial cystitis. *BJU Int.* 2020;126:549.

Hauser PJ, Buethe DA, Califano J, et al. Restoring barrier function to acid damaged bladder by intravesical chondroitin sulfate. *J Urol.* 2009;182:2477.

Holmes SA, Upadhyay J, Borsook D. Delineating conditions and subtypes in chronic pain using neuroimaging. *Pain Rep.* 2019;4:e768.

Huang L, Kutch JJ, Ellingson BM, et al. Brain white matter changes associated with urological chronic pelvic pain syndrome: multisite neuroimaging from a MAPP case-control study. *Pain.* 2016;157:2782.

Hunner GL. A rare type of bladder ulcer in women: report of cases. *Boston Med Soc J.* 1915;172:660.

Hurst RE, Zebrowski R. Identification of proteoglycans present at high density on bovine and human bladder luminal surface. *J Urol* 1994;152:1641.

Hurst RE, Roy JB, Min KW, et al. A deficit of chondroitin sulfate proteoglycans on the bladder uroepithelium in interstitial cystitis. *Urology* 1996;48:817.

Jhang JF, Ho HC, Jiang YH, et al. Electron microscopic characteristics of interstitial cystitis/bladder pain syndrome and their association with clinical condition. *PLoS One.* 2018;13:e0198816.

Logadottir Y, Delbro D, Lindholm C, et al. Inflammation characteristic in bladder pain syndrome ESSIC type 3C/classic interstitial cystitis. *Int J Urol.* 2014;21:75.

Kuhtz-Buschbeck JP, van der Horst C, Pott C, et al. Cortical representation of the urge to void: a functional magnetic resonance imaging study. *J Urol.* 2005;174:1477.

Kutch JJ, Labus JS, Harris RE, et al. Resting-state functional connectivity predicts longitudinal pain symptom change in urologic chronic pelvic pain syndrome: a MAPP network study. *Pain.* 2017;158:1069.

Maeda D, Akiyama Y, Morikawa T, et al. Hunner-type (classic) interstitial cystitis: a distinct inflammatory disorder characterized by pancystitis, with frequent expansion of clonal b-cells and epithelial denudation. *PLoS One.* 2015;10:e0143316.

Meriwether KV, Lei Z, Singh R, et al. The vaginal and urinary microbiomes in premenopausal women with interstitial cystitis/bladder pain syndrome as compared to unaffected controls: a pilot cross-sectional study. *Front Cell Infect Microbiol.* 2019;9:92.

Moisset X, Bouhassira D. Brain imaging of neuropathic pain. *Neuroimage.* 2007;37:S80.

Tadic SD, Griffiths D, Schaefer W, et al. Brain activity underlying impaired continence control in older women with overactive bladder. *Neurourol Urodyn.* 2012;31:652.

Nickel JC, Stephens-Shields AJ, Landis JR, et al. A culture-independent analysis of the microbiota of female interstitial cystitis/bladder pain syndrome participants in the MAPP Research Network. *J Clin Med.* 2019;8:415.

Pearce M, Zilliox M, Rosenfeld A, et al. The female urinary microbiome in urgency urinary incontinence. *Am J Obstet Gynecol.* 2015;347:1.

Peters KM, Killinger KA, Mounayer MH, Boura JA. Are ulcerative and nonulcerative interstitial cystitis/painful bladder syndrome 2 distinct diseases? A study of coexisting conditions. *Urology.* 2011;78:301.

Phillips K, Clauw DJ. Central pain mechanisms in chronic pain states—maybe it is all in their head. *Best Pract Res Clin Rheumatol.* 2011;25:141.

Whitmore KE, Fall M, Sengiku A, et al. Hunner lesion versus non-Hunner lesion interstitial cystitis/bladder pain syndrome. *Int J Urol.* 2019;26:26.

Clinical Phenotyping and Flares

Ahn ST, Jeong HG, Park TY, et al. Differences in urodynamic parameters according to the presence of a Hunner lesion in women with interstitial cystitis/bladder pain syndrome. *Int Neurourol J.* 2018;22:S55.

Clemens JQ, Mullins C, Ackerman AL, et al. Urologic chronic pelvic pain syndrome: insights from the MAPP Research Network. *Nat Rev Urol.* 2019;16:187.

Khullar V, Chermansky C, Tarcan T, et al. How can we improve the diagnosis and management of bladder pain syndrome? Part 1: ICI-RS 2018. *Neurourol Urodyn*. 2019;38:S66.

Lai HH, Krieger JN, Pontari MA, et al. Painful bladder filling and painful urgency are distinct characteristics in men and women with urological chronic pelvic pain syndromes: a MAPP Research Network study. *J Urol*. 2015;194:1634.

Lai HH, Vetter J, Song J, et al. Management of symptom flares and patient-reported flare triggers in Interstitial Cystitis/Bladder Pain Syndrome (IC/BPS)-findings from one site of the MAPP Research Network. *Urology*. 2019;126:24.

Logadottir Y, Fall M, Kåbjörn-Gustafsson C, Peeker R. Clinical characteristics differ considerably between phenotypes of bladder pain syndrome/interstitial cystitis. *Scand J Urol Nephrol*. 2012;46:365.

Naliboff BD, Stephens AJ, Lai HH, et al. Clinical and psychosocial predictors of urological chronic pelvic pain symptom change in 1 year: a prospective study from the MAPP Research Network. *J Urol*. 2017;198:848.

Nickel JC, Shoskes D, Irvine-Bird K. Clinical phenotyping of women with interstitial cystitis/painful bladder syndrome: a key to classification and potentially improved management. *J Urol*. 2009;182:155.

Nickel JC, Herschorn S, Whitmore KE, et al. Pentosan polysulfate sodium for treatment of interstitial cystitis/bladder pain syndrome: insights from a randomized, double-blind, placebo controlled study. *J Urol*. 2015;193:857.

Peters KM, Killinger KA, Mounayer MH, Boura JA. Are ulcerative and nonulcerative interstitial cystitis/painful bladder syndrome 2 distinct diseases? A study of coexisting conditions. *Urology*. 2011;78:301

Sutcliffe S, Colditz GA, Goodman MS, et al. Urological chronic pelvic pain syndrome symptom flares: characterisation of the full range of flares at two sites in the Multidisciplinary Approach to the Study of Chronic Pelvic Pain (MAPP) Research Network. *BJU Int*. 2014;114:916.

Sutcliffe S, Bradley CS, Clemens JQ, et al. Urological chronic pelvic pain syndrome flares and their impact: qualitative analysis in the MAPP network. *Int Urogynecol J*. 2015;26:1047.

Sutcliffe S, Jemielita T, Lai HH, et al. A case-crossover study of urological chronic pelvic pain syndrome flare triggers in the MAPP Research Network. 2018;199:1245.

van de Merwe JP, Nordling J, Bouchelouche P, et al. Diagnostic criteria, classification, and nomenclature for painful bladder syndrome/interstitial cystitis: an ESSIC proposal. *Eur Urol*. 2008;53:60.

Whitmore KE, Fall M, Sengiku A, et al. Hunner lesion versus non-Hunner lesion interstitial cystitis/bladder pain syndrome. *Int J Urol*. 2019;26:26.

Evaluation

Ackerman AL, Lee UJ, Jellison FC, et al. MRI suggests increased tonicity of the levator ani in women with interstitial cystitis/bladder pain syndrome. *Int Urogynecol J*. 2016;27:77.

Ahn ST, Jeong HG, Park TY, et al. Differences in urodynamic parameters according to the presence of a hunner lesion in women with interstitial cystitis/bladder pain syndrome. *Int Neurourol J*. 2018;22:S55.

Cameron AP, Gajewski JB. Bladder outlet obstruction in painful bladder syndrome/interstitial cystitis. *Neurourol Urodyn*. 2009;28:944.

Charlanes A, Boudghene F, Chesnel C, et al. Diffusion-weighted magnetic resonance imaging: a new tool for the diagnosis of bladder pain syndrome/interstitial cystitis. *Urol Int*. 2019;102:109.

Clemens JQ, Calhoun EA, Litwin MS, et al., Urologic Pelvic Pain Collaborative Research Network. Validation of a modified National Institutes of Health chronic prostatitis symptom index to assess genitourinary pain in both men and women. *Urology*. 2009;74:983.

Engeler D, Baranowski AP, Berghmans B, et al. *EAU Guidelines on Chronic Pelvic Pain*. Available at: https://uroweb.org/wp-content/uploads/EAU-Guidelines-on-Chronic-Pelvic-Pain-2020.pdf. Accessed October 6, 2020.

Hanno PM, Erickson D, Moldwin R, et al. Diagnosis and treatment of interstitial cystitis/bladder pain syndrome: AUA guideline amendment. *J Urol*. 2015;193:1545.

Humphrey L, Arbuckle R, Moldwin R, et al. The bladder pain/interstitial cystitis symptom score: development, validation, and identification of a cut score. *Eur Urol*. 2012;61:271.

Hunner G. A rare type of bladder ulcer. Further notes, with a report of eighteen cases. *JAMA*. 1918;70:203.

Koziol JA. Epidemiology of interstitial cystitis. *Urol Clin North Am*. 1994;21:7.

Kuo YC, Kuo HC. Videourodynamic characteristics of interstitial cystitis/bladder pain syndrome-The role of bladder outlet dysfunction in the pathophysiology. *Neurourol Urodyn*. 2018;37:1971.

Link CL, Pulliam SJ, Hanno PM, et al. Prevalence and psychosocial correlates of symptoms suggestive of painful bladder syndrome: results from the Boston area community health survey. *J Urol*. 2008;180:599.

Mayson BE, Teichman JM. The relationship between sexual abuse and interstitial cystitis/painful bladder syndrome. *Curr Urol Rep*. 2009;10:441.

Meister MR, Sutcliffe S, Ghetti C, et al. Development of a standardized, reproducible screening examination for assessment of pelvic floor myofascial pain. *Am J Obstet Gynecol*. 2019;220:255.e1.

O'Leary MP, Sant GR, Fowler FJ, et al. The interstitial cystitis symptom index and problem index. *Urology*. 1997;49:58.

Peeker R, Fall M. Toward a precise definition of interstitial cystitis: further evidence of differences in classic and nonulcer disease. *J Urol*. 2002;167:2470.

Ronstrom C, Lai HH. Presenting an atlas of Hunner lesions in interstitial cystitis which can be identified with office cystoscopy. *Neurourol Urodyn*. 2020;39:2394.

Shear S, Mayer R. Development of glomerulations in younger women with interstitial cystitis. *Urology*. 2006;68:253.

Shim JS, Kang SG, Park JY, et al. Differences in urodynamic parameters between women with interstitial cystitis and/or bladder pain syndrome and severe overactive bladder. *Urology*. 2016;94:64.

Tyagi P, Janicki J, Moon CH, et al. Novel contrast mixture achieves contrast resolution of human bladder wall suitable for T1 mapping: applications in interstitial cystitis and beyond. *Int Urol Nephrol*. 2018;50:401.

van de Merwe JP, Nordling J, Bouchelouche P, et al. Diagnostic criteria, classification, and nomenclature for painful bladder syndrome/interstitial cystitis: an ESSIC proposal. *Eur Urol*. 2008;53:60.

Waxman JA, Sulak PJ, Kuehl TJ. Cystoscopic findings consistent with interstitial cystitis in normal women undergoing tubal ligation. *J Urol*. 1998;160:1663.

Whitmore KE, Fall M, Sengiku A, et al. Hunner lesion versus non-Hunner lesion interstitial cystitis/bladder pain syndrome. *Int J Urol*. 2019;26:26.

Management of Interstitial Cystitis/Bladder Pain Syndrome

Bade JJ, Laseur M, Nieuwenburg A, et al. A placebo-controlled study of intravesical pentosanpolysulphate for the treatment of interstitial cystitis. *Br J Urol*. 1997;79:168.

Barua JM, Arance I, Angulo JC, Riedl CR. A systematic review and meta-analysis on the efficacy of intravesical therapy for bladder pain syndrome/interstitial cystitis. *Int Urogynecol J*. 2016;27:1137.

Bassaly R, Downes K, Hart S. Dietary consumption triggers in interstitial cystitis/bladder pain syndrome patients. *Female Pelvic Med Reconstr Surg*. 2011;17:36.

Cervigni M, Sommariva M, Tenaglia R, et al. A randomized, open-label, multicenter study of the efficacy and safety of intravesical hyaluronic acid and chondroitin sulfate versus dimethyl sulfoxide in women with bladder pain syndrome/interstitial cystitis. *Neurourol Urodyn*. 2017;36:1178.

Chennamsetty A, Khourdaji I, Goike J, et al. Electrosurgical management of Hunner ulcers in a referral center's interstitial cystitis population. *Urology*. 2015;85:74.

Cox M, Klutke JJ, Klutke CG. Assessment of patient outcomes following submucosal injection of triamcinolone for treatment of Hunner's ulcer subtype interstitial cystitis. *Can J Urol*. 2009;16:4536.

Crescenze IM, Gupta P, Adams G, et al. Advanced management of patients with ulcerative interstitial cystitis/bladder pain syndrome. *Urology*. 2019;133:78.

Crescenze IM, Tucky B, Li J, et al. Efficacy, side effects, and monitoring of oral cyclosporine in interstitial cystitis-bladder pain syndrome. *Urology*. 2017;107:49.

Daha LK, Lazar D, Simak R, et al. The effects of intravesical pentosanpolysulfate treatment on the symptoms of patients with bladder pain syndrome/interstitial cystitis: preliminary results. *Int Urogynecol J Pelvic Floor Dysfunct*. 2008;19:987.

Davis EL, El Khoudary SR, Talbott EO, et al. Safety and efficacy of the use of intravesical and oral pentosan polysulfate sodium for interstitial cystitis: a randomized double-blind clinical trial. *J Urol*. 2008;179:177.

Esteban M, Adot JM, Arlandis S, et al. Working group for recommendations on the diagnosis and management of bladder pain syndrome. Recommendations for the Diagnosis and Management of Bladder Pain Syndrome. Spanish Urological Association Consensus Document. *Actas Urol Esp*. 2015;39:465.

FitzGerald MP, Payne CK, Lukacz ES, et al. Randomized multicenter clinical trial of myofascial physical therapy in women with interstitial cystitis/painful bladder syndrome and pelvic floor tenderness. *J Urol*. 2012;187:2113.

Forrest JB, Payne CK, Erickson DR. Cyclosporine A for refractory interstitial cystitis/bladder pain syndrome: experience of 3 tertiary centers. *J Urol*. 2012;188:1186.

Foster Jr HE, Hanno PM, Nickel JC, et al. Effect of amitriptyline on symptoms in treatment naïve patients with interstitial cystitis/painful bladder syndrome. *J Urol*. 2010;183:1853.

Friedlander JI, Shorter B, Moldwin RM. Diet and its role in interstitial cystitis/bladder pain syndrome (IC/BPS) and comorbid conditions. *BJU Int*. 2012;109:1584.

Gafni-Kane A, Botros SM, Du H, et al. Measuring the success of combined intravesical dimethyl sulfoxide and triamcinolone for treatment of bladder pain syndrome/interstitial cystitis. *Int Urogynecol J*. 2013;24:303.

Giusto LL, Zahner PM, Shoskes DA. An evaluation of the pharmacotherapy for interstitial cystitis. *Expert Opin Pharmacother*. 2018;19:1097.

Han E, Nguyen L, Sirls L, Peters K. Current best practice management of interstitial cystitis/bladder pain syndrome. *Ther Adv Urol*. 2018;10:197.

Hanif AM, Armenti ST, Taylor SC, et al. Phenotypic Spectrum of Pentosan Polysulfate Sodium–Associated Maculopathy: A Multicenter Study. *JAMA Ophthalmol*. 2019;137:1275.

Hanno P, Dmochowski R. Status of international consensus on interstitial cystitis/bladder pain syndrome/painful bladder syndrome: 2008 snapshot. *Neurourol Urodyn*. 2009;28:274.

Hanno PM, Erickson D, Moldwin R, et al. Diagnosis and treatment of interstitial cystitis/bladder pain syndrome: AUA guideline amendment. *J Urol*. 2015;193:1545.

Hanno P, Cervigni M, Dinis P, et al. Bladder Pain Syndrome. In: Abrams P, Cardozo L, Wagg A, Wein A, eds. *Incontinence*. 6th ed. Tokyo: 6th International Consultation on Incontinence; 2017:2203.

Health Canada. *ELMIRON (Pentosan Polysulfate Sodium) and the Risk of Pigmentary Maculopathy.* December 15, 2020. Available at: https://healthycanadians.gc.ca/recall-alert-rappel-avis/hc-sc/2020/74549a-eng.php. Accessed July 13, 2021.

Hillelsohn JH, Rais-Bahrami S, Friedlander JI, et al. Fulguration for Hunner ulcers: long-term clinical outcomes. *J Urol*. 2012;188:2238.

Huckfeldt RM, Vavvas DG. Progressive maculopathy after discontinuation of pentosan polysulfate sodium. *Ophthalmic Surg Lasers Imaging Retina*. 2019;50:656.

Kim HJ, Lee JS, Cho WJ, et al. Efficacy and safety of augmentation ileocystoplasty combined with supratrigonal cystectomy for the treatment of refractory bladder pain syndrome/interstitial cystitis with Hunner's lesion. *Int J Urol*. 2014;21:69.

Kirk PS, Santiago-Lastra Y, Qin Y, et al. The effects of cystoscopy and hydrodistention on symptoms and bladder capacity in interstitial cystitis/bladder pain syndrome. *Neurourol Urodyn*. 2018;37:2002.

Khullar V, Chermansky C, Tarcan T, et al. How can we improve the diagnosis and management of bladder pain syndrome? Part 1: ICI-RS 2018. *Neurourol Urodyn*. 2019;38:S66.

Khullar V, Digesu GA, Veit-Rubin N, et al. How can we improve the diagnosis and management of bladder pain syndrome? Part 2: ICI-RS 2018. *Neurourol Urodyn*. 2019b;38:S71.

Linn JF, Hohenfellner M, Roth S, et al. Treatment of interstitial cystitis: comparison of subtrigonal and supratrigonal cystectomy combined with orthotopic bladder substitution. *J Urol*. 1998;159:774.

Lusty A, Kavaler E, Zakariasen K, et al. Treatment effectiveness in interstitial cystitis/bladder pain syndrome: do patient perceptions align with efficacy-based guidelines? *Can Urol Assoc J*. 2018; 12:E1.

Mahran A, Baaklini G, Hassani D, et al. Sacral neuromodulation treating chronic pelvic pain: a meta-analysis and systematic review of the literature. *Int Urogynecol J*. 2019;30:1023.

Malde S, Palmisani S, Al-Kaisy A, Sahai A. Guideline of guidelines: bladder pain syndrome. *BJU Int*. 2018;122:729.

Manning J, Dwyer P, Rosamilia A, et al. A multicentre, prospective, randomised, double-blind study to measure the treatment effectiveness of abobotulinum A (AboBTXA) among women with refractory interstitial cystitis/bladder pain syndrome. *Int Urogynecol J*. 2014;25:593.

Mateu Arrom L, Gutiérrez Ruiz C, Mayordomo Ferrer O, et al. Long-term follow-up after cystectomy for bladder pain syndrome: pain status, sexual function and quality of life. *World J Urol*. 2019;37:1597.

McKernan LC, Walsh CG, Reynolds WS, et al. Psychosocial co-morbidities in Interstitial Cystitis/Bladder Pain syndrome (IC/BPS): a systematic review. *Neurourol Urodyn*. 2018;37:926.

Neale A, Malik N, Taylor C, et al. Bladder pain syndrome/interstitial cystitis in contemporary UK practice: outcomes of phenotype-directed management. *Low Urin Tract Symptoms.* 2021;13:123.

Niimi A, Nomiya A, Yamada Y, et al. Hydrodistension with or without fulguration of hunner lesions for interstitial cystitis: Long-term outcomes and prognostic predictors. *Neurourol Urodyn.* 2016;35:965.

Nickel JC, Herschorn S, Whitmore KE, et al. Pentosan polysulfate sodium for treatment of interstitial cystitis/bladder pain syndrome: insights from a randomized, double-blind, placebo controlled study. *J Urol.* 2015;193:857.

Norus T, Fode M, Nordling J. Ileal conduit without cystectomy may be an appropriate option in the treatment of intractable bladder pain syndrome/interstitial cystitis. *Scand J Urol.* 2014;48:210.

Olson LE, Dyer JE, Haq A, et al. A systematic review of the literature on cystodistension in bladder pain syndrome. *Int Urogynecol J.* 2018;29:251.

Paredes Mojica JA, Mogica JAP, De EJB. Pentosan Polysulfate Maculopathy: What urologists should know in 2020. *Urology.* 2021;147:109.

Payne RA, O'Connor RC, Kressin M, Guralnick ML. Endoscopic ablation of Hunner's lesions in interstitial cystitis patients. *Can Urol Assoc J.* 2009;3:473.

Pearce WA, Chen R, Jain N. Pigmentary maculopathy associated with chronic exposure to pentosan polysulfate sodium. *Ophthalmology.* 2018;125:1793.

Peters KM, Carrico DJ, Kalinowski SE, Ibrahim IA, Diokno AC. Prevalence of pelvic floor dysfunction in patients with interstitial cystitis. *Urology.* 2007;70:16.

Porru D, Campus G, Tudino D, et al. Results of treatment of refractory interstitial cystitis with intravesical hyaluronic acid. *Urol Int.* 1997;59:26.

Pyo JS, Cho WJ. Systematic review and meta-analysis of intravesical hyaluronic acid and hyaluronic acid/chondroitin sulfate instillation for interstitial cystitis/painful bladder syndrome. *Cell Physiol Biochem.* 2016;39:1618.

Rahnama'i MS, Marcelissen T, Apostolidis A, et al. The efficacy of botulinum toxin A and sacral neuromodulation in the management of interstitial cystitis (IC)/bladder pain syndrome (BPS), what do we know? ICI-RS 2017 Think Thank, Bristol. *Neurourol Urodyn.* 2018;37:S99.

Rahnama'i MS, Javan A, Vyas N, et al. Bladder pain syndrome and interstitial cystitis beyond horizon: reports from the Global Interstitial Cystitis/Bladder Pain Society (GIBS) Meeting 2019 Mumbai - India. *Anesth Pain Med.* 2020;10:e101848.

Redmond EJ, Flood HD. The role of reconstructive surgery in patients with end-stage interstitial cystitis/bladder pain syndrome: is cystectomy necessary? *Int Urogynecol J.* 2017;28:1551.

Ryu J, Pak S, Song M, et al. Elimination of Hunner's ulcers by fulguration in patients with interstitial cystitis: is it effective and long lasting? *Korean J Urol.* 2013;54:767.

Sant GR, Propert KJ, Hanno PM, et al.. A pilot clinical trial of oral pentosan polysulfate and oral hydroxyzine in patients with interstitial cystitis. *J Urol.* 2003;170:810.

Shah R, Simonett JM, Lyons RJ, et al. Disease course in patients with pentosan polysulfate sodium-associated maculopathy after drug cessation. *JAMA Ophthalmol.* 2020;138:894.

Shorter B, Lesser M, Moldwin RM, Kushner L. Effect of comestibles on symptoms of interstitial cystitis. *J Urol.* 2007;178:145.

Taneja R. Current status of oral pentosan polysulphate in bladder pain syndrome/interstitial cystitis. *Int Urogynecol J.* 2021;32:1107.

Theoharides TC, Sant GR. Hydroxyzine therapy for interstitial cystitis. *Urology.* 1997;49:108.

Theoharides TC. Hydroxyzine in the treatment of interstitial cystitis. *Urol Clin North Am.* 1994;21:113.

Turner KJ, Stewart LH. How do you stretch a bladder? A survey of UK practice, a literature review, and a recommendation of a standard approach. *Neurourol Urodyn.* 2005;24:74.

Tutolo M, Ammirati E, Heesakkers J, et al. Efficacy and safety of sacral and percutaneous tibial neuromodulation in non-neurogenic lower urinary tract dysfunction and chronic pelvic pain: a systematic review of the literature. *Eur Urol.* 2018;73:406.

U.S. Food and Drug Administration. *ELMIRON-100 MG (Pentosan Polysulfate Sodium) Capsules: Prescribing Information.* FDA.gov. 2020. Available at: https://www.accessdata.fda.gov/drugsatfda_docs/label/2020/020193s014lbl.pdf.

van Ophoven A, Hertle L. Long-term results of amitriptyline treatment for interstitial cystitis. *J Urol.* 2005;174:1837.

Wang J, Chen Y, Chen J, et al. Sacral neuromodulation for refractory bladder pain syndrome/interstitial cystitis: a global systematic review and meta-analysis. *Sci Rep.* 2017;7:11031.

Whitmore KE, Fall M, Sengiku A, et al. Hunner lesion versus non-Hunner lesion interstitial cystitis/bladder pain syndrome. *Int J Urol.* 2019;26:26.

PART 7

Specific Conditions

36

Lower Urinary Tract Infection

Megan S. Bradley and Nazema Y. Siddiqui

CHAPTER OUTLINE

INTRODUCTION

Urinary tract infections (UTIs) are one of the most common bacterial infections, affecting 150 million people each year worldwide. Annually, UTIs result in 10.5 million office visits (constituting 0.9% of all ambulatory visits) and 2 to 3 million emergency department visits in the United States alone. Within the United States, societal costs, including health care costs and time missed from work, are approximately $3.5 billion per year. It is estimated that up to one out of every three women has had at least one episode of UTI requiring antimicrobial therapy by 24 years of age, with the lifetime risk being greater than 50%. The prevalence of UTIs among women is thought to increase even further with age, with 10% of women over 65 years and 30% of women older than 85 years reporting UTI within the prior 12 months. Clinicians managing urogynecologic patients need to be well-versed not only in management of acute UTIs, but also of recurrent UTIs (rUTIs) and asymptomatic bacteriuria (ASB) because of high incidence in this population (i.e., postmenopausal women and patients undergoing procedures that require instrumentation of the genitourinary tract).

By definition, UTIs include cystitis (infection of the bladder/lower urinary tract) and pyelonephritis (infection of the kidney/upper urinary tract) (Table 36.1). UTI is diagnosed based on the presence of a pathogen in the urinary tract and associated symptoms. Uncomplicated UTIs typically affect individuals who are otherwise healthy and have no structural or neurological urinary tract abnormalities; these infections are differentiated into lower tract UTIs (cystitis) and upper tract UTIs (pyelonephritis). In contrast, a complicated UTI refers to cystitis or pyelonephritis in a patient with a variety of factors including urologic abnormalities (such as nephrolithiasis, strictures, stents, or urinary diversions), immunocompromising conditions (such as neutropenia or advanced human immunodeficiency virus infection), or poorly controlled diabetes mellitus. Certain populations, such as pregnant women and renal transplant recipients, also have unique management considerations. There are multiple definitions for rUTI, but the most common is at least two episodes of culture-positive, symptomatic UTIs within 6 months, or at least three in 1 year. Finally, ASB is the presence of one or more species of bacteria growing in the urine at specified quantitative counts ($\geq 10^5$ colony-forming units [CFU]/mL), irrespective of the presence of pyuria, in the absence of signs or symptoms attributable to UTI.

ACUTE, SYMPTOMATIC, UNCOMPLICATED LOWER URINARY TRACT INFECTION

Definitions

Uncomplicated UTIs are differentiated into lower UTIs (cystitis) and upper UTIs (pyelonephritis) (Table 36.1). In this chapter we will discuss the diagnosis and management of lower UTIs (i.e., cystitis). Management guidelines for acute, symptomatic,

TABLE 36.1 Urinary Tract Infection Terminology

Diagnosis	Definition
Acute uncomplicated urinary tract infection	Infection of the lower and/or upper genitourinary tract that is diagnosed based on the presence of a urinary tract pathogen and its associated symptoms in an otherwise healthy individual without structural or neurological urinary tract abnormalities
Cystitis	Infection of the bladder/lower urinary tract
Pyelonephritis	Infection of the kidney/upper urinary tract
Complicated urinary tract infection	Cystitis or pyelonephritis in a patient with urologic abnormalities, immunocompromising conditions, or poorly controlled diabetes mellitus
Recurrent urinary tract infection	At least two episodes of culture-positive, symptomatic UTI in 6 months, or three or more in 1 year
Asymptomatic bacteriuria	The presence of bacterial growth on urine culture at $\geq 10^5$ colony-forming units/mL in the absence of signs or symptoms attributable to UTI
Urosepsis	Systemic response to uropathogen leading to organ dysfunction

UTI, Urinary tract infection.

uncomplicated UTI have been developed for nonpregnant premenopausal women without underlying structural urologic abnormalities, but they likely can be extrapolated to postmenopausal women without urological sequelae and/or recurrent infections.

Pathophysiology

UTIs can be caused by both gram-negative and gram-positive bacteria, but the most common causative agent for uncomplicated UTIs is uropathogenic *Escherichia coli*. UTI typically starts with periurethral contamination by a uropathogen residing in the gut, followed by colonization of the urethra and migration of the pathogen to the bladder. This process requires microbial virulence factors including flagellae, pili, and other adhesins that facilitate mucosal adherence and stimulation of the host immune response.

There are multiple factors that typically aid in UTI deterrence. These include: the acidic vaginal environment, the glycosaminoglycan (GAG) layer of the bladder, and immunoglobulins in the urine. The acidic pH of the vagina in premenopausal women inhibits the growth of enterobacteria such as *E. coli* and promotes the growth of *Lactobacilli*, a genus of microbes associated with health. The GAGs in the bladder lining and immunoglobulins in the urine restrict bacterial adherence. Tamm–Horsfall proteins secreted by the loop of Henle may also inhibit bacterial adherence to the urothelial cells, and antimicrobial peptides may serve to modulate the immune response during bacterial presence.

Diagnosis

There is currently no "gold standard" definition for an acute UTI, which poses a challenge not only for clinical care but also for epidemiologic research. Historically, establishing a diagnosis of symptomatic UTI requires a patient to have symptoms and signs of UTI with laboratory tests confirming the diagnosis (bacteriuria $\geq 10^5$ CFU/mL). Some experts advocate for relaxing these diagnostic criteria to include symptomatic patients with urine culture of 100 CFU/mL or more. Lower colony counts on culture may represent a partially treated infection, an earlier stage of infection, the effects of diluting the bacterial concentration with urination, or the mode of specimen collection (i.e., voided vs. catheterized sampling).

Cystitis in women usually causes dysuria, although it may also cause frequency, urgency, and suprapubic discomfort. Occasionally, mild incontinence and hematuria may occur. Gross hematuria is rare. Upper tract infections commonly present with fever, chills, malaise, flank pain, costovertebral angle tenderness, and occasionally nausea and vomiting. In young women, patients with dysuria and frequency without vaginal discharge or irritation have a 90% probability of a UTI. Dysuria remains the most discriminating symptom in older women seen in urogynecologic offices. However, in older women symptoms of frequency and urgency are less specific because of the high prevalence of other bladder symptom conditions like overactive bladder in aging populations.

Diagnostic Testing

Urine Dipstick. For many women with dysuria, lack of vaginal discharge, and classic acute simple cystitis (not in the setting of rUTI), no additional testing is warranted to make the diagnosis. For those with suggestive, but not clearly diagnostic, features, a urinary dipstick can be helpful to rule out an infection but may have less of a role in confirming an infection. In these settings, the absence of nitrites and leukocyte esterase lowers the probability of UTI. Nitrites are seen in the setting of gram-negative bacteria because these types of bacteria convert nitrates to nitrites. Leukocyte esterase on urinary dipstick corresponds to pyuria, or white blood cells in the urine. False-negative nitrite results could occur in the setting of gram-positive bacteria, but cystitis is uncommon in patients without pyuria. More commonly, false-positive urine dipstick results are seen, especially when voided specimens are used. In women, poor collection techniques and vaginal contamination with voided samples contribute to false-positive findings (Peach et al., 2016). Therefore, although urine dipsticks can provide clinical information, ultimately the provider should incorporate clinical judgment and/or additional diagnostic testing when making final decisions regarding treatment.

Microscopic Urinalysis. Microscopic examination of urine can detect the presence of bacteria, leukocytes, and red blood cells. Pyuria is defined as 10 or more leukocytes/mL or 3 or more leukocytes/high-powered field of unspun urine. As earlier, in the absence of pyuria, the diagnosis of UTI should be questioned. Pyuria has been proposed as a way to differentiate between acute UTI and ASB, but recent guidelines recommend that the diagnosis of ASB can be made even in the setting of pyuria. Patients could exhibit pyuria with negative urine culture (i.e., sterile pyuria) if urinalysis is performed after initiating antimicrobial therapy. Neither microscopic hematuria nor bacteriuria on urinalysis is a particularly sensitive finding for UTI. However, microscopic urinalysis is the gold standard for evaluation of hematuria outside of infection (see Chapter 40). Beyond this standard indication for testing, it is likely an unnecessary cost.

Urine Culture. Urine culture may not be necessary for acute cystitis, but the primary disadvantage of symptom-based diagnosis is that it may result in overtreatment and inappropriate antibiotic use. This is especially possible in older women, where symptoms of UTI overlap with other noninfectious bladder symptom conditions. Urine culture is considered the reference standard for diagnosis of UTI. Cultures should be submitted for scenarios such as negative urine dipstick test in a symptomatic patient, poor response to initial therapy, and recurrent symptoms less than 1 month after treatment for a previous UTI. As mentioned previously, although a culture result of 10^5 CFU/mL or more in a voided urine sample has historically been considered diagnostic for UTI, some feel that 100 CFU/mL or more should suffice in a patient who has symptoms consistent with UTI, as well as pyuria. If there is a suspicion for pyelonephritis (i.e., fever, costovertebral tenderness/flank pain), then a urine culture and antibiotic susceptibilities should always be obtained.

Clinical Management

Antibiotics for Simple Cystitis. The Infectious Diseases Society of America (IDSA) published an updated clinical practice guideline on the treatment of women with acute uncomplicated cystitis and pyelonephritis in 2010. They note that the focus of these guidelines is treatment of nonpregnant, premenopausal women with no known urological abnormalities. Postmenopausal women, those without rUTI, and/or those with well-controlled diabetes without urological sequelae can usually be treated with the same recommendations.

The three first-line antibiotics for UTI treatment are nitrofurantoin, trimethoprim-sulfamethoxazole (TMP-SMX), and fosfomycin (Table 36.2). Fluoroquinolones should only be used if there is any suspicion for early pyelonephritis.

Nitrofurantoin is bacteriostatic and therapeutically active only in the lower urinary tract. It is effective against *E. coli* and many gram-negative species with low levels of resistance. However, it can be ineffective against other uropathogens. TMP-SMX is a broad-spectrum antibiotic that covers gram-positive bacteria, including methicillin-resistant *Staphylococcus aureus,* and most gram-negative bacteria. In regions where there is greater than 20% local *E. coli* resistance to TMP-SMX, an alternative treatment should be given. Reported duration of TMP-SMX treatment has ranged from 3 to 14 days, with the 3-day course having similar efficacy to 5- to 10-day regimens. Finally, fosfomycin tromethamine, the stable salt form of fosfomycin, is taken in a single dose that becomes highly concentrated in the urine, resulting in urine levels that persist for 30 to 40 hours. Fosfomycin has activity against both gram-positive and gram-negative bacteria, including *S. aureus, Enterococcus, Pseudomonas aeruginosa,* and *Klebsiella pneumoniae.* There are relatively low levels of resistance to fosfomycin, making it a

TABLE 36.2 Antibiotic Regimen for Acute Cystitis

	Dose	Side Effects and Contraindications	Estimated Clinical Efficacy
First-Line Antibiotics			
Nitrofurantoin monohydrate/ macrocrystals	100 mg BID × 5 days	• GI distress • Minimal resistance propensity • Avoid if CrCl <30 mL/min • Rare pulmonary toxicity	79%–92%
Trimethoprim/sulfamethoxazole	160/800 mg BID × 3 days	• GI distress • Allergic response to sulfa component • Avoid if regional resistance >20%	79%–100%
Fosfomycin trometamol	3 g single dose	• Minimal resistance propensity • May have lower clinical efficacy than other medications	63%–91%
Second-Line Antibiotics			
β-lactams	Dose varies; typically 3- to 5-d regimen	• GI distress • Allergic response • Decreased efficacy compared with other options	
Fluoroquinolones	Dose varies; typically for 3–5 days	• High resistance prevalence • Possible risk of musculoskeletal adverse events	

BID, twice a day; *GI*, gastrointestinal; *CrCl*, creatinine clearance.

drug of choice in infections with multidrug-resistant organisms, but there is some suggestion that single-dose regimen may have less efficacy than other therapies. When first-line medications are not available or cannot be prescribed because of patient allergies, intolerances, or bacterial resistance, second-line antimicrobials, β-lactams, and fluoroquinolones can be used. Although 3-day fluoroquinolone regimens (i.e., ciprofloxacin and levofloxacin) are efficacious, they are not first-line agents because of increasing resistance, higher expense, and serious adverse events, as described in a 2016 Food and Drug Administration warning.

Antimicrobial-Sparing Strategies. Given that acute simple cystitis has a low risk of progression in patients without risk factors for serious infection (Peach et al., 2016), antimicrobial-sparing strategies are attractive to consider. Delaying antimicrobial therapy while awaiting urine culture results appears to be a reasonable approach in women without comorbidities, especially if empiric therapy is complicated by resistance or drug intolerance. In a randomized trial of nonpregnant women younger than 75 years of age with acute simple cystitis, symptom duration and severity were similar with immediate antimicrobial therapy compared with four other strategies, including delayed antimicrobial therapy and antimicrobial therapy based on a symptom score, urinalysis findings, or urine culture results (Little et al., 2010). One large, retrospective database analysis of patients 65 years of age or older with lower UTI suggested an association between delaying antimicrobial therapy and subsequent bloodstream infection within 60 days, but this study had significant limitations, including potential misdiagnosis of cystitis (Gharbi et al., 2019).

Substituting antiinflammatory agents for antimicrobial therapy has also been evaluated, but currently is not recommended as the initial approach to management of symptomatic acute simple cystitis. Two trials comparing nonsteroidal antiinflammatory drugs (ibuprofen and diclofenac) to antibiotics (fosfomycin and norfloxacin) showed that between 50% and 75% of women achieved symptom improvement, but there were higher incidences of pyelonephritis or additional therapy in the nonsteroidal antiinflammatory arms (Gágyor et al., 2015; Kronenberg et al., 2017).

COMPLICATED URINARY TRACT INFECTIONS

Definition

UTIs are considered to be "complicated" when there are host factors (e.g., poorly controlled diabetes or immunosuppression), anatomical abnormalities (e.g., outlet obstruction), or functional abnormalities (e.g., incomplete voiding because of detrusor muscle dysfunction) that lead to an infection that could be more difficult to eradicate than uncomplicated infections (Bonkat et al., 2018).

Pathophysiology and Clinical Management

Because the underlying comorbidities that may predispose to complicated UTI are heterogenous, there is not one unifying pathophysiologic mechanism. Important guiding principles include the continued necessity of assessing relevant clinical symptoms (e.g., dysuria, urgency, frequency, flank pain, costovertebral angle tenderness, suprapubic pain, and fever) to diagnose UTI. In some clinical situations, the symptoms may be atypical (i.e., neurogenic bladder disturbances, catheter-associated UTI), but it is important to maintain discretion regarding antibiotic usage and to remember that many lower urinary tract symptoms and systemic symptoms are not always attributed to UTI. Pretreatment urine cultures are an important component of management for patients with suspected complicated UTI, as bacteria are more likely to be resistant to antibiotics in this population.

Best practices include hospitalization for patients with suspected complicated UTI and associated systemic symptoms. The initial antimicrobial regimen should be chosen based on local resistance data and previous urine culture results from the patient, if available. Efforts should be made to improve contributing host factors and/or to mitigate or remove any structural or anatomic factors whenever possible. The antibiotic regimen should then be tailored on the basis of susceptibility results. Finally, longer courses of antibiotics (i.e., 7–14 days) are recommended for most cases.

RECURRENT SYMPTOMATIC URINARY TRACT INFECTION

Definition

There are multiple definitions for rUTI. We support the culture-based definition of at least two culture-proven episodes in 6 months, or at least three in 1 year (Table 36.1). It is assumed that these episodes are separate events; however, there is no consensus recommendation to document resolution of any episode with posttreatment culture. Generally, a recurrence is thought to be return of symptoms at least 2 weeks after prior treatment, or documentation of clearance. In the absence of documentation of clearance, a patient may also have a persistent infection that was not adequately cleared with initial therapy.

Diagnosis

When first seeing a patient with possible rUTI it is imperative to obtain clarification surrounding the details of UTI events, including UTI testing and culture results when available, as well as current prevention practices. The symptoms that the patient attributes to the UTI should be documented, including duration and response to therapy, because these may vary between patients. Symptoms are typically acute in onset and include dysuria, urinary frequency and urgency, suprapubic or flank pain, hematuria, and/or documented fever. Patients often attribute many nonspecific symptoms (i.e., foul-smelling urine, cloudy urine, general malaise, confusion) to UTI, although these are signs more consistent with ASB (see later).

Pathophysiology

Classically, major risk factors for UTI include sexual activity and a history of UTI, but the factors predisposing postmenopausal women to rUTI have been significantly less investigated than those for premenopausal women. Some women have a genetic predisposition to UTI owing to differences in mucosal bacterial binding properties, which could be related to certain red blood cell antigens.

Premenopausal. For premenopausal women, the pathogenesis of recurrent cystitis is assumed to be the similar to that of sporadic infection. Most uropathogens originate in the rectal flora, colonize the periurethral area and urethra, and ascend to the bladder. In studies of young women, frequency of sexual intercourse, spermicide exposure (with or without diaphragm use), a new sexual partner within the past year, a history of first UTI before the age of 15 years, and a maternal history of UTI have been demonstrated to increase risk of rUTI. Increasing evidence suggests that alteration of the normal vaginal flora, especially loss of hydrogen peroxide–producing lactobacilli, may predispose women to introital colonization with *E. coli* and ensuing cystitis (Beerepoot et al., 2013).

Postmenopausal. The urogenital microbiome undergoes changes as women age, often reducing a woman's natural defense mechanisms against UTI. The healthy premenopausal vagina is known to be largely colonized by *Lactobacilli*. After menopause, decreased systemic and local estrogen levels result in an elevated vaginal pH, which in turn results in fewer *Lactobacilli* in the vagina. Together, these factors increase the chance of microbes with uropathogenic capability establishing residence in the vagina and distal urethra. Recently, the discovery of the female urobiome has raised the possibility of alternatives to antibiotic treatment that modulate or boost the innate healthy commensal urinary microbiome. Despite sharing many bacterial species, the urinary microbiome is a unique niche that is related to, but not the same as, the vaginal microbiome. Ongoing studies will help clarify how components of the female urinary microbiome relate to the pathophysiology of UTIs in postmenopausal women.

In rUTI, similar to acute UTI, *E. coli* is the most common uropathogen. Preclinical data show that *E. coli* has the capacity to form intracellular bacterial communities (IBCs) that allow bacteria to survive in the urinary bladder after antibiotic treatment. These IBCs also shield bacteria from the host immune response. The detection of exfoliated urothelial cells with IBCs in the urine of women with UTI supports the hypothesis that intracellular bacterial niches persist, which may have important implications for UTI recurrence and treatment. Although *E. coli* remains the most common uropathogen, among postmenopausal women there is a higher proportion of non–*E. coli* bacteria, with up to 35% of rUTIs occurring in the setting of other microbes. *K. pneumoniae* and *Enterococcus faecalis* are other common uropathogens in postmenopausal UTIs, which raises questions as to whether rUTIs occur because of changes in the host immune response. Overall, risk factors for non–*E. coli* UTI include history of rUTI, recent pelvic surgery, and older age. Prolapse and urinary incontinence do not seem to be related to presence of non–*E. coli* uropathogens.

Evaluation

Initial physical examination should include abdominal and focused neurologic examinations, as well as pelvic examination, to detect manageable conditions, including genitourinary atrophy in postmenopausal women or urethral diverticulum. An assessment of bladder emptying should be considered by urethral catheterization or bladder scan (ultrasonography), especially in patients with neurologic disease, diabetes, or significant prolapse.

Radiographic imaging studies of the upper and lower urinary tract should only be considered in occasional scenarios, such as in patients with poor response to appropriate antimicrobial therapy, infections caused by unusual organisms such as *Proteus*, a history of calculi, potential ureteral obstruction, recurrent pyelonephritis, suspected urethral diverticula, or a history of many UTIs during childhood. The indications for cystourethroscopy in women with UTI are controversial, because findings often do not often alter management. However, it is reasonable to consider cystoscopy in patients with inadequate response to appropriate antimicrobial therapy, gross hematuria, suspected urethral diverticulum, and suspected mesh or nonabsorbable suture material in the bladder or urethra. It should also be considered in older patients for whom bladder cancer may be of concern for other reasons.

Acute Infections

Compared with uncomplicated UTI, the most important difference in management for those with rUTIs is that clinicians should obtain urine culture and sensitivity with each symptomatic acute cystitis episode before initiating treatment. This is because of the lower prevalence of *E. coli* and the higher chance of antibiotic resistance in this patient population, as well as the need for confirmation of UTI diagnoses in more complex clinical scenarios. Similar to patients without a history of rUTI, clinicians should offer hydration and urinary analgesics for patient comfort while awaiting urine culture results. Patients who have classic symptoms (i.e., dysuria, new-onset urinary urgency and/or frequency) and prefer prompt antibiotic therapy can provide urine samples for testing and initiate empirical therapy based on microbial history, allergy profile, and medical status. Two heterogeneous trials have evaluated this management strategy with different approaches. Zhong et al. (2011) studied single-dose versus short-course antibiotics after UTI-predisposing conditions, and Wong et al. (1985) compared intermittent TMP-SMX versus daily prophylactic TMP-SMX. Both trials were very small, and, with recent concerns for antimicrobial resistance, existing guidelines suggest that empiric or self-start therapy should at least be preceded by a urine culture collection to guide antibiotic management. Treatment refinements can follow final urine culture results. Management of symptomatic UTIs should be informed by microbial identification and susceptibility, as well as the local antibiogram, which provides clinicians with information regarding microbial resistance patterns in the local community. Most patients with rUTI can be prescribed 3 to 5 days of an appropriate antibiotic for each cystitis episode, but for those with refractory infections, short interval between infection, or multiple recent recurrent episodes, a longer course of antibiotics can be initiated. It is usually unnecessary to use antibiotics for longer than a 7-day period.

Prevention Strategies

The goal of rUTI prevention is to avoid or suppress subsequent infections. Although the most robust evidence is found with vaginal estrogen and antibiotics, alternative nonantibiotic options exist as well. In an era of antimicrobial stewardship, we generally consider starting with estrogen prophylaxis for appropriate candidates and adding antibiotics if needed for persistent rUTIs.

Vaginal Estrogen Prophylaxis. The pathogenesis of rUTIs in peri- and postmenopausal women may, in part, be related to the vaginal microbial changes associated with menopause. Lower systemic and local estrogen levels raise the vaginal pH and decrease the lactobacillus-dominant vaginal flora typical for premenopausal women. Together, these factors increase the chance that microbes with uropathogenic capability establish residence in the vagina.

In peri- or postmenopausal women, there is high-quality evidence that vaginal estrogen therapy can reduce the risk of rUTI, but there is little evidence recommending one formulation over another. Vaginal estrogen cream (17β-estradiol or conjugate equine estrogen), vaginal ring (17β-estradiol), or vaginal tablet (estradiol hemihydrate) could likely be used to prevent UTI recurrence, although one study suggests lower efficacy of the ring. The vaginal tablet has not technically been evaluated specifically for UTI prevention. In contrast to vaginal estrogen, oral estrogen has not been shown to decrease rUTI and has a much different risk and benefit profile.

Antibiotic Prophylaxis. There is a large body of evidence-based literature supporting antibiotic prophylaxis for treatment of rUTIs. The most recent systematic review identified 28 trials with sample sizes ranging from 26 to 308 ($n = 2758$) (Anger et al., 2019). Of the trials that compared prophylactic antibiotics to placebo, antibiotics were associated with a decreased likelihood of experiencing at least one UTI recurrence (relative risk [RR] 0.26, 95% confidence interval [CI] 0.18–0.37), and there was no difference when comparing nitrofurantoin to other antibiotics (RR 0.81, 95% CI 0.63–1.03). Unfortunately, the majority of trials were completed before 1995, and therefore do not necessarily consider growing antibiotic resistance.

The most common adverse events associated with antibiotic prophylaxis include gastrointestinal side effects, vaginal and/or oral candidiasis, and skin rash. Nitrofurantoin specifically has rare but potentially serious pulmonary and hepatic toxicity in the range of 0.001% to 0.7% of cases of long-term nitrofurantoin use. Current recommendations are to avoid nitrofurantoin use when creatinine clearance is below 30 mL/min, and the potential serious risks of long-term use should be discussed with patients.

There are scant data on the long-term impacts of antibiotic prophylaxis on antibiotic resistance. One study evaluating lactobacilli compared with antibiotics for UTI prevention showed that *E. coli* resistance in fecal and urine isolates increased to approximately 80% to 95% after only 1 month of trimethoprim-sulfamethoxazole prophylaxis (Beerepoot et al., 2012). The most common prophylactic options are presented in Table 36.3.

TABLE 36.3 Prophylactic Antibiotic Options

Medication	Dose
Trimethoprim	100 mg once daily
Trimethoprim-sulfamethoxazole	40/200 mg once daily
Nitrofurantoin monohydrate/macrocrystals	50 mg daily
	100 mg daily
Cephalexin	125 mg daily
	250 mg daily
Fosfomycin	3 g every 10 days

Given side effects, potential harm related to antibiotic resistance, and possible nonantibiotic alternatives, we recommend an initial 3- to 6-month trial of antibiotic suppression in appropriately selected patients, with cessation of antibiotics if UTIs cease over this period.

Postcoital Prophylaxis. If women note a temporal relationship of UTIs to sexual activity, a one-time dose of antibiotics, either before or after intercourse, has been shown to significantly reduce UTIs, with generally less antibiotic burden than once-daily dosing. This is likely to be a more effective option in premenopausal women, but, as it decreases total antibiotic burden, it is a reasonable option in postmenopausal women who report postcoital UTIs.

Increasing antimicrobial resistance has stimulated interest in nonantibiotic prophylaxis of rUTIs. The most commonly reported options were recently reviewed in a systematic review (Beerepoot et al., 2013).

Lactobacilli Supplements. Although there has been a lot of interest in lactobacilli probiotics for prevention of rUTI, current guidelines are unable to support their use, given the lack of data. Oral capsules of lactobacilli did not meet noninferiority criteria compared with TMP-SMX for prevention of UTIs, but there was less antibiotic resistance after *Lactobacillus* use. Although one trial showed a trend in UTI reduction after vaginal *Lactobacillus crispatus* suppositories, this trial was conducted in young women with a median age of 21 years, and the final results were not statistically significant when considering the confidence interval. It is possible that lactobacilli probiotics hold promise if administered in an optimal way to a targeted population, but, in general, pooled effects do not show significant benefits in the three available trials (RR 1.01, 95% CI 0.45–2.26).

Cranberry Supplements. Cranberry supplements have been used for decades as a preventative measure for UTI, with a proposed mechanism related to proanthocyanidins (PACs) that prevent adhesion of bacteria to the urothelium. Previous studies have used a wide variety of dosing protocols and cranberry formulations including tablets, juice, and more recently concentrated PACs. In a systematic review, cranberry was associated with decreased risk of at least one UTI recurrence as compared with placebo (five trials, RR 0.67, 95% CI 0.54–0.83), and the data comparing cranberry to antibiotics are limited (Beerepoot et al., 2013). More recently, a multicenter randomized controlled trial (RCT) in sexually active adult women suggested that a daily dose of 36 mg PACs or more provided an optimal antibacterial effect in the urine (Howell et al., 2010). This 36-mg dose is currently available under the trade name Ellura, and ongoing research may be able to determine whether this dosing significantly improves the rate of UTI recurrence.

Immunoactive Prophylaxis. Various bacterial lysates have been proposed for the indication of rUTI prophylaxis. To be effective, a bacterial extract must be able to stimulate the host's immune system to produce antibodies and cytokines. The oral immunostimulant OM-89 (Uro-Vaxom) is an extract of 18 different serotypes of heat-killed uropathogenic *E. coli* that stimulates innate immunity. It has been shown that, after repeated administration of OM-89, strain-specific immunoglobulin G and immunoglobulin A levels are increased in the urogenital tract of immunized mice. A total of four studies (n = 891) have evaluated the administration of oral OM-89 versus placebo capsule daily with a pooled RR for the development of at least one UTI of 0.61 and a 95% CI 0.48–0.78 (Naber et al., 2009). A similar number of adverse events were reported in the vaccine and placebo groups. Urovac is a vaginal vaccine that contains 10 heat-killed uropathogenic bacteria (six different serotypes of uropathogenic *E. coli* and one strain each of *Proteus vulgaris, K. pneumoniae, Morganella morganii,* and *E. faecalis*). No differences were found in the proportion of women with at least one UTI after primary immunization compared with placebo, but there is some suggestion that booster doses may decrease time to first reinfection. Up to 27.8% of women reported vaginal irritation shortly after suppository insertion, which may limit uptake of this method. Recent studies have begun to explore vaccine candidates with O-antigens of various serotypes of pathogenic *E. coli*. Although immunostimulants and vaccinations may play a future role in rUTI prevention, there is currently insufficient evidence to recommend clinical use.

Intravesical instillations. Nonantibiotic instillations, including hyaluronic acid and chondroitin sulfate along with gentamicin, have been studied, but are either not clinically available in the United States or do not have enough evidence to support their use in a nonneurogenic population.

D-mannose. D-mannose is a sugar that may inhibit bacterial adherence to uroepithelial cells by competitively binding to the type 1 pili of enteric bacteria. In a recent RCT of 308 women with acute UTIs and history of rUTI who were first treated for their acute UTI and then randomized to 2 g of D-mannose daily for 6 months, 50 mg of nitrofurantoin daily, or no prophylaxis, the rate of rUTI was 15%, 20%, and 60%, respectively (Kranjčec et al., 2014). The D-mannose group had significantly fewer side effects and equal adherence.

Methenamine salts. Hiprex (methenamine hippurate) is thought to have urinary antiseptic properties via conversion to formaldehyde in the urine, and therefore should not induce antimicrobial resistance. A 2012 Cochrane review demonstrated an acceptable side-effect profile, low reported adverse events, and likely some benefit (pooled RR for symptomatic UTI: 0.24, 95% CI 0.07–0.89) in patients without renal tract abnormalities (Lee et al., 2012).

ASYMPTOMATIC BACTERIURIA

Definition and Diagnosis

ASB is the presence of one or more species of bacteria growing in the urine at specified quantitative counts ($\geq 10^5$ CFU/mL), irrespective of the presence of pyuria, in the absence of signs or symptoms attributable to UTI (Table 36.1). For women, two consecutive specimens should be obtained, preferably within 2 weeks, to confirm the persistence of bacteriuria. Between 10% and 60% of women, varying with the population, do not have persistent bacteriuria on repeat screening after an initial positive specimen. ASB is a common finding in many healthy female populations. The incidence of ASB increases from 3.5% in the general population to 16% to 18% in women older than 70 years of age, and some longitudinal studies report that it affects up to 50% of older women.

Importantly, pyuria has previously been thought to be helpful in terms of discriminating between ASB and acute UTI. However, multiple studies have shown that pyuria is not a reliable discriminating factor. Ultimately, the presence or absence of urinary symptoms remains the most discriminating factor guiding therapy.

Pathophysiology

The microbiology of ASB is similar to that of symptomatic UTI, although some strains capable of producing ASB may have subtle adaptations that facilitate pathogenesis. For example, attachment of bacteria via fimbrial adhesins is thought to be important for the establishment and persistence of symptomatic infection. Some bacterial strains with reduced capability for fimbriae expression appear to have the capacity for relatively rapid growth, thus allowing them to cause ASB. Alternatively, strains implicated in ASB may simply be less virulent. The absence of symptoms in patients with ASB could also reflect differences in the host response, as studies in mice have shown a potential role for toll-like receptor inactivation in ASB carrier states.

Recently, it has been discovered that, in its normal healthy state, the bladder harbors a unique microbial community called the urinary microbiome. The human microbiome refers to the collective genomes of microorganisms that may augment their environment in a myriad of ways that are essential for human health. An imbalance of urinary microbiota may predispose women to certain bladder disorders. The study of the impact of the urinary microbiome on ASB and UTI is in its infancy, and its relevance to these conditions remains to be determined.

Clinical Management

In 2019, the IDSA published an updated guideline with recommendations for the management of ASB in adults (Nicolle et al., 2019). Since the previous guideline was published in 2005, antimicrobial stewardship programs have identified nontreatment of ASB as an important opportunity for decreasing inappropriate antimicrobial use.

For the general population, screening for ASB is not recommended. Historical studies failed to show differences in the frequency of subsequent UTI during 1 year of follow-up after treatment of bacteriuric women with a 1-week course of therapy of nitrofurantoin or placebo. Recent studies also refute the adage of a higher chance of symptomatic UTI in women with bacteriuria, and there does not seem to be an association between ASB and long-term morbidity such as chronic kidney disease or mortality.

Treatment of presumed UTI in long-term care facilities, despite absence of minimum signs and symptoms, is common. In general, the IDSA recommends against antibiotic therapy for older patients with functional and/or cognitive impairment, delirium, and/or falls who have bacteriuria in the absence of localizing urinary symptoms, although they state that this is based on very low-quality evidence. There is agreement that dysuria is the most discriminating factor of UTI, but other urinary symptoms such as urgency/frequency, especially in a population with chronic lower urinary tract symptoms, complicate diagnostic acumen. Specific biomarkers to help discriminate between ASB and acute UTI are needed.

This has been a significant paradigm shift over the last few decades from bacteriuria being considered a harmful clinical finding requiring identification and treatment to being considered a benign observation requiring no management in nonpregnant women. The optimal management of bacteriuria for most populations is well-characterized, although antibiotic stewardship programs and patient education are necessary to implement a "do not treat" approach.

SPECIAL CIRCUMSTANCES

Pregnancy

In pregnancy, approximately 20% to 35% of women with bacteriuria will progress to symptomatic UTI. The incidence of pyelonephritis is also higher than in the general population, likely as a result of physiologic changes in the urinary tract during pregnancy. Importantly, untreated bacteriuria has been associated with an increased risk of preterm birth and low birth weight at the time of delivery. In this population, *E. coli* remains the predominant uropathogen. Screening with urine culture should occur between 12 and 16 weeks of gestation, and treatment should be based on results. Nitrofurantoin, amoxicillin, and cephalexin are safe in pregnancy. Additionally, a single dose of fosfomycin trometamol (Monurol) also appears safe and effective in pregnancy (Keating, 2013). A urine culture should be completed approximately 1 week after treatment to document clearance of bacteriuria. Notably, women with group B streptococcus (GBS) bacteriuria early in pregnancy do not require additional GBS screening closer to delivery. Rather, GBS bacteriuria at any time during pregnancy is thought to be a sign of heavy anorectal colonization with GBS. Thus, women with GBS bacteriuria should receive intrapartum GBS prophylaxis at the time of delivery. Regardless of the microbe, for women with recurrent symptomatic cystitis or any instance of pyelonephritis during pregnancy, suppressive antibiotics should be continued for the remainder of the pregnancy.

Patients Undergoing Onabotulinum Toxin A Injection

UTI is very common after onabotulinum toxin A (BTX-A) injection, with reported rates ranging from 3.6% to 54.5% and four randomized trials reporting a rate of UTI of greater than 40.0% after injection. In terms of post–BTX-A UTI prevention, we adhere to the American Urological Association (AUA) guideline recommendations for the use of prophylactic antibiotics for cystoscopy with manipulation for all patients. These guidelines suggest administering antibiotics at the time of BTX-A injection, but specific recommendations are lacking. Dosages can range from a single dose to use for 3 days before and 3 days after injection (Lightner et al., 2019). A recent retrospective study of different prophylactic protocols found that starting antibiotics 1 day before BTX-A injection and continuing for 3 days afterwards decreased the odds of postinjection UTI compared with women who received postprocedure antibiotic prophylaxis only (odds ratio = 0.23; 95% CI 0.07–0.73; P = .01) (Bickhaus et al., 2020). Similarly, the largest, most recent RCT used ciprofloxacin 500 mg on the day of the procedure and for 3 days postprocedure (Amundsen et al., 2016). The aforementioned AUA guidelines recommend fluoroquinolones, trimethoprim-sulfamethoxazole, or even a second-generation cephalosporin, depending on patient allergies or intolerances.

Additionally, the FDA-provided safety instructions for BTX-A state that it should not be administered in a patient suffering from a UTI owing to concerns over adverse events. Although this recommendation may be considered, it should be noted that, with high rates of ASB in the elderly, current or recent bacteriuria may not be absolute contraindications to injection. In a cohort of patients undergoing BTX-A injection for either idiopathic or neurogenic detrusor overactivity, 38.8% of patients had ASB. There was a higher chance of postprocedure symptomatic UTI in the ASB group, but there were no differences in serious adverse events like urosepsis, and similar efficacy was observed among ASB and non-ASB patients. Furthermore, performing BTX-A injection within 30 days of a recent UTI does not increase the odds of postprocedure UTI. Our practice is to inquire about clinical symptoms and perform a urine dipstick analysis on the day of injection. Depending on degree of symptoms and presence of suspicious findings on dipstick analysis, we may proceed with injection or delay injection until a later date.

Patients Undergoing Urogynecologic Surgery

UTI is also common after surgery for either pelvic organ prolapse or stress urinary incontinence. Approximately 7% to 40% of these surgical patients will develop a postoperative UTI despite prophylactic antibiotics and other preventive measures.

Recent AUA guidelines for management of ASB recommend screening for ASB in patients undergoing endourological procedures, because of the concern for sepsis (Lightner et al., 2019). However, this is mostly based on high risk of infectious morbidity after procedures that breach the mucosal lining (i.e., transurethral surgery of the prostate or the bladder, ureteroscopy including lithotripsy, percutaneous stone surgery). Diagnostic or other urological procedures that do not breach the mucosal lining are considered low risk for infectious complications. Given the high incidence of UTI after urogynecologic surgery and the fact that a positive day-of-surgery urine culture may be associated with a higher chance of postoperative symptomatic UTI, it may be reasonable to screen for ASB before surgery. However, it is unclear if antibiotics above and beyond standard perioperative prophylactic antibiotics are necessary.

Finally, the frequency of postoperative UTI is compounded by the rate of postoperative urinary retention requiring short-term catheterization, which is up to 50%, depending on the procedures performed. Two high-quality RCTs have not shown a benefit of postoperative antibiotics for women who require short-term catheterization after urogynecologic surgery.

CONCLUSIONS

UTI and rUTI are common problems in urogynecologic patients. However, in this population diagnostic accuracy is not ideal when using symptoms alone. The combination of urinalysis and urine culture in symptomatic patients is useful to confirm the diagnosis of acute UTI. For prevention of rUTIs, evidence suggests that vaginal estrogen and judicious use of prophylactic antibiotics are helpful in reducing ongoing infections. Other supplements like cranberry and D-mannose have limited data but could be helpful. In urogynecologic patients, ASB is also common. Evidence-based guidelines state that ASB should not be treated. Therefore, laboratory testing including urine cultures should only be initiated when patients report symptoms of possible UTI. Ongoing studies in the urinary microbiome may be helpful to increase diagnostic precision and optimize preventative strategies in the future.

BIBLIOGRAPHY

ACOG Committee Opinion 797: Prevention of Group B streptococcal early-onset disease in newborns. *Obstet Gynecol.* 2020;135:e51.

Alperin M, Burnett L, Lukacz E, Brubaker L. The mysteries of menopause and urogynecologic health: clinical and scientific gaps. *Menopause.* 2019;26:103.

Amundsen CL, Richter HE, Menefee SA, et al. Onabotulinumtoxin A vs sacral neuromodulation on refractory urgency urinary incontinence in women: a randomized clinical trial. *JAMA.* 2016;31:1366.

Anger J, Lee U, Ackerman AL, et al. Recurrent uncomplicated urinary tract infections in women: AUA/CUA/SUFU Guideline. *J Urol.* 2019;202:282.

Aslam S, Albo M, Brubaker L. Recurrent urinary tract infections in adult women. *JAMA.* 2020;323:658.

Baird RC, Romich E, Holthaus E, et al. The effect of catheterization on susceptibility of uropathogens after pelvic reconstructive surgery. *Female Pelvic Med Reconstr Surg.* 2018;26:692.

Beerepoot MA, ter Riet G, Nys S, et al. Lactobacilli vs antibiotics to prevent urinary tract infections: a randomized, double-blind, noninferiority trial in postmenopausal women. *Arch Intern Med.* 2012;172:704.

Beerepoot MAJ, Geerlings SE, van Haarst EP, et al. Nonantibiotic prophylaxis for recurrent urinary tract infections: a systematic review and meta-analysis of randomized controlled trials. *J Urol.* 2013;190:1981.

Bickhaus JA, Vaughan M, Truong T, et al. A comparison of antibiotic prophylaxis regimens to decrease the risk of post-procedure urinary tract infection after onabotulinum toxin A injection. *Int Urogynecol J.* 2020;31:1907.

Bonkat G, Bartoletti RR, Bruyere F, et al. *EAU Guidelines on Urological Infections.* 2018. Available at: https://uroweb.org/wp-content/uploads/EAU-Guidelines-on-Urological-Infections-2018-large-text.pdf.

Brubaker L, Carberry C, Nardos R, et al. American Urogynecologic Society best-practice statement: recurrent urinary tract infection in adult women. *Female Pelvic Med Reconstr Surg.* 2018;24:321.

Brubaker L, Wolfe AJ. The new world of the urinary microbiota in women. *Am J Obstet Gynecol.* 2015;213:644.

Cai T, Koves B, Johansen TEB. Asymptomatic bacteriuria, to screen or not to screen - and when to treat? *Curr Opin Urol.* 2017;27:107.

Deville WL, Yzermans JC, van Duijn NP, et al. The urine dipstick test useful to rule out infections. A meta-analysis of the accuracy. *BMC Urol.* 2004;4:4.

Dune TJ, Price TK, Hilt EE, et al. Urinary symptoms and their associations with urinary tract infections in urogynecologic patients. *Obstet Gynecol.* 2017;130:718.

Flores-Mireles AL, Walker JN, Caparon M, Hultgren SJ. Urinary tract infections: epidemiology, mechanisms of infection and treatment options. *Nat Rev Microbiol.* 2015;13:269.

Foxman B. The epidemiology of urinary tract infection. *Nat Rev Urol.* 2010;7:653.

Gágyor I, Bleidorn J, Kochen MM, et al. Ibuprofen versus fosfomycin for uncomplicated urinary tract infection in women: randomised controlled trial. *BMJ.* 2015;351:h6544.

Gharbi M, Drysdale JH, Lishman H, et al. Antibiotic management of urinary tract infection in elderly patients in primary care and its association with bloodstream infections and all cause mortality: population based cohort study. *BMJ.* 2019;364:l525.

Griebling TL. Urologic diseases in America project: trends in resource use for urinary tract infections in women. *J Urol.* 2005;173:1281.

Gupta K, Hooton TM, Naber KG, et al. International clinical practice guidelines for the treatment of acute uncomplicated cystitis and pyelonephritis in women: a 2010 update by the Infectious Diseases Society of America and the European Society for Microbiology and Infectious Diseases. *Clin Infect Dis.* 2011;52:e103.

Gupta K, Trautner BW. Diagnosis and management of recurrent urinary tract infections in non-pregnant women. *BMJ.* 2013;346:f3140.

Hoang P, Salbu RL. Updated nitrofurantoin recommendations in the elderly: a closer look at the evidence. *Consult Pharm.* 2016;31:381.

Hooton TM. Uncomplicated urinary tract infection. *N Engl J Med.* 2012;366:1028.

Howell AB, Botto H, Combescure C, et al. Dosage effect on uropathogenic Escherichia coli anti-adhesion activity in urine following consumption of cranberry powder standardized for proanthocyanidin content: a multicentric randomized double blind study. *BMC Infect Dis.* 2010;10:94.

Keating GM. Fosfomycin trometamol: a review of its use as a single-dose oral treatment for patients with acute lower urinary tract infections and pregnant women with asymptomatic bacteriuria. *Drugs.* 2013;73:1951.

Kow N, Holthaus E, Barber MD. Bacterial uropathogens and antibiotic susceptibility of positive urine cultures in women with pelvic organ prolapse and urinary incontinence. *Neurourol Urodyn.* 2016;35:69.

Kranjčec B, Papeš D, Altarac S. d-mannose powder for prophylaxis of recurrent urinary tract infections in women: a randomized clinical trial. *World J Urol.* 2014;32:79.

Kronenberg A, Butikofer L, Odutayo A, et al. Symptomatic treatment of uncomplicated lower urinary tract infections in the ambulatory setting: randomised, double blind trial. *BMJ.* 2017;359:j4784.

Lavelle ES, Alam P, Meister M, et al. Antibiotic prophylaxis during catheter-managed postoperative urinary retention after pelvic reconstructive surgery: a randomized controlled trial. *Obstet Gynecol.* 2019;134:727.

Lee BSB, Bhuta T, Simpson JM, Craig JC. Methenamine hippurate for preventing urinary tract infections. *Cochrane Database Syst Rev.* 2012;10:CD003265.

Lightner DJ, Wymer K, Sanchez J, Kavoussi L. Best practice statement on urologic procedures and antimicrobial prophylaxis. *J Urol.* 2019;203:351.

Little P, Moore M V, Turner S, et al. Effectiveness of five different approaches in management of urinary tract infection: randomised controlled trial. *BMJ.* 2010;340:405.

Lo TS, Hammer KD, Zegarra M, Cho WC. Methenamine: a forgotten drug for preventing recurrent urinary tract infection in a multidrug resistance era. *Expert Rev Anti Infect Ther.* 2014;12:549.

Mazzulli T. Diagnosis and Management of Simple and Complicated Urinary Tract Infections (UTIs). *Can J Urol.* 2012;19(Suppl 1):42-48.

Mody L, Juthani-Mehta M. Urinary tract infections in older women: a clinical review. *JAMA.* 2014;311:844.

Muhleisen AL, Herbst-Kralovetz MM. Menopause and the vaginal microbiome. *Maturitas.* 2016;91:42.

Naber KG, Cho YH, Matsumoto T, Schaeffer AJ. Immunoactive prophylaxis of recurrent urinary tract infections: a meta-analysis. *Int J Antimicrob Agents.* 2009;33:111.

Nicolle LE, Gupta K, Bradley SF, et al. Clinical practice guideline for the management of asymptomatic bacteriuria: 2019 update by the Infectious Diseases Society of America. *Clin Infect Dis.* 2019;68:1611.

Nygaard I, Brubaker L, Chai TC, et al. Risk factors for urinary tract infection following incontinence surgery. *Int Urogynecol J.* 2011;22:1255.

Perrotta C, Aznar M, Mejia R, et al. Oestrogens for preventing recurrent urinary tract infection in postmenopausal women. *Cochrane Database Syst Rev.* 2008;2:CD005131.

Peach BC, Garvan GJ, Garvan CS, Cimiotti JP. Risk factors for urosepsis in older adults. *Gerontol Geriatr Med.* 2016;2: 233372141663898.

Pickard R, Bartoletti R, Bjerklund-Johansen TE, et al. *EAU Guidelines on Urological Infections.* 2016. Available at: https://uroweb.org/wp-content/uploads/EAU-Guidelines-Urological-Infections-2016-1.pdf.

Price JR, Guran LA, Gregory WT, McDonagh MS. Nitrofurantoin vs other prophylactic agents in reducing recurrent urinary tract infections in adult women: a systematic review and meta-analysis. *Am J Obstet Gynecol.* 2016;215:548.

Rowe TA, Juthani-Mehta M. Urinary tract infection in older adults. *Aging Health.* 2013;9:519.

Stapleton AE, Au-Yeung M, Hooton TM, et al. Randomized, placebo-controlled phase 2 trial of a Lactobacillus crispatus probiotic given intravaginally for prevention of recurrent urinary tract infection. *Clin Infect Dis.* 2011;52:1212.

Venuti K, Cabrera C, Burkett LS, Bradley MS. Impact of menopausal status on uropathogen prevalence and antimicrobial resistance profiles. *Female Pelvic Med Reconstr Surg.* 2019;27:e13.

Wong ES, McKevitt M, Running K, et al. Management of recurrent urinary tract infections with patient-administered single-dose therapy. *Ann Intern Med.* 1985;102:302.

Zhong YH, Fang Y, Zhou JZ, et al. Effectiveness and safety of patient-initiated single-dose versus continuous low-dose antibiotic prophylaxis for recurrent urinary tract infections in postmenopausal women: A randomized controlled study. *J Int Med Res.* 2011;39:2335.

37

Urethral Diverticula

Karina Pedersen and Sandip P. Vasavada

CHAPTER OUTLINE

INTRODUCTION

For years, investigators who described their experience with urethral diverticula stated that more general awareness of this condition must prevail to improve its identification. Urethral diverticula can be difficult to diagnose. They are often overlooked as a source of recurrent urinary tract infections, chronic pelvic pain, and voiding dysfunction. The standard evaluation for all patients with acute and chronic pelvic disorders should include urethral diverticula in the differential diagnosis so that diagnosis and, ultimately, therapy will not be prolonged. Most patients present with a constellation of nonspecific irritative and obstructive voiding symptoms, which makes the correct diagnosis challenging. It has been shown that there is a significant delay in the diagnosis of female urethral diverticula in most patients. Even now, many women may have had this diagnosis overlooked as a cause for their pelvic disorders, and many of these patients have seen more than one pelvic health specialist, either in urology or gynecology, for their symptoms. Changes in the standard evaluation of women with reports of pelvic pain disorders should be instituted, so that with a thorough history, physical examination, and appropriately selected radiologic imaging, an exact diagnosis of the correct urethral pathology can be made.

INCIDENCE

The true incidence of urethral diverticula is unknown, and the reported incidence varies. In 1967 Andersen showed that, of 300 women examined for cervical cancer, nine patients were diagnosed with urethral diverticula, for an incidence of 3%. The literature shows that the estimated incidence of urethral diverticula in women is 0.6% to 6%. It is the authors' belief that an incidence of 6% is high, and that the true incidence is probably at the lower end of that range.

ETIOLOGY

The female urethra is a short tubular structure that is surrounded by multiple periurethral ducts and glands, the largest of which are the Skene's glands; these are adjacent to the distal urethra and drain into the meatus. Congenital anomalies of the female urethra are rare. Infrequently, obstructing urethral valves have been identified; more often, an ectopic ureter is identified within the urethra, which may masquerade as a urethral diverticular communication site. Boyd and Raz (1993) reported a patient with an ectopic ureter that drained into a urethral diverticulum.

It is exceptionally rare to identify congenital urethral diverticula, although suburethral cysts have been identified in newborns. Even in those few instances, the urethral diverticula have ultimately been shown to be remnants of Gartner duct cysts. These diverticula are linked histologically to persistent cloaca, and even have been confused with possible urethral duplication. Nevertheless, the incidence of childhood female urethral diverticula is exceedingly low, and, as such, urethral diverticula are rarely diagnosed before the age of 20 years.

Female urethral diverticula are diagnosed most frequently in the third to fifth decades. Most diverticula are acquired, and a favored hypothesis regarding the etiology of female urethral diverticula begins in the paraurethral glands. Most diverticula of the female urethra are located dorsally or laterally and distally. It is believed that repeated infections and subsequent destruction of the paraurethral glands lead to abscess formation within the periurethral and urethral glands. These obstructed glands then rupture into the urethral lumen and remain as outpouchings off the urethra, which eventually epithelialize, becoming a true urethral diverticulum as opposed to a urethrocele or pseudodiverticulum.

Other possible etiologies of female urethral diverticula include obstetric trauma, trauma from urethral instrumentation, and postoperative urethral and vaginal surgery. Rarely, bulking agent injections for the treatment of stress urinary incontinence may result in a noncommunicating diverticulum with obstruction of a periurethral gland and persistent accumulation of secretions. Any patient who has had a bulking agent injection and subsequent pelvic imaging is more likely to have bulking agent adjacent to the urethra as opposed to a urethral diverticulum, as it is still uncommon to have an injection into a diverticulum or create the pseudoabscess.

Urethral diverticula are thought to be urothelial mucosa-lined sacs that lie outside the urethra within the periurethral fascia and lack surrounding muscle. They are prone to urine stasis and repeated infections. Inflammation and chronic irritation resulting from the presence of urine and debris may lead to malignant degeneration into adenocarcinoma, transitional cell carcinoma, or squamous cell carcinoma. More commonly, the stasis of urine causes repeated urinary tract infections and possible calculus formation. Recurrent urinary tract infections are a frequent problem in women with urethral diverticula; positive urine cultures (>100,000 colony-forming units/mL) often grow strains of *Escherichia coli*, other gram-negative bacilli, or gram-positive species such as *Streptococcus faecalis*.

Prolonged urinary stasis may result in the formation of calculi. Calculi in diverticula are uncommon, with stone formation occurring in only 1.5% to 10% of cases. Stones are usually caused by salt deposition, stagnant urine, and mucus from the epithelial lining of the diverticula.

The location, number, and extent of urethral diverticula have an impact on the choice of treatment. A classification system for female urethral diverticula described by Leach et al. (1993) considers location, number, size, configuration, communication, and continence factors. Although no classification system is commonly used, providing an accurate description of the diverticula under evaluation will facilitate therapy.

PRESENTATION

Women come to their physicians with a host of symptoms, and unfortunately the patient's description of each problem is not always textbook-clear. Therefore, the physician's task is to identify, evaluate, and treat the pathology. A history of recurrent urinary tract infections, stress urinary incontinence, and incomplete voiding are some of the most common presenting symptoms in women with urethral diverticula (Table 37.1). According to Hoffman and Adams (1965), the single most important problem is postmicturition dribbling. The addition of dysuria and dyspareunia complete the classic triad. These are all nonspecific problems, however, and are present less often than one may think. If the symptoms are also accompanied by urgency, urgency incontinence, frequency, and/or even a protruding vaginal mass, they are more highly suggestive of a urethral diverticulum. If pus can be expressed from the meatus with manual compression of the anterior vaginal wall, this strongly indicates the presence of a urethral diverticulum. Romanzi et al. (2000) reviewed their experience with diverse presentations of urethral diverticula and decided that, when symptoms mimic other disorders, and especially when they do not improve and respond with standard therapy, it is important to entertain the possibility of urethral diverticulum. In patients who have hematuria, difficulty voiding, and frank urinary retention, urethral diverticula may be the the cause of the voiding disorder, but these also represent more concerning findings for malignant changes within the diverticulum.

TABLE 37.1 Most Common Initial Problems in Women who came for Evaluation and were Ultimately Found to have Urethral DivertiCula, from 1964 to 2000

	Mean (%)	Range (%)
Recurrent urinary tract infections	47	9–83
Stress urinary incontinence	46	28–100
Incomplete voiding	33	28–38
Dysuria	29	4–58
Urgency	28	18–47
Urgency incontinence	27	11–35
Frequency	26	16–38
Postvoid dribbling	21	4–65
Lower abdominal pain	20	1–50
Pus per urethra	18	3–50
Protruding vaginal mass	18	7–17
Dyspareunia	13	1–24
Hematuria	10	5–18
Urine retention	10	3–21
Difficulty voiding	8	2–14

Many patients receive a variety of treatments that include antibiotics, anticholinergic and antidepressant medications, bladder hydrodistention, and urethral dilations for suspected pelvic disorders. Some of the more common presumed diagnoses are listed in Table 37.2. In summary, in any case of persistent lower urinary tract symptoms unresponsive to therapy, one should exclude a urethral diverticulum.

DIAGNOSIS

To establish the correct diagnosis in women with a myriad of symptoms, it is critical to perform a thorough history and physical examination. Included in a standard history are questions relating to stress urinary incontinence, urgency and urgency incontinence symptoms, and pad usage. Irritative voiding

TABLE 37.2 Initial Diagnoses and Treatment given to Patients Before the Diagnosis of Female Urethral Diverticulum is made

Diagnosis	Treatments
Chronic cystitis, trigonitis, cystitis cystica	Antibiotics
Stress urinary incontinence	Antiincontinence surgery
Urgency, frequency, urgency incontinence (overactive bladder, detrusor overactivity)	Anticholinergic therapy
Interstitial cystitis, idiopathic pain syndrome	Hydrodistention, dimethyl sulfoxide instillation, tricyclic antidepressant therapy
Urethral syndrome	Urethral dilation
Vulvodynia	Vaginal creams, antibiotic/antifungal therapy, physical therapy
Cystocele	Surgery
Psychosomatic disorder	Psychotherapy, pharmacotherapy

symptoms, such as frequency, nocturia, urgency, and dysuria, and obstructive voiding symptoms, such as poor urine stream, difficulty voiding, hesitancy, and double voiding, should be noted. A history of urinary tract infections, pyelonephritis, and hematuria should be queried. Obstetric history, neurologic history, and bowel patterns should be included in the questions. A complete medication list with allergies and medical and surgical histories are also important.

A focused genitourinary examination is performed with the patient in the lithotomy position. A half-speculum is placed into the vagina to expose the anterior vaginal wall. The urethra and bladder are then well-visualized, and the patient is asked to perform a Valsalva maneuver and cough, to evaluate for urethral hypermobility and stress urinary incontinence, as well as for the presence of a cystocele. Careful attention is given to palpation of the urethra, with attempts to express purulent material via the meatus and to evaluate for suburethral masses or tenderness. This step may be avoided in a patient with suspected acutely infected diverticulum to minimize systemic dissemination of bacteria. Not all patients will have a suburethral mass, and not all suburethral masses are urethral diverticula. The differential diagnosis of peri- or suburethral masses is extensive and includes urethral diverticulum, urethrocele, Skene's gland abscess, Gartner duct cyst, ectopic ureterocele, vaginal wall inclusion cyst, vaginal leiomyoma, and other, less frequent diagnoses (Box 37.1).

Postvoid residual volume measurement can be accomplished with an office ultrasound or with a urethral catheter. The catheterized urine specimen should be sent for urine culture. If the patient reports hematuria and irritative voiding symptoms, urine cytology should be obtained. Evidence of stress urinary incontinence may require urodynamic testing to assess the abdominal leak point pressure and to determine the need for a simultaneous sling with excision of the diverticulum and reconstruction of the urethra. It is important to distinguish stress incontinence from postvoid dribbling because dribbling

BOX 37.1 Differential Diagnosis of Suburethral Masses

Urethral diverticulum
Urethrocele
Skene's gland abscess
Gartner duct cyst
Ectopic ureterocele
Vaginal wall inclusion cyst
Urethral carcinoma
Vaginal carcinoma
Vaginal fibroma
Vaginal leiomyoma
Vaginal leiomyosarcoma

(Modified from Blaivas JG, Flisser AJ, Bleustein CB, Panagopolous G. Periurethral masses: etiology and diagnosis in a large series of woman. *Am J Obstet Gynecol.* 2004;103:842.)

will usually improve after diverticulectomy, whereas stress incontinence may persist or worsen. The use of urodynamics or perhaps videourodynamics may be helpful in discerning this. Furthermore, cystoscopy with a full bladder and subsequent close examination of the urethra with coughing may be sufficient to determine the etiology of leakage.

One must clinically suspect a urethral diverticulum to select the most appropriate procedures and imaging studies. Many patients with urethral diverticula undergo urodynamic testing to evaluate voiding dysfunction, in particular urinary incontinence symptoms, but not all patients will require urodynamic testing. Urethroscopy may help establish the diagnosis of urethral diverticula; it is easily performed, has minimal morbidity, and most often results in the correct diagnosis in experienced hands. Urethroscopy should be focused on the posterior wall in the 3 o'clock and 9 o'clock positions to try to identify the suspected communication sites. A standard rigid cystoscope with a zero-degree angle lens or a flexible cystoscope (authors' preference) may be used to evaluate the urethra.

RADIOLOGIC IMAGING

In addition to history-taking, thorough physical examination, urodynamic testing, and cystourethroscopy, radiologic imaging has clearly enhanced the detection rate of urethral diverticula. When a female urethral diverticulum is suspected, judicious selection of imaging techniques should correctly establish the diagnosis and provide details that aid in surgical excision. Traditionally, evaluation to confirm the diagnosis of female urethral diverticula was performed with positive-pressure urethrography (PPUG) and voiding cystourethrography (VCUG). However, currently multiple modalities are available to identify and characterize female urethral diverticula, including PPUG, VCUG, ultrasonography, and magnetic resonance imaging (MRI).

Positive-Pressure Urethrography

In the female, a retrograde urethrogram is performed with a double-balloon (Trattner) catheter. After catheterizing the urethra, both balloons are inflated with fluid, one inside the bladder and the other on the external meatus. Contrast is infused under pressure into a channel between the balloons to fill out any urethral communications. In a study by Fortunato et al. (1997), PPUG was found to have the highest accuracy and sensitivity in detecting urethral diverticula compared with all other imaging modalities. In another study by Neitlich et al. (1998), MRI was shown to be a more sensitive modality for detecting diverticula compared with PPUG. Although there are diagnostic benefits to PPUG, there is often hesitation in ordering this study because of patient discomfort, invasiveness, and lack of experience. Given these factors, PPUG is probably of historical significance more than anything.

Voiding Cystourethrography

Historically, VCUG was the radiologic study of choice, because it is easy to perform and can identify the number and location of any female urethral diverticula. The technique in performing the x-ray examination is important during a VCUG; if the initial plain abdominal x-ray (kidneys, ureters, and bladder [KUB]) does not show the inferior pubic rami, it is possible to miss the urethral pathology, because the urethra usually falls low on the KUB. Furthermore, many patients cannot void on the fluoroscopy table; accordingly, a postvoid film may not show the suspected diverticulum. To obtain the best study, both lateral and anteroposterior views of the pelvis during voiding delineate the position and number of diverticula in relation to the urethra. However, the success rates of VCUG vary compared with PPUG and MRI. Wang and Wang (2000) found that the sensitivity of VCUG was 51.3%, which was significantly lower than that of PPUG, which had a sensitivity of 84.6%. Another study showed that, in 22 of 30 cases, the VCUG failed to demonstrate a female urethral diverticulum that was seen on PPUG (Jacoby & Rowbotham, 1999). The cost of both tests was comparable. A comparison between endoluminal MRI and VCUG demonstrated that VCUG missed 7% of diverticula and underestimated their size and complexity. At present, VCUG is less useful as a diagnostic test for diverticula, as it does not have the spatial-describing ability nor the noninvasiveness of MRI.

Ultrasonography

The sonographic appearance of urethral diverticula was first described using a transabdominal approach, but the development of higher-frequency probes and enhanced detection rates led to the use of endovaginal, transperineal, and translabial approaches. The noninvasive nature of transperineal ultrasound is considered advantageous in screening for urethral diverticula. Translabial ultrasonography, which is done by placing the transducer against the labia minora and urethra, also has been described as a noninvasive approach to imaging the female urethra. An endorectal 5-MHz transducer can clearly show the presence of a urethral diverticulum; this may differ from endovaginal transducers, which tend to focus on the cervix and not the anterior vaginal wall. Chapter 13 describes in detail ultrasound imaging techniques for the lower urinary tract. The main limitation of ultrasonography as an imaging modality is that it is highly technician- and operator-dependent and, accordingly, does not have widespread acceptance at the present time.

Magnetic Resonance Imaging

MRI of the female urethra accurately demonstrates urethral pathology. There have been advances in MRI methods, including the development of endoluminal, endovaginal, endorectal, and external coils for MRI. All methods clearly distinguish urethral disorders. A standard protocol that is used extensively requires an external coil, T2-weighted, noncontrast study of the pelvis, which does not require premedication, instrumentation, or contrast opacification. Urine within the bladder has high signal intensity and appears bright white on T2-weighted images. A fluid-filled urethral diverticulum appears as a high–signal intensity sac, and the soft tissue of the urethra has low signal intensity. Midsagittal and axial views of the pelvis are requested with each study.

MRI clearly identifies urethral pathology, which provides a superior examination for surgical planning by accurately delineating the extent of the diverticula. Fig. 37.1 demonstrates an example of a large "saddlebag" urethral diverticulum with lateral extensions into the periurethral space. Urethral diverticula may contain debris, infected urine, calculi, and carcinoma. When additional lesions are suspected, tumors may show enhancement with intravenous gadolinium. The multiplanar capability and excellent soft tissue contrast of MRI allow demonstration of periurethral and diverticular anatomy. Furthermore, adjacent tissues can be evaluated, again, in cases of suspected (or not) malignant changes or adjacent pathology that may require a change in operative plans.

Kim et al. (1993) found that MRI had better sensitivity and better positive and negative predictive values than PPUG in diagnosing urethral diverticula in a study of 20 women with voiding symptoms. Clearly, MRI of the female pelvis provides excellent visualization of urethral diverticula, in addition to identifying other pelvic pathology and pelvic organ prolapse (Dwarkasing et al., 2011). Therefore, MRI is often the procedure of choice for evaluation of suspected urethral diverticula.

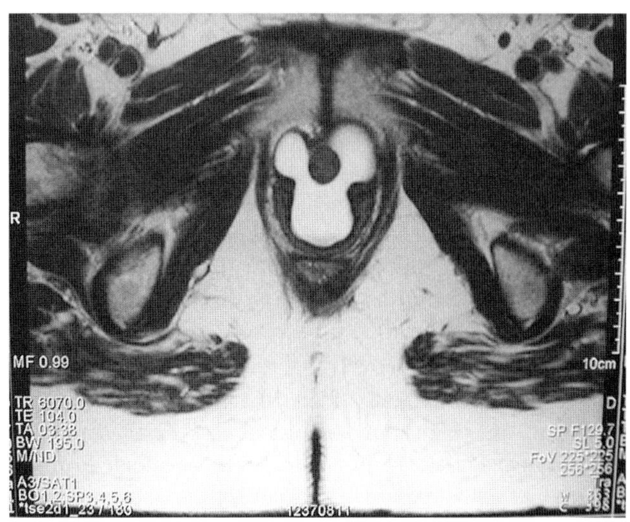

Fig. 37.1 Magnetic resonance image with coronal view of urethral diverticulum with large "saddlebag" appearance and extensions into lateral periurethral space. (Reprinted with the permission of The Cleveland Clinic Foundation.)

URETHRAL AND URETHRAL DIVERTICULAR PATHOLOGY

Benign

Pathology reports of urethral diverticula most often reveal chronic inflammation within transitional cell epithelium; however, there will be times when other lesions are discovered. Vaginal leiomyomata are rare anterior vaginal wall masses that may mimic urethral diverticula (see Box 37.1), and they may be removed during a vaginal exploration for a presumed urethral diverticulum. Careful histologic examination of the pathology specimen is needed to ensure the benign nature of the entity and rule out leiomyosarcoma. Case reports of benign pathology findings within urethral diverticula have shown calculi, Wegener granulomatosis, and nephrogenic adenoma.

Nephrogenic adenomas arise from chronic irritation and infection of transitional cell epithelium, creating a metaplastic response. These are more commonly reported from bladder biopsies in the trigone, the posterior or lateral bladder walls, and the bladder dome.

Malignant

Urethral diverticular malignancies are rare in women (Thomas et al., 2008). Until 1993, only 53 cases had been reported, with the first case report appearing in 1951. Adenocarcinoma is the most common histologic type (59%), followed by transitional cell carcinoma (30%) and squamous cell carcinoma (11%). This histologic pattern differs from malignancies of the urethra, in which the predominant cell type is squamous cell carcinoma. The most common presenting symptoms of patients with malignancy within a urethral diverticulum are dysuria, frequency, urethral bleeding, and urinary obstructive symptoms (O'Connor et al., 2018).

Clear cell adenocarcinoma has also been called mesonephric carcinoma because of its morphologic resemblance to clear cell carcinoma of the kidney. Three theories regarding the origin of urethral diverticular carcinoma are periurethral gland changes, metaplastic changes of the transitional cell epithelium, and embryonic remnants that undergo malignant change. The predominance of adenocarcinoma as the most common malignancy in urethral diverticula may best be explained by the diverticula arising from periurethral glands. The female paraurethral ducts are thought to be embryologically homologous to the male prostate gland and are the likely origin for diverticular cancer of the urethra. To date, it is unclear what is the best evaluation and follow-up in patients who may have the disease. The authors' practice is to closely observe older patients with diverticula after surgical therapy to avoid late presentations of cancer.

Diverticulectomy alone is inadequate treatment for a cancer because of the high rate of recurrence. Furthermore, the violation of the planes of spread make the oncologic principles of *en bloc* resection challenging. Adjuvant use of chemotherapy and/or radiation therapy may be required. Other therapy options may include anterior exenteration and diversion. The best treatment regimens for cancers within urethra diverticula are not well demonstrated, given the rarity of the diagnosis.

MANAGEMENT OF FEMALE URETHRAL DIVERTICULA

Nonsurgical

Patients who do not have significant symptoms from the diverticulum may be observed and treated with antibiotics and overactive bladder medications, thereby avoiding surgery if they remain asymptomatic. Small diverticula may be followed with conservative methods, which include observation, manual postvoid decompression, aspiration, or even older methods of diverticular packing or injection therapy, although anything but observation is done infrequently. Still, if observation is elected, our practice is to follow these patients to ensure that no issues develop with time. The natural history of the untreated urethral diverticulum is still unknown.

Female urethral diverticula identified during pregnancy should be managed conservatively during the antenatal period. Moran et al. (1998) reported four patients with urethral diverticulum during pregnancy who were all managed nonoperatively; three women underwent aspiration of the diverticulum for treatment of urethral symptoms, and one was treated with antibiotics alone, followed by excision postnatally. Aspiration can be performed easily using local anesthesia, gently inserting an 18-gauge needle into the diverticulum and slowly aspirating diverticular fluid with a syringe. Recurrence of the diverticulum after aspiration is common, and most patients will eventually need surgical intervention.

Thus, nonsurgical management of urethral diverticula ought to be considered in patients with few symptoms and in all patients in whom the risk of surgery might outweigh the benefits, as in pregnancy. Hemorrhage and surgical trauma to the vaginal and periurethral tissues could lead to wound breakdown, infection, and possible development of a urethrovaginal fistula. Surgical management of female urethral diverticula might be best delayed until conditions for adequate healing and satisfactory results are optimal, such as after the postnatal period or after antibiotic therapy has reduced inflammation.

Surgical Management

Marsupialization. Spence and Duckett (1970) advocated for a "generous meatotomy" to be employed for distal diverticula. This treatment was thought to be an effective treatment only for distal urethral diverticula, and required leaving the bladder neck area and proximal urethra completely untouched. It could result in incontinence if performed proximal to midurethral diverticula. The basic surgical technique involves incising along the floor of the urethra from the meatus to the diverticular ostia, trimming redundant tissue, and marsupializing the sac into the vagina. This is done uncommonly now, as surgical reconstruction is still the favored approach. Additionally, disruption of the distal urethra, which is simply a conduit for urine flow, can create problematic spraying of the urine stream or other changes in flow that can be distressing to the patient.

Endoscopic. Minimally invasive treatment options for female urethral diverticula have evolved from cauterization of the exposed urethral wall to transurethral electrocoagulation, always using urethroscopy as an intraoperative aid to verify the location and number of diverticular ostia. Lapides (1979), using electrocautery for transurethral incision of the diverticular ostia, was the first to describe endoscopic treatment of urethral diverticula. In continued attempts to simplify treatment, transurethral incision with a cold urethrotome in a longitudinal fashion, both proximally and distally, was used to widely open the roof of the diverticulum. Transurethral diverticulotomy promotes drainage of diverticular contents into the urethra. However, noting that recurrent urethral diverticula may develop, this was not considered as definitive a cure as transvaginal diverticulectomy.

Excision of Urethral Diverticula. Formal transvaginal excision of the urethral diverticulum is the treatment of choice for symptomatic women in most cases. A detailed description of diverticulectomy is included here and in Video 37.1 (note surgical footage starting at 3:00 minutes in this video). During the initial evaluation of a patient, if there is a considerable amount of inflammation and infection, incision and drainage of an infected urethral diverticulum may be needed before definitive excision and reconstruction.

After the patient is prepped and draped, a 16-French Foley catheter is inserted into the urethra. A suprapubic tube is placed (optional) using a Lowsley retractor through the lower midline anterior abdominal wall, and then placed on gentle traction to avoid extravasation of irrigation fluid. Our practice is to just use the Foley catheter, unless large diverticula and retention are a problem, in which case we place the suprapubic tube. Intraoperatively, the urethral Foley is replaced, and a Scott or Lonestar ring with hooks and a weighted vaginal speculum are used for retraction. Exposure of the anterior vaginal wall reveals a cystic mass in the midurethra (Fig. 37.2). An inverted-U incision that extends up to near the distal aspect of the urethral diverticulum and just proximal to the urethral meatus is outlined with a marking pen. A prepared solution of 0.5% lidocaine with 1:200,000 epinephrine is injected into the anterior vaginal wall to facilitate dissection and hemostasis.

A flap of the anterior vaginal wall is prepared and carefully dissected with Metzenbaum scissors (Fig. 37.3). Care should be taken to keep this dissection superficial over the periurethral fascia, to avoid entrance into the urethral diverticula. The hooks are then advanced to retract the edges of the anterior vaginal wall. The periurethral fascia should be opened transversely (Fig. 37.4). It is imperative that the dissection be carried out precisely and that each layer be identified and preserved to assist in later reconstruction of the periurethral fascia and vaginal wall flaps. The periurethral fascia is dissected posteriorly, and the distal dissection of this fascia further exposes the wall of the diverticulum (Fig. 37.5). This dissection is easier to do when the diverticulum is still full of fluid, because a full diverticular sac aids in identifying the edges of the sac and subsequently mobilizing it off the urethra and surrounding tissues. We tend to mobilize and dissect out the entire diverticulum before making any incision into the periurethral fascia. Another potential technique that can aid in the surgical dissection of a friable urethral diverticulum is placing a pediatric Foley catheter into

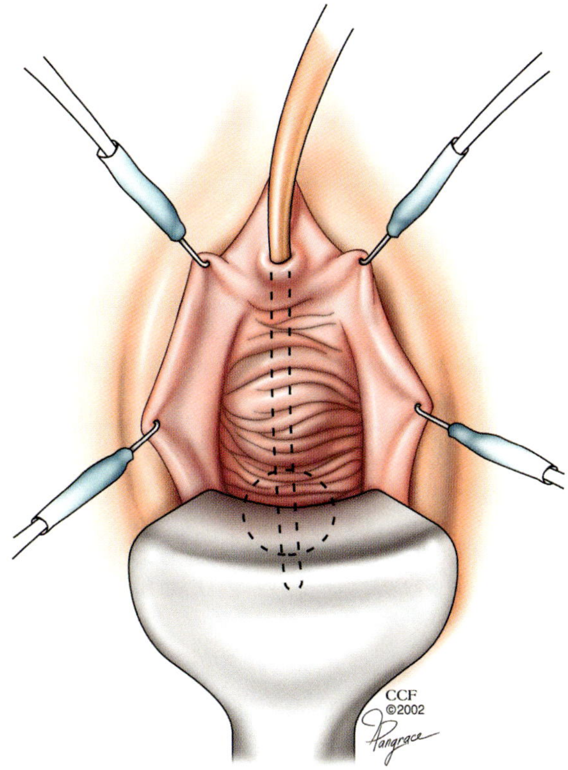

Fig. 37.2 Anterior vaginal wall mass (urethral diverticulum) exposed for surgery. The dashed lines indicate the location of the Foley catheter and balloon within the urethra and bladder. (Reprinted with the permission of The Cleveland Clinic Foundation.)

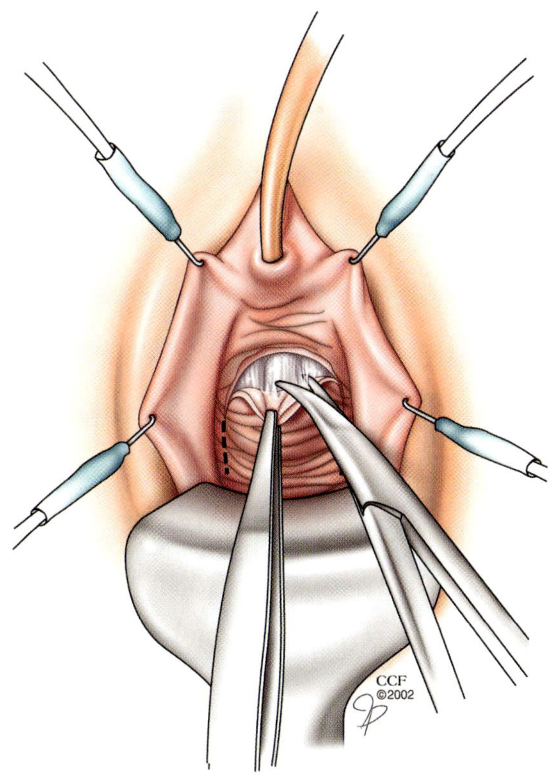

Fig. 37.3 The diverticulum is initially exposed by creating an inverted-U incision starting near the external urethral meatus and dissecting toward the diverticulum's most proximal extent. (Reprinted with the permission of The Cleveland Clinic Foundation.)

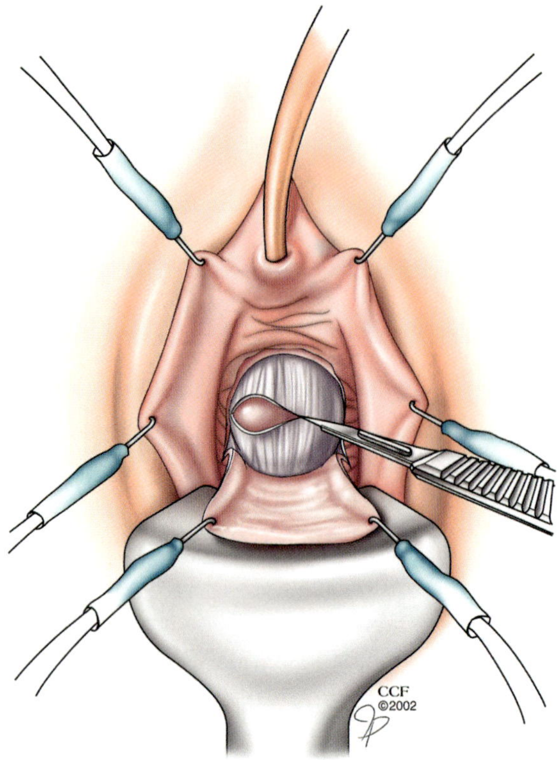

Fig. 37.4 The periurethral fascia is opened transversely to expose the diverticulum. (Reprinted with the permission of The Cleveland Clinic Foundation.)

the diverticulum and inflating the balloon, thereby distending the collapsed diverticulum.

In an intact urethral diverticulum, the diverticular wall is opened transversely, and a collection of pus and fluid is drained. This enables visualization of the lumen of the diverticular sac, after which the thick wall of the sac can be dissected free from the spongy tissue of the urethral wall. The diverticulum is excised flush to the point of entrance of the urethral wall (Fig. 37.6). The Foley balloon is deflated, and the catheter is brought into the urethral lumen, where irrigation of the urethra demonstrates the point of communication, the diverticular ostium (Fig. 37.7). The urethral communication site is identified and closed with fine synthetic absorbable suture in a longitudinal fashion before pressure-testing the urethra with fluid instilled through the partially removed catheter. The two flaps of the periurethral fascia and muscular wall of the urethra are identified, and the defect in the periurethral tissues is sutured adjacent to the urethra in a vertical manner to close the dead space and prevent a recurrence of the diverticulum. The periurethral fascial layers are then closed transversely with sutures applied in a figure-of-eight fashion and tied individually (Fig. 37.8). These layers are closed to avoid any overlapping suture lines that could lead to a dehiscence. Once again, the catheter is partially removed, and the urethra is irrigated to confirm a watertight closure. If a Martius flap or a pubovaginal sling is necessary, it may be placed after closure of the

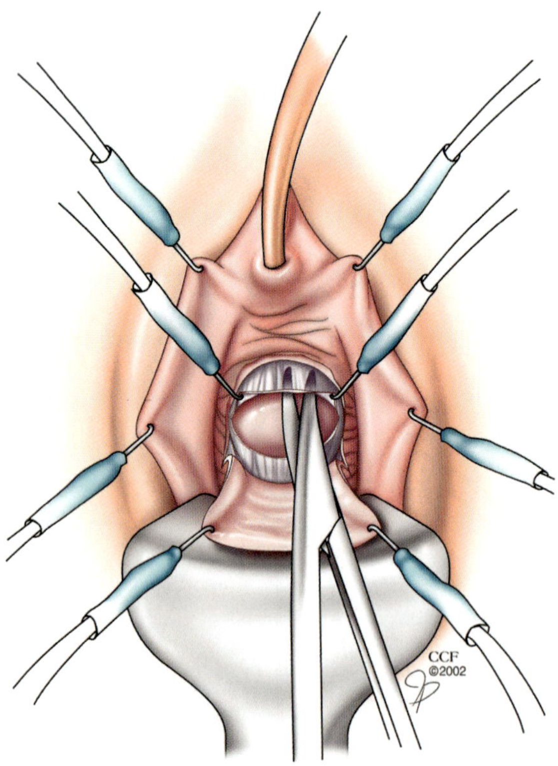

Fig. 37.5 The flaps of periurethral fascia are reflected anteriorly and posteriorly to expose the diverticulum. Good anterior, posterior, and lateral exposure are important at this step to allow the creation of a solid layer for reconstruction. (Reprinted with the permission of The Cleveland Clinic Foundation.)

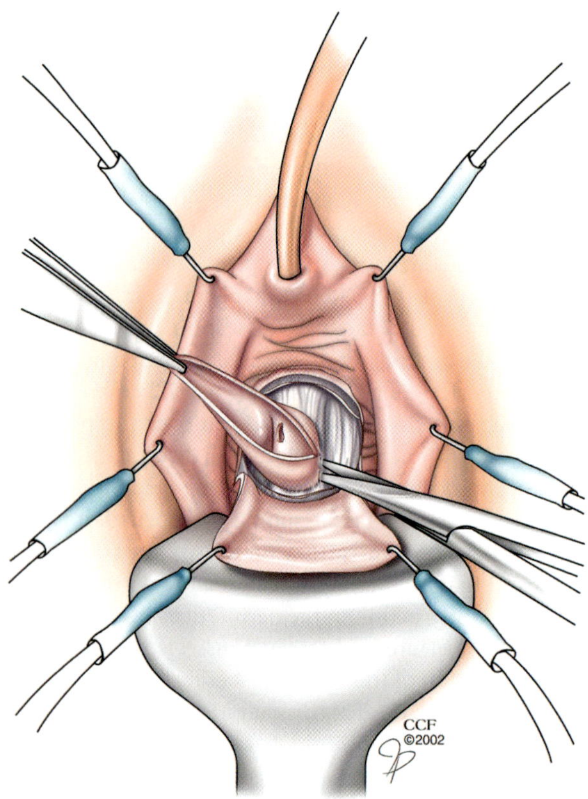

Fig. 37.6 The diverticulum is exposed completely and excised flush with the Foley catheter. One may elect not to excise much urethra, but the main point is to leave no residual diverticulum and to expose the ostium or ostia. (Reprinted with the permission of The Cleveland Clinic Foundation.)

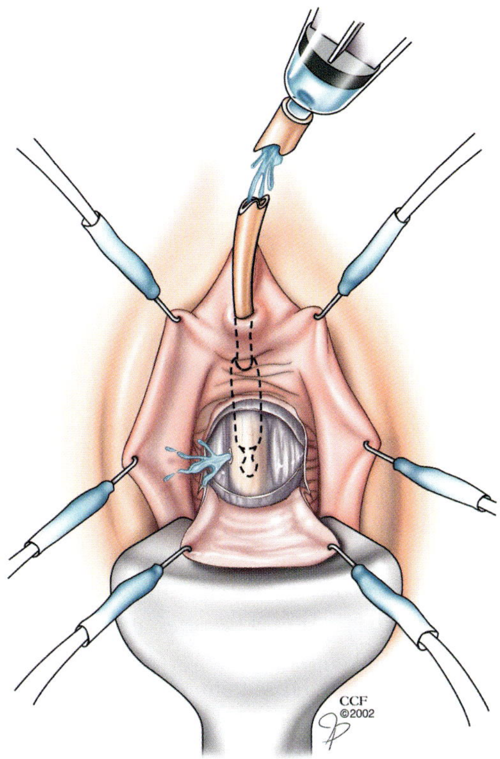

Fig. 37.7 Once the diverticulum is excised, the ostium may be located by displacing the Foley tip into the external urethral meatus and instilling saline to distend the urethra and identify the ostium or ostia. (Reprinted with the permission of The Cleveland Clinic Foundation.)

periurethral fascia, with the Martius fat pad graft most superficial, before closing the anterior vaginal wall flap. A Martius labial fat pad graft can be used between the urethra and the vaginal wall when there is an absence of adequate periurethral fascia for a second layer, when operating on recurrent diverticula, or in cases of poor-quality and inflamed tissues. Some authors prefer placement of a Martius flap if the diverticulum is large, recurrent, or circumferential to aid in prevention of recurrence.

The excess of vaginal wall is excised, and the anterior vaginal wall is advanced forward to cover the area of the reconstruction. Running No. 2-0 synthetic absorbable suture is used to complete the closure of the anterior vaginal wall (Fig. 37.9). An antibiotic or conjugated estrogen-based pack may be placed into the vagina, and the urethral and suprapubic catheters (if placed) are left to drain by gravity.

Optimal surgical results require absolute adherence to surgical principles and an understanding of the surgical anatomy of the layers of vaginal wall, periurethral fascia, and urethra. The most important factors in urethral diverticula operative success and avoidance of complications include a watertight anastomosis, precise dissection, anatomic closure of the urethral layers, and nonoverlapping suture lines.

Circumferential Urethral Diverticula

When the urethral diverticulum is circumferential, or a "saddlebag," it must be completely excised anterior to the urethra and behind the pubic ramus. This dissection can be unwieldy, and

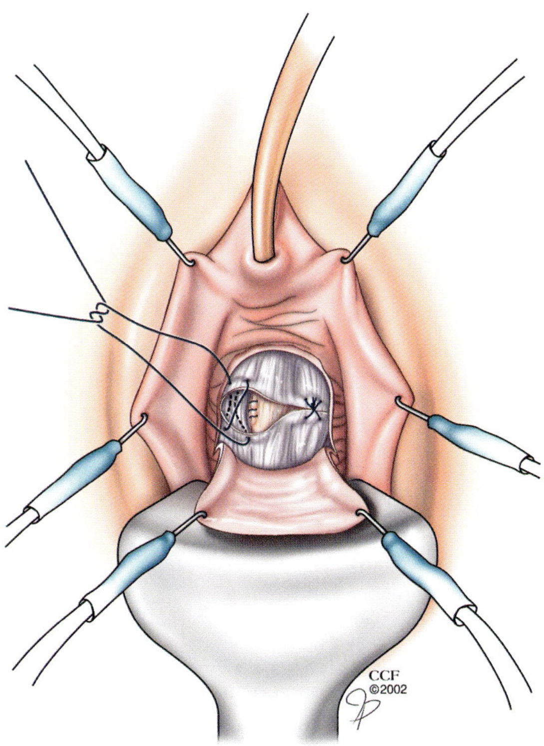

Fig. 37.8 Once the ostium is closed, the periurethral tissues are reapproximated to leave no dead space, and then the periurethral fascial flaps themselves are trimmed and closed with figure-of-eight sutures to reconstruct the urethral walls. (Reprinted with the permission of The Cleveland Clinic Foundation.)

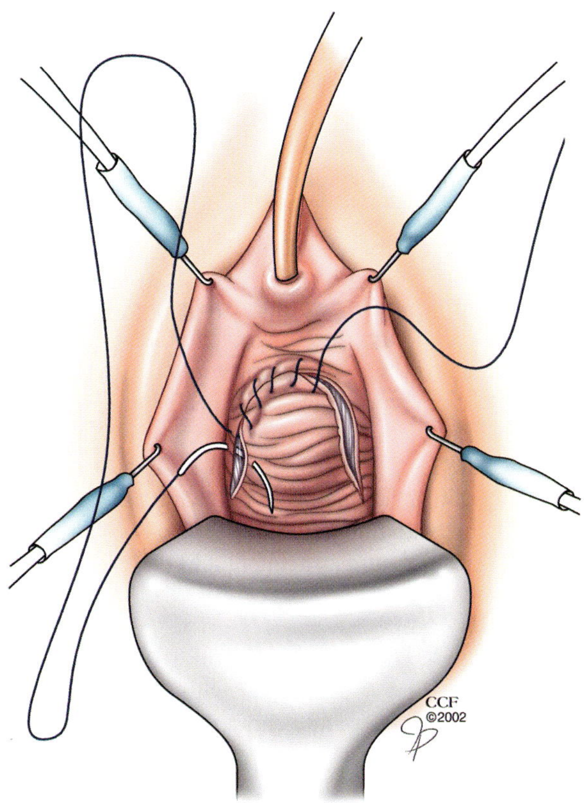

Fig. 37.9 The anterior vaginal wall closure is completed if no Martius flap or sling is required after the periurethral fascia flap is closed. (Reprinted with the permission of The Cleveland Clinic Foundation.)

visualization can be difficult. When a circumferential diverticulum is encountered, it may be necessary to completely divide the urethra and excise a segment to expose the dorsal wall of the diverticulum. Reconstruction of the urethra requires a tension-free end-to-end anastomosis; if the urethral ends will not meet the dorsal wall of the diverticulum, it can be tubularized to construct a neourethra (Rovner et al., 2001). Alternatively, a more anteriorly located diverticulum can be approached entirely suprameatally and excised accordingly. As previously mentioned, some authors suggest more routine use of the Martius flap in this situation, placed to "occupy" the space of the diverticulum, thereby reducing recurrent diverticula and potentially other complications (O'Connor et al., 2018).

Excision of Urethral Diverticula and Concomitant Pubovaginal Sling Surgery

Urethral diverticula are often present in women who have primary reports of stress urinary incontinence. Between 28% and 100% of patients have bona fide stress urinary incontinence and a coexisting urethral diverticula (Lee et al., 2008). Ganabathi et al. (1994) performed transvaginal needle suspension in 48% of patients to treat stress urinary incontinence intraoperatively before proceeding with the urethral diverticular dissection. Continence rates were high (80%) in that study in those patients who had a concomitant needle suspension and urethral diverticulum excision, but the recurrent stress incontinence rate was 20%. A pubovaginal sling procedure can be successfully performed at the time of urethral diverticulectomy in patients with urodynamic stress incontinence and may provide more durable continence rates. A recent retrospective multicenter study included 485 diverticulectomy cases, of which 96 (19.7%) had concurrent pubovaginal sling procedure (Bradley et al., 2020). Addition of the sling was associated with a somewhat greater resolution of stress urinary incontinence (79% vs. 66%) but also with higher rates of postoperative urinary retention and recurrent urinary tract infection compared with those patients who had diverticulectomy without a sling. Despite better stress urinary incontinence outcomes, the pubovaginal sling procedure did not seem to be protective against further urethral diverticula. These findings are congruent with those of Swierzewski and McGuire (1993), who found similar post–pubovaginal sling operation outcomes. It would be prudent to avoid using a synthetic graft under a fresh urethral reconstruction, to minimize the likelihood of graft erosion. Our practice, in most cases, is to stage the sling placement. We find that many patients have less incontinence with time, and the morbidity of the fascia harvest and sling placement may be more selectively considered.

Postoperative Care

Patients who undergo surgery for urethral diverticula are discharged the same day as surgery or within 23 hours, usually with both a urethral Foley and a suprapubic tube (if placed) for gravity drainage. Antibiotics and anticholinergics are used while the catheters remain in place. A VCUG 2 to 3 weeks after surgery is obtained to rule out extravasation. If a small amount of extravasation is seen, the urethral Foley is removed, and the suprapubic tube remains in place for gravity drainage, or the catheter is replaced. A repeat VCUG may be performed the following week to demonstrate the resolution of extravasation. The suprapubic tube is then plugged, and voiding trials are performed until the patient can void with low postvoid residual urine volumes, at which point the suprapubic tube is removed.

COMPLICATIONS

Intraoperative

During surgery, it is always possible to encounter an unexpected complication. Most important, it is necessary to be prepared for the unexpected, recognize errors, and understand the anatomy; this will help hasten correction and complete surgery successfully. Rarely is excessive bleeding noted in vaginal surgery; however, if this occurs, it is usually controlled with judicious use of electrocautery and timely wound closure with vaginal packing for a tamponade effect.

If the urethral diverticulum was large, and a large defect is noted in the urethra, this can be difficult to reapproximate. To close the urethral defect, it may be necessary to expose more of the urethral wall and suture the edges over a smaller catheter. Incomplete excision of the sac should be noted intraoperatively; the sac needs to be completely excised to prevent recurrence of urethral diverticula or urethrovaginal fistula.

Patients with long-standing urinary tract infections often have diverticula that are significantly inflamed and infected, even if they have been receiving antibiotic therapy. This often leaves poor-quality tissue for the urethral reconstruction. A vascularized Martius fat pad graft placed between the periurethral fascia and the vaginal wall adds a protective layer, helping to minimize the occurrence of a urethrovaginal fistula (Leach, 1991). If a large periurethral abscess is seen on exploration, a staged procedure may be required. First, incision and drainage of the abscess are needed, followed by excision of the urethral diverticulum at a later date, after a period of healing.

Large proximal urethral diverticula may extend into the trigone and bladder neck, and can be difficult to excise. It is essential to identify the location of the ureters ahead of periurethral fascial closure. Bladder and ureteral injury can occur and should be recognized promptly and repaired. Intravenous injection of indigo carmine or sodium fluorescein will help assess both ureteral and bladder integrity.

Postoperative

The most common complications recognized after urethral diverticular surgery are urethrovaginal fistula, urethral diverticulum recurrence, and new-onset urinary incontinence. In a review of the literature before 1995, Ganabathi et al. (1994) showed that the most common postoperative complications were urethrovaginal fistula (mean, 4.2%), recurrent diverticulum (mean, 12.2%), stress incontinence (mean, 8.5%), recurrent urinary tract infections (mean, 11.7%), and urethral strictures (mean, 2.1%).

Urethrovaginal fistula formation is the most difficult and dreaded complication of diverticular surgery and should be treated only after a reasonable period of healing, usually 3 months. Inflammation must be reduced before attempted reconstruction, to optimize the chance for a successful repair. A Martius fat pad graft is often used over the repair to improve vascularity and postoperative healing. Some believe that, because the urethra is a higher-pressure zone with urine flow, a Martius flap is essential.

Recurrent urethral diverticula occur in 10% to 12% of cases (Bradley et al., 2020; Ganabathi et al., 1994). Risk factors include active urethral infection at the time of surgery, difficult dissection, and excessive suture line tension (Ingber et al., 2011). Care must be taken during the primary repair to avoid these risk factors, even if mobilization of the urethra is necessary. As previously mentioned, the use of a Martius flap may help prevent diverticulum recurrence (O'Connor et al., 2018).

Secondary stress urinary incontinence that was not present before surgery is rare, but may develop in women because of dissection of the urethral support mechanisms (Barratt et al., 2019; Lee et al., 2008). Extensive dissection of the urethral wall can result in a nonfunctional urethral sphincter mechanism, and thus severe incontinence. Postoperative stress incontinence may require treatment with a subsequent pubovaginal sling or periurethral injection therapy, although these procedures must be done with caution. One can consider a synthetic sling perhaps several months postoperatively, assuming reconstruction was solid and no diverticular recurrence has occurred. There are no good data to suggest that synthetic slings are an optimal choice in this setting, but many surgeons have performed these procedures months after the initial diverticulectomy without incident.

SUMMARY

The key to successful treatment of female urethral diverticula is not only in surgical management, but also in the identification and evaluation of these patients who have a myriad of symptoms. Spence and Duckett (1970) noted that "recognition of this disorder is particularly gratifying." One needs to include urethral diverticula in the differential diagnosis when evaluating women who appear to have interstitial cystitis and urgency-frequency syndrome before these patients are misdiagnosed. The diagnosis may not be obvious, and the pathology not easily seen on physical exam; however, if the index of suspicion is high, and the proper radiologic imaging studies are acquired, the correct diagnosis will be made.

Evaluation of the female urethral diverticulum has evolved over the past 50 years; once the accurate diagnosis is made, the management is mostly straightforward. Strict adherence to the principles of surgical reconstruction will eradicate the diverticulum and prevent complications and recurrences. The identification, evaluation, and management of female urethral diverticula, as well as some of the surgical technical points, are described to help accomplish a successful reconstruction and avoid complications.

BIBLIOGRAPHY

Andersen MJF. The incidence of diverticula in the female urethra. *J Urol.* 1967;98:96.

Barratt R, Malde S, Pakzad M, et al. The incidence and outcomes of urodynamic stress urinary incontinence in female patients with urethral diverticulum. *Neurourol Urodyn.* 2019;38:1889.

Bass JS, Leach GE. Surgical treatment of concomitant urethral diverticula and stress incontinence. *Urol Clin North Am.* 1991;18:365.

Blaivas JG, Flisser AJ, Bleustein CB, Panagopolous G. Periurethral masses: etiology and diagnosis in a large series of women. *Am J Obstet Gynecol.* 2004;103:842.

Blander DS, Rovner ES, Schnall MD, et al. Endoluminal magnetic resonance imaging in the evaluation of urethral diverticula in women. *Urology.* 2001;57:660.

Boyd SD, Raz S. Ectopic ureter presenting in midline urethral diverticulum. *Urology.* 1993;41:571.

Bradley SE, Leach DA, Panza J, et al. A multicenter retrospective cohort study comparing urethral diverticulectomy with and without pubovaginal sling. *Am J Obstet Gynecol.* 2020;223:273.e1.

Catalano S, Jones I. Transitional cell carcinoma in a urethral diverticulum. *Aust N Z J Obstet Gynaecol.* 1992;32:85.

Clayton M, Siami P, Guinan P. Urethral diverticular carcinoma. *Cancer.* 1992;70:665.

Clemens JQ, Bushman W. Urethral diverticulum following transurethral collagen injection. *J Urol.* 2001;166:626.

Dwarkasing RS, Dinkelaar W, Hop WC, et al. MRI evaluation of urethral diverticula and differential diagnosis in symptomatic women. *AJR Am J Roentgenol.* 2011;197:676.

Fortunato P, Schettini M, Gallucci M. Diagnosis and therapy of the female urethral diverticula. *Int Urogynecol J.* 2001;12:51.

Fortunato P, Schettini M, Gallucci M. Diverticula of the female urethra. *Br J Urol.* 1997;80:628.

Ganabathi K, Leach GE, Zimmern PE, et al. Experience with the management of urethral diverticulum in 63 women. *J Urol.* 1994;152:1445.

Glassman TA, Weinerth JL, Glen JF. Neonatal female urethral diverticulum. *Urology.* 1975;5:249.

Goldman HB, Mandell BF, Volk EE, et al. Urethral diverticulum: an unusual presentation of Wegener's granulomatosis. *J Urol.* 1999;161:917.

Gousse AE, Barbaric ZL, Safir MH, et al. Dynamic half Fournier acquisition, single shot turbo spin-echo magnetic resonance imaging for evaluating the female pelvis. *J Urol.* 2000;164:1606.

Hickey N, Murphy J, Herschorn S. Carcinoma in a urethral diverticulum: magnetic resonance imaging and sonographic appearance. *Urology.* 2000;55:588.

Hoffman MJ, Adams WE. Recognition and repair of urethral diverticula. A report of 60 cases. *Am J Obstet Gynecol.* 1965;92:106.

Hricak H, Secaf E, Buckley DW, et al. Female urethra: MR imaging. *Radiology.* 1991;178:527.

Ingber MS, Firoozi F, Vasavada SP, et al. Surgically corrected urethral diverticula: long-term voiding dysfunction and reoperation rates. *Urology.* 2011;77:65.

Jacoby K, Rowbotham RK. Double balloon positive pressure urethrography is a more sensitive test than voiding cystourethrography for diagnosing urethral diverticulum in women. *J Urol.* 1999;162:2066.

Juang CM, Wang PH, Yu KJ, et al. Urethral diverticulum presenting with chronic pelvic pain: a case report. *Zhonghua Yi Xue Za Zhi (Taipei).* 1999;62:550.

Kato H, Ogihara S, Kobayashi Y, et al. Carcinoembyronic antigen positive adenocarcinoma of a female urethral diverticulum: case report and review of the literature. *Int J Urol.* 1998;5:291.

Keefe B, Warshauer DM, Tucker MS, et al. Diverticula of the female urethra: diagnosis by endovaginal and transperineal sonography. *AJR Am J Roentgenol.* 1991;156:1195.

Kim B, Hricak H, Tanagho EA. Diagnosis of urethral diverticula in women: value of MR imaging. *AJR Am J Roentgenol.* 1993;161:809.

Kohorn EI, Glickman MG. Technical aids in investigation and management of urethral diverticula in the female. *Urology.* 1992;40:322.

Lapides J. Transurethral treatment of urethral diverticula in women. *Trans Am Assoc Genitourin Surg.* 1979;70:135.

Leach GE, Sirls LT, Ganabathi K, et al. L N S C3: a proposed classification system for female urethral diverticula. *Neurourol Urodyn.* 1993;12:523.

Leach GE. Urethrovaginal fistula repair with martius labial fat pad graft. *Urol Clin North Am.* 1991;18:409.

Lee TG, Keller FS. Urethral diverticulum: diagnosis by ultrasound. *AJR Am J Roentgenol.* 1977;128:690.

Lee U, Goldman HB, Rackley RR, Moore C, Daneshgari F, Vasavada SP. De novo urinary incontinence after urethral diverticulectomy. *Urology.* 2008;71:849.

Leng WW, McGuire EJ. Management of female diverticula: a new classification. *J Urol.* 1998;160:1297.

Martensson O, Duchek M. Translabial ultrasonography with pulsed colour-doppler in the diagnosis of female urethral diverticula. *Scand J Urol Nephrol.* 1994;28:101.

Martinez-Maestre A, Gonzalez-Cejudo C, Canada-Pulido E, et al. Giant calculus in a female urethral diverticulum. *Int Urogynecol J.* 2000;1:45.

Moran PA, Carey MP, Dwyer PL. Urethral diverticula in pregnancy. *Aust N Z J Obstet Gynaecol.* 1998;38:102.

Neitlich JD, Foster HE, Glickman MG, et al. Detection of urethral diverticula in women: comparison of a high-resolution fast spin echo technique with double balloon urethrography. *J Urol.* 1998;159:408.

Nezu FM, Vasavada SP. Evaluation and management of urethral diverticula. *Tech Urol.* 2001;7:169.

O'Connor E, Iatropoulou D, Hashimoto S, et al. Urethral diverticulum carcinoma in females—a case series and review of the English and Japanese literature. *Transl Androl Urol.* 2018;7:703.

Oluyadi F, Ramachandran P, Gotlieb V. A rare case of advanced urethral diverticular adenocarcinoma and a review of treatment modalities. *J Investig Med High Impact Case Rep.* 2019;7:1.

Paik SS, Lee JD. Nephrogenic adenoma arising in a urethral diverticulum. *Br J Urol.* 1997;80:150.

Pallapattu G, Vasavada SP, Comiter CV, et al. Repair of urethral diverticulum. In: Raz S, ed. *Atlas of the Urologic Clinics of North America – Vaginal Surgery.* Baltimore: Williams and Wilkins; 2000.

Pathi SD, Rahn DD, Sailors JL, et al. Utility of clinical parameters, cystourethroscopy, and magnetic resonance imaging in the preoperative diagnosis of urethral diverticula. *Int Urogynecol J.* 2013;24:319.

Rajan N, Tucci P, Mallouh C, et al. Carcinoma in female urethral diverticulum: case reports and review of management. *J Urol.* 1993;150:19113.

Raz S. *Atlas of Transvaginal Surgery.* 2nd ed. Philadelphia: W. B. Saunders; 2002.

Romanzi LJ, Groutz A, Blaivas JG. Urethral diverticulum in women: diverse presentations resulting in diagnostic delay and mismanagement. *J Urol.* 2000;164:428.

Rovner E, Wein AJ. Diagnosis and reconstruction of the dorsal or circumferential diverticulum. *J Urol.* 2003;170:82.

Rovner ES, Banner M, Ramchandani P, et al. Diagnosis and reconstruction of the circumferential urethral diverticulum [abstract 815]. In: Program Abstracts of the American Urological Association Meeting, Anaheim 2001. *J Urol.* 2001;165:196.

Saito S. Usefulness of diagnosis by the urethroscopy under anesthesia and effect of transurethral electrocoagulation in symptomatic female urethral diverticula. *J Endourol.* 2000;14:455.

Seballos RM, Rich RR. Clear cell adenocarcinoma arising from a urethral diverticulum. *J Urol.* 1995;153:1914.

Seigelman ES, Banner MP, Ramchandani P, et al. Multicoil MR imaging of symptomatic female urethral and periurethral disease. *Radiographics.* 1997;17:349.

Shirvani AR, Winters JC. Vaginal leiomyoma presenting as a urethral diverticulum. *J Urol.* 2000;163:1869.

Spence HM, Duckett JW. Diverticulum of the female urethra: clinical aspects and presentation of a simple operative technique for cure. *J Urol.* 1970;104:432.

Swierzewski SJ, McGuire EJ. Pubovaginal sling for treatment of female stress urinary incontinence complicated by urethral diverticulum. *J Urol.* 1993;149:1012.

Thomas AA, Rackley RR, Lee U, et al. Urethral diverticula in 90 female patients: a study with emphasis on neoplastic alteration. *J Urol.* 2008;80:2463.

Vargas-Serrano B, Rodriguez-Romero R, Burgos F, et al. Nephrogenic adenoma in urethral diverticulum in a woman. *J Clin Ultrasound.* 1994;22:268.

Vasavada SP, Comiter CV, Rovner ES, et al. How to prevent complications in vaginal surgery. *J Bras Urol.* 1999;25:152.

Vergunst H, Blom JHM, De Spiegeleer AHVC, et al. Management of female urethral diverticula by transurethral incision. *Br J Urol.* 1996;77:745.

Wang AC, Wang CR. Radiologic diagnosis and surgical treatment of urethral diverticulum in women. *J Reprod Med.* 2000;45:377.

38

Lower Urinary Tract Fistulas

Neil Mendhiratta, Christopher Tarnay, and Victor W. Nitti

CHAPTER OUTLINE

HISTORIC PERSPECTIVES

The earliest evidence of gynecologic fistula dates back millennia, to Queen Henhenit, one of the wives of King Mentuhotep II of Egypt (11th Dynasty, c. 2050 bc). In his dissection of the mummy at the Cairo School of Medicine in 1923, Derry noted a large vesicovaginal fistula (VVF) in the presence of a severely contracted pelvis; he concluded that the fistula was a consequence of obstructed labor (Derry, 1935). In 1663, van Roonhuyse of Amsterdam published Medico-Chirurgical Observations About the Infirmities of Women, commonly thought of as the first textbook on operative gynecology. In it, van Roonhuyse proposed a revolutionary surgical technique for the closure of VVFs based on the following principles: lithotomy position, good exposure of the fistula with a vaginal speculum, marginal denudation of the fistula edge, use of a fine scissors or knife, and approximation of the denuded edges with "stitching needles of stiff swans' quills" (van Roonhuyse, 1676).

Centuries later, J. Marion Sims, advanced the surgical technique to repair vesicovaginal fistula. Sims practiced medicine at a time when treating women was considered distasteful and rarely done. With a modern lens his legacy is both complicated and divisive despite his contributions to the medical field. Sims published his classic paper "On the Treatment of Vesicovaginal Fistula" in 1852 in the *American Journal of Medical Sciences*, in which he deprecated the use of cautery and advocated for postoperative bladder drainage with a urethral catheter. His technique denuded the fistula edge, closing the defect in one layer with fine silver wire applied with leaden bars and perforated shot. From his work he developed novel surgical instruments including a vaginal speculum with a bent pewter spoon as a vaginal and utilized reflected light from a mirror. (Marion Sims, 1998). He later designed a silver sigmoid-shaped, self-retaining retractor for this purpose.

Sims is however a controversial figure as his research was conducted on enslaved Black women without anesthesia. This has led medical ethicists and historians to consider his use of enslaved Black bodies as medical test subjects falls into a long, ethically bereft history that includes the Tuskegee syphilis experiment and Henrietta Lacks. The American Medical Association recommends that if unethically acquired data are essential to science, any use or citation of these data should describe the unethical behavior and pay respect to the victims of the experimentation. A candid telling of the history of medicine can apply a new focus on the impact of the women and subjects in the narrative of Sims. Namely, the enslaved women, Lucy, Anarcha, and Betsy, who through their work, fortitude, and even suffering were equally responsible for the contemporaneous advances in surgical care. In this manner acknowledgment builds new ways to understand the history of medical research and to recognize the damage certain practices may continue to have as they reverberate over generations. (Reverby, 2017)

The discovery of antibiotics and the development of general and regional anesthesia contributed significantly to the surgical treatment of VVFs in the twentieth century. Other notable milestones included urethral reconstruction using lateral vaginal flaps and labium minus grafts (Noble, 1901); suprapubic intraperitoneal repair of posthysterectomy, high vesicovaginal and rectovaginal fistulas (Kelly, 1902); partial colpocleisis for posthysterectomy VVFs (Latzko, 1942); urethral reinforcement using pelvic floor muscles (Martius, 1928); pedicled gracilis muscle flap (Garlock, 1928); bulbocavernosus flaps (Martius,

1942); abdominal repair technique of VVFs involving bisection of the bladder (O'Conor & Sokol, 1951); pubococcygeus, bulbocavernosus, rectus abdominis, and gracilis flaps (Ingelman-Sundberg, 1960); the use of pedicled omental flaps in the repair of extensive VVFs (Kiricuta & Goldstein, 1972); and urethral reconstruction (Symmonds & Hill, 1978; Tanagho & Smith, 1972). Knowledge of effective repair of genitourinary fistulas became more widely disseminated with the publication of *The Vesico-Vaginal Fistula* (Moir, 1961). Greater international attention was brought to the immense problem of genitourinary fistulas in developing countries with the foundation of the Second Fistula Hospital in Addis Ababa, Ethiopia, in 1975, and the report of 1789 fistulas repaired during an 11-year period from Nigeria (Ward, 1980).

EPIDEMIOLOGY AND ETIOLOGY

Fistulas, including those in the lower urinary tract, occur secondary to an initial insult followed by a defect or vulnerability in the wound-healing process. Wounded tissue undergoes four phases of healing: coagulation, inflammation, fibroplasia, and remodeling. These phases do not occur independently, but overlap one another. During the fibroplastic phase, collagen is laid down, reaching its peak on the seventh day after injury and continuing for 3 weeks. Between the first and third weeks, healing is most vulnerable to hypoxia, ischemia, malnutrition, radiation, and chemotherapy, so this is the time when most fistulas present. Conditions known to interfere with wound healing are associated with an increased risk of fistula formation, including diabetes mellitus, smoking, infection, peripheral vascular disease, chronic steroid use, malignancy, and previous tissue injury.

Most of the literature on the etiology, diagnosis, management, and prevention of lower urinary tract fistulas consist of expert opinions, case series, or cohort studies, with few randomized controlled trials. Many of the studies are based on experiences with obstetric fistulas, which primarily occur in women in developing countries. Research in these environments is often limited by resource scarcity and plagued with short-term follow-up periods. It is important to review the information presented in this chapter with these limitations in mind.

Obstetric Fistulas

The vast majority of urogenital fistulas that occur in women in developing countries are caused by obstetric trauma, accounting for an estimated 95% of genitourinary fistulas (Hillary et al., 2016). Obstetric fistula occurs when women experience prolonged, obstructed labor, typically associated with young childbearing age and lack of access to emergency obstetric care allowing cesarean section (Wall et al., 2005). Prolonged pressure of the fetal head within the maternal pelvis results in ischemia and necrosis of tissue trapped between the fetal head and the maternal bony pelvis, with consequent tissue breakdown and eventual fistula formation. The consequences of obstetrical fistula can be severe and life-altering. The obstructed labor injury complex described by Wall et al. (2006) includes urinary incontinence that is typified by constant urinary leakage from the vagina. Additional devastating symptoms of the resultant fistula include gynecologic injury such as vaginal stenosis, chronic pelvic infection, secondary infertility, cutaneous manifestations such as vulvar urinary dermatitis, and neurologic injury such as foot drop or complex neuropathic bladder dysfunction (Mellano & Tarnay, 2014). Tragically, the cruelest outcome is high rates of fetal loss, with over 90% of pregnancies in women who develop fistulas resulting in stillbirth. Because of the intractable urine loss, associated odor, and lack of feminine hygiene resources, women who develop fistulas often suffer ostracism from their communities and families (Ahmed et al., 2016). There is a subsequent loss of psychological and social support resulting in limited means to access appropriate care. In some series, over 50% of affected women were divorced by or separated from their husbands, and over 70% experienced depression attributed to their symptoms. See Video 38.1 for an example of an obstetrical fistula.

Obstetric fistula is estimated to affect 2 to 3.5 million women in the developing world, including sub-Saharan Africa and South Asia. Prevalence estimates of obstetric fistula from demographic health surveys and other population-based surveys range widely from 0.16% to 4.7% in sub-Saharan Africa and 0.08% to 2.7% in South Asia. The World Health Organization estimates that between 50,000 and 100,000 women develop obstetric fistula annually (Tunçalp et al., 2015). However, the true disease burden is unknown and believed to be significantly underreported. Most estimates are based on models that combine extrapolations from facility-based studies, which include only individuals with access to health care, and from cross-sectional community-based surveys, which lack standardization and validation for fistula diagnosis and suffer from both potential overestimation attributed to other causes of incontinence and underreporting because of embarrassment associated with incontinence.

Commonly described physical and social risk factors for development of obstetric fistula in developing countries include prolonged labor, early marriage and pregnancy (mean age 15.5 years), short stature (<150 cm), and limited access to emergency obstetric care (Wall et al., 2004). In a retrospective review of 93 patients treated for obstetric fistula in Central Uganda, the average time spent in labor was 2.56 days, with an average of 1.3 days' delay in seeking medical care (McCurdie et al., 2018). Barageine et al. (2014) concluded in a case control study that postprimary education was associated with a protective effect against development of fistula. Women at risk for and with obstetric fistula commonly live in rural areas, deliver at home without access to established medical care, and may go unnoticed by public health officials or health care providers. Many women are unaware that the condition is treatable, and thus lack appropriate care because of social isolation as a result of their urine leakage symptoms. Poverty, lack of knowledge, long travel distances, and waiting lists deter women from traveling to major centers and receiving care. As a result, many of these women live with fistula symptoms for years and face abandonment by their families and isolation from society (Shallon et al., 2018).

The commonly accepted archetype of the fistula patient is a poor and malnourished young woman with limited formal education, from a rural area, who attempts a home delivery without a trained birth attendant, which results in prolonged, obstructed labor and delivery of a stillborn infant. In various hospital-based case series, the mean age of women with obstetric fistula ranges from 19 to 35 years, and in approximately half (31%–81%) of women, the fistula developed during their first delivery. Female circumcision has not been shown to be associated with an increased risk for fistula development; however, Gishiri cutting (i.e., longitudinal cuts in the vagina, made for various obstetric and gynecologic disorders) and the use of traditional postpartum vaginal caustic agents are associated with fistula development. Fistula resulting from obstructed labor is often associated with cephalopelvic disproportion. Supporting this concept are several case series that have documented the prevalence of short stature in women with fistulas, with average heights of 149 to 156 cm, and smaller foot sizes. The concomitant anthropomorphic factors of reduced pelvic inlet with inadequate obstetrical conjugate distance as a result of early childbearing, chronic disease, malnutrition, and even rickets can increase dystocia risk. VVFs can also follow cesarean delivery or peripartum hysterectomy, particularly after a prolonged and difficult labor. Endometritis and postpartum hemorrhage also increase the incidence. Furthermore, labor management with an operative vaginal delivery utilizing forceps or vacuum can increase risk of fistula formation.

That obstetric fistula is still a public health problem in some countries demonstrates the enormous gap in maternal health care between high-income and low-income countries. Women with obstetric fistula are indicators of health system shortcomings in terms of the ability to deliver accessible, timely, and appropriate intrapartum care. Obstetric fistula consistently and disproportionately affects the poorest women, whose voices are hardly heard.

Nonobstetric Genitourinary Fistulas

VVFs represent the majority of lower urinary tract gynecologic fistulas. In developed countries, obstetric causes are rare. The majority of genitourinary fistulas in high-income countries are associated with iatrogenic factors, specifically surgery and pelvic radiation. The most common surgeries associated with fistula development are benign gynecologic procedures, specifically hysterectomy. A recent meta-analysis describing 35 years of reported cases in the literature concluded that, among 2055 reported urogenital fistulas in developed countries, 46% were attributed to abdominal hysterectomy (with a total of 62% associated with hysterectomy by any route). Overall, over 96% of urogenital fistulas were attributed to surgery (83.2%) or radiation therapy (13%) (Hillary et al., 2016). Minimally invasive approaches have gained in popularity in recent years, and a meta-analysis of outcomes from laparoscopic versus abdominal hysterectomy demonstrated a higher risk of intraoperative and postoperative urologic complications associated with a laparoscopic approach. However, this difference was not seen in the subgroup of studies published after 2012, suggesting that increasing experience with minimally invasive approaches may lead to a comparable complication rate (Hwang, 2012).

Genitourinary fistulas that result from gynecologic surgery occur secondary to either direct urinary tract injuries or devascularization, often with the use of diathermy (electrocautery). Bladder injuries resulting from hysterectomy occur primarily during blunt dissection of the bladder off the lower uterine segment. Devascularization or an unrecognized tear in the posterior bladder wall subsequently results in tissue ischemia, necrosis, and fistula formation. Operative risk factors for lower urinary tract fistulas include intraoperative cystotomies that extend into the trigone or bladder neck, hysterectomy for a large uterus, pelvic adhesions from prior surgery, and intraoperative blood loss greater than 1000 mL (Duong et al., 2009). Patient risk factors can include previous pelvic operations including cesarean section, history of pelvic inflammatory disease, prior pelvic irradiation, endometriosis, body mass index greater than 30, diabetes mellitus, tobacco use, and concurrent infection (Harmanli et al., 2013).

In a study in Finland, Harki-Siren et al. (1998) reviewed the incidence of urinary tract injury on a national scale. During the study period, 62,379 hysterectomies were performed, and 142 urinary tract injuries were reported. The incidence of bladder injury was 1.3 per 1000 hysterectomies. The incidence of VVF was 1 in 1200 procedures: 1 in 455 after laparoscopic hysterectomy, 1 in 958 after total abdominal hysterectomy, and 1 in 5636 after vaginal hysterectomy. Notably, the risk of ureteral injury was greater with laparoscopic procedures than with open or vaginal procedures.

Bladder and urethral injury are also known complications of antiincontinence procedures and repair of pelvic organ prolapse. Broad adoption of synthetic mesh slings for the treatment of urinary incontinence can carry risk of mesh-related complications. Whether because of intraoperative injury or postoperative erosion of synthetic material into the bladder or urethra, vesicovaginal and urethrovaginal fistula (UVF) formation after antiincontinence sling procedures have been reported to occur in up to 0.5% to 1% of cases (Goujon et al., 2018). There are also case reports of UVF development after urethral diverticulectomy and periurethral injection of a bulking agent.

Radiation therapy, used for carcinoma of the cervix or other pelvic malignancies, may also result in fistula formation. Healthy tissues of the anterior vaginal wall tolerate radiation doses as high as 8000 cGy. Fistulas may first appear during the course of radiotherapy, usually from necrosis of the tumor itself, or after treatment is completed. Late fistulas arise secondary to endarteritis obliterans, usually within the first 2 years, but they can occur anytime from 6 months to 5 years after treatment completion.

A subset of genitourinary fistulas occur secondary to advanced malignancy, with estimates ranging between 3% and 5%. The most common types of associated malignancies include cervical, vaginal, and endometrial carcinoma (Penalver & Angioli, 2000).

Ureterovaginal fistulas occur uncommonly, but generally have a similar etiological profile and risk factors as VVFs. Although the majority are attributed to gynecologic surgery, other reported causes include obstetric surgery, vaginal delivery, infertility treatment with oocyte retrieval, pelvic radiation, and retained pessary (Chen et al., 2019).

PRESENTATION AND DIAGNOSIS

Patients with genitourinary fistulas present in many ways, but virtually all share the symptom of some form of persistent insensate urinary leakage from the vagina. The timing of symptom onset and the severity of symptoms coincide with the size, location, and nature of the injury. After surgery, radiation, or other inciting insult or injury to the tissue, symptoms may develop after an interval of days, weeks (surgical and obstetric fistulas), months, or even years (radiotherapy-related fistulas). Postsurgical fistulas, the most common type in developed countries, usually present in the first 14 days after surgery. The classic presentation is a patient who describes continuous urinary leakage (day and night) or persistent watery vaginal discharge. If the fistula is very small, leakage may be intermittent, occurring only at maximal bladder capacity or with particular body positions, such as lying supine. Other associated signs and symptoms include unexplained fever, hematuria, recurrent cystitis or pyelonephritis, vaginal pain, suprapubic pain, flank pain, and abnormal urinary stream.

The size, location, and number of fistulous connections should be ascertained to facilitate the best curative measures. Office evaluation, cystourethroscopy, and imaging studies such as intravenous urography permit the localization and characterization of suspected fistula, and additional exclusion or identification other types of urinary tract injury. The initial evaluation of all patients with symptoms of genitourinary fistulas starts with a complete physical examination. In a patient with vaginal leakage, a thorough speculum examination of the vagina may reveal the source. Oftentimes, the first examination finding consistent with fistula is urine pooling in the vaginal vault. Depending on the patient's anatomy, the fistula may best be seen using a full speculum to retract both the anterior and posterior vaginal wall. This is particularly true when the fistula is located at the vaginal cuff, which is most common for VVFs occurring as a result of hysterectomy. When the fistula is more distal, it is useful to use the bottom blade of a Grave's speculum to allow careful visualization of the anterior vaginal wall. During examination, the surrounding tissue should be assessed for signs of inflammation, edema, and necrosis, which portend poor wound healing and should be addressed before repair.

If a urethral fistula is suspected but not immediately seen, it may be necessary to place a urethral catheter to elongate the urethra and allow for inspection of the entire vaginal epithelium overlying the urethra. If any portion of the catheter becomes visible on vaginal examination, a sizable fistula is present.

If leakage is seen, and a fistula suspected without certainty based on exam, the fluid may be analyzed for urea or creatinine concentrate to confirm the presence of urine. If leakage is not immediately demonstrated, the bladder may be filled (with saline or methylene blue saline), and provocative maneuvers, such as Valsalva or manual pressure over the bladder, may be used to reproduce and confirm the patient's symptoms.

Further office-based evaluation to confirm the presence of a small-diameter VVF and/or evaluate for ureteral involvement includes the tampon test. Instillation of methylene blue or indigo carmine into the bladder typically stains a vaginal swab or tampon blue in the presence of a VVF. If instillation volume is inadequate because of urethral leakage, a transurethral Foley catheter should be placed to prevent any staining of the distal tampon from leakage of fluid through the urethral meatus. Unstained but wet swabs may indicate a ureterovaginal fistula. If a ureterovaginal fistula is suspected, oral phenazopyridine can be administered at the time of methylene blue bladder instillation, which will cause orange-colored staining of the tampon. Other options include intravenous indigo carmine, which would stain the tampon blue, and sodium fluorescein. Sodium fluorescein (25 mg of 10% intravenous sodium fluorescein [0.25 mL]) is quickly renally excreted and stains the urine a greenish hue (Lea et al., 2018). However, both of these dyes require intravenous access, and may be most appropriate if performing an examination without anesthesia. Intravenous methylene blue must be used with caution because of the risk of methemoglobinemia, a rare but serious complication.

Cystourethroscopy or combined cystoscopy-vaginoscopy is recommended to further characterize the fistula size, number, complexity, and location within the bladder, along with associated lesions and condition of surrounding tissue. Key observations include the fistula's size and proximity to the bladder neck, urethral sphincter, and ureteral orifices, as well as the presence of tissue edema, slough, infection, induration, stones, foreign material (sutures, mesh), and scarring. An additional benefit is the opportunity to perform retrograde pyelogram in order to assess for ureteral involvement. Cystoscopy can be difficult with large fistulas because of leakage of irrigation; in such cases, a Foley catheter may be placed within the fistula tract to decrease leakage and observe the rest of the bladder. Bladder biopsy should be performed as needed if there is a history or suspicion of malignancy or lesions suspicious for infectious agents, such as tuberculosis, contributing to the development of fistula.

There is no clear consensus on the optimal imaging modality that should be performed to diagnose and determine the extent of a urinary tract fistula. In fact, imaging is frequently not required to make a diagnosis and treat a vesicovaginal or UVF, but it may be helpful. In a multiinstitutional study of 226 VVFs diagnosed in the United States, 23% of fistulas were diagnosed and managed based on physical examination alone, while the other 77% were assessed with some form of imaging or cystoscopy (Oakley et al., 2014).

If one chooses to pursue imaging, the choice of study should be tailored to maximize the likelihood of detecting the fistula based on suspected location. Suspected bladder injuries can be evaluated using retrograde cystourethrography, but for suspected urethral injuries, voiding cystourethrogram is better. However, we prefer intravenous urography with cross-sectional imaging, such as computed tomography (CT) or magnetic resonance urogram, which evaluates not only the bladder but also the ureters for fistula or obstruction (Fig 38.1). However, this technique may not be optimal for suspected concomitant ureteral and bladder fistulas, as they are sometimes difficult to distinguish and, under distension of the bladder, may lead to poor or no visualization of a small VVF. If the fistula is clearly seen on physical exam, imaging may be of less value. In the uncommon setting of vesicouterine fistula, hysterosalpingography may be useful. Other advanced imaging techniques include subtraction magnetic resonance fistulography and endocavitary ultrasound with or without Doppler and contrast (Dwarkasing et al., 2004; Volkmer et al., 2000).

CONSERVATIVE MANAGEMENT

Various conservative or minimally invasive therapies are available for lower urinary tract fistulas, although the true viability

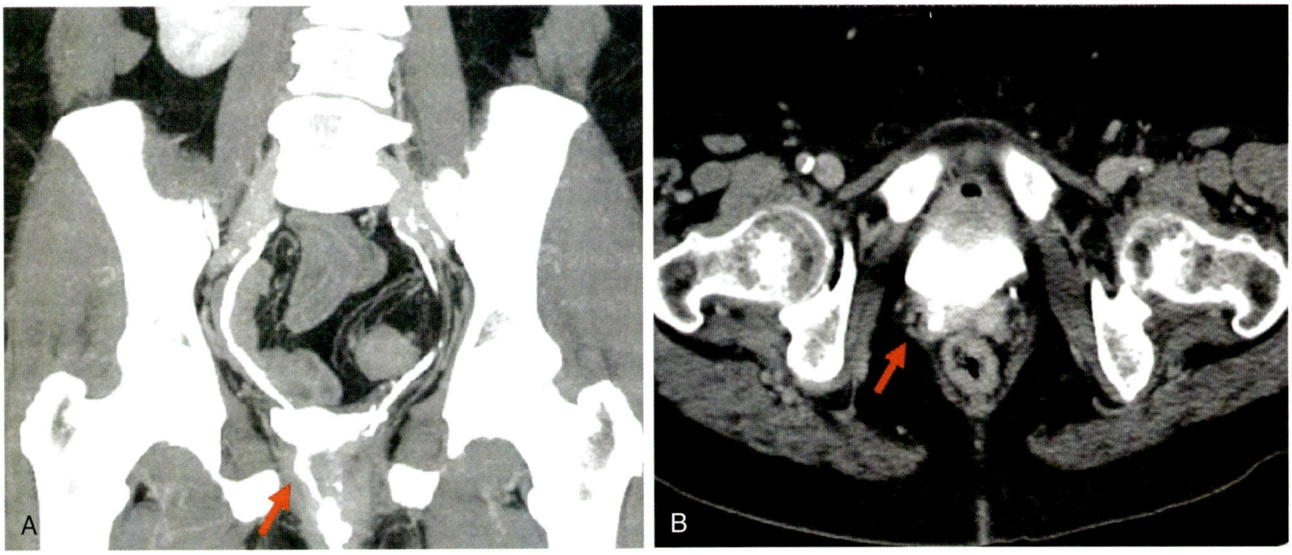

Fig. 38.1 Computed tomography (CT) urography can be useful to demonstrate ureterovaginal fistulas that are not identified on physical exam. Coronal (**A**) and axial (**B**) cuts of a CT urogram demonstrate a distal right ureterovaginal fistula (*red arrow*).

and success of these treatment modalities are unknown, as the literature consists mostly of case reports and small retrospective series. The most conservative treatment of a VVF is simply prolonged bladder drainage with a Foley catheter. In a retrospective analysis of 1716 women with obstetric VVF, continuous catheter drainage resulted in spontaneous fistula closure in 15% of patients. Spontaneous closure occurred in 50% to 60% of patients with fistulas that were 2 cm or less and who presented for care no later than 4 to 6 weeks after delivery (Waaldijk, 1994; Waaldijk, 2004). Because it may be logistically difficult to repair a VVF immediately, and/or there may be tissue factors such as necrosis preventing immediate repair, it is reasonable to proceed with a trial of continuous bladder drainage for 4 weeks in fistulas that are less than 1 cm in diameter and unrelated to malignancy or radiation, as these fistulas may spontaneously resolve in 12% to 80% of cases.

Other less invasive options include curetting, electrofulguration, and laser ablation to deepithelialize the fistula tract and allow it to spontaneously heal while the bladder is continuously drained. Once the fistula tract has been deepithelialized, injection of agents such as fibrin glue and collagen into the fistula tract has been shown to successfully promote closure. Most of these studies report successful treatment in small fistulas (≤5 mm) resulting from gynecologic surgery. There have also been reports of using these methods to successfully close radiation-induced fistulas. Agents such as cyanoacrylic glue administered percutaneously, endoscopically, or vaginally have been used in a series of 13 urinary tract fistulas of differing etiology, with an 85% success rate after a mean follow-up period of 35 months (Muto et al., 2005). The failures were in larger fistulas (>1 cm). Nonsurgical fistula closure is best attempted in a patient who has a small fistula, who is a poor surgical candidate, or who desires to first try less invasive options.

Since the 1990s, the recommended initial management of an isolated ureterovaginal fistula has been ureteral stenting when feasible. In 1995, Selzman et al. reported 100% successful curative treatment of ureterovaginal fistula among seven patients in whom stent placement was feasible. More recently, Chen et al. (2019) described their 13-year experience with ureteral stent placement. Among 12 patients who underwent conservative management, 11 (92%) were able to be successfully stented (8 retrograde, 3 antegrade). At a median stent duration of 10 weeks, all patients had successful closure of ureterovaginal fistula. Stenting may be more successful when performed sooner rather than later. In a series by Shaw et al. (2014), stent failure occurred in two patients who underwent stent placement at 90 and 390 days after initial surgery. However, one patient who was stented 780 days after surgery experienced full resolution of symptoms.

Patients who undergo stent placement should be counseled about the risks of infection, stone formation, and ureteral stricture formation. After 8 to 12 weeks, a retrograde pyelogram can be performed to evaluate for persistence of the fistula. If the fistula has healed, the stent may be removed, and a renal ultrasound, CT urogram, or nuclear renogram may be performed after 4 to 6 weeks to rule out subsequent stricture formation and obstruction.

If stenting is not possible, or the patient fails treatment, interval management with percutaneous nephrostomy may be used until inflammation has subsided and the patient can safely undergo surgery.

TIMING OF SURGICAL REPAIR

The timing of surgical repair for a lower urinary tract fistula has long been a point of contention (early vs. delayed attempt at closure). We believe timing primarily depends on the condition and quality of the tissue and surgeon experience. There is little objective evidence to suggest optimal timing for repair or a significant benefit to waiting 3 to 6 months after fistula formation.

Most contemporary studies have shown that there is little advantage to delaying treatment, and that repair can be equally successful without a 3- to 6-month waiting period. This can spare the patient the devastating physical, psychological, and social impacts on quality of life from prolonged high-grade urinary incontinence. Blaivas et al. (1995) recommended that the timing of repair be individualized and based on examination or endoscopic evidence of healing. We would add surgeon experience/expertise to that. When the fistula site and adjacent tissue are pliable, noninflamed, epithelialized, and free of granulation tissue and necrosis, little is gained by waiting longer. Corticosteroids and nonsteroidal antiinflammatory drugs have been used by some to facilitate early surgery, but their efficacy has not been proven, and their use is not routine. We recommend transurethral catheter for continuous bladder drainage for management of small fistulas during this time, as the fistula may spontaneously close. Studies have shown successful repair rates of 91% to 100% in posthysterectomy VVFs that were closed within 35 days of surgery (Cruikshank, 1988; Shelbaia & Hashish, 2007). In a large series of obstetric VVFs in which 88% of the fistulas were repaired within 60 days, more than 90% of fistulas were successfully closed (Waaldijk, 1994; Waaldijk, 2004).

PRESURGICAL MANAGEMENT

Once the decision has been made to proceed with surgical correction of the fistula, patients awaiting surgical repair should be given perineal and urinary care instructions. Leakage from small fistulas may be controlled by frequent voiding and the use of tampons, perineal pads, or silica-impregnated incontinence pants. A vaginal diaphragm with a watertight attachment to a urinary catheter can collect urine from larger fistulas in a leg bag. Perineal care is important and makes the patient more comfortable and tolerant of delayed closure. Frequent pad changes are required to minimize inflammatory edema and vulvar irritation. The addition of bidet-style toilet seats to home toilets can improve compliance with and convenience of perineal care. The dermatitis that can result from the constant urinary leakage can additionally be treated with Sitz baths and zinc oxide barrier ointments. Before surgical repair, vaginal estrogen can be given to women who are surgically or naturally postmenopausal to improve urogenital tissue integrity. In malnourished patients, a high-protein diet, vitamin and trace elements supplements, and correction of anemia are essential before surgical repair. Many experts recommend that surgery not be performed during menstruation because of the increased tissue vascularity.

We recommend administration of one dose of antibiotic prophylaxis, usually a first-generation cephalosporin, at the time of surgical repair. In a placebo-controlled randomized trial of 79 obstetric fistula patients who underwent repair via abdominal, vaginal, or combined routes, antibiotic prophylaxis (ampicillin 500 mg) administered intraoperatively did not improve repair success or decrease incontinence; however, fewer patients who received antibiotics developed a urinary tract infection on postoperative day 10 (40% vs. 90%, odds ratio 0.07, 95% confidence interval 0.01–0.55) (Tomlinson & Thornton, 1998). More recently, another randomized trial compared one dose of intraoperative antibiotics (gentamicin 80 mg) with extended use of antibiotics started 2 to 3 hours after completion of surgery and continued for 7 days in 722 obstetric fistula patients. No differences were found in repair success (95% for the gentamicin group vs. 89% for the extended antibiotic group), length of hospital stay, rates of incontinence, fever, or postoperative infection (Muleta et al., 2010). In cases of long-term chronic catheter drainage with associated catheter cystitis, catheter removal 1 to 2 weeks prior to surgery can be considered. Furthermore, if an indwelling catheter does not significantly reduce incontinence and improve quality of life for patients while awaiting fistula repair, we would prefer that it be removed.

SURGICAL REPAIR

The following important principles for a successful repair apply to all types of fistula: adequate exposure and mobilization of the fistula tract; reapproximation of healthy tissue in several layers to ensure a watertight closure; tension-free suture lines; interposition of a healthy, well-vascularized tissue flap when necessary; and adequate bladder drainage of urine in the postoperative period to allow complete healing.

Lower urinary tract fistulas can be repaired vaginally, abdominally, laparoscopically, or robotically. Most studies report high fistula closure rates, with highest success after the first attempt and decreased success with subsequent attempts. There is limited level I evidence recommending one surgical technique over another, with very little information on topics such as the optimal technique, route of surgery, or suture type or size. Therefore, much of what is presented regarding techniques for surgical repair is based on the experiences of the authors, expert opinions, and published study findings. Risk factors for failure include complete loss of the posterior wall of the urethra, severe vaginal scarring, large fistula replacing anterior vaginal wall, circumferential fistula, and irradiated tissue. Other factors that may contribute to repair failure include the surgeon's experience, health facility availability, patient's general health, and number of attempted repairs.

Vaginal Repair of Vesicovaginal Fistula

The majority of VVFs can be closed transvaginally, although examination under anesthesia may be necessary to identify tissue edges and to plan surgical approaches in certain situations such as large fistulas, restricted vaginal access because of small genital hiatus, or patients with a very long vagina (>10 cm) with limited descent. There are numerous advantages of a vaginal over an open abdominal approach, including decreased operative time, blood loss, and postoperative pain, as well as shorter hospital stays. Additionally, because many of these procedures are performed in developing countries under regional anesthesia, patients are able to better tolerate vaginal surgery.

When performing a VVF repair, it is important to assess the location of the fistula from the vaginal side as well as the bladder side. Examination of the vagina allows the surgeon to determine the quality of the tissues and the mobility of the vaginal cuff and anterior vaginal wall and to estimate the proximity of the peritoneum. It is critical to identify the fistula before starting the procedure, and filling the bladder with a solution of indigo carmine or methylene blue can facilitate identification. The bladder side of the VVF is assessed cystoscopically. Often, the fistula is larger than it appears on the vaginal side. If the fistula encroaches on one or both ureteral orifices, stents can be placed in the ureters at the outset of surgery. As a general rule,

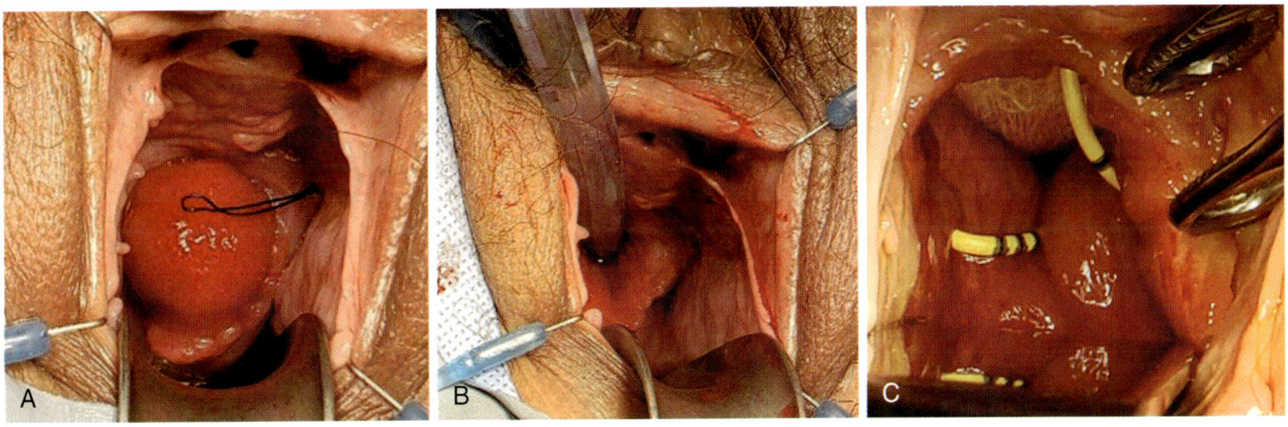

Fig. 38.2 A large vesicovaginal fistula after prior vaginal surgery is visualized. **A**, Bladder herniation through the fistula. **B**, Herniation is reduced to visualize the fistula margin. **C**, Ureteral orifices are cannulated using 5-French ureteral catheters under direct vision.

stents should be placed if the fistula is within 0.5 to 1 cm of a ureteral orifice. If the fistula is large, the ureteral orifices may be cannulated under direct visualization (Fig 38.2).

Most VVFs will be located along the anterior vaginal wall or at the vaginal cuff following prior hysterectomy. The first step in a successful repair is to control the fistula. This can be done by placing a transurethral catheter or ureteral catheter into the tract from the vagina into the bladder. Then, gentle traction can be applied to expose the fistula and facilitate mobilization. Stay sutures can also be placed through the vaginal epithelium on the margins of the fistula to allow traction on the tissue and make the fistula more accessible. If needed, very small fistulas can be gently dilated using lacrimal duct probes and small dilators to allow insertion of a catheter through the fistula tract (Fig. 38.3). Another technique is to pass a wire through the fistula, in either direction, to allow dilation with sequential catheters. Alternatively, small-caliber vascular catheters such as the Fogarty Arterial Embolectomy Catheter (Edwards Lifesciences, Irvine, CA), which range from 2- to 7-French, with an inflatable catheter balloon at the tip, can be placed within the fistula tract to improve descent and stability for dissection.

Although not commonly needed, placement of a suprapubic tube at this time can be considered in cases where a transurethral catheter may sit on the site of repair or if prolonged urinary drainage is expected. Suprapubic tube placement may be done in a percutaneous or open fashion. To allow distension of the bladder, the fistula catheter balloon may be inflated to prevent leakage.

The Latzko technique is commonly used for repair of posthysterectomy VVFs, with reported cure rates between 93% and 100%. Because it is a relatively simple procedure, it has the advantage of a short operating time, minimal blood loss, and low postoperative morbidity. Inadequate vaginal length is not typically a problem unless the vagina is already foreshortened. The vaginal epithelium is mobilized around the fistula margin for at least 2.5 cm in all directions, with closure of the vesicovaginal fibromuscular connective tissue and then placement of interrupted absorbable sutures (Fig 38.4). Because the fistula tract is not typically excised, the vaginal tissue in contact with the bladder reepithelializes as

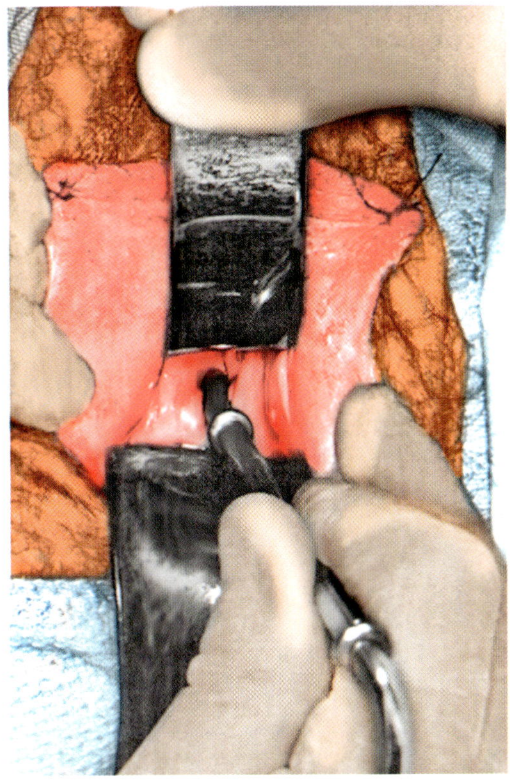

Fig. 38.3 The vesicovaginal fistula is dilated to allow insertion of a pediatric Foley catheter through the fistula and into the bladder. Use of a catheter helps evert the fistula edge, thus improving descent and stability for dissection.

transitional epithelium. See Video 38.2 for a demonstration of a modified Latzko VVF repair.

For complicated or larger fistulas, such as fistulas typically seen after obstructed labor, a classic fistula closure technique may be best. Infiltration of tissues with normal saline or a dilute solution of epinephrine (1:200,000) or vasopressin may aid in dissection in the appropriate plane and maintenance of local hemostasis. A circumscribing incision is then made around the fistula. This incision can be extended anteriorly for a more proximal fistula, or posteriorly for a more distal fistula. The

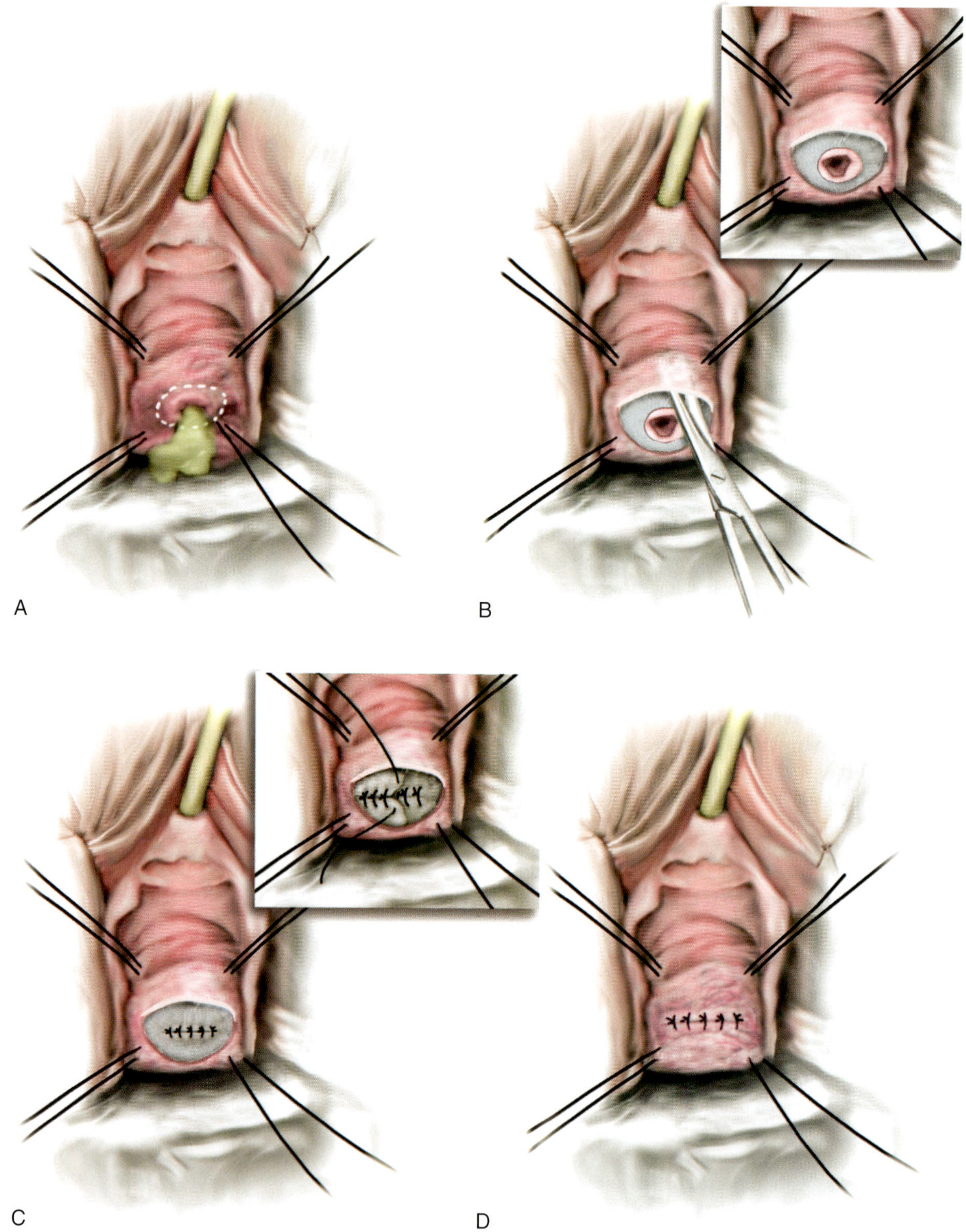

Fig. 38.4 The Latzko technique of partial colpocleisis. **A**, Stay sutures are placed in the vaginal wall to assist in exposing the fistula. An initial circumferential incision is made around the fistulous tract (dotted circle). **B**, Sharp dissection mobilizes the vaginal mucosa for a distance of 2.5 cm in all directions. **C**, The vaginal edges are then approximated with delayed absorbable sutures. Note that no attempt is made to excise the fistulous tract or freshen the edges of the fistula. If possible, a second layer of pubocervical fascia is approximated over the initial layer *(inset)*. **D**, The vaginal mucosa is approximated, thus completing the repair.

vaginal epithelium surrounding the fistula is then dissected off the underlying vesicovaginal fibromuscular connective tissue to permit a tension-free closure of the fistula in layers (Fig. 38.5). In our experience, after the immediate scarred area is mobilized, more lateral vaginal dissection progresses with more ease, and ample fibromuscular layer mobility can be achieved. Depending on the size of the fistula, this may require a fair amount of mobilization of the vagina. To assist this process, traction is applied to the scar tissue surrounding the fistula, and countertraction is placed on the edges of the vaginal epithelium to facilitate accurate plane identification and undermining of the vaginal epithelium.

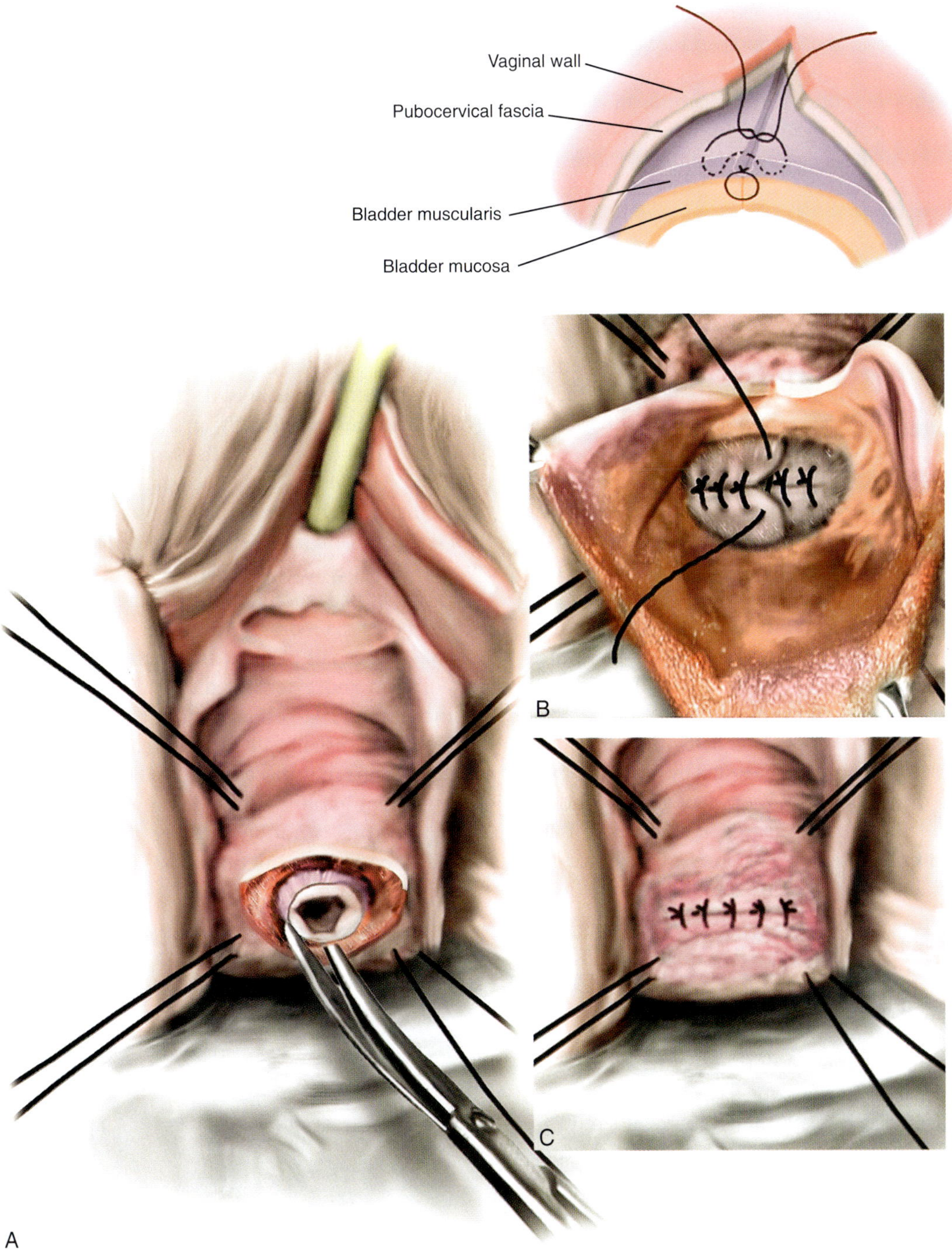

Fig. 38.5 The classic method of vaginal repair of vesicovaginal fistula. **A**, Stay sutures are placed to help expose the fistula. After an initial circumferential incision is made around the fistula, either the fistulous tract is excised completely (smaller fistulas), or the scarred edges are cut back until fresh vascular tissue is identified (larger fistulas). **B**, The vaginal mucosa is widely mobilized in all directions, and the fistula is closed in layers. The initial layer involves placement of No. 4-0 delayed absorbable sutures in the extramucosal portion of the bladder edge. The second layer is placed through the muscular portion of the bladder wall, imbricating the first layer. **C**, The repair is completed by closure of the vaginal epithelium.

Traditionally, the fistula tract is excised or the fistula edges freshened to improve healing after fistula closure. This may be especially relevant in obstetric fistulas, where there is often a wide area of ischemia and fibrosis surrounding the fistula. However, we generally do not advocate for excision of the fistula tract itself, because of the risk of enlarging the existing fistula and thereby potentially compromising the residual bladder size, as well as increasing bleeding and possibly requiring cauterization, which may affect vascularity and healing. In a randomized controlled trial of 64 women with obstetric VVFs who underwent vaginal fistula repair with Martius graft, the authors found similar success rates regardless of whether the fistula edges were trimmed or not (Shaker et al., 2011). The authors did not report on the extent of local fibrosis/scarring in these patients, and all of these patients had fistula repairs augmented with Martius graft; therefore, these findings may not be generalizable. As with much of the discussion regarding management strategies, deciding whether to trim the fistula edges is often individualized and will typically depend on the experience of the surgeon.

Once the fistula is adequately mobilized from the vaginal epithelium, a layered closure is performed. If the fistula tract is not excised, the perivesical fascia surrounding the fistula is dissected and mobilized widely to allow complete imbrication of the first suture line (Fig 38.5B). The fistula itself is closed with a suture line in a simple interrupted fashion. Once the surgeon is ready to tie these sutures, the fistula catheter (if present) is removed. We generally use a delayed absorbable suture like polyglactin 910 (PGA). The needle size and shape will depend upon the location of the fistula and the extent of mobilization. We prefer to use No. 2-0 or 3-0 PGA circle taper (CT-2) sutures for the layered closure. The second layer of repair is accomplished by placing interrupted sutures in the surrounding perivesical fascia to completely imbricate the first suture line. The integrity of these two layers can then be tested by distending the bladder with saline or a solution of methylene blue or indigo carmine. Additional sutures can be placed at any sites of fluid extravasation. The third layer of VVF repair may be accomplished by interposition of well-vascularized tissue, either a local peritoneal flap or a Martius flap. For posthysterectomy fistulas, a peritoneal flap, generally harvested beneath the posterior vaginal flap, is sutured in place to cover the first two layers of VVF repair. This can be done extraperitoneally by mobilizing the peritoneum off of the posterior vaginal flap or intraperitoneally if the peritoneum is entered during the dissection. For more mid- or proximal VVF, a Martius flap must first be tunneled from the harvest site beneath the vaginal epithelium to the VVF site. This is generally accomplished by dissecting a tunnel beneath the ipsilateral vaginal wall and passing a right-angle or tonsil clamp beneath to pull the Martius flap in. Finally, the vaginal epithelium is closed with delayed absorbable sutures to cover the entire repair (Fig. 38.5C). Some experts recommend closing the vaginal epithelium in a perpendicular direction to the fistula closure to avoid overlapping suture lines only if there is adequate tissue laxity to do so.

Regarding the vaginal repair technique, most advocate repairing the bladder in two layers. In cases of large fistula or obstetric fistula, potential disadvantages of two-layer closure include longer operative time and decreased bladder size in cases of large fistula. Although there are no randomized controlled trials addressing this issue, a retrospective review of 832 patients with obstetric fistula undergoing vaginal repair found similar repair success rates with one-layer closure (91%) compared with two-layer closure (93%) in patients with similar-sized fistulas (Nardos et al., 2009). See Video 38.2 for a demonstration of an obstetrical fistula repair.

Repair of Urethrovaginal Fistula

Most UVFs result in urinary incontinence and require surgical repair (Fig 38.6). Occasionally, a fistula distal to the external sphincter may be asymptomatic and not require repair. A nonirradiated, primary fistula can usually be repaired successfully with a layered, tension-free closure, similar to the techniques presented earlier. If the surrounding tissue appears to be devascularized, the tissue has been irradiated, or the fistula is recurrent, interposing a labial fat pad between the urethra and the anterior vagina may be beneficial. If the fistula is in the proximal urethra or in the bladder neck, the continence mechanism may have been compromised. In this case an antiincontinence procedure, most commonly an autologous fascial suburethral sling, may be performed at the same time as the fistula repair. Unless certain of the continence status outcome after repair, we recommend the two procedures be staged and the sling placed at a different time as a separate procedure. Because the blood supply to the urethra may be limited, or the defect may be large, a labial fat pad should be considered and may be placed between the repaired urethra and sling.

The UVF repair begins with urethroscopy to further define the location and extent of the fistula and its relation to the sphincter complex. Following this, a transurethral Foley catheter is placed, usually 14- or 16-French. To optimally identify the fistula, one may place a small catheter (ureteral catheter or feeding tube) into the fistula. Because UVFs are generally easy to identify, this is not always necessary. The anterior vaginal wall is then injected with normal saline or a diluted hemostatic

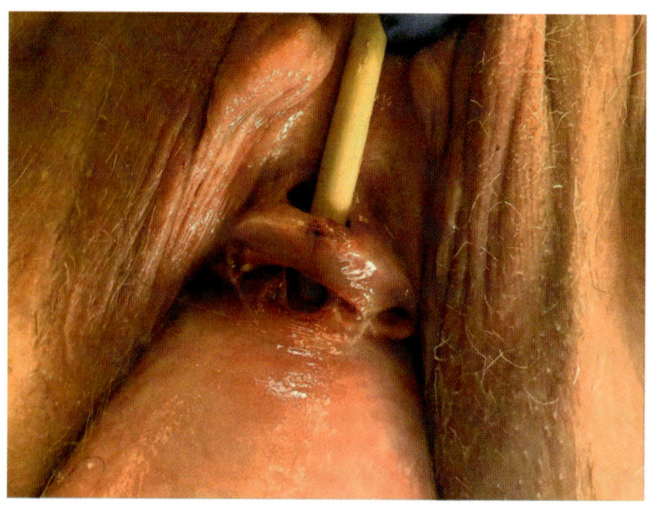

Fig. 38.6 Urethrovaginal fistula caused by prolonged catheterization in a patient with high-grade prolapse.

solution to facilitate dissection in the appropriate plane and decrease bleeding.

As with any vaginal approach to fistula repair, to optimize vaginal exposure we often use a ring retractor with sharp hooks. A midline anterior vaginal wall incision is made, which can either circumscribe or extend on both sides of the urethral defect (Fig. 38.7B). Alternatively, an inverted U-shaped vaginal epithelial flap can be created and separated from the underlying vesicovaginal fibromuscular connective tissue and later used to cover the fistula repair at the end of the case. Sharp dissection with a fine scissor is used to separate the vaginal epithelium from the underlying urethrovaginal and vesicovaginal fibromuscular connective tissue. This dissection should be extended laterally to the inferior pubic ramus to allow the urethra to be

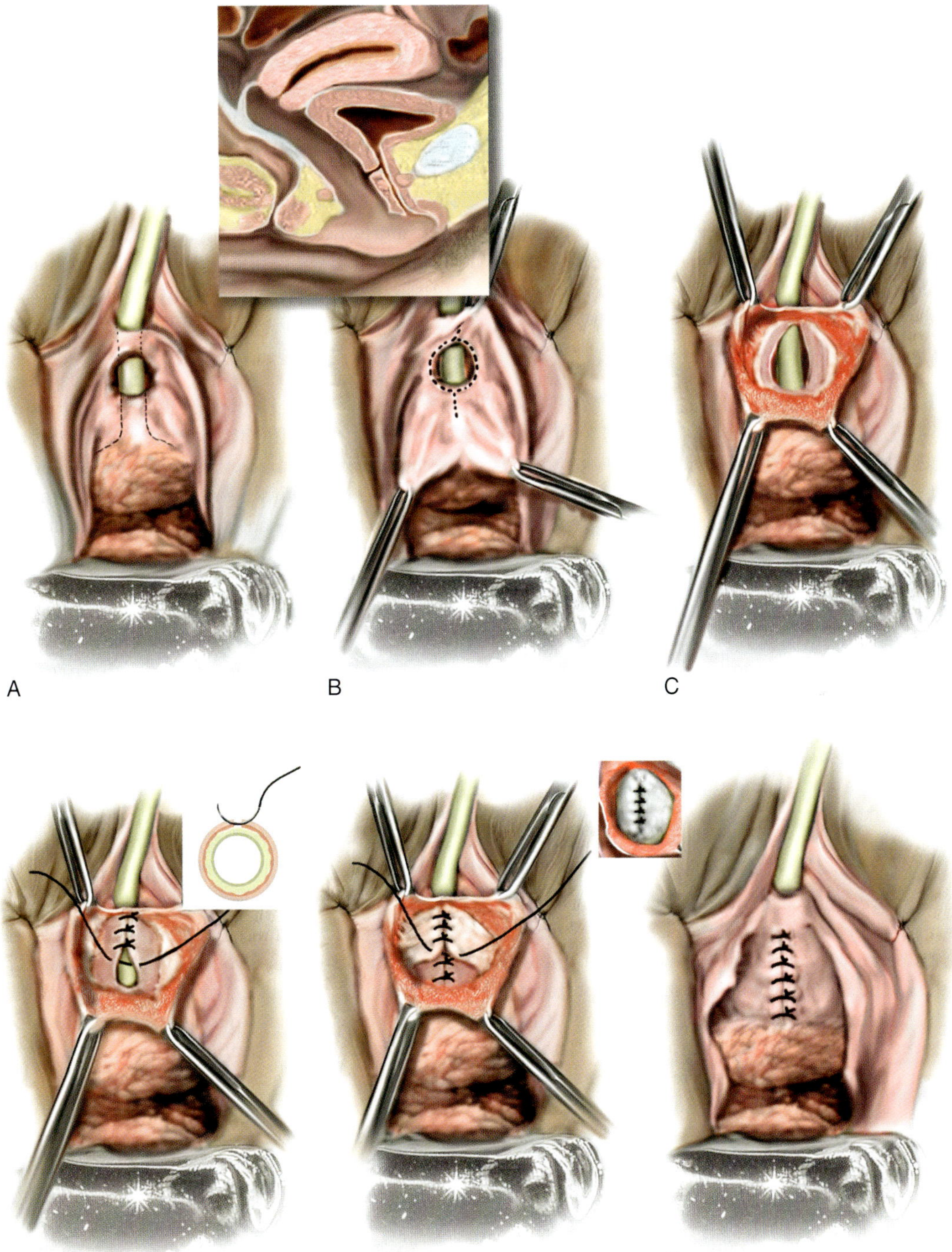

A B C D E F

Fig. 38.7 Repair of urethrovaginal fistula. **A**, Urethrovaginal fistula. **B**, Anterior vaginal wall incision is made and extended on both sides of the urethral defect. **C**, Vaginal wall is sharply separated from underlying pubocervical fascia. **D**, Fine delayed absorbable interrupted sutures are placed in an extramucosal fashion. **E**, The initial suture line is then inverted with a second suture incorporating the pubocervical fascia. **F**, Vaginal incision is closed with interrupted No. 2-0 delayed absorbable sutures.

completely mobilized, thus allowing a tension-free closure (Fig. 38.7C). Depending on the extent of the fistula, the retropubic space may be entered vaginally to facilitate urethral mobility. Vaginal flaps may be retracted widely using the hooks on the ring retractor to visualize the periurethral fascial edges. As with VVF, we do not advocate for excision of the fistula itself because this only enlarges the caliber of the defect. The edges of the urethra are then approximated with fine delayed absorbable suture (PGA) in an interrupted fashion with full-thickness urethral bites to close the fistula (Fig. 38.7D). The initial suture line is then inverted with a second suture line incorporating the periurethral tissue using delayed absorbable suture (Fig. 38.7E). At this point, the integrity of the repair may be interrogated using methylene blue or indigo carmine instilled directly into the urethra using an angiocatheter or small Foley catheter. The decision for tissue interposition, for example with a Martius flap, can be made at this time (Fig 38.8). If the fistula is located in the proximal urethra or bladder neck, an autologous fascial sling can be placed at the time of repair as an additional layer of tissue, as well as a supportive hammock, to improve any stress incontinence/intrinsic sphincter deficiency. The sling can be sutured over the periurethral fascial suture line as a third layer of tissue. The vaginal incision is closed with interrupted or delayed absorbable sutures (Fig. 38.7F). A Foley catheter is typically left in place for 10 to 14 days at the surgeon's discretion.

In cases of mesh erosion leading to UVF, it is critical to remove all of the involved intervening mesh, as well as all adjacent mesh to the extent possible. In a series of 10 patients who developed urinary fistula(s) secondary to synthetic midurethral sling (one ureterovaginal, one enterovesical, six vesicovaginal, and seven urethrovaginal), Blaivas and Mekel (2014) reported successful fistula repair in seven when maximum mesh removal was prioritized.

A circumferential VVF involves complete detachment of the bladder from the urethra and is one of the most challenging types of obstetric fistulas to repair (Genadry et al., 2007). The principles of the repair technique are similar to what has already been presented here; however, the reanastomsis of the urethra to the bladder requires vigilance and expertise. Not only must the distal bladder, which is completely detached from the proximal urethra, be mobilized from the vaginal epithelium posteriorly, but also the endopelvic fascia must be perforated and the retropubic space (space of Retzius) entered vaginally so that the bladder can be mobilized anteriorly and laterally, allowing for circumferential tension-free reattachment to the proximal urethra. Because the defect in the distal bladder is much larger than the opening of the proximal urethra, the anterior portion of the distal bladder is wrapped around the proximal urethra to reestablish the connection between the urethra and the bladder. The remaining bladder defect is reapproximated vertically.

Abdominal Repair of Vesicovaginal Fistulas

Relative indications for abdominal repair of VVFs include high or retracted fistulas that are not accessible vaginally, a vagina that is inaccessible because of severe scarring and stenosis, multiple fistulas that cannot all be accessed vaginally, involvement of the uterus, cervix, or bowel, the need for ureteral reimplantation, the need for other concurrent transabdominal procedures, the need for extensive bladder reconstruction like augmentation cystoplasty, and surgeon experience or preference. This section discusses the surgical considerations for an open abdominal approach; for laparoscopic and robotic approaches, see the following section.

Some surgeons find it valuable to vaginally cannulate the fistula tract before an abdominal repair. A midline or transverse skin incision can be used. A midline incision can allow easier access to the abdomen for retrieval and mobilization of omentum. Once the peritoneum has been opened, the bowel is packed posteriorly, and a self-retaining retractor is usually placed and the bladder exposed. The classic O'Conor technique involves complete bisection of the bladder intraperitoneally or extraperitoneally, carrying the incision down to the fistula tract (Fig. 38.9). If the fistula tract is in close proximity to the ureteral orifice, a ureteral stent should be placed. Of note, the ureteral stent can also be placed before the incision is made, via a cystoscopic approach. Any necrotic or fibrotic tissue surrounding the fistulous tract can be excised, and the vagina is sharply mobilized off the posterior bladder. Modification of this technique may include making an intentional cystotomy large enough to access the fistula tract through the cystotomy but not include the fistula tract within the cystotomy. From within the bladder, the fistula tract is excised and dissected off the underlying vaginal tissue. The vagina and bladder are closed separately. Most experts would recommend placement of an interposing flap of tissue, such as omentum or a flap of peritoneum between the vagina and bladder. The bladder cystotomy is closed last.

Alternatively, without making an intentional cystotomy or bisecting the bladder, the posterior bladder may be dissected off the anterior vagina intraperitoneally until the fistula tract is encountered. A Foley catheter can be placed within the fistula tract vaginally to facilitate locating the fistula tract during dissection. The bladder with the fistula tract is then completely mobilized from the vagina. A vaginal pack, sponge stick, or end-to-end anastomosis sizer or similar device can be placed in the vagina to facilitate dissection and accurate separation of the bladder and vagina. The dissection should be extended well beyond any scarring produced by the fistula. The vagina is then closed with interrupted or running absorbable sutures, in one or two layers. Some experts have recommended that the vagina be closed transversely and the bladder closed longitudinally so that the suture lines do not overlap. The bladder is closed with a delayed absorbable suture such as PGA in a running or interrupted fashion, typically in two layers. We recommend mobilizing a piece of omentum or peritoneum and interposing it between the repaired bladder and vagina. The omentum is sutured to the anterior wall of the vagina or posterior wall of the bladder to provide additional blood supply and act as a tissue barrier between the two suture lines (Fig. 38.9). Sigmoid epiploica has also been used as an extra layer. In a small retrospective series of 24 patients undergoing abdominal repair, use of an omental flap was shown to be associated with higher rates of successful repair than peritoneal flap or no tissue

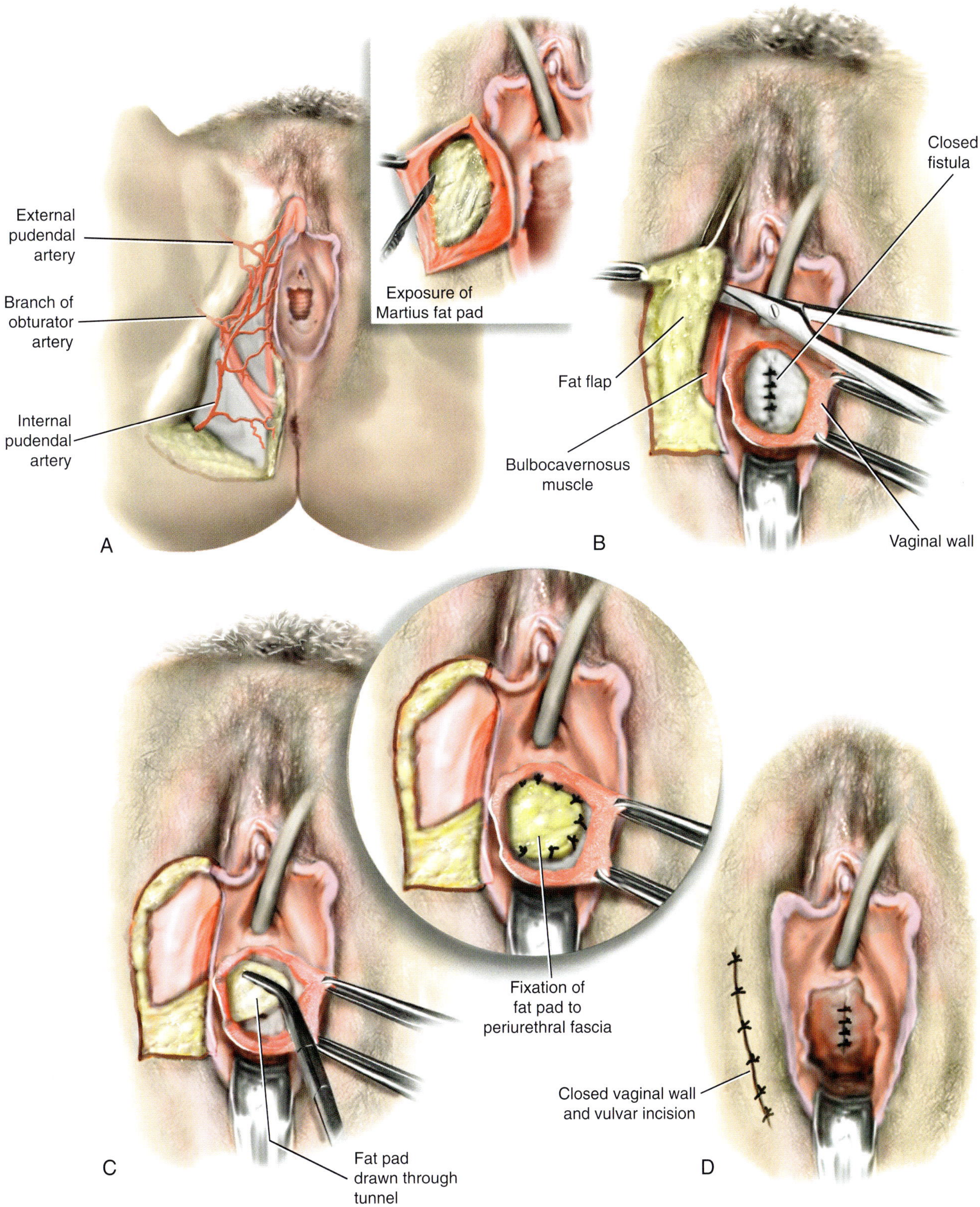

Fig. 38.8 Technique of modified Martius graft for vesicovaginal fistula repair. **A**, Blood supply of labia majora. **B**, Exposed fat pad with clamp passing underneath anterior portion of fat pad before detachment and mobilization. **C**, Fat pad has been tunneled into anterior vaginal wall and fixed over the closed fistula (*inset*). **D**, Labial and vaginal incisions have been closed.

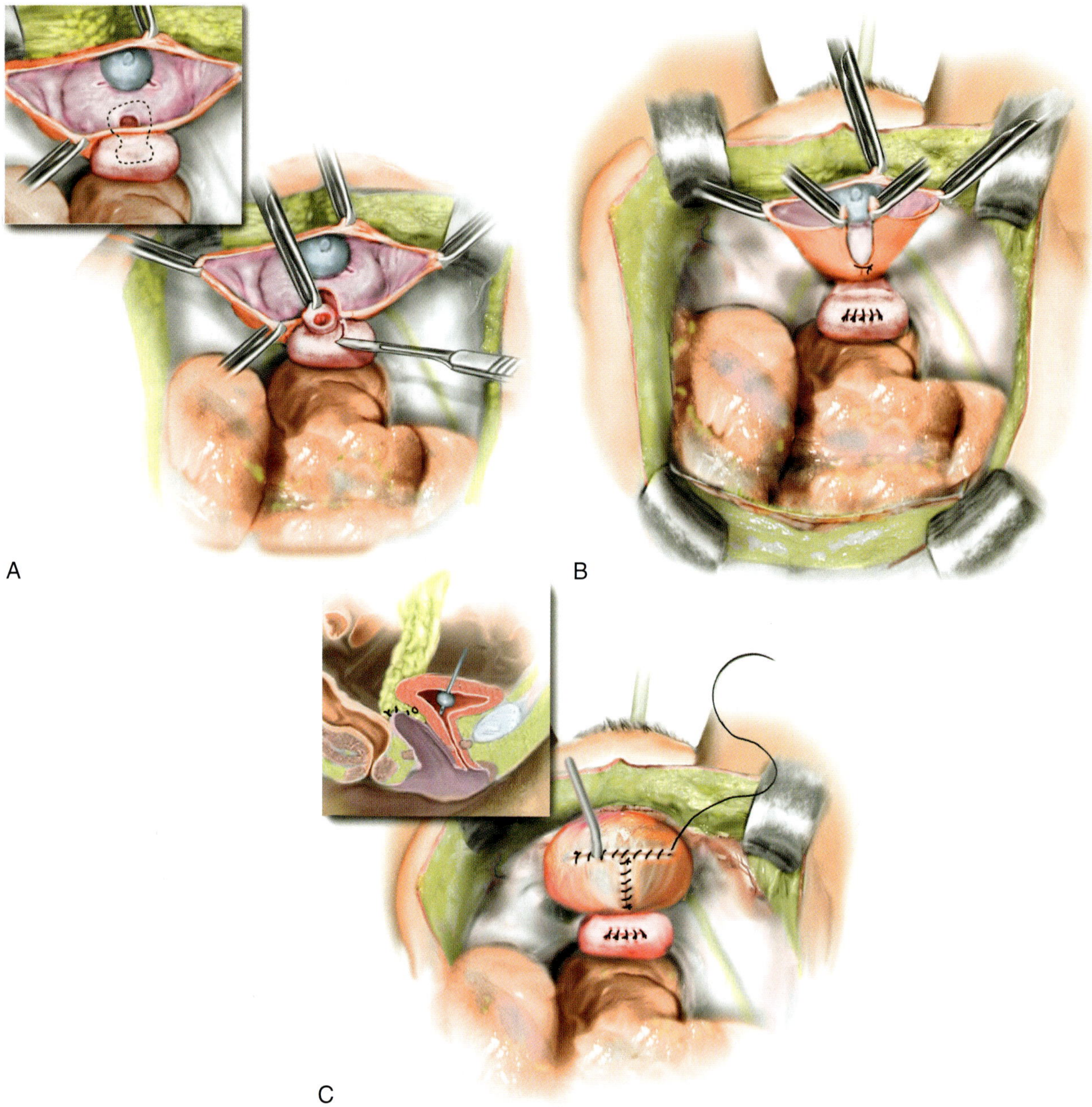

Fig. 38.9 Abdominal repair of vesicovaginal fistula. **A**, Fistulous tract and scarred vagina and bladder are excised. **B**, Dissection has been completed, and the fistulous tract has been excised. The vagina has been closed, and closure of the back of the bladder has been initiated. Note that the dissection is extended well below the level of the fistula. **C**, Closure of the bladder and vagina with interposition of omental flap (*inset*).

interposition (94% vs. 38%). Catheter drainage for 10 to 14 days may be accomplished with a transurethral or suprapubic approach, or both, depending on the extent and circumstances of the repair.

Laparoscopic and Robotic-Assisted Laparoscopic Repair of Vesicovaginal Fistula

Laparoscopic or robotic routes can be used by an experienced laparoscopic/robotic surgeon for the repair of urinary tract fistulas that require an abdominal approach. A laparoscopic approach was first described by Nezhat and colleagues in 1994 to reduce the morbidity associated with the open operation. However, because of the steep learning curve and challenging nature of intracorporeal suturing and dissection between the bladder and vagina, a conventional laparoscopic approach had slow adoption. Since the first robotic repair described by Melamud and colleagues in 2005, there have been many published small case series of robotic experiences with 93% to 100% success rates, minimal blood loss, low complication rates, and operative times of 95 to 305 minutes (Sharma et al., 2018).

Robotic approaches have been described using a four-port transperitoneal approach with the DaVinci platform (Intuitive Surgical, Sunnyvale, California). The patient may be positioned in low lithotomy position to allow access to the vagina and urethra during the case. Cystoscopy should be performed initially, and stents placed if necessary. To facilitate identification of the fistula tract, multiple techniques have been described, including focusing the light of the cystoscope on the area of the fistula with the robotic camera light turned off, tugging a transurethral catheter placed across the fistula, or placing an angiocath across the fistula that can be identified by the scrubbed surgeon. Thereafter, the principles of laparoscopic/robotic repair are the same as for open surgery. However, the major modification and advantage of a minimally invasive approach is the ability to perform a limited posterior cystotomy rather than completely bivalving the bladder, allowing minimal trauma to the bladder and a smaller suture line for closure. Similar to the laparotomy route, procedures involving the ureter, such as ureteroneocystostomy with psoas hitch, can also be performed laparoscopically or robotically.

Although there are no randomized controlled trials comparing laparoscopic/robotic techniques to open techniques, the commonly cited advantages of laparoscopic or robotic routes include decreased intraoperative blood loss, decreased postoperative pain and hospital stay, and faster recovery. Limitations include surgeon experience and expertise, specialized operative instruments and operating room setup, general anesthesia, and possibly longer operative times. Gupta et al. (2010) reported on a retrospective study from India that matched 12 recurrent VVF cases repaired robotically with 20 recurrent fistula cases repaired via laparotomy by factors such as fistula size and cause and route of previous repair. The authors found statistically similar success rates (100% for robotic vs. 90% for open), operative times (140 minutes for robotic vs. 149 minutes for open), and rates of complications (0% for robotic vs. 10% for open), with significantly decreased mean blood loss (88 mL for robotic vs. 170 mL for open) and hospital stays (3.1 days for robotic vs. 5.6 days for open) in the robotic group.

Bladder Drainage after Vesicovaginal Fistula Repair

In most cases, transurethral drainage using a 16- to 18-French transurethral catheter for 10 to 14 days is adequate. In some instances, it may be appropriate to use two drainage catheters in the postoperative period (transurethral and suprapubic) to allow maximum bladder drainage in the event that one of the catheters becomes plugged. Also, if there are excessive bladder spasms or discomfort from the urethral catheter, it can be removed, leaving only the suprapubic catheter. In cases of small fistulas, or in high-risk situations, we will forgo suprapubic tube placement. We also often employ anticholinergic agents to prevent bladder spasms during the healing process.

Although the optimal duration of drainage is not clear, many experts advocated a range of 10 to 21 days of continuous drainage at the discretion of the surgeon, depending on the size and complexity of the fistula. In resource-limited countries, prolonged catheter duration may lead to increased hospital stay and risk of complications, as fistula patients often stay in the hospital until catheter removal. One randomized controlled trial demonstrated no differences in repair success and postoperative infection in 189 obstetric fistula patients randomized to 10 days of continuous bladder drainage compared with 14 days of continuous bladder drainage (Nardos et al., 2012).

Repair of Ureterovaginal Fistula

Surgery for ureterovaginal fistula depends on the site of involvement of the ureter and how best a repair can be accomplished with minimal tension. Typically, to address fistulas involving the distal third of the ureter, the ureter can be reimplanted into the bladder (ureteroneocystostomy). If there is tension at the reimplantation site, a psoas hitch or Boari flap can be performed. Fistulas that involve more proximal parts of the ureter usually require more advanced reconstructive techniques. See Chapter 24 for further discussion of ureteral injuries and their management.

Repair of Vesicouterine Fistula

Vesicouterine fistulas are rare, accounting for 1% to 4% of genitourinary fistulas, and are usually complications of cesarean section or other obstetrical surgery. Extravasation of urine, superimposed infection, and subsequent dehiscence of the uterine incision can constitute the most likely sequence of events and formation of a fistula. Risk factors for vesicouterine fistula development include uterine rupture, severe uterine infection, placenta percreta, manual removal of the placenta, excessive intraoperative bleeding, and previous cesarean section (Alkatib et al., 2005). The clinical presentation of vesicouterine fistula may vary. A fistula above the internal uterine orifice may be associated with cyclic hematuria, amenorrhea, and lack of urinary leakage, referred to as Youssef's triad. However, fistulas involving the uterine cervix may be characterized by continuous urinary leakage without menstrual anomalies (Milani et al., 2018).

Conservative management has been attempted using catheterization, antibiotics, and hormone therapy. However, reported results show limited success rates, with spontaneous closure occurring in only 5% of cases (Porcaro et al., 2002). The surgical repair of vesicouterine fistulas through various techniques, including transvaginal, transvesical, and transabdominal (open, laparoscopic, and robotic) has been described (Fig. 38.10). Early repair is typically done within 2 to 3 days of cesarean section, whereas delayed repair is typically done after 2 to 3 months to allow the uterus to involute and inflammation to resolve. For an abdominal approach, a transverse or longitudinal skin incision is made. The peritoneum is opened, and a high cystotomy is made in the extraperitoneal portion of the bladder. The fistulous tract is then identified, and sharp dissection is used to dissect between the bladder and the uterus. As mentioned earlier, this can also be done without first performing a cystotomy. Once the bladder is completely mobilized off the uterus and the fistulous tract has been excised, the bladder is closed in two layers of interrupted or continuous absorbable sutures. This is followed by an interrupted or continuous closure of the defect in the uterus. Interposition of omentum or peritoneum between the two suture lines may be placed.

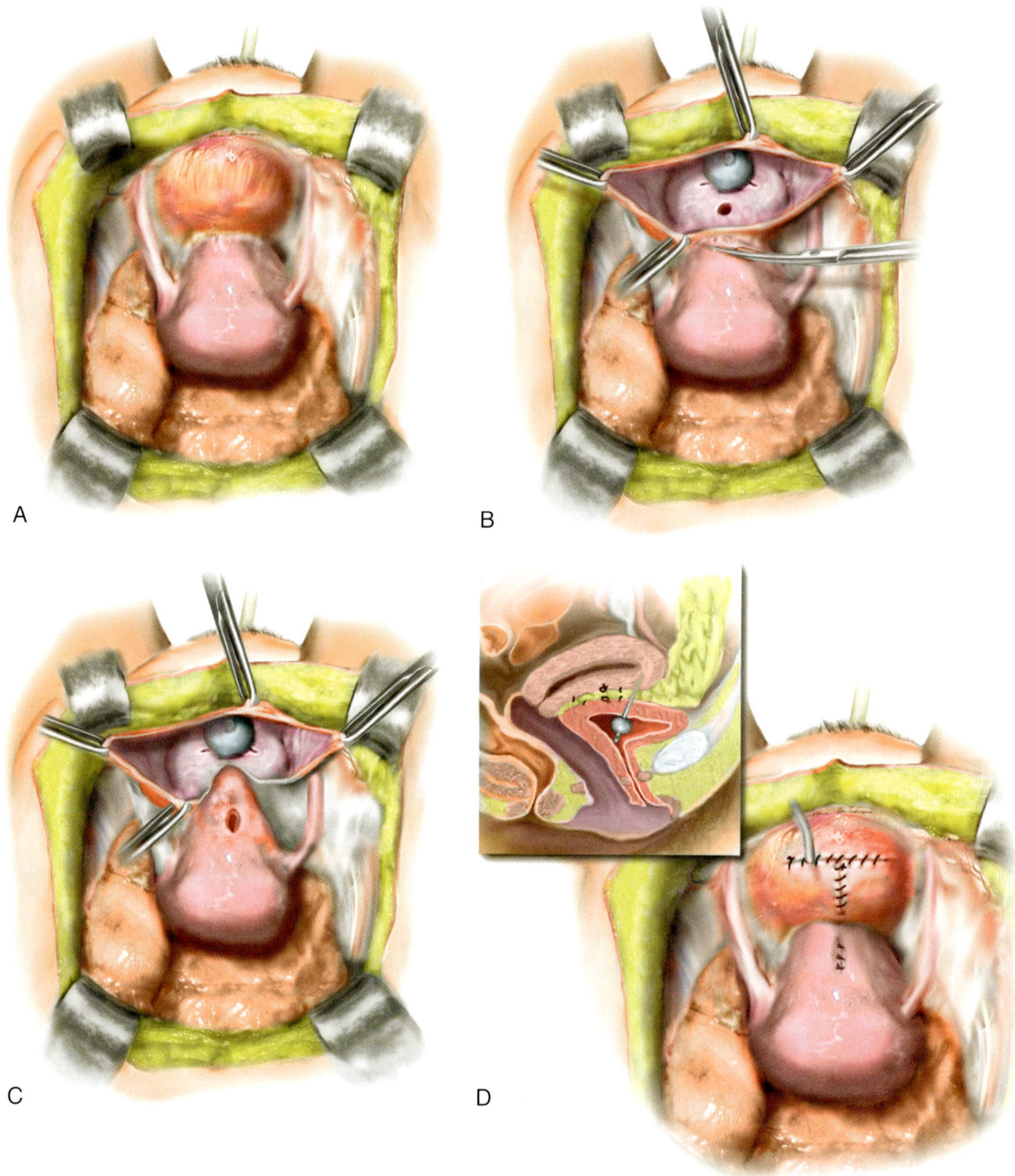

Fig. 38.10 Repair of vesicouterine fistula. **A**, Vesicouterine fistula involving the lower uterine segment and upper cervix and the back of the bladder. **B**, A high cystotomy has been made, and sharp dissection is used to separate the bladder from the uterus. **C**, Sharp dissection has been completed, and there is complete separation of the bladder and uterus. **D**, Bladder and uterus are each closed in two layers; omental flap is interposed between the two structures (*inset*).

Robotic techniques have also been used to repair these fistulas abdominally. If the fistula involves the cervix and bladder and can be identified and accessed through the vagina, the fistula can be closed vaginally by dissecting the cervix and lower uterine segment off the bladder and identifying the fistula tract. The bladder can then be closed in layers as described earlier, followed by reapproximation of the uterus/cervix. If the patient does not desire future fertility, abdominal hysterectomy with closure of the bladder defect can be a definitive therapy for a vesicouterine fistula.

Repair of Neobladder-Vaginal Fistula

Orthotopic neobladder construction after radical cystectomy was initially performed in men until an improved understanding of the female continence mechanism facilitated its use in women. Neobladder-vaginal fistula is an uncommon

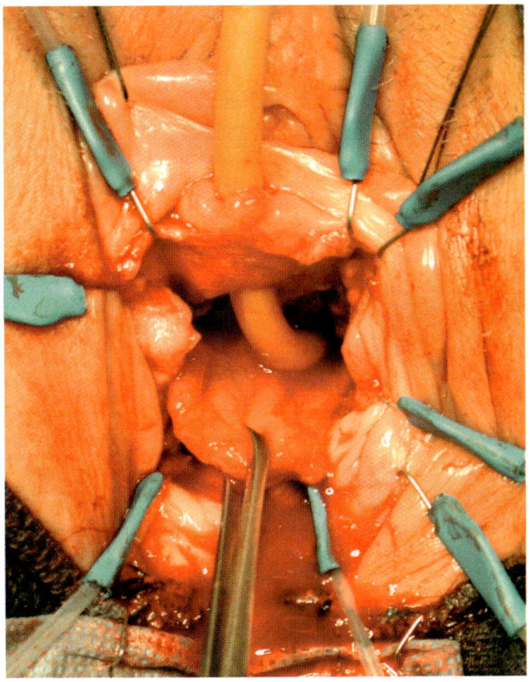

Fig. 38.11 Neobladder-vaginal fistulas have been reported to occur in 0% to 10% of patients after radical cystectomy and neobladder creation. While some can be repaired using a vaginal approach, larger or more complex fistulas may require conversion to an incontinent diversion.

complication reported to occur in 0% to 10% of cases (Fig 38.11). Associated risk factors for fistula development include injury or devascularization of the anterior vaginal wall during dissection, overlying suture lines of neobladder and vaginal wall repair, pelvic radiation, local recurrence, and the use of bulking agents in patients with postoperative incontinence (Ali-El-Dein et al., 2008; Rapp et al., 2004). Conservative management with catheter drainage is unlikely to be effective, and few to no data exist to assess the efficacy of endoscopic fulguration or injectable agents.

Techniques for repairs have been described using abdominal and vaginal approaches, with similar considerations to VVF repair. In one series of 13 neobladder-vaginal fistulas repaired over a 20-year period, Rosenberg et al. (2018) reported successful fistula repair in eight (61.5%) patients using a vaginal approach. The remaining patients underwent conversion to a nonorthotopic diversion. Another series reported successful repair without recurrence of fistula in eight patients using a transvaginal approach, although five (63%) required interventions for stress urinary incontinence following repair (Carmel et al., 2016). However, some authors advocate for an abdominal approach to facilitate adequate dissection and placement of adequate tissue interposition, especially in cases of large fistulas or vaginal fibrosis.

Strategies for prevention of neobladder-vaginal fistulas include rigorous closure of the vaginal cuff, vascular flap interposition, limited blunt dissection near the bladder neck, and avoidance of overlapping suture lines (Kaufman, 2019). As fistulas may occur as a result of urethral bulking agent injections for postoperative stress incontinence, some authors have advocated for limiting injected volume, aiming away from the bladder neck, and concentrating injections anteriorly in the 12 o'clock position.

URINARY DIVERSION

Most patients requiring urinary diversion because of genitourinary fistulas have had previous radiation therapy, one or more failed prior fistula closure attempts, complete sphincteric compromise leading to persistent incontinence (especially in developing countries), or extensive tissue compromise from obstructed labor. In those with radiation history, the bladder capacity may be severely compromised from fibrosis. Urinary conduits and reservoirs can be constructed from small or large bowel; they may be continent or incontinent. The major continent diversions are the Kock pouch, Indiana pouch, and the Miami pouch. The Kock pouch uses ileum with intussusception techniques, and the Indiana and Miami pouches use right hemicolon and a tapered terminal ileum. Both continent conduits have similar continence rates of 93% to 94%. Patients must be able and motivated to catheterize the stoma every 4 to 8 hours. Complications include stone formation, conduit leak and reflux, and metabolic disturbances. Early and late complications in continent diversions occur in 13% to 15%; reoperation is necessary in 1% to 4%. In many cases a simpler incontinent diversion like an ileal conduit with an external collection device is the best option.

COMPLICATIONS OF FISTULA REPAIR

The surgical repair of genitourinary fistulas may be complicated by risks common to all operations, such as hemorrhage, infection, and thromboembolism. The main challenge is recurrence or persistence of the fistula. Nonwatertight repair and/or undue tension may cause tissue breakdown at the vaginal or bladder suture lines. Other delayed surgical complications include vaginal stenosis and small-bladder syndrome, as well as post–fistula repair urethral urinary incontinence (see later). Dyspareunia attributed to vaginal scarring, stenosis, or tenderness over the site of Martius grafts has been reported. Metabolic disturbances and recurrent pyelonephritis may develop after ureterosigmoidostomy. After successful repair of a genitourinary fistula, elective cesarean delivery is strongly recommended for all subsequent births.

Although most series report a high cure rate of obstetric fistula closure, persistent urinary incontinence remains a significant clinical issue in these patients, and has been reported to occur in 10% to 55% of women after successful fistula closure. The same ischemic damage that led to the development of the fistula may also compromise continence mechanisms, with either direct urethra/urethral sphincter damage or local soft tissue destruction and nerve damage resulting in extensive local fibrosis. Many experts believe that a urethral length of at least 1.5 to 2.0 cm is needed to preserve continence (Waaldijk, 2004). Risk factors associated with incontinence include urethral involvement, small, contracted bladder or large fistula, increased vaginal scarring or fibrosis, or recurrent fistulas (Browning,

2006; Sjøveian et al., 2011). In a few small case series of urodynamic findings in obstetric fistula patients who present with urinary incontinence after successful fistula repair, 31% to 56% had stress incontinence, 37% to 41% had mixed incontinence, and 4% to 13% had voiding dysfunction, with a mean bladder capacity of 200 mL found in one study (Carey et al., 2002; Murray et al., 2002).

When patients present with incontinence symptoms after fistula surgery, it is critical to first ensure the fistula has not recurred or persisted. Women with incontinence after successful fistula repair are surgically challenging, because these patients will often have a scarred and fixed urethra, instead of one that is hypermobile (84% in one small series; Murray et al., 2002). Techniques such as periurethral injection of bulk-enhancing agents have been reported for women with stress incontinence symptoms after successful repair of a fistula. Autologous rectus or fascia lata slings and synthetic slings have been used, with similar rates of stress incontinence resolution or improvement (64%–90%) but with significantly higher rates of erosion (20%) in the synthetic sling group (Ascher-Walsh, 2010; Murray et al., 2002). Another autologous sling that has been reported in the literature is the pubococcygeus sling, created by identifying the pubococcygeus muscle and surrounding connective tissue bilaterally (Browning, 2004; Browning, 2006). The muscle is detached posteriorly while leaving the anterior attachment intact on both sides. Sufficient muscle must be detached posteriorly to allow for tension-free approximation under the urethra. The freed posterior ends of the muscle are then sutured in the midline under the urethra. In two small case series (12 women and 32 women, respectively) with short-term follow-up periods (2–3 weeks), 67% to 69% of women were continent, with 13% to 16% experiencing urinary retention.

PREVENTION

Because the majority of lower urinary tract fistulas in developed countries arise from iatrogenic causes, prevention efforts have been focused on mitigating the risk of fistula formation during inciting surgery or radiation. VVFs that occur as a result of hysterectomy are usually found in the posterior wall of the bladder superior to the interureteric ridge. Tancer (1992), in a retrospective review of 151 urogenital fistulas, presented suggestions and observations on avoiding injury to the bladder during total abdominal hysterectomy. These included the use of a two-way indwelling catheter; sharp dissection of the bladder off the uterus, cervix, and upper vagina; careful placement of sutures and clamps during vaginal cuff closure; use of an extraperitoneal cystotomy when the dissection is difficult; retrograde filling of the bladder to define the border or when injury is suspected; and attention to repair of an overt bladder injury only after mobilization of the injured area. Judicious and careful use of electrical diathermy is imperative during dissection and electrocautery near the vaginal cuff and bladder margin. Delayed tissue necrosis owing to lateral spread of thermal injury is a major etiology of fistula formation. These types of injuries are difficult to detect at time of surgery because they often have a delayed presentation. Another method of preventing bladder injury is by performing an intrafascial hysterectomy. The vesicocervical space must be completely developed, and the bladder must be thoroughly mobilized inferiorly and laterally. In theory, the bladder has been mobilized from the site of entry into the vagina and is less likely to be compromised, because it rests on the dissected fascia. In a review of 867 women who underwent an intrafascial abdominal hysterectomy, a bladder injury incidence of 0.4% was reported (Conde-Agudelo, 2000).

It is paramount to recognize and repair bladder and ureteral injury intraoperatively to prevent fistula development. In an older meta-analysis, only 52% of bladder injuries and 12% of ureteral injuries were detected intraoperatively, with an increase in detection rate to 85% and 90%, respectively, if routine cystoscopy was performed intraoperatively (Gilmour et al., 1999). Studies by Pettit and Petrou (1994) and Wiskind and Thompson (1995) have shown a significant prevalence of unsuspected ureteral injuries (0.1%–2%) and advocate routine cystoscopy at all pelvic operations. When a cystotomy occurs, the first priority is to determine the proximity of the cystotomy to the ureteral orifices and if the ureter is also compromised. This is best done via cystoscopy, by extending the cystotomy or by creating a separate extraperitoneal cystotomy during an abdominal case. The authors prefer to tag the opposing poles of the cystotomy with delayed absorbable sutures, and usually a No. 2-0 or a No. 3-0 absorbable suture is used to close the cystotomy. The cystotomy may be closed with interrupted or continuous sutures. We prefer to include the mucosa in the closure of high, nondependent cystotomies; however, we attempt to place sutures extramucosally in lower, dependent cystotomies. A second layer is usually included to imbricate the bladder muscularis over the first layer. One can ensure complete closure of the cystotomy and ensure that the repair is watertight by instilling dilute methylene blue, indigo carmine, or sterile milk into the bladder. Low intraperitoneal cystotomies usually require a minimum of 7 days of continuous drainage, whereas a high extraperitoneal cystotomy in a nondependent portion of the bladder may require as little as 24 to 48 hours of drainage. Some surgeons advocate routinely obtaining a cystogram before removal of the catheter.

Routine preoperative ureteral stenting in gynecologic surgery has not been shown to result in a statistically significant reduction in ureteral injury rate (Chou et al., 2009). However, in difficult cases where the anatomy is likely to be obscured, such as severe endometriosis, history of pelvic infection, or multiple previous pelvic/abdominal surgeries, prior stent placement may be prudent to prevent or recognize ureteral injury.

Careful dosage calculation, administration, source insertion, and shielding, together with appropriate bladder drainage, can reduce the risk of radiation-induced lower urinary tract fistulas. This complication may nonetheless arise many years after a symptom-free interval and may not be completely preventable.

Prevention of obstetric fistulas in developing countries is a critical but very challenging approach to mitigating the devastation caused by this condition. Epidemiologic research is urgently needed to identify communities with a high prevalence of fistulas and to determine the characteristics of women at high risk for bladder or urethral injury during childbirth. Preventive strategies must be directed systemically at several levels to achieve a meaningful reduction in the occurrence of genitourinary fistulas caused by neglected obstructed labor. Strategies to improve outreach and prenatal education for women in rural areas are essential to remove barriers to access to adequate safe peripartum care. Additional sociocultural changes are necessary to promote delayed childbearing until pelvic maturity. For example, one study using logistic regression models on delivery data from Niger, Nigeria, and Tanzania found that 11% to 13% of obstructed labor can be prevented if women 17 years or younger do not bear children (Tsui et al., 2007). Increased availability of prenatal care and establishment of maternity waiting homes would improve care during pregnancy and identify conditions such as abnormal fetal presentation before labor. Trained birth attendants could perform bladder drainage in labor and identify abnormal labor patterns using portographs. Emergency transport for women in prolonged labor to centers staffed by skilled personnel could enable abdominal delivery when vaginal delivery is impossible.

One potentially low-cost and community-based strategy that has been proposed is the use of prolonged urinary catheterization after obstructed labor to prevent fistula formation. Although scant data exist to support the safety and efficacy immediate catheterization, the duration of catheterization necessary, and patient selection criteria, this measure was nonetheless recommended by several developing nations and in 2013 by Fistula Care, a fistula repair and prevention project from the US Agency for International Development. Unless significant further investigation into prevention strategies is undertaken, genitourinary fistulas will continue to occur, and women will continue to need advanced care for surgical management.

BIBLIOGRAPHY

Ahmed S, Anastasi E, Laski L. Double burden of tragedy: stillbirth and obstetric fistula. *Lancet Glob Health*. 2016;4:e80.

Ali-el-Dein B, Shaaban AA, Abu-Eideh RH, et al. Surgical complications following radical cystectomy and orthotopic neobladders in women. *J Urol*. 2008;180:206.

Alkatib M, Franco AV, Fynes MM. Vesicouterine fistula following Cesarean delivery—ultrasound diagnosis and surgical management. *Ultrasound Obstet Gynecol*. 2005;26:183.

Ascher-Walsh CJ, Capes TL. Robot-assisted laparoscopic myomectomy is an improvement over laparotomy in women with a limited number of myomas. *J Minim Invasive Gynecol*. 2010;17:306.

Barageine JK, Tumwesigye NM, Byamugisha JK, et al. Risk factors for obstetric fistula in Western Uganda: a case control study. *PLoS One*. 2014;9:e112299.

Blaivas JG, Heritz DM, Romanzi LJ. Early versus late repair of vesicovaginal fistulas: vaginal and abdominal approaches. *J Urol*. 1995;153:1110.

Blaivas JG, Mekel G. Management of urinary fistulas due to midurethral sling surgery. *J Urol*. 2014;192:1137.

Browning A. Prevention of residual urinary incontinence following successful repair of obstetric vesico-vaginal fistula using a fibro-muscular sling. *BJOG*. 2004;111:357.

Browning A. Lack of value of the Martius fibrofatty graft in obstetric fistula repair. *Int J Gynaecol Obstet*. 2006;93:33.

Carey MP, Goh JT, Fynes MM, Murray CJ. Stress urinary incontinence after delayed primary closure of genitourinary fistula: a technique for surgical management. *Am J Obstet Gynecol*. 2002;186:948.

Carmel ME, Goldman HB, Moore CK, et al. Transvaginal neobladder vaginal fistula repair after radical cystectomy with orthotopic urinary diversion in women. *Neurourol Urodyn*. 2016;35:90.

Chen YB, Wolff BJ, Kenton KS, Mueller ER. Approach to ureterovaginal fistula: examining 13 years of experience. *Female Pelvic Med Reconstr Surg*. 2019;25:e7.

Chou MT, Wang CJ, Lien RC. Prophylactic ureteral catheterization in gynecologic surgery: a 12-year randomized trial in a community hospital. *Int Urogynecol J Pelvic Floor Dysfunct*. 2009;20:689.

Conde-Agudelo A. Intrafascial abdominal hysterectomy: outcomes and complications of 867 operations. *Int J Gynaecol Obstet*. 2000;68:233.

Cruikshank SH. Early closure of posthysterectomy vesicovaginal fistulas. *South Med J*. 1988;81:1525.

Derry, DE. Note on five pelves of women of the eleventh dynasty in Egypt. *BJOG*. 1953;42:490.

Duong TH, Gellasch TL, Adam RA. Risk factors for the development of vesicovaginal fistula after incidental cystotomy at the time of a benign hysterectomy. *Am J Obstet Gynecol*. 2009;201:512.e1.

Dwarkasing S, Hussain SM, Hop WC, Krestin GP. Anovaginal fistulas: evaluation with endoanal MR imaging. *Radiology*. 2004;231:123.

Garlock JH. The cure of an intractable vesicovaginal fistula by the use of pedicled muscle graft. *Surg Gynecol Obstet*. 1928;47:255.

Genadry RR, Creanga AA, Roenneburg ML, Wheeless CR. Complex obstetric fistulas. *Int J Gynaecol Obstet*. 2007;99:S51.

Gilmour DT, Dwyer PL, Carey MP. Lower urinary tract injury during gynecologic surgery and its detection by intraoperative cystoscopy. *Obstet Gynecol*. 1999;94:883.

Goujon E, Jarniat A, Bardet F, et al. Retrospective study on the management and follow-up of 18 patients with a mid-urethral sling penetrating the urethra or bladder. *J Gynecol Obstet Hum Reprod*. 2018;47:289.

Gupta NP, Mishra S, Hemal AK, et al. Comparative analysis of outcome between open and robotic surgical repair of recurrent supra-trigonal vesico-vaginal fistula. *J Endourol*. 2010;24:1779.

Harki-Siren P, Sjoberg J, Titinen A. Urinary tract injuries after hysterectomy. *Obstet Gynecol*. 1998;92:113.

Harmanli O, Esin S, Knee A, et al. Effect of obesity on perioperative outcomes of laparoscopic hysterectomy. *J Reprod Med*. 2013;58:497.

Hillary CJ, Osman NI, Hilton P, Chapple CR. The aetiology, treatment, and outcome of urogenital fistulae managed in well- and low-resourced countries: a systematic review. *Eur Urol*. 2016;70:478.

Hwang JH. Urologic complication in laparoscopic radical hysterectomy: meta-analysis of 20 studies. *Eur J Cancer*. 2012;48:3177.

Ingelman-Sundberg A. Pathogenesis and operative treatment of urinary fistula in irradiated tissue. In: Youssef AF, ed. *Gynecological Urology*. Springfield, IL: Charles C. Thomas; 1960.

Kaufman MR. Neobladder-vaginal fistula: surgical management techniques. *Curr Urol Rep*. 2019;20:67.

Kelly HA. The treatment of vesico-vaginal and recto-vaginal fistulae high up in the vagina. *Johns Hopkins Hosp Bull*. 1902;13:73.

Kiricuta I, Goldstein AM. The repair of extensive vesicovaginal fistulas with pedicled omentum: a review of 27 cases. *J Urol.* 1972;108:724.

Latzko W. Postoperative vesicovaginal fistulae: genesis and theory. *Am J Surg.* 1942;58:211.

Lea D, Annie-Kim GL, Eve-Lyne L, et al. Sodium fluorescein for ureteral jet detection: a prospective observational study. *JSLS.* 2018;22:e2018.00019.

Martius H. Die operative Wiederher-stellung der Volkommen fehlenden Harnrohre und des Schliessmuskels derselben. *Zentralbl Gynakol.* 1928;8:480.

Martius H. Zur Auswahl der harnfistel-und inkontinenz Operation. *Zentralbl Gynakol.* 1942;32:1250.

McCurdie FK, Moffatt J, Jones K. Vesicovaginal fistula in Uganda. *J Obstet Gynaecol.* 2018;38:822.

Mellano EM, Tarnay CM. Management of genitourinary fistula. *Curr Opin Obstet Gynecol.* 2014;26:415.

Milani R, Cola A, Frigerio M, Manodoro S. Repair of a vesicouterine fistula following cesarean section. *Int Urogynecol J.* 2018; 29:309.

Moir JC. *The Vesico-Vaginal Fistula.* London: Balliere Tindall; 1961.

Muleta M, Tafesse B, Aytenfisu HG. Antibiotic use in obstetric fistula repair: single blinded randomized clinical trial. *Ethiop Med J.* 2010;48:211.

Murray C, Goh JT, Fynes M, Carey MP. Urinary and faecal incontinence following delayed primary repair of obstetric genital fistula. *BJOG.* 2002;109:828.

Muto G, D'Urso L, Castelli E, et al. Cyanoacrylic glue: a minimally invasive nonsurgical first line approach for the treatment of some urinary fistulas. *J Urol.* 2005;174:2239.

Nardos R, Browning A, Chen CC. Risk factors that predict failure after vaginal repair of obstetric vesicovaginal fistulae. *Am J Obstet Gynecol.* 2009;200:578.e1.

Nardos R, Menber B, Browning A. Outcome of obstetric fistula repair after 10-day versus 14-day Foley catheterization. *Int J Gynaecol Obstet.* 2012;118:21.

Noble CP. The new formation of the female urethra with report of a case. *Am J Obstet Gynecol.* 1901;43:170.

Oakley SH, Brown HW, Greer JA, et al. Management of vesicovaginal fistulae: a multicenter analysis from the Fellows' Pelvic Research Network. *Female Pelvic Med Reconstr Surg.* 2014;20:7.

O'Conor VJ, Sokol JK. Vesicovaginal fistula from the standpoint of the urologist. *J Urol.* 1951;66:579.

Penalver M, Angioli R. Urinary Diversion. In: Hurt WG, ed. *Urogynecologic Surgery.* Lippincot-Raven Press; 2000:193.

Pettit PD, Petrou SP. The value of cystoscopy in major vaginal surgery. *Obstet Gynecol.* 1994;84:318.

Porcaro AB, Zicari M, Zecchini Antoniolli S, et al. Vesicouterine fistulas following cesarean section: report on a case, review and update of the literature. *Int Urol Nephrol.* 2002;34:335.

Rapp DE, O'Connor RC, Katz EE, Steinberg GD. Neobladder-vaginal fistula after cystectomy and orthotopic neobladder construction. *BJU Int.* 2004;94:1092.

Reverby SM. *Memory and Medicine: A Historian's Perspective on Commemorating J. Marion Sims.* 2017. https://www.historians.org/publications-and-directories/perspectives-on-history/september-2017/memory-and-medicine-a-historians-perspective-on-commemorating-j-marion-sims.

Rosenberg S, Miranda G, Ginsberg DA. Neobladder-vaginal fistula: The University of Southern California experience. *Neurourol Urodyn.* 2018;37:1380.

Science must acknowledge its past mistakes and crimes. Nature. 2017 Sep 4;549(7670):5-6. Erratum in: *Nature.* 2017 Sep 13;549(7671):144.

Shaker H, Saafan A, Yassin M, et al. Obstetric vesico-vaginal fistula repair: should we trim the fistula edges? A randomized prospective study. *Neurourol Urodyn.* 2011;30:302.

Shallon A, Ojengbede OA, Mugisha JF, Odukogbe AA. Social reintegration and rehabilitation of obstetric fistula patients before and after repair in sub-Saharan Africa: a systematic review. *Nepal J Obstet Gynaecol.* 2018;13:5.

Sharma AP, Mavuduru RM, Bora GS, et al. Robot-assisted vesico-vaginal fistula repair: a compilation. *Urology.* 2018;119:1.

Shaw J, Tunitsky-Bitton E, Barber MD, Jelovsek JE. Ureterovaginal fistula: a case series. *Int Urogynecol J.* 2014;25:615.

Sims JM. On the treatment of vesico-vaginal fistula. 1852. *Int Urogynecol J Pelvic Floor Dysfunct.* 1998;9:236.

Shelbaia AM, Hashish NM. Limited experience in early management of genitourinary tract fistulas. *Urology.* 2007;69:572.

Sjøveian S, Vangen S, Mukwege D, Onsrud M. Surgical outcome of obstetric fistula: a retrospective analysis of 595 patients. *Acta Obstet Gynecol Scand.* 2011;90:753.

Symmonds RE, Hill LM. Loss of the urethra: a report on 50 patients. *Am J Obstet Gynecol.* 1978;130:130.

Tanagho EA, Smith DR. Clinical evaluation of a surgical technique for the correction of complete urinary incontinence. *J Urol.* 1972;107:402.

Tancer ML. Observations on prevention and management of vesicovaginal fistula after total hysterectomy. *Surg Gynecol Obstet.* 1992;175:501.

Tomlinson AJ, Thornton JG. A randomised controlled trial of antibiotic prophylaxis for vesico-vaginal fistula repair. *Br J Obstet Gynaecol.* 1998;105:397.

Tsui AO, Creanga AA, Ahmed S. The role of delayed childbearing in the prevention of obstetric fistulas. *Int J Gynaecol Obstet.* 2007;99:S98.

Tunçalp Ö, Tripathi V, Landry E, et al. Measuring the incidence and prevalence of obstetric fistula: approaches, needs and recommendations. *Bull World Health Organ.* 2015;93:60.

Van Roonhuyse H. *Medico-chirurgical observations by Henry Van Roonhuyse practitioner of Physick and cirurugery in Amsterdam, Englished out of the Dutch by a careful hand.* London: Moses Pitt; 1676.

Volkmer BG, Kuefer R, Nesslauer T, et al. Colour Doppler ultrasound in vesicovaginal fistulas. *Ultrasound Med Biol.* 2000;26:771.

Waaldijk K. The immediate surgical management of fresh obstetric fistulas with catheter and/or early closure. *Int J Gynaecol Obstet.* 1994;45:11.

Waaldijk K. The immediate management of fresh obstetric fistulas. *Am J Obstet Gynecol.* 2004;191:795.

Ward A. *Vesicovaginal Fistulas: A Report of 1789 Cases.* Paper presented to the meeting of the Federation of International Gynaecology and Obstetrics World Congress, San Francisco, 1980.

Wall LL, Arrowsmith SD, Briggs ND, et al. The obstetric vesicovaginal fistula in the developing world. *Obstet Gynecol Surv.* 2005;60:S3.

Wall LL, Karshima JA, Kirschner C, Arrowsmith SD. The obstetric vesicovaginal fistula: characteristics of 899 patients from Jos, Nigeria. *Am J Obstet Gynecol.* 2004;190:1011.

Wall LL. Obstetric vesicovaginal fistula as an international public-health problem. *Lancet.* 2006;368:1201.

Wiskind AK, Thompson JD. Should cystoscopy be performed at every gynecologic operation to diagnose unsuspected ureteral injury? *J Pelvic Surg.* 1995;1:134.

39

Bladder Drainage and Urinary Protective Methods

Ellen R. Solomon and Deepali Maheshwari

CHAPTER OUTLINE

INTRODUCTION

Patients who undergo surgery for urinary incontinence or pelvic organ prolapse may require catheterization postoperatively because of voiding difficulty. Patients with neurogenic bladder, dysfunctional voiding, or intractable incontinence may require intermittent or indwelling catheterization for long-term management. Three catheterization methods—transurethral, suprapubic, and intermittent self-catheterization (ISC)—can be used. Surgeons may also recommend voiding trials for their patients postoperatively. Failure to void with voiding trials usually requires catheterization for a period of days to weeks.

Incontinent patients may use protective products to aid with urine loss. These appliances may be helpful when medical or surgical management is not entirely successful, or when treatment is not an option or is more objectionable to the patient than continued incontinence. This chapter will discuss indwelling catheterization, voiding trials, and various protective products.

BLADDER DRAINAGE

Obstetricians and gynecologists often encounter the need for bladder drainage in patients after surgery and obstetric deliveries. Urinary retention is common after anesthesia and surgery, with a reported incidence of as high as 70%. General anesthesia can cause bladder atony by relaxing smooth muscle cells and by interfering with autonomic detrusor regulation. Intrathecal anesthetics interfere with the micturition reflex by blocking the afferent nerve supply to the bladder. Local anesthesia does not interfere with voiding function. Surgery for stress incontinence or pelvic organ prolapse also increases this risk by increasing urethral resistance to flow, which places the patient at risk for postoperative retention requiring temporary or prolonged bladder drainage. The risk of this retention after midurethral, vaginal, and retropubic procedures ranges from 3% to 25% and may be up to 47% for pubovaginal sling procedures. Adequate postoperative bladder drainage is important because overdistension is not only uncomfortable, but may lead to infection, as well as difficulty in resuming normal voiding. If overdistension or retention persists, patients may experience secondary myogenic damage attributable to changes in bladder architecture and function.

Transurethral Catheterization

The first self-retaining transurethral catheter was described in 1937 by Frederic Foley. A saline-inflated intravesical balloon holds the catheter in place. The transurethral catheter is commonly used after many gynecologic procedures. In a prospective cohort study by Ghezzi et al. (2007) that evaluated urinary retention after laparoscopic and vaginal surgery, 21% of the study population developed urinary retention, with the risk of retention greater in vaginal hysterectomy versus laparoscopic hysterectomy. In another study, conducted by Hakvoort et al. (2009), it was found that urinary retention was increased in patients who underwent high-grade cystocele repairs, levator plication, and Kelly plication.

Transurethral catheters may be used for short periods of time and are made of silicone/silastic or latex. Catheters are measured using the Charriere or French scale, where 0.33 mm equals 1 French. The rule of placing a catheter is to use the smallest catheter that will still allow for unobstructed drainage. In female patients, the usual size of transurethral catheter used during and after procedures is 14- to 16-French.

The major difficulty with use of transurethral drainage is the potential for infection. Urinary tract infections account for about 40% of hospital-acquired (nosocomial) infections, and about 80% of urinary tract infections occurring in hospitals are associated with urinary catheters. Pelvic surgery is frequently complicated by urinary tract infection. The risk of infection after incontinence surgery is approximately 33% to 47%. Some 45% of women who undergo obliterative procedures for prolapse develop urinary tract infection within 3 months of surgery. Factors that are associated with development of a urinary tract infection after surgery for prolapse and/or stress urinary incontinence include postoperative catheterization because of inability to void, longer operative times, history of recurrent urinary tract infection, and concomitant procedures. Bacterial colonization of a closed system is unavoidable, with a rate of 5% to 10% per day. The bacteria within the catheter system form an ever-changing biofilm that colonizes the catheter tubing and bag. Once these biofilms have developed, it is impossible to eradicate the organism from the urinary system, and the biofilms will persist until the catheter is removed. It is not recommended to treat asymptomatic bacteriuria in the presence of an indwelling catheter. Urinary tract infections will be eliminated in one third of patients who have their Foley catheter removed.

Medicare rules that took effect in October of 2008 deny reimbursement for treatment of inpatient catheter-associated urinary tract infections (CAUTIs) and any associated complications. Box 39.1 lists the Centers for Disease Control and Prevention guidelines for prevention of CAUTI.

There have been some advances, such as the development of catheters impregnated with various metals or antibiotics to try to decrease risk of infection. In a prospective randomized trial performed by Regev-Shoshani et al. (2010), it was shown that impregnation with nitric oxide decreased the incidence of formation of *Escherichia coli* biofilms on catheters. In a Cochrane review by Lam et al. (2014), silver alloy–impregnated catheters did not statistically decrease CAUTI. Catheters impregnated with nitrofurazone were found to reduce the risk of symptomatic CAUTI and asymptomatic bacteriuria in patients catheterized for 1 week or less, although the overall benefit was small. No catheters decreased the rate of urinary tract infections beyond 1 week of catheterization.

BOX 39.1 United States Centers for Disease Control and Prevention Guidelines for Placing Catheters in Patients

Examples of Appropriate Indications for Indwelling Catheter Use

- Patient has acute urinary obstruction or bladder retention
- Need for accurate measurement of urinary function in critically ill patients
- Perioperative use for selected surgical procedures
  - Patients undergoing urologic surgery or other surgery on contiguous structures of the genitourinary tract
  - Anticipated prolonged duration of surgery (catheters inserted for this reason should be removed in the postanesthesia care unit)
  - Patients anticipated to receive large-volume infusions or diuretics during surgery
  - Need for intraoperative monitoring of urinary output
- To assist in healing of open sacral or perineal wounds in incontinent patients
- Patient requires prolonged immobilization (e.g., potentially unstable thoracic or lumbar spine, multiple traumatic injuries such as pelvic fractures)
- To improve comfort for end-of-life care if needed

Examples of Inappropriate Uses of Indwelling Catheters

- As a substitute for nursing care of the patient or resident with incontinence
- As a means of obtaining urine for culture or other diagnostic tests when the patient can voluntarily void
- For prolonged postoperative duration without appropriate indications (e.g., structural repair of urethra or contiguous structures, prolonged effect of epidural anesthesia, etc.)

(From Gould CV, Umscheid CA, Agarwal RK, et al. Guideline for prevention of catheter-associated urinary tract infections. *Infect Control Hosp Epidemiol.* 2010;31:319.)

Other problems with prolonged use of transurethral catheters include periurethral discomfort and irritation of the trigone, against which the balloon rests. Once the catheter is removed, repeated catheterization is needed if the patient does not void spontaneously.

Indwelling urethral catheters are generally contraindicated for long-term control of urinary incontinence in women. The Omnibus Reconciliation Act of 1987 lists three acceptable indications:

- Retention (leading to problems) that cannot be surgically corrected or managed with ISC
- Prevention of contamination of skin wounds with urine
- The care of impaired or terminally ill patients for whom bedding and clothing changes are disruptive

The risks of long-term urethral catheterization include chronic urinary tract infection, urethral abscess and fistula, bladder stones, bladder spasms, bladder neck erosion, leakage around the catheter, and blockage caused by calcium encrustation.

An infrequent complication of transurethral catheterization that may occur is difficulty removing the catheter from the bladder. This may occur because of encrustation, entrapment by sutures, or inability to deflate the balloon. Reasons for inability to deflate the balloon include problems with the valve mechanism, crystallization of the balloon, or problems with the balloon channel. If this occurs, the first thing to do is try to inflate the catheter balloon with an additional 1 to 2 mL of fluid. If this does not work, then the balloon port may be cut; if the port is the problem, this will allow the balloon to empty its contents. If the balloon continues to remain inflated, there is a problem with the inflation lumen of the catheter; therefore, a surgical steel wire or the stiff end of a guidewire should be inserted along the valve inflation lumen and be used to perforate the balloon. If these maneuvers do not work, a spinal needle can be inserted vaginally or suprapubically under ultrasound guidance and used to perforate the balloon.

Suprapubic Catheterization

Hodgkinson and Hodari (1966) demonstrated a lower incidence of bacteriuria and shorter time to reestablish normal voiding with suprapubic bladder drainage compared with transurethral drainage after surgical procedures for incontinence. Other studies have supported these findings. Suprapubic catheters have been shown to decrease urethral injury and stricture with long-term use compared with transurethral catheterization and have similar rates of upper tract injury and bladder calculi. Suprapubic catheters also improve patient comfort and ease of nursing care. However, there are few data comparing suprapubic catheters with transurethral catheters with respect to quality of life and user preference. These catheters allow patients to control voiding, and they eliminate the need for transurethral catheterizations to check postvoid residual urine volumes. This makes them preferable for longer-term (more than a few days) use and for use in patients in whom postoperative retention is expected, such as the elderly. Suprapubic tubes are used less frequently than in the past because of their invasive nature, and because most patients who undergo prolapse and incontinence surgery generally do not need a catheter for longer than 72 hours. See Fig. 39.1 for common types of transurethral and suprapubic catheters that are available.

As with transurethral drainage, the main problem with suprapubic catheterization is infection, but to a lesser degree. When suprapubic tubes were used for long-term drainage in patients with spinal cord injuries, 51% developed infections, and 100% had asymptomatic bacteriuria. However, additional studies and meta-analyses seem to show a lower risk for infection from suprapubic tubes versus transurethral catheters. There are other risks associated with suprapubic catheter use. Urinary deposits and blood clots may obstruct the smaller-caliber catheters, necessitating frequent irrigation. The invasive nature of insertion can lead to rare complications such as hematuria, cellulitis, bowel injury, urine extravasation, and catheter fracture. However, suprapubic catheters can be useful in patients who undergo gynecologic procedures that require long-term bladder drainage. In a case series, suprapubic catheters were placed in patients who underwent surgery for stress incontinence using midurethral slings. These patients were able to measure their voiding function and conduct voiding trials at home, which was convenient and time-saving for the patients. In a randomized double-blind trial by Rogers et al. (2004), it was suggested that prophylaxis with nitrofurantoin until the catheter was removed decreased the rate of positive urine cultures, without selection for resistant organisms; however, after 6 weeks postoperatively there was no difference between groups that took antibiotics and groups that did not take antibiotics.

Contraindications to suprapubic insertion, especially closed insertion, include extensive abdominal adhesions from previous surgeries, ventral hernia, extensive intraoperative bladder reconstruction, carcinoma of the bladder, and postoperative anticoagulation therapy. Despite these potential problems, suprapubic catheters are preferred to transurethral catheters when prolonged drainage is anticipated or when significant dissection around the urethra has been performed. In a systematic review and meta-analysis by Healy et al. (2012), it was found that suprapubic catheterization significantly reduced postoperative urinary tract infections, although there was increased risk of iatrogenic injury and catheter-associated complications.

Suprapubic catheters can be inserted using an open or closed technique. Cystotomy into the bladder dome under direct visualization is the safest method for use during open abdominal approach surgery. It is preferred when distension of the bladder is difficult, when gross hematuria is present, when there has been a recent cystotomy, or in the presence of gynecologic malignancy. To perform this procedure, the bladder is filled with saline. A stab incision is made through the skin above or below the surgical incision (the suprapubic catheter incision should be separate from the surgical incision) with a scalpel. The catheter and introducer are passed through the skin, muscle, and fascia. The bladder is then punctured through the dome, taking care to avoid large vessels. The catheter is advanced through the

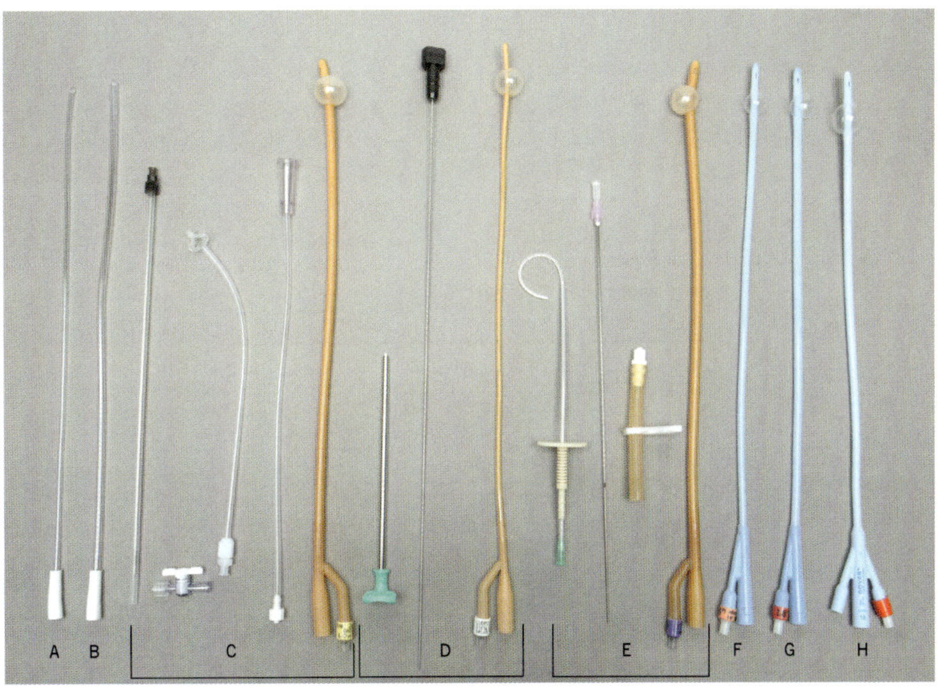

Fig. 39.1 Common types of catheters and catheter systems used during and after surgical procedures. 12-French (**A**) and 18-French (**B**) Kendall Seamless Robinson plastic urethral catheters. **C**, Cook Stamey percutaneous suprapubic catheter set. **D**, Bard Suprapubic Introducer Foley catheter set. **E**, BD Bonanno Suprapubic Bladder Drainage catheter. 16-French (**F**) and 18-French (**G**) Kendall Dover 100% silicone Foley catheters. **H**, Kendall Dover 3-Way 100% silicone Foley catheter.

sheath or over the needle guide, which is simultaneously withdrawn. Efflux of urine or saline should be ensured. If the catheter has a balloon, it is inflated. The catheter is sutured in place on the skin.

Closed insertion can be performed using a variety of catheters, including an ordinary Foley catheter through an introducer, when there is no abdominal incision (see Video 39.1 for closed insertion technique). To insert a catheter, the surgeon should place the patient in the Trendelenburg position and fill the bladder through a transurethral catheter or cystoscope with at least 400 to 500 mL sterile saline or water until the bladder is easily palpable abdominally. This positioning helps ensure that no bowel lies between the bladder and the anterior abdominal wall. After the usual skin prepping, the needle or trocar should be inserted through the skin and fascia into the bladder, at a point no more than 3 cm above the pubic symphysis, and at an angle directed downward toward the pubic symphysis (Fig. 39.2A). The trocar or needle is removed, and the catheter is secured (Fig. 39.2B and C). The transurethral catheter is then removed. Correct placement can be verified with a cystoscope.

Intermittent Self-Catheterization

The technique of clean ISC was evaluated initially by Lapides et al. (1972) in patients with incontinence or voiding dysfunction

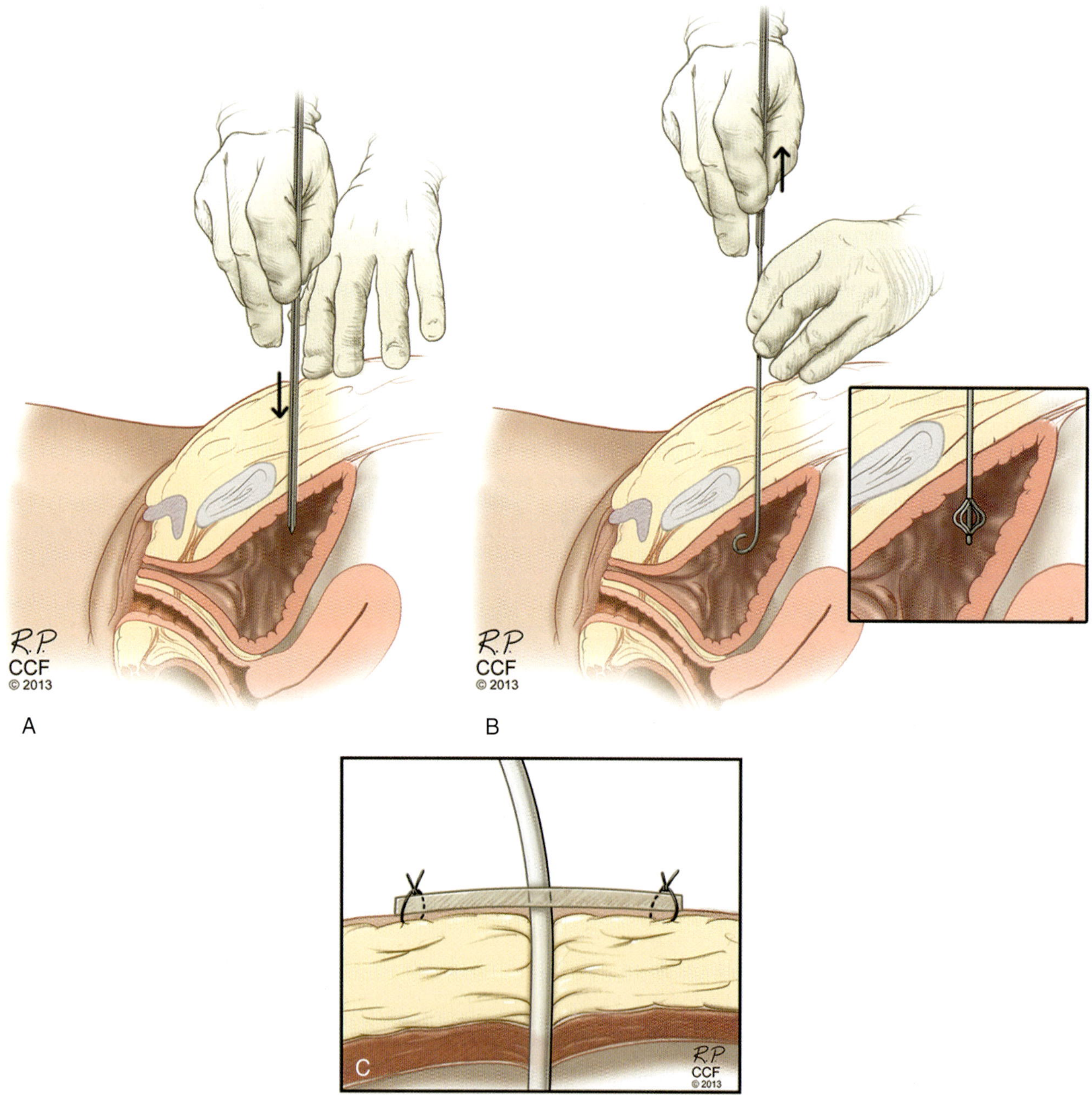

Fig. 39.2 Typical method of insertion of a suprapubic catheter. **A**, Insertion of suprapubic catheter via trocar. **B**, Withdrawal of trocar with insertion of pigtail catheter. *Inset,* Mallecot type of catheter tip. **C**, Catheter sutured to skin.

because of neurogenic bladder disease. ISC allows the patient to insert a short plastic catheter into the urethra as needed to empty the bladder. Studies suggest that women using ISC after hysterectomy have lower bacteriuria rates than women with a transurethral Foley.

The rationale for nonsterile, clean ISC is based on the theory that functional abnormalities of the lower urinary tract lead to infection. Decreased blood flow resulting from overdistension is cited as one of the most common causes of infection. The benefits of eliminating overdistension outweigh the disadvantages of intermittent insertion of a nonsterile catheter. Each catheterization event carries a 3% to 4% infection rate, and bacteriuria occurs in most patients within 2 to 3 weeks. Despite this, clinical studies of ISC have shown its safety with long-term follow-up in children with neurogenic bladder dysfunction. Ninety percent of these children were free of major kidney infection after 10 years, despite a 56% rate of intermittent bacteriuria. Since then, ISC has been evaluated in patients with spinal cord injury and multiple sclerosis. A recent review of ISC in spinal cord patients suggests that prophylactic antibiotics should only be used for a short time during the initiation of ISC. Elderly persons have experienced infection rates of up to 12.5% per year with ISC. The frequency of catheterization is the most important factor as far as prevention of infection. There is no difference in colonization or infection rates between sterile catheters and clean catheters. Meatal cleansing offers no advantage either.

The complication rate for postoperative use of ISC should be lower than that for long-term ISC because it is seldom used for longer than 6 weeks. ISC can be started immediately postoperatively, or a Foley catheter can be used for the first 24 hours. To use ISC the patient must have the manual dexterity and mental ability to perform self-catheterization. The bladder capacity should be at least 100 mL. Complications other than infection are rare; they include retention of the catheter and perforation of the urethra, creating a false passage. A Cochrane review by Moore et al. (2007) found little evidence to suggest that the incidence of urinary tract infections is affected by sterile, single-use, cleaned and reused, or coated catheters.

The technique of ISC can be taught to patients preoperatively or postoperatively by direct demonstration (Fig. 39.3 and Box 39.2). The patient should be supplied with a device to measure urine and with short plastic or rubber catheters. There are newer hydrophilic low-friction catheters that may be more comfortable than the standard plastic catheters. Patients should be instructed to carry catheters at all times, with separate containers for clean and used catheters. Catheterization can be performed anywhere, and the importance of emptying the bladder often enough to keep the urine volumes obtained below 400 to 500 mL should be stressed to the patient.

Most patients catheterize every 3 to 4 hours and then as needed during the night. The need to catheterize should take priority over the availability of soap and water. The urethra does not need to be cleansed before catheterization. Voiding should be attempted before every catheterization, and the residual urine volume measured and recorded, if possible.

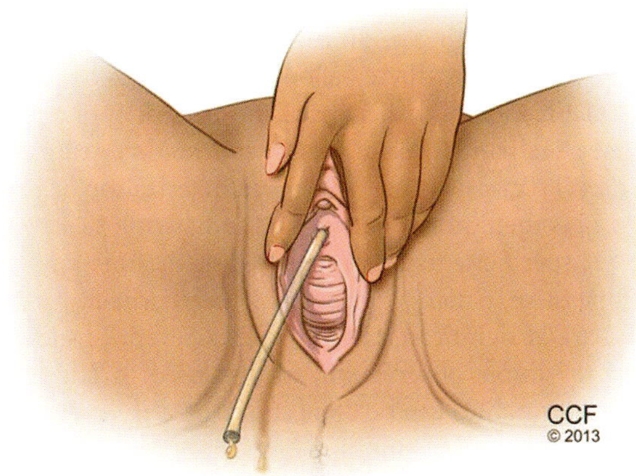

Fig. 39.3 Illustration of instructions for patient self-catheterization.

BOX 39.2 Instructions to Patient on Performing Intermittent Self-catheterization

1. Wash your hands with soap and water.
2. Use a clean (soap and water) catheter, with water-soluble lubricant if needed.
3. Attempt to empty your bladder before catheterization.
4. Position yourself lying in bed or straddling a toilet.
5. Spread the labia with the fourth and index fingers of one hand and use the middle finger to locate the urethra.
6. Insert the catheter 1 to 2 inches and drain until all urine flow stops.
7. Measure and record the amount of urine ("residual") obtained.

When residual volumes are consistently less than 20% of the total voided volume, ISC can be stopped. Prophylactic antibiotics can be given, if desired, for short periods of ISC, although equivocal benefit has been shown in patients using ISC for a long time.

Voiding Trials After Surgery

It is common to have postoperative voiding dysfunction after prolapse or incontinence surgery. It is estimated that 3% to 40% of patients who undergo urogynecologic procedures will have postoperative voiding dysfunction. There are many factors contributing to voiding dysfunction postoperatively, including type of anesthesia used during the surgery, type of surgery, type of analgesia used, and fluid status of the patient. Several retrospective studies have analyzed preoperative risk factors. In a prospective study conducted by Kim et al. (2012), the risk factors of age, parity, and concomitant cystocele repair appeared to increase risk of voiding dysfunction after midurethral sling surgery.

To establish if patients have return of voiding function after surgery, it is common to have the patient perform a voiding trial. There are many different methods that can be used to perform voiding trials. One technique is to retrograde fill the patient's bladder with normal saline or sterile water, remove the catheter, and have the patient void. The voided amount is measured, and if the patient can void more than 50% of the fluid placed in the bladder, he or she can remain catheter-free. This method has been found to have 94.4% sensitivity and 58.1% specificity for predicting voiding dysfunction. An alternate process is to remove the catheter, allow the patient to naturally fill his or her bladder, and then have the patient spontaneously void. Once the patient has urinated, the residual urine in the bladder can be measured via straight catheterization or bladder scanner. This method has been found to have 100% sensitivity and 25.8% specificity to determine voiding dysfunction.

Postoperative patients who have their urinary catheters removed are at significant risk of cystitis. Several strategies, in addition to simple observation, can be used to address this problem. A urinalysis can be done and, if positive, cultures sent or empiric short-course antibiotics given. A study of hospitalized patients who underwent short-term urinary catheterization suggested that they might benefit from antimicrobial prophylaxis when the catheter is removed, as the patients given antimicrobial prophylaxis experienced fewer subsequent urinary tract infections (Marschall et al., 2013). This concept was also supported by a 2013 Cochrane review (Lusardi et al., 2013); however, the review included nonsurgical studies. A recent randomized controlled trial found that daily nitrofurantoin did not reduce the incidence of urinary tract infection among women requiring catheter management of urinary retention after pelvic reconstructive surgery (Lavelle et al., 2019).

When a suprapubic catheter is used, some hematuria on the first day is common. Narrow-diameter catheters may require periodic irrigation to remove blood clots. The catheter is left to straight drainage until the patient is able to get up and begin voiding trials. The catheter is clamped, and the patient allowed to void with the catheter clamped at least once every 2 to 4 hours. If the patient cannot void, the clamp is opened, the bladder drained, and the catheter reclamped until the next voiding trial. If the patient seems to be voiding well, a postvoid residual volume can be obtained by unclamping the tube for 15 minutes after a voiding episode and measuring the amount of urine obtained. The catheter can be left open overnight for convenience. When the residual volume is less than 20% to 50% of the total voided volume, the catheter can be removed. If voiding trials are unsuccessful, the patient should be discharged with the catheter and given written instructions and diary forms to continue the voiding trials at home. The patient should follow up in the office a few days to 1 week later, or when the postvoid residual is less than 100 mL.

Catheter and Drainage Bag Management

In general, care of the drainage bag is similar for both suprapubic and transurethral catheters. The most common route of bacterial entry into the bladder is via ascension of bacterial biofilm along the tubing and the catheter. To prevent ascending infection, disconnection of the catheter and bag should be avoided. A bag with a urometer helps to break the urine column between the bag and catheter. The bag should be below the level of the bladder at all times, and the drainage port should be kept clean. Prophylactic antibiotics are of no benefit in preventing colonization of the system, and patients should not be treated for bacterial infection unless they are symptomatic. If patients are more mobile, they may be able to use a leg bag, which is a smaller catheter bag that attaches to the upper leg. Leg bags can hold less urine than the standard catheter bags and may necessitate more frequent drainage. If patients experience leakage around the catheter tubing, it may be because of bladder spasm. Treatment may include anticholinergics and phenazopyridine for comfort.

URINE LOSS APPLIANCES AND ABSORPTIVE PRODUCTS

Patients whose incontinence is not correctable with bladder training, physical therapy, medical therapy, or surgical therapy have a variety of choices for protective options. These choices range from shields resembling ordinary sanitary pads to disposable briefs to washable garments designed to hold pads, as well as menstrual sanitary pads. Absorbent products that are disposable are the most commonly used devices for incontinence. Absorbent products are made of many different designs; however, they can be classified into two general groups: products used for "light" incontinence and products used for "moderate" or "heavy" incontinence. The Cochrane review of available randomized trials in 2008 noted that there are significant and substantial differences between the designs of absorbent products, and that a blanket policy of using washable garments alone is not recommended for patients with moderate to heavy leakage. The review also found that women prefer "pull-up" type protective garments; however, these are more expensive than inserts. The selection of products should be based on the individual patient's fit, skin condition, ability to use the product independently, volume of leakage, and living situation, as well as convenience to caregivers and financial considerations (Box 39.3).

Multiple different brands of disposable shields are available. These are shaped like sanitary pads but contain a powder (such as sodium polyacrylate) and a fluffed cellulose wood pulp that absorbs liquid to form a gel, thus preventing clothing wetness. They are available in different absorbencies and are ideal for patients who experience small amounts of urine loss (e.g., only with exercise). Reusable underwear that hold disposable pads or

BOX 39.3 Criteria for Selection of Incontinence Products

The ideal product should meet the following criteria:

- It contains urine (and stool) completely and prevents leakage onto clothing, bedding, and furniture.
- It is comfortable to wear and protects vulnerable skin from maceration, chafing, and pressure sores.
- It is easy for the incontinent person to use. If this is not feasible because of physical or mental disability, it should be easy for a caregiver to use.
- It disguises or contains odor.
- It is inconspicuous under clothing, without bulk or noise.
- It is easy to dispose of or clean, as required.
- It is reasonably priced and readily available.

(From Jeter KF, Faller N, Norton C, eds. *Nursing for Continence*. Philadelphia: WB Saunders; 1990:210.)

shields snugly against the perineum are available. A randomized crossover trial comparing disposable pads to reusable underwear found no difference in quality-of-life measures between the two options, but did find that reusable underwear was preferred with respect to measures such as discreteness, comfort, and fit (Alam et al., 2018). Use of superabsorbent material is associated with less leakage; however, no product is currently leak-proof.

Disposable fitted briefs are suitable for moderate to heavy leaking and are available in a variety of absorbencies. Fitted briefs are bulkier than undergarments because they wrap around the hips; they are held in place with front-to-back reusable elastic straps or adhesive panels. For severe incontinence, rubber and vinyl underpants to wear over regular underpants, as well as reusable, washable, absorbent underpants with waterproof outer barriers, are available.

Quality of life with regard to women who use these products is an important factor. In a qualitative analysis of 99 women with light incontinence, pad use and "treatment effects" were measured in the context of quality of life (Gertliffe et al., 2007). In this study, five subthemes were developed regarding pad characteristics that were important for use: the ability of the pad to hold urine, to contain smell, and to stay in place; discreteness; and comfort when wet. High levels of anxiety were associated with use of pads that were not satisfactory with regard to the five subthemes.

Consideration should also be given to use of products to clean, moisturize, and protect skin from urine. Incontinence-associated dermatitis is an inflammation of the perineal skin that occurs when it comes into contact with urine or stool. Perineal skin cleansing should be performed after each incontinence episode. Perineal skin in patients who have incontinence should be moisturized with humectants. Barrier lotions can be used that contain petroleum jelly or silicone. The National Association for Continence publishes a *Resource Guide of Continence Products and Services* (National Association for Continence, n.d.). This publication is cross-referenced by product categories and manufacturers and contains an index of mail and phone order information.

BIBLIOGRAPHY

Alam PA, Burkett LS, Clark BA, et al. Randomized cross-over comparison of icon reusable underwear to disposable pads for the management of mild to moderate urinary incontinence. *Female Pelvic Med Reconstr Surg.* 2018;24:161.

Albo ME, Richter HE, Brubaker L, et al. Burch colposuspension versus fascial sling to reduce urinary stress incontinence. *N Engl J Med.* 2007;356:2143.

Anderson JT, Heisterberg L, Hebjoren S, et al. Suprapubic vs. transurethral bladder drainage after colposuspension/vaginal vault repair. *Acta Obstet Gynecol Scand.* 1985;64:139.

Anger JT, Litwin MS, Wang Q, et al. Complications of sling surgery among female medicare beneficiaries. *N Engl J Med.* 2007;109:707.

Bakke A, Vollset SE. Risk factors for bacteriuria and clinical urinary tract infection in patients treated with clean intermittent catheterization. *J Urol.* 1993;149:527.

Baldini G, Bagry H, Aprikian A, et al. Postoperative and perioperative considerations: anesthetic and perioperative considerations. *Anesthesiology.* 2009;110:1139.

Beeckman D, Schoonhoven L, Verhaeghe S, et al. Prevention and treatment of incontinence-associated dermatitis: literature review. *J Adv Nurs.* 2009;65:1141.

Bergman A, Matthews L, Ballard CA, Roy S. Suprapubic vs. transurethral bladder drainage after surgery for stress urinary incontinence. *Obstet Gynecol.* 1987;69:546.

Boccola MA, Sharma A, Taylor C, et al. The infusion method trial of void vs standard catheter removal in the outpatient setting: a prospective randomized trial. *BJU Int.* 2011;107:43.

Brazelli M, Shirran E, Vale L. Absorbant products for containing urinary and/or fecal incontinence in adults. *J Wound Ostomy Continence Nurs.* 2002;29:45.

Breitenbucher RB. Bacterial changes in the urine samples of patients with long-term indwelling catheters. *Arch Intern Med.* 1984;144:1585.

Britt MR, Garibaldi RA, Miller WA, et al. Antimicrobial prophylaxis for catheter associated bacteriuria. *Antimicrob Agents Chemother.* 1977;11:240.

Brown J, Doloresco F, Mylotte JM. Never events: not every hospital-acquired infection is preventable. *Clin Infect Dis.* 2009;49:743.

Clark-O'Neill S, Pettersson L, Fader M, et al. A multicenter comparative evaluation: washable pants with an integral pad for light incontinence. *J Clin Nurs.* 2002;11:79.

Cottenden AM. Incontinence pads: clinical performance, design, and technical properties. *J Biomed Eng.* 1988;10:506.

Cravens DD, Zweig S. Urinary catheter management. *Am Fam Phys.* 2000;61:369.

Darrah DM, Griebling TL, Silverstein JH. Postoperative urinary retention. *Anesthesiol Clin.* 2009;27:465.

De Souza GM, Costa WS, Bruschini HE, Sampaio FJ. Morphological analysis of the acute effects of overdistension on the extracellular matrix of the rat urinary bladder wall. *Ann Anat.* 2004;186:55.

Dieter AA, Amundsen CL, Visco AG, Siddiqui NY. Treatment for urinary tract infection after midurethral sling: a retrospective study comparing patients who receive short-term postoperative catheterization and patients who pass a void trial on the day of surgery. *Female Pelvic Med Reconstr Surg.* 2012;18:175.

Diokno AC, Mitchell BA, Nash AJ, Kimbrough JA. Patient satisfaction and the Lofric catheter for clean intermittent catheterization. *J Urol.* 1995;153:349.

Dobbs SP, Jackson SK, Wilson AM, et al. A prospective, randomized trial comparing continuous bladder drainage with catheterization at abdominal hysterectomy. *Br J Urol.* 1997;80:554.

Dunn S, Kowanko I, Paterson J, Pretty L. Systematic review of the effectiveness of urinary continence products. *J Wound Ostomy Continence Nurs.* 2002;29:129.

Fader M, Cottenden A, Getliffe K, et al. Absorbent products for urinary/faecal incontinence: a comparative evaluation of key product designs. *Health Technol Assess.* 2008;12:iii.

Fader M, Cottenden AM, Getliffe K. Absorbent products for moderate-heavy urinary and or faecal incontinence in women and men. *Cochrane Database Syst Rev.* 2008;4:CD0074808.

Faller N, Jeter KF. The ABC's of product selection. *Urol Nurs.* 1992;12:52.

Fitzgerald MP, Richter HE, Bradley CS, et al. Pelvic support, pelvic symptoms, and patient satisfaction after colpocleisis. *Int Urogynecol J Pelvic Floor Dysfunct.* 2008;19:1603.

Foley FEB. A self-retaining bag catheter. *J Urol.* 1937;38:140.

Garibaldi RA, Burke JP, Dickman ML, Smith CB. Factors predisposing to bacteriuria during indwelling urethral catheterization. *N Engl J Med*. 1974;291:215.

Geller EJ, Hankins KJ, Parnell BA, et al. Diagnostic accuracy of retrograde and spontaneous voiding trials for postoperative voiding dysfunction. *Obstet Gynecol*. 2011;118:637.

Gertliffe K, Fader M, Cottenden A, et al. Absorbent products for incontinence: 'treatment effects' and impact on quality of life. *J Clin Nurs*. 2007;16:1936.

Ghezzi F, Cromi A, Uccella S, et al. Immediate Foley removal after laparoscopic and vaginal hysterectomy: determinants of postoperative urinary retention. *J Minim Invasive Gynecol*. 2007;14:706.

Gould CV, Umscheid CA, Agarwal RK, et al. Guideline for prevention of catheter-associated urinary tract infections. *Infect Control Hosp Epidemiol*. 2010;31:319.

Hakvoort RA, Dijkgraff MG, Burger MP, et al. Predicting short-term urinary retention after vaginal prolapse surgery. *Neurourol Urod*. 2009;28:225.

Harding GK, Nicolle LE, Ronald AR, et al. How long should catheter-acquired urinary tract infection in women be treated? A randomized controlled study. *Ann Intern Med*. 1991;114:713.

Harlass FE, Magelssen DJ. Benefits of posturethropexy bladder conditioning: fact or fiction? *J Reprod Med*. 1988;33:961.

Healy EF, Walsh CA, Cotter AM, Walsh SR. Suprapubic compared with transurethral bladder catheterization for gynecologic surgery: a systematic review and meta-analysis. *Obstet Gynecol*. 2012;120:678.

Hicklin K. Lessons learned: adult urine incontinence protective wear. *Urol Nurs*. 2002;22:129.

Hodgkinson CP, Hodari AA. Trocar suprapubic cystotomy for postoperative bladder drainage in the female. *Am J Obstet Gynecol*. 1966;96:773.

Hunter KF, Bharmal A, Moore KN. Long-term bladder drainage: suprapubic catheter versus other methods: a scoping review. *Neurourol Urodyn*. 2013;32:944.

Hu TW, Kaltreider DL, Igov J. Incontinence products: which is best? *Geriatr Nurs*. 1989;10:184.

Jeter KF, Faller N, Norton C, eds. *Nursing for Continence*. Philadelphia: WB Saunders; 1990.

Karram MM, Segal JL, Vassallo BJ, Kleeman SD. Complications and untoward effects of the tension-free vaginal tape procedure. *Obstet Gynecol*. 2003;101:929.

Kass EJ, Koff SA, Diokno AC, Lapides J. The significance of bacilluria in children on long-term intermittent catheterization. *J Urol*.1981;126:223.

Kasturi S, Cassiere EK, Bently-Taylor M, Woodman PJ, Hale DS. Use of suprapubic tube to assess voiding function after synthetic midurethral slings. *Female Pelvic Med Reconstr Surg*. 2012;18:179.

Kim JK, Moon DG, Shin JH, et al. Predictors of voiding dysfunction after mid-urethral sling surgery for stress urinary incontinence. *Int Neurourol J*. 2012;16:30.

King RB, Carlson CE, Mervine J, et al. Clean and sterile intermittent catheterization methods in hospitalized patients with SCI. *Arch Phys Med Rehabil*. 1992;73:798.

Kleeman S, Goldwasser S, Vassallo B, Karram M. Predicting post-operative voiding efficacy after operation for incontinence and prolapse. *Am J Obstet Gynecol*. 2002;187:49.

Lam TBL, Omar M, Fisher E, et al. Types of indwelling urethral catheters for short-term catheterization in hospitalized adults. *Cochrane Database Syst Rev*. 2014;9:CD004013.

Lapides J, Diokno AC, Silber SJ, Lowe BS. Clean, intermittent self-catheterization in the treatment of urinary tract disease. *J Urol*. 1972;107:458.

Lavelle ES, Alam P, Meister M, et al. Antibiotic prophylaxis during catheteter-managed postoperative urinary retention after pelvic reconstructive surgery: a randomized controlled trial. *Obstet Gynecol*. 2019;132:727.

Lian CJ, Bracken RB. Urinary catheter sterilization with microwave oven. *Int Urogynecol J*. 1991;2:94.

Lusardi G, Lipp A, Shaw C. Antibiotic prophylaxis for short-term catheter bladder drainage in adults. *Cochrane Database Syst Rev*. 2013;7:CD005428.

MacDiarmid SA, Arnold EP, Palmer NB, Anthony A. Management of spinal cord injured patients by indwelling suprapubic catheterization. *J Urol*. 1995;154:492.

Marschall J, Carpenter CR, Fowler S, Trautner BW. CDC Prevention Epicenters Program. Antibiotic prophylaxis for urinary tract infections after removal of urinary catheter: meta-analysis. *BMJ*. 2013;346:f3147.

Maynard FM, Diokno AC. Urinary infection and complications during clean intermittent catheterization following spinal cord injury. *J Urol*. 1984;132:943.

McClish DK, Wyman JF, Sale PG, et al. Use and costs of incontinence pads in female study volunteers. Continence Program for Women Research Group. *J Wound Ostomy Continence Nurs*. 1999:26:207.

McPhail MJW, Abu-Hilial M, Johnson CD. A meta-analysis comparing suprapubic and transurethral catheterization for bladder drainage after abdominal surgery. *Br J Surg*. 2006:93:1038.

Mendez-Probst CE, Razvi H, Denstedt JD. Fundamentals of instrumentation and urinary drainage. In: Wein AJ, Kavoussi LR, Novick AC, et al., eds. *Campbell-Walsh Urology*. 10th ed. New York: Elsevier; 2012:e177.

Moore KN, Fader M, Getliffe K. Long-term bladder management by intermittent catheterisation in adults and children. *Cochrane Database Syst Rev*. 2007;4:CD006008.

National Association for Continence. (n.d.). *Ordering Printed Patient Resources*. Retrieved August 15, 2021, from https://www.nafc.org/resource-center/resource-guide-products-and-services-for-incontinence.

Novara G, Galfano A, Boscolo-Berto R, et al. Complication rates of tension-free midurethral slings in the treatment of female stress urinary incontinence: a systematic review and meta-analysis of randomized controlled trials comparing tension-free midurethral tapes to other surgical procedures and different devices. *Eur Urol*. 2008;53:288.

Nacey JN, Tulloch AG, Ferguson AF. Catheter induced urethritis: a comparison between latex and silicone catheter in a prospective clinical trial. *Br J Urol*. 1985;57:325.

Nicolee LE. Urinary catheter-associated infections. *Infect Dis Clin North Am*. 2012;26:13.

Nix D, Haugen V. Prevention and management of incontinence-associated dermatitis. *Drugs Aging*. 2010;27:491.

Nygaard I, Brubaker L, Chai TC, et al. Risk factors for urinary tract infection following incontinence surgery. *Int Urogynecol J*. 2011;22:1255.

O'Brien WM. Percutaneous placement of a suprapubic tube with peel away sheath introducer. *J Urol*. 1991;145:1015.

Regev-Shoshani G, Ko M, Miller C, Av-Gay Y. Slow release of nitric oxide from charged catheters and its effect on biofilm formation by Escherichia coli. *Antimicrob Agents Chemother*. 2010; 54:273.

Richter HE, Albo ME, Zyczynski HM, et al. Retropubic versus transobturator midurethral slings for stress incontinence. *N Engl J Med.* 2010;362:22.

Rogers RG, Kammerer-Doak DN, Olsen A, et al. A randomized double-blind placebo controlled comparison of the effect of nitrofurantoin monohydrate macrocrystals on the development of urinary tract infections following surgery for pelvic organ prolapse and/or stress urinary incontinence with suprapubic catheterization. *Am J Obstet Gynecol.* 2004;191:182.

Stekkinger E, Van der Linden PJQ. A comparison of suprapubic and transurethral catheterization on postoperative urinary retention after vaginal prolapse repair: a randomized controlled trial. *Gynecol Obstet Invest.* 2011;72:109.

Stickler DJ, Zimakoff J. Complications of urinary tract infections associated with devices used for long-term bladder management. *J Hosp Infect.*1994;28:177.

Terpenning MS, Allada RA, Kauffman CA. Intermittent urethral catheterization in the elderly. *J Am Geriatr Soc.* 1989;37:411.

Van der Wall E, Verkooyen RP, Mintjes-DeGroot J, et al. Prophylactic ciprofloxin for catheter associated urinary tract infection. *Lancet.* 1992;339:946.

Waller L, Johnsson O, Norlén L, Sullivan L. Clean intermittent catheterization in spinal cord injury patients: long-term follow-up of a hydrophilic low friction technique. *J Urol.* 1995;153:345.

Wanick CK, Reilly NJ. Incontinence care products: non-surgical management of urinary incontinence. *Ostomy Wound Manage.* 1991;34:43.

Warren JW. Catheter-associated urinary tract infections. *Infect Dis Clin North Am.* 1997;11:609.

Warren JW, Anthony WC, Hoopes JM, Muncie HLJ. Cephalexin for susceptible bacteriuria in afebrile, long term catheterized patients. *JAMA.* 1982;248:454.

Webb RJ, Lawson AL, Neal DE. Clean intermittent self-catheterization in 172 adults. *Br J Urol.* 1990;65:20.

Wyndaele JJ. Complications of intermittent catheterization: their prevention and treatment. *Spinal Cord.* 2002;40:536.

40

Urology for the Urogynecologist

Elizabeth R. Mueller and Thythy T. Pham

CHAPTER OUTLINE

Basics of Urinary Stone Disease

Introduction

One out of 13 women will become symptomatic with a kidney stone in her lifetime; that incidence is rising in the United States resulting from the increasing prevalence of obesity and diabetes. Often, the symptoms are acute and painful, and require a visit to the emergency room. Unfortunately, half of patients who pass a kidney stone will have a recurrence within 5 years. This section will provide a brief review of urinary tract stone disease and recommendations for prevention in women with known stone disease, as well as when to refer a patient with an asymptomatic stone found on an evaluation for microscopic or gross hematuria.

Epidemiology/Gender Differences

The incidence of asymptomatic stones is 8% to 10% of the population. In a study of over 5000 patients undergoing a screening computed tomography colonography, asymptomatic stones were found in 9.7% of men and 6.3% of women. The average number of stones found was 2.1, with a mean stone size of 3 mm (Boyce et al., 2010). Survey studies are used to assess the prevalence of symptomatic stones. The National Health and Nutrition Examination Survey (NHANES) conducted in 2007 to 2010 (n = 12,100) included questions about a history of kidney stones. The prevalence was found to be 8.8% overall, at 10.6% in men and 7.1% in women (Scales et al., 2012). This was a marked increase from the NHANES III cohort (1976–1994), in which the prevalence was 6.3% among men and 4.1% among women (Stamatelou et al., 2003). Scales et al. (2012) found that kidney stones were more prevalent among obese individuals compared with normal-weight individuals (11.2% vs. 6.1%). Black, non-Hispanic and Hispanic individuals were less likely to report a history of stone disease than White, non-Hispanic individuals. Obesity and diabetes were strongly associated with a history of kidney stones in multivariate analysis.

Pathophysiology

The pathophysiology of stone formation is complex; however, there are a few concepts that are important in understanding renal stone formation. Urinary supersaturation is the driving force for the phase change of minerals from a dissolved salt to a solid. Although supersaturation is essential, by itself it does not result in the formation of a stone. The solid precipitates out of the urine and forms crystals in the urine that are often identified by a clinical laboratory with urine microscopy. The process of stone formation requires nucleation, crystal growth, crystal aggregation, and crystal retention. Once formed, the crystals may flow in the urine or become retained in the urinary tract at sites that promote growth, leading to stone formation.

The majority of stones seen in the United States contain calcium, most commonly calcium oxalate (60%), followed by hydroxyapatite (20%) and brushite (2%). Of the non–calcium-containing stones, uric acid (7%) and struvite stones (7%) are the most common. Along with low urine volume and low urine pH, urinary calcium and oxalate are important and equal contributors to calcium oxalate stone formation. Inhibitors of stone formation include high urinary volume, higher urinary pH, citrate, and magnesium.

Radiologic Imaging for the Presence of Stones

Noncontrast computed tomography (CT stone protocol) is the gold standard for imaging urinary tract stones because of its lower radiation exposure (85% decrease) as compared with three-phase CT. It is also beneficial because it can assess renal anatomy and other associated findings such as hydronephrosis and perinephric stranding. An alternative imaging modality includes the use of renal ultrasound in combination with a plain film of the kidneys, ureters, and bladder (KUB). KUB imaging is typically required with ultrasound imaging because ultrasound measurements of renal stone size are not as accurate and are less able to visualize stones in the ureter.

Treatment

There is not much evidence on how or when to treat asymptomatic stones. Stones that are asymptomatic in the kidney can become symptomatic while passing through the ureter. Ureteral stones usually become impacted at three distinct ureteral sites: at the ureteropelvic junction, crossing the iliac vessels, and at the ureterovesical junction. Stone passage rates are dependent on the size of the stone and will be discussed in detail later. Stones that are 2 mm or less have excellent passage rates and require intervention less than 5% of the time. That said, the average time to passage could be a week. Renal stones 2 mm or greater should be referred to a urologist, who can clearly state the risk and benefits of a stone removal from the kidney. Kidney stones larger than 1 cm are less likely to traverse the ureteropelvic junction and result in acute pain. Although asymptomatic, they should be addressed, because the stone will continue to enlarge. Stones less than 2 cm may be amenable to more conservative surgical treatments, such as extracorporeal shock wave lithotripsy and ureteroscopic interventions. Stones greater than 2 cm require percutaneous nephrolithotomy or open/laparoscopic stone removal, which are more morbid procedures.

Upper urinary tract stones can be the cause of pain, infection, obstruction, active stone growth, or hematuria. In a study of 180 women presenting to the emergency room with a symptomatic upper tract stone, one-third had kidney stones, and two-thirds had ureteral stones (Dall'era et al., 2005). Of those with a kidney stone on presentation, the average stone size was 7.9 mm. The majority (45%) required no intervention other than medications and a urology referral, whereas 33% required ureteroscopy, 10% required a stent, and 12% required percutaneous nephrolithotomy. Ureteral stones had an average size of 4.3 mm. The majority (86%) of the stones were located in the distal ureter, 11% were in the proximal ureter, and 3% were located in the midureter. The majority of the women (77%) were managed without surgical intervention. Of the individuals for whom follow-up information was obtained (41%), the average size of the stones that passed spontaneously was 3.3 mm.

Spontaneous passage rates of stones in the ureter are dependent on the stone size and location. In a study of 850 male and female patients with acute flank pain, 172 (13.5%) were found to have ureteral stones (Coll et al., 2002). The majority of stones (67%) passed spontaneously, and the rest required intervention. The spontaneous passage rate for stones 1 mm in diameter was 87%; for stones 2 to 4 mm, 76%; for stones 5 to 7 mm, 60%; for stones 7 to 9 mm, 48%; and for stones larger than 9 mm, 25%. Spontaneous passage rates as a function of the stone location were 48% in the proximal ureter, 60% for midureteral stones, 75% for distal stones, and 79% for ureterovesical junctional stones. Limited studies have demonstrated that 84% of pregnant women with ureteral colic spontaneously pass renal calculi when treated conservatively with hydration, analgesics and, if infected, antibiotics. If stents are required, they can be done cystoscopically using ultrasound or minimal radiographic imaging (Stothers & Lee, 1992).

Time to passage of stones is also dependent on stone size. In a study of 75 men and women who were prospectively followed for stone passage, stones smaller than 2 mm passed in 8.2 days, with 4.8% requiring intervention, whereas stones between 2 and 4 mm took an average of 12 days and up to 40 days to pass, with 17% requiring intervention (Miller & Kane, 1999). Stones that were larger than 4 mm took 22 days to pass, and 11% needed an intervention, whereas intervention was required for 50% of patients with ureteral calculi greater than 5 mm. Factors that predicted a spontaneous stone passage were right-sided stones, distal location in the ureter, and smaller size.

Recurrence

The recurrence rate for patients who have passed their first stone is approximately 50%. Risk factors for stone recurrence are anatomic upper tract abnormalities (pelvic kidney), a family history of renal stones, intestinal diseases that result in chronic diarrhea, osteoporosis, urinary tract infections, and gout. There is some debate if a complete metabolic work-up for stone disease should be undertaken after passage of the first stone. Many experts advocate fluid and dietary recommendations until patients suffer a recurrence. A metabolic work-up may be required if a woman has the previously listed risk factors, is premenopausal, has a solitary or transplanted kidney, or has stones that were composed of cystine, uric acid, or struvite. Blood tests such as a basic metabolic panel, serum calcium, serum uric, and intact parathyroid hormone are relatively inexpensive and can be performed in first-time stone formers as a simple screen for underlying metabolic issues.

Dietary Recommendations for Individuals With Stones

The following dietary recommendations should be reviewed with women who have a history of kidney stones:

- Increase fluid intake to achieve a urine output of 2 L or more a day. Carbonated water is preferred to still water because it has been found to increase urinary citrate levels, which inhibit stone formation.
- Increase the dietary intake of citrate to increase urinary citrate levels, which inhibit stone formation. Natural juices that are highest in citrate are grapefruit, lemon, and orange juice. Of the commercially available citrus-based beverages,

Crystal Light (Kraft Foods) has the highest concentration of citrate.
- Abstain from high protein diets, because protein increases urinary calcium, oxalate, and uric acid excretion and can increase the probability of stone formation even in normal subjects.
- Reduce dietary sodium, because dietary sodium and not dietary calcium restriction has been found to prevent recurrent nephrolithiasis.
- Reduce dietary oxalate by limiting foods that are rich in oxalate, such as spinach, beets, chocolate, nuts, and tea. There is debate about the conversion of ascorbic acid to urinary oxalate; however, most experts agree that daily vitamin C intake should be limited to less than 2 grams.

Bladder Stones

Women have 5% of the bladder stones seen in adults, and these stones are typically associated with foreign bodies (sutures, synthetic meshes) or urinary stasis (Stav & Dwyer, 2012). Bladder stones can be asymptomatic or can be the source of recurrent urinary tract infections, hematuria, and irritable symptoms. Bladder stones typically result from an underlying issue, such as urinary retention or foreign body in the bladder; therefore, the treatment must address the stone and the underlying issue. In cases of urinary retention caused by pelvic organ prolapse, the placement of a pessary or surgical intervention should be considered at the same time as bladder stone removal.

The stone can usually be fragmented manually with the use of a mechanical stone-crushing forceps bridge, requiring the use of a 26-/28-French resectoscope sheath and 30-degree lens. Care should be taken when using a crushing forceps; the stone is picked up and positioned away from the bladder mucosa when the jaws of the crushing forceps are engaged, because they can cause significant damage. When the stone is attached to mesh, it may be impossible to elevate the stone sufficiently; however, holding the forceps horizontally and parallel to the bladder mucosa will allow for the stones to be crushed safely into fragments. Typically, stones attached to a foreign body are soft and easily crushed.

Although there are numerous reports discussing the use of cystoscopic removal of stone and underlying foreign body, most experts recognize that the stone will recur unless the offending material is completely removed from the bladder wall. The most difficult cases of stone/foreign body removal from the bladder typically involve a mesh sling arm on the anterior lateral bladder wall, which often requires a combined transvaginal and retropubic approach. Cystoscopic access to the lateral anterior bladder wall is limited, and endoscopic transvesical procedures are usually best approached through the anterior bladder wall or bladder dome.

BLADDER CANCER

Introduction

Bladder cancer is the most common malignancy of the urinary tract and ranks as the seventeenth most common cancer in women based on worldwide cancer data (Bray et al., 2018). There are approximately 19,000 newly diagnosed cases of bladder cancer in women annually, and the incidence in men outnumbers that in women by a ratio of 3.2:1 owing to the higher rates of cigarette use and occupational exposures in men (American Cancer Society, 2020). Bladder cancer is 1.5 times more common in White women than in Black women. Despite women having higher health care utilization than men, by the time bladder cancer is diagnosed, women have more distant metastasis and, as a result, a higher mortality rate (Najari et al., 2013). Delay in bladder cancer diagnosis in women may be attributed to delay in the evaluation of associated symptoms that mimic common lower urinary tract symptoms (Cohn et al., 2014).

In the United States and Western Europe, the most common histological type (>90%) is urothelial carcinoma, whereas in other parts of the world squamous cell carcinoma is more prevalent, because of schistosomiasis. This distinction is important, because squamous carcinoma is more aggressive and has a mortality rate that is significantly higher than that of urothelial carcinoma. There is also a non–schistosomiasis-associated squamous cell carcinoma that has been reported in patients with spinal cord injury, particularly following long-term use of an indwelling catheter. These patients are generally diagnosed at a late stage and present with poor prognosis (Kalisvaart et al., 2010).

Risk Factors

Bladder cancer risks increase with age. Nine out of ten individuals diagnosed are over the age of 55 years; the average age at diagnosis is 73 years (American Cancer Society, 2020). External risk factors include tobacco use in the form of cigarettes, which accounts for 30% of urothelial cancers in women and 46% of all bladder cancer deaths in high-income countries (Boffetta, 2008; Brennen et al., 2001; Gandini et al., 2008). The risk of bladder cancer decreases 15 years after quitting, but the risk remains and is dependent on the number of years smoked and the number of cigarettes smoked per day (IARC Working Group, 2004; Wynder & Goldsmith, 1977). The risk of secondhand smoke in promoting bladder cancer formation is considered to be negligible but has not been well studied.

Occupational carcinogens, such as aromatic amines, diesel engine exhaust, paints, dyes, chlorinated hydrocarbons, metals, and industrial oils that affect the lung and skin, are associated with approximately 30% of bladder cancers. Occupations associated with environmental risks include aluminum process painters, machinists and other metal workers, leather workers, shoemakers, printers, hairdressers, dry cleaners, and transport workers (Kogevinas & Garcia-Closas, 2014). Although dietary factors such as artificial sweeteners have been associated with the development of bladder cancers in animals, there has been no evidence in humans. Medical interventions associated with bladder cancer include pelvic radiation exposure and cyclophosphamide chemotherapy. The latency period for bladder cancer development is often 15 to 30 years after the exposure.

Clinical Presentation

Few studies have looked at lower urinary tract symptoms at the time of evaluation for hematuria. As a result, the literature regarding urinary symptoms, degree of hematuria, and diagnosis of bladder cancer is often based on the retrospective analysis of patients referred to a urology clinic. The limitations of these studies are based on the reality that compliance with guidelines for referral is low. In a survey of primary care physicians, 64% of microscopic hematuria findings were not routinely referred for urologic evaluation (Nieder et al., 2010).

Hematuria is the most common presenting symptom of patients with bladder cancer, noted in approximately 85% of those who are subsequently diagnosed. Men and women may also present with common lower urinary tract symptoms such as dysuria, urgency, and nocturia before the first-time diagnosis of bladder cancer (Aziz et al., 2015). A prospective study looking at gender disparities regarding clinical symptoms and referral patterns before a diagnosis of bladder cancer found that, although clinical symptoms did not differ between the sexes, there might be a difference in referral patterns (Henning et al., 2013). Even when presenting with gross hematuria, one study showed that men are 65% more likely to receive a urologic referral than women (Johnson et al., 2008). Women were more likely to receive symptomatic treatment for alleged urinary tract infections without further investigation or referral, resulting in diagnostic delay.

Gross hematuria is the most prognostic clinical sign of underlying urologic disease; up to 23% of patients with gross hematuria have a malignancy, and another 44% might have other urological conditions (Khadra et al., 2000). In patients 40 to 59 years of age, gross hematuria carries a positive predictive value for urologic cancer that is higher for women than for men (6.4% vs. 3.6%; Bruyninckx et al., 2003). Microscopic hematuria is less commonly associated with malignancy than gross hematuria; however, hematuria can occur in apparently normal individuals and is, most often, the result of benign causes. In a prospective study of 736 women with a mean age of 59 years who presented to a hematuria clinic, 252 (34%) had gross hematuria, with a cancer detected in 40 (15.9%), compared with a 3.5% cancer detection rate in women with microscopic hematuria (≥3 red blood cells [RBC]/high power field [HPF]). Richards et al. (2016) report that 115 (15.6%) had the finding of urinary tract infection, and that 34% had irritative voiding symptoms. There were no pathological findings in 68% and 52% of the patients evaluated for microscopic and gross hematuria, respectively.

Asymptomatic Microscopic Hematuria Guidelines in Women

Asymptomatic microscopic hematuria (AMH) is commonly encountered, although the risk of associated malignancy is low. In a retrospective cohort study using a large, integrated health care system database of 3,742,348 urinalyses performed on 2,705,696 women over a 6-year span, 20% of the urinalyses had microscopic hematuria, including those of patients with an identified benign cause of microscopic hematuria, such as urinary tract infection (Lippmann et al., 2017). The overall rate of urologic cancer in this cohort was 1.3%.

Screening of healthy asymptomatic patients with urinalysis for cancer detection is not currently recommended by any major health organization. The US Preventative Services Task Force concludes that the evidence is "insufficient to determine the balance of benefits and harms of screening for bladder cancer in asymptomatic adults" (Moyer, 2011). Despite the lack of evidence for screening, annual urinalysis screening by primary care practitioners (including obstetrics/gynecologists) who care for women continues, and, as a result, urogynecologists and urologists receive referrals for women with AMH. Until recently, the only published guidelines directing the work-up for microscopic hematuria were the 2016 American Urological Association (AUA) Guidelines for AMH. These 2016 guidelines outlined the principles and recommendations for AMH and gross hematuria in men and women. The guidelines were not gender-specific and recommended that AMH (≥3 RBC/HPF) in a single specimen in a patient over the age of 35 years warrants a cystoscopy and CT urography, whereas persistent or recurrent AMH should have a repeat evaluation within 3 to 5 years. Contrary to common practice, urine cytology was not recommended as part of the microscopic hematuria work-up.

Recent studies in women suggest that the 2016 AUA guidelines may result in unnecessary evaluations. In 2011, Gleason et al. published a study of 210,000 women with AMH (≥3 RBC/HPF) and gross hematuria (>100 RBC/HPF) on microscopic analysis who were enrolled in an institutional health plan and followed for 3 years after their diagnosis of AMH. The authors found low rates of urologic cancers (0.02%) in women younger than 40 years, independent of the degree of hematuria. The rates of urologic cancers in women older than 40 years were dependent on the degree of hematuria (from 0.16% in women with 0–2 RBC/HPF to 1.77% in those with 100+ RBC/HPF [representing gross hematuria]). The authors proposed that an alternative approach to the AUA guidelines is to perform hematuria evaluation in women over the age of 40 years with one urinalysis that demonstrates greater than 25 RBC/HPF.

In light of this study and others, the American College of Obstetricians and Gynecologists (ACOG) and the American Urogynecological Society (AUGS) published AMH guidelines for women in 2017 based on studies that only included women. The guidelines state the following conclusions:

- In low-risk, never-smoking women younger than 50 years without gross hematuria and with fewer than 25 RBC/HPF, the risk of urinary tract malignancy is less than or equal to 0.5%.
- Asymptomatic, low-risk, never-smoking women aged 35 to 50 years should undergo evaluation only if they have more than 25 RBC/HPF.
- Age over 60 years, history of smoking, and gross hematuria are the strongest predictors of urologic cancer.
- ACOG and AUGS encourage organizations producing future guidelines on the evaluation of microscopic hematuria to perform sex-specific analysis of the data and produce practical sex-specific recommendations.

In 2020, the AUA, in conjunction with the Society of Urodynamics, Female Pelvic Medicine & Urogenital Reconstruction, updated their guidelines to use a risk-stratified approach for evaluation of AMH based upon a patient's risk factors for urinary tract cancer (Barocas et al., 2020). Based on these updated guidelines, once diagnosed, clinicians should categorize patients as low-, intermediate-, or high-risk for genitourinary malignancy, which will determine next steps: See Fig. 40.1 for the algorithm. The AUA guideline panel suggests that physicians and patients engage in a shared decision-making process to select the best option for each individual patient. The new clinical guidelines include the following principles:

- When diagnosing, clinicians should not define microhematuria by a positive dipstick test alone. Rather, the dipstick test should prompt formal microscopic evaluation of the urine to determine microhematuria.
- During the initial evaluation of microhematuria, clinicians should consider such factors as genitourinary malignancy, medical renal disease, and gynecologic or nonmalignant genitourinary disease as potential causes of microhematuria.
- After evaluation, clinicians should categorize patients based on risk to determine next steps, including repeating urinalysis, cystoscopy, renal ultrasound, or axial imaging (e.g., CT urogram).

Use of Urinary Markers and Cytology

Urine cytology is the examination of cells in urine under a microscope. Low-grade bladder lesions typically have normal cellular morphology; thus, urine cytology does not reveal an abnormality. Cytology is very sensitive (99%) in the detection of high-grade bladder cancers, including carcinoma *in situ* (CIS). However, because most bladder cancers are low grade, the use of cytology does not aid in the initial diagnosis and is no longer routinely required with AMH work-up. Cytology is indicated during office cystoscopy if bladder lesions are irregular or are associated with red, raised, velvety patches of urothelium indicating CIS. Although urinary markers for bladder cancers are often marketed to urogynecology practices, they are intended for patients who have been diagnosed with bladder cancer and are undergoing bladder cancer surveillance. A systematic review of 18 urine markers, including cytology, found no evidence that urine markers could be used as a substitution for cystoscopy because of their low sensitivity and specificity (van Rhijn et al., 2005).

Grading and Staging

The histological grading of bladder cancer is based on the microscopic appearance of the tumor, and the pathologist typically reports one of three grades based on the World Health Organization (WHO) 1973 classification. Grade 1 lesions look like normal bladder cells, are well-differentiated, tend to grow slowly, rarely invade past the urothelium, and are associated with a lower likelihood of recurrence. Grade 2 cancers are moderately differentiated and associated with invasion into the detrusor muscle and higher rates of recurrence. Grade 3 (high-grade) bladder cancer cells are poorly differentiated and, as a result, are more likely to be invasive and associated with higher recurrence.

The staging of bladder cancer is based on the depth of invasion of the tumor into the bladder wall (Fig. 40.2). Lesions that are limited to the urothelium are high-grade CIS (T_{is}) and noninvasive papillary carcinomas (T_a). A special note about CIS tumors is that, although confined to the urothelium, they are high grade and are associated with high recurrence rates, progression into the bladder wall, and decreased survival as compared with T_a tumors. Tumors that invade into the layer that separates the urothelium from the detrusor muscle (lamina propria) are T_1 tumors. Tumors that invade into the detrusor muscle (T_2) are staged based on the level of invasion to the inner half (T_{2a}) or outer half (T_{2b}) of the muscle. T_3 tumors invade past the boundary of the detrusor muscle into the perivesical fat, whereas T_4 tumors invade past the fat and into adjacent organs such as the uterus or vagina.

The WHO in 2004 developed a grading system for non–muscle-invasive urothelial cancers that is being increasingly used by pathologists when reporting bladder tumors (Montironi & Lopez-Betran, 2005). A tumor with a particularly good prognosis (papillary urothelial neoplasm of low malignant potential) no longer carries the label of "cancer" and avoids the use of ambiguous grading such as "1 and 2" or "2 and 3" (as done in the 1973 WHO classification). This classification allows for clearer clinical guidelines for counseling. Papillary neoplasms of low malignant potential will recur 27% to 47% of the time, occasionally progress to a higher grade (11%), and rarely invade deeper tissues (0%–4%; Montironi & Lopez-Betran, 2005). In sharp contrast, high-grade papillary T_a and T_{is} will recur 50% of the time and advance to a higher-stage tumor with their recurrence 27% to 61% of the time (Fig. 40.3). As a result, high-grade lesions are associated with decreased survival (74%–90%) compared with papillary neoplasms of low malignant potential (93%–100%).

Tumor Resection

Fortunately, 80% of urothelial cancers are non–muscle-invasive tumors at initial presentation. To characterize a bladder cancer, tumor resection is needed to obtain the histological grade and stage of the tumor. Critical to staging is the ability of the pathologist to gauge the depth of invasion of the bladder tumor. Recognition of the lamina propria and underlying detrusor muscle can be challenging for the pathologist owing to poor specimen quality, such as a specimen lacking the lamina propria or muscularis mucosa, or having been subjected to thermal injury during collection. The goals of tumor resection should be to (1) remove the tumor with minimal thermal injury; (2) collect a tissue sample below the tumor to measure the depth of invasion; (3) biopsy any CIS-appearing lesions at the same time; and (4) ensure hemostasis at the end of the case using cautery. Tumors that are clearly papillary in nature, and thus low grade, can be easily resected using a rigid biopsy forceps (Fig. 40.3). The specimen should be placed into two distinct collection containers: the first should include the bladder tumor fragments, and the second should be the base of the tumor. Each of the containers should be specifically marked "tumor" and "base." Large, sessile tumors with bleeding, calcifications, and necrotic appearance are often high-grade lesions that cannot be easily resected (Fig. 40.4 and Fig. 40.5). When large or high-grade tumors are found on office cystoscopy, the patient is best served by obtaining urine cytology and a CT urogram (to look for ureteral involvement) and referring to a

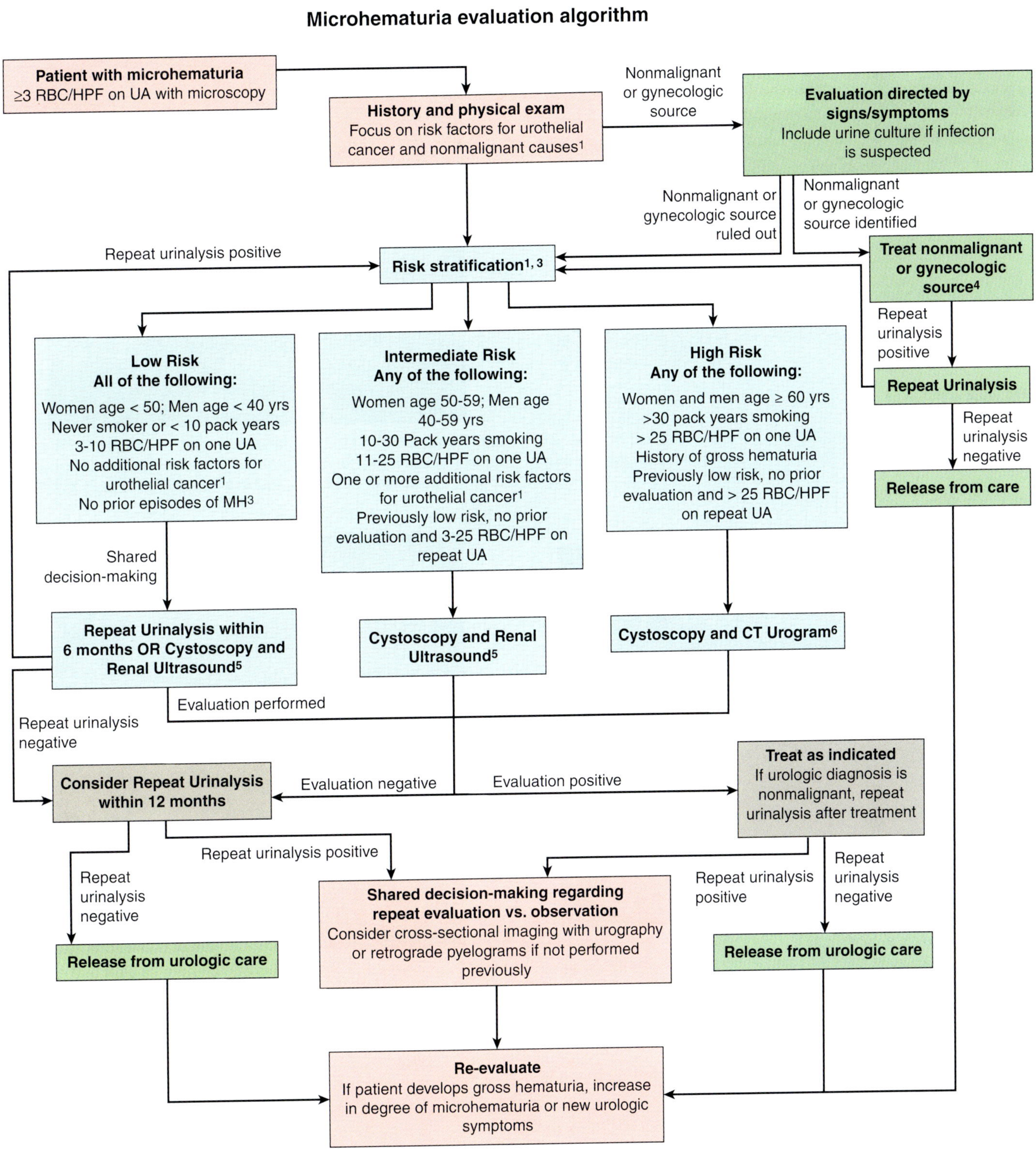

1. Main risk factors for urothelial cancer are those in the AUA risk stratification system (age, male sex, smoking, degree of microhematuria and history of gross hematuria). Additional risk factors for urothelial carcinoma include but are not limited to irritative lower urinary tract voiding symptoms, history of cyclophosphamide or ifosfamide chemotherapy, family history of urothelial carcinoma or Lynch syndrome, occupational exposures to benzene chemicals or aromatic amines, history of chronic indwelling foreign body in the urinary tract.
2. If medical renal disease is suspected, consider nephrologic evaluation, but pursue concurrent risk-based urological evaluation.
3. Patients may be low risk at first presentation with microhematuria, but may only be considered intermediate- or high-risk if found to have persistent microhematuria.
4. There are nonmalignant and gynecologic sources of hematuria that do not require treatment and/or may confound the diagnosis of MH. Clinicians can consider catheterized urine specimen in women with vaginal atrophy or pelvic organ prolapse. Clinicians must use careful judgment and patient engagement to decide whether to pursue MH evaluation in the setting of chronic conditions that do not require treatment, such as the aforementioned gynecologic conditions, non-obstructing stones or BPH.
5. Clinician may perform cross-sectional imaging with urography or retrograde pyelograms if hematuria persists after negative renal ultrasound.
6. MR urogram or Non-contrast imaging plus retrograde pyelograms if contraindications to CT urogram.

Fig. 40.1 2020 American Urological Association microhematuria evaluation algorithm. *RBC,* Red blood cells; *HPF,* high-power field; *UA,* urinalysis; *MH,* microhematuria; *CT,* computed tomography; *MR,* magnetic resonance.

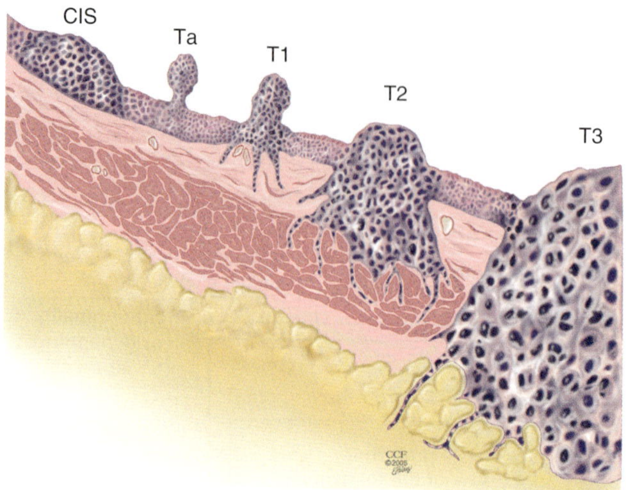

Fig. 40.2 Carcinoma *in situ* (*CIS*) and papillary tumors (T_a) are confined to the urothelium. T_1 tumors invade the lamina propria, while T_2 tumors invade the detrusor muscle. T_3 tumors are in the extravesical fat. (Reprinted with permission from Jones SJ. Non-muscle invasive bladder cancer. In: Wein AJ, Kavoussi LR, Partin AW, Peters CA, eds. *Campbell's Urology*. 11th ed. Philadelphia: Elsevier; 2016.)

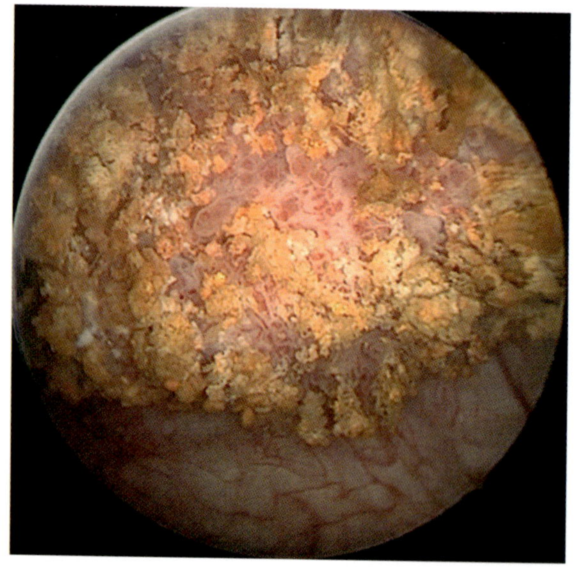

Fig. 40.4 High-grade T_a bladder tumor with calcifications. Bladder tumors can be a source of recurrent urinary tract infection. (Photograph courtesy of Marcus Quek, MD, Loyola University Chicago, IL.)

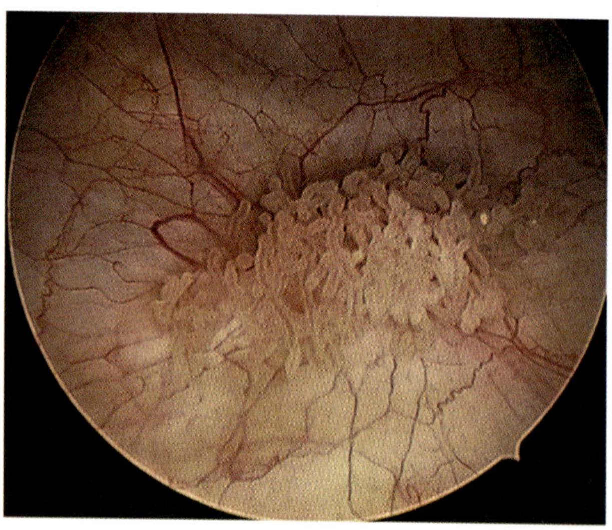

Fig. 40.3 Low-grade superficial bladder tumor. The tumor should be grasped at its base and resected using a rigid or flexible biopsy forceps. A second biopsy of the base should be obtained before any cautery defect to control hemostasis.

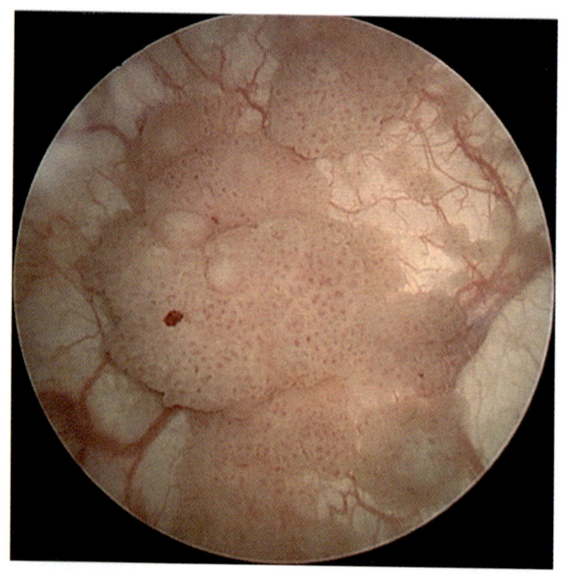

Fig. 40.5 High-grade T_1 bladder tumor. Note the disorganized appearance and the numerous satellite lesions. (Photograph courtesy of Marcus Quek, MD, Loyola University Chicago, IL.)

urologic oncologist. Before any tumor resection, a vaginal examination under anesthesia should be performed and documented, with attention paid to the characteristics of the bladder neck and anterior vaginal wall.

RETROGRADE URETEROGRAM AND STENT PLACEMENT

Introduction

The recognition of ureteral injuries at the time of surgery is aided by the intravenous use of indigo carmine or sodium fluorescein and Lasix, as well described in Chapter 24. When a ureteral stent is warranted, an understanding of upper urinary tract anatomy and landmarks can ensure that the stent has been properly placed in the renal pelvis. The same landmarks can be used when reviewing a plain film of the abdomen outside of the operating room. In this section we will review the equipment and procedures for retrograde ureterogram/pyelogram and ureteral stent placement and how to interpret retrograde images.

Equipment Needed for Retrogrades and Stent Placement

Box 40.1 lists the equipment needed to perform a retrograde pyelogram and ureteral stent placement. Because fluoroscopy is needed to visualize contrast during the retrograde pyelogram

BOX 40.1 Equipment Needed for Retrograde Ureterogram and/or Stent Placement

Equipment	Notes
Cystoscope	Allows passage of a 6-French ureteral stent and wire
21-French sheath (or larger)	
30-degree lens *or*	Aids in the visualization of the ureteral orifice and the stent in the same visual field of the scope
70-degree lens with Albarron bridge	
Fluoroscopy	Visualizes the anatomy before the procedure
	Visualizes the ureter and renal pelvis
	Confirms ureteral stent placement in the renal pelvis and the urinary bladder
Radiopaque contrast	Typically diluted 50/50 with sterile saline or water (20–30 mL)
Double open-ended ureteral catheter	A hollow open-ended catheter (5- to 6-French) used to pass the guidewire through the cystoscope and direct the wire through the ureter and into the renal pelvis
Guidewires	Hydrophilic wires (typically 3-French, with use specifically intended for stent placement)
Double-J ureteral stent	6-French in diameter; length in cm is determined by the patient's height in inches minus 42. Example: 5′6″ women would typically require a 24-cm stent length (66 inches – 42 = 24 cm)

and to confirm wire and stent placement, it would be prudent to ensure that the operative bed can accommodate the C-arm of the fluoroscope and allow for the necessary images. Because of the radiation emitted, lead aprons and thyroid shields should be used by all of the staff in the operating room.

For orientation, before introducing the cystoscope, a single fluoroscopic image of the pelvis is obtained, and the radiology technician adjusts the image so that the spinal column is vertical. Place a metal object on the pelvis with the tip of the instrument directed to the left or right shoulder and obtain an image to make sure the tip is being directed to the correct side on the image. It would also be helpful to take the time to let the technician know the purpose of the study so that he or she can work with you to move the image frame as needed during the procedure. Finally, it is important to inform the technician that you will specifically review the images obtained during the case and choose the ones that should be saved from the procedure.

Anatomic Landmarks on Fluoroscopy

As demonstrated in Fig. 40.6A, the right kidney is lower than the left, and, as a result, the right renal pelvis lies across from the L3 vertebra. The normal renal pelvis has three to five major calyces. Calyces that are directed anterior and posterior are not visible in plain films or fluoroscopy. A line drawn between the upper-pole and lower-pole calyces should lie in the same direction as the ipsilateral psoas muscle (Fig. 40.6B and C). A malrotated kidney or a single pole of a duplicated kidney will not lie in the correct position (Figs. 40.7 and 40.8). When performing a retrograde pyelogram for a noneffluxing ureter, starting with the side that is effluxing properly will allow for the establishment of a normal "control" for comparison.

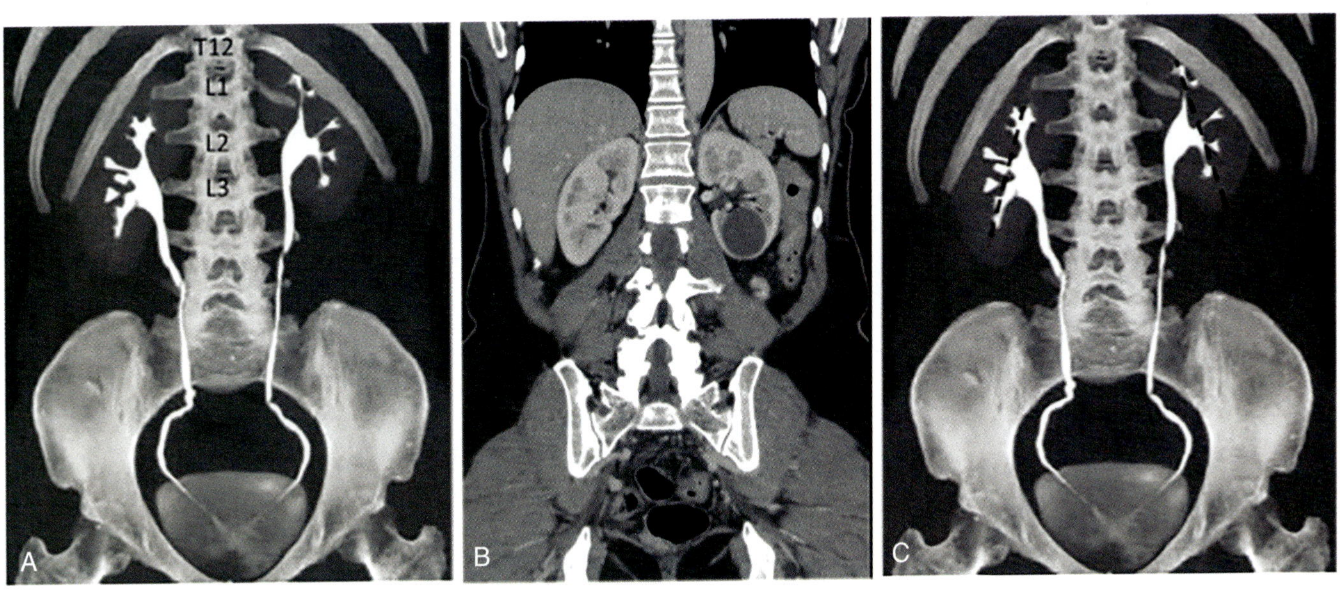

Fig. 40.6 A, Reconstruction of computed tomography (CT) urogram demonstrating the anatomic landmarks associated with retrograde imaging. The last attached rib easily identifies T12. The right renal pelvis lies across from L3, whereas the left lies at L2. **B**, The lie of the kidney follows the psoas muscle on its respective side, as demonstrated by this CT with contrast. A simple renal cyst in seen in the left lower pole parenchyma. **C**, A line drawn from the upper pole to lower pole calyx is parallel to the psoas muscle, as can be seen in this image.

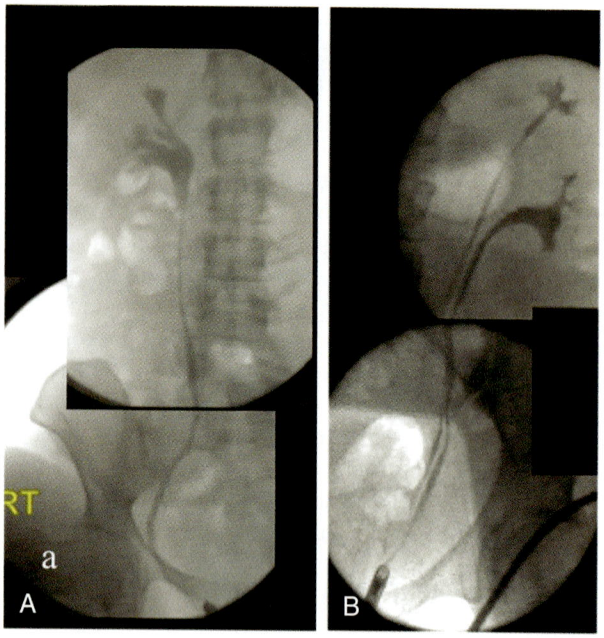

Fig. 40.7 **A**, Normal right-sided retrograde image of the ureter and renal pelvis. **B**, The lower renal unit in this left retrograde image of a duplicated kidney has a line from the upper and lower pole that is angled away from the psoas muscle, demonstrating the classic "drooping lily" appearance. In duplicated renal systems, the upper-pole ureteral orifice can be easily missed, and the only clue to the presence of a duplicated system is the abnormal lie of the lower-pole calyces.

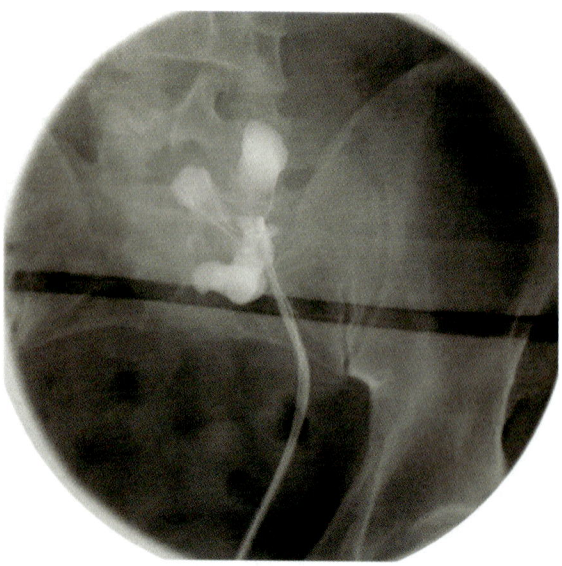

Fig. 40.8 Retrograde image of a pelvic kidney. A double open-ended catheter was placed inside the renal pelvis to visualize the anatomy.

Performing a Retrograde Ureterogram/Pyelogram

Performance of the retrograde pyelogram begins with introducing the cone-tip catheter into the cystoscope with a 21-French or larger sheath. Once the scope is in the bladder, the tip of the catheter is brought into view. Turning the cystoscope light cord attachment toward the ureteral orifice of interest while keeping the camera upright aligns the cone-tip catheter in the direction of the ureteral orifice. Once aligned, a 20-mL syringe filled with 50/50 contrast media is attached to the cone-tip catheter, and contrast is injected until the air bubbles have been flushed from the catheter. The cone-tip catheter is guided into the ureteral orifice so that the cone tip occludes the orifice (Fig. 40.9). A single fluoroscopic image is then obtained with full visualization of the distal and midureter because this is typically the area of interest. The contrast media is slowly injected while watching under fluoroscopy. If there is no evidence of obstruction or extravasation, the contrast is tracked up to the renal pelvis. The volume of the renal pelvis and ureter is 3 to 10 mL but can be higher with hydronephrosis. During the pyelogram, we look for any filling defects, ureteral kinking, or contrast extravasation. Once the ureter and renal pelvis have been filled with contrast, there is no need to inject further contrast. An image of the contrast-filled renal pelvis is captured and saved. The cone-tip catheter is then removed, and the bladder is emptied through the cystoscope. This allows the contrast to be expelled from the ureter.

If the ureter is constricted following a surgical procedure, and the contrast is not draining, the characteristics of the contrast emptying from the affected side can be compared with that emptying from the other side, which is effluxing normally. An intravenous injection of 20 mg of Lasix can be administered to help the contrast drain from the kidney. If the ureter is not effluxing urine or contrast, there may be a significant obstruction, which should then be further addressed. It is important to remember that, when you find ureteral dilation on a retrograde pyelogram, dilation by itself does not necessarily mean obstruction. There are many reasons for a ureter to be dilated from events in the past. A dilated ureter that effluxes urine briskly is not obstructed.

Performing a Retrograde Stent Placement

Once the decision to place a ureteral stent has been made, appropriate equipment should be made available. A retrograde ureterogram should be performed first to assess the ureteral

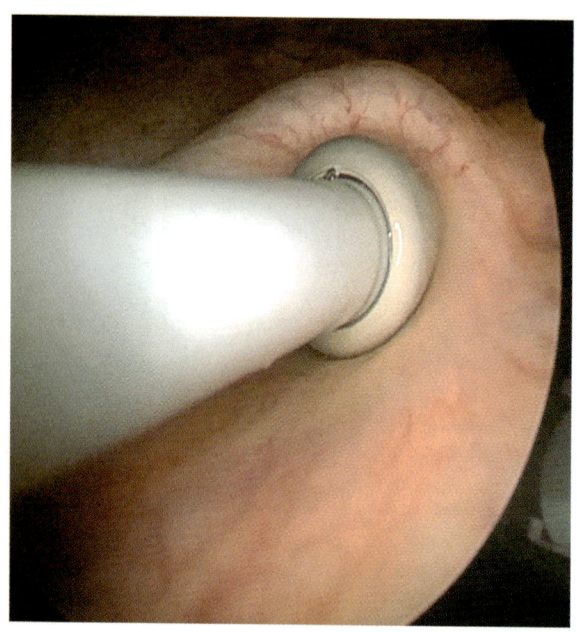

Fig. 40.9 Cone-tip catheter placed in left ureteral orifice. When placed appropriately, the cone tip occludes the orifice.

anatomy unless the stent is being placed prophylactically. Placement of a ureteral stent begins with the introduction of the double open-ended ureteral catheter into the cystoscope with a 21-French sheath (at a minimum). Once the scope is in the bladder, the tip of the open-ended ureteral catheter is brought into view. The guidewire (floppy tip first) is advanced until the tip of the guidewire is visualized at the opening of the double open-ended catheter. Turning the light cord attachment toward the ureteral orifice that you are trying to cannulate aligns the wire and ureteral catheter to the ureteral orifice.

The guidewire and the double open-ended ureteral catheter are advanced together through the ureter using fluoroscopic imaging. The wire should be kept ahead of the double open-ended catheter by a couple of centimeters to reduce ureteral trauma. The purpose of the double open-ended ureteral catheter is to guide the wire into the renal pelvis, so the catheter does not need to make its way to the renal pelvis. Resistance will be felt when the wire has reached one of the upper calyces of the kidney. At this point, a fluoroscopic image is obtained to visualize the wire in the kidney. In most cases, the wire will be higher than the renal pelvis (L3 on the right and L2 on the left). Once the position of the wire is confirmed, the double open-ended ureteral catheter is retracted while placing forward pressure on the wire. This will ensure that the wire does not lose its position in the renal calyx. Fluoroscopic images can be obtained for reassurance that the position of the wire in the renal pelvis is maintained during retraction of the open-ended catheter. Holding firmly to the wire as it exits the cystoscope port, the open-ended catheter is removed and placed on the operative table.

Taking the patient's height in inches and subtracting 42 can determine the stent size in centimeters. For example, for a woman who is 5'6", the height in inches is 66, and after subtracting 42, the stent size would be calculated to be 24 cm. Exceptions to this rule are pelvic tumors, hydroureter and renal abnormalities such as a pelvic kidney, or ureteral reimplant. The double open-ended catheter can also be used to measure the appropriate stent size using the markings on the side of the catheter. With one end of the open-ended catheter in the renal pelvis, noting the markings on the ureteral catheter at the level of the ureteral orifice allows for estimation of the ureteral stent size needed. To place the ureteral stent, the tapered end of the ureteral stent is introduced over the wire and advanced to the cystoscope port. As the surgeon advances the stent 1 cm at a time, the assistant holds tension on the guidewire to aid stent passage. Appropriate tension on the wire is needed, while taking care to not pull the proximal end of the wire out of the kidney. Fluoroscopic images of the wire in the kidney can be obtained to ensure that the wire keeps its position. It is also critical to position the sheath end of the cystoscope right at the ureteral orifice opening (Video 40.1) to keep the wire from curling between the ureteral orifice and the end of the cystoscope.

The stent is advanced until its proximal end can be seen at the ureteral orifice. The stent pusher arm should now be advanced over the guidewire and will be used to push the stent through the cystoscope. Fluoroscopic images can be obtained periodically. The ureteral stent is advanced until the final marking of the stent is at the ureteral orifice. An image at the level of the renal pelvis is obtained to ensure that the stent is correctly positioned. If it is in position, the cystoscope can then be backed out from the pusher arm by holding the pusher arm steady and sliding the cystoscope back to the bladder neck until the end of the pusher arm is visualized. The guidewire is removed as the pusher arm is held in place. With the removal of the guidewire, the distal curl of the stent will then retract into the bladder. The bladder is emptied, and the cystoscope is withdrawn. An image of the ureteral stent, with a proximal curl in the renal pelvis and a distal curl in the bladder, is obtained and saved.

There are times when a stent is passed without fluoroscopic guidance using the same method as above. It is critical during these instances that a KUB image is obtained in the operating room or the recovery room to ensure that the stent is in the correct position. A well-placed and well-sized stent will have a curl at the renal pelvis or higher and will not cross the midline in the bladder (Fig. 40.10).

Counseling a Patient With a Ureteral Stent

Indwelling ureteral stents can significantly affect patients' quality of life, and, similar to indwelling Foley catheters, they should only be used for a limited time. Joshi et al. (2003) studied 39 men and 23 women 1 week and 4 weeks following stent placement using a validated stent symptoms questionnaire. The authors found that the majority of patients experienced one or more of the following urinary symptoms: daytime voiding every 2 hours or less, nocturia, gross hematuria, urinary urgency, and dysuria. Stent pain varied considerably, with 7% having pain at rest, and a minority (15%) reporting no pain even with vigorous activity. The remainder of patients had pain with moderate or vigorous activity. More than 60% reported pain that occurred primarily in the flank region, and 38% in the bladder. Over a 4-week period, 26% of patients spent more than 2 days in bed, whereas 42% reduced their daily activities. Over

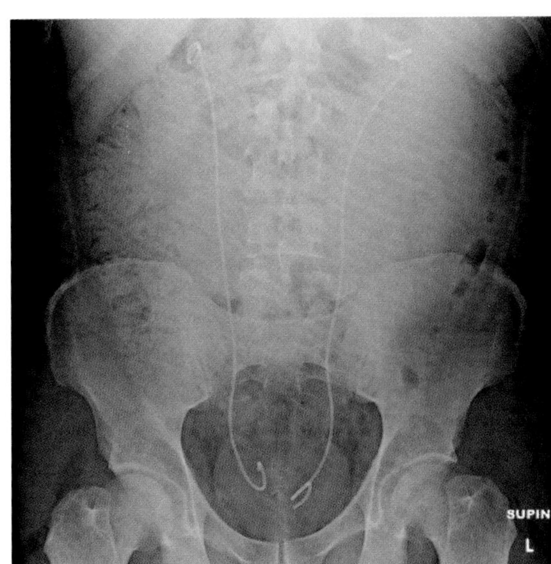

Fig. 40.10 Bilateral ureteral stent placement with both proximal curls in the upper calyces and distal curls in the bladder, not crossing the midline in the bladder.

two-thirds of patients developed urinary tract infections after 4 weeks of stent insertion and received at least one course of antibiotics. Although dysuria improved over 4 weeks, urge incontinence symptoms worsened. Stent pain and urinary symptoms can be treated prophylactically with an α-1 antagonist (tamsulosin hydrochloride 0.4 mg orally every night) and an anticholinergic medication while the stent remains in place.

Ureteral Stents for Ureterovaginal Fistula

Ureteral stent placement with a Foley catheter placement is a conservative and successful first-line treatment option for women who present with ureterovaginal fistula following a surgical procedure. It is not indicated for fistulas following radiation treatment. The success rates of stent placement are higher than for percutaneous nephrostomy tube placement, most likely caused by urine passing across the stent and injured ureter, which is associated with lower stricture rates. Chen et al. (2019) reported on a series of 19 women treated for ureterovaginal fistula. Ureteral stenting was attempted in 12 women and was successful in 11 (92%). Three stents had to be placed antegrade by interventional radiology after failed retrograde attempts. Urine leakage from the vagina stopped in 48 hours; the median indwelling stent time was 73 days. One patient (9%) developed a ureteral stricture, consistent with published rates of ureteral stricture following stent placement for ureterovaginal fistula.

Important considerations in using a ureteral stent for ureterovaginal fistula include the use of a Foley catheter for a week after the vaginal leakage has ceased, prophylactic antibiotics, and retrograde ureterogram assessment of the ureter when the stent is being removed to detect a ureteral stricture (Fig. 40.11). The Foley catheter allows the urine from both kidneys to drain from the bladder, reducing the amount of urine that can reflux up to the stented kidney and potentially out the fistula tract. Once the fistula tract has closed, usually within a week after vaginal leakage has ceased, the catheter is no longer needed. However, the possibility of pyelonephritis continues; therefore, prophylactic antibiotics are recommended for the duration of the stent placement.

Although it is customary to remove a ureteral stent in the office following a ureteral reimplant, it is not recommended

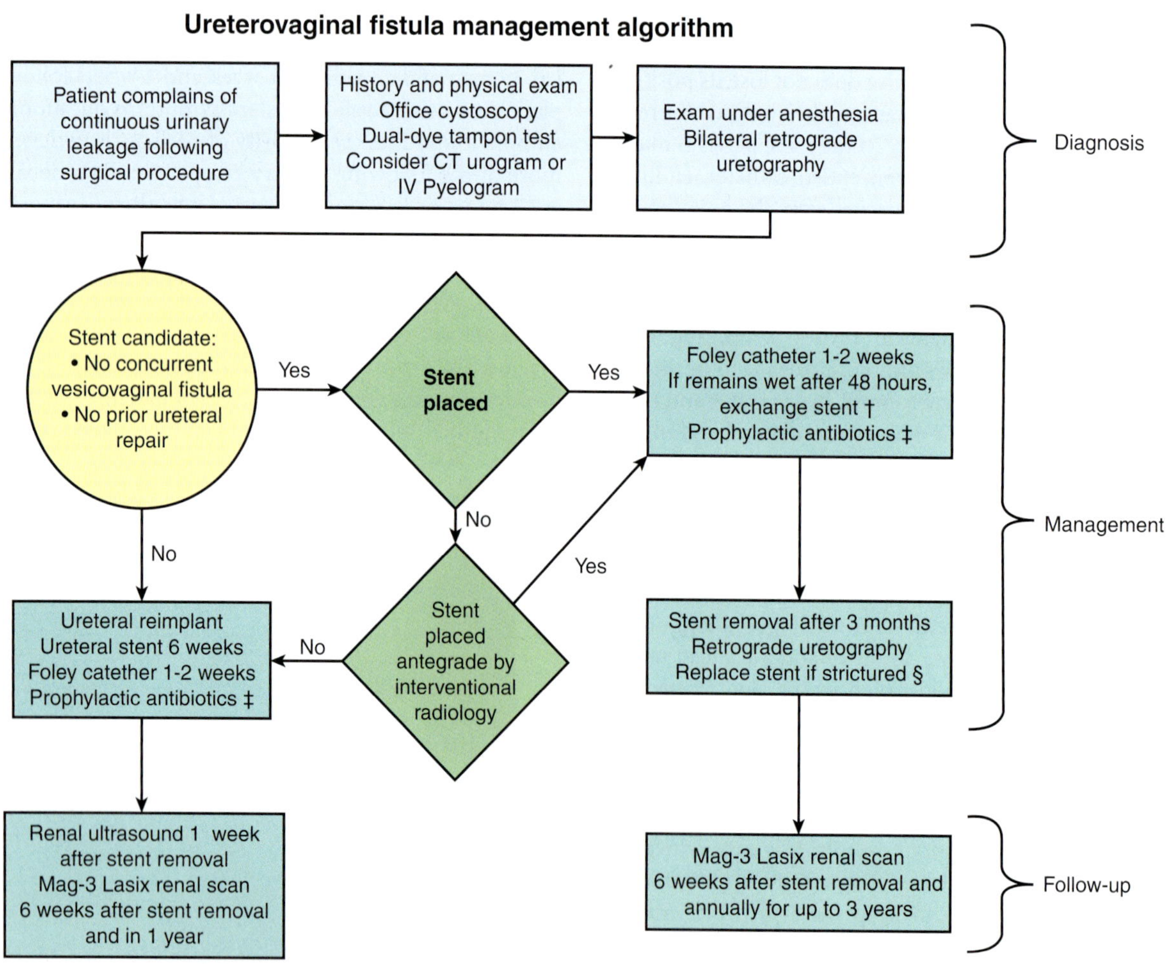

† If leakage occurs for more than 48 hours after stent placement, return to OR for stent exchange with 6-Fr lumen double-J stent
‡ For pyelonephritis prevention while ureteral stent is in place
§ We repeat retrograde pyelogram in 2-3 months after a second stent. Attempt balloon dilation or reimplant ureter if persistently strictured.

Fig. 40.11 Algorithm for ureterovaginal fistula management. *CT,* computed tomography; *IV,* intravenous; *OR,* operating room. (Reprinted with permission from Chen YB, Wolff BW, Kenton KS, Mueller ER. Approach to ureterovaginal fistula: examining 13 years of experience. *Female Pelvic Med Reconstr Surg.* 2019;25:e7.)

following a ureterovaginal fistula. Stricture rates following a ureteral reimplant are less than 2% owing to the excellent blood supply from the bladder; this is not the case with a ureterovaginal fistula, which most likely is caused, in part, by an ischemic event. Pyelonephritis and urosepsis commonly occur in patients with an obstructed ureteral stricture; therefore, the detection of a ureteral stricture is best not left to chance. On the day of stent removal, the preoperative antibiotic given should have excellent gram-negative coverage. If the retrograde imaging of the ureter is reassuring, the stent is not replaced, and follow-up imaging can include a renal ultrasound in 1 week if desired. At 6 weeks after stent removal, we perform a Lasix renal scan to document that there is no ureteral obstruction. Although CT urograms can detect upper urinary tract dilation, they are anatomic studies, not functional studies. As a result, they cannot distinguish dilation from obstruction.

BIBLIOGRAPHY

American Cancer Society. *Key Statistics for Bladder Cancer*. Revised January 8, 2020. Available at: https://www.cancer.org/cancer/bladder-cancer/about/key-statistics.html. Accessed February 8, 2020.

Aziz A, Madersbacher S, Otto W, et al. Comparative analysis of gender-related differences in symptoms and referral patterns prior to initial diagnosis of urothelial carcinoma of the bladder: a prospective cohort study. *Urol Int.* 2015;94:37.

Barocas D, Boorjian S, Alvarez, R et al. *Microhematuria: AUA/SUFU Guideline 2020*. Revised May, 2020. Available at: https://www.auanet.org/guidelines/microhenaturia. Accessed July 7, 2020.

Boffetta P. Tobacco smoking and the risk of bladder cancer. *Scand J Urol Nephrol Suppl.* 2008;218:45.

Boyce CJ, Pickhardt PJ, Lawrence EM, et. al. Prevalence of urolithiasis in asymptomatic adults: objective determination using low dose noncontrast computerized tomography. *J Urol.* 2010;183:1017.

Bray F, Ferlay J, Soerjomataram I, et al. Global Cancer Statistics 2018: Globocan estimates of incidence and mortality worldwide for 36 cancers in 185 countries. *CA Cancer J Clin.* 2018;68:394.

Brennen P, Bogillot O, Greiser E, et al. The contribution of cigarette smoking to bladder cancer in women (pooled European data). *Cancer Causes Control.* 2001;12:411.

Bruyninckx R, Buntinx F, Aertgeerts B, Van Casteren V. The diagnostic value of macroscopic haematuria for the diagnosis of urological cancer in general practice. *Br J Gen Pract.* 2003;53:31.

Chen YB, Wolff BW, Kenton KS, Mueller ER. Approach to ureterovaginal fistula: examining 13 years of experience. *Female Pelvic Med Reconstr Surg.* 2019;25:e7.

Cohn JA, Vekhter B, Lyttle C, et al. Sex disparities in diagnosis of bladder cancer after initial presentation with hematuria: a nationwide claims-based investigation. *Cancer.* 2014;120:555.

Coll DM, Varanelli MJ, Smith RC. Relationship of spontaneous passage of ureteral calculi to stone size and location as revealed by unenhanced helical CT. *AJR Am J Roentgenol.* 2002;178:101.

Committee on Gynecological Practice, American Urogynecological Society. Asymptomatic Microscopic Hematuria in Women. *Female Pelvic Med Reconstr Surg.* 2017;23:228.

Dall'era JE, Kim F, Chandhoke PS. Gender differences among Hispanic and Caucasians in Symptomatic Presentation of Kidney and Ureteral Stones. *J Endourol.* 2005;19:283.

Gandini S, Botteri E, Iodice S, et al. Tobacco smoking and cancer: a meta-analysis. *Int J Cancer.* 2008;122:155.

Gleason JH. Association of hematuria on microscopic analysis and risk of urinary tract cancer. *J Urol.* 2011 May;185:1698.

Henning A, Wehrberger M, Madersbacher S, et al. Do differences in clinical symptoms and referral patterns contribute to the gender gap in bladder cancer? *BJU Int.* 2013;112:68.

IARC Working Group on the Evaluation of Carcinogenic Risks to Humans. Tobacco smoke and involuntary smoking. *IARC Monogr Eval Carcinog Risks Hum.* 2004;84:1.

Johnson EK, Daignault S, Zhang Y, Lee CT. Patterns of hematuria referral to urologists: does a gender disparity exist? *Urology.* 2008;72:498.

Jones SJ. Non-muscle invasive bladder cancer. In: Wein AJ, Kavoussi LR, Partin AW, Peters CA, eds. *Campbell's Urology.* 11th ed. Philadelphia: Elsevier; 2016.

Joshi HB, Stainthorpe A, MacDonagh RP, et al. Indwelling ureteral stents: evaluation of symptoms, quality of life and utility. *J Urol.* 2003;169:1065.

Kalisvaart JF, Katsumi HK, Ronningen LD, Hovey RM. Bladder cancer in spinal cord injury patients. *Spinal Cord.* 2010;48:257.

Khadra MH, Pickard RS, Charlton M, et al. A prospective analysis of 1930 patients with hematuria to evaluate current diagnostic practice. *J Urol.* 2000;163:524.

Kogevinas M, Garcia-Closas M. Bladder cancer. In: Antitla S, Boffetta P, eds. *Occupational Cancers.* London: Springer Nature; 2014.

Lippmann QK, Slezak JM, Menefee SA, et al. Evaluation of microscopic hematuria and risk of urologic cancer in female patients. *Am J Obstet Gynecol.* 2017;216:146.e1.

Miller OF, Kane CJ. Time to stone passage for observed ureteral calculi: a guide for patient education. *J Urol.* 1999;162:688.

Montironi R, Lopez-Betran A. The 2004 WHO classification of bladder tumors: a summary and commentary. *Int J Surg Pathol.* 2005;13:143.

Moyer VA. Screening for bladder cancer: U.S. Preventative Services Task Force recommendation statement. *Ann Intern Med.* 2011;155:246.

Najari BB, Rink M, Li PS, et al. Sex disparities in cancer mortality: the risks of being a man in the United States. *J Urol.* 2013;189:1470.

Nieder AM, Lotan Y, Nuss GR, et al. Are patients with hematuria appropriately referred to urology? A multi-institutional questionnaire based survey. *Urol Oncol.* 2010;28:500.

Richards KA, Ham S, Cohn JA, Steinberg GD. Urinary tract infection-like symptom is associated with worse bladder cancer outcomes in the Medicare population: implications for sex disparities. *Int J Urol.* 2016;23:42.

Scales CD, Smith AC, Hanley JM, et al. Prevalence of kidney stones in the United States. *Eur Urol.* 2012;62:160.

Stamatelou KK, Franics ME, Jone CA, et al. Time trends in reported prevalence of kidney stones in the US 1976-1994. *Kidney Int.* 2003;63:1817.

Stav K, Dwyer PL. Urinary bladder stones in women. *Obstet Gynecol Surv.* 2012;67:715.

Stothers L, Lee LM. Renal colic in pregnancy. *J Urol.* 1992;148:1383.

van Rhijn BW, van der Poel HG, van der Kwast TH. Urine markers for bladder cancer surveillance: a systematic review. *Eur Urol.* 2005;47:736.

Wynder EL, Goldsmith R. The epidemiology of bladder cancer: a second look. *Cancer.* 1977;40:1246.

PART 8

Research Methods

Outcomes and Quality-of-Life Measures in Pelvic Floor Research

Matthew D. Barber

CHAPTER OUTLINE

INTRODUCTION

Outcome measures are the tools used to determine the efficacy, safety, and side effects of a treatment. Researchers assess outcome measures before and after treatments to determine their relative efficacy. Clinicians can use outcome measures to track the success of their treatments and/or longitudinally to follow the outcomes of individual patients. Urinary incontinence, fecal incontinence, pelvic organ prolapse (POP), and other pelvic floor disorders are multidimensional phenomena that can impact a patient in a wide variety of ways. They rarely result in severe morbidity or mortality; rather, they cause symptoms that can impact a woman's daily activities and negatively affect her quality of life (QOL). No single measure can fully characterize the outcome of an intervention for these conditions. Therefore, outcomes of treatment should be evaluated in multiple areas or domains. A number of organizations, including the International Continence Society (ICS), International Urogynecologic Association (IUGA), National Institutes of Health (NIH), and World Health Organization (WHO) -sponsored International Consultation on Incontinence (ICI), have made recommendations to standardize outcome measures in studies of pelvic floor disorders. In general, all agree on several basic principles: (1) outcome assessments should be made using the same measures before and after the intervention; (2) both subjective and objective measures should be included, incorporating improvements and deterioration in function, as well as complications of the intervention; and (3) pelvic floor disorders should be assessed from multiple domains, including some or all of the following:

- The subject's observations (symptoms)
- Quantification of symptoms
- The clinician's observations (anatomic and functional)
- QOL
- Socioeconomic measures

In particular, patient-reported outcomes (PROs) have been increasingly incorporated into the practice and study of pelvic floor disorders. Because of the nature of these disorders, inclusion of the patient's perspective is essential. PROs measure patient perceptions at four levels of increasing complexity: symptoms, functioning, general health perceptions, and health-related QOL (HRQOL).

A good outcome measure should be valid, reliable, simple to implement, easy to interpret, and able to detect clinically meaningful change. When planning a study, outcome measures should be selected within the context of the specific study's hypothesis or goal. In general, they should be chosen so that they will be clinically relevant and so that the results may be incorporated into practice at the end of the study. For a clinical trial, researchers will typically define a primary outcome and several secondary outcomes. The primary outcome is of central interest and should be tied directly to the study's primary hypothesis. It is the primary outcome that is used for sample size determination. Secondary outcomes are the remaining outcome measures being assessed in the study. They are not the focus of the main study objective but provide additional data that are complementary to the primary outcome measure. Because of the desire to assess pelvic floor disorders in multiple domains, typically several secondary outcome measures are used in studies of these conditions.

In this chapter, many of the currently available outcome measures available to clinicians and researchers to assess treatment outcomes for pelvic floor disorders will be reviewed, including symptom diaries, pad tests, physical examination, physiologic tests (such as urodynamics, symptom severity, or bother questionnaires), QOL questionnaires, and socioeconomic measures. The chapter will conclude by discussing the current challenges and recommendations for defining treatment success in patients with urinary incontinence and POP.

SYMPTOM DIARIES

Physicians often attempt to determine the presence and severity of a patient's symptoms by history-taking or administering a questionnaire. These methods depend upon the patient's ability to accurately recall and report her recent health experiences. Research has shown, however, that recall is often unreliable and can result in inaccuracies and bias. For instance, in one study, more than half of women overestimated their daytime urinary frequency when compared with a bladder diary. The use of symptom diaries has been advocated to limit recall bias by capturing experiences prospectively close to or at the time of occurrence. The bladder or urinary diary is perhaps the most common outcome measure used in studies of urinary incontinence and other forms of lower urinary tract dysfunction. It is also a useful clinical tool (see Chapters 9 and 14). In its simplest form, a patient is asked to prospectively record the time and number of voluntary voids and incontinence episodes over a specified period of time, usually 1 to 7 days. In more complex forms, a subject may be asked to record pad usage, type and amount of fluid intake, voided volumes, frequency and severity of urinary urgency, and/or activities that occur in relation to their lower urinary tract symptoms (LUTS). Subjects are also often asked to record the time that they go to bed and the time they awaken to distinguish daytime from nighttime symptoms. For research studies of urinary incontinence, the NIH recommends a 3-day bladder diary that records and reports, at a minimum, pad usage, urinary incontinence episodes, and voiding frequency. Diaries in which patients are asked to report fluid intake and record voided volume using a graduated toilet insert are often called frequency-volume charts. Although more cumbersome for patients, frequency-volume charts provide a significant amount of additional data about lower urinary tract function not available from simpler bladder diaries, including average daily fluid intake, total daily voided volume, mean voided volume, largest single void (functional bladder capacity), and daytime and nighttime voided volumes. Although diaries have been used primarily as an outcome measure for studies of urinary symptoms in the gynecology and urology literature, symptom diaries are used extensively in many areas of clinical research as well. For instance, they have been used frequently in studies of bowel dysfunction to record the frequency of bowel movements, fecal incontinence episodes, and so on. Similarly, pain diaries are a standard outcome measure in studies of acute and chronic pain management.

The accuracy of symptom diaries depends upon the subject's ability to follow instructions. The circumstances under which a diary is kept should approximate everyday life and should be similar before and after the intervention to allow for meaningful comparison. Reproducibility depends upon the nature of the diary and the parameters being measured. In general, the reproducibility of symptom diaries improves as the duration of self-reporting increases. However, as diary duration increases, patient compliance tends to decrease. The most appropriate duration for bladder diaries has not been established. Although some have advocated the use of a single 24-hour diary, the reliability of diaries using this short duration is poor, limiting its use in research. The most commonly used duration is 7 days. Studies have demonstrated a high reliability for incontinence episodes, urinary frequency, urgency, and nocturic episodes in both men and women with either stress urinary incontinence (SUI) or overactive bladder (OAB) with this diary duration. In women with SUI, a 3-day diary appears to have similar reproducibility compared with a 7-day dairy with regard to number of incontinence episodes and voiding frequency. Similarly, in patients with OAB, the reliability of urgency incontinence episodes, urgency episodes, and daytime and nighttime frequency was adequate with a 3-day diary, but not as good as with a 7-day diary. Although a survey of clinicians and patients suggests that 4 days is the optimal diary duration, Bright et al. (2014) found that a 3-day dairy explains at least 94% of the variance of a 4-day diary. As mentioned, the NIH recommends a dairy duration of at least 3 days for the evaluation of LUTS.

The primary strength of symptoms diaries, at least in theory, is that they avoid the biases and inaccuracies of memory recall and record a subject's symptoms in her normal day-to-day environment. There is evidence, however, that many patients may not actually complete their diary as events occur. In a study of adults with chronic pain by Stone et al. (2003), subjects were asked to complete a pain diary for 21 consecutive days. Each of these "paper and pen" diaries was fitted with an unobtrusive photosensor that detected light and recorded when the diary was opened and closed. Subjects were asked to record their pain at three set time periods each day and were not informed of the presence of the photosensor. At the end of the study, subjects reported a greater than 90% compliance with the diary; however, the photosensor revealed that only 11% of subjects had filled out their diaries at the prescribed times. For most subjects, the records were marked by long periods, from days to weeks, when the diary was not opened, even although entries were made for those days when the diary was turned in at the end of the study, suggesting that subjects frequently backfilled their diary to complete missing days. Such backfilling is particularly subject to retrospective biases. In this study, a parallel group of patients were given computer diaries that prompted them to complete their diary at the specified times, and 94% true compliance was noted in this group, suggesting an advantage of computer diaries over paper ones. However, such computer prompting would not be useful for recording spontaneous events like voiding or incontinence episodes. In spite of this concern about retrospective completion of symptom diaries, they remain an important outcome measure in the study of pelvic floor disorders because of their widespread use, general acceptance, and proven reproducibility, particularly for studying lower urinary tract dysfunction. When using a bladder diary or similar symptom diary in a study, time should be spent instructing the subject in the proper use of the diary and the importance of completing the diary in a prospective manner.

Another strength of symptom diaries is that they provide information on symptom frequency and, in some cases, severity in a way that is quantifiable. This is particularly useful in studies of an intervention in which patients are not commonly "cured," but may show an improvement in symptoms, such as studies of medical or behavioral therapy for urinary incontinence. In fact, bladder diaries are the most common primary outcome measure used in studies of this type. Furthermore, outcome measures that are continuous variables tend to provide greater statistical power than a dichotomous variable, so using a variable from a bladder diary, such as number of incontinence episodes per week, rather than a dichotomous outcome such as "cure/failure," will usually allow for a smaller study sample size. An additional strength of bladder diaries in particular is that normal population values for variables like voiding frequency, mean voided volume, and daytime and nighttime urine output have been published, providing useful reference values for defining study populations and estimating treatment goals.

In addition to the possibility that symptom diaries may not always be completed contemporaneously, another potential weakness of this outcome tool is lower patient compliance with completing symptom diaries when compared with simpler measures like questionnaires. In large pharmaceutical trials in which subjects are carefully selected and often financially compensated to participate, compliance with symptom diaries is typically high, often over 90%, but high compliance may be difficult to achieve in other settings. A multicenter NIH-funded cohort study of 1064 participants with urinary symptoms included a 3-day voiding and fluid intake diary at baseline. Some 902 (85%) participants returned the diary, 796 diaries (75%) were considered usable, and only 448 (42%) were considered complete (Cameron et al., 2019). Younger participants were more likely to have missing or incomplete diaries. In smaller, less well-funded studies, patient compliance with symptom diaries may be even lower. Singh et al. (2004) prospectively studied 107 women who underwent pubovaginal sling procedures. They used the Simplified Urinary Incontinence Outcome Score, a composite outcome that combines the results of a questionnaire, a 24-hour pad test, and a 24-hour bladder diary into a single score, as their primary outcome. Although all patients completed the questionnaire postoperatively, only 52% completed the symptom diary and/or the pad test even after repeated telephone contacts, reducing the number of subjects for whom the primary outcome was available to half the original study population. When considering using a symptom diary as an outcome measure, the advantages of this tool must be weighed against the possibility of poor patient compliance.

Another important consideration when using a bladder diary as an outcome measure is the therapeutic effect that dairy completion in itself may have on lower urinary tract function. As described in Chapter 14, bladder retraining using diaries is an effective intervention for both SUI and urgency urinary incontinence (UUI). Several authors have suggested that the high improvement rates seen in the placebo groups in pharmaceutical trials of OAB and other similar trials (often >40%) are caused, in part, by a "bladder retraining effect" that occurs just by using diaries throughout the trial. Some studies suggest that this effect can occur as early as 4 days after starting diary use. When using a bladder diary to evaluate the effect of an intervention, the only certain way of accounting for the therapeutic effect of the diary itself is to include a control group in the study.

In recent years, there has been increased interest in electronic diaries, particularly those that use a mobile phone app interface. Electronic diaries have several advantages over patient diaries, including the ability to automatically calculate various parameters, the ability to remind or prompt patients to complete the diary input, and the ability to record the exact time of data entry. Also, patients tend to prefer electronic over paper entry. Disadvantages of electronic diaries include the potential cost, although most apps currently available are free or have a nominal cost, as well as concerns that the presence of a device that may include reminders may distort the diary results. One study comparing paper diary to mobile app found that participants recorded more voids and leaks on the paper diary than they entered into the app; the reasons for this difference are unclear (Sussman et al., 2016). Currently, there are over a dozen bladder diary mobile apps available on iPhone or Android platforms. Unfortunately, although often based on validated paper-based bladder diaries, none of the apps that are publicly available appear to have been specifically validated for this format. Mateu Arrom et al. (2019) validated a Spanish-language 3-day bladder diary mobile app, demonstrating it to be a reliable, valid method of assessing symptoms in patients with OAB and nocturia who have a smart phone. The National Institute of Diabetes and Digestive and Kidney Diseases (NIDDK) Prevention of Lower Urinary Tract Symptoms Consortium developed a mobile app (Where I Go+) to study healthy bladder habits in women and girls that includes geo-location tracking; currently this app is only available to study participants.

PAD TESTING

Pad testing attempts to objectively quantify the volume of urine loss by weighing a perineal pad before and after a specified time and/or group of activities. It is currently the only incontinence severity measure that captures the actual volume of leakage. Pad testing also has been used to attempt to distinguish continent from incontinent women. Numerous pad test protocols have been described, but in general they can be divided into short-term and long-term tests.

The short-term pad tests each ask subjects to perform a set of standardized provocative maneuvers in the office that, depending upon the protocol, can last from 10 minutes to 2 hours. In an attempt to standardize bladder volumes, most short-term pad tests specify that subjects start the pad test with a symptomatically full bladder, drink a standardized volume of liquid, or have a standard volume of fluid instilled in the bladder before the test. A preweighed pad is then worn while performing a predefined group of activities that typically includes such things as walking, climbing stairs, jumping, bending, coughing, and washing hands over a specified period of time. The volume of urine loss is obtained by weighing the pad at the completion of the test. For short-term tests, a change in pad weight of greater than 1 g is considered positive. When using a short-term pad test as a study outcome, the specific protocol used should be described. In 1983, the ICS recommended the 1-hour pad test described in Box 41.1 in an attempt to standardize this outcome measure across studies. Compared with long-term tests, short-term pad tests are easy and quick, and patient compliance can be directly monitored. Because of this, they are used frequently in clinical trials. However, a significant disadvantage of short-term pad tests is that they lack authenticity. These office tests do not necessarily reproduce the activities or situations that result in urine loss in a patient's everyday life. In fact, some patients may not be physically capable of completing all of the prescribed activities in the protocol. Another limitation of short-term pad tests is their poor test-retest reliability. Although some studies have demonstrated good correlation between short-term pad tests performed in the same subject on two separate occasions, many have found poor repeatability with this test. Lose et al. (1988) demonstrated differences of up to 24 g between two test results in the same subject 1 to 15 days apart using the ICS 1-hour pad test, and concluded that this test is not precise enough to allow reliable quantitation of urinary incontinence. This variation within subjects is largely attributable to differences in bladder volumes at the time of the test, and protocols that standardize pretest bladder volumes tend to have higher reliability.

Long-term pad tests are performed by giving a patient several preweighed pads to take home and wear for 24 to 48 hours. Patients are encouraged to mimic their regular daily activities and change the pads as they wish during the study period. Subjects should be instructed to place the pads in a sealed plastic bag after use to avoid evaporation. Afterward, pads are mailed to the clinic to be weighed on a precision scale to determine the total urine loss over the specified time period. Studies have shown that, as long as sealed bags are used, evaporation loss is minimal for up to 2 weeks. A bladder diary is often completed concurrently with the pad test to provide a comprehensive lower urinary tract evaluation. Changes in pad weights up to 7 g per 24 hours can be seen in healthy continent women, so values less than this should be considered insignificant. The primary advantage of long-term pad tests is that their results reflect everyday life. Also, the reproducibility of long-term tests is generally higher than that of short-term pad tests. Increasing the duration of the test from 24 hours to 48 to 72 hours increases the reliability further but decreases patient compliance. Of note, in patients with SUI, 24-hour pad test was inferior to cough stress test for diagnosis (Henderson et al., 2018). Not surprisingly, compliance with long-term pad tests varies considerably from study to study. As with bladder diaries, in large trials in which patients are carefully selected and are compensated for study participation, compliance with long-term pad tests tends to be high, whereas in smaller, less well-funded studies, compliance is often lower.

BOX 44.1 Steps of the 1-Hour Pad Test Recommended by the International Continence Society

- Test is started without the patient voiding.
- Preweighed pad is put on, and the first 1-hour test period begins.
- Subject drinks 500 mL of sodium-free liquid within a short period (maximum 15 minutes), then sits or rests.
- Half-hour period: subject walks, including stair-climbing equivalent to one flight up and down.
- During the remaining period, the subject performs the following activities:
  - Standing up from sitting, 10 times;
  - Coughing vigorously, 10 times;
  - Running on the spot for 1 minute;
  - Bending to pick up small object from floor, 5 times;
  - Washing hands in running water for 1 minute.
- At the end of the 1-hour test, the pad is removed and weighed.
- If the test is regarded as representative, the subject voids, and the volume is recorded.
- Otherwise, the test is repeated, preferably without voiding.

(From Abrams P, Blaivas JG, Stanton SL, Andersen JT. The standardisation of terminology of lower urinary tract function. The International Continence Society Committee on Standardisation of Terminology. *Scand J Urol Nephrol Suppl.* 1988;114:5.)

ANATOMIC OUTCOMES

Physical Examination

Outcome measures that assess changes in anatomy have an essential role in studies of pelvic floor disorders, particularly POP. Anatomic outcomes can be assessed by physical examination or radiographic studies. Currently, the presence and magnitude of POP are most often determined by physical examination. Although imaging studies have a role in evaluating women with prolapse, and may, in fact, be more accurate in determining which organs are involved in prolapse, the current lack of standardization, validation, and universal availability precludes their use as the "gold standard" for evaluating pelvic organ support.

Accurately evaluating the anatomic effects of prolapse surgery requires a standardized, reliable, validated, and reproducible system for describing the topographic anatomy of the pelvic floor and vaginal support. The Pelvic Organ Prolapse Quantitation (POPQ) system was introduced in 1996 jointly by the Society of Gynecologic Surgeons, the American Urogynecologic Society, and the ICS as the accepted method for describing pelvic support and comparing examinations over time and after interventions. This system has since been similarly adopted by the NIH, the IUGA, and the ICI. Details of the POPQ system can be found in Chapter 8. This prolapse grading system has been shown to have good inter- and intraexaminer reproducibility in a number of studies in the United States and Europe, and, although other prolapse grading systems are still used by some, POPQ has become the most commonly used system in the peer-reviewed literature.

In addition to its widespread adoption and proven reproducibility, another advantage of the POPQ system is its relative precision (nine site-specific measurements in 1-cm increments), which has allowed an improved understanding of the relationship between the anatomic characteristics of POP and the development of specific pelvic floor symptoms. Disadvantages include its relative complexity and the exclusion of some anatomic findings that some investigators believe to be essential for complete patient description, such as vaginal caliber, status of paravaginal support, pelvic floor descent, and urethral mobility. When evaluating pelvic organ support in a study, investigators should perform a standardized evaluation including the POPQ before and after the intervention. Details of this evaluation should be reported, including the position in which the examination was performed, the fullness of the bladder, the type of vaginal specula, retractors, and measuring devices used, and the method used to ensure that the maximal extent of prolapse is seen. It is critical that the examiner sees and describes the maximum protrusion noted by the individual during her daily activities. Ideally, the examiner should not be the subject's surgeon and should be blinded to the treatment assignment to limit observer bias.

Other anatomic outcomes that are often assessed by physical examination include pelvic floor and anal sphincter muscle strength, for which several valid and reliable grading scales exist, and urethral mobility measurements using the cotton swab test, ultrasound, or similar system.

Radiology

Imaging techniques, including evacuation proctography or defecography, magnetic resonance imaging (static and dynamic), and ultrasonography, can be used to assess anatomic outcomes in studies of women with pelvic floor disorders. These techniques may provide a more accurate picture of the location, support, and integrity of the pelvic visceral structures than does a simple physical examination. The use of dynamic imaging techniques can provide functional, as well as structural, information about an individual subject and may be useful in providing insights into the pathogenesis of many pelvic floor disorders, including urinary incontinence, fecal incontinence, defecatory dysfunction, and POP. Details of the various imaging studies that can be used to assess anatomic outcomes in the investigation of pelvic floor disorders, including their relative advantages and disadvantages, can be found in the previous chapters of this text. All research using imaging studies as an outcome should report: (1) the position of the patient; (2) specific verbal instructions given to the patient; (3) bladder and bowel content, including prestudy preparations; and (4) specific details of the imaging technique and equipment. See Chapter 13 for a detailed description of radiologic studies in the evaluation and outcome assessment of pelvic floor disorders.

PHYSIOLOGIC TESTING

Physiologic testing attempts to describe or quantify the underlying function of the pelvic viscera and pelvic floor, often including an assessment of whether such function is normal or pathologic. Physiologic testing serves two principal roles in pelvic floor research: to describe subjects at study entry, and to help define or understand treatment outcome. The most common physiologic test of the lower urinary tract is urodynamics. Physiologic tests of the lower gastrointestinal tract include anal manometry and colon transit studies. Other physiologic tests of the pelvic floor include such things as vaginal pressure transducers to measure levator ani contraction strength and electromyography of the pelvic floor muscles and urinary and anal sphincters to evaluate neuromuscular function. In addition to defining subjects at baseline and evaluating treatment outcomes, the use of physiologic testing in pelvic floor research can provide valuable insight into the underlying pathophysiology of the condition and into the mechanisms of treatment success or failure. Additionally, physiologic testing allows correlation between changes in symptoms and changes in physiology. The primary disadvantage of using physiologic tests in research is that they are often costly and time-consuming, and many can be uncomfortable for the patient.

Historically, urodynamic testing was considered the "gold standard" treatment outcome for studies evaluating the treatment of urinary incontinence because it is one of the only means of objectively assessing lower urinary tract function or dysfunction in incontinent patients. Unfortunately, few physiologic tests of pelvic floor function, including urodynamics, have undergone a rigorous evaluation of their reproducibility or validity. In 2009, a panel of international experts convened to evaluate the ability of urodynamics to improve or predict outcome of incontinence treatment concluded that, other than in children and in patients with neurogenic bladder, the evidence supporting each component of urodynamic testing and anal manometry was generally weak (grade C or D recommendations), and many components of the tests were considered investigational. Nygaard (2004), in a review for the International Foundation of Functional Gastrointestinal Diseases Consensus Conference on Advancing Treatment of Fecal and Urinary Incontinence, concluded that more clinical evidence is needed to establish the reproducibility of many components of urodynamic testing before the tests can be used as primary outcome measures in incontinence treatment studies. Recent clinical trial data suggest that multichannel urodynamics does not provide clinical benefit over basic office testing in patients with uncomplicated SUI, and that urodynamic parameters correlate poorly with outcomes. Thus, although physiologic outcome measures provide unique insight into pelvic floor function and are essential in explanatory trials, they should not be considered the gold standard by which patient-oriented outcomes are judged but should instead constitute one element of a range of patient responses to therapy. When using physiologic testing in pelvic floor research, investigators should use generally accepted standardized terminology and methods, such as those recommended by the ICS and/or NIH, whenever possible.

QUESTIONNAIRES

Pelvic floor symptoms can be assessed in a number of ways. Obviously, taking a thorough clinical history is an important method of assessing a patient's symptoms and their effect on daily life. However, in a situation in which a standardized, reproducible assessment is desired, clinical histories can be problematic, because they typically take on a different form for each clinician and patient encounter. The most valid way of measuring the presence, severity, and impact of a symptom or condition on a patient's activities and well-being is using psychometrically robust self-administered questionnaires. An increasing number of questionnaires and other PROs for women with pelvic floor disorders is now available. Most are intended to evaluate LUTS, but, over the last two decades, questionnaires have been developed for women with fecal incontinence and POP. In general, the two most commonly used and clinically relevant categories of questionnaires are: (1) those that measure the presence of particular symptoms and their severity (symptom questionnaires); (2) those that measure HRQOL. Other types of questionnaires are available for women with pelvic floor disorders, including those that measure sexual function, pain, physical functioning, and surgical complications.

Properties of a Good Patient-Reported Outcome Measure

PRO development is a complex process that is governed by the principles of psychometrics. Psychometrics is the science of the measurement of responses to phenomena that are not easily quantifiable. Ideally, the items on a questionnaire or PRO are based upon a conceptual framework that is constructed with direct input from patients and experts, usually using cognitive interviews, focus groups, and/or similar qualitative methods. For a questionnaire to be useful in research or in practice, it must demonstrate three important psychometric properties: validity, reliability, and responsiveness. Put in the simplest terms, the validity of a questionnaire is whether it measures what is intended. The reliability of a questionnaire refers to its ability to measure in a reproducible fashion. Responsiveness refers to a questionnaire's ability to reliably detect the overall effect of treatment and clinically meaningful change. When studies have been performed to demonstrate that a particular questionnaire has good psychometric properties, that questionnaire is said to "validated." Some important aspects of validity, reliability, and responsiveness that should be assessed when evaluating the psychometric properties of a PRO are listed in Table 41.1. Other characteristics that are desirable in a questionnaire include being easy to understand and being feasible to implement.

Most PROs used for pelvic floor disorders have been developed using the principles of classic test theory. In recent years, there has been increased emphasis on developing PROs using more state-of-the-art methods, specifically Item Response Theory (IRT). This effort has been spearheaded by the NIH Patient-Reported Outcomes Measurement Information System (PROMIS) initiative (http://www.nihpromis.org). The goal of PROMIS is to build and validate item banks of self-reported measures that assess key health concepts for adults for functions, symptoms, behaviors, and feelings using IRT psychometrics. Item banks created from IRT are content-valid, cover all aspects of the construct being measured, and have enough items to attain high measurement precision. Once items are calibrated using IRT, they can either be administered as a static short form, or the calibrations can be used to guide computerized adaptive testing (CAT). In CAT, a seed item is delivered to the patient and based upon her response, the most relevant

TABLE 41.1 Psychometric Properties of a Questionnaire

Psychometric Property	Description
Validity	
Face validity	Subjective assessment by an expert panel and/or patient focus group as to whether the instrument appears to measure what it intends to measure.
Content validity	Subjective assessment by an expert panel and/or patient focus group as to the extent that the domain of interest is comprehensively sampled by the questions in the instrument.
Construct validity	An assessment as to whether the instrument has appropriate relationships with other variables or measures. That is, the instrument correlates or agrees with other tests or measures of the same construct (convergent validity) and has little or no correlation or agreement with measures of different constructs (discriminant or divergent validity).
Criterion validity	Extent to which an instrument correlates with an established criterion standard (or "gold standard"). For HRQOL questionnaires, no gold standard exists; thus, criterion validity cannot be assessed. Criterion validity is assessed for diagnostic and prognostic tests and other measures where an established criterion standard exists.
Reliability	
Internal consistency	The extent to which the items on a scale are related to one another; often assessed with the Cronbach's alpha statistic (values of >0.70 demonstrate adequate internal consistency).
Test-retest reliability	An assessment of the repeatability; the correlation between instrument scores on two separate occasions. Repeat measurements should be made far enough apart in time so earlier responses are forgotten, yet not so far apart that the construct being measured might have changed.
Responsiveness	
	Assessment as to whether the instrument can detect clinically meaningful change. Methods for assessing responsiveness can broadly be separated into groups: distribution-based methods that measure the relative amount of change from baseline of an instrument after treatment (i.e., paired *t*-test, effect size) and anchor-based methods that compare the change in an instrument to some other measure that has clinical relevance (example: a 5-point improvement in IQOL score is associated with a 25% or greater decrease in number of incontinence episodes on bladder diary).

HRQOL, Health-related quality of life; *IQOL*, incontinence quality of life questionnaire.

items from the bank are selected for further administration. Two individuals taking a CAT may receive different items, but because items are all calibrated along a common dimension, the scores are comparable, without patients needing to answer non-relevant questions (Sung et al., 2011). The principal advantage of a short form or CAT is decreasing question burden (typically by ~50%) while maintaining precision. CAT administration requires the patient/subject to have access to a computer, tablet, or mobile phone app, however. Sung et al. (2016) developed and validated a CAT for women with urinary incontinence based on the PROMIS framework. Further details of PROMIS PROs and other condition-specific PROs for women with pelvic floor disorders that have used IRT methodology are detailed later.

Choosing a Patient-Reported Outcome Measure

When choosing a questionnaire for use in clinical practice or in research, the first step is to determine if the questionnaire actually measures what you desire. A brief review of the questionnaire's content and structure will provide important information in this regard. It is important to keep in mind the purpose for which a questionnaire was originally designed and the population in which it was validated. Before questionnaires are used in populations or contexts other than those they were designed for, further validation is usually necessary. The second step is to assess the reliability, validity, and responsiveness of the questionnaire. Use of nonvalidated questionnaires may provide misleading information or fail to detect important clinical changes. Whenever possible, it is desirable to use a validated questionnaire that is widely accepted and has been used many times in the population you wish to evaluate. The final step is to determine whether the length and construct of the questionnaire, as well as mode of administration (e.g., paper, phone, computer, mobile app, etc.), are such that it is feasible to administer in your practice or research study. Long questionnaires may be desirable for research studies in which lots of detail is desirable but are likely to be too burdensome and time-consuming to be used effectively in clinical practice. In general, in PROs developed using classic test theory, using only part of a validated questionnaire or changing the order or content of a questionnaire is discouraged because this can change its psychometric properties. PROs developed using IRT offer more flexibility in terms of question order and ease of developing short forms or even CAT, as previously discussed.

Symptom Questionnaires

Symptom questionnaires are used to assess the presence, severity, and impact of particular symptoms or groups of symptoms. A list of valid and reliable symptom questionnaires developed for women with various pelvic floor disorders is shown in Box 41.2. One of the most widely used symptom questionnaires in the study of pelvic floor disorders is the Urogenital Distress Inventory (UDI). The UDI contains 19 questions about LUTS separated into three scales: irritative symptoms, obstructive/discomfort symptoms, and stress symptoms. Respondents are asked if they have a particular symptom and, if they do, to assess the degree it bothers them on a four-point scale from "not at all" to "greatly." The shortened version of the UDI is the UDI-6, a six-question instrument that correlates well with the longer version and has been widely used.

BOX 41.2 Recommended Symptom Questionnaires for Women with Pelvic Floor Disorders[a]

Urinary Incontinence/Lower Urinary Tract Symptoms

Incontinence Severity Index
International Consultation on Incontinence Questionnaire short form (ICIQ-SF)
Urogenital Distress Inventory (UDI)
Urogenital Distress Inventory short form (UDI-6)
Lower Urinary Tract Dysfunction Research Network Symptom Index-29 (LURN SI-29)
Lower Urinary Tract Dysfunction Research Network Symptom Index-10 (LURN SI-10)
King's Health Questionnaire
Bristol Female Lower Urinary Tract Symptom Questionnaire (BFLUTS)

Fecal Incontinence

St. Mark's (Vaizey) score
Fecal Incontinence Severity Index (FISI)
Accidental Bowel Leakage Evaluation (ABLE)

Pelvic Organ Prolapse

Pelvic Floor Distress Inventory (PFDI)
Pelvic Floor Distress Inventory short form (PFDI-20)

All Pelvic Floor Disorders (UI, FI, POP)[b]

Pelvic Floor Distress Inventory (PFDI)
Pelvic Floor Distress Inventory short form (PFDI-20)

[a]All instruments listed have been shown to be valid, reliable, and responsive.
[b]The PFDI and its short form (PFDI-20) have been used primarily in women with pelvic organ prolapse (grade A recommendation from 6th International Consultation on Incontinence) and have demonstrated good psychometric properties in all forms of pelvic floor disorders. Each has urinary, anorectal, and pelvic organ prolapse scales.
UI, Urinary incontinence; *FI*, fecal incontinence; *POP*, pelvic organ prolapse.

A simple urinary incontinence symptom severity questionnaire that has been used frequently, particularly in epidemiology studies, is the Incontinence Severity Index developed by Sandvik et al. (1993) (Box 41.3). This index has been shown by multiple authors to have good validity and reliability and is responsive to both behavioral and surgical treatments. It is able to accurately distinguish between women with and without incontinence and has good correlation with pad test and bladder diary results. The brevity and simplicity of this questionnaire makes it ideal for use in clinical practice. Another brief urinary incontinence severity questionnaire is the International Consultation on Incontinence Questionnaire–Urinary Incontinence Short Form (ICIQ-UI Short Form) (Box 41.4). This four-item questionnaire was developed by the WHO-sponsored ICI in an effort to provide a brief, robust urinary incontinence symptom questionnaire that could be applied widely in clinical practice and research. It has been evaluated in both men and women and has been shown to be valid, reliable, and responsive in numerous studies.

BOX 41.3 Incontinence Severity Index

How Often do you Experience Urinary Leakage?
0 Never
1 Less than once a month
2 Once or several times a month
3 Once or several times per week
4 Every day and/or night

How Much Urine do you Lose Each Time?
0 None
1 Drops or little
2 More

Scoring: Multiply the score for question 1 by the score for question 2. The total score is then used to classify patients into one of four severity categories:

0 = Dry 1–2 = Slight 3–4 = Moderate 6–8 = Severe

(Modified from Sandvik H, Hunskaar S, Seim A, et al. Validation of severity index in female urinary incontinence and its implementation in an epidemiological survey. *J Epidemiol Community Health.* 1993;47:497.)

It is currently available in over 30 languages. The ICIQ-UI Short Form contains three scored items (assessment of the frequency, severity, and perceived impact of incontinence) and an unscored self-diagnostic item. ICI has developed several other scales (http://www.iciq.net) that are intended to be modular in nature, including a more comprehensive female LUTS questionnaire, questionnaires for patients with nocturia and OAB, a questionnaire that assesses vaginal symptoms/sexual function, and a bowel/fecal symptoms questionnaire, among others.

With a goal of capturing the full spectrum of LUTS in both men and women with interpretable scales that can be used for outcome measurement, the NIDDK's Symptoms of Lower Urinary Tract Dysfunction Research Network (LURN) developed the Comprehensive Assessment of Self-reported Urinary Symptoms (CASUS) using the state-of-the-art methodology of NIH PROMIS. CASUS assesses a comprehensive set of 93 manifestations of LUTS in both men and women. Two short forms, the 29-item LURN Symptom Index (LURN SI-29) and the 10-item LURN Symptom Index (LURN SI-10), have subsequently been developed for use as clinical or research outcome questionnaires that capture aspects of LUTS relevant to both sexes. The LURN SI-29 comprises five scales—incontinence, urgency, voiding difficulty, bladder pain, and nocturia—and has demonstrated internal consistency and construct validity. The LURN SI-10 is a brief questionnaire intended to be used in clinical practice to assess urinary frequency, nocturia, urgency, incontinence, bladder pain, voiding, and postmicturition symptoms. Test-retest reliability and responsiveness has not been assessed for either of these instruments. Additionally, only patients seeking treatment were included in the validation of these scales, so use should be limited to this population until further studies are available.

Urinary urgency is the essential symptom of OAB, and, although varying techniques have been used to assess the level of urgency in OAB studies, the most commonly used method incorporates a rating of urgency recorded with each void on a voiding diary. Valid and reliable urgency rating scales incorporated as part of a bladder diary include the Indevus Urgency

BOX 41.4 International Consultation on Incontinence Questionnaire (ICIQ)–Urinary Incontinence Short Form

Many people leak urine some of the time. We are trying to find out how many people leak urine, and how much this bothers them. We should be grateful if you could answer the following questions, thinking about how you have been, on average, over the PAST FOUR WEEKS.

1 Please write in your date of birth: ☐☐ DAY ☐☐ MONTH ☐☐ YEAR

2 Are you *(tick one)*: Female ☐ Male ☐

3 How often do you leak urine? *(Tick one box)*
never ☐ 0
about once a week or less often ☐ 1
two or three times a week ☐ 2
about once a day ☐ 3
several times a day ☐ 4
all the time ☐ 6

4 We would like to know how much urine you think leaks. How much urine do you usually leak (whether you wear protection or not)? *(Tick one box)*
none ☐ 0
a small amount ☐ 2
a moderate amount ☐ 4
a large amount ☐ 6

5 Overall, how much does leaking urine interfere with your everyday life?
Please ring a number between 0 (not at all) and 10 (a great deal)

0 1 2 3 4 5 6 7 8 9 10
not at all ... a great deal

ICIQ score: sum scores 3+4+5 ☐☐

6 When does urine leak? *(Please tick all that apply to you)*
never – urine does not leak ☐
leaks before you can get to the toilet ☐
leaks when you cough or sneeze ☐
leaks when you are asleep ☐
leaks when you are physically active/exercising ☐
leaks when you have finished urinating and are dressed ☐
leaks for no obvious reason ☐
leaks all the time ☐

Thank you very much for answering these questions.

Severity Scale, the Sensation-Related Bladder Diary, the Patient Perception of Intensity of Urgency Scale (PPIUS), and the Urinary Sensation Scale (USS) (Table 41.2). In each scale, patients rate their degree of urgency for that void on a three-, four-, or five-point scale. Each places urinary urgency on a continuum ranging from no desire to void, to normal desire to void, to pathologic urgency. Generally, only the highest rating (or in the case of the PPIUS and USS, the top two ratings) indicate pathologic urgency.

There are four commonly used severity scores for fecal incontinence: the Pescatori Incontinence Score, Wexner (Cleveland Clinic) Score, St. Mark's (Vaizey) Score, and Fecal Incontinence Severity Index (FISI). FISI is a questionnaire that was developed with the support of the American Society of Colon and Rectal Surgeons (Table 41.3). It is based on a type-by-frequency matrix that assigns values to various frequencies and

TABLE 41.2 Urinary Urgency Scales

Indevus Urgency Severity Scale	Sensation-related Bladder Diary	Patient Perception of Intensity of Urgency Scale	Urinary Sensation Scale
0: None—No urgency.	Grade 1—No desire to void.	0—No urgency: I felt no need to empty my bladder but did so for other reasons.	1—No urgency: No feeling of urgency. Can continue activities until it is convenient to use the bathroom.
1: Mild—Awareness of urgency, but it is easily tolerated, and you can continue with your usual activity or task.	Grade 2—Desire to void, but voiding can be delayed for at least 30 min.	1—Mild urgency: I could postpone voiding for as long as necessary without fear of wetting myself.	2—Mild urgency: Feel urgency. Can easily tolerate. Can finish usual activity and task quickly, and then go right to the bathroom.
2: Moderate—Enough urgency or discomfort that it interferes with or shortens your usual activity or tasks.	Grade 3—Desire to void, and voiding cannot be delayed for more than 15 min.	2—Moderate urgency: I could postpone voiding for a short while without fear of wetting myself.	3—Moderate urgency: Enough urgency discomfort. Need to stop usual activity and task and go right to the bathroom.
4: Severe—Extreme urgency discomfort that abruptly stops all activity or tasks.	Grade 4—Desire to void, and voiding cannot be delayed for more than 5 min.	3—Severe urgency: I could not postpone voiding, but had to rush to the toilet in order not to wet myself.	4—Severe urgency: Strong urgency discomfort. Almost cannot hold urine. Need to stop usual activity and tasks immediately, and run to bathroom to avoid wetting accident.
		4—Urge incontinence: I leaked before arriving at the toilet.	5—Urge incontinence: Extreme urgency discomfort. Cannot hold urine, and have a wetting accident before arriving at the bathroom.

(Modified from Cartwright R, Srikrishna S, Cardozo L, et al. Validation and reliability of the patient's perception of intensity of urgency scale in overactive bladder. *BJU Int.* 2010;107:1612.)

TABLE 41.3 Fecal Incontinence Severity Scales

Fecal Incontinence Severity Index	2 or more times a day	Once a day	2 or more times a week	Once a week	1–3 times a month	Never
Gas	❑	❑	❑	❑	❑	❑
Mucus	❑	❑	❑	❑	❑	❑
Liquid stool	❑	❑	❑	❑	❑	❑
Solid stool	❑	❑	❑	❑	❑	❑
Weights[a]						
Gas	12	11	8	6	4	0
Mucous	12	10	7	5	3	0
Liquid stool	19	17	13	10	8	0
Solid stool	18	16	13	10	8	0

St. Mark's (Vaizey) Score	Never[b]	Rarely[b]	Sometimes[b]	Weekly[b]	Daily[b]
Incontinence for solid stool	0	1	2	3	4
Incontinence for liquid stool	0	1	2	3	4
Incontinence for gas	0	1	2	3	4
Alteration in lifestyle	0	1	2	3	4
				No	Yes
Need to wear a pad or plug				0	2
Taking constipating medicines				0	2
Lack of ability to defer defecation for 15 minutes				0	4

Fecal Incontinence Severity Index Score: Sum the weights associated with the boxes that are checked in each row (range 0–61).
St. Mark's (Vaizey) Score: Add one score from each row: minimum score = 0 = perfect continence; maximum score = 24 = totally incontinent.
[a]Patient-derived weights shown.
[b]Never, no episodes in the past 4 weeks; rarely, one episode in the past 4 weeks; sometimes, >1 episode in the past 4 weeks but <1 a week; weekly, one or more episodes a week but <1 a day; daily, one or more episodes a day.
(Modified from Rockwood TH, Church JM, Fleshman JW, et al. Fecal incontinence quality-of-life scale: quality-of-life instrument for patients with fecal incontinence. *Dis Colon Rectum.* 2000;43:9; Vaizey CJ, Carapeti E, Cahill JA, et al. Prospective comparison of faecal incontinence grading systems. *Gut.* 1999;4:477.)

types of incontinence based on a subjective rating of severity. The scoring algorithm was developed through independent interviews with patients and colorectal surgeons. The severity ratings of both groups were very highly correlated, although, interestingly, patients tended to rate liquid incontinence as most severe, whereas surgeons rated solid stool incontinence as most severe. The authors do not endorse the use of the values of one group over another (patient-derived weights or surgeon-derived weights); but an argument can be made that the subjective experience of the patients should be more important. The FISI needs further psychometric testing, particularly with regard to reliability and responsiveness. It has, however, demonstrated significant correlations with QOL and with extent of anal sphincter injury as measured by endoanal ultrasound in women with other pelvic floor disorders. The St. Mark's (Vaizey) Score, like the FISI, assesses frequency of incontinence by type (solid, liquid, gas); however, it also assesses alterations in lifestyle, need to use pads or a plug, use of constipating medications, and ability to defer defecation (e.g., fecal urgency) (Table 41.3). Several studies have demonstrated the reliability and validity of the St. Mark's score and, unlike the FISI, it has demonstrated responsiveness, and the minimum important difference (MID) has been established. Improvement in St. Mark's score is highly correlated with fecal incontinent episodes ($r = 0.79$, $P < .001$). There is also a moderate correlation with the St. Mark's score and changes in maximum incremental squeeze pressure ($r = -0.30$, $P < .05$). The Pescatori Incontinence Score and the Wexner Score have not been as rigorously validated as the FISI or St. Mark's score.

In addition to these commonly used fecal incontinence symptom questionnaires, the Accidental Bowel Leakage Evaluation (ABLE) questionnaire was recently developed and introduced by the Pelvic Floor Disorders Network (Rogers et al., 2020). This measure improves upon existing questionnaires because it is based on a comprehensive conceptual framework created through state-of-the-art qualitative methods to identify symptoms important to patients suffering from fecal incontinence and, therefore, is more patient-centered. Specifically, it includes items that cover areas not included in the existing measures but that were found to be important to patients, such as predictability, awareness, control, emptying, and discomfort. The ABLE questionnaire has 18 items and demonstrates good reliability and validity.

To date, the only valid, reliable, and responsive symptom questionnaire designed specifically for use in women with POP is the Pelvic Floor Distress Inventory (PFDI). This comprehensive symptom questionnaire is intended for women with all forms of pelvic floor disorders. It assesses 46 pelvic floor symptoms and has three scales: a urinary scale (identical to the UDI), a colorectal scale, and a POP scale. Its structure is similar to that of the UDI; patients are asked to indicate if they have a particular symptom and, if so, are asked to assess how much it bothers them on a four-point scale. A short version of the PFDI is also available, the Pelvic Floor Distress Inventory Short Form 20 (PFDI-20), which also has urinary, colorectal, and POP scales. The urinary scale of the PFDI-20 is identical to the UDI-6. Both the PFDI and the PFDI-20 have good reliability and validity and have demonstrated excellent responsiveness in patients undergoing surgical and nonsurgical treatment for POP.

Quality-of-Life Questionnaires

HRQOL refers to a person's total sense of well-being and considers multiple dimensions, including (but not limited to) their social, physical, and emotional health. Measures of HRQOL can be classified into two types: generic and condition-specific. Generic HRQOL instruments are used to assess QOL in a broad range of illnesses or populations. Generic instruments have the advantage of allowing comparisons across different groups or illnesses but may lack sensitivity to the unique aspects of a specific disease and how it impacts the life of an affected patient. The two generic HRQOL instruments that have been used frequently in women with pelvic floor disorders are the Short Form–36 (SF-36) and EuroQOL-5D (EQ-5D) (Box 41.5). Both instruments are widely used, have been translated into several languages, and have reached the highest levels of evidence relating to psychometric testing. Although these instruments are relatively unresponsive to change in women with pelvic floor disorders, larger surgical trials, as well a smaller study of elderly women with severe prolapse, have demonstrated statistically significant and clinically relevant improvements in the mental and physical components of the SF-36 after surgery (Barber et al., 2007; Lukacz et al., 2016).

The PROMIS Global-10 is a publicly available 10-item generic global health assessment tool developed through the NIH PROMIS initiative that allows measurements of symptoms, functioning, and HRQOL for a wide variety of chronic diseases and conditions. The questionnaire consists of 10 items that assess general domains of health and functioning, including overall physical health, mental health, social health, pain, fatigue, and overall perceived QOL. Scoring of the PROMIS Global-10 provides a mental health and physical health summary score. Additionally, each of the individual items can be examined separately to provide specific information about perceptions of physical function, pain, fatigue, emotional distress, social health, and general perceptions of health. Additionally, a two-item PROMIS Global Mental Health and two-item PROMIS Global Physical Health are available that provide a "bottom-line" assessment of mental and physical health, respectively. In addition to the PROMIS Global questionnaires, there are over 300 questionnaires or CATS available through the NIH PROMIS initiative to assess a broad range of aspects of physical, mental, and social health, including fatigue, pain, physical function, sleep, anxiety, depression, social health, and sexual function (https://www.healthmeasures.net/explore-measurement-systems/promis/intro-to-promis/list-of-adult-measures). The PROMIS Global questionnaires, SF-36, and EQ-5D can each be converted to a T-score metric allowing for comparisons to a general (norm) population.

Condition-specific HRQOL instruments are designed to measure the impact of a specific disease on HRQOL. Condition-specific instruments provide a more in-depth assessment of specific issues and concerns critical to the disease process they were designed for. They also tend to be more responsive to

BOX 41.5 Recommended Quality-of-Life and Sexual Function Scales for Women with Pelvic Floor Disorders*

Generic Quality-of-Life Questionnaires
SF-36
EuroQOL-5D (EQ-5D)
PROMIS Global Health–10

Condition-Specific Quality-of-Life Questionnaires
Urinary Incontinence
Incontinence Impact Questionnaire (IIQ)
Incontinence Impact Questionnaire short form (IIQ-7)
Incontinence Quality-of-Life Questionnaire (I-QOL)
King's Health Questionnaire
Urge Incontinence Impact Questionnaire (Urge IIQ)

Overactive Bladder
Overactive Bladder Questionnaire (OAB-q)

Fecal Incontinence
Fecal Incontinence QOL Scale (FIQL)
Manchester Health Questionnaire

Pelvic Organ Prolapse
Pelvic Floor Impact Questionnaire (PFIQ)
Pelvic Floor Impact Questionnaire Short Form 7 (PFIQ-7)
Prolapse Quality-of-Life Questionnaire (P-QOL)

All Pelvic Floor Disorders (UI, FI, POP)
Pelvic Floor Impact Questionnaire (PFIQ)
Pelvic Floor Impact Questionnaire Short Form 7 (PFIQ-7)

Sexual Function Questionnaires
Female Sexual Function Index (FSFI)
Prolapse and Incontinence Sexual Function Questionnaire (PISQ)
Prolapse and Incontinence Sexual Function Questionnaire short form (PISQ-12)
Prolapse and Incontinence Sexual Function Questionnaire—IUGA Revised (PISQ–IR)
PROMIS Sexual Function and Satisfaction Instruments (PROMIS SF)

PROMIS, National Institutes of Health Patient-Reported Outcomes Information System; *SF-36*, Short Form 36; *IUGA*, International Urogynecological Association.

change than generic instruments. Their primary disadvantage is that they can only be used in the particular patient group they were designed for, and the data cannot be compared with norms for a general population or other groups. Condition-specific HRQOL questionnaires for women with pelvic floor disorders with established reliability and validity are listed in Box 41.5.

The Incontinence Impact Questionnaire (IIQ) is a condition-specific QOL questionnaire for women with urinary incontinence that is a companion to the UDI. This questionnaire has 30 questions and assesses the degree to which LUTS affect a range of daily activities and emotions. It has four scales: travel, social, emotional, and physical activity. Like the UDI, it is a valid, reliable, and responsive questionnaire that was originally designed for use in women with urinary incontinence, and has been used extensively to measure the effect of LUTS on the HRQOL of women with POP. The IIQ-7 is a shortened version of the IIQ that is a companion to the UDI-6.

The Incontinence Quality of Life Questionnaire (I-QOL) is a 22-item questionnaire with three scales (avoidance/limiting behavior, psychosocial impact, and social embarrassment) designed for use in clinical trials to measure impact of incontinence on men and women. It is available in several languages and has demonstrated reliability and validity in multiple different populations. Although the I-QOL has only moderate responsiveness, unlike many questionnaires for women with pelvic floor disorders, the minimum change in score that should be considered clinically significant (the MID) has been evaluated. The MID of the I-QOL is an improvement in score of approximately 2% to 5%. A 2% to 5% improvement in I-QOL score is associated with a 25% reduction in pad weight and a 25% reduction in incontinence episodes in the bladder diary, and was the change in score noted in patients who stated that they were "a little better" after treatment.

The King's Health Questionnaire is a 32-item questionnaire that assesses 10 domains related to HRQOL and urinary incontinence. It was originally developed in Britain, but eight validated cultural adaptations of the questionnaire are available in 26 languages. It has demonstrated good psychometric properties, and, like the I-QOL, its MID has been determined. A change from baseline of at least 5 points (out of 100) on any of the questionnaire's 10 domains indicates clinically meaningful improvement in that domain.

The Overactive Bladder Questionnaire was developed to assess symptom bother and the impact of OAB on HRQOL. The instrument was developed and validated in both continent and incontinent patients with OAB, including both men and women. It includes eight items that evaluate symptom bother and 25 items that evaluate impact of OAB on HRQOL, and has demonstrated reliability, validity, and responsiveness to pharmacotherapy in both continent and incontinent patients.

As with the symptom severity questionnaires, condition-specific HRQOL instruments for women with fecal incontinence are less well established than those for women with urinary incontinence. The Fecal Incontinence Quality of Life (FIQOL) scale is a 29-item instrument developed with the support of the American Society of Colon and Rectal Surgeons that measures the impact of anal incontinence over four domains: lifestyle, coping/behavior, depression/self-perception, and embarrassment. The Manchester Health Questionnaire is an adaptation of the King's Health Questionnaire for women with fecal incontinence. It includes items in eight domains of QOL and a symptom severity scale. Both the FIQOL scale and the Manchester Health Questionnaire have demonstrated adequate validity and reliability, but their responsiveness has yet to be established.

The Pelvic Floor Impact Questionnaire (PFIQ) and the Prolapse Quality of Life Questionnaire (P-QOL) are currently the only condition-specific questionnaires with demonstrated reliability, validity, and responsiveness that assess the impact of POP on QOL. The PFIQ is a companion questionnaire to the PFDI and can be used by clinicians and researchers to measure the extent to which lower urinary tract, lower gastrointestinal tract, and POP symptoms affect the QOL of women who suffer from the full spectrum of pelvic floor disorders. Like the PFDI, it has urinary, colorectal, and POP scales and has good reliability and validity. It also has demonstrated responsiveness in women receiving surgical and nonsurgical management for POP. The PFIQ-7 is a short version of the PFIQ that includes within it the IIQ-7 and colorectal and prolapse scales. The P-QOL is a 20-item questionnaire that covers nine QOL domains, including general health, prolapse impact, role, physical and social limitations, personal relationships, emotional problems, and sleep/energy disturbance, as well as measurements of symptom severity.

Sexual Function Questionnaires

Sexual function is an important outcome to consider when evaluating a treatment of pelvic floor disorders (see also Chapter 10). Although a number of valid and reliable generic sexual function questionnaires exist, their use in women with POP or other pelvic floor disorders has been limited. A systematic review by Daker-White performed in 2002 identified 14 valid and reliable self-reported sexual function measures for men or women; however, only two met the highest standards and were recommended for general use: the McCoy Female Sexuality Questionnaire (MFSQ) and the Female Sexual Function Index (FSFI). The MFSQ is a 19-item questionnaire for use in postmenopausal women that aims to assess a woman's level of sexual interest and response. The FSFI is also a 19-item questionnaire and has six domains: desire, arousal, lubrication, orgasm, satisfaction, and pain. The FSFI can be used in any age group and is the general sexual function questionnaire that has been used most frequently in studies of pelvic floor disorders. The main difference between these questionnaires is that the MFSQ includes social and relationship factors, whereas the FSFI is more focused on individual function. Both measures contain questions that are only applicable for people with a current sexual partner.

Other generic measures have been developed since the Daker-White review, but most lack psychometric rigor (Cartagena-Ramos et al., 2018; Flynn et al., 2013). To fill this gap, the NIH PROMIS initiative developed the NIH PROMIS Sexual Function and Satisfaction (PROMIS SexFS) measure. The initial version was directed specifically to patients with cancer, but a second version has been developed and validated for use in diverse populations of both men and women (Flynn et al., 2013; Weinfurt et al., 2015). PROMIS SexFS version 2.0 has 11 scored scales (interest in sexual activity, lubrication, vaginal discomfort, clitoral discomfort, labial discomfort, erectile function, orgasm ability, orgasm pleasure, oral dryness, oral discomfort, satisfaction) and is applicable for both men and women and those sexually active with a partner and without, and scoring allows comparisons to population norms. Importantly, the PROMIS SexFS is customizable, allowing users to select relevant domains and items for their study.

Currently, the only condition-specific sexual function questionnaire for women with POP or urinary incontinence is the Pelvic Organ Prolapse and Incontinence Sexual Function Questionnaire (PISQ). The PISQ is valid and reliable and contains 31 items and three domains: behavioral/emotive, physical, and partner-related. It is designed for use in sexually active women with POP and/or urinary incontinence and assesses the impact of these diseases on sexual function. The PISQ-12 is a short version of the PISQ that correlates well with its long form. More recently, IUGA established a working group to improve the PISQ with the goals of refining its measurement properties, enhancing the ability to assess outcomes in women who are not sexually active and in women with anal incontinence, and developing an instrument ultimately intended for international use (Rogers et al., 2013). The Pelvic Organ Prolapse and Incontinence Sexual Questionnaire—IUGA Revised is a 20-item questionnaire with demonstrated reliability, validity, and responsiveness in women with urinary incontinence, anal incontinence, and POP that has sections for those who are sexually active and those who are not sexually active. It is available in multiple international languages and contexts.

Global Indices

A global index is a simple, usually single-item, instrument that asks an individual patient to rate the severity of a specific condition or to rate the response of her condition to treatment. As the name implies, the goal of a global index is to get an overall appraisal of a complex phenomenon, not to evaluate every component of the phenomenon. Global indices are simple, direct, and easy to interpret. Additionally, global indices provide the single best measure of significance of change from the individual perspective. They take into account more information that may affect HRQOL than other methods for assessing clinically meaningful change. The principal disadvantage of global indices is their lack of information and specificity regarding the precise aspects or manifestations of disease severity or improvement that result in an individual patient selecting a specific rating. A common global index used in pelvic floor research is the visual analog score (VAS), where respondents are asked to indicate the severity of their disease on a 10-cm VAS scale, with 0 representing no complaint and 100 indicating unbearable urinary symptoms or something similar.

A validated global index for urinary incontinence is the Patient Global Impression of Improvement (PGI-I), a single-item questionnaire that asks subjects to rate their improvement after treatment on a seven-point scale (Box 41.6). The PGI-I responses demonstrate significant correlation with changes in pad testing, urinary incontinence frequency, and I-QOL score

BOX 41.6 Patient Global Impression of Improvement

Check the one number that best describes how your urinary tract condition is now, compared with how it was before your treatment.

1. Very much better
2. Much better
3. A little better
4. No change
5. A little worse
6. Much worse
7. Very much worse

(Modified from Yalcin I, Bump R. Validation of two global impression questionnaires for incontinence. *Am J Obstet Gynecol.* 2003;189:98.)

after treatment for urinary incontinence. Thus, this simple tool appears to be a valid global assessment of a patient's response to treatment for urinary incontinence. Interestingly, data from Yalcin and Bump (2003) using the PGI-I suggest that patients begin to perceive themselves as being at least a little better with treatment when their incontinence episodes decrease by about 45% or more, or when their 1-hour pad test improves by approximately 25% or more.

Additionally, a PGI-I scale for urogenital prolapse has been developed and shown to have excellent test-retest reliability and construct validity (Srikrishna et al., 2010). In a study of over 2000 prolapse surgery patients, 90% of patients reported improvement in comparison with their preoperative state on PGI-I (Mattsson et al., 2020a). Changes in PGI-I 2 years after surgery were found to correlate more strongly with the PFDI-20 than with the generic QOL measure 15D (Mattsson et al., 2020b). However, overall correlations between all three instruments were weak, leading the authors to conclude that quantified health gains after prolapse surgery are strongly dependent on the chosen PRO and to emphasize the importance of using condition-specific measures for this condition.

Patient-Selected Goals

Patient-selected outcome measures, also called goal attainment scaling (GAS), is a technique for measuring goal achievement after therapy that has been commonly used in psychiatry, physical therapy, and nursing, and has also been applied to pelvic floor disorders. It seems particularly suited for fields in which the goal of therapy is to improve QOL and where success is subjective and individualized. Before therapy, subjects are asked to list the goals they wish to achieve from the intervention. Patient goals are not stated in terms of traditional outcome measures, but rather in terms that are specific and personal to the individual subject. Examples might include such things as "spending less time getting up at night to the bathroom," "being able to play tennis without leaking," or "getting rid of my uncomfortable bulge." After therapy, goal achievement, or lack thereof, is measured using VAS or Likert-type responses. Hullfish et al. (2002) found that women scheduled for surgery for pelvic floor dysfunction had, on average, 3.6 goals that could be broadly separated into five categories: urinary/bowel symptoms, improving activity, general/other health, social relationships/self-image, and physical appearance. Twelve weeks after surgery, 85% felt that all or some of their prespecified goals had been met, 46% had all of their goals met 12 weeks postoperatively, and 42% felt that all of their preoperative goals had been met at 2-year follow-up (Hullfish et al., 2004). Srikrishna et al. (2015) found in a long-term prospective cohort that 83% of goals achieved were maintained 10 years following prolapse and/or incontinence surgery. They also noted that goals differed between patients and surgeons. Goal achievement correlates with both improvements in QOL and satisfaction with treatment, often better than objective outcome measures do. Goal assessment is not, however, identical to QOL assessment, as each provides complementary, but independent, indications of long-term subjective treatment success.

Patient-selected goal assessment is a valuable clinical tool when applied to the individual patient. It can assist in understanding and managing a patient's expectations, provide treatment goals, and be used to direct therapy. In the evaluation of a therapy, GAS provides a unique insight into the components that make up a successful intervention and helps explain why two subjects who have similar treatment outcomes from an objective standpoint may have differences in terms of satisfaction with treatment. Unfortunately, the application of GAS to clinical research is challenging, primarily because of the heterogeneous nature of subject-selected goals. Potentially large differences in the number, magnitude, and characteristics of individual subjects' goals within a study can make analysis and interpretation of study results difficult. Furthermore, the application of GAS to surgical research or to the evaluation of drug therapy is in its infancy. Further research is necessary to determine how best to apply GAS to therapeutic trials for pelvic floor disorders.

SOCIOECONOMIC OUTCOMES

Public policy decisions and socioeconomic evaluations require an assessment of treatment cost in relation to treatment outcome. A detailed discussion of cost-effectiveness studies and their ilk are beyond the scope of this chapter; however, attempts at capturing treatment cost should be an important consideration in any well-designed clinical trial. Such assessments should attempt to quantify both direct and indirect costs. Direct medical costs should include personnel costs/time (physician, nurse, technician), diagnostic and laboratory tests, hospital costs, treatment costs (drugs, operating room time, etc.), treatment of side effects, and outpatient visits. Indirect costs are often more difficult to quantify, but should include things such as loss of productivity, time lost from work, loss of service to family and community, and premature mortality. In economic evaluations, it is important to consider the *perspective* of the evaluation, as the perspective (e.g., patients, hospital, third-party payer, government, and society) will have significant influence on which costs should be included in the analysis.

DEFINING TREATMENT SUCCESS

In contrast to trials evaluating treatment of cancer or cardiovascular disease, in which mortality is an obvious clinically relevant primary outcome measure, choosing the appropriate primary outcome measure for clinical trials of pelvic floor disorders can be challenging, because treatment "success" is often difficult to define. Despite the recent effort by national and international organizations to standardize outcomes in studies of pelvic floor disorders, there is currently no clearly established single best outcome measure or group of measures for any of these conditions; hence the emphasis on assessing outcomes in many domains. Historically, there has been a tendency to use objective physician or test-based measures, such as urodynamic outcomes for studies of urinary incontinence and physical examination for studies of POP, as the primary outcome variables in intervention trials of pelvic floor disorders.

However, in the last two decades there has been increasing emphasis on patient-based outcomes, such as symptom questionnaires and QOL assessments. In fact, a survey of physicians, nurses, and patients performed by Tincello and Alfirevic (2002) found that subjective measures and improvement in QOL were regarded by all groups as the most important outcomes in urogynecology studies. In spite of this, subjective outcomes alone are often inadequate to accurately characterize the effects of treatment on disorders of the pelvic floor. Both subjective and objective outcome measures should be assessed, and the primary outcome should be chosen based on the study's goal.

Clinical trials can broadly be separated into explanatory trials and pragmatic trials. In explanatory trials, the intent is to determine not only if one treatment is superior to another, but also why it is superior, and to determine the mechanism of success or failure. In explanatory trials, the inclusion/exclusion criteria tend to be strict to capture an "ideal" patient population. There is an emphasis on objective outcome measures that study mechanism of disease and treatment; these might include physiologic tests (i.e., urodynamics, anal manometry), radiologic evaluation, biochemical measures, etc. The goal of a pragmatic trial is to determine which treatment is superior in a real-world setting, without consideration of why it is superior or how it works. The inclusion/exclusion criteria of these trials tend to be liberal to mimic clinical practice, and the emphasis is on subjective patient-driven outcomes, such as questionnaires or symptom diaries. When choosing outcome measures during the planning of a trial, a good first step is to determine whether the intent of the trial is to be explanatory or pragmatic. The next step should be to identify valid, reliable outcome measures that will appropriately meet the study's objectives.

Urinary Incontinence

For a condition such as urinary incontinence, it might seem obvious that the primary outcome measure for a therapeutic trial should be "continence," but unfortunately it is not that simple. No clear consensus exists on how best to define continence. Should a therapy be considered "successful" if the patient reports that she no longer leaks urine, but has developed voiding dysfunction or new-onset urinary urgency? Similarly, should a patient be considered "continent" if she reports no urinary leakage after treatment on a voiding diary but leaks urine on multiple occasions during a urodynamic evaluation or has a positive pad test? The outcome or outcomes chosen as the primary outcome measure of a study can have a profound impact on the study's results. This is nicely illustrated in a multicenter randomized controlled trial performed in the United Kingdom comparing tension-free vaginal tape (TVT) to Burch colposuspension for treatment of SUI (Ward & Hilton, 2002). The authors of this study defined "cure" as the absence of stress incontinence at urodynamics and a negative 1-hour pad test (both criteria had to be satisfied to be considered a cure). Using this definition, 66% of subjects receiving TVT and 57% of those receiving colposuspension were cured. Fig. 41.1 illustrates how varying the definition of cure would have resulted in different cure rates. Using the absence of stress incontinence at urodynamic testing alone as the definition of cure would have resulted in cure rates of 81% and 65% for TVT and

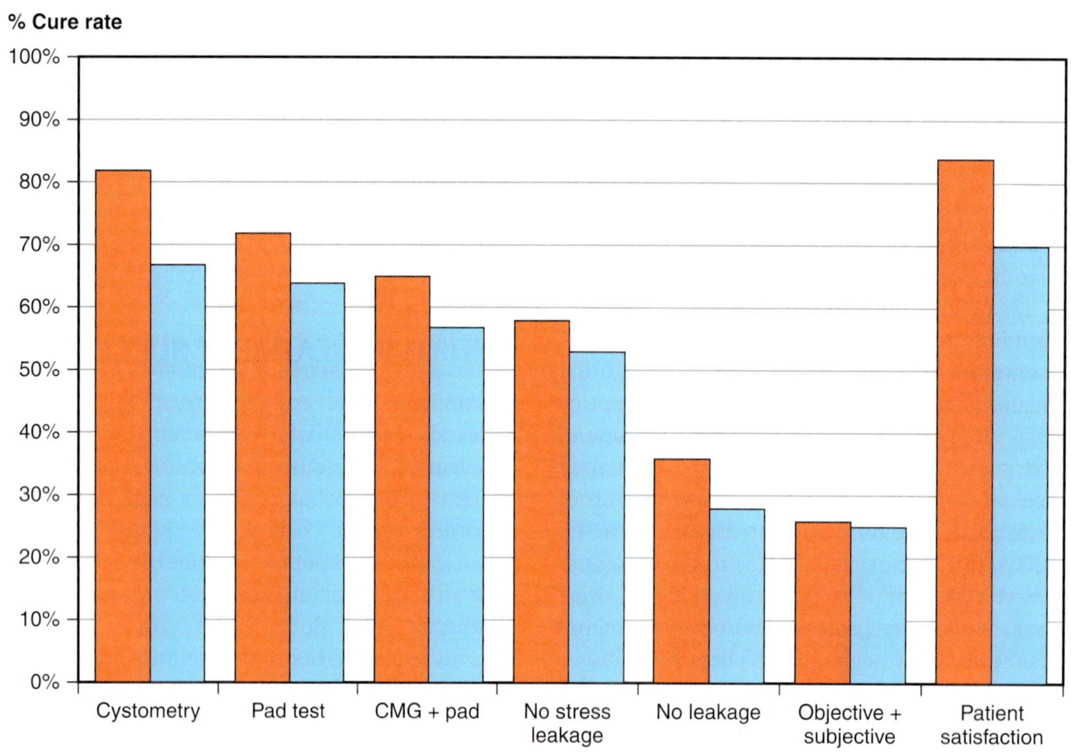

Fig. 41.1 Cure rates of the UK randomized controlled trial of tension-free vaginal tape (*red*) versus Burch colposuspension (*blue*) for stress urinary incontinence, based on various definitions of cure. *CMG*, Cystometrogram. (From Hilton P. Trials of surgery for stress incontinence—thoughts on the 'Humpty Dumpty principle'. *BJOG*. 2002;109:1081. With permission.)

colposuspension, respectively, which is consistent with previous reports in the literature. In contrast, the cure rate would have been less than 40% for both procedures if the authors had chosen a patient report of "no urinary leakage" on a symptom questionnaire as the primary outcome measure. This example not only illustrates the impact of choice of outcome measure on study results, but also emphasizes the importance of choosing the outcome measure before the onset of the study. To wait until completion of a study to define "success" or "cure" would allow for considerable manipulation of results.

The IUGA guidelines on the evaluation and outcome measures for female SUI provide no specific recommendation for defining cure after SUI treatment, although they note that definitions of SUI treatment outcome "should include all aspects of disease, usually a combination of subjective and objective measures, and patient's degree of satisfaction/quality-of-life" (Ghoniem et al., 2008). In a more recent review of the literature, Castillo et al. (2010) found that the definition of cure after SUI surgery was widely variable, with 4% using solely objective outcome measurements, 33% assessing only subjective outcome measurements, and 63% including both subjective and objective outcome measurements in the outcome assessments. Subjective cure was most often determined by patient self-assessment (34%), followed by patient questionnaires (19%). Objective cure was most frequently assessed by a cough stress test, with one-third of studies using this parameter as part of their definition of cure. Carmel et al. (2016), in a systematic review of studies evaluating outcomes after surgery for SUI or voiding dysfunction published between 2010 and 2015, found that the most frequently used parameters for objective success were a negative cough stress test, a negative pad test, and the absence of retreatment for SUI. The definition of subjective success most often involved questionnaires. The questionnaires most frequently used were the PGI-I, the UDI/UDI-6, the ICIQ-UI Short Form, and the Medical Epidemiologic and Social Aspects of Aging (MESA).

Increasingly, researchers are using a combination of outcome measures to create a composite measure of cure when assessing SUI surgeries. The Trial of Midurethral Slings study was a multicenter, randomized equivalence trial comparing the effect of the retropubic midurethral sling (RMUS) and the transobturator midurethral sling (TMUS) for the treatment of SUI (Richter et al., 2010). The composite primary outcome included objective measures (negative 300-mL retrograde fill stress test, negative 24-hour pad test, and no retreatment) and subjective measures (no stress symptoms on the MESA questionnaire, no leakage noted on a 3-day bladder diary, and no retreatment) assessed at 12 months. An equivalence margin of 12 percentage points was chosen on the basis of clinical importance, accounting for 80% power and feasibility. Unadjusted objective and subjective cure rates were similar between RMUS and TMUS (80.8% and 77.7%, respectively, and 62.2% and 55.8%, respectively). If a single definition had been used to define the primary outcome (either an objective or a subjective outcome), urinary incontinence cure rates would have varied between 65% and 95%.

When choosing an outcome or composite set of outcomes for defining cure, it is important that those measures, whether objective or subjective, are valid and can be reliably measured. Ideally, it is also useful to know how much change in a particular outcome is clinically relevant or considered important to the patient. For pharmacologic treatment of stress incontinence, it appears that patients recognize reductions of incontinence episode frequency of approximately 50% as having clinical value (Yalcin et al., 2010). Reductions of less than 40% do not appear to be clinically relevant to women. Whether this is also true for surgery for SUI or for treatment of UUI is unknown. Frick et al. (2010) evaluated the relative responsiveness of outcome measures used to evaluate surgery for SUI and found that the Incontinence Severity Index, PFDI-20, UDI-6, and bladder diary had the greatest responsiveness when compared with other measures and suggested that these measures may be preferable as primary outcome measures in trials of SUI treatment. Identifying responsive outcome measures is important when designing trials for incontinence treatment. More responsive outcome measures detect change better, thus increasing study power and potentially decreasing the number of participants required for enrollment.

As with SUI, outcome measures used in studies of therapy for UUI are heterogeneous. In the Cochrane review on bladder training, treatment outcomes consist of patient perception of cure or improvement of incontinence, quantification of symptoms (number of incontinence episodes and/or micturitions per day on a diary), and QOL (IIQ and SF-36). Similarly, outcomes used in trials evaluating pelvic muscle exercises with or without biofeedback included quantification of symptoms by diary and urodynamic outcomes. The Agency for Healthcare Research and Quality evidence report on treatment of OAB noted that the most consistently reported outcome measures were number of incontinence episodes and voids per day (Hartmann et al., 2009). Campbell et al. (2009) evaluated definition of treatment success in trials of UUI refractory to antimuscarinic medications and noted that, in 48 trials, success outcomes included complete continence in 44%, 50% or more improvement in incontinence episodes in 31%, and subjective improvement/patient satisfaction in 25%. These authors found that the treatment success outcome of 50% or more improvement in incontinence episodes was associated with clinically meaningful improvement in disease-specific HRQOL. They recommended this definition of treatment success be used in future UUI trials, as it was less restrictive than complete continence but included patients who were satisfied with treatment and experienced meaningful improvement in symptoms. Payne and Kelleher (2007) noted that, in studies of OAB, urgency, frequency, and nocturia should be important components of treatment response along with UUI. In particular, they emphasized that, according to the ICS definition, urinary urgency, not incontinence, is the fundamental symptom of OAB. They evaluated three composite outcome measures of treatment response for OAB and identified two definitions that appear to capture change in HRQOL most effectively: (1) reduction by half or more of all four baseline symptoms (episodes of urgency, incontinence, nocturia, and voiding frequency per 24 hours), and

(2) reduction by half or more in urgency and at least one other symptom (incontinence, frequency, or nocturia). Payne and Kelleher (2007) concluded that establishing the most appropriate definition to capture treatment-related changes in OAB will require further investigation but noted that the use of a composite clinical endpoint appears to be a valid approach when assessing OAB symptom changes.

Pelvic Organ Prolapse

POP, like all pelvic floor disorders, is a multidimensional phenomenon, and "success" of treatment is often difficult to define. Historically, most studies evaluating the treatment of POP have focused exclusively on anatomic success, without considering other important areas, such as symptoms, QOL, or socioeconomic outcomes. A systematic review by Kowalski et al. (2018) evaluating outcome measures used in studies of POP surgery from 1996 to 2016 found that 68% of studies reported an anatomic-only definition of success, 31% included a subjective component to their definition of success, and 16% reported a composite definition of success, including 8% containing anatomic, symptomatic, and retreatment components. The most common definition of anatomic success was POPQ stage I or lower.

For an individual patient, the most important outcomes of a surgical procedure are relief of symptoms and improvement in QOL (Barber et al., 2009). Fortunately, over the last 20 years, measures to evaluate POP have improved; there is now an internationally accepted and reliable assessment of the anatomic support of the uterus and vagina (POPQ), as well as a number of valid, reliable, and responsive symptom questionnaires and condition-specific HRQOL instruments. A 2012 joint report from ICS and IUGA recommended that the following outcomes be reported in studies of prolapse surgery: objective (e.g., POPQ), PROs (particularly the presence or absence of vaginal bulge symptoms), satisfaction, QOL, and perioperative data (e.g., operative time, hospital stay, etc.) (Tooz-Hobson et al., 2012). A careful report of short- and long-term complications is also essential to properly weigh the risk-benefit ratio of each procedure.

Traditionally, researchers have defined surgical success using the NIH satisfactory anatomic outcome (POPQ stages 0–I) and defined surgical failure as POPQ stage II or greater. More recently, it has been suggested that these anatomic definitions are too strict, as over 75% of women presenting for annual gynecologic examinations without symptoms of POP would not meet the definition of "optimal anatomic outcome," and almost 40% would not meet the definition of "satisfactory anatomic outcome." Thus, a substantial number of women considered "surgical failures" by these definitions would be within the normal distribution of vaginal support for parous women. The hymen may be a more clinically relevant anatomic threshold for surgical success, and some researchers have begun defining anatomic failure after surgery as prolapse that extends beyond the hymen. Another challenge is that the five-level staging system of the current POPQ (stages 0–IV) may be insufficient to discriminate among clinically important groups of women with POP, placing virtually all such women into stage II or III. Although the staging may facilitate comparisons, it may not provide as much detail as the individual POPQ measurements. A third area of uncertainty is whether or not apical prolapse should be considered by the same anatomic standards as prolapse of the anterior or posterior vaginal wall.

We have gained an improved understanding of the relationship between pelvic organ support and the development of symptoms. Most symptoms often attributed to prolapse have, at best, weak to moderate correlations with worsening pelvic organ support; however, the one symptom that is almost consistently acknowledged by patients with advanced prolapse is the presence of a vaginal bulge that can be seen or felt. The absence of vaginal bulge symptoms postoperatively has a significant relationship with a patient's assessment of overall improvement and improvement in QOL after surgery, whereas anatomic success alone does not (Barber et al., 2009). The hymen seems to be an important "cutoff point" for symptom development (Swift & Barber, 2010). Women with prolapse beyond the hymen have more pelvic floor symptoms and are more likely to report a vaginal bulge than women with prolapse at or above the hymen.

Reoperation after POP surgery for recurrence is an important measure of procedure efficacy. It is important to realize that reoperation rates likely represent the "tip of the iceberg" in terms of unsuccessful surgical outcomes, as many women with recurrence of symptomatic prolapse may not elect another surgery. Nonetheless, repeat surgery for recurrent prolapse is an undesirable outcome that should, in most cases, be considered a surgical failure. The rates of reoperation after prolapse surgery reported in the literature vary widely, in large part because of varying definitions and timeframes. Olsen et al. (1997), using administrative data from a large US health care system, reported a lifetime reoperation rate of 29.2%. Importantly, this study included both prolapse and stress incontinence surgery and did not distinguish between reoperation for incontinence or POP in their report. Moreover, the authors did not distinguish between reoperation for prolapse in the same compartments originally operated versus the development of prolapse in a new segment of the vagina ("*de novo* pelvic organ prolapse"). More recently, several investigators have looked specifically at the issue of site-specific recurrence, with reoperation rates ranging from 3.4% to 9.7%. In a meta-analysis of 258 studies evaluating reoperation rates after apical prolapse repairs, Diwadkar et al. (2009) reported a reoperation rate of 3.9% (95% confidence interval [CI] 3.5–4.4) for traditional vaginal vault suspensions (sacrospinous ligament suspension and uterosacral vault suspensions) after a mean of 32 months, 2.3% (95% CI 1.9–2.7) for sacrocolpopexy with a mean follow-up of 26 months, and 1.3% (95% CI 1.0–1.7) after transvaginal mesh procedures at a mean follow-up of 17 months. Notably, the total reoperation rate (if one includes reoperations for recurrent prolapse and for complications) was highest in the transvaginal mesh group (8.5%).

To provide some clarity for future studies reporting reoperation rates after pelvic organ prolapse surgery, the joint ICS/IUGA report (Tooz-Hobson et al., 2012) on reporting outcomes after prolapse surgery has proposed the following standardized terminology for prolapse surgery studies:

Primary surgery: For POP, this is the first procedure required for the treatment of prolapse in any compartment.

Further surgery: This gives a global figure for the number of subsequent procedures the patient undergoes, directly or indirectly relating to the primary surgery. This is subdivided into:

1. Primary prolapse surgery/different site: A prolapse procedure in a new site/compartment following previous surgery in a different compartment (e.g., anterior repair following previous posterior repair).
2. Repeat surgery: A repeat operation for prolapse arising from the same site. Where combinations of procedures arise (e.g., new anterior repair plus further posterior repair), these should be reported separately (i.e., repeat posterior repair and primary anterior repair).
3. Surgery for complications: Some complications include: mesh exposure, extrusion, pain, patient compromise, and hemorrhage.
4. Surgery for non–prolapse-related conditions: Some conditions include subsequent surgery for SUI or fecal incontinence.

The definition of success substantially affects treatment success rates following surgery for POP. Since the publication of the NIH workshop recommendations, considerable variability in defining treatment success still persists in studies evaluating surgery for prolapse. A number of trials define success as POPQ stage 0 or I consistent with the workshop's "satisfactory anatomic outcome" definition, with one reporting success rates as low as 30% using standard surgical techniques. Some have used the Baden–Walker prolapse grading system rather than the POPQ system. Other studies have used a combination of anatomic criteria and the presence or absence of symptoms to define treatment success. Such variability makes it difficult to compare study results. Moreover, there are many unknowns, including the clinical relevance of these definitions or how different outcome definitions might affect the comparison between treatment arms within a study.

A secondary analysis of the Colpopexy And Urinary Reduction Efforts (CARE) trial described prolapse surgical success rates after sacrocolpopexy using 18 different definitions of treatment success with differing requirements for anatomic, symptomatic, and/or retreatment outcomes (Barber et al., 2009). Treatment success rates varied widely depending upon the definition used (19.2%–97.2%). Overall, 71.4% considered their surgery "very successful," and 85.2% considered themselves "much better" than before surgery. Definitions of success requiring all anatomic support to be proximal to the hymen had the lowest treatment success rate (19.2%–57.6%), and 94.3% achieved surgical success when it was defined as the absence of prolapse beyond the hymen. Subjective cure (absence of bulge symptoms) occurred in 92.1% of patients, whereas absence of retreatment occurred in 97.2% of patients. Subjective cure was associated with significant improvements in the patient's assessment of both treatment success and overall improvement, more so than any other definition considered ($P = .0002$ and $P < .0001$, respectively). Similarly, the greatest difference in symptom burden and HRQOL between treatment successes and failures was noted when success was defined as subjective cure (absence of vaginal bulge symptoms; $P < .0001$). The authors concluded that the absence of vaginal bulge symptoms postoperatively has a significant relationship with a patient's assessment of overall improvement, whereas anatomic success alone does not. Based on this analysis, along with the currently available literature on the distribution of pelvic support loss in the general population and on data on the relationship between pelvic organ support loss and symptom development, authors from the National Institute of Child Health and Human Development (NICHD) Pelvic Floor Disorders Network have recommended that: (1) any definition of success after POP surgery should include the absence of bulge symptoms in addition to anatomic criteria and the absence of retreatment, and (2) using the hymen as a threshold for anatomic success seems a reasonable and defensible approach.

In 2001, Weber et al. published the results of a randomized trial of three methods of anterior colporrhaphy and reported failure rates of 58% to 70% using the NIH workshop's definition (failure was defined as POPQ stage ≥II). Recently, this study has been reanalyzed using the more clinically relevant criteria for treatment success proposed above (Chmielewski et al., 2011). Treatment success, a composite outcome defined as absence of prolapse beyond the hymen, symptomatic recurrence (absence of bulge symptoms), and retreatment, was achieved in 88% of patients at 1 year. Only 10% of patients developed anatomic recurrence beyond the hymen, 5% developed symptomatic recurrence, and less than 1% underwent retreatment at 23 months. This study highlights the importance of defining treatment success from the patient's perspective rather than using strict anatomic outcomes that may not have clinical relevance.

A recent analysis from the NICHD Pelvic Floor Disorders Network evaluated 1250 patients undergoing surgery for prolapse in four clinical trials followed for up to 5 years and considered how different outcomes identify success and failure during longitudinal follow-up. The investigators found that the overlap between anatomic and subjective success and failure is less than previously thought, and, importantly, that outcomes after surgery are dynamic over time, frequently transitioning from success to failure and back without intervening treatment (Jelovsek et al., 2020). Surgical failure was defined in this analysis by a composite measure requiring one or more of the following: (1) anatomic failure (any prolapse beyond the hymen), (2) subjective failure (presence of bothersome vaginal bulge symptoms), or (3) retreatment for POP with either pessary or surgery. Among the 433 of 1250 women (34.6%) who had surgical failure outcomes at more than one time point, 85.5% (370 of 433) met only one component of the composite outcome at the assessment of failure (anatomic failure, 46.7%; subjective failure, 36.7%; retreatment, 2.1%). Only 13% met the criteria for both anatomic and subjective failure. The authors note that the substantial discordance between symptoms and vaginal anatomy seen in their analysis and others' analyses suggests that it may be more valuable to evaluate these outcomes independently, rather than as a composite outcome, for POP surgery, because a single composite outcome may muddle our understanding of a patient's experience. Moreover, they suggest that single-composite outcomes likely overestimate failure relative to the entirety of the patient's postoperative experience.

Perhaps the most interesting finding of the analysis by Jelovsek et al. (2020) is that, with long-term longitudinal follow-up, subjective and objective measures of success are dynamic, fluctuating between success and failure for many patients without intervening treatment (Fig. 41.2A). Patients were followed every 6 months for up to 5 years, and 65% met the composite definition of success at all time points. However, one-quarter of patients who met the criteria for "failure" at some time point transitioned between success and failure over time ("intermittent success/failure"), with 84% of these meeting all criteria for success at their last follow-up (Fig. 41.2B). Women with intermittent success/failure had mean Pelvic Organ

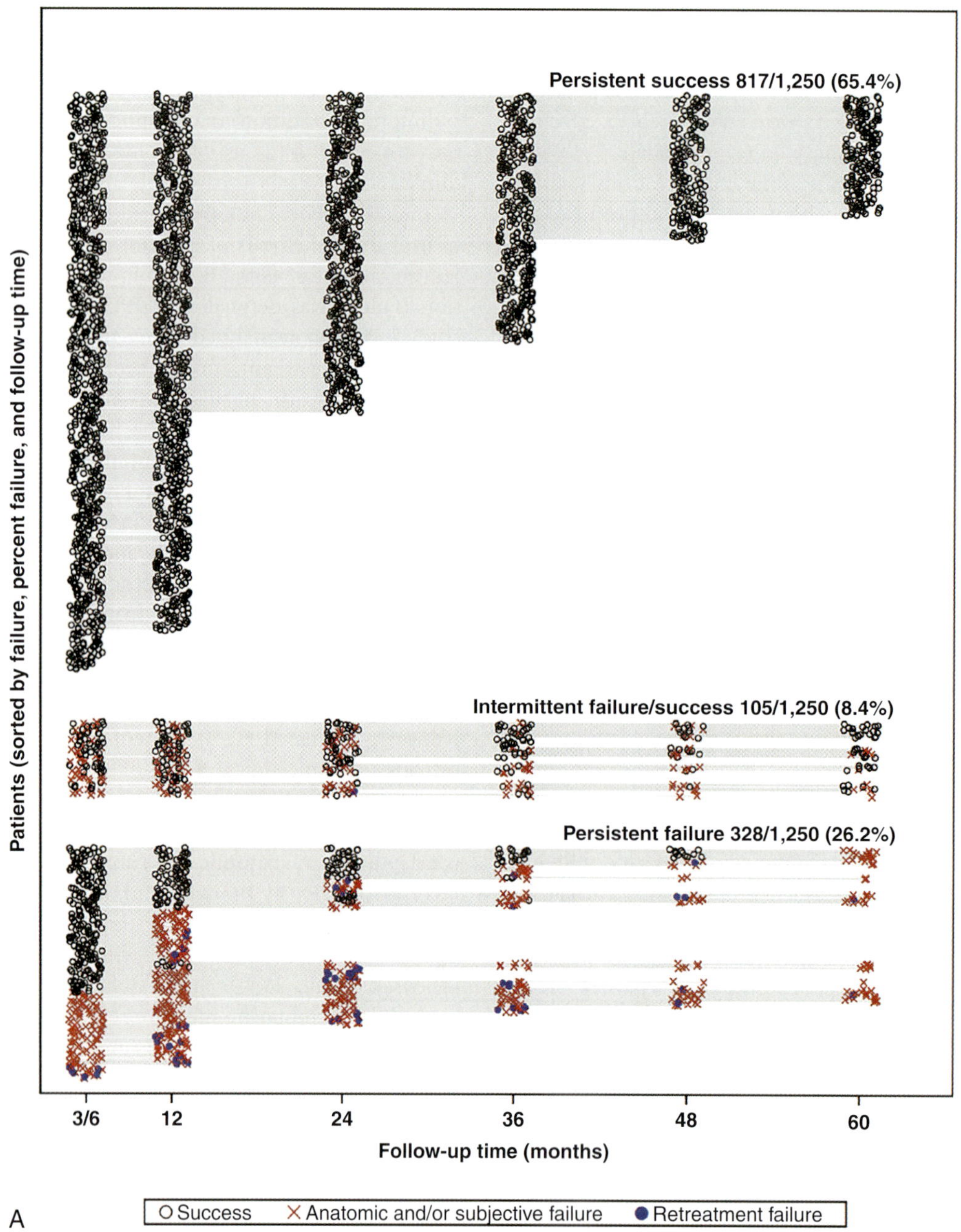

Fig. 41.2 A, Success and failure outcomes after pelvic organ prolapse surgery in 1250 patients enrolled in four Pelvic Floor Disorders Network trials. Success is indicated by a black circle, failure is indicated by a red X, and retreatment for pelvic organ prolapse is indicated by a blue circle. The top group is the "persistent success" participants who met the definition of success at all time points. The bottom group is the "persistent failure" participants who met the definition of failure at all follow-up visits. The middle group is participants who moved back and forth between success and failure states over the follow-up period.

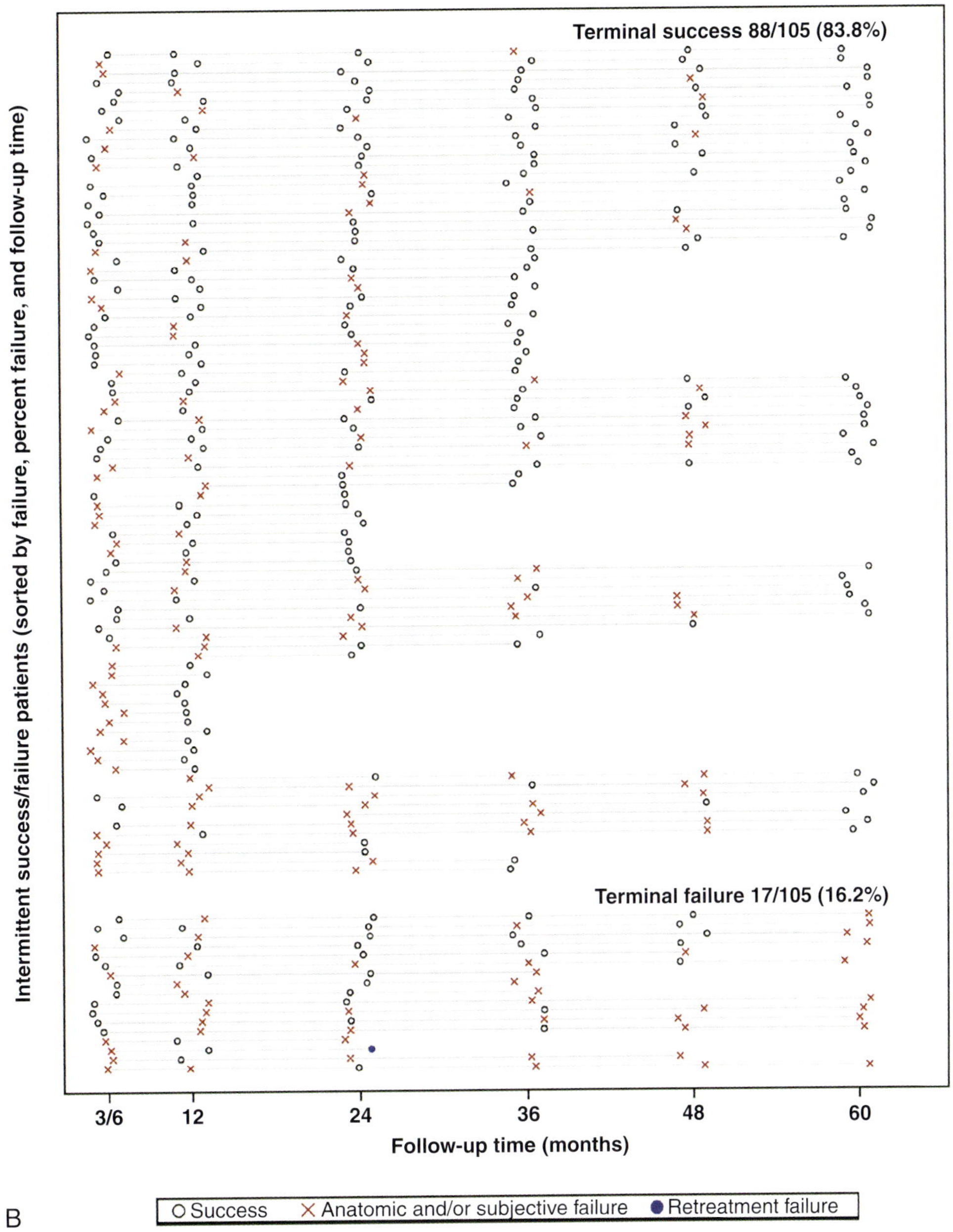

Fig. 41.2, cont'd **B**, Intermittent success and failure outcomes after pelvic organ prolapse surgery. Success is indicated by a black circle, failure is indicated by a red X, and retreatment for pelvic organ prolapse is indicated by a blue circle. The top group is the "terminal success" participants who met the definition of success at the last follow-up visit. The bottom group is the "terminal failure" participants who met the definition of failure at their last follow-up visit. (From Jelovsek JE, Gantz MG, Lukacz E, et al. Success and failure are dynamic, recurrent event states after surgical treatment for pelvic organ prolapse. *Am J Obstet Gynecol.* 2021;224:362.e1. With permission.)

Prolapse Distress Inventory scores in between those meeting persistent failure and persistent success definitions at each year of follow-up, suggesting they are an intermediate group. As most studies of POP assess outcomes at a single time point or use standard survival analysis, where "once a failure, always a failure," these results suggest that current studies likely do not truly reflect the patient experience long-term and may overestimate failure rates. These novel findings are likely to impact choice of outcomes and type of analysis used for future studies.

BIBLIOGRAPHY

Introduction

Abrams P, Blaivas JG, Stanton SL, Andersen JT. The standardisation of terminology of lower urinary tract function. The International Continence Society Committee on Standardisation of Terminology. *Scand J Urol Nephrol Suppl.* 1988;114:5.

Hilton P. Trials of surgery for stress incontinence—thoughts on the 'Humpty Dumpty principle'. *BJOG.* 2002;109:1081.

Lose G, Fantl JA, Victor A, et al. Outcome measures for research in adult women with symptoms of lower urinary tract dysfunction. *Neurourol Urodyn.* 1988;17:255.

Mattiasson A, Djurhuss JC, Fonda D, et al. Standardization of outcomes studies in patients with lower urinary tract dysfunction. *Neurourol Urodyn.* 1998;17:249.

Payne C, Blaivas J, Brown J, et al. Research methodology. In Abrams P, Cardozo L, Khoury S, Wein A, eds. *3rd International Consultation on Incontinence.* Paris: Health Publication; 2005.

Proceedings of International Foundation of Functional Gastrointestinal Disorders Consensus Conference on advancing treatment of fecal and urinary incontinence through research. *Gastroenterol Suppl.* 2004;126:S1.

Wall LL, Versi E, Norton P, Bump R. Evaluating the outcome of surgery for pelvic organ prolapse. *Am J Obstet Gynecol.* 1998;178:877.

Weber AM, Abrams P, Brubaker L, et al. The standardization of terminology for researchers in female pelvic floor disorders. *Int Urogynecol J Pelvic Floor Dysfunct.* 2001;12:178.

Symptom Diaries and Pad Testing

Abrams P, Klevmark B. Frequency/volume charts: an indispensable part of lower urinary tract assessment. *Scand J Urol Nephrol.* 1985;179:47.

Al Afraa T, Mahfouz W, Campeau L, et al. Normal lower urinary tract assessment in women: I. Uroflowmetry and post-void residual, pad tests, and bladder diaries. *Int Urogynecol J.* 2012;23:681.

Amundsen CL, Parsons M, Tissot B, et al. Bladder diary measurements in asymptomatic females: functional bladder capacity, frequency and 24-hr volume. *Neurourol Urodyn.* 2007;26:341.

Bright E, Drake MJ, Abrams P. Urinary diaries: evidence for the development and validation of diary content, format and duration. *Neurourol Urodyn.* 2011;30:348.

Bright E, Cotterill N, Drake M, et al. Developing and validating the International Consultation on Incontinence Questionnaire bladder diary. *Eur Urol.* 2014;66:294.

Cameron AP, Wiseman JB, Smith AR, et al. Are three-day voiding diaries feasible and reliable? Results from the Symptoms of Lower Urinary Tract Dysfunction Research Network (LURN) cohort. *Neurourol Urodyn.* 2019;38:2185.

Fitzgerald MP, Brubaker L. Variability of 24-hour voiding diary variables among asymptomatic women. *J Urol.* 2003;169:207.

Groutz A, Blaivas J, Chaikin D, et al. Noninvasive outcome measures of urinary incontinence and lower urinary tract symptoms: a multicenter study of micturition diary and pad test. *J Urol.* 2000;164:698.

Henderson JW, Kane SM, Mangel JM et al. A Randomized comparative study evaluating various cough stress tests and 24-hour pad test with urodynamics in the diagnosis of stress urinary incontinence. *J Urol.* 2018;199:1557.

Lose G, Rosenkilde P, Gammelgaard J, et al. Pad-weighing test performed with standardized bladder volume. *Urology.* 1988;32:78.

Mateu Arrom L, Peri Cusi L, López-Fando L, et al. Validation of a 3 day electronic bladder diary as an app for smart-phone. *Neurourol Urodyn.* 2019;38:764.

Nygaard I, Holcomb R. Reproducibility of the seven-day voiding diary in women with stress urinary incontinence. *Int Urogynecol J Pelvic Floor Dysfunct.* 2000;11:15.

Ryhammer AM, Djurhuus JC, Laurberg S. Pad testing in incontinent women: a review. *Int Urogynecol J.* 1999;10:111.

Singh M, Bushman W, Clemens JW. Do pad tests and voiding diaries affect patient willingness to participate in studies of incontinence treatment outcomes? *J Urol.* 2004;171:316.

Stav K, Dwyer PL, Rosamilia A. Women overestimate daytime urinary frequency: the importance of the bladder diary. *J Urol.* 2009;181:2176.

Stone A, Shiffman S, Schwartz J, et al. Patient compliance with paper and electronic diaries. *Control Clin Trials.* 2003;24:182.

Sussman RD, Richter LA, Tefera E, et al. Utilizing technology in assessment of lower urinary tract symptoms: a randomized trial of electronic versus paper voiding diaries. *Female Pelvic Med Reconstr Surg.* 2016;201:224.

Wyman JF, Choi SC, Harkins SW, et al. The urinary diary in evaluation of incontinence women: a test-retest analysis. *Obstet Gynecol.* 1988;71:812.

Anatomic and Physiologic Outcomes

Bharucha AE. Outcome measures for fecal incontinence: anorectal structure and function. *Gastroenterology.* 2004;126:S90.

Bump RC, Mattiasson A, Bo K, et al. The standardization of terminology of female pelvic organ prolapse and pelvic floor dysfunction. *Am J Obstet Gynecol.* 1996;175:10.

Hosker G, Rosier P, Gajewski J, et al. Dynamic testing. In: Abrams P, Cardozo L, Khoury S, et al., eds. *4th International Consultation on Incontinence.* Paris: Health Publication; 2009.

Muir TW, Stepp KJ, Barber MD. Adoption of the pelvic organ prolapse quantitation system in the peer review literature. *Am J Obstet Gynecol.* 2003;189:1632.

Nager CW, Brubaker L, Litman HJ, et al. A randomized trial of urodynamic testing before stress incontinence surgery. *N Engl J Med.* 2012;336:1987.

Nager CW, Sirls L, Litman HJ, et al. Baseline urodynamic predictors of treatment failure 1 year after mid-urethral sling surgery. *J Urol.* 2011;186:597.

Nygaard I. Physiologic outcome measures of urinary incontinence. *Gastroenterology.* 2004;126:S99.

Questionnaires

Avery K, Donovan J, Peters T, et al. ICIQ: A brief and robust measure for evaluating the symptoms and impact of urinary incontinence. *Neurourol Urodyn.* 2004;23:322.

Barber MD, Kuchibhatla MN, Pieper CF, et al. Psychometric evaluation of two comprehensive condition-specific quality-of-life instruments for women with pelvic floor disorders. *Am J Obstet Gynecol.* 2001;185:1388.

Barber MD, Walters MD, Bump RC. Short forms for two condition-specific quality-of-life questionnaires for women with pelvic floor disorders (PFDI-20 & PFIQ-7). *Am J Obstet Gynecol.* 2005;193:103.

Barber MD, Walters MD, Cundiff GW, PESSRI Trial Group. Responsiveness of the pelvic floor distress inventory and pelvic floor impact questionnaire in women undergoing surgical and non-surgical treatment for pelvic organ prolapse. *Am J Obstet Gynecol.* 2006;194:1492.

Barber MD. Symptoms and outcome measures of pelvic organ prolapse. *Clin Obstet Gynecol.* 2005;48:648.

Barber MD, Amundsen CL, Paraiso MF, et al. Quality of life after surgery for genital prolapse in elderly women: obliterative and reconstructive surgery. *Int Urogynecol J.* 2007;18:799.

Baxter NN, Rothenberger DA, Lowry AC. Measuring fecal incontinence. *Dis Colon Rectum.* 2003;46:1591.

Bland JM, Altman DG. Validating scales and indexes. *BMJ.* 2002;324:606.

Boreham MK, Richter HE, Kenton KS, et al. Anal incontinence in women presenting for gynecologic care: prevalence, risk factors, and impact upon quality-of-life. *Am J Obstet Gynecol.* 2005;192:1637.

Cartagena-Ramos D, Fuentealba-Torres M, Rebustini F, et al. Systematic review of the psychometric properties of instruments to measure sexual desire. *BMC Med Res Methodol.* 2018;18:109.

Cartwright R, Srikrishna S, Cardozo L, et al. Validation and reliability of the patient's perception of intensity of urgency scale in overactive bladder. *BJU Int.* 2010;107:1612.

Cella D, Riley W, Stone A, et al., on behalf of the PROMIS Cooperative Group. The Patient Reported Outcomes Measurement Information System (PROMIS) developed and tested its first wave of adult self-reported health outcome item banks: 2005-2008. *J Clin Epidemiol.* 2010;63:1179.

Cella D, Smith AR, Griffith JW, et al. A new outcome measure for LUTS: symptoms of lower urinary tract dysfunction research network symptom index-29 (LURN SI-29) questionnaire. *Neurourol Urodyn.* 2019;38:1751.

Cella D, Smith AR, Griffith JW, et al. A new brief clinical assessment of lower urinary tract symptoms for women and men: LURN SI-10. *J Urol.* 2020;203:164.

Coyne KS, Margolis MK, Hseih R, et al. Validation of the urinary sensation scale. *Neurourol Urodyn.* 2011;30:360.

Crosby RD, Kolotkin RL, Rhys Williams G. Defining clinically meaningful change in health-related quality-of-life. *J Clin Epidemiol.* 2003;56:395.

Daker-White G. Reliable and valid self-report outcome measures in sexual (dys)function: a systematic review. *Arch Sex Behav.* 2002;31:197.

Diaz DC, Robinson D, Bosch R, et al. Patient reported outcome assessment. In: Abrams P, Cardozo L, Wagg A, et al., eds. *6th International Consultation on Incontinence.* Tokyo: ICUD ICS; 2017.

Flynn KE, Lin L, Cyranowski JM, et al. Development of the NIH PROMIS ® Sexual Function and Satisfaction measures in patients with cancer. *J Sex Med.* 2013;10:43.

Guyatt GH, Feeny DH, Patrick DL. Measuring health-related quality-of-life. *Ann Intern Med.* 1993;118:622.

Hanley J, Capewell A, Hagen S. Validity study of the severity index, a simple measure of urinary incontinence in women. *BMJ.* 2001;322:1096.

Hays RD, Bjorner JB, Revicki DA, et al. Development of physical and mental health summary scores from the patient-reported outcomes measurement information system (PROMIS) global items. *Qual Life Res.* 2009;18:873.

Jorge JM, Wexner SD. Etiology and management of fecal incontinence. *Dis Colon Rectum.* 1993;36:77.

Kelleher CJ, Cardozo LD, Khullar V, et al. A new questionnaire to assess the quality-of-life of urinary incontinent women. *Br J Obstet Gynaecol.* 1997;104:1374.

Lubeck DP, Prebil LA, Peebles P, et al. A health related quality-of-life measure for use in patients with urge urinary incontinence: a validation study. *Qual Life Res.* 1999;8:337.

Lukacz ES, Warren LK, Richter HE, et al. Quality of life and sexual function 2 years after vaginal surgery for prolapse. *Obstet Gynecol.* 2016;127:1071.

Mattsson NK, Karjalainen PK, Tolppanen AM, et al. Pelvic organ prolapse surgery and quality of life-a nationwide cohort study. *Am J Obstet Gynecol.* 2020;222:588.e1.

Mattsson NK, Karjalainen P, Heikkinen AM, et al. Agreement between patient global impression scale of improvement, pelvic floor distress inventory and 15D in measuring the outcome of pelvic organ prolapse surgery. *Neurourol Urodyn.* 2020;39:2171.

McCoy NL, Matyas JR. McCoy female sexuality questionnaire. In Davis CM, Yarber WL, Fisher TD, et al. *Handbook of Sexuality-Related Measures.* London: Sage; 1988.

National Institutes of Health Patient-Reported Outcomes Measurement Information System (PROMIS). Available at: http://www.nihpromis.org. Accessed December 27, 2020.

Naughton MJ, Donovan J, Badia X, et al. Symptom severity and QOL scales for urinary incontinence. *Gastroenterology.* 2004;126:S114.

Nichols NM, Gill EJ, Nguyen T, et al. Anal sphincter injury in women with pelvic floor disorders. *Obstet Gynecol.* 2004;104:690.

Patrick DL, Martin ML, Bushnell DM. Quality-of-life of women with urinary incontinence: further development of the incontinence quality-of-life instrument (I-QOL). *Urology.* 1999;53:71.

Rockwood TH. Incontinence severity and QOL scales for fecal incontinence. *Gastroenterology.* 2004;126:S106.

Rockwood TH, Church JM, Fleshman JW, et al. Fecal incontinence quality-of-life scale: quality-of-life instrument for patients with fecal incontinence. *Dis Colon Rectum.* 2000;43:9.

Rogers RG, Kammerer-Doak D, Villarreal A, et al. A new instrument to measure sexual function in women with urinary incontinence and pelvic organ prolapse. *Am J Obstet Gynecol.* 2001;184:552.

Rogers RG, Coates KW, Kammerer-Doak D, et al. A short form of the Pelvic organ prolapse/urinary incontinence sexual questionnaire (PISQ-12). *Int Urogynecol J.* 2003;14:164.

Rogers RG, Rockwood TH, Constantine ML, et al. A new measure of sexual function in women with pelvic floor disorders (PFD): the pelvic organ prolapse/incontinence sexual questionnaire, IUGA-revised (PISQ-IR). *Int Urogynecol J.* 2013;24:1091.

Rogers RG, Sung VW, Lukacz ES, et al. Accidental bowel leakage evaluation: a new patient-centered validated measure of accidental bowel leakage symptoms in women. *Dis Colon Rectum.* 2020;63:668.

Rosen RC, Brown C, Heiman J, et al. The female sexual function index (FSFI): a multidimensional self-report instrument for the assessment of female sexual function. *J Sex Marital Ther.* 2000;26:191.

Sandvik H, Hunskaar S, Seim A, et al. Validation of severity index in female urinary incontinence and its implementation in an epidemiological survey. *J Epidemiol Community Health.* 1993;47:497.

Sandvik H, Seim A, Vanvik A, et al. A severity index for epidemiological surveys of female urinary incontinence: comparison with 48-hour pad-weighing tests. *Neurourol Urodyn.* 2000;19:137.

Srikrishna S, Robinson D, Cardozo L. Validation of the Patient Global Impression of Improvement (PGI-I) for urogenital prolapse. *Int Urogynecol J.* 2010;21:523.

Shumaker SA, Wyman JF, Uebersax JS, et al. Health-related quality-of-life measures for women with urinary incontinence: the incontinence impact questionnaire and the urogenital distress inventory. *Qual Life Res.* 1994;3:291.

Sung VW, Marques F, Rogers RR, et al. Content validation of Patient Reported Outcome Measurement Information System (PROMIS) framework in patients with urinary incontinence. *Neurourol Urodyn.* 2011;30:503.

Sung VW, Griffith JW, Rogers RG, et al. Item bank development, calibration and validation for patient-reported outcomes in female urinary incontinence. *Qual Life Res.* 2016;25:1645.

Todd R, Church J, Fleshman J, et al. Patient and surgeon ranking of the severity of symptoms associated with fecal incontinence: the fecal incontinence severity index. *Dis Colon Rectum.* 1999;42:1525.

Uebersax JS, Wyman JF, Shumaker SA, et al. Short forms to assess life quality and symptom distress for urinary incontinence in women. *Neurourol Urodyn.* 1995;14:131.

Vaizey CJ, Carapeti E, Cahill JA, et al. Prospective comparison of faecal incontinence grading systems. *Gut.* 1999;4:477.

Weinfurt KP, Lin L, Bruner DW, et al. Development and initial validation of the PROMIS sexual function and satisfaction measures version 2.0. *J Sex Med.* 2015;12:1961.

Weinfurt KP, Griffith JW, Flynn KE et al. The comprehensive assessment of self-reported urinary symptoms: a new tool for research on subtypes of patients with lower urinary tract symptoms. *J Urol.* 2019;201:1177.

Wren PA, Janz NK, Brubaker L, et al. Reliability of health-related quality-of-life measures one year after surgical procedures for pelvic floor disorders. *Am J Obstet Gynecol.* 2005;192:780.

Yalcin I, Bump R. Validation of two global impression questionnaires for incontinence. *Am J Obstet Gynecol.* 2003;189:98.

Patient-Selected Goals

Brubaker L, Shull B. EGGS for patient-centered outcomes, *Int Urogynecol J.* 2005;16:171.

Elkadry EA, Kenton K, FitzGerald MP, et al. Patient-selected goals: a new perspective on surgical outcome. *Am J Obstet Gynecol.* 2003;189:1551.

Hullfish KL, Bovbjerg VE, Gibson J, et al. Patient-centered goals for pelvic floor dysfunction surgery: what is success, and is it achieved? *Am J Obstet Gynecol.* 2002;187:88.

Hullfish KL, Bovberg VE, Steers WD. Patient-centered goals for pelvic floor dysfunction surgery: long-term follow-up. *Am J Obstet Gynecol.* 2004;191:201.

Srikrishna S, Robinson D, Cardozo L, et al. Patient and surgeon goal achievement 10 years following surgery for pelvic organ prolapse and urinary incontinence. *Int Urogynecol J.* 2015;26:1679.

Defining Treatment Success

Barber MD, Brubaker L, Nygaard I, et al. Defining success after surgery for pelvic organ prolapse. *Obstet Gynecol.* 2009;114:600.

Campbell JD, Gries KS, Watanabe JH, et al. Treatment success for overactive bladder with urinary urge incontinence refractory to oral antimuscarinics: a review of published evidence. *BMC Urol.* 2009;9:18.

Carmel ME, Deng DY, Greenwell TJ, et al. Definition of success after surgery for female stress incontinence or voiding dysfunction: an attempt at standardization. *Eur Urol Focus.* 2016;2:231.

Castillo PA, Espaillat-Rijo LM, Davila GW. Outcome measures and definition of cure in female stress incontinence surgery: a survey of recent publications. *Int Urogynecol J.* 2010;21:343.

Chmielewski L, Walters MD, Weber AM, et al. Reanalysis of a randomized trial of 3 techniques of anterior colporrhaphy using clinically relevant definitions of success. *Am J Obstet Gynecol.* 2011;205:69.e1.

Diwadkar GB, Barber MD, Feiner B, et al. Complication and reoperation rates after apical vaginal prolapse surgical repair: a systematic review. *Obstet Gynecol.* 2009;113:367.

Frick AC, Ridgeway B, Ellerkmann M, et al. Comparison of responsiveness of validated outcome measures after surgery for stress urinary incontinence. *J Urol.* 2010;184:2013.

Ghoniem G, Stanford E, Kenton K, et al. Evaluation and outcome measures in the treatment of female urinary stress incontinence: International Urogynecological Association (IUGA) guidelines for research and clinical practice. *Int Urogynecol J.* 2008;19:5.

Hartmann KE, McPheeters ML, Biller DH, et al. *Treatment of Overactive Bladder in Women. (Evidence Reports/Technology Assessments, No. 187.)* Rockville, MD: Agency for Healthcare Research and Quality (US); 2009.

Jelovsek JE, Gantz MG, Lukacz E, et al. Success and failure are dynamic, recurrent event states after surgical treatment for pelvic organ prolapse. *Am J Obstet Gynecol.* 2021;224:362.e1.

Kowalski JT, Mehr A, Cohen E, et al. Systematic review of definitions for success in pelvic organ prolapse surgery. *Int Urogynecol J.* 2018;29:1697.

Olsen AL, Smith VJ, Bergstrom JO, et al. Epidemiology of surgically managed pelvic organ prolapse and urinary incontinence. *Obstet Gynecol.* 1997;89:501.

Parker-Autry CY, Barber MD, Kenton K, et al. Measuring outcomes in urogynecology: "perspective is everything." *Int Urogynecol J.* 2013;24:15.

Payne CK, Kelleher C. Redefining response in overactive bladder syndrome. *BJU Int.* 2007;99:101.

Richter HE, Albo ME, Zyczynski HM, et al. Retropubic versus transobturator midurethral slings for stress incontinence. *N Engl J Med.* 2010;362:2066.

Swift SE, Barber MD. Pelvic organ prolapse: defining the disease. *Female Pelvic Med Reconstr Surg.* 2010;16:201.

Tincello DG, Alfirevic Z. Important clinical outcomes in urogynecology: views of patients, nurses and medical staff. *Int Urogynecol J.* 2002;13:96.

Tooz-Hobson P, Freeman R, Barber M, et al. An International Urogynecological Association (IUGA)/International Continence Society (ICS) joint report on terminology for reporting outcomes of surgical procedures for pelvic organ prolapse. *Int Urogynecol J.* 2012;23:527.

Ward K, Hilton P, United Kingdom and Ireland Tension-free Vaginal Tape Trial Group. Prospective multicentre randomised trial of tension-free vaginal tape and colposuspension as primary treatment for stress incontinence. *BMJ.* 2002;325:67.

Weber AM, Walters MD, Piedmonte MR, et al. Anterior colporrhaphy: a randomized trial of three surgical techniques. *Am J Obstet Gynecol.* 2001;185:1299.

Yalcin I, Peng G, Viktrup L, et al. Reductions in stress urinary incontinence episodes: what is clinically important for women? *Neurourol Urodyn.* 2010;29:34.

INDEX

Note: Page numbers followed by *f* indicate figures; *t*, tables; *b*, boxes.

A

B

C

K

L

M

Q

R

S

V